D0944671

Pharmacology

Pharmacology: Principles and Practice

Edited by

Miles Hacker

University of Toledo College of Pharmacy, Toledo, OH

William Messer

University of Toledo College of Pharmacy, Toledo, OH

Kenneth Bachmann

CeutiCare, LLC and University of Toledo College of Pharmacy (Emeritus), Toledo, OH

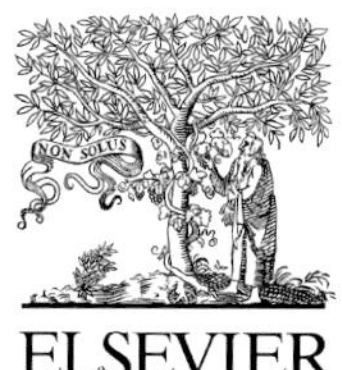

AMSTERDAM • BOSTON • HEIDELBERG • LONDON
NEW YORK • OXFORD • PARIS • SAN DIEGO
SAN FRANCISCO • SINGAPORE • SYDNEY • TOKYO
Academic Press is an imprint of Elsevier

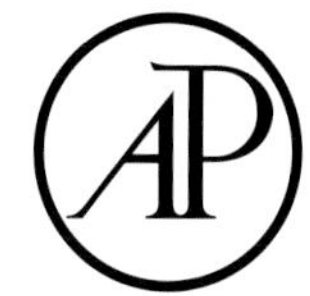

Academic Press is an imprint of Elsevier
30 Corporate Drive, Suite 400, Burlington, MA 01803, USA
525 B Street, Suite 1900, San Diego, California 92101-4495, USA
84 Theobald's Road, London WC1X 8RR, UK

Library of Congress Cataloging-in-Publication Data
APPLICATION SUBMITTED

British Library Cataloguing-in-Publication Data
A catalogue record for this book is available from the British Library.

ISBN: 978-0-12-369521-5

For information on all Academic Press publications
visit our Web site at www.elsevierdirect.com

Printed in China
09 10 9 8 7 6 5 4 3 2 1

This textbook is dedicated to the memory of three of our close colleagues and friends, Gerald Sherman, Timothy Sullivan, and James Byers, and their efforts to help students understand and appreciate pharmacology and pharmacokinetics.

Accompanying Web site with additional materials available at
http://www.elsevierdirect.com/companions/9780123695215.

Kenneth Alexander (Ch. 2)
University of Toledo College of Pharmacy, Toledo, OH

Kenneth Bachmann (Ch. 8, 12)
CeutiCare, LLC and University of Toledo College of Pharmacy (Emeritus), Toledo, OH

James Bigelow (Ch. 11)
Department of Biomedical and Pharmaceutical Sciences, Idaho State University, Pocatello, ID

William Bress (Ch. 14)
Vermont Department of Health, Burlington, Vermont

James P. Byers (Ch. 10)
University of Toledo College of Pharmacy, Toledo, OH

Edward Calabrese (Ch. 5)
Environmental Health Sciences Division, School of Public Health, University of Massachusetts, Amherst, MA

Jen-Fu Chiu (Ch. 20)
Open Laboratory for Molecular Biology, Shantou University Medical College, Shantou, China

Paul Erhardt (Ch. 19)
University of Toledo College of Pharmacy, Toledo, OH

Aaron Grabovich (Ch. 17)
University of Toledo, Toledo, OH

Martin Holcik (Ch. 18)
Children's Hospital of Eastern Ontario Research Institute, Ottawa, ON, Canada

Miles Hacker (Ch. 1, 13, 15)
University of Toledo College of Pharmacy, Toledo, OH

Lori Hazlehurst (Ch. 15)
H. Lee Moffitt Cancer Center & Research Institute

Qing-Yu He (Ch. 20)
University of Hong Kong, Hong Kong, SAR, China

Terry Kenakin (Ch. 4)
GlaxoSmithKline Research and Development, Research Triangle Park, NC

Eric C. LaCasse (Ch. 18)
Children's Hospital of Eastern Ontario Research Institute, Ottawa, ON, Canada

John S. Lazo (Ch. 21)
Allegheny Foundation Professor, Department of Pharmacology & Chemical Biology, Drug Discovery Institute, The University of Pittsburgh, Pittsburgh, PA

Markos Leggas (Ch. 7)
Department of Pharmaceutical Sciences, College of Pharmacy, University of Kentucky, Lexington, KY

Karen Lounsbury (Ch. 6)
University of Vermont, Burlington, VT

Patrick J. McNamara (Ch. 7)
Department of Pharmaceutical Sciences, College of Pharmacy, University of Kentucky, Lexington, KY

Georgi V. Petkov (Ch. 16)
Department of Pharmaceutical and Biomedical Sciences, South Carolina College of Pharmacy, University of South Carolina, Columbia, SC

George S. Robertson (Ch. 18)
Dalhousie University, Halifax, NS, Canada

Jeffrey G. Sarver (Ch. 10)
University of Toledo College of Pharmacy, Toledo, OH

David R. Taft (Ch. 9)
Long Island University, Brooklyn, NY

Pei Tang (Ch. 3)
University of Pittsburg School of Medicine, Pittsburgh, PA

William R. Taylor (Ch. 17)
University of Toledo, Toledo, OH

Tommy S. Tillman (Ch. 3)
University of Pittsburg School of Medicine, Pittsburgh, PA

Ying Wang (Ch. 20)
University of Hong Kong, Hong Kong, SAR, China

Yan Xu (Ch. 3)
University of Pittsburg School of Medicine, Pittsburgh, PA

Several years ago we noted a paucity of textbooks that dealt with the principles of pharmacology as a science, rather than pharmacology as a therapeutic entity. In an attempt to remedy this, we organized a textbook designed to meet the needs of students interested in pharmacology at the advanced undergraduate and early graduate level. This text addresses the many facets that form the foundation of pharmacology.

Students will find extensive discussions by leaders in the field are written in clear and straightforward manner. Illustrations are included to help further the reader's understanding of the material covered in each chapter. The editors and authors have focused on the science of pharmacology and use drugs for illustrative purposes only.

As pharmacology is a field of science that encompasses science from various arrays, we have included chapters dealing with each level of biological organization, both biology and chemistry which has been included in discussion of each chapter and how they related to one another. The material in this textbook will provide the student and the practicing pharmacology scientist excellent education and reference materials. Each chapter is written in a matter similar to Scientific American, where the text is not interrupted by referencing, but an extensive bibliography is provided for the reader at the end of each chapter.

The editors are grateful for the dedication and cooperation of the authors and recognize the efforts put forth by each to create a textbook that is not only first rate, but also a useful resource to students and researchers alike. The editors are also deeply grateful for the assistance that we received from the highly talented and professional staff of the publisher, Elsevier.

Chapter

1

History of Pharmacology—From Antiquity to the Twentieth Century

Miles Hacker

OUTLINE

1.1 WHAT IS PHARMACOLOGY?

Obviously, a discussion of all the ancient remedies would require more space than possibly could be allotted for one chapter in a textbook. In this chapter we will discuss a few of the more fascinating examples of how ancient civilization was able to treat disease with available natural products. We will then discuss the progression of pharmacology from the science of testing crude extracts of plants, animals, and minerals for their medicinal properties, to the science it is today, in which isolated chemicals are examined for their effects on live tissue. This begs the question, what is a good working definition for modern pharmacology? On the surface, this seems like an easy task, but as we peruse the textbooks and articles pertaining to pharmacology we rapidly realize that the definition of pharmacology varies greatly, depending on who is defining the discipline.

A dictionary defines pharmacology as:

> **1. Study of drugs**: the science or study of drugs, especially of the ways in which they react biologically at receptor sites in the body
>
> **2. Drug's effects**: the effects that a drug has when taken by somebody, especially as a medical treatment

Yet another source defines pharmacology in this way:

> Branch of **medicine** dealing with the actions of **drugs** in the body—both therapeutic and toxic effects—and development and testing of new drugs and new uses of existing ones.

Though the first Western pharmacological treatise (a listing of herbal plants) was compiled in the first century AD, scientific pharmacology was possible only from the eighteenth century on, when drugs could be purified and standardized. Pharmacologists develop drugs from plant and animal sources and create synthetic versions of these, along with new drugs based on them or their chemical structure. They also test drugs, first *in vitro* for biochemical activity and then *in vivo* for safety, effectiveness, side effects, and interactions with other drugs and to find the best dose, timing, and route.

When reading textbooks, we find such definitions as:

> Pharmacology is the science of drugs, their chemical composition, their biological action and their therapeutic application to man and animal. It includes toxicology, which encompasses the harmful effects of chemicals, whether it is used therapeutically or not.
>
> Pharmacology is the study of the interaction of chemicals with biological entities.
>
> Pharmacology is the study of substances that interact with living systems through chemical processes, especially by binding to regulatory molecules and thereby activate or inhibit biological activities in the body.

There are as many definitions of pharmacology as there are those defining the science. Given the breadth and scope of the discipline it is hardly surprising that there is such a variance in definitions. For the purposes of this chapter we will define the field in as simple yet inclusive terms as possible:

Pharmacology is the study of the effects of chemicals and the mechanism of these effects on living organisms (pharmacodynamics), and the effects of the living organisms on the chemicals including absorption, distribution, metabolism, and excretion (pharmacokinetics).

1.2 WHAT IS THE POSITION OF PHARMACOLOGY IN THE FIELD OF THERAPEUTICS?

Briefly, the medicinal chemist works in concert with the pharmacologist in determining the efficacy of the chosen target molecule. The lead molecule then is identified following a series of chemical modifications of the target molecule (structure activity relationship, or SAR). The analytical chemist works with both the medicinal chemist and the pharmacologist to assure the chemical structure and purity of the chemical product. The pharmacodynamics group works closely with pharmacology while performing the SAR studies. The pharmacokinetics group works with pharmacology and analytical chemistry to assess how the body affects a chemical once administered. The pharmaceutics group works with the pharmacokinetics/pharmacodynamics groups and the pharmacologist to determine how best to formulate the drug for maximum efficacy. Once the lead compound, formulation, and route(s) of administration have been selected, the toxicology group works with the pharmacologist to determine potential sites of toxicity in experimental animals.

Once preclinical toxicology studies have been completed, an application is submitted to the FDA for approval to perform clinical trials for efficacy and toxicity in human subjects. Finally, if efficacy and toxicology warrant it, another application is submitted to the FDA for drug marketing approval. As we can see from the brief description, the pharmacologist plays a pivotal role in every aspect of the drug discovery and development process. A thorough discussion of this process can be found in Chapter 15 of this textbook.

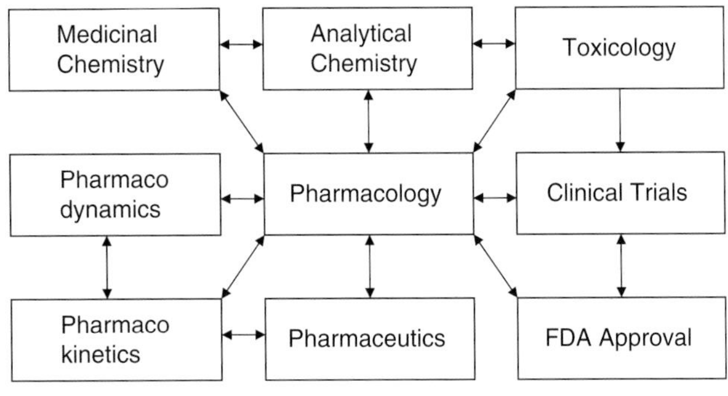

Figure 1.1 Pharmacology: A multifacted discipline.

1.3 THE BEGINNINGS OF PHARMACOLOGY

Pharmacology is both an ancient science and a relatively new science. Since the beginning of mankind there has been a search for ways to alleviate the pain and suffering associated with life. To the ancient pharmacologist this meant painstaking observations and experimentation with natural products such as plants, animals, and minerals. Substances like fruits, leaves, bark, roots, dirt, and animal parts were rubbed on to the human body, boiled in hot water and drunk, smelled, or consumed in the physical state that they were gathered. The effects of these preparations on the human were noted and discussed and thus tribal folklore evolved. Slowly a knowledge base developed regarding what to use for a given malady.

As different tribes comingled, exchange of tribal folklore more than likely occurred and an ever-increasing compendium of useful, not so useful, and even horribly dangerous remedies developed. A good example of how these ideas and concepts grew into understanding the need of specific items in our diet and health was common salt. Long before recorded time, salt trade routes were established between the hot dry climates near the sea where salt deposits flourished, and the areas where salt was scarce. Why did salt become an essential ingredient in the lives of the ancients? Perhaps by ancients observing animal behavior and dietary activities in and around natural salt flats. The practice of mimicking animal behavior aided in the evolution of both foodstuffs and potential remedies for disease.

Diet was then and remains today a vital component of maintaining good health and battling disease. Various foods were scrutinized for their possible health values and were passed from culture to culture and generation to generation. Those who were charged with maintaining the health of a given tribe or population were expected to know the values of different foods, medicinal plants, minerals, and even such esoteric things as the healing properties of smoke and chants. Equally importantly these individuals had to know how and when to administer these healing agents. Records from ancient China, India, Sumeria, Egypt, and Greece are full of suggestions, often in great detail, of the health benefits of every known fruit, grain, tuber, berry, or vegetable. Other records describe different soil and mineral preparations, as well as animal parts, for medicinal properties. In certain cultures, many of these preparations remain in vogue and are still used.

Consider one example and how important it may have been in maintaining the health of early hunter/gatherer societies, especially nomadic tribes constantly moving into new uncharted territories. Having no extensive knowledge of the new area these people relied heavily on trial and error when it came to gathering plants for food. Using observational information obtained by watching what the indigenous animal ate helped somewhat. Given what we now know about species variation among animals, plants that are edible for a given animal could prove to be a devastating poison to the humans who recently moved into the new region. From careful observations the ancients also knew that certain plants or parts of plants could induce vomiting. If the consumption of an unknown foreign plant resulted in unpleasant sensations in the GI tract they knew to consume a medicinal plant to rid themselves of the new plant. In fact, one of the most widely described medicinal purposes of plants was that of a purgative.

One of the oldest medicinal preparations made by man was alcohol. Here again careful observations provided the basis for the development of this ancient and important drug. Recipes for beer, wine, and mead are found in the oldest of recorded literature from cultures worldwide. Not only were these liquids used in ceremonial practices, their medicinal properties of decreasing pain sensation and the ability to induce sleep were greatly appreciated. As the cultures became more sophisticated these alcoholic beverages were used as tinctures of herbs to enhance the medicinal effectiveness of herbs and plants.

1.4 PHARMACOLOGY OF THE GRECO-ROMAN ERA

Probably the best recognized of all the ancient Greek physicians is Hippocrates. It is likely that much of the writings attributed to this man came from a group of health professionals of whom Hippocrates was the most prominent member. During this time rationality was introduced in the healing process as they began to understand the importance of careful descriptions of diseases, symptoms, and geographical locations. In spite of the importance of this group in the field of medicine they really had little to do with drugs. Rather, Hippocrates and his followers relied much more on the healing power of nature, known as *Vis medicatrix naturae*. It is of interest that even today there is evidence of the placebo effect in which the patient cures him- or herself though the belief in the curing effects of the drug even though no drug is present in their medicine. Is this not an example of the healing power of nature?

The evolution of the healing practices was transferred to the Roman empire as Greek doctors came to Rome, many times as slaves. It is here where interest in medicines grew rapidly. Celsus wrote eight books on disease, containing significant references to the use of drugs in the treatment of disease. As in Greece, the health professionals of Rome felt it necessary to maintain excellent records and perform careful observations. One of the most important records of that time was kept by Dioscorides, a Roman surgeon, who traveled with Nero's armies compiling all the information on drugs that he could. This compendium, entitled *Materia Medica*, included some 600 plants, also including illustrations, how to find the plant, where to find the plant, and how and when to use the plant.

With the growth of knowledge of the medicinal properties associated with plants came the fear of accidental or intentional poisoning. Rulers of Rome were especially fearful as it was clearly established that ascension along the political ranks was best accomplished by assassination of those above you. An interesting undertaking was that of Mithridates, King of Pontus, in which he described a "universal antidote" called mithridatium, a concoction of 35 different ingredients. An interesting myth associated with this universal antidote is that a ruler taking mithridatium was given the opportunity to kill himself rather than suffer the embarrassment of being killed by his captors. To do this he had to use his sword because none of the available poisons were effective against mithridatium.

An important physician during the second century AD was Galen, who solidified the concept of the four humors first championed by Hippocrates into the workings of the healthcare providers. These humors were blood, phlegm, yellow bile, and black bile. So powerful was the influence of Galen, that Galenic principles of medicine were practiced to the eighteenth century, much to the detriment of medical evolution. It must be noted however that Galen was an excellent experimentalist and observationalist. Galen first described that blood occupied the arterial system, that the heart provided the power to move blood, and that the heart isolated from the body continued to beat.

As time progressed, the Byzantine and Muslim worlds added to the base of knowledge concerning drugs. Most of the information gained during this period was a continuation of the efforts started in Greece and Rome, that being the production of further compendia of medicinal plants. The Muslims provided such contributions as the development of syrups for respiratory ailments, the use of mercurial formulations for skin diseases and the process of distillation to obtain concentrates of beer and wine. In addition, important refinements were made in the record keeping and organization of medical plants. However during this time the alchemists came into fashion and worked diligently on such projects as turning lead into gold and the search for the universal "elixir of life" to cure all diseases and prolong a healthy life. The concept behind the elixir arose from the observations that wine made the ill feel better, brought on a feeling of euphoria, and made the elders feel young again. Thus, it was believed that with proper distillation techniques the important elixir or spirit could be isolated and used. Unfortunately for all, this was never accomplished.

1.5 PHARMACOLOGY AND THE MIDDLE AGES

The middle ages of Europe (*ca* 10–15 centuries AD) were a time of feudalism, authoritarianism, and dogmatic religious leaders. During this period intellectual thought and discovery were hampered terribly by the intellectual complexity of the times. The Roman era of peace and security was gone and was replaced by epidemics, squalor, poverty, and ignorance throughout Europe. All teachings revolved around salvation through the church. The health professional virtually disappeared and the use and understanding of drugs fell back to pre-Greco-Roman times. Civilization and learning were almost the exclusive provenance of the monasteries, monks skillfully copying manuscripts for dispersal to other monasteries. Monks maintained drug-herbal gardens to assure at least a semblance of plant drug supply.

If one city can be highlighted as the most important in bringing Greco-Roman medicine back to Europe it must be Salerno, an important trading center on the southwest coast of Italy. Here traders from all over the world came to trade their goods and bring information and knowledge back to Europe. It is here where a hospital not under the thumb of the church sprang up. The caretakers of the sick sought reference works from the foreign traders and back came the drug information that had been all but lost during the middle ages. The task of converting these compendia from their native languages of Greek and Arabic to Latin fell onto the shoulders of a few, with one of the most notable being Constantinus Africanus. Born in Carthage and widely traveled, Constantinus took on the onerous responsibility of manuscript translation including a major compendium on Greco-Roman and Muslim plant- and animal-based drugs. So influential was his work that he was asked to translate classical literature, which may have played a role in the recovery of universities in Europe.

The medical school in Salerno slowly became quite successful. Members of the school were allowed to think freely and question authority, providing an intellectual atmosphere for growth. During this time a rebirth in codifying medical plants occurred. New approaches to treating disease were developed such as the use of seaweed (high in iodine) to treat goiter, cleaning a wound using alcohol distillates, and the rediscovery of mercurial ointments to treat skin sores and lice. So successful was this school of medicine that the churches began to build medical schools modeled after that in Salerno. Toward the end of the middle ages drug use and drug trade were firmly reestablished, thus paving the way for growth during the Renaissance.

1.6 PHARMACOLOGY AND THE RENAISSANCE

Several important events occurred during the Renaissance that drove the growth of pharmacology. First was the development of the movable type printing press. With this machine came the availability of books that could be dispersed and read. Knowledge could be obtained and spread with relative ease, enabling those interested to learn about medicinal plants and animals. Further, new knowledge could be dispersed far more easily and rapidly than ever before. At the same time glorious new geographical explorations were leaving from Europe to the far reaches of the Earth. The adventurers returned with exotic plants and stories on how these plants were used medically. Finally, the mind of the European was now open after centuries of religious constraints and new ideas and concepts began to evolve.

Herbalists in every country were gathering plants and knowledge in attempts to develop new medicines to treat disease. With the gain of medical knowledge came the birth of a formalized botany. German herbalists are considered to be the fathers of botany. One German physician condemned his fellow German herbalists for using names on their drug receptacles with Greek names that were no longer applicable. He authored a short poetic piece that expressed the feelings of society of that day toward the healers (come to think of it, many today still hold this belief):

> Three faces has the doctor:
> A god's when first he's sought
> And then an angel's, cures half wrought:
> But when comes due the doctor's fee,
> Then Satan looks less terrible than he!

What was the crowning achievement of this enlightened period? Probably a continuation of what had preceded this era—care in cataloguing plant medicines, how to prepare them, and how to use them. The printing press enabled these cataloguers to widely disperse their work. Two important names are associated with this period, Cordus and Vesalius. Valerius Cordus, during his relatively short life, edited and expanded the pivotal work of Dioscorides. His work marked the transition from magic, spells, and alchemy to a rational approach to chemical experimentation. In addition, Cordus developed the first true pharmacopeia, the *Dispesatorium pharmacopolarum*, which received wide use and served as the format for plethora of pharmacopeias that arose following the publication of his work. Vesalius's major contribution was the standardization of drug preparation in order to assure to some degree a uniformity in expected results following the use of any given drug.

One of the most important experimentalists of the time was a Swiss named Auerrolus Theophrastus Bombastus von Hohenheim, or Paracelsus as he called himself. His father was a physician and he, too, became a trained physician. After earning his degree he traveled extensively, learning the art of medicine from a number of different sources. An interesting character, he was appointed professor of medicine at Basel and shortly thereafter was erroneously thought to have been killed in a tavern brawl in Salzburg. A gruff, bombastic, but brilliant individual, he first described the concept of dose response relationship when he said (paraphrased), "Everything is a poison and nothing is a poison, it is only the dose that counts." As an experimentalist he noted a correlation between exposure to dust in mines and lung damage, he studied the effect of mineral baths on skin disorders, and the role of heavy metals in the treatment of disease. He may well have been the first to use pure chemicals as drugs.

Along with the growing appreciation for careful observations and record keeping came the increased interest in and the use of poisons. The most fascinating family of the era was the Borgias, an Italian family who manipulated the papacy and the empire in large part through their expertise in poisoning. An interesting aspect of this was the fact that they used arsenic trioxide, a water-soluble white powder without taste or aroma. The compound often was mixed with wine and was virtually nondetectable. It is often said that the Borgias gave rise to experimental toxicology. Although arsenic trioxide was used during the Renaissance, just recently the drug has been approved by the FDA for the treatment of cancer!

1.7 PHARMACOLOGY AND THE BAROQUE PERIOD

The next two centuries brought about changes in medicine and the developing field of pharmacology too numerous to discuss in detail. An attempt will be made to select some of the more important highlights of this interesting era. This period can be considered a groundbreaking time with respect to experimentalism. A motivating factor in drug discovery during this period was the introduction of new plants (and drugs) from places far away for this was the time of extended geographical exploration. The Spaniards brought back a variety of plant samples from South America, and the Portuguese discovered a trade route to the Far East and brought back many medicinal plants and spices.

The introduction of these highly acclaimed and important new sources of drugs to European medicine was slow because each country carefully guarded their findings. However, two of the most important drugs had to be ipecacuanha and cinchona bark. The former was shown to have significant but relatively safe emetic properties. The drug became an important treatment for diarrhea and dysentery. In the decoction was a drug emetine that became the treatment of choice for amebic dysentery and amebic abscess. It wasn't until the twentieth century that newer drugs to treat amebiasis were introduced. The cinchona bark was important in treating fevers as an extract of the bark; often referred to simply as *The Bark*, it seemed to treat all fevers regardless of origin. The use of The Bark became so widespread throughout Europe that the cinchona tree became scarce. It is of interest that a similar situation occurred quite recently when the bark of old-growth Yew trees was shown to contain taxanes, which proved effective in treating cancer. So effective in fact that there was a very real fear that there were insufficient trees to support the production of the drug. We encourage you to read the story of taxol and how this problem was overcome.

Cinchona remained a very valuable medicine even up to WWII, when Allied soldiers in the South Pacific were exposed to malaria. Cinchona bark (quinine) was used extensively to treat the disease. After the Japanese invaded and controlled Java, an important source of the bark was lost, which necessitated the development of alternative medicines to treat this horrid disease.

In addition to the introduction of many new medicines, many important discoveries were made by scientists of the time. For example, William Withering, a British physician, first described the effects of an extract of the leaves of the purple foxglove on cardiac dropsy (congestive heart failure). From his careful experimentation, the dose-related difference in the effects of digitalis on the human body were first described and still remain pertinent today. Edward Jenner noted that milkmaids seldom got small pox but instead suffered a far less severe form of the disease known as cow pox. From this observation, soon he was inoculating an individual with the pus from a cow pox pustule and then later challenged that individual with small pox. Cow pox protected the person from small pox! William Harvey first reported that the circulatory system was a closed system using the heart to pump blood through the vasculature system. He also suggested that drugs taken orally entered the body through the gastrointestinal tract and were distributed throughout the body via the blood.

Work done during this period was severely hampered by the lack of chemical isolation and characterization techniques. However, it was during this time that the foundations for such approaches were developed. Individuals such as Robert Boyle, Joseph Priestly, and Antoine-Laurent Lavoisier were actively investigating the principles of physics, gasses, and chemical isolation. This time period provided the basis for the explosion of scientific investigation and the birth of modern pharmacology that occurred during the next century.

1.8 THE BIRTH OF MODERN PHARMACOLOGY

The basics of analytical chemistry had been introduced in the late eighteenth century and were rapidly applied to pharmacology. The seminal work in the field of active ingredient isolation was that of Friedrich Wilhelm Serturner, a German pharmacist with a deep interest in opium. Extracting opium with an acid, he isolated a water soluble compound that induced sleep in dogs and himself. He called the chemical *morphine*, in honor of the god of sleep. Within a relatively short period of time a variety of chemicals were isolated from crude plant sources and the beginnings of testing isolated chemicals, rather than a crude extract of a plant, for pharmacological activities began in earnest.

Francois Magendie studied a variety of chemical extracts of plants, focusing primarily on the newly defined class of chemicals called the alkaloids. He became so impressed with the chemicals that he developed a compendium of alkaloids that described the actions and indications of a variety alkaloids recently isolated and described. More importantly, Magendie laid down the basic principles that remain unique to pharmacology today:

- Dose response effect, explored from the beginning but not quantitated until 1927
- Factors involved in ADME
- Identification of the drug site of action
- The mechanism of action of the drug
- Structure activity relationship

Much of the work done regarding the use of these principles in the scientific laboratory was done first by Magendie's pupil Claude Bernard, a gifted physiologist/early pharmacologist. He developed a number of theories—some proved wrong, such as the coagulation theory of anesthesia, and some proved quite valid, such as the use of morphine before chloroform to enhance the anesthetic properties of chloroform. This latter observation was one of the first to describe drug–drug interactions.

Magendie's other student, equally gifted as Bernard but less well known, was James Blake. Enamored with technology of the time, Blake used newly developed instrumentation to determine blood pressure, blood circulation time, and was probably the first to report on structure activity relationships as they pertain to drug discovery. He was truly a renaissance man as he was involved in a variety of pharmacological, medical, and veneologic enterprises. He even served as president of the California Academy of Science, where he reported on his studies in meteorology, geology, and biochemistry to name a few. The contributions of Magendie and his students Bernard and Blake laid the groundwork for modern pharmacology.

A significant advance made during the first half of the nineteenth century was research into anesthesiology. Surgical techniques developed far faster than did methods to decrease or eliminate the pain associated with surgery. As a result the mark of a good surgeon was the speed with which he could complete a given procedure. The first anesthetic to gain popularity was nitrous oxide, although it must be said that the interest in this gas was more at medical side shows than medical practice. A dentist, Horace Wells, demonstrated that tooth extraction could be completed painlessly if the patient were under the influence of nitrous oxide. Unfortunately, when the procedure was performed at the Massachusetts General Hospital, in front of the medical leaders of the time, the demonstration was a failure as the patient squawked and fought the extraction. As is the case all too often in science, the establishment attacked Wells for the failure and Wells retired in disgrace.

William Morton, a colleague and partner of Wells, the man who set up the nitrous oxide demonstration at Massachusetts General, feared that nitrous oxide was not reproducibly strong enough to provide the needed anesthesia and sought a more powerful anesthetic. Ether was selected as the next anesthetic for testing. Morton developed the technique for ether delivery and provided a demonstration again at Mass. General, and this time the demonstration was a total success. He also reported on ether-induced vomiting in children, an experience this author is all too familiar with following tonsil extraction in the early 1950s.

James Young Simpson was dissatisfied with the time required for ether-induced anesthesia and received from a chemist friend of his, three chloroform-based liquids. He then tested these products on his friends and family for anesthetic potential! Of the samples tested, chloroform provided the most rapid and effective anesthesia. Simpson went on to use chloroform with great success in controlling pain of childbirth but this did not come without controversy. The church fought the use of anesthetics in something so divine as childbirth. Even at this time fundamentalism was still supreme but Simpson ultimately won the day by arguing that the Bible states clearly how Adam was put to sleep before Eve was born from him.

The success of both ether and chloroform resulted in much debate about the merits of each. Chloroform was preferred in England and Europe, whereas ether was preferred in the United States. A great deal of work was done on which anesthetic was better, and although no true conclusion was attained, this scientific undertaking was one of the first in comparative pharmacology addressing the risks and benefits of different drugs.

During this time the fathers of modern pharmacology were establishing their laboratories in Germany. Rudolf Buchheim, recognized as the first German pharmacologist, was able to eliminate a number of old and ineffective therapies, and produced a new compendium of drugs based on the proven effects of the drugs. He taught pharmacology out of his home and studied the pharmacokinetics of minerals and heavy metals and ascribed to the belief that drugs must be studied in a systematic way to provide a rational background for drug therapy. His pupils then established the field of pharmacology throughout the Germanic countries. One of his students, Oswald Schmiedeberg, has been credited with training all the Americans who established pharmacology in the United States.

During the nineteenth century, the concept of isolating pure chemicals with bioactivities was established. The pure chemical then could be characterized structurally and could be evaluated carefully and accurately for varying biological activities. The success of this approach meant that health practitioners could provide their patients the benefits of these isolated characterized bioactive natural products. As pharmacology matured further, the concept of making synthetic drugs through chemical synthesis began to take hold.

The rise of chemistry at this time made this approach possible. John Dalton described the atomic theory, making it possible to understand how inorganic molecules fit together. Kekule described the aromatic ring of organic compounds. In addition, synthetic chemistry was coming of age. A driving force for the production of synthetic drugs was the economic problem with quinine and the bark of the cinchona tree and the hope for safer more effective drugs coming from the chemist's bench.

In 1872, Schmiedeberg established his laboratories in a newly renovated building in Strassburg, which became the first well-equipped modern laboratory for pharmacology. As stated before, these new and up-to-date facilities attracted many of the brightest young U.S. students of pharmacology. His research included investigations on the similarities between the chemical muscarine and electrical stimulation and that the effects of both could be blocked by atropine. As can be seen, the ability to study single drug entities greatly enhanced the quantity and quality of the pharmacological research being done in the latter portion of the nineteenth century.

Another important contribution of the Schmiedeberg lab was the careful studies on how drugs were "detoxified" and removed from living tissue. He showed the importance of glucuorinic acid and the liver in removal of drugs from the body via the kidney. His laboratory and the students within it were so prolific that a journal, often referred to as *Schmiedeberg's Archives* (formally known as *Archives for Experimentelle Pathlogie and Pharmakologie*), was established. The importance of this event rests in the fact that it established pharmacology as an independent field of investigation and the important role pharmacology would play in medical education.

Schmiedeberg's successor, Rudolf Bohm, isolated and characterized anti-helmentic therapy. Of interest, Bohm also demonstrated that there are times when a crude preparation on a botanical is safer and more effective than the chemically pure isolate.

The number of exciting findings made during the latter portion of the nineteenth century are too numerous to describe, as are the scientists involved in this research. Suffice it to say that the latter part of the nineteenth century was an amazing time in pharmacology, bringing together all the advances made in the recent past and utilizing them to propel pharmacology into the twentieth century, and the importance of this exciting field in the next 108 years. The advances made during the twentieth century provide the basis of this textbook, and the ever-growing importance of pharmacology as a discipline. Hopefully, this chapter provided an interesting read and new insight into how the field of pharmacology developed into the discipline it is today.

REFERENCES

Holmstedt, B., & Liljestrand, G. (1963). *Readings in pharmacology*. New York: MacMillan.

Leake, C. D. (1975). *An historical account of pharmacology to the 20th century*. Springfield, IL: Charles C. Thomas.

Oldham, F. K., Kelsey, F. E., & Geiling, E. M. K. (1955). *Essentials of pharmacology*. Philadelphia: Lippincott.

Sneader, W. (1985). *Drug discovery: The evolution of modern medicines*. New York: Wiley.

Chapter

2

Dosage Forms and Their Routes of Administration

Kenneth Alexander

OUTLINE

2.1 INTRODUCTION

Drug substances are seldom administered in their natural or pure state, as they once were when families cultivated medicines that in their gardens or native peoples of the land collected in the wild.

The pharmaceutical industry combines the active ingredient, which was either synthesized in a laboratory or extracted from its source, with those nonmedicinal agents that serve varied and specialized pharmaceutical functions. These latter ingredients usually are referred to as pharmaceutical ingredients, aides, adjuncts, necessities, or excipients, which result in a variety of pharmaceutical dosage forms. These ingredients are added to solubilize, stabilize, preserve, color, flavor, suspend, thicken, dilute, emulsify, and produce efficacious and appealing dosage forms.

Each pharmaceutical preparation is unique in its physical and pharmaceutical characteristics as well as the final form in which the drug is presented for patient acceptance.

The pharmaceutical industry thus is challenged to produce a dosage form that provides therapeutics for the patient, which a physician can deem acceptable. The potent nature and low dosage for most drugs used in practice usually precludes any expectation that the general public could safely obtain the appropriate dose of the drug from the bulk material. The vast majority of drug substances are administered in milligrams, which usually requires the use of a very sensitive laboratory balance. When the dose of a drug is minute, solid dosage forms such as tablets and capsules must be prepared with the diluents or fillers so that the resultant dosage unit may be large enough to be handled.

In addition to providing the mechanism for a safe and convenient delivery of an accurate dose, the dosage form must provide:

1. Protection of the drug from destructive influences of atmospheric oxygen or moisture (e.g., coated tablets, sealed capsules, etc.)
2. Protection of a drug from the destructive influences of gastric acid after oral administration
3. Concealment of the bitter, salty, or obnoxious taste or odor of a drug substance (e.g., capsules, coated tablets, flavored syrups)
4. Liquid dosage forms for soluble substances in a desired vehicle (e.g., solutions)
5. Liquid dosage forms for either the insoluble or the unstable in the desired vehicle (e.g., suspensions)
6. Extended drug action through the use of special controlled release mechanisms
7. Optimal drug action from topically applied sites (e.g., ointments, creams, ophthalmic, ear, and nasal preparation)

8. The ability to insert the drug into one of the body's orifices
9. The ability to place drugs within body tissues (e.g., injections)
10. Drug actions through inhalation

In addition, many dosage forms include appropriate markings to permit ease of drug identification by the use of distinctive color, shape, or packaging.

2.2 THERAPEUTIC RAMIFICATIONS IN SELECTING THE APPROPRIATE DOSAGE FORMS

2.2.1 Overview

The nature of the disease or illness for which the drug substance is intended is essential in deciding which dosage forms of that drug should be prepared and marketed. Is the disease state better when treated locally or systematically? Which dosage forms should be prepared and evaluated by clinical trials? What assessments are to be made as to whether the disease state is best treated with prompt, slow, short, or long acting dosage forms? Is there a chance that a given drug may have applications to an emergency situation as to whether the patient is comatose, unlikely, or unwilling to take oral medication, thus necessitating the administration of an appropriate parental dosage that would need to be developed? Is the illness of such a nature that self-administration of an appropriate dosage form (e.g., tablets, capsules, administered liquid) can treat it safely?

In the majority of the cases the drug manufacturer will prepare a single drug substance into several dosage forms to satisfy the personal preferences of physicians or patients, or to partly meet the specific needs or requirements of a certain situation.

Medication may be given prophylactically (e.g., to combat nausea and vomiting from motion sickness or pregnancy). It should be noted that this therapy would have little value during the course of the illness for which it was taken to prevent. Suppositories are also prepared and available for use when required, and can be extremely useful when treating infants or small children.

Each drug administered has its own characteristics relating to drug absorption. Some drugs may be well absorbed from a given route of administration whereas others may be poorly absorbed. Each drug must be individually evaluated with the most effective routes determined and dosage forms prepared.

Drugs intended for localized effects are generally applied directly to the intended site of action. These products include those intended for use in the eyes, ears, nose, and throat, as well as applied to the skin or placed into, on, or around the other body cavities. They may even be applied to the oral cavity or swallowed to treat any localized diseases within the gastrointestinal tract.

2.2.2 The Patient's Age

The patient's age has a profound influence on the types of dosage forms in which a drug may be given. Pharmaceutical liquids rather than solid dosage forms should be considered for infants and children who are under the age of five years. The liquid dosage forms are generally flavored aqueous solutions, syrups, hydroalcoholic solutions, suspensions, or emulsions, which are administered directly into the oral cavity or administered with food to aid consumption.

When the infant or child cannot swallow, due to a crisis such as vomiting, gagging, or rebellion, there may be a question as to how much of the drug has been ingested or expectorated. A single liquid, *pediatric,* dosage form can be used for infants and children of all ages. The dose of the drug can be varied by the volume administered. Rectal suppositories may also be administered to infants and children using smaller sized dosage units. It should be realized that drug absorption from the rectum is erratic and often unpredictable.

2.2.3 Factors Affecting Dosage

Drug dosing has been described as a quantity of an entity that is just enough but not too much, with the intended idea to produce an optimum therapeutic effect in a given patient with the lowest possible dose. Many things in nature can be considered poisons if the dose is uncontrolled. Those poisons that have their dose controlled are called drugs. This concept becomes evident if the patient consumes too much drug per dose and becomes toxic.

During the evolution of European society, aspiring enemies or family routinely killed nobility with poisons. In order to avoid this demise, many nobles instituted two general procedures: one, tasters who consumed some of the food prior to the nobility, and two, the gradual consumption of the common poisons of their time in an increasing dosage to build up tolerance and avoid death by poison.

The dose of a drug is an individual consideration with many factions contributing to the size and effectiveness of that given. The correct drug dose would be the smallest effective amount. This would probably vary among individuals. It could also vary in that same individual on different occasions. A normal distribution or bell-shaped curve would be indicative of these scenarios, and would produce an average effect in the majority of individuals.

A portion of the patients will see little effect from the drug whereas another group of similar size could see a greater effect from the same dose of drug. The majority will exhibit the average effect. The dosage that will provide the average effect will be the drug's usual dosage.

In order to produce systemic effects, the drug must be absorbed from its route of administration at a suitable rate. It must also be distributed in adequate concentration to the receptor sites, and must remain at the receptor site for a sufficient duration of time. A measurement of a drug's absorption characteristics can be determined by the blood serum concentration over a specific time interval. Blood samples usually are taken at specific points within this time frame. For systemic drugs a correlation can be made between the blood serum concentration and the presentation of a therapeutic effect. The average blood serum concentration of a drug can be determined, which represents the minimum in concentration expected to produce the desired patient response (also known as the Minimum Effective Concentration or MEC). The second level of blood serum concentration is that of Minimum Toxic Concentration (MTC).

Drug concentrations above this level would produce dose-related toxicity effects while challenging patient safety. Ideally, serum drug concentration is usually well maintained between the MEC and MTC for the period of time that the desired drug effects are in force. The time–blood level will usually vary among patients and will be dependent upon the drug itself, the drugs physicochemical characteristics, the dosage form type, the pathological state of the patient, the patient's diet, the patient's ethnicity, concomitant drug therapy, as well as other factors.

The median effective dose of a drug is that quantity that will produce 50% of the desired therapeutic intensity. The median toxic dose is that quantity of drug that will produce a defined toxic effect in 50% of the individuals tested. The relationships between the desired and undesired effects of a drug are expressed as its therapeutic index. It is defined as the ratio between a drug's median toxic dose and its median effective dose (TDSO/EDSO).

The therapeutic index is usually viewed as a general guide to the margin of safety. It must be judged with respect to each patient and the patient's response to a given drug; these should be considered separately.

Factions that can influence giving the proper dose of a drug for a given patient include the patient's age, weight, sex, pathological state, tolerance to the drug, time of drug administration, route of administration, concurrent administration of one or more other drugs, and a wide variety of physiologic and psychological factors.

2.2.3.1 Age

The age of the patient who is being treated must be considered, especially if the patient is very young or very old. Newborns, particularly if born premature, are abnormally sensitive to certain drugs due to the immature state of their hepatic and renal function, which would normally inactivate and eliminate the drugs from the body. Failure to detoxify and eliminate drugs results in their accumulation in the tissues to toxic levels. Aged individuals may also respond abnormally to drugs due to their impaired ability to inactivate or excrete drugs because of other concurrent pathogens. Prior to current concepts of the physiologic difference among adults, children, and infants, these last two patients were treated is if they were miniature adults. Various rules of dosage in which pediatric dosing has been prominent, specify the child's dose (CD) and the adult dose (AD) as follows:

Young's Rule

$$CD = \frac{Age}{Age + 12}(AD)$$

Clark's Rule

$$CD = \frac{\text{Weight (in pounds)} \times AD}{150}$$

Cowling's Rule

$$CD = \frac{\text{Age at next birthday (in years)} \times AD}{24}$$

Fried's Rule

$$CD = \frac{\text{Age (in month)} \times AD}{150}$$

Today, these rules are not often used since age alone is no longer considered to be a valid criterion by itself for use in the determination of children's dosage. This stems from the fact that the adult dose itself provides wide clinical variations in response. The usual clinical pediatric dose is now determined for specific drugs and dosage for through clinical evaluation.

2.2.3.2 Body Weight

When considering body weight, the usual doses for infants and children is given by the following rule:

Clark's Rule

$$CD = \frac{\text{Weight (in pounds)} \times AD}{150}$$

Adult doses for drugs generally are considered suitable for those individuals who are 70 kilograms (150 pounds). This weight does not match with today's average adult weight; females average between 120 to 220 pounds, and males average between 180 to 360 pounds. The ratio between the amount of drug administered and the size of the body influences the drug concentration at its site of action.

Drug dosage may require adjustment for those individuals who are abnormally thin or obese. We must also consider the drug to be administered as well as the patient's pathology and physiological state.

The dosage of a number of drug substances is based on body weight and can be expressed in a milligram (mg) of a drug per kilogram (kg) of the body weight, or mg per pound basis.

2.2.3.3 Body Surface Areas

There is a close correlation between a large number of physiological processes and body surface area (BSA). A formula for determining a child's dose based

Table 2.1 Nomogram for Children

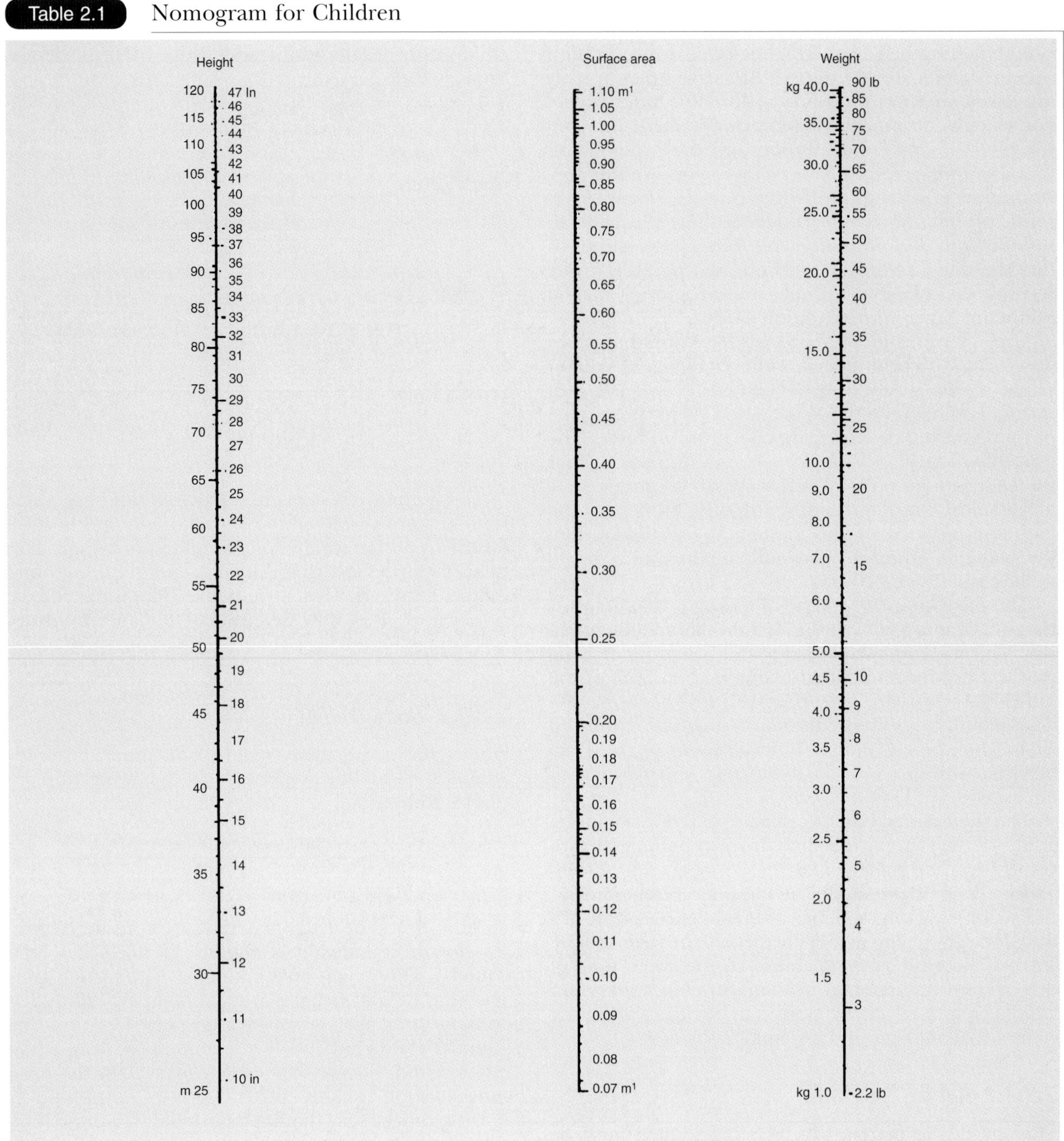

on relative body surface area and the adult dose is as follows:

$$\mathrm{CD} = \frac{\text{Surface area of child's body}}{\text{Surface area of adult's body}} \times \mathrm{AD}$$

This equation provides the approximate child's dose without considering any other factors. The surface area for an individual may be determined using one of the methods described in Tables 2.1 and 2.2, and by using Table 2.3. Tables 2.1 and 2.2 compare the approximate relationship of surface area and weights of individuals of average body dimensions, and are based on an average BSA of 1.73 square meters. Table 2.3 compares the BSA of both children and adults based on their body weight and heights. The nomogram is based on the formula of DuBois and Dubois,[1] where $S = W^{0.25} \times H^{0.725} \times 71.84$ or $\log S = 0.425 \log W + 0.725 \log H + 1.8564$ where S = body surface area in cm^2, W = weight in kg, and H = height in cm.

[1]DuBois and Dubois (1916). *Arch Intern Med* **17**: 863.

Table 2.2 Nomogram for Adults

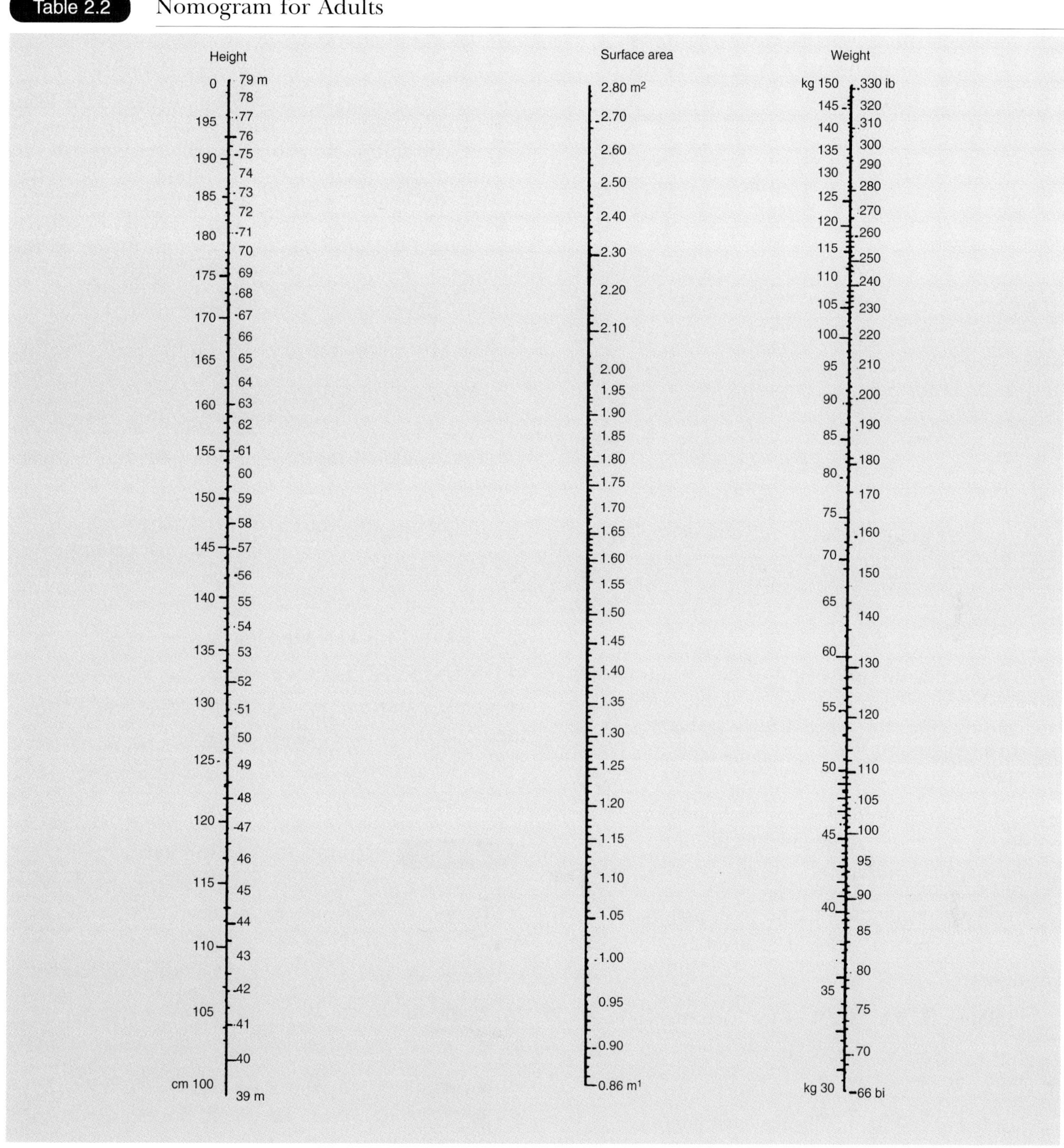

It has long been recognized that a relationship exists between physiological processes and BSA; practitioners have advocated the use of BSA as a parameter for calculating doses for both adults and children. Upon determining the BSA for either an adult or child the dose can be calculated as follows:

$$(\text{BSA}(\text{m}^2)/1.73\text{m}^2) \times \text{usual adult dose} = \text{dose administered}$$

2.2.4 Dose Based on Creatinine Clearance

There are two major mechanisms by which drugs are eliminated from the body, hepatic (liver) metabolism and renal (kidney) excretion. Kidney functions will dramatically affect the rate of drug loss when renal excretion is the major elimination route. Polar drugs are eliminated predominately renally.

For most drugs, a specific drug concentration must be reached in the blood to maintain a proper therapeutic effect. The initial serum concentration attained by a specific dose is usually dependent on the weight of the patient and the volume of body fluids into which the drug is distributed. This volume is usually a theoretical volume based on the serum concentration and the initial dose.

The lean body mass (LBM) provides an excellent estimation of the distribution volume, especially for

Table 2.3 Approximate Relations of Surface Area and Weights of Individuals of Average Body Dimensions

Kilograms	Pounds	Surface Area in Square Meters	Percent of Adult Dose
2	4.4	0.15	9
3	6.6	0.2	11.5
4	8.8	0.25	14
5	11	0.29	16.5
6	13.2	0.33	19
7	15.4	0.37	21
8	17.6	0.4	23
9	19.8	0.43	25
10	22	0.46	27
15	33	0.63	36
20	44	0.83	48
25	55	0.95	55
30	66	1.08	62
35	77	1.2	69
40	88	1.3	75
45	99	1.4	81
50	110	1.51	87
55	121	1.58	91

those drugs that are not well distributed into body fat (adipois) tissue. Lean body mass can be readily calculated using the following formulas based on the patient's height and sex.
For males:

$$LBM = 50kg + 2.3 \text{ kg for each inch over 5 feet of height}$$

or

$$LBM = 110 \text{ lbs} + 5 \text{ lbs for each inch over 5 feet of height}$$

For females:

$$LBM = 45.\ 5 \text{ kg} + 2.3 \text{ kg for each inch over 5 feet of height}$$

or

$$LBM = 100 \text{ lbs} + 5 \text{ lbs for each inch over 5 feet of height}$$

The kidneys receive about 20% of the cardiac output (blood flow) and filters approximately 125 ml of plasma per minute. As the patient loses kidney function, the quantity of plasma filtered per minute decreases with an accompanying decrease in clearance. The most useful estimation of creatinine clearance rate (CC_R) is obtained using the following empirical formula based on the patient's age and serum creatinine level.
For males:

$$CC_R = [98 - 0.8 \text{ (patients age in years} - 20)] / \text{serum creatinine as mg\% (mg/100ml)}$$

For females:

$$CC_R = [(0.9) \times (CC_R \text{ determined for males})]$$

Normal CC_R may be considered as 100ml/minute; once the CC_R and LBM have been calculated the loading dose (initial dose) required to reach a certain serum concentration and the maintenance dose to maintain the specified concentration can be calculated. The loading dose (LD) is based solely on the LBM of the patient. The maintenance dose (MD) is based on LBM and the renal clearance rate of the drug.

$$LD = LBM \text{ (mg, kg, or lbs.)} \times \text{drug dose (kg or lbs)}$$

The MD can be calculated for a "normal" patient:

$$MD_{normal} = LBM(kg) \times \text{dose per kg per dosing interval}$$

For renally impaired patients the MD can be calculated as:

$$MD_{impaired} = [CC_R(\text{patient})/CC_R(\text{normal})] \times \text{dose for a normal patient}$$

2.3 ROUTES OF DRUG ADMINISTRATION

Tables 2.4 and 2.5 show sites of routes of administration and the primary dosage forms.

Table 2.4 Routes of Administration

Term	Site
Oral	Mouth
Peroral (per os 1)	Gastrointestinal tract via mouth
Sublingual	Under the tongue
Parenteral	Other than the gastrointestinal tract (by injection)
Intravenous	Vein
Intraarterial	Artery
Intracardiac	Heart
Intraspinal/intrathecal	Spine
Intraosseous	Bone
Intraarticular	Joint
Intrasynovial	Joint-fluid area
Intracutaneous/intradermal	Skin
Subcutaneous	Beneath the skin
Intramuscular	Muscle
Epicutaneous (topical)	Skin surface
Conjuctival	Conjuctiva
Intraocular	Eyes
Intranasal	Nose
Aural	Ear
Intrarespiratory	Lung
Rectal	Rectum
Vaginal	Vagina
Urethral	Urethra

Table 2.5 Primary Dosage Forms

Route of Administration	Primary Dosage Forms
Oral	Tablets
	Capsules
	Solutions
	Syrups
	Elixirs
	Suspensions
	Magmas
	Gels
	Fast dissolve stips
	Fast dissolve tablets
	Powders
Sublingual	Tablets
	Troches/lozenges
Parenteral	Solutions
	Suspensions
Epicutaneous	Ointments
	Creams
	Pastes
	Powders
	Aerosols
	Lotions
	Solutions
Conjuctival	Ointments
Intraocular	Solutions
Intraaural	Suspensions
Intranasal	Solutions
	Sprays
	Inhalants
	Ointments
Intrarespiratory	Aerosols
Rectal	Solutions
	Ointments
	Suppositories
Vaginal	Solutions
	Ointments
	Emulsion foams
	Tablets
	Suppositories
Urethral	Solutions
	Suppositories

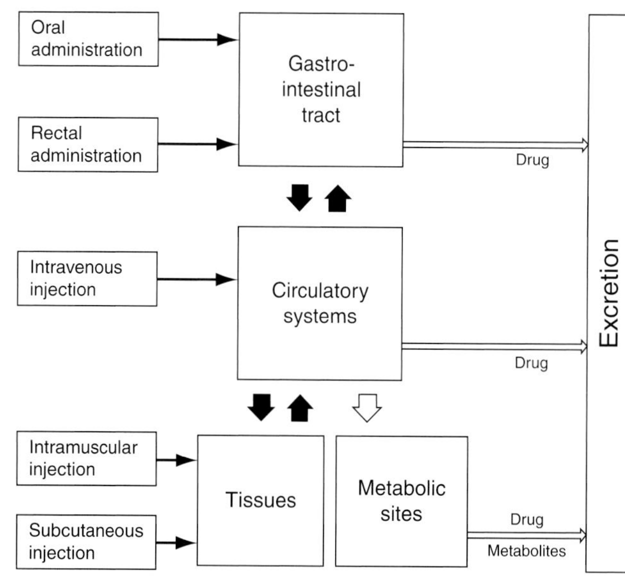

Figure 2.1 Diagram for absorption along the GI tract.

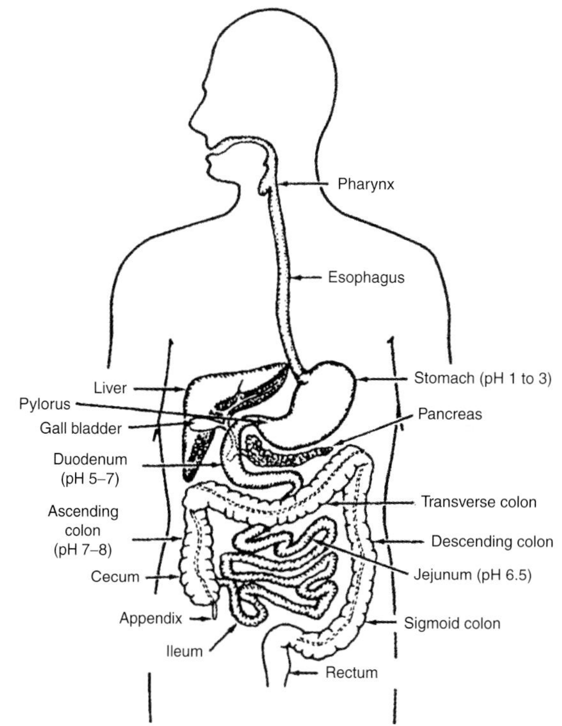

Figure 2.2 Various organs of the GI tract.

2.3.1 Oral Route

2.3.1.1 Introduction

In the United States, drugs are most often taken orally. There are only a few drugs that are intended to be dissolved within the mouth, in sublingual (under-the-tongue) and buccal (against-the-cheek) tablet dosage forms. The vast majority are intended to be swallowed. The majority of these dosage forms are taken for their systemic effects resulting after absorption from the various surfaces along the gastrointestinal (GI) tract. A very few drugs are taken orally for their local action within the confines of the GI tract due to their insolubility and/or poor absorbability from this route. Figure 2.1 provides a diagram for the absorption of drugs along the GI tract, and Figure 2.2 shows the various organs that must be taken into account in the GI tract.

Compared to alternate routes, the oral route is the most natural, uncomplicated, convenient, and safe for administering drugs. Disadvantages include slow response (as compared to parenteral and sublingual dosage forms), chance of irregular absorption of drugs (depending upon such factors as constitutional gut make-up, the amount and/or type of food present at time of ingestion), and destruction of the drug by acid reaction in the stomach and/or by GI enzymes.

The uncertainty of drug maintenance is in the hands of the patient and can lead to over- or underdosage with self-administered drugs.

2.3.1.2 Dissolution and Drug Absorption

In order for a drug to be absorbed, it must be dissolved in the fluid at the absorption site. A drug administered orally in a tablet or capsule dosage form cannot be absorbed until the drug particles are solubilized by the fluids at some point within the GI tract. When the solubility is dependent upon either an acidic or basic medium, the drug would be solubilized in the stomach or intestines, respectively. Drug dissolution is described by the Noyes-Whitney Equation:

$$dC/dt = KS(C_s - C)$$

where

dC/dt = rate of dissolution
K = dissolution rate constant
S = surface area of the dissolving solid
C_s = concentration of the drug in the diffusion layer
C = concentration of the drug in the dissolution medium at time (t)

Factors that can influence bioavailability of oral drugs are summed up in Table 2.6.

2.3.1.3 Ionization of Drugs

Most drugs are either weak acids or bases. Only the unionized species of the drug (unless it is a small molecule, ~ 100 daltons or less) can be absorbed by biological membranes. Therefore knowledge of their individual ionization or dissociation characteristics are important as it governs their absorption by the degree of ionization they present to the absorbing membrane barrier. Cell membranes are more permeable to the unionized form of the drug due to its greater lipid solubility. It is the highly charged cell membrane that results in binding or repelling the ionized form, thus decreasing cell penetration. Ions can become hydrated through their association with covalent molecules. This results in larger particles than the undissociated molecule and decreases penetration capability.

The degree of drug ionization depends upon both the *pH* of the solution in which it is presented to the biological membrane and on the *pKa* (dissociation constant) of the drug (whether it is an acid or base). The entire concept of *pKa* is derived from the Henderson-Hasselbalch equation for both acids and bases as follows:
Acids:

$$pH = pKa + \log[(\text{salt concentration(ionized)}/\text{acid concentration(unionized)}]$$

Bases:

$$pH = pKw - pKb + \log[(\text{base concentration (unionized)}/\text{salt concentration(ionized)}]$$

where

pKa = acid dissociation constant
pKb = base dissociation constant
$pKw \approx 14$ = dissociation of water at 25°C

It should be noted that *pKw* is temperature-dependent and can affect the calculation. Table 2.7 presents the effect of *pH* on the ionization of weak electrolytes (acids and bases) and is taken from Doluisis and Somtoskz.[2]

Table 2.6 Factors That Can Influence the Bioavailability of Orally Administered Drugs

1. Drug substance characteristics
   A. Particle size
   B. Crystalline or amorphous form
   C. Salt form
   D. Hydration
   E. Lipid/water solubility
   F. pH
2. Pharmaceutic ingredients and dosage form characteristics
   A. Pharmaceutic ingredients
      1. Fillers
      2. Binders
      3. Coatings
      4. Disintegrating agents
      5. Lubricants
      6. Suspending agents
      7. Surface active agents
      8. Flavoring agents
      9. Coloring agents
      10. Preservative agents
      11. Stabilizing agents
   B. Disintegration rate (tablets)
   C. Product age and storage conditions

III. Patient characteristics
   A. Gastric emptying time
   B. Intestinal transit time
   C. Gastrointestinal abnormality or pathologic condition
   D. Gastric contents
      1. Other drugs
      2. Food

Table 2.7 The Effect of pH on the Ionization of Weak Electrolytes

pKa-pH	If Weak Acid	If Weak Base
-3	0.1	99.9
-2	0.99	99
-1	9.09	90.9
-0.7	16.6	83.4
-0.5	24	76
-0.2	38.7	61.3
0	50	50
0.2	61.3	38.7
0.5	76	24
0.7	83.4	16.6
1	90.9	9.09
2	99	0.99
3	99.9	0.1

[2] Doluisis and Somtoskz (1965). *Amer J Pharm* **137**: 149.

2.3.1.4 Dosage Forms

Drugs in Solution Drugs in solution represent a number of different dosage forms and include waters, solutions, syrups, elixirs, tinctures, and fluid extracts. Because the drug is already dissolved in the solvent system of the dosage form, absorption begins immediately after ingestion. The rate of absorption depends upon the *pKa* of the drug and the *pH* of the stomach. It is also possible that the environment of the stomach could cause precipitation of the drug, which would delay absorption. This delay would be dependent upon the rate of dissolution of the precipitated drug.

Drugs in Suspension This dosage form contains finely dissolved drug particles (suspensoid) distributed somewhat uniformly throughout the vehicle (suspending medium) in which the drug exhibits a minimum degree of solubility. There are two types of products available commercially:

1. Ready-to-use: A product that is already dispersed throughout a liquid vehicle with or without stabilizers and other pharmaceutical additives.
2. Dry Powders intended for suspension in liquid vehicles: A powder mixture containing the drug and suitable suspending and dispersing agents, which upon dilution and agitation with a specified quantity of vehicle (usually purified water) results in the formation of the final suspension suitable for administration.

There are several reasons for preparing an oral suspension:

1. Certain drugs are chemically unstable when in solution but stable when in suspension.
2. For many patients, the liquid form is preferred over the solid forms (tablets and capsules) due to ease of swallowing.
3. A greater flexibility in dose administration especially for exceedingly large doses.
4. Safety and convenience of liquid doses for infants and children.

The disadvantages of a disagreeable taste for certain drugs given in solution are negligible when the same drug is administered as a suspension. Chemical forms of certain poor-tasting drugs have been developed specifically for the sole purpose of attaining a palatable finished product. Suspensions also include magmas and gels.

2.3.1.5 Emulsion Dosage Form

Emulsions are dispersions in which the dispersed phase (internal phase) is composed of small globules of a liquid distributed throughout a liquid vehicle (external or continuous phase) in which it is immiscible. Emulsions having an oleagenous internal phase and an aqueous external phase are designated oil-in-water (o/w) emulsions, whereas water-in-oil (w/o) emulsions have an aqueous internal phase and an oleaginous external phase. The o/w emulsion can be diluted with water. In order to prepare a stable emulsion an emulsifying agent as well as energy in the form of work is required. Orally administered o/w emulsions permit the administration of a palatable product that normally would be distasteful by adjusting the flavor and sweetener in the aqueous vehicle. The reduced particle size of the oil globules may render the oil more digestible and therefore more readily absorbed.

2.3.1.6 Tablet Dosage Form

Tablets are solid dosage forms prepared by compression on molding. They contain medicinal substances as well as suitable diluents, disintegrants, coatings, colorants, flavors, and sweeteners, if and when needed. These latter ingredients are necessary in preparing tablets of the proper size, consistency, proper disintegration, flow of powders, taste, and sweetness. Various coatings are placed upon tablets to permit safe passage through the acid stomach environment where the acidity or enzymes can destroy the drug. Other coatings can be employed to protect drugs from destructive environmental influences such as moisture, light, and air during storage. Coatings can also conceal a bad or bitter taste of the drug from the patient. Commercial tablets have distinctive colors, shapes, monograms, and code numbers to facilitate their identification and serve as added protection to the public. Figure 2.3 shows several tablet shapes.

2.3.1.7 Capsule Dosage Form

Capsules are solid dosage forms in which the drug and such appropriate pharmaceutical adjuncts, such as fillers, antioxidants, flow enhancers, and surfactants are enclosed in a gelatin shell. A "hard" gelatin capsule is composed of gelatin, glycerin, sugar, and water, whereas a "soft" gelatin capsule is composed of only gelatin, glycerin, and water. Capsules vary in size from 000 to 5. As the number increases the capsule size becomes smaller. The sizes provide a convenient container for the amount of drug to be administered and can be of distinctive shapes and colors when produced commercially. Figure 2.4 shows various capsule sizes.

Generally drugs are released from capsules faster than from tablets because the powdered drug has not been compressed and can dissolve at faster rates. The gelatin (a protein) is acted upon rapidly by the enzymes of the GI tract, which permits gastric juices to penetrate and reach the contents to promote dissolution.

2.3.1.8 Miscellaneous Oral Dosage Forms

Included in this category are lozenges (medicated and nonmedicated), fast dissolving cellulosic strips (Listerine®), and mini melt granules (Mucosin D Pediatric®).

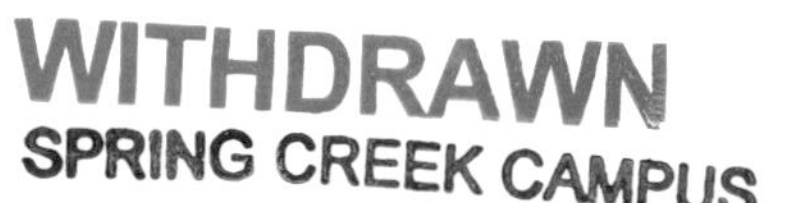

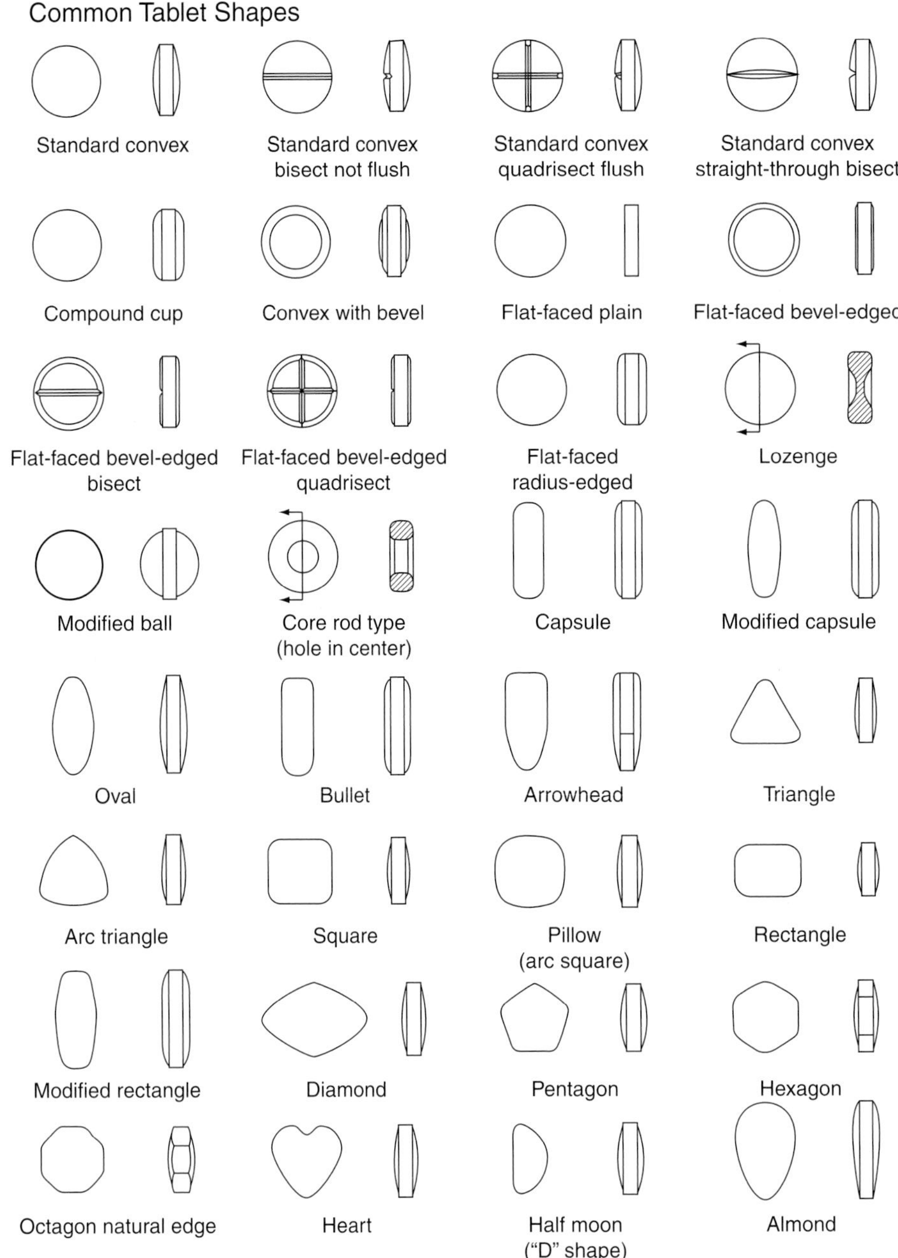

Figure 2.3 Various common tablet shapes. (Used with permission from CSC Publishing. Tablets and Capsules Annual Buyers Guide.)

2.3.2 Rectal Route

Drugs are administered rectally either for their local, or less frequently, for their systemic effects. The dosage forms given rectally include solutions, suspensions, suppositories, and ointments.

The rectum and colon are capable of absorbing many soluble drugs. Rectal administration of drugs intended for systemic action may be preferred for those drugs that are destroyed or inactivated by the stomach or intestines. The rectal route is also preferred when the oral route is precluded due to vomiting or when the patient is unconscious or incapable of swallowing drugs safely without choking. Drugs absorbed rectally do not pass through the liver before entering the systemic circulation. Compared to oral administration, rectal administration of drugs is inconvenient and absorption is frequently irregular and difficult to predict. As a rule of thumb the rectal dose is usually twice the oral dose.

Suppositories are solid bodies of various weights and shapes intended for introduction into various body orifices (rectal, vaginal, or urethral) where they soften or melt, release their medication, and exert their therapeutic effect. These effects include the promotion of laxation (glycerin), the relief of discomfort (pain or hemorrhoids) from inflamed tissue, or the promotion of systemic effects (analgesic or antifebrile) in infants, children, and adults.

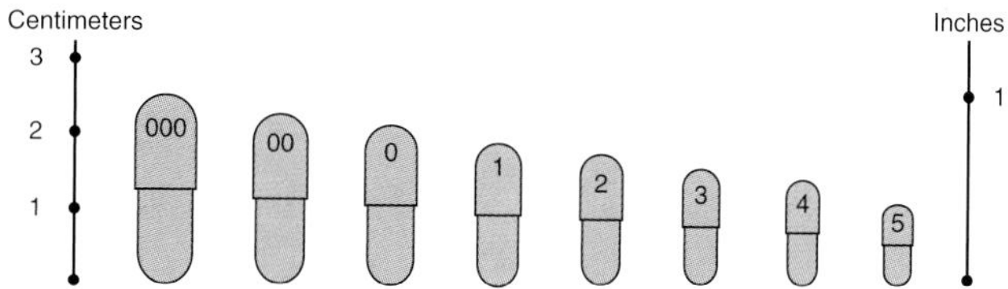

Table 1 Dimensions (in Millimeters) and Volumes (in Milliliters) of Coni-Snap Two-Piece Hard Capsules by Capsugel Division of Pfizer

Capsule Size	Cap Length	Body Length	Cap Diameter	Body Diameter	Locked Length	Capsule Volume
000	12.95	22.20	9.91	9.55	26.10	1.37
00el	12.95	22.20	8.53	8.18	25.30	1.02
00	11.74	20.22	8.53	8.18	23.30	0.91
0el	11.68	20.19	7.65	7.34	23.10	0.78
0	10.72	18.44	7.64	7.34	21.70	0.68
1el	10.49	17.70	6.91	6.63	20.42	0.54
1	9.78	16.61	6.91	6.63	19.40	0.50
2	8.94	15.27	6.35	6.07	18.00	0.37
3	8.08	13.59	5.82	5.57	15.90	0.30
4	7.21	12.19	5.32	5.05	14.30	0.21
5	6.20	9.30	4.91	4.68	11.10	0.13
Tolerance	±0.46	±0.46	±0.46	±0.46	±0.30	N/A

Table 2 Dimensions (in Millimeters) and Posilok Two-Piece Hard Capsules by Qualicaps

Capsule Size	Cap Length	Body Length	Cap Diameter	Body Diameter	Locked Length
00	11.70	20.40	8.56	8.21	23.60
0E	12.00	20.90	7.66	7.36	24.00
0	10.90	18.60	7.66	7.36	21.80
1E	10.60	18.40	6.95	6.65	21.20
1	9.70	16.70	6.95	6.65	19.50
2	8.90	15.30	6.38	6.08	17.80
3	7.90	13.50	5.85	5.60	15.80
4	7.20	12.40	5.34	5.07	12.40
Tolerance	±0.30	±0.30	±0.30	±0.30	±0.30

Figure 2.4 Common capsule sizes. (Used with permission from CSC Publishing. Tablets and Capsules Annual Buyers Guide.)

The composition of the suppository base can generally influence the degree and rate of drug release. It should be selected on an individual basis of each drug.

The use of rectal ointments is generally limited to the treatment of local conditions. Rectal solutions are employed as enemas or cleansing solutions.

2.3.3 Parenteral Route

A drug administered parenterally is one that is injected through the hollow of a fine needle into the body at various sites and to various depths. The three primary routes are subcutaneous (SC, SubQ), intramuscular (IM), and intravenous (IV). Strict sterility requirements make this dosage form more expensive and require competent trained personnel for administrations.

Drugs destroyed or inactivated in the GI tract or that are too poorly soluble to provide a satisfactory response may be administered parenterally. Rapid absorption is essential in emergency situations, when the patient is uncooperative, unconscious, or otherwise unable to accept the medication. The major disadvantage of parenteral administration is that once injected there is no return. Removal of the drug, which may be warranted by an untoward or toxic effect or an inadvertent overdose, is very difficult. Other routes of administration provide more time between administration and absorption, allowing for intervention, which becomes a safety factor to allow the extraction of the unabsorbed drug.

Injectable preparations are usually either sterile suspensions or solutions of a drug in water or in a suitable vegetable oil. Solutions act faster than drugs in suspensions with an aqueous vehicle, providing faster action than an oleaginous vehicle. Drug absorption occurs only after the drug has dissolved. Thus a suspension must first allow the drug to dissolve to be absorbed. The body is more foregoing to an aqueous vehicle and permits faster absorption than an oleaginous vehicle. A depot or repository (long acting) effect may be obtained either from a suspension or oleaginous solution since it will act as a storage reservoir within the body for the drug. This type of injection is usually limited to the IM type. Drugs injected intravenously do not encounter absorption barriers and produce rapid drug effects. Therefore, IV preparations must not interfere with blood components or with circulation and are limited to aqueous solutions of drugs. On rare occasions, IV lipids can be administered as an emulsion and is still mandated to be sterile.

2.3.3.1 Subcutaneous Administrations

Subcutaneous injections are usually aqueous solutions or suspensions administered in small volumes of 2mL or less. They are generally given in the forearm, upper arm, thigh, or abdomen. The site should be rotated if frequent injections are to be given, to reduce tissue irritation.

2.3.3.2 Intramuscular Injections

Intramuscular injections are performed deep into the skeletal muscles at either the deltoid, gluteal, or lumbar muscles. The site is chosen to minimize danger of hitting a nerve or blood vessel. Aqueous or oleaginous solutions or suspensions may be used with rapid effects or depot activity selected to meet the requirements of the patient. Drugs that are irritating to subcutaneous tissue are often administered intramuscularly with volumes of 2 to 5 mL or more. When a volume of 5 mL or more is to be injected it should be in divided doses using two injections.

2.3.3.3 Intravenous Injections

Intravenous administration of drugs (as an aqueous solution) is injected directly into a vein at a rate that is commensurate with efficiency, safety, comfort for the patient, and desired duration of the drug response. The drug may be administered via a slow drip to maintain the blood level or to provide nutrients and drugs after surgery. The drug must be maintained in solution after injection so that no precipitation occurs to produce emboli. Injections with oleaginous bases are not given IV as they might produce pulmonary embolisms.

2.3.3.4 Intradermal Injections

These are administered into the conium of the skin, usually in volumes of about a tenth of a milliliter. Common sites are the arm and back, where there is no hair. They are frequently done for diagnostic measures (tuberculin and allergy testing).

2.3.3.5 Ocular, Aural, and Nasal Routes of Administration

Drugs are frequently applied topically to the eye, ear, and mucus membranes of the nose. In these instances ointments, suspensions, and solutions are generally employed. They are generally not employed for systemic effects. Nasal preparations may be absorbed and a systemic effect may be seen.

Ophthalmic preparations (solutions and suspensions) are sterile aqueous preparations with other qualities essential to the safety and comfort of the patient. Ophthalmic ointments must be sterile and free from grittiness.

Nasal preparations are usually solutions or suspensions administered by drops or as a fine mist from a nasal spray container, which could include an aerosol with a metered valve.

Otic or ear preparations are usually very viscous so that they may have contact with the affected area. They can be employed to soften ear wax, relieve an earache, or combat an infection.

2.3.4 Transdermal Drug Delivery Systems

These are dosage forms designed to be applied to the skin and include ointments, creams, lotions, liniments, topical solutions, tinctures, pastes, powders, aerosols, and transdermal delivery systems.

The applications of these dosage forms can be used for their physical effects, in that they act as protectants, lubricants, emollients, drying agents, and such. They may also be used for the specific effect of the medicinal agent present. Preparations that are sold over-the-counter (OTC) often must contain a mixture of medicinal substances for the treatment of minor skin infections, itching, burns, diaper rash, insect stings and bites, athlete's foot, corns, calluses, warts, dandruff, acne, psoriasis, eczema, pain, arthritis, and to supply warmth to aching joints.

Absorption of the medicament may occur on the epidermis; however it is possible that other drugs may go deeper to penetrate the upper dermis, and still others may find themselves in proximity to blood capillaries that feed on the subcutaneous tissues and exhibit a systemic effect.

Absorption of substances from outside the skin to positions beneath the skin, including entrance into the blood stream, is referred to as percutaneous absorption. This is shown in Figure 2.5. The absorption of a medicament present in a dermatological such as a liquid, gel, ointment, cream, paste, among others depends not only on the physical and chemical properties of the medicament but also on its behavior in the vehicle in which it is placed and upon the skin conditions. The vehicle influences the rate and degree of penetration, which varies with different drugs and vehicles.

The skin is composed of three tissue layers: epidermis, dermis, and subcutaneous. The epidermis is a laminate of five types of tissues:

- Stratum Corneum (Horney Layer)
- Stratum Lucidum (Barrier Zone)

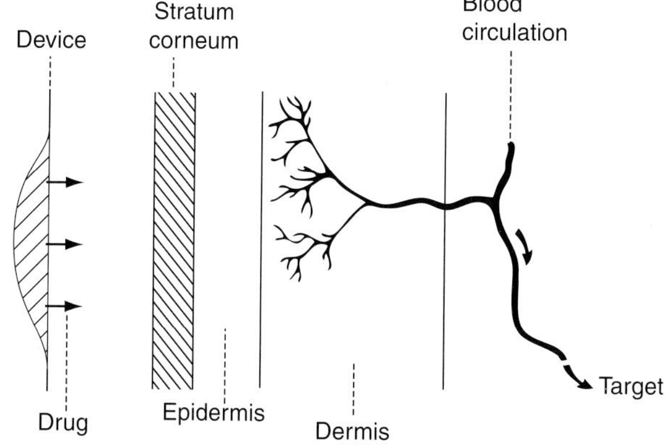

Figure 2.5 Schematic of the path of transdermally delivered drug to the systemic circulation.

- Stratum Granulosum (Granular Layer)
- Stratum Spinosum (Prickle Cell Layer)
- Stratum Germinativum (Basal Cell Layer)

The following factors affect percutaneous absorption:

- The drug itself
- The drug concentration
- Surface area to which it is applied
- Attraction of the drug to the base, which slows absorption, or for the skin, which speeds absorption
- Solubility of the drug as demonstrated by the partition coefficient
- Ability of the base to cover, mix with the sebum, and bring the drug in contact with the skin
- Vehicle composition
- Hydration of the skin
- Types of bandage covering the skin and preparations
- Amount of rubbing or energy (inunctions) applied
- Thickness of the skin
- Amount of time permitted in contact with the skin

These factors pertain to normal skin. If an injury or disease state should prevail of a varying dimension, then differences in drug absorption will occur. If the skin has been abraded, cut, or broken, this will facilitate drugs and any other foreign matter to gain direct access to the subcutaneous tissues.

The various dosage forms that are applied transdermally will be defined as follows:

- Ointments are semisolid preparations intended for external application and can be either medicated or nonmedicated. They are used for their emollient or lubricating effect.
- Creams are viscous liquid or semisolid emulsions of either the o/w or w/o type, which are employed as emollients or as medicated applications to the skin.
- Pastes are intended for external application to the skin. They differ from ointments in that they contain high percentages of solid material and are thicker and stiffer than an ointment.
- Lotions are liquid preparations intended for external application to the skin. They usually contain finely powdered substances that are insoluble in the dispersion medium and are suspended through use of suspending and dispersing agents. Lotions are intended to be applied to the skin for the protective or therapeutic value of their constituents. Their fluidity allows for rapid and uniform application over a large surface area. They are intended to dry rapidly on the skin after application to leave a thin coat of medicament on the surface. Because they are biphasic (fine particles dispersed in a liquid vehicle) and tend to separate on standing, they should be shaken vigorously before each use to redistribute any matter that has separated.

2.3.5 Topical Solutions and Tinctures

In general, topical solutions employ an aqueous vehicle, whereas topical tinctures employ an alcoholic vehicle. Cosolvents or adjuncts may be required to enhance stability or solubility of the solute (drug).

Topical solutions and tinctures are prepared mainly by simple solution of the solute in the solvent or solvent blend. Certain solutions are prepared by chemical reaction. Tinctures for topical use may be prepared by maceration (soaking) of the natural components in the solvent whereas others are prepared by simple solution.

Liniments are alcoholic or oleaginous solutions or emulsions of various medicinal substances intended for external application to the skin with rubbing. Alcoholic or hydroalcoholic liniments are useful as rubefacients, counterirritants, or where penetrating action is desired. Oleaginous liniments are employed primarily when massage is desired, and are less irritating to the skin than the alcoholic liniments. Solvents for the oleaginous liniments include such fixed oils (nonvolatile) as almond, peanut, sesame, or cottonseed or volatile oils (those that evaporate at room temperature and are odoriferous) like wintergreen (methyl salicylate) or turpentine. Combinations of fixed and volatile oils are also acceptable.

Collodions are liquid preparations composed of pyroxylin (soluble gun cotton, collodion cotton) dissolved in a solvent mixture composed of alcohol (94% ethanol) and ether with or without added medicinals. Pyroxylin is obtained by the action of nitric and sulfuric acids on cotton or other cellulosic material to produce cellulose tetranitrate. Pyroxylin is completely soluble in 25 parts of a mixture of 3 volumes of ether and 1 volume of alcohol. It is extremely flammable and must be stored in a well-closed container away from flame, heat, and light. Collodions are intended for external use as a protective coating to the skin. When medicated, it leaves a thin layer of that medication firmly placed against the skin.

Glycerogelatins are described as plastic masses intended for topical application containing gelatin, glycerin, water, and a medicament including zinc oxide, salicylic acid, resorcinol, and other appropriate agents. This dosage form is usually melted prior to application, cooled to above body temperature, and then applied to the affected area with a fine brush.

Plasters are solid or semisolid adhesive masses spread upon a suitable backing material that is intended for external application to an area of the body to provide prolonged contact at that site. The backing materials commonly used include paper, cotton, felt, linen, muslin, silk, moleskin, or plastic. Plasters are adhesive at body temperature and are used to provide protection or mechanical support (nonmedicated) or localized or systemic effects (medicated). The backings onto which the masses are applied are cut into various shapes to approximate the contours and extent of the body surface to be covered. These products commonly are used as back plasters, chest plasters, breast plasters, and corn plasters. This product has been commercialized today to provide warmth and protection. Adhesive tape was once known as adhesive plaster.

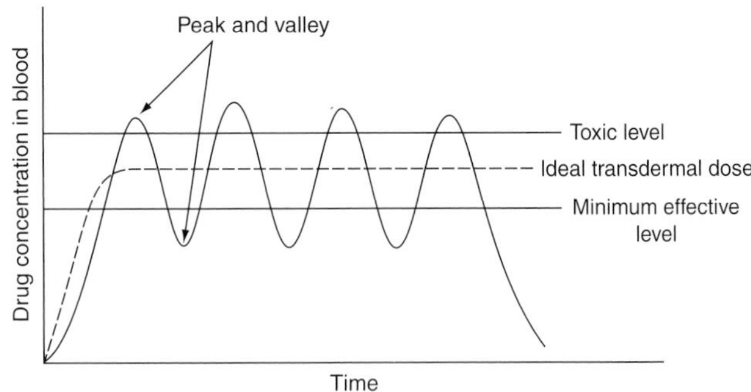

Figure 2.6 Hypothetical blood level pattern from a conventional multiple dosing schedule, and the idealized pattern from a transdermal controlled release system.

2.3.5.1 Miscellaneous Preparations for Topical Application to the Skin

These preparations include:

- Rubbing Alcohol, which is 70%v/v of ethyl alcohol and water. It contains denaturants with or without color additives and perfume oils and stabilizers.
- Isopropyl Rubbing Alcohol, which is 70%v/v isopropyl alcohol and water with or without color additives, stabilizers, and perfume oils.
- Hexachlorophene Liquid Cleanser, which is an antibacterial sudsing emulsion containing a colloidal dispersion of 3%w/w hexachlorophene in a special stable vehicle.
- Chlorhexidine Liquid Cleanser, which is an antibacterial liquid cleanser containing 4%w/w chlorhexidine in a special stable vehicle.

2.3.6 Transdermal Drug Delivery Systems

Transdermal drug delivery is designed to provide the passage of drug substances from the surface of the skin, through its various layers, and into the systemic circulation.

Figure 2.6 provides a hypothetical blood level pattern from a conventional oral multiple dosing schedule superimposed on an idealized pattern from a transdermal release system.

The basic objectives of transdermal dosage form design are to:

1. Optimize drug therapy by establishing relatively constant blood levels.
2. Release the drug according to pharmacokinetically rational rate to the intact skin for systemic absorption.
3. Optimize the selectivity of drug action and minimizing the number of undesirable side effects as well as their severity and incidence.
4. Provide a predictable and extended duration of action.
5. Reduce the disincentives to regimen compliance by patients.
6. Minimize the inconvenience of patient remedication.
7. Provide a therapeutic advantage over other drug delivery systems.
8. Stimulate innovation and therapeutic use of established but unpatented drugs and natural substances.

When the transdermal patch is applied to the skin, the steady state systemic dosage may not be reached for some time due to the slow absorption of the drug by the skin. It is not possible simply to equate the rate of drug delivery with the rate of appearance of drug in the systemic circulation. When the skin absorption sites are saturated steady state is reached. It is at this point that the rate of drug release equals the rate of appearance in the blood.

Criteria for drug selection for transdermal systems include:

1. Physicochemical properties of the drug including molecular size (100–800 daltons) as dictated by the patient's skin type, oil-to-water solubility (K^{o}_{w}) as well as the hydration state; melting point is a major contributor to drug absorption and may require enhancers or electrical potential driving forces partitioning between the delivery system and stratum corneum as well as the stratum corneum and the viable epidermis.
2. Drug potency as indicated by low dose in order for this route to be a feasible option.
3. Biological half-life should be short rather than long. Long half-lived drugs delay steady state levels and plasma concentration will rapidly decline following termination.
4. Must lead to plasma levels above the minimum effective concentration (MEC) but below the minimum toxic concentration (MTC).
5. The drug must not include a cutaneous irritation or allergic response.
6. There must be a clinical need for this mode of administration, especially if oral administration is adequate for the delivery of the drug.

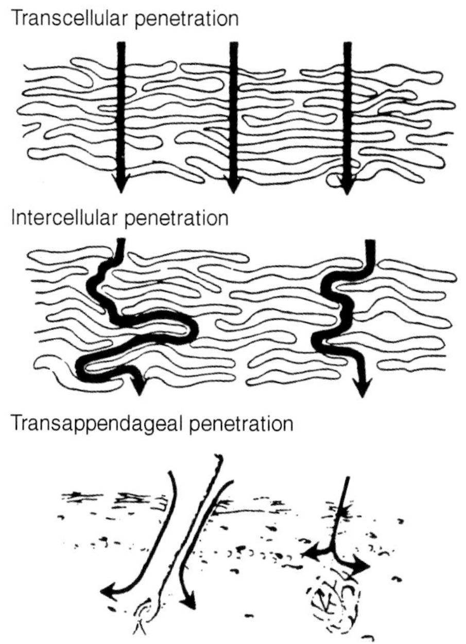

Figure 2.7 Possible routes of penetration of drugs through skin.

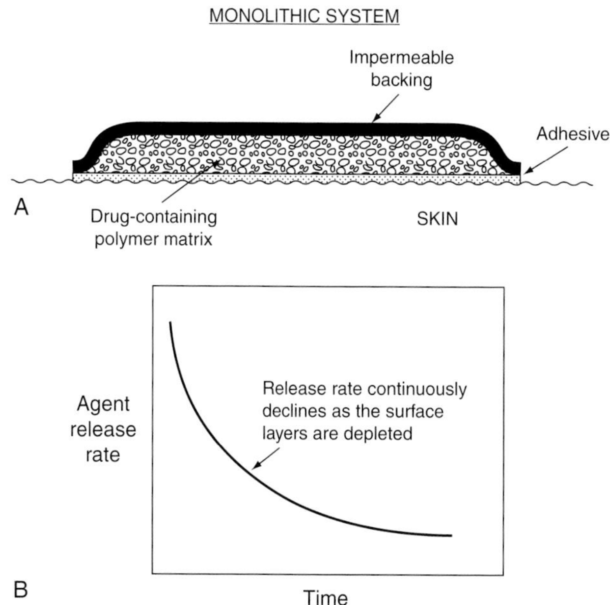

Figure 2.8 Schematic of a monolithic transdermal drug-delivery system (A) and the drug-release rate obtained (B).

Permeation of the skin can occur via passive diffusion by the three processes given in Figure 2.6. Absorption results from the direct penetration of the drug through the stratum conium, which, being keratinized, behaves as a semipermeable membrane that allows for passive drug diffusion (Figure 2.7).

The amount of material passing through the skin per unit area is given by:

$$J = K_m D(\Delta C/h)$$

where:

J = flux of the drug in g/cm/sec

K_m = partition coefficient based on the affinity of the drug for the skin from the vehicle that is applied

D = the diffusion coefficient and is a reflection of the degree of interaction of the drug with the skin barrier

$(\Delta C/h)$ = the driving force for drug penetration (drug concentration) versus stratum conium thickness (h)

There are two basic types of transdermal dosing systems:

- Those that allow the skin to control the rate of drug absorption (Figure 2.8) and are known as the Monolithic type
- Those that control the rate of drug delivery (Figure 2.9) and are of the Reservoir type

Monolithic systems incorporate a polymeric drug matrix layer between the impermeable backing and the adhesive that is contacting the skin. The matrix is of two types:

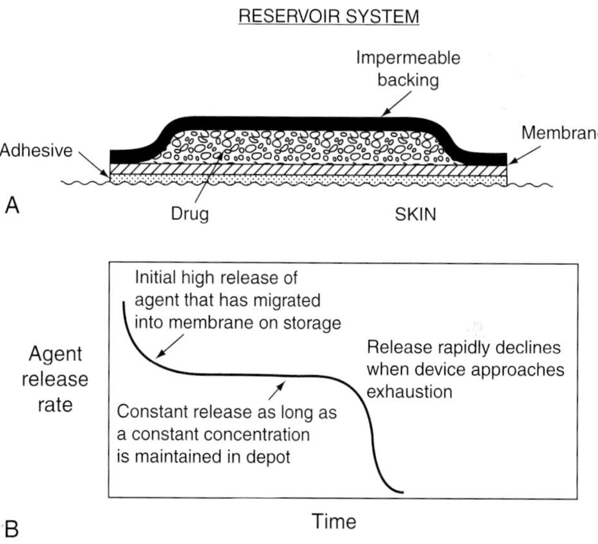

Figure 2.9 Schematic of a reservoir transdermal drug-delivery system (A) and the drug-release rate obtained (B).

- With or without an excess of drug with regard to its equilibrium solubility and steady state concentration
- Those having no excess drug to maintain the saturation of the stratum cornium

Reservoir systems also have a backing and adhesive layer, but are contained by a rate-controlling membrane. The drug is contained within the reservoir as a suspension in a liquid or gel phase. The drug is released rapidly when the device is placed on the skin to give an initial burst effect. Thereafter, drug release is controlled by the rate of drug diffusion through the membrane and adhesive layers as seen in Figure 2.9B. The release rate can be controlled by changing the membrane thickness and permeability.

Enhancers and other excipients may be used in these devices to promote skin permeation. The mechanisms by which enhancers exert their effects include:

- Solvent action to directly plasticize or solubilize the skin tissue components
- Interaction with intercellular lipids to disrupt the highly ordered lamellar structure to increase the diffusivity through the membrane.
- Interaction with intracellular proteins to promote permeation through the corneocyte layer
- Increasing the partitioning of the drug or coenhancer into the membrane

Enhancer systems include:

- Lipophilic solvents (ethanol, polyethylene glycol, dimethylsulfoxide (DMSO) and azone)
- Fatty acid esters and long chain alcohols
- Water-enhanced transport
- Sulfoxide enhanced transport (DMSO and Decylmethylsulfoxide (DCMS))
- Aprotic solvent enhanced transport (n-Methyl-2-Pyrrolidone, Pyrrolidone, Dimethyl acetamide, Dimethyl formamide, Dimethyl isosorbide)
- Propylene glycol enhanced transport
- Azone related compounds for enhanced transport (parent compound being 1-dodecyl-azaclycloheptane-2-one)
- Amines and amides as enhancers (chlorpheneramine, diphenhydramine, 3-phenoxypyridine, nicotine, alkyl n,n-dialkyl amino acetate)
- Alcohol and acids as enhancers (methanol, ethanol, decyl alcohol, dodecyl alcohol, capric acid, lauric acid, myristic acid) that have been mixed with hydrophobic cosolvents such as n-hexane, n-dodecane, and n-hexadecane
- Esters as enhancers (methyl acetate, ethyl acetals, butyl acetals, methyl propionate, ethyl propionate, methyl valerate, isopropyl myristate, and glucol monolaureate)
- Organic acids and salicylates as enhancers (salicylic acid, citric acid, succinic acid, and glycol derivatives such as methyl, ethyl and propyl) of salicylic acid

The advantages obtained by using transdermal delivery include:

1. Avoidance of GI drug absorption difficulties associated with *pH*, enzymatic activity, drug interactions with food drink, or other orally administered drugs
2. Avoidance of the first-pass effect (deactivation by digestive and liver enzymes)
3. Acts as a substitute for oral administration when this route is not suitable (e.g., diarrhea and vomiting)
4. Increased patient compliance due to the elimination of multiple dosing schedules
5. Termination of drug effects rapidly, if clinically desired, by simple removal of the patch
6. Minimization of the inter- and intrapatient variation, as is the case with oral products, where differences arise due to the variability in:
   - Drug absorption
   - Gastric emptying
   - Transit time in the small intestine
   - Blood flow in the absorption area
   - Differences in first-pass effect
   - Small fluctuations due to individual activities such as eating, sleeping, and physical activity
7. Reduced side effects due to optimization of the blood concentration profile
8. Reproducible and extended duration of action

The disadvantages for this dosage form include:

1. Unsuitable for drugs that irritate or sensitize the skin
2. Difficulty with skin penetration
3. Unsuitable for the delivery of large doses of the drug
4. Unsuitable for drugs that are extensively metabolized in the skin
5. Technical difficulties can arise during the manufacture of the patch that can cause erratic absorption; environmental and adhesive problems can cause variable rate-controlling drug delivery problems

2.3.7 Aerosol Delivery Devices for Inhalation, Inhalants, and Sprays

Aerosols are primarily pressurized packaging of a drug product. Pharmaceutical aerosols depend upon the container, valve assembly, and propellant. The physical form in which the contents are emitted is dependent upon the product formulation and type of valve and actuator employed to produce the following:

- Fine mists: Space spray
- Coarse wet mist: Surface coating sprays
- Dry powders
- Steady stream
- Foams: Quick breaking or stable (shave cream)

The aerosol dosage form provides several distinct advantages including:

- A portion of the medication can be withdrawn easily from the package without contaminating or exposing the remaining product.
- The packaging prevents environmental oxygen, light, and moisture from adversely affecting the product.
- The medication can be applied in a uniform thin layer without touching the affected area.
- It is possible to control the physical form, dose, and particle size of the emitted product through a metered valve.
- It is a clean process requiring little or no clean-up by the user.

There are two delivery mechanisms used for these products. The first utilizes either a compressed or liquefied gas system and the second relies on Bernoulli's Principle. Compressed gases operate on the Laws of Boyles, Charles, and Guy Lussac over two sets of conditions to give:

$$(P_1V_1)/T_1 = (P_2V_2)/T_2$$

and when $T_1 = T_2$ then

$$P_1V_1 = P_2V_2$$

and the equation of state becomes

$$P_{(\text{atm})}V_{(\text{Liters})} = nR_{(\text{molar gas constant})}T_{(\text{deg K})}$$

and $R = 0.08205$ L atm/mole degree, or as $R = 1.987$ Cal/mole degree.

Liquefied gases operate under the principle of Raoult's Law, which states that the total pressure of a system is equal to the sum of the partial pressures of the volatile ingredients. The partial pressure of each ingredient is equal to the mole fraction of that ingredient in the mixture times its own pure vapor pressure. The equation becomes

$$P_T = p_A^0X_A + p_B^0X_B + p_C^0X_C \ldots + p_N^0X_N$$

where

P_T = total pressure
p_A^0 = pure vapor pressure of component A, B, C, etc.
X_A = mole fraction of component A, B, C, etc.

The partial pressure equation is written as

$$P_T = p_A + p_B + p_C \ldots + p_N$$

In compressed gas systems, when the actuator (button) is pressed to permit the exit of product, gas is also emitted. This loss of gas causes a decrease in pressure. As the product is used the pressure will continue to decline until the pressure inside equals the pressure outside the container and no more product can be obtained. This is demonstrated in Figure 2.10. In contrast, liquefied gas propellants form an equilibrium between the liquefied gas and the gas to maintain a constant pressure. Therefore, when the actuator is pressed and both products, liquefied gas and gas, escape, the pressure inside the container remains constant and almost all of the product can be made available to the patient. This is demonstrated in Figure 2.11.

The compressed gases used today include nitrogen, carbon dioxide, and nitrous oxide. The liquefied gases that once were used include the Freons® and Gentrons®, which were fluorinated chlorinated hydrocarbons. Today most of these products have been replaced by chlorinated hydrocarbons, which are predominantly inert.

The presence of the aerosol is critical to its performance and is controlled by the type and amount of propellant as well as the nature and amount of material compressing the product concentrate. Pressure can be provided from 11 psig (pounds per square inch gauge) up to 90 psig.

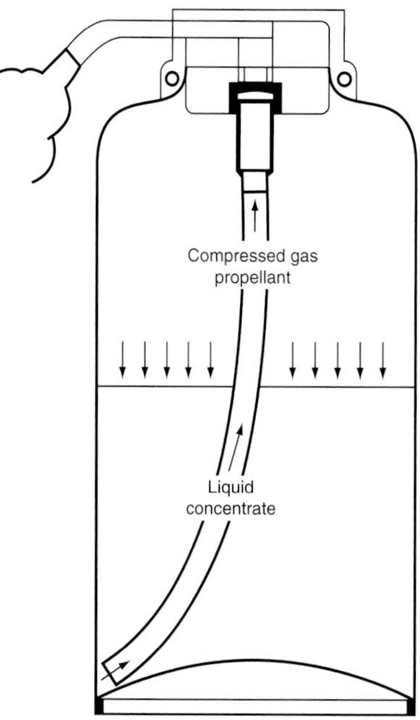

Figure 2.10 Compressed gas aerosol. (Printed with permission from Lippincott Williams & Wilkins. Copyright 1974. Dittert, LW.)

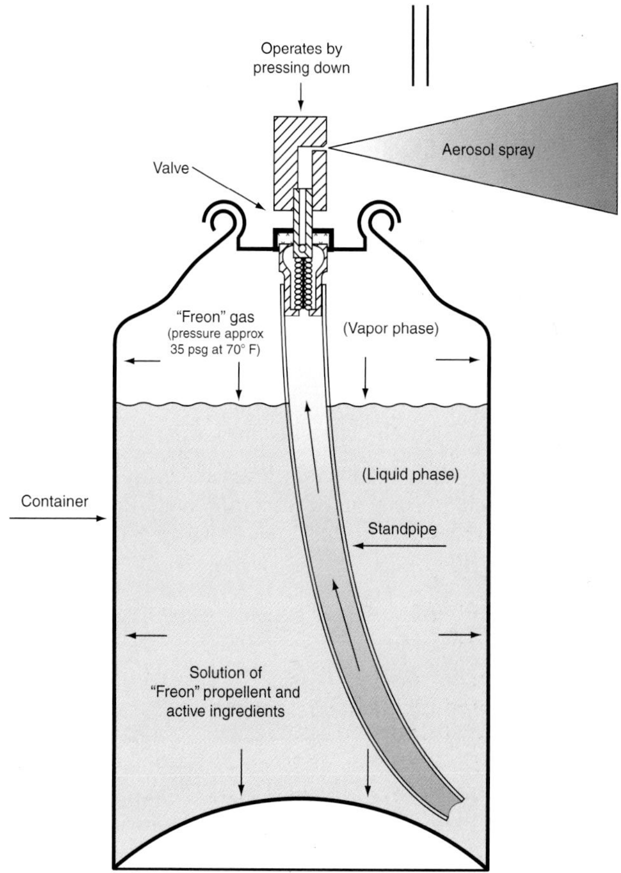

Figure 2.11 Cross-section of a typical two-phase package. (Printed with permission from Lippincott Williams & Wilkins. Copyright 1974. Dittert, LW.)

Aerosol containers can be any of the following:

- Glass: uncoated or plastic coated
- Metal: Tin-plated steel, aluminum, or stainless steel
- Plastic and resins

Pharmaceutical and nonpharmaceutical aerosol products are used as convenient forms of delivery and include personal deodorant sprays, cosmetic hair lacquers and sprays, perfume and cologne sprays, shaving lathers, toothpaste, surface pesticide sprays, and paint sprays. Also included are various household products such as spray starch, waxes, polishers, cleaners, and lubricants. A number of veterinary and pet products have been put into aerosol form. Food products and dessert toppings and food spreads are also available.

2.3.8 Inhalations

These are drugs or solutions of drugs administered by the nasal or respiratory route. The drugs are administered for their local action on the bronchial tree or for their systemic effects through absorption from the lungs. Certain gases such as oxygen and ether are administered as finely powdered drug substances and as solutions administered as fine mists.

A number of devices are available for the delivery of medications for inhalation therapy. Among these are the nebulizer, atomizer, and insufflator, which operate under Bernoulli's Principle.

Bernoulli demonstrated that as air passes through a structure in a glass tube, or any tube, the pressure drops only to increase again after leaving the structure (Figure 2.12). This can be further demonstrated by preparing a glass tube in the shape of a "T" such that when air or any gas is passed through a vacuum it is produced at the perpendicular tube. If this tube is inserted into a liquid, the liquid will rise in the perpendicular tube until it reaches the moving gas. At this point the liquid will be carried by the moving gas and exit the tube as fine droplets. This is seen in Figure 2.13 for a nebulizer and in Figure 2.14 for a vacuum atomizer. An offshoot of this principle is demonstrated by Figure 2.15 for a pressure atomizer, in which the air puts pressure on the liquid and when the liquid equalizes the pressure the air can thus produce a fine spray at the end of the tube. The same principle can be used in a powder insufflator (Figure 2.16).

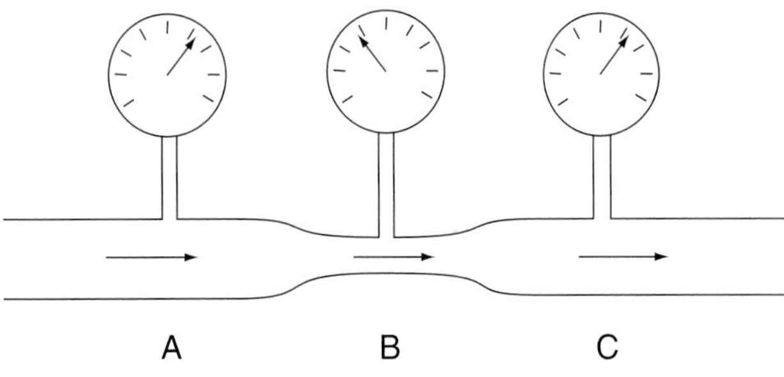

Figure 2.12 Illustration of Bernoulli's theorem. The fluid (or gas) flows more rapidly at B than A or C, and the pressure is less at B than A or C.

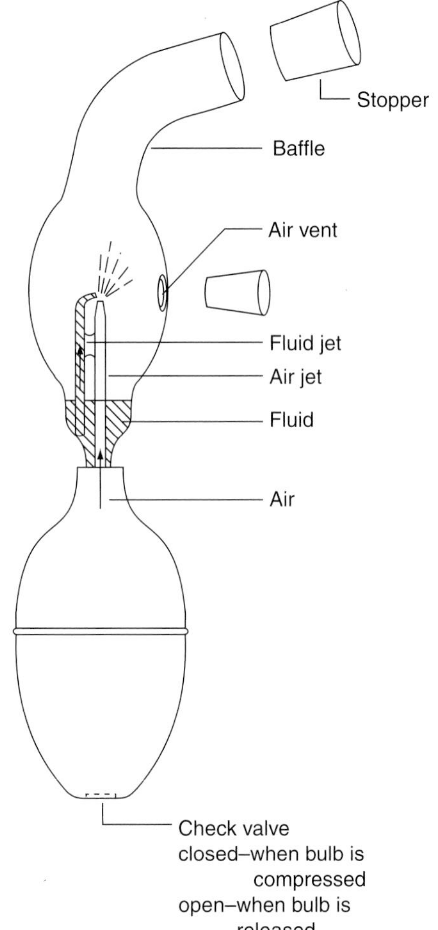

Figure 2.13 Sketch of a commercially available nebulizer. (Printed with permission from Lippincott Williams & Wilkins. Copyright 1974. Dittert, LW.)

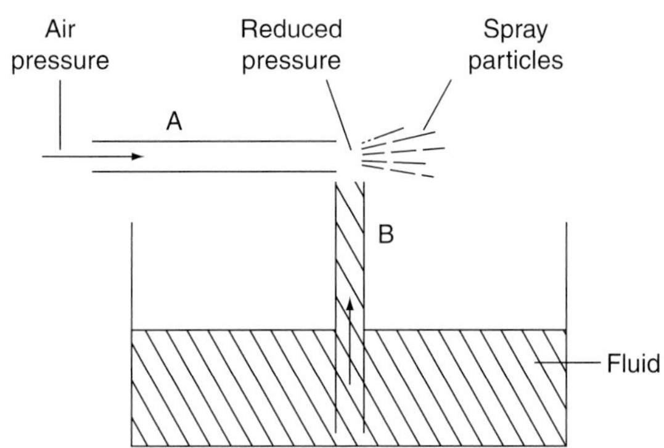

Figure 2.14 Operation of a simple vacuum atomizer.

2.3.9 Vaporizers and Humidifiers

The common household vaporizer produces a fine mist of water (as steam or droplets of water) to humidify a room. Confusion has persisted since there are both steam and cool mist humidifiers. Vaporizers actually boil the water, utilizing an electric current passing between two electrodes. The addition of an electrolyte (e.g., NaCl)

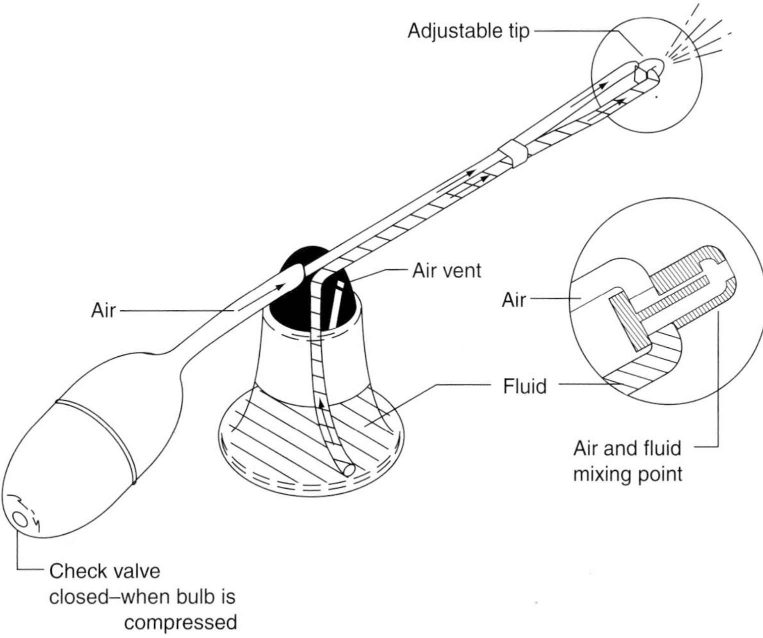

Figure 2.15 Sketch of a commercially available atomizer that operates on the vacuum principle. (Printed with permission from Lippincott Williams & Wilkins. Copyright 1974. Dittert, LW.)

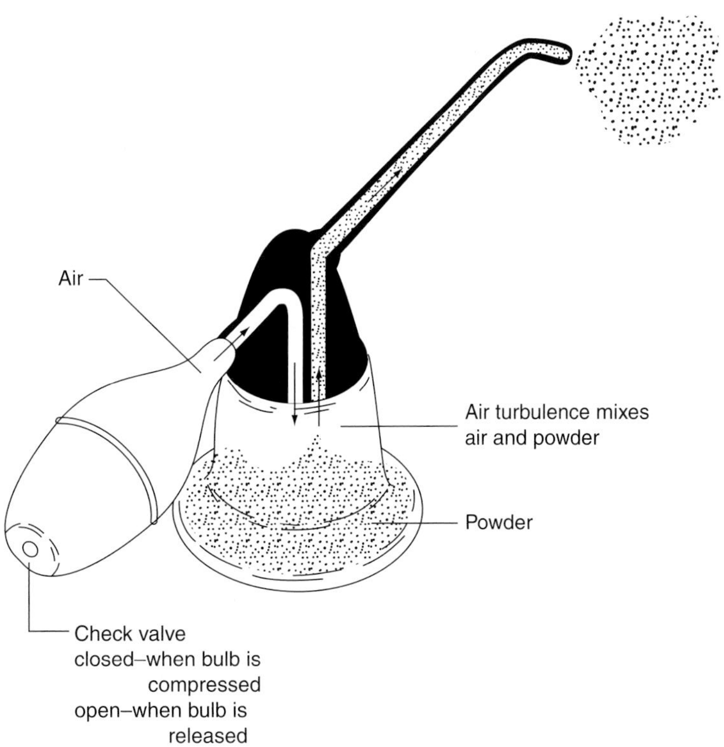

Figure 2.16 Sketch of a commercially available powder blower or powder insufflator. (Printed with permission from Lippincott Williams & Wilkins. Copyright 1974. Dittert, LW.)

can facilitate this process. When a volatile medication is added to the vaporizer both steam and the aromatic volatilizes, which is then inhaled by the patient.

A true humidifier does not boil water, but rather operates by one of two principles. Ultrasound can be used to produce a mist of cool water, which is emitted as fine droplets, and the smallest of these evaporate. The larger droplets fall and eventually cause wetness beneath the humidifier.

Moisture in the air is important to prevent mucous membranes of the nose and throat from becoming dry and irritated. Vaporizers and humidifiers are used commonly in adjunctive treatment of colds, cough, and chest congestion.

2.3.10 Inhalants

Inhalants are drugs or combinations of drugs that by virtue of their high vapor pressure can be carried by an air current into the nasal passage where they exert their effect. The device in which the medication(s) is contained and from which it is administered is called an *inhaler* (e.g., Vicks® Inhaler; Benzedrex® Inhaler).

2.3.11 Vaginal and Urethral Drug Administration

Drugs can be inserted into the vagina and urethra for local effects. Drugs are presented to the vagina in the form of tablets, suppositories, creams, ointments, gels or jellies, emulsion foams, or solutions.

Urethral medication for both males and females present themselves as either suppositories or solutions. Systemic drug effects are generally undesired from the mucous membranes of these sites.

Vaginal preparations are designed for two purposes: (1) to combat infections occurring in the female genitourinary tracts and (2) to restore the vaginal mucosa to its normal state. Powders are used to prepare solutions for vaginal douching (irrigation and cleansing). These bulk powders are admixed with an appropriate volume of aqueous vehicle until dissolved. Commercialization of this product has ready-to-use product available in disposable self-administration units. Among the components of douche powders are:

- Boric acid or sodium borate
- Astringents (potassium alum, ammonium alum, zinc sulfate)
- Antimicrobials
- Quaternary ammonium compounds
- Detergents (sodium lauryl sulfate)
- Oxidizing agents (sodium perborate)
- Salts (sodium citrate, sodium chloride)
- Aromatics (menthol, thymol, eucalyptol, methyl salicylate, phenol).

These products are generally employed for their hygienic effects.

2.3.12 Nanoparticle

Nanotechnology is the study of extremely small particles. The National Nanotechnology Initiation defines nanotechnology as the research and technology development at the atomic, molecular, or macro-molecular scale, leading to the controlled creation and use of structures, devices, and systems with a length scale of approximately 1 to 100 nanometers (nm). This size has been expanded to include 1–1000 nanometers. Extensive work in nanotechnology has provided a tremendous opportunity for the pharmaceutical and biotechnology industries. These industries have seen the role of these various particles as delivery systems that can opportunistically incorporate more than one drug into the nanosystem to obtain beneficial therapeutic effects. Strategies are being developed to get various kinds of drug molecules to overcome drug resistance both in cancer and infectious disease as well as into the brain to treat debilitating diseases.

Nanoparticles such as liposome, dendrimers, gold nanoshells, quantum dots, and fullerenes have a number of potential advantages over classic drug delivery methods. These advantages include a greatly altered absorption, distribution and length of time that drugs stay in the body, as well as allowing for targeted drug delivery to diseased sites. Its application to cancer therapeutics to improve drug targeting and avoid toxic systemic effects is well known. The exploration of applications in the areas of cardiology and infectious disease is currently under way. The field is not without its challenges. Some scientists cite liability concerns, still others challenge taking this type of particle from the laboratory to scaling them up from chemical studies and commercial production.

First-generation nanodrug delivery was considered in the use of lipid-based drugs and nanopowders. Nanoparticles allow for multiple functionalities. Liposomes have been around for approximately 20 years and were the first nanoparticles to be used for drug delivery. Liposomes are phospholipids (e.g., polylactic-coglycolic acid) with a proven safety record and are used pharmaceutically. Other phospholipids are being synthesized but must go through safety screens. Abraxane (a liposome-based drug) from Abraxis Bioscience Inc., Los Angeles, California was approved in 2005 for metastatic breast cancer. It is a formulation of the cancer drug paclitaxel that uses nanoparticles made of human protein albumin. Due to the interaction of the nanoparticle with two biochemical processes in tumors, they are capable of boosting the amount of paclitaxel delivered to the body at a 50% higher dose over 30 minutes. The standard paclitaxel administration must be given as an infusion for up to three hours. Binding the paclitaxel to albumin avoids the toxic effects. However, due to its poor solubility in blood, paclitaxel, if given unbound, must be mixed with various solvents, which can result in serious hypersensitivity reactions and other side effects. This necessitates steroid treatment before chemotherapy, which has been suspected to result in hyperglycemia, immunosuppresion, and insomnia. Abraxane, being less toxic, can be given in higher doses, which may explain a response rate almost double that of plain paclitaxel in clinical trials.

Nanopowders are the second approach to enhanced drug delivery. The four drugs on the market, all reformulators, use Nano Crystal® technology from Elan Pharmaceuticals, Dublin Ireland, which decreases drug particle size to typically less than 1000 nanometers in diameter. This increases surface area and dissolution rates for poorly water soluble compounds to improve activity. The Nano Crystals® are produced using a proprietary, wet milling technique. They are then stabilized from agglomeration by surface adsorption of a selected stabilizer, which results in an aqueous dispersion of the drug substance that behaves like a solution.

The second generation of nano-enabled drugs are being enabled by the Nanotechnology Characterization Laboratory (NCL) in Frederick, Maryland.

The National Cancer Institute (NCI) established the NCL to perform preclinical efficacy and toxicity testing of nanoparticles to accelerate the transition of nano scale particles and devices into clinical application. The NCL has characterized about 65 different particles and as of 2006 there are about 150 nanoparticle cancer therapies in development and thousands of other potential candidates waiting in the wings.

Some of these key particles investigated to date include:

- *Dendrimers*, which have well-defined chemical structures and exhibit monodispersity with potential applications in targeting cancer cells, drug delivery, and imaging.
- *Gold Nanoshells*, which are actually a gold shell surrounding a semiconductor that can be irradiated when reaching their target. This heats the nanoshell, which in turn kills the cancer cells.
- *Fullerenes*, which are a form of carbon (C-60) composed of carbon atoms arranged in a soccer ball-like configuration, hence their name, *bucky balls*. They are easily manufactured in quantity and appear to be ideal drug delivery vehicles due their size and shape.

These particles and others have a great deal of potential. Another concern that arises is the potential for toxicity. Of the 65 particles characterized so far by the NCI, all but one has been very benign. The future seems bright for this next generation of drug delivery systems.

REVIEW QUESTIONS

1. Describe the reasons why drug encapsulation is used in the preparation of a drug formulation.
2. Although oral administration of a drug is by far the easiest route of drug administration, describe situations in which this is not an acceptable route.
3. What role does age play in the selection of a drug formulation to be used?
4. What is meant by the MEC and the MTC? These concepts gave rise to the therapeutic drug monitoring. What role would TDM play in proper drug therapy and why would this be more important when dealing with drugs having a small therapeutic index?
5. What is the difference in dose calculation using drug weight/body weight and drug weight/body surface area? What are the advantages of each approach?
6. Why would one consider creatinine clearance in dose calculation?
7. A drug causes extreme irritation to soft tissues when the drug comes in contact with these tissues. What is the more likely route of administration to be used and why?
8. If a drug is given by the oral route one must consider the first-pass effect. When the same drug is given sublingually, first-pass effect is far less important. What is first-pass effect and why is the oral route so susceptible to this phenomenon?
9. What is bioavailability? Why is this concept important to understanding the efficacy (and toxicity) of a drug?
10. What is the Henderson-Hasselbach equation and why is it an important consideration if a drug crossed membranes by simple passive diffusion? Why is it far less important if a drug utilizes either facilitated transport or active transport carrier systems to cross membranes?
11. Compare and contrast tablet formulation and gelatin capsule formulation. What might consequences be to the overall bioavailability of a drug if one formulation dissolves four times faster in the gut than another tablet formulation of the same drug?
12. What is the blood–brain barrier and what role does it play in drug entering the cerebral spinal fluid? Would you predict that a drug that is highly lipid soluble would be more or less likely to enter the CSF than a highly water soluble drug? Why? How might you administer a drug that enters the CSF poorly or not at all?
13. What is transdermal drug administration? What are the theoretical advantages of this route of administration? What considerations must be taken into account when using this route?
14. How does the monolithic formulation differ from the reservoir system?
15. What are advantages of inhalational drug administration? Why might an inhalant administered corticosteroid be preferred over a systemically administered corticosteroid in an asthmatic patient, whereas the reverse might be true in a patient suffering from severe inflammatory disease?
16. What are nanoparticles and why are they considered to be the next important form of drug preparation and drug administration?

REFERENCES

Annual Buyer's Guide Reference. Tablets and Capsules (Vol. 4, No. 8, p. 35). St Paul, MN: CSC Publishing.

Ansel, H. C., Allen, R., & Popovich, N. G. (1999). *Pharmaceutical dosage forms and drug delivery systems* (7th ed.). Baltimore, MD: Lippincott, Williams and Wilkins.

Dittert, L. W. (Ed.). (1974). *Sproul's American pharmacy. Introduction to pharmaceutical technique and dose forms* (7th ed.). Philadelphia, PA: Lippincott Co.

Martin, A. (1993). *Physical pharmacy* (4th ed.). Baltimore, MD: Lippincott, Williams and Wilkins.

Martin, E. M. (Ed.). (1971). *Dispensing of medication* (7th ed.). Easton, PA: Mack Publishing.

Stoklosa, M. J., & Ansel, H. C. (1980). *Pharmaceutical calculations* (7th ed.). Philadelphia, PA: Lea and Febriger.

Chapter

3

Membranes and Drug Action

Yan Xu ▪ Tommy S. Tillman ▪ Pei Tang

OUTLINE

3.1 INTRODUCTION

In the discussion of drug distribution in Chapter 4, pharmacokinetics in Chapter 7, signal transduction and second messengers in Chapter 12, and ion channels and transport in Chapter 13, membranes are treated as boundaries and barriers to divide living cells into organizational compartments. In this chapter, we will direct our attention to the membranes themselves. We will focus on the molecules that make up biological membranes, the ways in which these molecules are organized, the influence of the microscopic and macroscopic properties of membranes on biological processes, and the unique dynamic environment formed by membranes that support and regulate the function of membrane-associated and integral membrane proteins. Because more than 50% of the drugs currently on the market target membrane proteins and the vast majority of drugs interact with membranes at one point or another before reaching their intended sites of action, membranes are central to modern drug design and studies of the molecular and cellular mechanisms of drug actions.

3.1.1 Membranes Define Life

In the strictest sense, life starts quite literally with the separation of matters by membranes. Having a membrane is not a sufficient definition of life, but it is a necessary one. Cells are the basic unit of life on Earth, and a cellular membrane encloses and maintains a highly regulated state distinguishable from the surrounding environment. More importantly, biological membranes establish discrete regions within the cell that create complex intracellular environments essential for important cellular functions. Though only two molecules thick—as little as about 5 nm or 5 hundred-thousandths the thickness of a typical piece of paper—membranes represent the largest structural component of a cell by mass. In an average human, membranes are estimated to provide about 100 square kilometers of coverage, an area equivalent to approximately 19,000 U.S. football fields.

The ubiquitous nature of biological membranes results from the fact that oil and water do not mix. Water, because of its unique structure, is widely appreciated as being essential to life. Oils from biological sources, or *lipids*, are intimately associated with life because of their tendency to self-aggregate in water and form closed boundaries separating aqueous compartments. It is within these membrane boundaries that life evolves.

3.1.2 Membranes Characterize the Process of Life

The permeability barrier formed by lipids separating one aqueous environment from another is the defining characteristic of a biological membrane. This barrier enables maintenance of different concentrations of solutes on the two sides of the membrane. Control over these concentration gradients is the essential work of the life process and is provided by various membrane components. Most essential among these components are membrane proteins, which make up 30 to 80% of a biological membrane depending on where the membrane is derived. Whereas some proteins regulate cellular transport mechanisms, either allowing a solute to equilibrate along its concentration gradient or actively transporting the solute against its gradient, others are involved in signal transduction events with which a cell senses changes in its environment. Modulation of membrane proteins is the primary means by which a cell regulates molecular traffic across and between membranes. Membrane proteins are also a key structural element of a biological membrane, maintaining membrane domains and forming a framework for specialized functions.

As we shall learn in the following sections of this chapter, the lipid and protein compositions of membranes and changes to these compositions are among the most essential characteristics that distinguish membranes derived from different species, different cells, and different subcellular structures. For example, the membranes of the cell nucleus, where the genetic information of eukaryotic cells is stored, are connected to, but distinguishable from, the membranes of the endoplasmic reticulum, where many gene products—proteins—are synthesized. Mitochondria, which form the powerhouse of the cell, contain intertwined and highly convoluted inner and outer membranes that support the cell machinery vital for energy production. Differences among membranes directly reflect their distinct and specialized functions, and the proteins within them are sensitive to particular lipid compositions. Thus biological membranes function as an integrated whole to perform such tasks as maintaining a constant internal environment (homeostasis), energy production and transduction (metabolism), cell–cell communication, response to external stimuli, adaptation, reproduction, and myriad other processes that define the state of being alive.

3.1.3 Membranes Are Essential to Drug Action

Given that a biological membrane surrounds all living cells, it should come as no surprise that the vast majority of drugs must interact with a membrane to reach their target. Exceptions are rare and often involve an extracellular site of action. For example, an antacid exerts its pharmaceutical effect by neutralizing gastric acid within the alimentary canal without passing through a membrane. As another example, in cases of severe lead poisoning, a chelating agent administered intravenously renders lead dissolved in the blood biologically inert. In most cases, however, a drug is administered to an extracellular space remote from a cellular site of action. Between the drug and its site of action there are typically multiple layers of anatomical barriers comprised by cells in tight association. To cross such barriers, the drug must either pass between the cells through *filtration* (*paracellular*) transport, or more typically, across the cell membranes through *transcellular* transport. Since life processes are cellular in nature, a drug usually interacts with a specific cellular component once arriving at its site of action. Thus most drugs must interact with biological membranes, either during transport to the target within the cell or at the specific cellular component within the membrane that produces their biological effect.

From the drug design point of view, drugs with high *efficacy* and *specificity* often are those that target certain proteins (particularly membrane receptors) or specific intracellular components. Approximately 50% of the drugs currently available and nearly 90% of cancer drugs target *integral membrane proteins*. Many of these drugs also have strong interactions with membrane lipids. Since membrane proteins are sensitive to lipid composition, these interactions may also play an important role in producing the desired and undesired physiological effects of the drugs. Similarly, drugs with intracellular targets must transverse the cell membrane, either by partitioning into the membrane or by taking advantage of the transport mechanisms the cell uses for transmembrane trafficking. These same considerations apply to excretion of the drug and its metabolites. In practice, many drugs are lipid soluble and readily cross the membrane barrier. Often these drugs are metabolized to forms that are less soluble in lipid. Once removed from the cell by membrane transport proteins, the lipid membrane prevents the metabolite from reentering the cell.

Thus, membranes are key to drug action. Understanding biological membranes and the way that drugs interact with them is essential to understanding the way the majority of drugs work.

3.2 WHAT IS A MEMBRANE?

3.2.1 The Lipid Molecules

Despite its immense complexity, the biosphere seems to have selected a very limited number of simple organic molecules as building blocks. DNA, encoding the genetic information passed from one generation to the next during cell reproduction, is constructed with a linear sequence of only four major types of *nucleotides* in a *polynucleotide chain*. The backbone of a polynucleotide is invariant, joined by a repeating phosphodiester linkage of sugar phosphates (Figure 3.1A). The part that varies along the sequence is the nitrogenous base covalently attached to the repeating sugar phosphate. Similarly, proteins—the primary products of genes—are formed from linear polymers composed from a library of 20 different *amino acids* joined by identical peptide bonds to form *polypeptide chains* (Figure 3.1B). The complexity of proteins and their functions are achieved through the arrangement of these amino acid polymers in three-dimensional space.

The situation with membranes is considerably more complicated, both in terms of the number of chemical species and in the manner in which they form

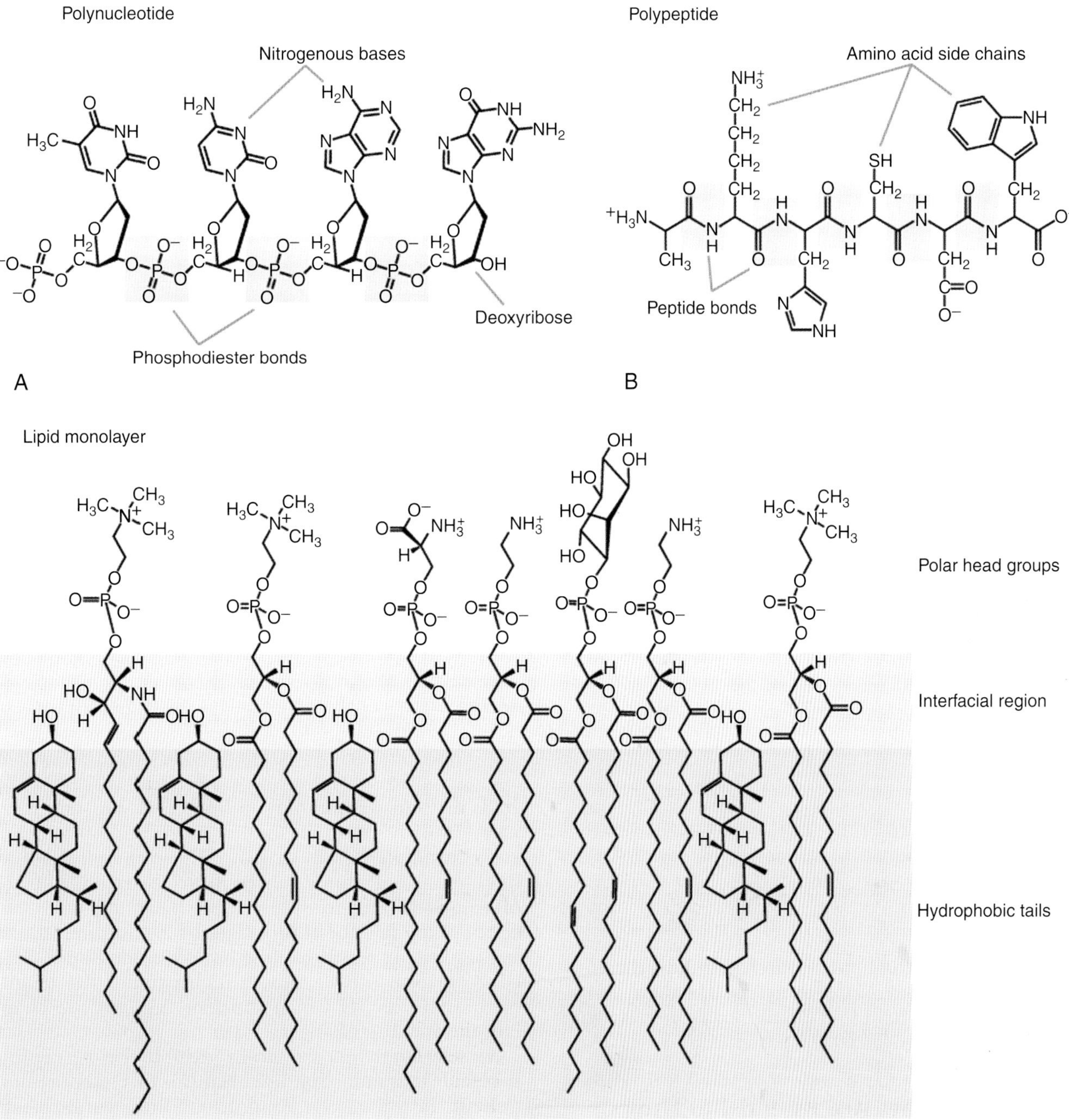

Figure 3.1 Macromolecular structures in biological molecules. Most biological macromolecules are composed of a limited number of building blocks joined by covalent bonds, as shown for deoxyribonucleic acid (A) and proteins (B). Membranes (C) are composed of a large diversity of molecules sharing similar physical properties that allow for noncovalent self-association.

macromolecular structures. There are literally hundreds of different types of lipids within each cell. These lipids do not form covalent polymers, rather, they self-associate with each other and with protein components to form dynamic, but stable, aggregates. Membrane-forming lipids share a bipartite structure consisting of a polar region (head) covalently connected to a hydrocarbon region (tail). These distinct chemical differences between the head and tail regions govern the self-assembly of lipid molecules into macromolecular structures with the head and tail regions of each lipid molecule aligned with one another (Figure 3.1C).

Although lipids are derived from different pathways and each pathway produces many different species, they share a similar overall structure (Figure 3.2 and Table 3.1). Structurally, lipid molecules can be classified into five categories based upon the backbone from which they are derived:

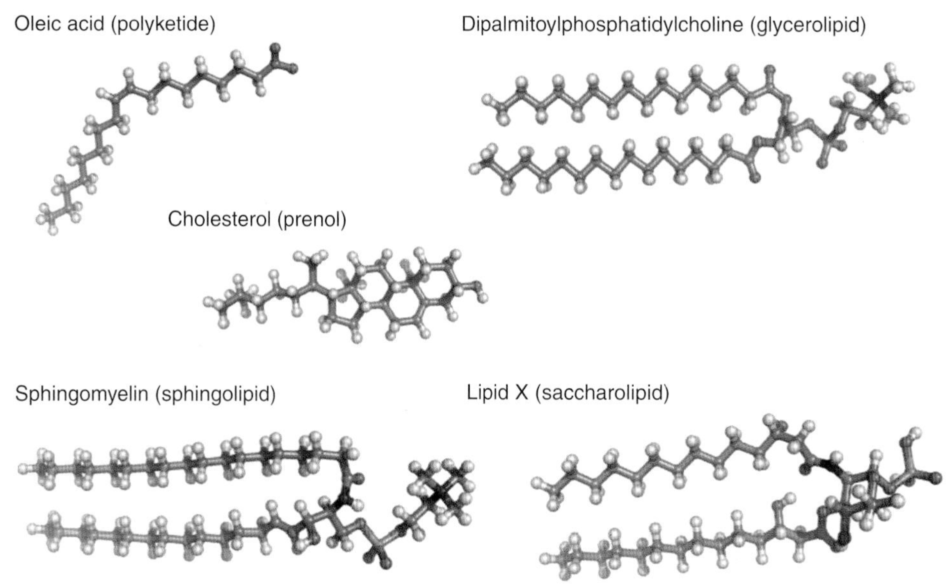

Figure 3.2 Anatomy of a lipid molecule. Lipid molecules found in membranes all share a bipartite structure consisting of a hydrophilic region (head) covalently connected to a hydrophobic region (tail). Structurally, these fall into five major categories distinguished by their overall structure: polyketides, represented here by the fatty acyl derivatives that form the hydrocarbon tails of more complex lipids; glycerolipids, where the tail is joined to the head through a common glycerol backbone; sphingolipids, containing a long chain sphingoid base at their core; the diverse prenols, derived biosynthetically from five carbon isoprene units; and the saccharolipids, in which fatty acyl groups are linked directly to sugar backbones. A representative member of each of the five categories of lipid molecules is shown. Carbon is colored violet, hydrogen is white, oxygen is red, phosphorous is orange, and nitrogen is blue. The similarity between classes is easy to see; each is a bipartite structure with a hydrocarbon tail and a polar head group.

- Polyketides
- Glycerolipids
- Sphingolipids
- Prenols
- Saccharolipids

A comprehensive classification system for lipids with broad support in the lipid research community can be found at the Lipid Maps Structure Database (www.lipidmaps.org). The Lipid Maps Structure Database currently catalogs over 10,000 structures.

Polyketides include a wide variety of hydrocarbon metabolites, but the most relevant in discussions of membrane structure are the fatty acids. Fatty acids are long-chain hydrocarbons with a carboxyl group (-COOH) attached at one end. Free fatty acids are found only transiently in membranes, but they are important as signaling molecules, and as the covalently attached hydrocarbon tails of glycerolipids, sphingolipids, and saccharolipids, where they form the bulk of membrane lipid. A few of the typical fatty acids found in membranes are shown in Table 3.1. Much of the complexity found in membrane lipids comes from the diverse chemical composition of the long-chain fatty acid tails. The chain lengths of fatty acids can range from 4 to 36 carbons, but in most membranes the chain lengths are between 12 and 24 carbons, with 16 and 18 carbon chains dominating.

Due to the way fatty acids are synthesized, nearly all fatty acids have an even number of carbons. These fatty acids are most commonly unbranched, but considerable diversity exists in nature, including branched, cyclic and heteroatom structures. The chemical bonds linking carbon atoms can be fully saturated, but are often unsaturated to different degrees. Fatty acids can adopt many flexible conformations around methylene bonds, but are less flexible around double bonds. The conformation can be *trans*, which extends the length of the lipid, or *cis*, which shortens the effective chain length while increasing its width.

Unsaturated lipids typically exhibit the *cis* conformation. A standard nomenclature to describe acyl chains is a numeric representation with two numbers separated by a colon. The first number denotes the number of carbons in the chain, and the second number represents the number of double bonds in the chain. The positions of the double bonds are denoted by numbers as superscripts preceded by the Greek letter Δ. For example, the 18-carbon saturated *stearic* (or *octadecanoic*) acid is represented by 18:0, whereas the 18-carbon unsaturated *oleic* (or *octadecenoic*) acid is written as 18:1 or more completely, 18:1(Δ^9).

Glycerolipids are defined by the presence of a glycerol backbone. The three carbons of glycerol are designated according to a stereospecific number system, *sn*-1, *sn*-2, and *sn*-3. The most important membrane-forming glycerolipids are the *glycerophospholipids*, which are the most common components of the lipid bilayer. The term *phospholipid* is often used, but this term would also include the *phosphosphingolipids*, discussed later.

Table 3.1 Representative Lipids of Biological Membranes

Polyketides (Fatty Acyls)

Common Name	Systematic Names	Structure
Palmitic acid	hexadecanoic acid; 16:0 fatty acid	
Oleic acid	9Z-octadecenoic acid; 18:1 Δ^9 fatty acid; 18:1 (9Z) fatty acid	
Arachidonic acid	5Z,8Z,11Z,14Z-eicosatetraenoic acid; 20:4 $\Delta^{5,8,11,14}$ fatty acid; 20:4 (5Z,8Z,11Z,14Z) fatty acid	

Glycerolipids

Common Name	Systematic Names	Structure
1-palmitoyl 2-oleoyl phosphatidic acid	16:0-18:1Δ^9-*sn*-glycero-3-phosphate; 1-hexadecanoyl-2-(9Z-octadecenoyl)-*sn*-glycero-3-phosphate; GPA(16:0/18:1(9Z))	
1-palmitoyl 2-oleoyl phosphatidyl choline (POPC)	16:0-18:1Δ^9-*sn*-glycero-3-phosphocholine; GPCho(16:0/18:1(9Z)); 1-hexadecanoyl-2-(9Z-octadecenoyl)-*sn*-glycero-3-phosphocholine	
1-palmitoyl 2-oleoyl phosphatidyl ethanolamine (POPE)	16:0-18:1Δ^9-*sn*-glycero-3-phosphoethanolamine; GPEtn(16:0/18:1(9Z)); 1-hexadecanoyl-2-(9Z-octadecenoyl)-*sn*-glycero-3-phosphoethanolamine	
1-palmitoyl 2-oleoyl phosphatidyl serine (POPS)	16:0-18:1Δ^9-*sn*-glycero-3-phosphoserine; GPSer(16:0/18:1(9Z)); 1-hexadecanoyl-2-(9Z-octadecenoyl)-*sn*-glycero-3-phosphoserine	
1-palmitoyl 2-oleoyl phosphatidyl glycerol (POPG)	16:0-18:1Δ^9-*sn*-glycero-3-[phospho-rac-(1-glycerol)]; GPGro(16:0/18:1(9Z)); 1-hexadecanoyl-2-(9Z-octadecenoyl)-*sn*-glycero-3-phospho-(1′-sn-glycerol)	

Continued

Table 3.1 Representative Lipids of Biological Membranes—cont'd

Common Name	Systematic Names	Structure
1-palmitoyl 2-oleoyl phosphatidyl inositol (POPI)	16:0-18:1Δ^9-*sn*-glycero-3-phosphoinositol; GPIns(16:0/18:1(9Z)); 1-hexadecanoyl-2-(9Z-octadecenoyl)-*sn*-glycero-3-phospho-(1′-myo-inositol)	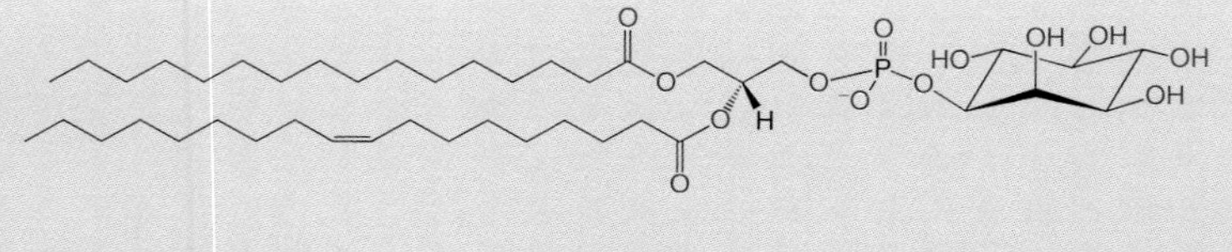
1-palmitoyl 2-oleoyl phosphatidyl inositol glycan	16:0-18:1Δ^9-*sn*-glycero-3-phosphoinositolglycan; EtN-P-6Manα1-2Manα1-6Manα1-4GlcNα1-6GPIns(14:0/14:0); 1-hexadecanoyl-2-(9Z-octadecenoyl)-*sn*-glycero-3-phosphoinositolglycan	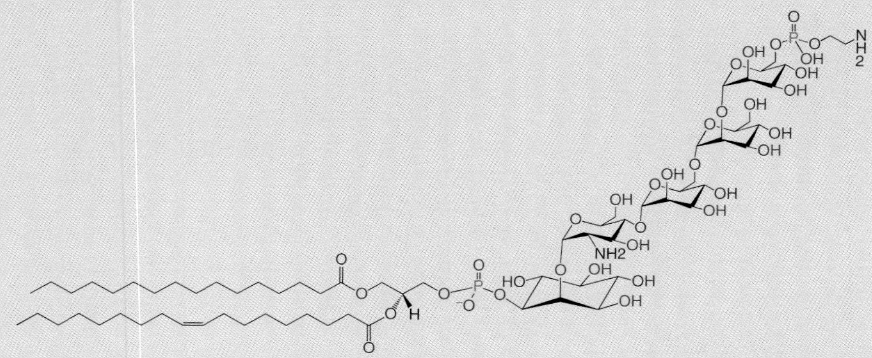
1-palmitoyl 2-oleoyl diacylglycerol	16:0-18:1Δ^9-*sn*-glycerol; DG(16:0/18:1(9Z)); 1-hexadecanoyl-2-(9Z-octadecenoyl)-*sn*-glycerol	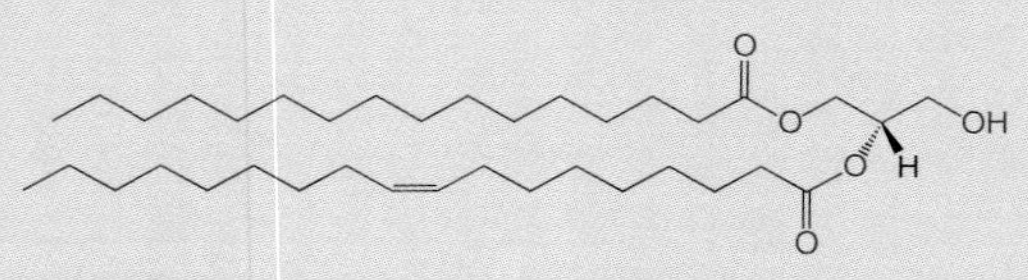

Sphingolipids

Common Name	Systematic Names	Structure
Sphingosine	D-*erythro*-sphingosine; sphing-4-enine; (2S,3R,4E)-2-aminooctadec-4-ene-1,3-diol	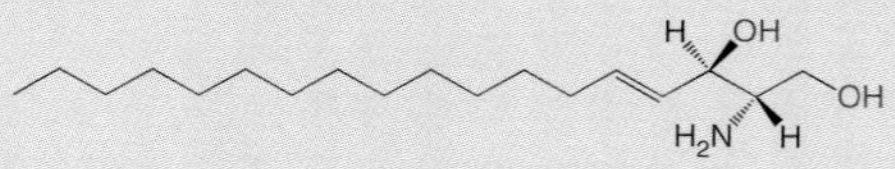
N-palmitoyl sphingosine (a ceramide)	Cer(d18:1/16:0); N-(hexadecanoyl)-sphing-4-enine	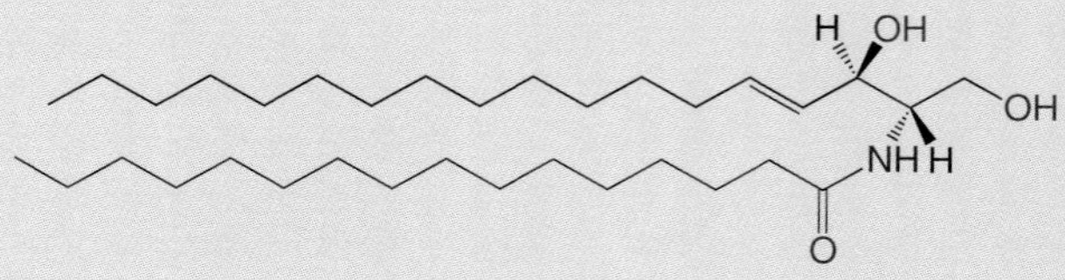
N-stearyl-sphingomyelin	SM(d18:1/18:0); N-(octadecanoyl)-sphing-4-enine-1-phosphocholine	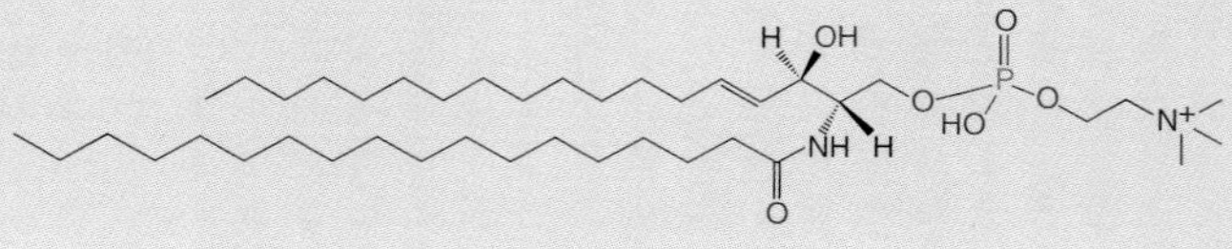

glucosyl(ß) Lauroyl ceramide (a cerebroside)	C12 ß-D-Glucosyl Ceramide GlcCer(d18:1/12:0); N-(dodecanoyl)-1-β-glucosyl-sphing-4-enine	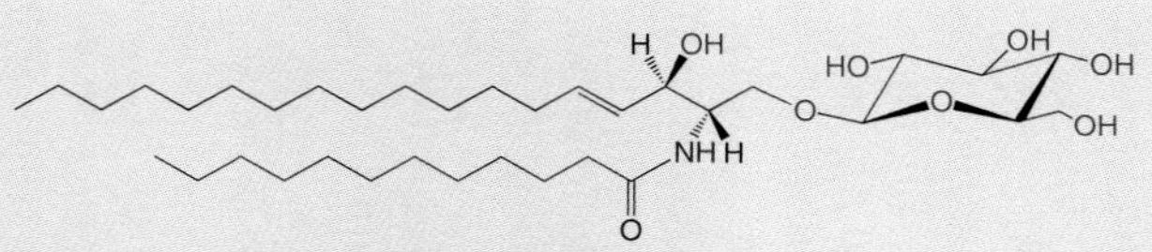

Prenols (Sterols)

Common Name	Systematic Names	Structure
Cholesterol	Cholest-5-en-3β-ol	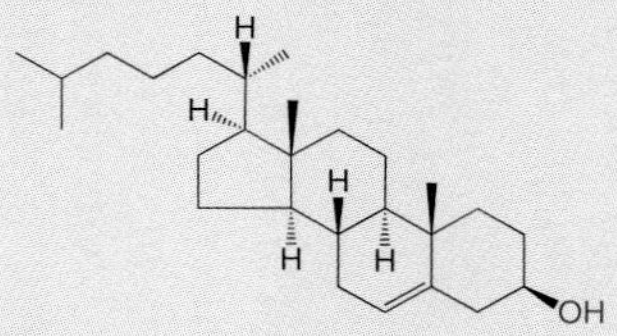
Lauroyl cholesterol	12:0 Cholesterol ester; cholest-5-en-3β-yl dodecanoate	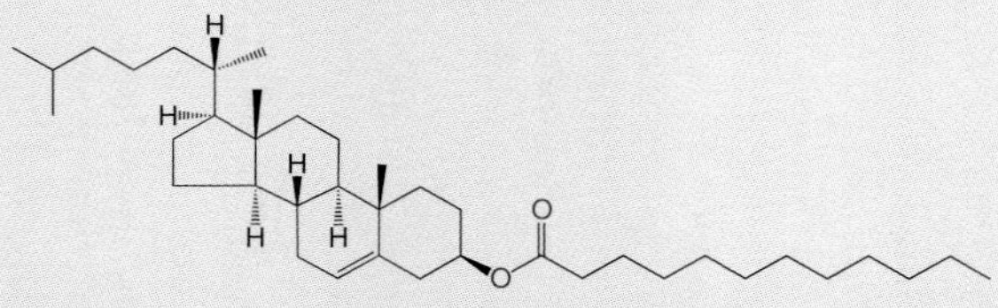

Saccharolipids

Common Name	Systematic Names	Structure
Lipid X	2,3-bis-(3R-hydroxy-tetradecanoyl)-αD-glucosamine-1-phosphate	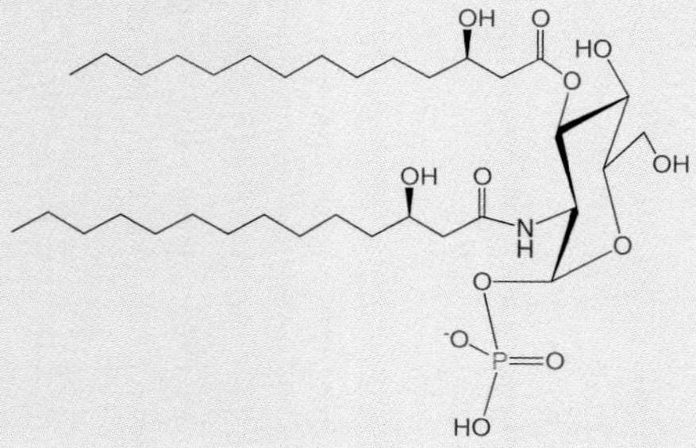

In a typical glycerophospholipid, the *sn*-1 and *sn*-2 positions are esterified (or sometimes ether-linked) with fatty acyl groups. The *sn*-3 position is linked through an ester bond to a phosphate or a phosphorylated alcohol. If it is a phosphate, the molecule is known as a *phosphatidic acid* (or *phosphatidate*).

Phosphatidic acids are present at low concentrations in biological membranes where they serve transiently as signaling molecules and precursors to other phospholipids. The most abundant glycerophospholipids found in animals and plants have various alcohol derivatives attached to the phosphate group, including phosphatidylcholine (PC), phosphatidyl-ethanolamine (PE), phosphatidylserine (PS), phosphatidylinositol (PI), and phosphatidylglycerol (PG). A glycerophospholipid is usually named using the names of the two fatty acid tails, followed by the name of the phosphatidate derivatives of the head group. If there is only one fatty acid tail, the prefix *lyso-* precedes the name. For example, a glycerol esterified with 16:0 and 18:1 fatty acids at carbons 1 and 2, respectively, and a phosphatidylcholine at carbon 3 is called 1-palmitoyl-2-oleoyl-phosphatidylcholine (POPC). Table 3.1 lists some common glycerophospholipids by their name, systematic representations, and structure. Also shown in Table 3.1 is a derivative of a phosphatidylinositol with a chain of additional sugar groups attached to inositol by a glycosidic linkage. Similarly, chains of sugar groups can be attached directly to the glycerol backbone at the *sn*-3 position, forming a class of glycerolipids referred to as *glycerolglycans*. Lipids with one or more sugars attached via glycosidic linkages are referred to as *glycolipids*. These glycan modifications can vary greatly, contributing to the overall diversity of lipid molecules. Glycolipids occur in every lipid category.

Two other important subclasses in the glycerolipid category include the *diacylglycerols*, in which the *sn*-3 carbon of the glycerol backbone is unmodified (-OH is the head group), and the *triacylglycerols* (*triglycerides*), in which the *sn*-3 position is linked to a third fatty acid. Diacylglycerols are present only transiently in membranes but serve an important role in signal transduction as activators of protein kinase C signaling pathways. Triacylglycerols are a major form of energy storage, but are not present in significant amounts in membranes due to a structure that favors phase separation. A high level of triacylglycerols in the human bloodstream is associated with atherosclerosis, a disease manifested by hardening of the arteries.

Sphingolipids make up a third major category of lipids. These lipids differ from the glycerolipids in that their backbone is a long chain amino alcohol base synthesized from serine and a long chain fatty acyl-CoA. The major sphingoid base of mammals is sphingosine, but sphingoid bases vary in alkyl chain length, unsaturation, branching, and other features. Representatives of several major classes of sphingolipids are shown in Table 3.1. Most sphingolipids contain an amide-linked fatty acid, forming a ceramide. More complex ceramides are defined based on the head group substitution at the 1-hydroxyl group in the sphingoid base.

The major subclasses include *phosphosphingolipids*, with head groups attached through phosphodiester linkages, and *glycosphingolipids*, with head groups attached through glycosidic bonds. Most phosphosphingolipids found in mammals are ceramide phosphocholines (*sphingomyelins*). Ceramide phosphoethanolamines and ceramide phosphoinositols can also be found in nature. Glycosphingolipids are a subclass of sugar-containing glycolipids, in which the head group substitution at the 1-hydroxyl position of a ceramide is either a single sugar or an oligosaccharide. Sphingolipids with an uncharged single sugar head group are called *cerebrosides*. In the plasma membranes of neural cells, cerebrosides typically have galactose as the head group, whereas in the nonneural tissues, the head group is glucose.

Two important subclasses of glycosphingolipids with oligosaccharide head groups include *globosides* and *gangliosides*. The former has two or more uncharged sugars, usually galactose, glucose, or N-acetyl-D-galactosamine, whereas the latter has more complex oligosaccharides with at least one sialic acid, which is negatively charged at pH 7.

Sphingolipids have many functions; some important ones have been identified only recently. One of these functions is the biological recognition of different cell surfaces. Therefore, sphingolipids play a critical role in cell signaling and immune responses. For example, blood types in humans are determined partially by the oligosaccharides in the head groups of glycosphingolipids. As will be discussed later, sphingolipids, along with cholesterols, are involved in the inhomogeneous distribution of different lipids in the membranes and are responsible for the formation of *phases* or *domains* in the cell membranes. Synthesis of complicated gangliosides can be induced during tumor formation, and trace amounts of gangliosides have been shown to trigger differentiation of neuronal tumor cells in culture. Even simple ceramides have been found to function as second messengers to mediate signal cascades in cell proliferation and apoptosis. Thus, these lipids are potential drug targets.

Prenols make up a major category of lipids derived from 5-carbon isoprene units, with cyclic or long chain carbon skeletons and varying functional groups. These are probably the most diverse group of lipids and are the source for some of the scents and flavors in various spices and herbs. Many key ingredients in traditional herbal remedies may actually be prenols. A systematic investigation is still needed to understand the mechanisms of their pharmacological effects. Other important prenols include vitamins, steroids, bile acids, and the polyprenols involved in the transport of oligosaccharides across membranes. However, the most important prenols involved in membrane structure and function are the sterols, which, along with glycerophospholipids and sphingomyelins, form the bulk of eukaryotic membrane lipid.

Sterols have a carbon skeleton of three 6-carbon rings and one 5-carbon ring fused together. This gives them a relatively rigid structure compared to the other major lipid classes, along with a unique role in membrane formation. Membrane sterols do not exhibit the wide diversity of other lipid classes, with a single species predominating in a particular organism; cholesterol in animals, sitosterol in plants, and ergosterol in fungi. Sterols are not common in prokaryotes, though exceptions do exist. In eukaryotes, sterols distribute very differently in different membranes. For example, the weight percentage of cholesterol is 30 to 50% in plasma membranes, but only 8% in Golgi, 6% in endoplasmic reticulum, and 3% in mitochondria. This gradient of cholesterol content in the membranes of different subcellular compartments is believed to contribute to protein trafficking and sorting in cells.

Using the same nomenclature as for glycerolipids and sphingolipids, the -OH group in sterols is equivalent to the head group of other lipids. Similarly, the fused carbon rings and attached hydrocarbon groups form the tail region. The most pronounced characteristic that sets sterols apart from glycerolipids and sphingolipids is their small polar head combined with a rigid tail. As will be discussed later, this feature is essential for membranes to provide support for the specific functions of many membrane proteins.

Saccharolipidsm, where fatty acids are linked in ester and amide linkages directly to sugar molecules. This is a relatively small class of molecules, best described in bacteria and plants. The most well known of these are the acylated glucosamine precursors of the lipid A component of the endotoxin thought to be responsible for the toxicity of Gram-negative bacteria. A simple monosaccharide precursor, Lipid X, is shown in Table 3.1.

3.2.2 Organization of Lipid Molecules

3.2.2.1 The Amphipathic Property of Lipid Molecules

In order to understand how lipid molecules are organized when surrounded by water, let us first examine some interesting physical properties of lipid and water molecules. One of the principal differences between the head and tail regions of lipid molecules is their ability to mix with water. It is well known that water and oil (i.e., the hydrocarbon region forming the tail of a lipid) do not mix, but the hydroxyl group, the phosphate, the phosphorylated alcohols, and the sugar groups in the lipid head region are readily dissolvable in water. The terms describing solubility in water are *hydrophobic* (water-avoiding) and *hydrophilic* (water-liking). Molecules that cannot dissolve in water are *hydrophobic*, meaning they have an aversion to water. Molecules that are polar or polarizable are hydrophilic. Molecules that have both hydrophobic and hydrophilic properties are called amphipathic (or amphiphilic). Lipids that form membranes are amphipathic molecules, and lipids that do not, like triacylglycerols, are predominantly hydrophobic.

The hydrophobic effect is an aggregate phenomenon, distinguished from all other molecular forces (e.g., covalent, ionic, dipolar, hydrogen bonding, π interactions, van der Waals, and London forces) in that it arises from the collective behavior of many molecules by disruption of the hydrogen-bonded structure of water.

Water is an extremely cohesive fluid because of its ability to form an extended three-dimensional network of hydrogen bonds in addition to dipole–dipole interactions. Each water molecule can engage in up to four hydrogen bonds with neighboring water molecules. These bonds are dynamic, constantly being exchanged for new ones with different neighbors. Many different arrangements are possible, and thus entropic effects stabilize the entire hydrogen-bonding network. Although the precise structure of water is still under investigation, the resulting cohesive forces are easily seen on a macroscopic scale. For example, water is liquid under conditions where hydrogen compounds of similar mass, such as methane and ammonia, are gas. The density of solid water under normal conditions (i.e., ice) is smaller than that of liquid water. Most relevant to the discussion is the fact that water exhibits high surface tension relative to most other fluids.

The surface tension of water is defined as the energy required to increase the surface area of a water interface with air or with a hydrophobic medium. It is a measure of the cohesive forces between water molecules. The strength of these forces can be seen in the way a drop of pure water defies gravity by forming a semi-spherical bead on a smooth waxed surface instead of flattening over a large area, as we would expect in the absence of strong attractive forces holding the water droplet together. A comparison of a drop of water with a drop of methanol is shown in Figure 3.3. Water molecules in bulk water can interact with other water molecules in a dynamic fashion, forming up to four hydrogen bonds at any given time. Water molecules at the interface have much fewer options and form fewer hydrogen bonds, resulting in a loss of degrees of freedom and hence entropy. To minimize the loss of entropy, the hydrogen-bonding network can be stabilized only by minimizing the number of water molecules at the interface, or, in other words, minimizing the surface area.

In fact, hydrophobic molecules such as hydrocarbons are excluded from water through the same mechanisms as outlined above. Because they cannot dissolve in water they must form an interface. The same forces that defy gravity to minimize the surface area of a water droplet drive the segregation of hydrophobic compounds to minimize their interfacial contact with water. This is the macroscopic manifestation of the hydrophobic effect. It is a complex phenomenon with both enthalpic and entropic components, but under physiological conditions the

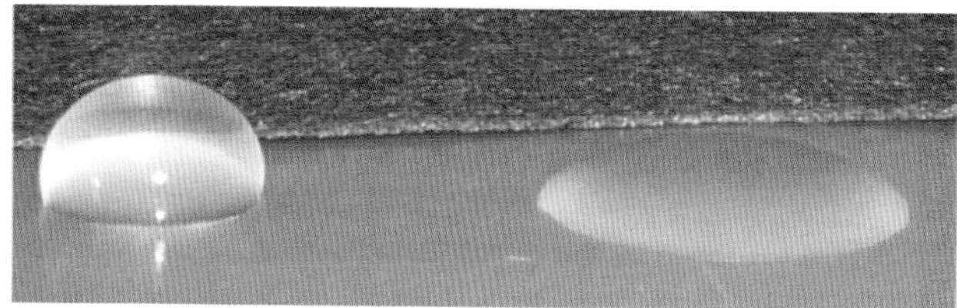

Figure 3.3 Surface tension of a water droplet. A water droplet is shown on the left. A methanol droplet of the same volume is shown on the right. Water is capable of forming a much more extensive hydrogen-bond network than methanol, giving it much greater cohesive forces and allowing it to defy the force of gravity.

entropic component dominates. The hydrophobic effect is moderated by the same parameters affecting hydrogen bond formation and dipole–dipole interactions. These include temperature, pH, ionic strength, and cooperativity.

The possible aggregate structures that minimize interfacial contact depend upon the structure of the hydrophobic compounds being aggregated. For a truly hydrophobic substance, such as any of the simple hydrocarbons, the minimal interface is provided by phase separation into a bulk aqueous phase and a bulk hydrocarbon phase. Amphipathic molecules form much more interesting structures. At a water interface, amphipathic molecules will orient such that their polar regions face the water phase while their nonpolar regions are excluded. The presence of a water-interactive polar region at the interface accommodates the extended structure of water much better than air, or the dewetted surface of a hydrocarbon phase; in effect, softening the edge of the interface. This reduces interfacial tension, which increases the stability of dispersions of hydrophobic compounds. Examples of this phenomenon are found in the effect of emulsifiers and surfactants.

In the same way, amphipathic compounds are arranged by the hydrophobic effect to minimize abrupt water-hydrophobic interfaces. Proteins, for example, are amphiphathic, composed of both hydrophobic and hydrophilic amino acids. One of the primary forces for the proper folding and self-assembly of protein molecules is the hydrophobic effect. For a water-soluble protein, the polar regions dominate the exterior of a properly folded protein, and hydrophobic regions dominate the interior. This effect is modulated by other interactions of the protein with itself, including electrostatic interactions, hydrogen bonding, and disulfide bonds. For integral membrane proteins, the situation is more complex—the protein folds in an environment with both hydrophobic and hydrophilic regions.

As mentioned earlier, lipids are typically amphipathic molecules. Their so-called self-assembly is to a large degree an assembly driven by water. Lipid molecules, much shorter than proteins, cannot fold individually to minimize the water-hydrocarbon interface. Instead they are driven by the hydrophobic effect into aggregated structures to minimize the water-hydrocarbon interface by helping each other as a "society." Likewise, it is energetically unfavorable to bury the polar head group within the hydrophobic phase. The structures therefore must also keep the head group region in a polar environment—either in contact with water or with other head groups. Several stable arrangements are possible to satisfy the separation of the hydrophobic and hydrophilic phases. In biological membranes, the so-called bilayer is by far the most common arrangement.

3.2.2.2 The Bilayer

Long before we had an in-depth understanding of the molecular properties of lipid molecules, the question arose of how these molecules are organized in biological membranes. The experimental investigation started around the turn of the twentieth century. The work of Ernest Overton was among the first to indicate that a biological membrane is a lipid-formed boundary layer. He found that the permeability of organic solutes across a cell membrane could be predicted by the oil-water partition coefficient of the solute more than any other characteristic. Overton concluded that the membrane must be a lipid-impregnated boundary layer with properties similar to those of cholesterol esters and lecithin. He was—as we now know—exactly right. The details, however, are still being established over a hundred years later.

Shortly thereafter, Gorter and Grendel advanced the idea that lipids in a membrane must be arranged as a bimolecular film. By measuring the surface area of a monolayer of lipids extracted from a known number of red blood cells, they calculated that there was a sufficient amount of lipid molecules to form a double layer of lipid around each cell. Ironically, they were wrong. Hampered by the early technologies, they underestimated the surface area of the red blood cells from which they extracted the lipids. Modern measurements indicate that there is a sufficient amount of lipids to cover roughly only half the surface area of the red blood cells as a bilayer. The remaining surface area is covered by the protein component of the membrane, of which nothing was known at the time. Nonetheless, the 2:1 ratio they described between the surface areas of the lipid monolayer and of the red blood cells was striking, providing the insight necessary to propose the bilayer model of a biological membrane. That model forms the basis of our understanding today.

The bilayer model was not immediately accepted as the general description for biological membranes. In particular, it was difficult to see how all the functions occurring at the boundary of a cell could be regulated with such a simple arrangement. The emergence of electron microscopy in the 1950s established that all cellular membranes shared a similar structure. This was true not only for the plasma membrane surrounding many different types of cells, but also for the boundaries of subcellular organelles. In cross-sections, the boundaries appeared as two dense outer bands separated by a lighter central region. This was called the *unit membrane.* Since all the cellular membranes shared a similar structure, the unit membrane had to be sufficiently adaptable to handle such disparate processes as electron transport and glucose uptake. The imaging studies at that time, however, did not have sufficient resolution to distinguish the molecular composition of the unit membrane. Since it had already been established from biochemical studies that the unit membrane was composed of mixtures of lipids and proteins, there was a debate about whether the basic structure of the unit membrane was composed of subunits of lipoproteins or a lipid bilayer with attached proteins. Work with model membrane systems—purified and synthetic lipids—resolved this debate, as it was shown that the purified lipids could reproduce many of the characteristics of biological membranes. Even more intriguingly,

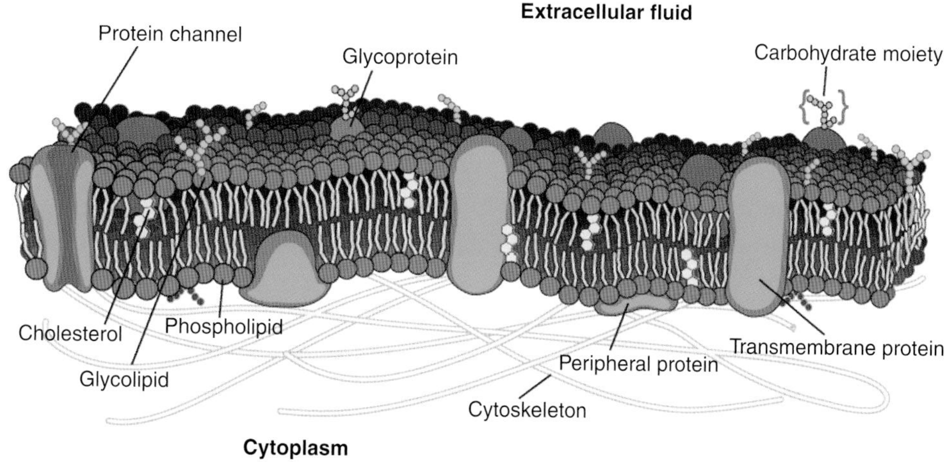

Figure 3.4 Fluid mosaic model of a biological membrane. This model represents a biological membrane as a sea of lipids with a mosaic of associated proteins either floating on the surface or embedded within a fluid bilayer of lipids. This model is sufficient to describe many phenomena associated with membranes. It has been modified more recently to include the concept of membrane domains constrained over different timescales by interactions among lipids, between lipids and proteins, and between membrane proteins and the cytoskeletal network. (Modified from a public-domain image created by Mariana Ruiz Villarreal.)

protein components could be added back to model membranes to reconstitute additional function. Some of these proteins were accessible from both sides of the membrane, establishing that at least some proteins must span the membrane.

About the same time, advances in magnetic resonance spectroscopy allowed a measure of the dynamics of biological membranes, demonstrating that lipids behaved more like a fluid constrained to two dimensions than a solid. This finding, combined with experiments demonstrating the lateral diffusion of proteins in membranes, generated the concept of the membrane as a sea of lipids with a mosaic of associated proteins either floating on the surface or embedded within a bilayer of lipids. The concept is known as the *fluid mosaic model* of biological membranes, as depicted in Figure 3.4.

3.2.2.3 Trans-bilayer Structure

The fluid mosaic model is supported and has been further developed by measurements with modern techniques, including nuclear magnetic resonance spectroscopy, X-ray and neutron scattering, and computer simulations. Details with molecular resolutions have now been revealed. Figure 3.5 depicts a snapshot of a fully hydrated ternary membrane patch composed of a 3:1:1 ratio of POPC:POPA:cholesterol from a large-scale, all-atom computer simulation. Several structural

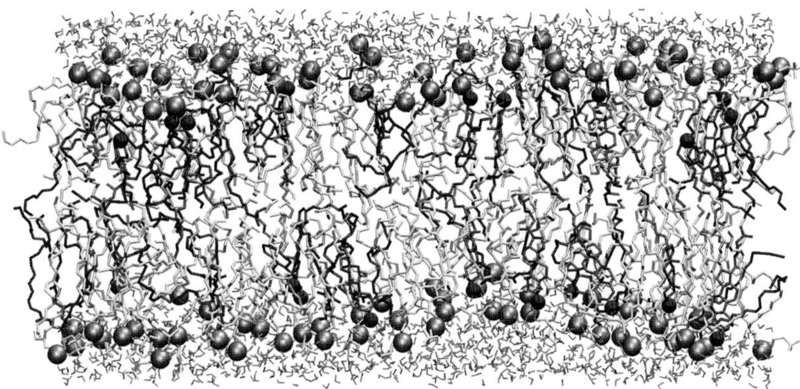

Figure 3.5 Molecular dynamics simulation of a membrane bilayer. This is a snapshot of a fully hydrated ternary membrane patch composed of 3:1:1 ratio of POPC:POPA:cholesterol from a large-scale, all-atom computer simulation. Only a thin slab is depicted for display clarity. Heterogeneity perpendicular to the bilayer is evident in the broadened head group and interfacial regions, and in the diverse conformations found in the tail region. The gray angles represent water molecules. For clarity, only single atoms from each of the head groups are shown: the phosphorous from POPC (gold) and POPA (violet), and the oxygen from cholesterol (red). The hydrocarbon tails are shown for POPC (yellow), POPA (blue), and cholesterol (red).

characteristics are notable. First, the lipids in the bilayer are very dynamic. Although many of the fatty acyl tails can be seen approaching the lowest energy extended conformation, others are bent and twisted to varying degrees. Second, the head groups are not aligned perfectly into two flat planes. There is a significant degree of undulation perpendicular to the bilayer. Thus, the interface between the aqueous phase and the lipid interior is not a smooth or sharp transition, but a region with a rough surface and dynamic thickness. Third, because of the undulation of the interface, the thickness of the bilayer, typically measured from the head groups of one leaflet to the head groups of the other leaflet, is not a single number but a distribution around an averaged number. Fourth, the water molecules penetrate deeply from the head group region to the glycerol bridge.

These dynamic features in the trans-bilayer direction can be averaged for the collective behavior of many lipid molecules and plotted as the averaged electron density profiles of various lipid groups and segments. In computer simulations, the electron density profile can be calculated on the basis of the atomic number and the so-called partial charges for all heavy atoms (i.e., C, O, N, and P). The summation of all components gives the total electron density profile, which is typically what is measured experimentally by X-ray diffraction. Figure 3.6 shows an example of an electron density profile for a simulated dimyristoyl phosphatidylcholine (DMPC) bilayer showing the distance of each component from the center of the bilayer. By looking at the profiles for each component, it is easy to see that each component occupies a range rather than a unique position in space. For example, the carbonyls from fatty acid esters in this experiment ranged from about 7 to 20 Å from the center of the bilayer, with an average distance of about 14 Å.

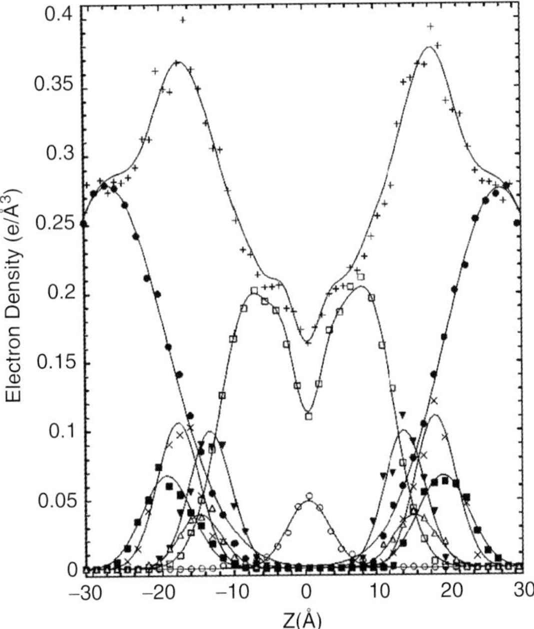

Figure 3.6 Electron density profile for a DMPC bilayer. A calculated electron density profile for a dimyristoyl phosphatidylcholine (14:0-14:0-sn-glycero-3-phosphocholine) bilayer showing the averaged thicknesses of bilayer density regions. Legend: terminal methyl (open circle); long-chain methylene (open square); carbonyl (inverted solid triangle); glyceryl (open triangle); phosphate (X); choline (solid square); and water (solid circle). (Adapted with permission from Zubrzycki, Xu et al. (2000).)

3.2.2.4 Lateral Structure of a Bilayer

A molecular picture of the two-dimensional structure in the membrane plane, or the lateral relationship among lipid molecules, has started to emerge only in recent years. Only a few biophysical techniques, including atomic force microscopy and cryo-electron microscopy, can directly probe the distribution of lipid molecules in the membrane plane with sufficient resolution. Advances in single particle tracking using fluorophores or colloidal particles attached to lipids and membrane proteins allow assessment of the lateral mobility of these membrane components. Results from recent investigations using these and various indirect techniques suggest that the fluid mosaic model oversimplifies the structural role of lipids. The fluid mosaic model relegates the function of the lipid bilayer to a passive permeability barrier that provides a laterally homogeneous environment for protein constituents. The homogeneity arises from the fluidity of the membrane; there are no barriers to lateral diffusion in the fluid mosaic model. In reality, it has become clear that there are barriers to the rate of lipid diffusion, both through specific and nonspecific interactions with proteins, and through interactions among lipid molecules. These interactions, combined with the action of enzymes that alter lipid compositions within the membrane, serve to create regions with physicochemical properties distinct from what would be predicted if the bilayer were truly homogeneous.

The importance of the microheterogeneity of the lipid bilayer is not yet fully understood. Because the bilayer is an aggregate structure whose properties depend not on an individual molecule, but on the sum of the dynamic interactions among molecules, we expect that the nature of the aggregation must in some way depend on the shape of the individual lipid molecules, the chemical and physical properties of these molecules, and the aggregate structure of the surrounding water. Indeed, as will be discussed later, the presence of sphingolipids and cholesterols has been correlated with the formation of two-dimensional domains on micro-, meso-, and macroscales. The microdomains are called lipid rafts. Although the existence of lipid rafts in living cells is still a subject of debate due to the lack of truly noninvasive (nondisturbing) detection methods, it has become clear from recent studies that certain lateral organizations of lipids are important for cell–cell communication, cell recognition, and protein trafficking and sorting. We will return to this topic later.

3.2.2.5 Other Possible Lipid Organizations

The hydrophobic effect discussed earlier acts to segregate hydrophobic regions away from water, aligning head groups and compressing the hydrocarbon tails. Additional attractive forces such as hydrogen bonds between lipid head groups and dispersion forces between the hydrocarbon chains also play a role. Countering these forces are the repulsive forces between lipid head groups and between lipid hydrophobic regions. The flexible fatty acyl chains, adopting many different conformations, are sterically constrained by their neighbors. This results in an entropic repulsion somewhat larger than expected from the width of the extended acyl chain. The head group repulsions are both steric and electrostatic in origin and head groups may recruit other molecules that contribute to these forces. Because of these interacting forces, the shape of a lipid molecule is dynamic and is influenced by many factors that alter the strength of these forces, including temperature, ionic strength, pH, and the inclusion of other molecules. It is the average shape of a lipid molecule under a specific set of conditions that determines its tendency to form a variety of aggregate structures.

When gangliosides with their large, negatively charged oligosaccharide head groups and flexible long hydrocarbon chains are compared to cholesterol with its tiny head group and rigid ring structure, it is easy to appreciate the difference in bulkiness and rigidity of various lipid molecules. If the ranges of interaction are taken into consideration, the abstract view of lipid heads and tails immediately carries a geometric meaning. Charged head groups have a larger effective size than neutral head groups due to electrostatic repulsion, and lipid tails with *cis* double bonds take more lateral space than *trans* double bonds or the saturated hydrocarbon chains. The rigid ring structure of cholesterol gives it a very specific shape that has profound effects on the packing of other lipids. In general, the effective shape of a lipid molecule, especially in relation to the size of its polar region, determines the physicochemical effect of that lipid on lipid packing. Orienting the lipid molecule with the head group at the top, lipids with charged head groups and saturated tails (e.g., gangliosides) and lysolipids with only a single tail typically have an ice cream cone shape. Phospholipids with uncharged head groups and saturated or lightly unsaturated hydrocarbon chains usually have a cylindrical shape. Cholesterols and simple ceramides with their small head groups or other phospholipids with multiple unsaturated hydrocarbon chains appear as upside-down cones.

The aggregate structures that pure lipids can adopt based on geometric considerations are shown in Figure 3.7. At the extremes, lipids with a large head and a small tail produce a micelle, and lipids with a small head and a large tail produce an inverted micelle. Essentially, cylindrical lipids produce perfect bilayers. Natural biological membranes consist of mixtures of a wide variety of lipids along with proteins of varying shapes. It is easy to see that the *curvature stress*, or tendency to form nonlamellar structures, introduced into a bilayer by cone-shaped lipids or proteins may be relieved by lipids with an inverted cone shape. Similar stresses can be introduced in many ways, including the presence of other hydrophobic compounds, proteins, distortion of the bilayer by cytoskeletal components, and chemical changes to lipids in the bilayer. This can be purposeful; destabilized bilayers are important for functions such as membrane fusion and proper functioning of some membrane proteins.

The inverted hexagonal phase (H_{II}) in Figure 3.7 deserves special mention. Total lipids extracted from the bilayers of many different types of cells, when purified away from other cellular components, form H_{II} structures instead of bilayers, suggesting that the H_{II} structure is energetically more favorable for these lipids. Lipids with a tendency to form nonlamellar (H_{II}) phases have been shown to modulate protein activity as well as processes involving membrane fusion and other regions of high curvature. Because of their tendency to mediate fusion processes, these lipids are of great interest in designing drug delivery vehicles. Various lipid-soluble drugs also increase the tendency toward nonlamellar phases and it has been hypothesized that this tendency is intrinsic to the action of these drugs. For example, the nonsteroidal anti-inflammatory drug flufenamic acid induces nonlamellar phases, enhancing the trans-bilayer flip-flop of lipids. It has been suggested that this is the basis for its inhibition action on phopholipase activity.

3.2.3 The Role of Proteins in a Bilayer

Proteins are not needed in order for lipids to form a bilayer. Many lipids can spontaneously form closed bilayers, or *lipid vesicles*, when hydrated at low ionic strength. However, all natural biological membranes include a substantial amount of protein. Proteins make up about 30 to 70% of a biological membrane, depending on the cell and the specific membrane. The protein components alter the nature of the biological membrane, changing its permeability and giving rise to structural and functional heterogeneity.

The proteins intrinsic to membranes are diverse. About 30% of the genome encodes for integral membrane proteins, and possibly more than that for membrane-associated proteins. Protein constituents of a membrane are the primary means to regulate molecular traffic, effect cellular communication, and alter membrane structure. These processes are involved in many different aspects of cell function. In addition, many different enzymatic pathways are associated with cellular membranes, ranging from the metabolism of lipid molecules to the synthesis of carbohydrates. Membrane proteins define specialized membrane structures. Examples include subcellular organelles and the specialized regions of polarized cells like neurons and epithelial cells, as well as smaller domains like clathrin-coated pits. Supramolecular assemblies are often anchored to membranes. The largest of these is the cytoskeletal network that defines the shape of the cell, and together with connections to integral membrane proteins, divides the bilayer into a mosaic of diffusionally restricted regions.

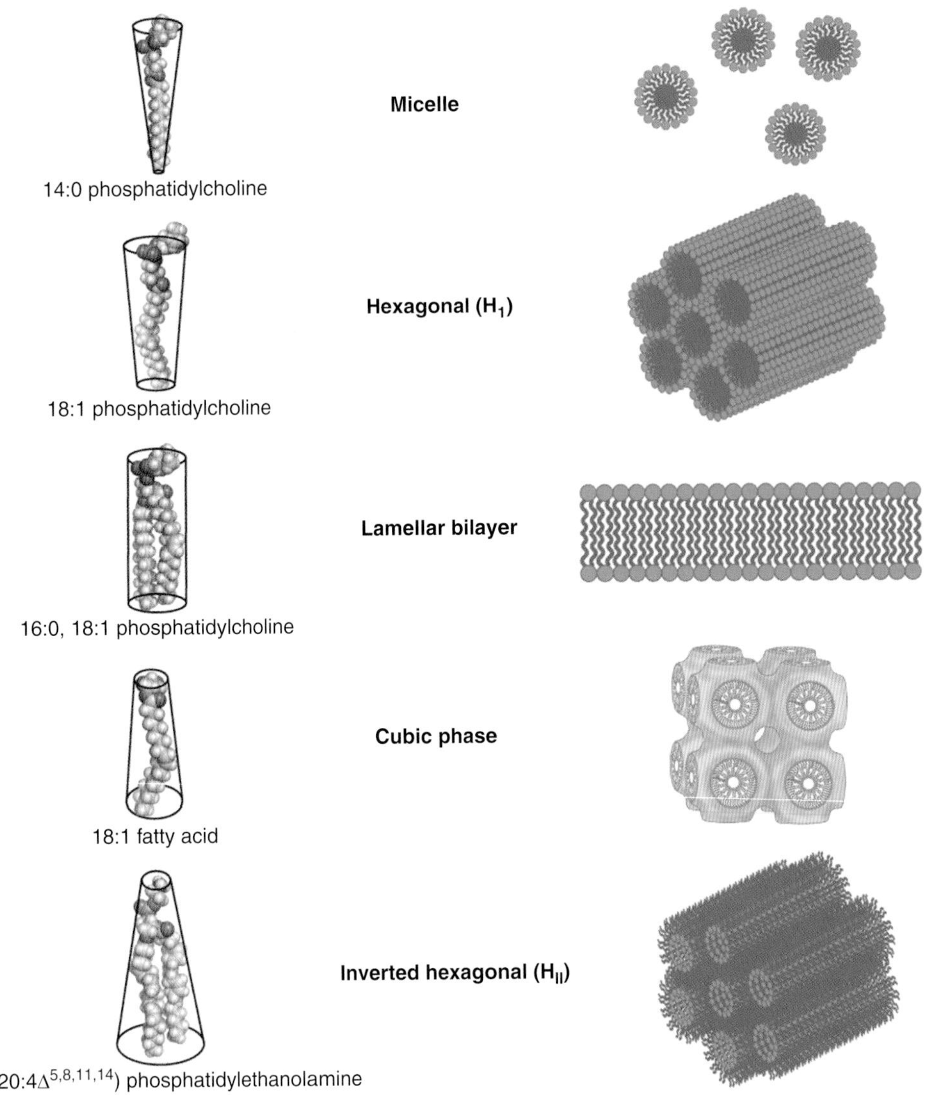

Figure 3.7 Aggregate structures adopted by lipid molecules in aqueous solution. Schematic illustration of how the shape of a lipid determines its tendency to form nonlamellar structures. The lipid forming the structure on the right is depicted as a space-filling model on the left. The cubic phase has multiple forms. The inverted micelle is not shown, since it does not form in aqueous solutions. The inverted hexagonal phase is comprised essentially of cylinders of inverted micelles packed with the hydrocarbon tails adjacent.

Traditionally, membrane proteins are classified according to how they are solubilized away from lipids. Integral membrane proteins require detergent to be solubilized from membranes, whereas peripheral membrane proteins are released by high salt or pH changes. Peripheral membrane proteins are anchored to the membrane primarily through ionic interactions with lipid head groups or other protein components. Integral membrane proteins are inserted into the hydrocarbon core of the bilayer. Other membrane proteins do not fall neatly into either category. Some of these proteins are modified with isoprenyl, fatty acyl or glycolyl-phosphotidylinositol (GPI) moieties. These moieties serve to anchor the protein to the hydrocarbon core of the membrane. The interaction with the membrane often strengthened by sequence motifs on the protein that interact with negatively charged lipid head groups or specifically with cholesterol. Another type of interaction may be represented by protein kinase C, where a phospholipid acyl chain is proposed to extend up from the membrane to occupy a hydrophobic cavity in the protein. Seven different ways that a protein may interact with a biological membrane are represented schematically in Figure 3.8.

Integral membrane proteins represent a particularly interesting problem in protein folding and structure stabilization. A water-soluble protein folds and is stabilized in a relatively isotropic environment. In contrast, an integral membrane protein is exposed to a structured environment divided into regions with different properties, including the aqueous compartments on either side of the bilayer, the bilayer interfaces (including the lipid head groups and associated molecules), and the hydrocarbon core. Neither the aqueous compartments nor the bilayer interfaces are identical

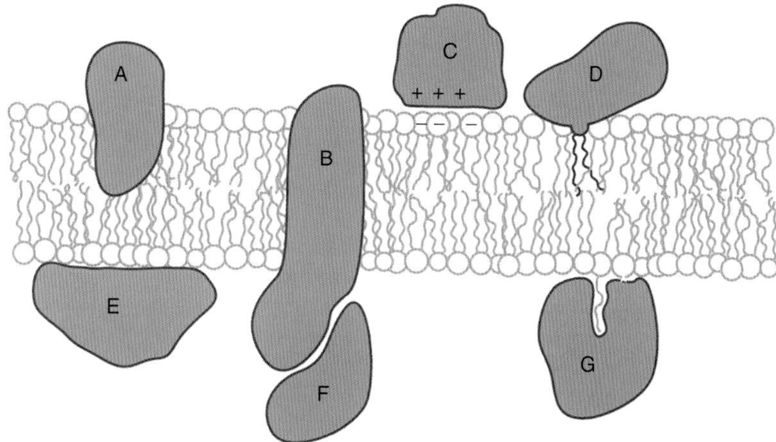

Figure 3.8 Protein interactions with biological membranes. A protein may interact with biological membranes in seven different ways, as illustrated here. A: The hydrophobic domain of a protein penetrating into the hydrocarbon bilayer. B: A protein with a transmembrane domain. C: Electrostatic interactions with lipid head groups. D: Lipid anchor covalently attached to the protein. E: Nonspecific binding of the protein to the head group region by weak physical forces. F: Interaction with a membrane-anchored protein. G: Lipid extension into a hydrophobic pocket within the protein.

on two sides of the bilayer, and the hydrocarbon core is also anisotropic, with different physical parameters at different depths. Within the hydrocarbon core, the protein is almost always fully hydrogen-bonded, usually in the form of helices but sometimes as beta sheets. Helical structure is more favorable than the beta sheets for the transmembrane domains because the hydrogen-bonding requirement can be satisfied locally with residues close to each other in the sequence. Hydrophobic amino acids dominate the lipid-facing regions of the transmembrane domains, as we might expect. Interestingly, they also dominate contacts between transmembrane segments, just as protein–protein contacts are largely hydrophobic for the interior of soluble proteins. In the hydrophobic core, however, packing effects, rather than the hydrophobic effect, drive the association.

Given this highly structured environment, it is not surprising that integral membrane proteins are specifically adapted to the membrane environment in which they reside. Changes to this environment can have a profound effect on the functions of these proteins. Perhaps this is one reason lipid composition, and therefore the physicochemical properties of membranes, are maintained by highly regulated lipid metabolizing enzymes. Disturbances in lipid metabolism have been associated with numerous disease states, such as neurodegenerative diseases and schizophrenia. Amphiphilic and hydrophobic drugs will partition into the bilayer, and may cause sufficient changes in membrane composition to affect protein function.

3.3 THE MEMBRANE ENVIRONMENT

3.3.1 Lateral Heterogeneity

The fluid mosaic model is a gross oversimplification of a biological membrane, but is surprisingly useful and sufficient to explain many aspects of membrane biology. It is useful on a sufficiently small scale up to about 10 nm. At larger scales, however, it is insufficient. Barriers to diffusion must exist in membranes; otherwise a cell would quickly become homogeneous, with every region of every membrane having the same protein and lipid constituents. This is known not to be the case. Specialized membrane regions are evident in terms of large stable assemblies of lipids and proteins that can be visualized microscopically and sometimes preferentially purified away from other membranes. These assemblies include the membranes of subcellular organelles, plasma membrane domains like the membranes of polarized cells (e.g., the axonal and somatodendritic membranes of axons or the apical and basolateral membranes of epithelial cells), and specialized regions like cell adhesion structures, caveolae, or clathrin coated pits. These assemblies are stable in the sense that their overall morphology exists long enough—at least under the specialized measuring conditions—to be identified by light or electron microscopy, ranging from a few hundred seconds to the lifetime of the cell. The individual lipid and protein molecules in these aggregates may be much more dynamic, exchanging with bulk pools and undergoing metabolic turnover. Overall, however, these structures are maintained by low affinity attractions between the involved molecules combined with high local concentrations and limited diffusion. Diffusion is limited by specific and nonspecific interactions of proteins and lipids with each other and with the cytosolic components forming the cytoskeletal network.

In addition to these stable structures, it has become clear that there are much more transient interactions in the membrane that nonetheless create regions of distinct physicochemical properties. The largest of these is created by the interaction of the actin-based cytoskeleton with membrane proteins, both through direct binding and through steric interactions. Tracking techniques have established that lipid and proteins tend to diffuse freely within a compartment between

30 and 400 nm depending on the molecule and the cell type. Because of the dynamic nature of the fluid bilayer, the molecules are not trapped in one compartment, but can hop to the adjacent compartment on a time scale of 1 to 100 ms, where they again diffuse freely before hopping to the next compartment. The membrane cytoskeletal network thus creates a mosaic of regions on the cell surface separated by a reduced rate of diffusion. This, in combination with rapid changes in membrane components due to metabolic processes, can create regions that, dynamically, are quite distinct from surrounding regions.

Lipids do not form an ideal fluid, but exist as a mixture of diverse species that show preferences in associating with each other as a result of head group attractions or repulsions, and packing effects in the hydrocarbon core. Small transient microdomains are formed by specific and nonspecific protein–protein, protein–lipid, and lipid–lipid interactions. A variety of techniques have shown that membrane proteins are surrounded by a dynamic boundary layer of lipids with an average composition distinct from the bulk phase. Membrane proteins, through their preferential association with specific lipids, can induce microdomains consisting of these boundary lipids and the lipids that interact preferentially with the boundary lipids. In turn, these microdomains enhance the formation of protein clusters.

It should be pointed out that microdomains are difficult to study in biological membranes because of their small size and dynamic nature. In model systems, interactions between cholesterol and the saturated hydrocarbons of sphingolipids and certain glycerolipids can form rafts of lipids separated from unsaturated lipids, both because of better packing of the rigid cholesterol backbones with saturated hydrocarbons and because of hydrogen bonding between cholesterol and sphingolipid head groups. These lipid rafts are stable enough to be probed by atomic force microscopy. In biological systems, with a greater diversity of lipids and the influence of membrane proteins, the lipid rafts are much smaller and must be detected indirectly. Accumulating evidence seems to confirm their existence. Lipid rafts are thought to be important for clustering of specific proteins, intracellular trafficking, and signal transduction.

The existence of microdomains within a membrane creates lateral heterogeneity that has consequences in terms of local concentrations of membrane-associated compounds, including membrane-active drugs, and the cooperativity between membrane proteins. It also causes fluctuations in the physicochemical properties of bilayers, including chemical interactions in the interfacial head group regions. These fluctuations can have profound effects on protein function and drug availability.

3.3.2 In Support of Protein Function

Interactions with the interfacial head group region usually anchor and stabilize integral membrane proteins in the bilayer. They are also the primary attractive force for the initial adsorption of peripheral membrane proteins. Intracellular membranes contain up to 10% anionic lipids (lipids with negatively charged head groups), and most membrane targeting domains of peripheral membrane proteins contain cationic surfaces. This initial adsorption to the membrane effectively enhances the concentration of the protein at the membrane, increasing its probability of forming more specific interactions with particular lipids or membrane proteins. A large number of cytoplasmic proteins involved in signal transduction or membrane trafficking reversibly bind to specific lipids or particular regions of the membrane. This reversible binding can be induced by conformational changes in the protein or by other factors such as calcium release or phosphorylation. Changes in the membrane can also lead to stabilization of these structures.

Other interfacial chemistries are found in *juxtamembrane* domains of certain proteins that show a preferential interaction with specific lipids in their head group region. Important lipids involved in these interactions include the polyphosphate phosphatidylinositol lipids, cholesterol, gangliosides, and sphingomyelin. Interfacial chemistries play a role in the formation of microdomains and can determine the effective concentration of certain amphiphilic drugs in different membranes or even in different leaflets of the same membrane.

Another important membrane environmental variable that has strong impact on protein function is lipid packing. *Packing efficiency* describes how well membrane constituents come together to minimize abrupt interfaces. Though ultimately driven by the hydrophobic effect, at close range London dispersion forces also become significant, especially when viewed as a sum of multiple interactions. In general, the better molecular surfaces fit one another, the more stable the aggregate structure. This has obvious implications in terms of membrane permeability; membranes become most permeable at disordered interfaces where there are dramatic packing defects. Other parameters affected by packing efficiency include phase formation, membrane fluidity, membrane lateral pressure profile, and membrane thickness.

Pure lipids form phases with tight transitions between one another depending on temperature and the physicochemical properties of the particular lipids. The lowest energy structure is achieved by saturated phospholipids with fully extended chains, which pack tightly. This tight packing forms the so-called *gel phase*, which is highly ordered and distinctly different from a fluid. In the gel phase, lipids are no longer free to sample different conformations. Their lateral diffusion is extremely slow and membrane proteins cease to function within them. At higher temperatures, the increased energy state of the system allows the hydrocarbon chains to sample many different conformations. The lipids no longer pack together as tightly and the gel phase melts into the so-called *liquid disordered* phase, characterized by a high degree of lateral movement as well as conformational freedom of the hydrocarbon chains. In biological membranes, lipids occur as mixtures of different hydrocarbon lengths and saturation. The different species do not fit together neatly, so at physiological temperatures, membranes exist mostly in the liquid disordered state.

The lipid rafts described earlier, with their high concentrations of cholesterol and saturated hydrocarbons, are thought to exist in an intermediate state called the *liquid ordered* state. The rigid ring structure of cholesterol packs better with the extended conformation of saturated lipids, and thus tends to associate with saturated lipids in a nonideal mixture and stabilize the extended conformation. The packing is not as tight as with pure saturated lipids, so the gel state does not form. Saturated lipids tend to remain conformationally ordered, but the lipids are still free to diffuse laterally. Cholesterol is present at a level of 20 to 50% in the plasma membranes of all animals, and one of its important roles is to prevent the formation of the gel phase in biological membranes, along with the leaky gel-liquid phase transitions at physiological temperatures. Cholesterol has only a slight preference for saturated lipids, and readily partitions into the liquid disordered phase. It tends to increase order, thus softening the difference between phases.

In the absence of clear delineated phases in real biological membranes, the concept of *membrane fluidity* is useful. Membrane fluidity is a measure of microviscosity—the freedom of movement of a lipid or solute within its immediate region of the bilayer. Lipids with a high degree of unsaturation or saturated lipids at high temperatures are fluid and can easily accommodate multiple conformations of a solute. Fluidity varies in both trans-bilayer and lateral directions in the bilayer and is thought to affect the internal dynamics of membrane proteins as well as the rate of protein association.

The effects discussed earlier of the shape of lipid molecules on curvature stress in the membrane can also influence membrane fluidity. The more general description of these effects is the *lateral pressure profile*, which is a measure of several counteracting forces exerted at different depths across the bilayer. Three major contributors to the lateral pressure can be considered. At the outmost surface of the bilayer there is a repulsion force among the head groups that tends to push the lipid molecules apart from each other. This force has the tendency to increase the surface area of the bilayer and is defined by convention as a positive force. Likewise, in the lipid tail region, the flexibility of the hydrocarbon chains creates an entropic force that also tries to push lipid molecules apart (thus also positive). When the bilayer is in equilibrium, the net forces across the bilayer must be zero. The negative force pulling all lipid molecules together is the hydrophobic force that acts at the interface between the head groups and hydrocarbon tails.

As we already know, the hydrophobic forces try to minimize the exposure of lipid tails to the aqueous environment. Because the thickness of this interfacial layer is very thin, the strain built up at this interface is very large. It can be estimated that the lateral pressure in a lipid bilayer can amount to several hundred atmospheres. This is a tremendous amount of pressure, which is highly sensitive to lipid compositions and changes in the amount of nonlamellar lipids and solutes such as drugs in the bilayer. The lateral pressure profile can influence protein conformation directly by mechanical pressure, or indirectly by stabilizing nonlamellar structures or by changing membrane thickness.

Membrane thickness is of particular importance for a wide range of membrane proteins. The average thickness of a membrane is about 3 nm for the hydrocarbon core, and another 3 nm for the interfacial region, but this can vary considerably in time and space. The highly structured environment provided by a biological membrane requires a matching protein structure for proper folding and functioning. This phenomenon is termed *hydrophobic matching*, reflecting that it is energetically unfavorable to immerse polar or charged residues within the hydrocarbon core or to expose a hydrophobic surface to the aqueous milieu. As a consequence, membrane thickness varies dynamically to match the length of a protein's transmembrane domain. As we have discussed, the thickness of a membrane is determined by the length of the hydrocarbon chains in the two leaflets of the bilayer and the degree of unsaturation, the temperature, the lateral pressure profile, and the hydration of head groups (changing their effective average size).

Another common variable affecting membrane thickness is cholesterol content. Cholesterol alters the lateral pressure profile, extending hydrocarbon chains and thus thickening the bilayer. The thickness can also be altered by interactions with proteins, which cannot only stabilize lipids in certain conformations but can also recruit special lipids to provide the desired thickness. In this way, hydrophobic matching initiates the formation of microdomains, which can in turn recruit other proteins and lipids attracted to that particular membrane thickness. This process is thought to be the mechanism of protein clustering and targeting to specific membranes. For example, proteins resident in the Golgi apparatus have transmembrane helices about five residues shorter than those in the plasma membrane, reflecting the thinner membrane of the Golgi apparatus. Alternatively, some proteins can undergo a shift in structure to accommodate the hydrophobic mismatch. One mechanism involves the tilting of transmembrane helices to accommodate a thinner membrane.

The activity of a number of membrane proteins has been linked to the thickness of the membrane, including channels, ion pumps, and sugar transporters. For example, the Na^+K^+-ATPase (sodium pump) is an integral membrane protein that shows maximal activity in synthetic bilayers with longer chain saturated lipids. In the presence of cholesterol, the maximum shifts to shorter chain saturated lipids, consistent with the fact that cholesterol thickens a bilayer by encouraging the extended chain conformation.

3.4 ROLE OF DRUG POLARITY

In order to reach its target or site of action, a drug must be absorbed and distributed through the body. Usually this involves interacting with or crossing a biological membrane. A drug can thus be amphiphilic, with solubility in both aqueous and lipid phases; hydrophilic, with its site of action accessible from the extracellular space or being passed through the membrane by special transport mechanisms to reach its site of action; or hydrophobic, with special measures needed to deliver the drug to the desired membrane target.

Not surprisingly, amphiphilic drugs make up the largest class of drugs. Amphiphilic drugs don't require specific transport mechanisms to cross the membrane. Soluble in both aqueous biological fluids and in lipid membranes, they simply diffuse throughout the body. For many amphiphilic drugs, efficacy is determined by how fast the drug can partition into or cross the membrane. The rate of drug clearance through metabolism or specific pathways opposes the rate of accumulation. Thus, faster exchange and equilibration between the aqueous and lipid phases means that less drug is needed to produce a desired effect.

The classic experiments were those performed by Ernest Overton and Hans Meyer at the turn of the twentieth century, where tadpoles were placed in solutions containing alcohols of increasing hydrophobicity. They found a correlation between the concentration of the alcohol required to cause cessation of movement and the concentration of the alcohol distributed into the lipid phase of a lipid-water mixture. The ratio of the concentration in the lipid phase to the concentration in the aqueous phase at equilibrium is known as the Overton-Meyer or lipid-water *partition coefficient.* The higher the partition coefficient, the less alcohol was needed to cause cessation of movement.

Since then, many different studies have shown that these early findings are broadly applicable to a wide range of amphiphilic drugs and cell types. The partition coefficient is still a valuable parameter in predicting the efficacy of a drug. Octanol is typically used as the nonpolar phase and partitioning is expressed as the log of the partition coefficient, *log P.* Chromatographic methods used to assess *lipophilicity* typically are calibrated to log P using standards. There are also *in silico* methods for predicting lipophilicity.

It is very difficult for an ion to diffuse across the hydrocarbon core of a membrane. Nonetheless, many drugs are organic compounds that do form ions in solution. These drugs, however, are weak electrolytes that exist in equilibrium between ionized and unionized forms. It is the unionized form of the electrolyte that can diffuse across the membrane. The relative amount of ionized and unionized forms depends on the ionization constant of the electrolyte and the pH. The pH dependence of the partition coefficient is incorporated into the lipophilicity measurement known as *log D.* An interesting effect of amphiphiles that are also weak electrolytes is the interaction of the charged moiety with the interfacial head group region. Given the asymmetry of bilayer leaflets and lateral heterogeneity, this can cause drugs to concentrate based on interfacial chemistries.

Although the efficacy of many drugs can be predicted using log P or log D, many exceptions exist. In some cases the efficacy is anomalously low relative to analogous drugs. This can result from several factors, including retention of the drug in nonproductive membranes due to large size or specific interactions, reduced potency of the analog at the active site, greater vulnerability to degradation, or metabolic conversion or active efflux from the target cell by drug transporters. High lipophilicity reduces water solubility and increases nonspecific binding to hydrophobic surfaces.

An anomalously high efficacy is usually the result of the action of a protein transporter or endocytotic mechanism. Biological membranes contain protein components evolved specifically for transporting hydrophilic nutrients across the membrane. Cellular models that directly measure permeability from both passive diffusion and transport mechanisms have been developed for screening purposes using monolayers of Caco-2 intestinal adenocarcinoma cells or MDK canine kidney cells.

The earliest screenings for effective drugs were herbal folk remedies, particularly in China and other East Asian countries where generations of trial and error established which plant extracts were effective as drugs. The bioavailability and potency of various ingredients at their putative sites of action were tested using recurring illness and diseases in humans as bioassays. Most of the key ingredients identified as effective were either amphipathic and thus could diffuse past membrane barriers, or mimicked natural nutrients, so that transport mechanisms designed to transport nutrients or endogenous substrates would transport the herbal medicine as well. Caffeine, arguably the most widely consumed drug in the world, is a good example. It is a water-soluble compound with poor lipophilicity. It is readily absorbed from the gastrointestinal tract, however, by nucleoside transporters and passed into the bloodstream. Caffeine's stimulating effects on the central nervous system are thought to derive from competition with adenosine at cell surface adenosine receptors leading to changes in the intracellular concentration of cyclic AMP. This is a common theme for hydrophilic drugs. The similarity of the drug to an endogenous substrate underlies both its mechanism of action and the means by which the drug traverses across the biological membranes.

Modern methods of drug screening and design focus on structure–activity relationships (SAR). Various assays are used to screen drug libraries for the desired effect, and those drugs identified as positive are used as the starting point for the synthesis of analogues that explore physicochemical parameters that improve the desired effect. Unlike early screening techniques, the barriers to drug delivery innate to a human being are not considered until potency at the therapeutic site is established. Thus many more potentially effective drugs are identified, but problems of drug delivery past biological membrane barriers remain. *Pharmaceutical profiling* refers to the screening of drug candidates for physicochemical properties relevant for drug delivery, including solubility, lipophilicity, and stability. This profiling step usually precedes any sort of bioassay where such physicochemical properties may have an effect. If *in vivo* systems establish a problem with pharmacokinetics, these properties may be altered to improve drug availability.

One strategy to improve drug availability is to include parameters necessary for uptake by endogenous transport mechanisms in the design of the drug, while maintaining efficacy at the therapeutic site. However, the necessary parameters are not typically known, and sometimes it may not be possible to achieve high availability and efficacy at the same time. Alternatively, it is often possible to chemically add a moiety to increase the drug's lipophilicity, thus taking advantage of passive diffusion across lipid bilayers. Another strategy is to conjugate the drug to a natural substrate or nanoparticle, taking advantage of endogenous transport mechanisms already developed by evolution to breach membrane barriers. The different strategies employed by drugs crossing a biological membrane are reviewed in the next section.

3.5 CROSSING THE MEMBRANE

3.5.1 Passive Diffusion

As discussed earlier, nearly all drugs have to cross multiple cellular membranes to reach their targets. These membranes vary in protein and lipid content, but share a bilayer structure, thereby creating a tight hydrophobic barrier composed predominately of phospholipids and cholesterol. An artificial membrane composed only of phospholipids and cholesterol is impermeable to strong electrolytes (molecules that carry a charge over the physiological range of pH) and large molecules (molecules in excess of ~300 daltons). Thus, this artificial membrane would block the drugs that fall into these categories. However, because membrane barriers are dynamic and heterogeneous in nature, small polar molecules like water can slowly find their way across through temporary defects in hydrocarbon packing. For these molecules the membrane is a semipermeable barrier, allowing a slow equilibration to occur in the absence of any other factors. For drugs that can partition into the lipid bilayer, the barrier ranges from semipermeable to permeable, depending not only on the solubility of the drugs in the hydrocarbon region, but, especially for large organic molecules, also on their ability to pass through the interfacial region of the bilayer. All these scenarios describe *passive diffusion* across the lipid bilayer, where kinetic energy drives the distribution of molecules to equalize the concentration everywhere.

3.5.2 Transporters

The importance of passive diffusion in drug efficacy is underlined by how often the lipid-water partitioning coefficient can be used to predict the relative efficacy of a series of related drugs. The permeability of a biological membrane to many compounds correlates well with the lipid-water partition coefficient of the compound, but the exceptions are remarkable. Most noticeable among these exceptions are: water; ions such as sodium, potassium, calcium, and chloride; metabolites such as glucose; even large complexes of peptides and other molecules—in short, all the molecules for which the living cell has an interest in regulating the molecular traffic.

The cell controls the expression and activity of membrane proteins that increase the movement of specific molecules across the membrane. These proteins can be classified broadly according to the energy consumed as those governing *facilitated diffusion* or *active transport*. They may also be categorized as *channels* that form an aqueous pore in the membrane through which solutes can pass or *carriers* that selectively bind a molecule to effect its translocation. The term *transporter* is currently used to refer to both channels and carriers, although some authors use it synonymously with carrier.

A comprehensive classification of all protein and nonprotein components that can transport molecules across the membrane is provided by the Transport Classification Database (www.tcdb.org/tcdb), largely the work of Milton H. Saier Jr. of the University of California in San Diego and adopted by the Nomenclature Committee of the International Union of Biochemistry and Molecular Biology (IUBMB). The Transport Classification Database currently has 3000 protein sequences categorized into 550 transporter families. The Human Genome Organization's Gene Nomenclature Committee (HGNC) provides an alternative classification system. Though originally designed to provide unique and meaningful names to every human gene, it is sometimes convenient to refer to a protein by its genetic nomenclature.

Channels, by virtue of opening a "hole" in the membrane, are necessarily a form of facilitated diffusion. In facilitated diffusion the driving force is the concentration gradient of the solute just like passive diffusion, but the solute no longer has to partition into the hydrophobic bilayer. Instead, a protein complex opens a hydrophilic pore in the membrane to allow solutes to pass. Channels can be open constantly, such as those found in ion channels that help establish the resting membrane potential. Channels can also be *gated*, opening or closing in response to external stimuli such as voltage, light, membrane stress, or ligand binding. Nerve transmission, heart contraction, kidney excretion and reabsorption, and a diverse range of other functions in many organs are controlled and regulated by voltage-gated and ligand-gated ion channels. Thus, ion channels represent a very large class of targets for novel drugs, as well as the targets for various toxins and venoms. Ion channels will be examined in depth in Chapter 13.

This category also includes a large number of families of toxic or apoptotic molecules that form pores in the membrane, typically killing the cell. One family of these pore-forming molecules is comprised of simple ceramides that can form pores in membranes at physiological concentrations. At low concentrations these molecules serve as second messengers through sphinogomyelin hydrolysis, but as their concentration increases they disrupt the integrity of the membrane. This process is thought to play a role in cytochrome release from mitochondria during apoptosis. At intermediate concentrations these ceramides are thought to induce nonlamellar phase transitions, allowing bilayer lipids to diffuse across the membrane, destroying bilayer asymmetry, and participating in membrane fusion processes. Other peptides and molecules in this category are synthesized specifically by bacteria, plants, and animals as a form of interspecies biological warfare, many of which have been coopted for use as antimicrobials or antibiotics. Also included in this category are neurodegenerative molecules like the amyloid β-protein (Aβ) peptides in Alzheimer's disease and the polyglutamine channels involved in the neurotoxicity of Huntington's and other diseases caused by unstable CAG codon expansions in human genes.

Carriers are a diverse group of integral membrane proteins that bind a specific (usually stereospecific) substrate and undergo a conformational change to release the substrate on the other side of the membrane. This process is typically several orders of magnitude slower than diffusion through a channel, though some carriers approach a channel in their rate of transport. Most channels are oligomeric complexes with multiple subunits, however carriers can be monomeric or oligomeric. There are four major classes of carriers: electrochemical potential-driven transporters, primary active transporters, transport electron carriers, and group translocators. Transporters that facilitate diffusion of a single substance across a membrane are categorized with the electrochemical potential-driven transporter class, since transport is driven by the substrate's own electrochemical gradient. For example, glucose uptake by a cell typically has a favorable concentration gradient—the only barrier to uptake is the lipid membrane. The glucose transporters are a homologous family of proteins, each with about 500 amino acids and 12 transmembrane spanning segments. The rate of diffusion facilitated by these transporters can be 50,000 times greater than passive diffusion through the bilayer.

The other members of the electrochemical potential-driven transporter class and all members of the other classes expend metabolic energy to transport a molecule with or against its electrochemical gradient, and thus represent *active transport* mechanisms. When coupled with the electrochemical energy arising from ion gradients (typically sodium or proton gradients), the process is termed *secondary transport,* since the ion gradients are created by other (primary) active transporters coupled with chemical, electrical, or solar energy. Secondary active transporters make up the rest of the electrochemical potential-driven transporters class, emphasizing the close relationship between facilitated diffusion and secondary active transporters. Secondary active transporters are often categorized into uniporters (a single charged substrate), symporters (the substrate and the coupled ion move in the same direction), or antiporters (the substrate and the coupled ion move in opposite directions). These classifications are subordinate to phylogenetic classifications as described in the Transport Classification Database.

Other active transport classes are divided according to the vectorial nature of the energy linked to membrane transport. *Primary active transporters* couple the energy of a chemical reaction (including oxidoreduction reactions) or light on one side of the membrane to the transport of a solute. *Transport electron carriers* catalyze electron flow across a biological membrane, from donors localized on one side of the membrane to acceptors localized on the other side. These carriers and processes are important in membrane energetics. *Group translocators* alter the solute during its passage across the membrane in a vectorial enzymatic reaction. Originally speculated to be a major mechanism of membrane transport, the only known example of group translocators consists of the bacterial phosphoenolpyruvate: sugar phosphotransferase.

The primary active transporters class includes 30 families and superfamilies of most of the proteins involved in primary active transport. Important examples include the photosynthetic reaction center family, which converts solar energy to chemical energy, the general secretory pathway family, which governs the insertion of membrane proteins and the passage of secreted proteins across the membrane, and the P-type ATPase superfamily, which includes the Na^+K^+-ATPase. The Na^+K^+-ATPase, also called the sodium pump, couples the hydrolysis of ATP to the simultaneous movement of three sodium ions out of the cell for every two potassium ions moved into the cell against their concentration gradients. This is an electrogenic reaction, establishing the resting membrane potential and providing gradients for subsequent secondary transport. The Na^+K^+-ATPase has been estimated to consume some 25% of the energy-yielding metabolism of a person at rest.

3.5.3 Vesicle-mediated Transport

In addition to passive diffusion, channels, and carrier proteins, a fourth mechanism of breaching biological membranes is provided by *vesicle-mediated transport,* which can also be used for drug delivery. *Endocytosis* refers to the uptake of cell surface constituents by the formation of vesicles from the plasma membrane. This process can be subclassified into *phagocytosis,* the engulfment of particles, and *pinocytosis,* the engulfment of fluid.

Phagocytosis is a form of ingestion common to protozoa and specialized cell types in animals, such as white blood cells, where it provides protective and scavenging roles, or in the epithelium of the gut where it functions in nutrient uptake. Phagocytosis is triggered by particles binding to receptors on the membrane. The details of the interactions are not well understood, but appear to operate by both negative and positive signals. Transport mediated by this process is relatively nonspecific; even inanimate particles such as glass beads can be internalized.

Pinocytosis occurs in virtually all cells as the invagination of special regions of the plasma membrane along with small amounts of fluid and solutes form vesicles generally less than 200 nm in diameter. These processes can be constitutive or triggered in response to stimuli, and in many cells a large fraction of the plasma membrane is internalized every hour. Much of what is internalized is recycled back to the plasma membrane by fusion of intracellular vesicles to the plasma membrane in a process called *exocytosis. Macropinocytosis* refers to the formation of large vesicles up to 5 microns in diameter by extensions of the plasma membrane (ruffles) found in some cell types such as dendritic cells and macrophages.

There are multiple mechanisms for endocytosis, distinguished by the proteins that make up the necessary scaffolding. Distinct pathways dependent on the cytoplasmic protein *clathrin* or the membrane protein *caveolin* have been relatively well studied, but other mechanisms independent of these two proteins are just beginning to be defined. Different mechanisms of uptake lead to different pathways once internalization occurs, determining the ultimate fate of the absorbed solute. The specific solutes transported by these pathways are largely determined by receptors in the respective specialized structures. These receptors are usually proteins, but the carbohydrate domains of the negatively charged gangliosides also serve to bind ligands in a relatively specific manner.

The main route of endocytosis is through the clathrin-mediated pathway. Specialized transient pits about 100 nm in diameter and coated by the structural protein clathrin can cover up to 2% of the cytosolic face of a plasma membrane. Roth and Porter first described these pits in 1964 as invaginations of the plasma membrane covered with bristle-like projections. The same bristles could be seen covering vesicles just inside the membrane; deeper in the cell the vesicles had lost their bristles. They correctly hypothesized that the bristle-coated pits invaginated to form coated vesicles, which then lost their coat and fused to form a storage granule.

The work of Brown and Goldstein in the late 1970s on low density lipoprotein (LDL) uptake definitively established the function of clathrin-coated vesicles as an endocytotic process. Clathrin-coated pits are enriched with a wide variety of receptors, and internalization of these receptors with their ligands is the primary method of entry of many types of molecules, including iron complexed to transferrin and cholesterol microencapsulated into LDL lipoprotein particles. Clathrin-coated pits are continually invaginating and pinching off to form vesicles, which then lose their clathrin coat and fuse as early endosomes. The early endosomes undergo a series of sorting and transforming events that lead to recycling of membrane components and eventual lysosomal hydrolysis of internal constituents.

Another important mechanism of vesicle-mediated transport is defined by the structural protein caveolin. Caveolins are a family of integral membrane proteins that self-associate and also specifically bind to cholesterol and glycosphingolipids in a relatively stable microdomain. These microdomains are an important component of lipid rafts, though it is clear that there are other cholesterol and sphingolipid microdomains forming lipid rafts that do not have caveolin. *Caveolae* can be visualized in the electron microscope as 50 to 100 nm wide flask-shaped invaginations in the plasma membrane, independently described in the mid 1950s by Palade and Yamada. The caveolae close off to form vesicles and fused endosomes (*caveosomes*) distinct from those of the clathrin receptor mediated pathway. In particular, caveosomes do not acidify and their contents are delivered to the cytosol and to the ER. This type of endocytosis is sometimes called *potocytosis* to distinguish it from clathrin-dependent receptor-mediated endocytosis, even though receptors are still involved.

Although specific protein receptors are involved in the process, gangliosides also play an important role in substrate recognition. Caveolin-mediated endocytosis has been shown to be a pathway for uptake of nutrients including folate, albumin, and cholesterol esters; toxins such as cholera toxin; and a pathway for virus attack such as Simian virus 40. It also has been shown to function in efflux pathways and transcellular transport. Caveolae are enriched in efflux transporters, and cholesterol uptake from cells by HDL lipoprotein particles in the plasma can be mediated by caveolae. Particles as large as 500 nm in diameter have been reported to be ingested by a clathrin-dependent mechanism, blurring the distinction between phagocytosis and pinocytosis.

These pathways are not absolute. There is a substantial degree of variability among different cell types. A number of studies have shown that certain ligands (and drugs) undergo endocytosis by multiple pathways, indicating multiple receptors, a wide distribution of receptors in the plasma membrane, or some degree of pathway crossover once internalized. In addition, transporters sometimes transport compounds also absorbed by endocytotic mechanisms. There is some confusion in the literature; the criteria needed to distinguish between different endocytotic mechanisms are still being defined. For example, many studies have assumed that isolated lipid rafts are synonymous with caveolae, but now it is clear that there are at least two additional endocytotic pathways associated with cholesterol and sphingolipid microdomains that are independent of both caveolin and clathrin. Also, both phagocytosis and macropinocytosis are actin-mediated processes covering a relatively large area of the plasma membrane. Both processes have been shown to be independent of caveolin and clathrin. They are distinct processes, however, in terms of their morphology and regulation, although the distinctions between the two processes are not fully understood.

Size can also be a factor determining which endocytotic pathways are involved in ligand absorption. For example, in nonphagocytotic cells, latex beads with diameters less than 200 nm were taken up by the clathrin-dependent pathway, and latex beads with diameters between 200 and 500 nm were taken up by a caveolin-dependent process. Similarly, absorption of DNA-polycation complexes showed clear size dependence: sizes greater than 200 nm were internalized by macropinocytosis. Intermediate size complexes between 100 and 200 nm were internalized by clathrin-coated pits. Small complexes less than 100 nm were internalized through caveolae. This size-dependent selection of pathways has a clear implication in the development of treatment strategies with gene therapies.

Vesicle-mediated transport is a promising method of drug delivery because it is relatively insensitive to the nature of the conjugate attached to the carrier molecule. Whereas a transporter may be fairly restrictive as to the size or chemical nature of a conjugate in its active site, vesicle-mediated transport is much more promiscuous. Extremely hydrophilic or hydrophobic drugs encapsulated in nanoparticles or conjugated with carrier ligands or antibodies can be efficiently targeted to cells and taken up by endocytosis. The down side of using the endocytosis pathways for drug delivery is that when the conjugates cross the plasma membrane they are still bound by the vesicle membrane. In the majority of cases they are headed to the lysosomal acid hydrolases for potential degradation. Developing strategies to recover an active drug in sufficient quantity from its endocytotic vesicle and transport it to its intended intracellular site of action is an area of vigorous research.

3.5.4 Membrane Permeant Peptides

Cationic *membrane permeant peptides* derived from viral proteins and their derivatives are capable of translocating conjugated cargo molecules ranging from small drugs to nanoparticles across the cell membrane. The mechanisms of translocation are not well established, but multiple repeating lysines and especially arginines, combined with the negative charge on the cell surface and a transmembrane potential, seem to be the key components for translocation to occur. The size of the conjugate seems to determine whether uptake is vesicle-mediated or goes directly into the cytosol.

One of the best studied of these permeation peptides is the basic amino acid region from the HIV-1 transactivator of transcription (TAT) protein. The TAT peptide binds to cellular membranes through strong ionic interactions between multiple lysines and arginines, and negatively charged plasma membrane components, such as heparin or negatively charged lipids. What happens next depends on the size and perhaps nature of the cargo. In a recent study utilizing peptides of different lengths, it was found that cargo consisting of greater than 50 amino acids drove the fusion protein through an endocytotic pathway. The fusion protein largely restricted to intracellular vesicles, although the exact nature of the pathway was not determined. Interestingly, for cargos of less than 50 amino acids, the translocation occurred through a vesicle independent mechanism directly into the cytosol. The mechanism of this transfer is unknown, but may represent either a transient membrane perturbation (a hexagonal phase transition was proposed, with the cargo confined to the aqueous lumen) or lipophilic ion pair diffusion driven by the membrane potential.

This is another promising area of drug delivery research, both in the characterization of permeation peptides and in the analysis of the mechanism by which the membrane is transiently breached. Membrane permeation peptides are highly effective in drug delivery, even breaching traditionally difficult barriers such as the skin and the blood–brain barrier. Cell selectivity is one of the important limitations of this system—the nonspecific mechanism leaves all cells open to exposure by the conjugated drug. New strategies being investigated include ways to reversibly shield the permeation peptide or to alter the drug to be active only in targeted cells.

3.6 THE MEMBRANE AS A DRUG TARGET

The original concept of the fluid mosaic model of biological membranes emphasized the protein and lipid components of the membrane as independent entities. Current understanding recognizes the interdependence of these components in defining the nanostructure of a biological membrane. Thus, the idea of treating membranes as a drug target includes drugs that act on myriad channels, carriers, receptors, enzymes, and structural proteins that reside in the membrane as well as those drugs that interact directly with the lipid components of the membrane. As mentioned earlier, most of the drugs currently on the market belong to this category. Several chapters in this book are devoted to the important classes of drugs that act on membrane targets such as receptors, signal transduction molecules, and ion channels. Therefore, we will focus here only on drugs that act through bilayer lipids to exert their effects on cellular functions.

3.6.1 Pore-forming Peptides

The most obvious of the drugs that exert their pharmaceutical effects directly through bilayer lipids are the pore-forming antimicrobial peptides. Endogenous peptide antibiotics are expressed as a form of biological warfare in all organisms, including humans. Antimicrobial peptides are highly divergent 9-100 amino acid peptides typically characterized by positive or negative charges and high hydrophilicity with the potential to form some sort of self-associating amphipathic structure in membranes. Note that the latter characteristic distinguishes these pore forming peptides from the membrane permeant peptides discussed earlier. There have been over 800 native pore-forming sequences identified and thousands of derived synthetic structures. Whereas some of these peptides are active in the nanomolar range toward specific types of cells, most are active in the micromolar range, with broad specificity. The latter class has been demonstrated to bind to the membrane lipids without the need for a protein receptor or a specific glycolipid.

A good example of this class is the principle active component in bee venom, melittin. Melittin is a 26 amino acid water-soluble peptide with a highly cationic carboxyl terminus. It forms electrostatic interactions with the interfacial region of a membrane, where it is induced to form an amphipathic helix parallel to the plane of the bilayer with the hydrophobic face buried toward hydrocarbon core and the hydrophilic face toward the extracellular milieu. The peptide also self-associates, and when the local concentration is high enough the peptide permeates the membrane. The exact structure permeating the membrane is unclear, and may be membrane dependent.

In one possible structure, the so-called *barrel-stave* model, the hydrophilic faces come together to create a hydrophilic pore, which increases in size as more monomers aggregate. The barrel-stave model has been established only for the peptide alamecithin. Melittin is more likely to form a toroidal pore, in which its hydrophilic face remains associated with the polar head groups of lipids. Peptide aggregation induces the associated lipid to form tight bends, such that the pore is lined by both the peptides and the associated lipid headgroups. Melittin may also function by a variation of this mechanism called the *carpet* model. Toroidal pores are also formed in the carpet model, but the carpet model emphasizes a loose peptide arrangement oriented parallel to the bilayer surface, which at sufficiently high concentrations disrupts the bilayer in a manner similar to detergents. Both of these types of mechanisms are thought to occur among the diverse species of pore-forming peptides, including those involved in apoptosis and neurodegenerative disease. Binding is separate from pore formation, and both are affected by the lipid composition of the membrane. A schematic illustrating the mechanisms of pore-forming peptides is shown in Figure 3.9.

The pharmacological interest in these pore-forming peptides comes from the fact that they do exhibit some cellular specificity. Peptides such as melittin are toxic to many cells, however similar peptides like magainin are toxic only to bacteria. Magainin differs from melittin mostly in its charge distribution; the cationic amino acids are spread across the entire peptide. Apparently the localized cationic charge on peptides like melittin helps permeabilize the eukaryotic membrane. Permeabilizaton of the eukaryotic membrane has other structural requirements not important for permeablizing bacteria. For example, melittin can be modified by cyclization or incorporation of D-amino acids to be much less toxic to mammalian cells while retaining its activity against bacteria. The ability to discriminate between these membranes appears to be based entirely on lipid composition. Bacterial bilayers lack sterol and carry a negative charge from high concentrations of phosphatidylglycerol. Eukaryotic plasma membranes are asymmetric with high levels of sterols and zwitterionic lipids and varying amounts of negatively charged glycoproteins and glycolipids in the extracellular leaflet. The inner leaflet has a negative charge due to high amounts of phosphatidylserine.

Interestingly, some antimicrobial peptides specific for bacteria will also attack cancer cells characterized by increased levels of phosphatidylserine and negatively charged glycoproteins. Studies with model membranes show similar effects of charge and cholesterol content for both melittin and magainin. In addition to charge, it is clear that the lateral pressure of the bilayer plays an important role. Incorporation of cholesterol or other nonlamellar lipids with a negative curvature inhibits the ability of these peptides to form pores, whereas lipids with a positive curvature enhance pore-forming ability. Establishing the precise mechanisms of these pore-forming peptides and the related membrane permeant peptides should reveal much about membrane nanostructure and dynamics.

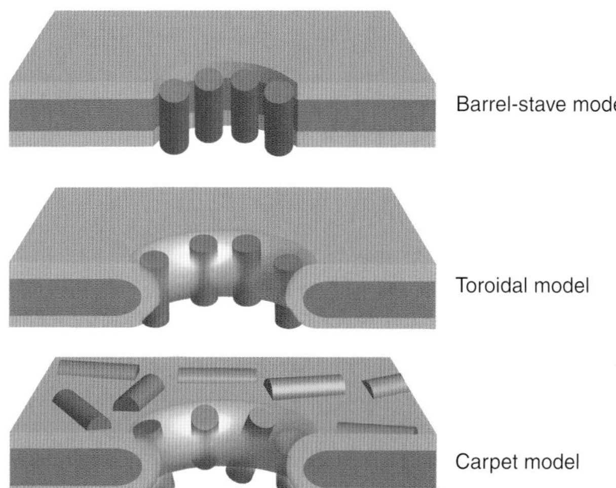

Figure 3.9 Models of pore-forming peptides. This schematic illustrates the differences between three models for pore formation by pore-forming peptides, showing the peptides in blue, the lipid headgroup region of the bilayer in gray, and the hydrocarbon core in purple. In the barrel-stave model, the aggregating peptides form a peptide-lined pore, much like any channel protein. In the toroidal model, the peptide induces bending of lipid monolayers, forming a pore lined by both peptides and lipid headgroups. In the carpet model, toroidal pores also form, but this model emphasizes the detergent-like properties of these amphipathic peptides rather than the specific structures they form. Although peptide accumulation on the membrane surface is a feature of all three models, it is an inherent property of the carpet model, which at high enough concentrations essentially solubilizes the membrane.

3.6.2 General Anesthesia

Perhaps the largest class of drug interactions with the bilayer is the least understood. As mentioned previously, amphipathic drugs will dissolve into membranes and change the properties of bilayers in ways that are just beginning to be identified. In addition to physicochemical changes caused by the presence of drugs in the membrane, chronic exposure can induce changes in lipid content through homeostatic mechanisms controlling membrane composition. These changes have effects on the functions of proteins that interact with the membrane. The fact that many membrane proteins are affected by the lipid composition of the bilayer is now well established. The submolecular details of lipid–lipid and lipid–protein interaction are still unresolved and are a subject of active investigation. The extent to which a particular protein is affected by an amphipathic drug directly through protein binding or indirectly through the drug's interaction with the membrane is often unclear.

A good example of this type of drug is ethanol. In addition to its use as a disinfectant, which essentially acts on membranes to kill bacteria, ethanol is perhaps one of the most commonly consumed drugs worldwide. Its popularity has contributed a huge amount of data on the acute and chronic effects of ethanol consumption. Ethanol is a member of the class of nerve-acting drugs that also include diverse molecules such as short- to medium-chain alcohols, halogenated alkanes, ethers, nitric oxide, and even the heavy noble gases. These molecules can induce general anesthesia at concentrations that are strongly correlated with their oil-gas partition coefficients, as predicted by the Meyer-Overton rule. The concentrations needed for general anesthesia are fairly high compared to other drugs, typically in the micromolar to millimolar range.

Ethanol is entirely miscible in water and reasonably soluble in lipid. The amphiphilic nature of this small, weakly polar molecule allows it to incorporate readily into the structure of water while at the same time partitioning into hydrophobic environments such as the lipid bilayer. At the concentrations needed to produce a cognitive effect, ethanol will distribute fairly evenly throughout the aqueous and hydrophobic regions of the body, easily crossing the gut, blood–brain and placental barriers.

The most obvious effect of ethanol consumption is that it depresses central nervous system responses. The depression of psychological inhibitions makes it a recreational favorite. Chronic moderate consumption of ethanol is believed to provide protective effects against cardiovascular disease, involving changes in membrane lipids and lipid metabolism. Ethanol is also a potent toxin, causing all sorts of uncomfortable side effects such as headaches and gastrointestinal upset. Chronic overuse of ethanol produces a host of medical complications including hemorrhagic esophagitis and gastritis, liver disease, pancreatitis, ataxia, dementia, cerebrovascular lesions, and cardiomyopathy.

The range of effects caused by ethanol consumption reflects its wide tissue distribution and general interactions with many different protein targets. However, even though specific proteins are involved in the different effects caused by ethanol, in many cases these effects do not appear to be specific for ethanol. In isolated systems where ethanol can be shown to have an effect on a particular protein or pathway, other members of this class of drugs can often be demonstrated to have a similar effect, with a potency predicted by the Meyer-Overton rule. This low specificity of interaction, combined with the high lipophilicity necessary to produce an effect, suggests that the active sites are likely hydrophobic or amphipathic with low binding affinity and broad specificity. The lipid bilayers of biological membranes are one of the obvious targets meeting these criteria. Proteins sensitive to the lipid composition of the membrane may be sensitive to drug-induced changes in the physicochemical properties of the bilayer. This idea forms the basis of the physicochemical or lipid theory of general anesthesia, which dominated anesthesia research for nearly a century since the first public demonstration of general anesthesia in the Ether Dome in 1846. It was an attractive theory in that a single mechanism of action could account for the similar effects of a chemically diverse group of drugs.

The lipid theory of general anesthesia met considerable challenges when it was discovered that many of the physicochemical effects produced by general anesthetics on lipid bilayers could be reproduced by small temperature increases. The same elevation in body temperature does not cause general anesthesia. Moreover, it was found that some of the physical changes to the lipid bilayer caused by general anesthetics persisted even after awakening from general anesthesia. Thus, a pure lipid theory does not explain the action of general anesthetics.

There are other low-affinity amphipathic sites in the cell. Both membrane-bound and soluble proteins contain amphipathic crevices and pockets that are of appropriate size for anesthetic occupancy. Lipids make up a dynamic part of many integral proteins, inserting themselves into crevices at the protein-lipid interface or slipping between subunits or domains of multidomain protein receptors. The protein theory of general anesthesia started with an important discovery by Issaku Ueda in 1965 that the bioluminescence of a water-soluble (thus lipid-free) protein, firefly luciferase, could be inhibited in a concentration-dependent manner by different anesthetics. He and Henry Eyring expanded the study to include more anesthetic molecules, and in 1973 proposed a protein theory of anesthetic action based on protein conformational changes. In 1984, Nicholas Franks and William Lieb repeated virtually identical experiments using more anesthetic molecules to establish a correlation between the anesthetic concentration for luciferase inhibition and the anesthetic potency in animals. This correlation resembles the Meyer-Overton correlation, suggesting that proteins—not lipids—can be the primary targets for general anesthetics. It was proposed that anesthetics could compete with native ligands for hydrophobic binding pockets in proteins to produce anesthesia.

With the advent of modern molecular biology techniques and various functional assays, particularly mutagenesis and electrophysiology, many soluble and integral receptor proteins implicated in signal transduction have now been subjected to functional measurements in the presence of general anesthetics. One particular superfamily of postsynaptic neurotransmitter-gated ion channels, the Cys-loop receptors, has drawn a great deal of attention because of the hypersensitivity of its members to volatile and gaseous anesthetics. This superfamily of receptors includes γ-aminobutyric acid type A ($GABA_A$) receptors, nicotinic acetylcholine (nAChR) receptors, glycine receptors, and 5-hydroxytryptamine type 3 (5-HT_3) receptors. $GABA_A$ receptors are the major inhibitory receptors in the brain, and glycine receptors are the primary inhibitory receptors in the spinal cord and brain stem. Nicotinic acetylcholine receptors are the major excitatory receptors at neuromuscular junctions. Thus, it is conceivable that potentiation or inhibition of these receptors by general anesthetics can in some way cause general anesthesia.

Indeed, mutagenesis studies have identified an amphipathic pocket in the transmembrane domains where point mutations can alter the $GABA_A$ receptor's response to anesthetics. Although it is entirely possible that the effects are allosteric, a series of experiments, in which the volume of the mutation was systematically related to the size of the anesthetic that could affect channel activity, seems to support the idea that anesthetics might bind directly to this pocket. It was argued that anesthetic binding to this pocket was both necessary and sufficient to mediate the anesthetic effect on the $GABA_A$ receptor at clinical concentrations. This is particularly noteworthy given that there is subunit specificity to this interaction. The $GABA_A$ receptor, like other members of the Cys-loop superfamily, consists of a pentamer of homologous subunits arranged around a central ion channel. For the $GABA_A$ receptor, the subunits are broadly classified into α, β, and γ subunits, with variants for each class for a total of 19 different subunit genes. Mutations in the α subunits seem to mediate response to ethanol and volatile anesthetics, whereas mutations in the β subunits seem to mediate response to propofol and entomidate, two intravenous anesthetics. It is remarkable that the pockets in different subunits have different specificities of interaction with general anesthetics, implying that although anesthetics bind at low affinity to similar sites, they do exhibit considerable specificity.

Transgenic animal experiments, replacing specific subunits of the $GABA_A$ receptor with mutated forms exhibiting near normal $GABA_A$ receptor activity but with modified anesthetic sensitivities, have been important tools to help dissect the targets of anesthetic action. These studies, in combination with analysis of the differential effects of anesthetics and anesthetic analogues on different targets, have resulted in different results for different anesthetics, leading to the proposal that there are multiple mechanisms and multiple sites for different anesthetics. A direct inference is that the major components of anesthesia—sedation, hypnosis (unconsciousness), analgesia, paralysis, and amnesia—can be mediated by the same drug acting at different ion channels.

Resorting to multiple mechanisms to explain different—and sometimes contradicting—results of different anesthetics on different proteins may simply reflect the limitation of our current knowledge on membrane and membrane protein assemblies. The protein theory of general anesthesia based on anesthetics fitting into protein pockets in order to compete with endogenous ligands does not explain the phenomenon of anesthetic *additivity*, where half a dose of one drug and half a dose of another drug provide the full effect of general anesthesia. The two drugs can be structurally completely different, with one being a structureless noble gas and the other a complicated steroid. Likewise, receptors within the same superfamily, of which the structural basis of function is expected to be similar due to sequence homology, can be both potentiated (as in the case of $GABA_A$ and glycine receptors) and inhibited by the same volatile anesthetics. Moreover, nearly all anesthetics are low-affinity drugs without absolute stereoselectivity, meaning that even though potency differences exist for enantiomers of some anesthetics, all enantiomers *are* nevertheless anesthetics. All this seems to argue against a mode of anesthetic action on the basis of a structure-function paradigm.

Recently, a new protein theory of general anesthesia based on protein global dynamics was proposed by Pei Tang and Yan Xu. They argue that anesthetic binding to hydrophobic or amphipathic pockets in proteins is a sufficient but not necessary condition for anesthetics to produce anesthesia. According to this theory, the most essential element in the anesthetic-protein interaction is the modulation of the protein global dynamics that matches the timescale of protein function. For example, ion permeation across an open channel is on a timescale of tens to hundreds of microseconds. Anesthetic modulation on this time scale will manifest as a functional change in the single-channel current or channel conductance. This dynamics-function paradigm can potentially unify the action of a diverse range of anesthetics on a diverse range of receptors without the need for specific binding. Indeed, the majority of mutations that can change receptor sensitivity to general anesthetics are located near the membrane-water interface, where most transmembrane proteins are anchored and where changes in dynamics have the most profound effect on proteins due to sharp variations in the lateral pressure as discussed previously. Experimental validation of this theory requires structure and dynamics measurements at atomic resolution, for which the only method currently suitable is nuclear magnetic resonance spectroscopy.

When protein global dynamics are considered, many integral proteins have been shown to respond to changes in the lipid composition. This has been studied in depth for nAChR, for which the activity depends on the presence of cholesterol and phosphatidic acid. A similar dependence might also be found in other receptors. In the case of nAChR, the receptor forms strong interactions with phosphatidic acid, recruiting it from a complex mixture to form a lipid domain enriched in receptor and phosphatidic acid. The detailed effect of anesthetics on this interaction has not been reported, though anesthetics have been shown to disrupt the partitioning of phosphatidic acid induced by the antibiotic peptide polymyxin B. Labeling studies indicate that nAChR has several binding sites for anesthetics, including the ligand-binding site in the extracellular domain and sites near the transmembrane pore and at the periphery of the lipid-protein interface. Mutations in any of these regions can cause similar changes in acetylcholine receptor function, reflecting the fact that these ion channels are allosterically regulated. The anesthetic binding at all these sites seems to have relatively low affinity; and at clinical concentrations of anesthetics, all these sites could be occupied and the effective local concentration of anesthetics in the membrane, again, is determined by the anesthetic partition coefficient in the membrane. In this and all other transmembrane receptors that have multiple low-affinity interaction sites for general anesthetics, the question remains as to which of the interactions is necessary for the effect of anesthetics on the activity of the receptors. Functional studies alone based solely on a receptor's sensitivity to anesthetics will not be able to answer this question. Again, a complementary approach from a structural viewpoint delineating anesthetic effects on the structure and dynamics of the protein may hold the key to this question.

3.7 DRUG TRANSPORTERS

We now return to membrane transporters to consider their role in drug transportation. As discussed earlier, membrane transporters maintain cellular and organism homeostasis by importing nutrients, facilitating the release and uptake of signaling molecules, regulating ion gradients, and exporting proteins, lipids, carbohydrates, and toxic compounds. Transporters also play a crucial role in drug response, serving as the drug targets and setting the drug levels inside the cells. Transporters are a very diverse group of proteins, typically consisting of multiple (often 12) helical transmembrane domains but having many unrelated families. It is difficult to estimate the total number of proteins involved, given the lack of sequence homology between families, but it has been estimated to be about 4 to 5% of all expressed proteins. Only a fraction of the transporters are known, and only a fraction of the known transporters have established drug responses. This section deals with two aspects of drug transport mediated by carriers: multiple drug resistance and carrier-mediated drug delivery.

3.7.1 Multiple Drug Resistance

The lipid bilayer serves as a poor barrier to amphipathic molecules, but a class of transporters that actively exports a wide array of structurally unrelated amphipathic compounds protects cells from the negative effects of amphipathic toxins. Unfortunately, this protection also works against amphipathic drugs, providing a dynamic but very effective barrier to drug action. The best studied of these transporters is the P-glycoprotein, belonging to the multiple drug resistance (MDR) family of the ATP-binding Cassette (ABC) superfamily of transporters. The ABC transporters are transmembrane proteins that bind ATP and use the energy of hydrolysis to drive transport of various molecules across the membrane. Functional ABC transporters contain two ATP binding domains (also called NBFs or nucleotide binding folds) with the unique signature sequence LSGGQ, and two transmembrane domains, typically with six transmembrane helices each. Some exist as a protein with single NBF and transmembrane domains (half transporters) but must form homo- or heterodimers to form functional transporters. Translocation of the substrate occurs by a conformational change accompanied by hydrolysis of ATP. Other important members of the ABC transporter superfamily include the ABCA1 protein responsible for cholesterol and phospholipid secretion and the cystic fibrosis transmembrane conductance regulator (CFTR) chloride transporter, in which a defect causes cystic fibrosis.

P-glycoprotein is a very large (170 kD) integral phosphorylated glycoprotein found in the plasma membrane of essentially all tissues. It is believed to function specifically to remove endogenous and exogenous toxins, and export peptides not exported by the secretion pathway. The ATP sites are allosterically linked; both are needed to effect the translocation. There are two nonidentical active transport sites apparently accessible from the inner leaflet of the bilayer; some substrates appear to act allosterically to affect binding at the other transport site and the nucleotide binding sites. The substrate specificity of P-glycoprotein varies among individuals, and P-glycoprotein expression can be induced by chronic exposure to high levels of substrates. This has become one of the major obstacles for successful chemotherapy of tumors, accounting for up to a 100-fold increase in drug resistance. These variations also account for some of the differences seen in appropriate dosing for different individuals over time for a wide range of therapies.

Substrates for P-glycoprotein are amphipathic and often cationic, but otherwise the parameters leading to substrate selection are not clear. Sizes range from 250 daltons to 1800 daltons. Other important parameters for transport activity appear to be the ability of the substrate to form hydrogen bonds, insertion of the substrate into the membrane, and the membrane lipid environment. A drug that is a substrate for P-glycoprotein is effectively excluded from cells that express substantial P-glycoprotein, unless the drug's rate of diffusion across the bilayer is greater than its rate of efflux by P-glycoprotein. This greatly reduces the amount of drug available for an intracellular drug target. Many drug substrates also induce an increased expression of P-glycoprotein, making the situation worsen over time. Thus, pharmaceutically, the goal is usually to inhibit P-glycoprotein as an adjuvant therapy to the therapeutic drug.

The largest class of P-glycoprotein inhibitors is formed by substrates capable of very rapid membrane permeation by passive diffusion. The rate of P-glycoprotein mediated efflux is about 900 molecules per minute, much faster than most of its substrates can cross the membrane unaided. However, those substrates that do passively permeate the bilayer more rapidly will form a nonproductive cycle competing with other substrates for P-glycoprotein binding. Another class of inhibitors includes those that bind to P-glycoprotein, but are transported and released very slowly. Examples are cyclosporine A and its derivatives. Most inhibitors become toxic at high doses; after all, all of these are capable of crossing membranes by passive diffusion, and thus have a wide distribution in the body. Interestingly, clinically achievable concentrations of some surfactants apparently alter membrane properties sufficiently to inhibit transporter efflux. Although a synergistic effect from combinations of suboptimal doses of multiple inhibitors has been reported, current strategies for inhibiting P-glycoprotein as an adjuvant therapy focus on inhibitors that bind tightly, but transport slowly.

P-glycoprotein inhibitors often induce greater toxicities of the substrate drugs due to the compromised permeability barriers for tissues other than the targeted tissues. For example, the antidiarrheal drug loperamide is a substrate of P-glycoprotein and is normally excluded from the blood–brain barrier (BBB) by that mechanism. Inhibition of P-glycoprotein allows loperamide to breach the BBB, resulting in serious neurotoxicity. Similarly, when coadministered drugs are both substrates of P-glycoprotein, pharmacokinetic interactions are common. In addition to toxicity and undesirable pharmacokinetic interactions, another obstacle for adjuvant therapy is the presence of other transporters contributing to multidrug resistance depending on the drug and tissue involved.

Although P-glycoprotein enjoys a wide distribution and is clearly the primary efflux path for some drugs, at least 10 other transporters involved in multiple drug resistance have been identified. Intense research in this area has produced second-generation inhibitors that appear to inhibit P-glycoprotein with minimal toxicity, do not induce increases in P-glycoprotein expression, and have minimal undesirable pharmacokinetic interactions. However, clinical trials have yielded mixed results, indicating that additional understanding of these drug efflux pathways is needed.

3.7.2 Carrier-mediated Drug Transport

As mentioned earlier, targeting drugs into cells using carrier-mediated drug transport is a strategy being vigorously pursued. Some of the transporters responsible for the uptake of nutrients exhibit broad specificity and can also transport pharmacologically active compounds similar to the natural substrates. Other transporters are targeted because of their ability to transport surprisingly large drug molecules conjugated to natural substrates or their derivatives. An example is the sodium-dependent multivitamin transporter (SMVT). SMVT is a 635 amino acid, 12 transmembrane domain sodium symporter responsible for the uptake of the water-soluble vitamins biotin, pantothenate, and lipoic acid at micromolar concentrations. It has wide tissue distribution and is capable of transporting drug-biotin conjugates as large as 29 kd. Biotin conjugates targeting SMVT have been used successfully to increase the uptake of drugs treating HIV and cancer.

Similar approaches have been applied successfully to a wide variety of nutrient transporters, including sugar, amino acid, nucleoside, and peptide transporters. However, the physicochemical parameters leading to efficient transport are not well defined for any of these transporters. For example, the PepT1 oligopeptide transporter mediates the cellular uptake of dietary dipeptides and tripeptides. It shows a broad specificity in that it is also a natural transporter of peptide-like drugs such as β-lactam antibiotics, ACE inhibitors, and renin inhibitors. Amino acid esters of nucleoside drugs are also efficiently transported. Recently, however, it has become clear that this apparent broad specificity may simply reflect a lack of understanding at the molecular level. Most dipeptides bind to PepT1, but surprisingly, some are not transported at all, and for others the rate of transport varies considerably. Molecular volume, hydrophobicity, electrostatics, and the side chain flexibility all play a role in efficient transport. The molecular details leading to this specificity are not yet known.

Delivering drugs to specific targets using endogenous transporters is still in its infancy. Although many transporters have been identified, few are understood in detail. As with most large integral proteins, only a few crystallographic structures are available. For the most part, specificity and efficacy of transport is determined by trial and error approaches rather than by rational designs. Currently, criteria affecting the choice of transporter for targeted transport include the similarity of the drug to the defining characteristics of an endogenous substrate, the physicochemical limitations of the drug as a conjugate, and the tissue distribution of the targeted transporter. None of these parameters have been fully established for the drug transporters.

3.8 KEY POINTS AND CONCLUSION

Biological membranes are, in their simplest form, a dynamic mixture of proteins and lipids organized to exclude and be excluded from water. The coarse structure of the membrane is driven almost entirely by the hydrophobic effect. The fine structure, however, is governed by interactions among membrane-associated proteins, membrane proteins, and lipids, including polar interactions and packing effects at the lipid-water interfacial region and packing effects at the hydrocarbon core. Although lipids represent the most diverse group of biological molecules in living systems, all lipids share certain common molecular features. The most fundamental property of lipid molecules is their amphiphilicity, each molecule having distinct hydrophilic and hydrophobic moieties that govern its association with other lipid molecules to form macromolecular structures. Formation of a stable membrane structure by the "social" behavior of many lipid molecules is not an accident but a natural process by which order emerges from chaos.

The fluid mosaic model of biological membranes is an adequate description of the static organization of the membrane on a small scale, but fails to capture the dynamic characteristics that underlie the function of biological membranes to sustain life. A real biological membrane is a nonideal mixture of a wide variety of components that interact with each other to form specialized domains on various scales of time and space. Thus, a biological membrane exhibits heterogeneity in its properties, both within the plane of the membrane and within the bilayer normal. Although some of these features are understood in detail, most are areas of ongoing research.

Both membrane lipids and membrane proteins are potential targets for pharmaceutical agents. Nearly all drugs interact with membranes before reaching their intended site(s) of action. The modern art of drug design must consider strategies to circumvent the natural barrier created by biological membranes. These include strategies that take advantage of the physicochemical properties of a membrane, like fine-tuning amphipathic properties of a drug to increase its passive diffusion through the membrane, conjugating drugs to membrane permeant peptides, or altering the specificity of a drug by taking advantage of differences between cell membranes. They also include strategies that take advantage of endogenous transport systems to transport the drug, such as designing chemical derivatives mimicking natural substrates, conjugating drugs to natural substrates, or hijacking the endocytotic pathways.

REVIEW QUESTIONS

1. Why are membranes essential to drug action? Are there any drugs that do not interact with a membrane?
2. What is unique about the structures formed by lipids?
3. How is the hydrophobic effect different from other molecular forces?
4. What are the five major types of lipid? How are they similar, and how are they different?
5. What lipids are included in the term phospholipid? What lipids are included in the term glycolipid?
6. Why is the fluid mosaic model of biological membranes inadequate?
7. Describe the environment in which an integral membrane protein resides.
8. How do weak electrolytes get across a membrane?
9. What are the four major routes to breach the membrane barrier?
10. What is the difference between primary and secondary active transport?
11. What is the difference between a passive transporter and an active secondary transporter?
12. What is the difference between a membrane permeant peptide and a pore-forming peptide?
13. In models of mechanisms of pore forming peptides, how is the pore of a barrel stave different from a toroidal pore?
14. How does an organism protect itself from amphipathic molecules? Why is this necessary?
15. What are the two major approaches to delivering drugs across biological membrane barriers?

GLOSSARY

Active transport Transport across a membrane using metabolic energy.

Amino acid Compound with both an amino group and a carboxylic acid. Amino acids form the building blocks of proteins.

Amphipathic Molecule with both hydrophobic and hydrophilic regions, synonymous with *amphiphilic*.

Amphiphilic Molecule with both hydrophobic and hydrophilic regions, synonymous with *amphipathic*.

Anesthetic additivity Phenomenon where half-doses of two unrelated anesthetic drugs provide the full effect of amnesia.

Barrel-stave model Model for pore-forming amphipathic peptides in which the polar face forms a hydrophilic pore.

Carpet model Model for pore-forming amphipathic peptides in which the peptide behaves much like a detergent.

Carrier protein Protein that selectively binds a molecule to effect its translocation.

Caveolae Flask-shaped invaginations of the plasma membrane mediated by caveolin.

Caveolin Family of proteins mediating caveolin-dependent endocytosis.

Caveosomes Endosome formed from fused caveolae vesicles.

Ceramide Sphingolipid with an amide-linked fatty acid and an unsubstituted 1-hydroxyl.

Cerebroside Sphingolipid with an uncharged monosaccharide headgroup.

Channel protein Transmembrane protein that opens a pore in the membrane.

Clathrin One of the main scaffolding proteins mediating clathrin-dependent endocytosis.

Curvature stress Stress generated by the presence of a nonlamellar lipid in a lamellar membrane.

Diacylglycerol Glycerolipid with two fatty acyl groups esterified to two of the three alcohol moieties of glycerol.

Efficacy In pharmaceuticals, the ability of a drug to produce its desired effect.

Electrochemical potential-driven transporters Group of transporters driven by electrochemical gradients using facilitated or (secondary) active transport mechanisms.

Endocytosis Uptake of cell surface constituents by the formation of vesicles from the plasma membrane.

Exocytosis Fusion of intracellular vesicles to the plasma membrane.

Facilitated diffusion Passive diffusion across a membrane facilitated by membrane transporter proteins.

Filtration In biology, the process by which matter passes between cells in a tissue.

Fluid mosaic model Model of a biological membrane that depicts a fluid sea of lipids with a mosaic of proteins floating within.

Ganglioside Sphingolipid with one or more sialic acids in the oligosaccharide headgroup.

Gated channel Channel protein that opens and closes in response to external stimuli.

Gel phase In lipids, a meso-phase state in which the lipid molecules are tightly packed, diffuse slowly, and sample fewer conformational states.

Globoside Sphingolipid with an uncharged oligosaccharide headgroup.

Glycerolglycan Glycerolipid with a sugar attached to the sn-3 hydroxyl of the glycerol backbone.

Glycerolipid Lipid containing glycerol as a backbone.

Glycerophospholipid Lipid with a glycerol backbone and a phosphate group, usually linked to the sn-3 carbon by a phosphoester bond.

Glycolipid Lipid containing a sugar moiety; these occur in all classes of lipid.

Glycosphingolipid Sphingolipid with a sugar moiety.

Group translocators Group of carriers that alter the solute during its passage across the membrane in a vectorial enzyme reaction.

Hydrophilic Easily dissolved in water.

Hydrophobic Insoluble in water, hydrophobic surfaces tend to minimize contact with water.

Hydrophobic matching Match between the length of the hydrophobic region of a transmembrane protein and the thickness of the bilayer.

Integral membrane protein Protein stabilized by its association with the hydrocarbon core of a bilayer.

Juxtamembrane Near the membrane surface, used to refer to regions of proteins near the membrane interface.

Lateral pressure profile Measure of several counteracting forces exerted at different depths across the bilayer.

Lipid domain Region in a bilayer with distinct lipid constituents and physicochemical properties.

Lipid phase Distinct physical state defined by the interaction between lipid molecules.

Lipid vesicle Closed bilayer structure.

Lipids Oils from biological sources.

Lipophilicity Solubility in lipids.

Liquid disordered phase In lipids, a meso-phase state in which lipid molecules are loosely packed together, diffuse rapidly, and sample many conformational states.

Liquid ordered phase In lipids, a meso-phase state with properties between the liquid disordered state and the gel state, in which lipid molecules diffuse rapidly but have somewhat restricted conformational freedom.

Log D Log of the sum of the equilibrium ratios for both ionized and unionized species of an electrolyte partitioned between two or more phases.

Log P Log of the partition coefficient.

Macropinocytosis Formation of large vesicles internalizing extracellular fluids by extensions of the plasma membrane.

Membrane fluidity Measure of microviscosity or the freedom of movement of a lipid or solute within its immediate region of the bilayer.

Membrane permeant peptide Cationic peptides capable of breaching the biological membrane without causing cell lysis.

Nucleotide Compounds with a nitrogenous base linked to a pentose phosphate that form the building blocks of nucleic acids such as DNA.

Octadecanoic 18-carbon hydrocarbon with a carboxylic acid at one end; a synonym for stearic.

Octadecenoic 18-carbon hydrocarbon with a carboxylic acid at one end and one or more double bonds.

Oleic acid 18-carbon hydrocarbon with a carboxylic acid at one end and a double bond at the ninth carbon.

Packing efficiency Refers to the way membrane constituents pack together to minimize abrupt interfaces.

Paracellular Process by which matter passes between cells in a tissue.

Partition coefficient Equilibrium ratio of a solute partitioned between two or more phases.

Passive diffusion Translocation driven by kinetic energy down electrochemical gradients.

Phagocytosis Ingestion of particles into a cell by extensions of the plasma membrane.

Pharmaceutical profiling Screening of drug candidates for physicochemical properties relevant for drug delivery, including solubility, lipophilicity, and stability.

Phosphatidate Glycerophospholipid with only a phosphate at the sn-3 hydroxyl on the glycerol backbone.

Phospholipid Lipid containing a phosphorous, including glycerophospholipids and sphingophospholipids.

Phosphosphingolipid Lipid containing a sphingoid base and a phosphorous.

Pinocytosis Invagination of specialized regions of the cell membrane, internalizing a vesicle of extracellular fluid and solutes.

Polyketide Hydrocarbon metabolite formed of repeating methylenes in pathways analogous to fatty acid biosynthesis.

Polynucleotide Polymer of nucleotides.

Polypeptide Polymer of amino acids, often forming a protein.

Potocytosis Caveolin-mediated endocytosis, or, potentially, clathrin-independent endocytosis.

Prenol Lipid derived from 5-carbon isoprene units.

Primary active transporters Group of transporters that couple the energy of a chemical reaction or light on one side of the membrane to the transport of a solute.

Saccharolipid Lipid derived from fatty acids linked in ester or amide linkages directly to sugar molecules.

Specificity In pharmaceuticals, the degree to which a drug avoids undesired side effects.

Sphingolipid Lipid containing a long chain amino alcohol as a backbone.

Sphingomyelin Sphingolipid with an amide-linked fatty acid and a phosphocholine headgroup, a ceramide phosphocholine.

Stearic acid 18-carbon hydrocarbon with a carboxylic acid at one end, a synonym for octadecanoic.

Toroidal pore model Model for pore-forming amphipathic peptides in which the polar face remains associated with the polar headgroups of lipids, bending the bilayer such that the pore is lined with both peptide and associated lipid headgroups.

Transcellular Process by which matter passes through the cell membranes to reach the other side of a tissue.

Transport electron carriers Group of carriers that catalyze electron flow across a membrane.

Transporter protein Channel or carrier protein, sometimes used to refer exclusively to carriers.

Triacylglycerol Glycerolipid with three fatty acyl groups esterified to the three carbons of glycerol.

Unit membrane Morphology of a membrane as described by electron microscopy showing two electron-dense layers enclosing a less dense layer.

Vesicle-mediated transport Transport of a substance between cellular membranes with the substance either within or enclosed by a vesicle.

REFERENCES

Books

Amidon, G. L., & Sadâee, W. (1999). *Membrane transporters as drug targets.* New York: Kluwer Academic/Plenum Publishers.

Lash, L. H. (2005). *Drug metabolism and transport: Molecular methods and mechanisms.* Totowa, N.J.: Humana Press.

Lu, D. R., & ¢ie, S. (2004). *Cellular drug delivery: Principles and practice.* Totowa, N.J.: Humana Press.

Mouritsen, O. G. (2005). *Life—As a matter of fat: The emerging science of lipidomics.* Berlin; New York: Springer.

Tamm, L. K. (2005). *Protein-lipid interactions: From membrane domains to cellular networks.* Weinheim: Wiley-VCH.

Walsh, C. T., Schwartz-Bloom, R. D., et al. (2005). *Levine's pharmacology: Drug actions and reactions.* London; New York: Taylor & Francis.

Monographs, Review Articles, and Original Papers

Allende, D., Simon, S. A., et al. (2005). Melittin-induced bilayer leakage depends on lipid material properties: Evidence for toroidal pores. *Biophysical Journal, 88*(3), 1828–1837.

Borghese, C. M., Werner, D. F., et al. (2006). An isoflurane- and alcohol-insensitive mutant GABA(A) receptor alpha(1) subunit with near-normal apparent affinity for GABA: Characterization in heterologous systems and production of knockin mice. *The Journal of Pharmacology and Experimental Therapeutics, 319*(1), 208–218.

Brogden, K. A. (2005). Antimicrobial peptides: Pore formers or metabolic inhibitors in bacteria? *Nature Reviews. Microbiology, 3*(3), 238–250.

Cantor, R. S. (2001). Breaking the Meyer-Overton rule: Predicted effects of varying stiffness and interfacial activity on the intrinsic potency of anesthetics. *Biophysical Journal, 80*(5), 2284–2297.

Cardelli, J. (2001). Phagocytosis and macropinocytosis in Dictyostelium: Phosphoinositide-based processes, biochemically distinct. *Traffic, 2*(5), 311–320.

Cheng, Z. J., & Singh, R. D. et al. (2006). Membrane microdomains, caveolae, and caveolar endocytosis of sphingolipids. *Molecular Membrane Biology, 23*(1), 101–110.

Cheng, Z. J., & Singh, R. D. et al. (2006). Distinct mechanisms of clathrin-independent endocytosis have unique sphingolipid requirements. *Molecular Biology of the Cell, 17*(7), 3197–3210.

Colloc'h, N., Sopkova-de Oliveira Santos, J., et al. (2007). Protein crystallography under xenon and nitrous oxide pressure: Comparison with in vivo pharmacology studies and implications for the mechanism of inhaled anesthetic action. *Biophysical Journal, 92*(1), 217–224.

Edidin, M. (2003). Lipids on the frontier: A century of cell-membrane bilayers. *Nature Reviews. Molecular Cell Biology, 4*(5), 414–418.

Franks, N. P., & Lieb, W. R. (2004). Seeing the light: Protein theories of general anesthesia. 1984. *Anesthesiology, 101*(1), 235–237.

Grage, S. L., Gauger, D. R., et al. (2000). The amphiphilic drug flufenamic acid can induce a hexagonal phase in DMPC: A solid state 31P- and 19F-NMR study. *Physical Chemistry Chemical Physics, 2*, 4574–4579.

Grasshoff, C., Drexler, B., et al. (2006). Anaesthetic drugs: Linking molecular actions to clinical effects. *Current Pharmaceutical Design, 12*(28), 3665–3679.

Grosse, S., Aron, Y., et al. (2005). Potocytosis and cellular exit of complexes as cellular pathways for gene delivery by polycations. *The Journal of Gene Medicine, 7*(10), 1275–1286.

Gullingsrud, J., & Schulten, K. (2004). Lipid bilayer pressure profiles and mechanosensitive channel gating. *Biophysical Journal, 86*(6), 3496–3509.

Hemmings, H. C., Jr., Akabas, M. H., et al. (2005). Emerging molecular mechanisms of general anesthetic action. *Trends in Pharmacological Sciences, 26*(10), 503–510.

Lee, A. G. (2004). How lipids affect the activities of integral membrane proteins. *Biochimica et Biophysica Acta, 1666*(1-2), 62–87.

Lee, M. T., Hung, W. C., et al. (2005). Many-body effect of antimicrobial peptides: On the correlation between lipid's spontaneous curvature and pore formation. *Biophysical Journal, 89*(6), 4006–4016.

Liu, Z., Xu, Y., Tang, P. (2005). Molecular dynamics simulations of C2F6 effects on gramicidin A: Implications of the mechanisms of general anesthesia. *Biophysical Journal, 88*(6), 3784–3791.

Liu, Z., Xu, Y., & Tang, P. (2006). Steered molecular dynamics simulations of Na^+ permeation across Gramicidin A channel. *The Journal of Physical Chemistry, 110*, 12789–12795.

Lobo, I. A., Trudell, J. R., et al. (2006). Accessibility to residues in transmembrane segment four of the glycine receptor. *Neuropharmacology, 50*(2), 174–181.

Marrink, S. J., & Mark, A. E. (2004). Molecular view of hexagonal phase formation in phospholipid membranes. *Biophysical Journal, 87*(6), 3894–3900.

Mineo, C., & Anderson, R. G. (2001). Potocytosis. Robert Feulgen Lecture. *Histochemistry and Cell Biology, 116*(2), 109–118.

Mueller, P., Chien, T. F., et al. (1983). Formation and properties of cell-size lipid bilayer vesicles. *Biophysical Journal, 44*(3), 375–381.

Pelkmans, L., Burli, T., et al. (2004). Caveolin-stabilized membrane domains as multifunctional transport and sorting devices in endocytic membrane traffic. *Cell, 118*(6), 767–780.

Rejman, J., Oberle, V., et al. (2004). Size-dependent internalization of particles via the pathways of clathrin- and caveolae-mediated endocytosis. *The Biochemical Journal, 377*(Pt 1), 159–169.

Royle, S. J. (2006). The cellular functions of clathrin. *Cellular and Molecular Life Sciences: CMLS, 63*(16), 1823–1832.

Rudolph, U., & Antkowiak, B. (2004). Molecular and neuronal substrates for general anaesthetics. *Nature Reviews. Neuroscience, 5*(9), 709–720.

Sachs, J. N., & Engelman, D. M. (2006). Introduction to the membrane protein reviews: The interplay of structure, dynamics, and environment in membrane protein function. *Annual Review of Biochemistry, 75*, 707–712.

Saier, M. H., Jr., Tran, C. V., et al. (2006). TCDB: The Transporter Classification Database for membrane transport protein analyses and information. *Nucleic Acids Research, 34*(Database issue), D181–D186.

Stoeckenius, W., & Engelman, D. M. (1969). Current models for the structure of biological membranes. *The Journal of Cell Biology, 42* (3), 613–646.

Swanson, J. A., & Watts, C. (1995). Macropinocytosis. *Trends in Cell Biology, 5*(11), 424–428.

Tang, P., & Xu, Y. (2002). From the Cover: Large-scale molecular dynamics simulations of general anesthetic effects on the ion channel in the fully hydrated membrane: The implication of molecular mechanisms of general anesthesia. *Proceedings of the National Academy of Sciences of the United States of America, 99*(25), 16035–16040.

Torchilin, V. P. (2006). Recent approaches to intracellular delivery of drugs and DNA and organelle targeting. *Annual Review of Biomedical Engineering, 8*, 343–375.

Tunnemann, G., Martin, R. M., et al. (2006). Cargo-dependent mode of uptake and bioavailability of TAT-containing proteins and peptides in living cells. *The FASEB Journal, 20*(11), 1775–1784.

Ueda, I. (1965). Effects of diethyl ether and halothane on firefly luciferin bioluminescence. *Anesthesiology, 26*(5), 603–606.

Ueda, I., Kamaya, H., et al. (1976). Molecular mechanism of inhibition of firefly luminescence by local anesthetics. *Proceedings of the National Academy of Sciences of the United States of America, 73*(2), 481–485.

Vereb, G., Szollosi, J., et al. (2003). Dynamic, yet structured: The cell membrane three decades after the Singer-Nicolson model. *Proceedings of the National Academy of Sciences of the United States of America, 100*(14), 8053–8058.

Werner, D. F., Blednov, Y. A., et al. (2006). Knockin mice with ethanol-insensitive alpha1-containing gamma-aminobutyric acid type A receptors display selective alterations in behavioral responses to ethanol. *The Journal of Pharmacology and Experimental Therapeutics, 319*(1), 219–227.

Xu, Y., & Tang, P. (1997). Amphiphilic sites for general anesthetic action? Evidence from 129Xe-{1H} intermolecular nuclear Overhauser effects. *Biochimica et Biophysica Acta, 1323* (1), 154–162.

Yamakura, T., Bertaccini, E., et al. (2001). Anesthetics and ion channels: Molecular models and sites of action. *Annual Review of Pharmacology and Toxicology, 41*, 23–51.

Yang, L., Harroun, T. A., et al. (2001). Barrel-stave model or toroidal model? A case study on melittin pores. *Biophysical Journal, 81*(3), 1475–1485.

Ziebell, M. R., Nirthanan, S., et al. (2004). Identification of binding sites in the nicotinic acetylcholine receptor for [3H]azietomidate, a photoactivatable general anesthetic. *The Journal of Biological Chemistry, 279*(17), 17640–17649.

Zubrzycki, I. Z., Xu, Y., et al. (2000). Molecular dynamics simulations of a fully hydrated dimyristoylphosphatidylcholine membrane in liquid-crystalline phase. *Journal of Chemical Physics, 112*(7), 3437–3441.

Chapter

4 Ligand-Receptor Binding and Tissue Response

Terry Kenakin

OUTLINE

4.1 INTRODUCTION

Pharmacology is unique because it involves the indirect study of molecular events through changes in cellular behavior; in essence, the cell becomes the translator for those events. The object of this study is to define the molecular events since these define the action of drugs in all systems and, if quantified correctly, these can be used to predict drug effect in all systems including the therapeutic one(s). Drug activity can be summarized concisely in a graphical display of biological effect and drug concentration in the form of a dose-response curve. It is first worth considering dose-response curves as descriptors of drug action.

4.2 DOSE-RESPONSE CURVES

If drug effect can be observed directly, then the magnitude of effect can be displayed as a function of drug concentration in the form of a dose-response curve. Figure 4.1A shows a typical dose-response curve and some characteristic parameters that describe it. A curve is characterized by a threshold, maximal effect, and slope. The quantifiable parameters of a curve are the location along the abscissal (concentration) axis and the maximal effect. On a semi-logarithmic scale, dose-response curves are characteristically sigmoidal in shape; this is a function of the mathematical relationship between the parameters describing the induction of biological effect (*vide infra*). The location parameters of such curves denote the potency of the drug; a convenient parameter to numerically quantify potency is to report the pEC_{50} of the curve, literally the negative logarithm of the molar concentration of the drug that produces half the maximal response to the drug.

It is worth describing some general drug nomenclature at this point; this nomenclature is based on the behavior of a drug in a particular system and this may change in a different system (tissues). In general, a drug that causes a cellular system to change its state and that produces a measurable biological response is referred to as an *agonist*. A drug that produces the maximal response of the system (a maximal response equal to the maximal capability of the system to report cellular response) is termed a *full agonist* (Figure 4.1B). It should also be noted that a drug need not produce response equal to the maximal response capability of the system; that is, a given drug may only produce a maximal response that is below the maximal capability of the system. When this occurs, the drug is referred to as a *partial agonist*. A drug that reduces the biological effect of another drug is called an *antagonist*. An antagonist may itself produce a low level of direct response (i.e., a partial agonist can produce antagonism of responses to full agonists). Finally, there are cases where the tissue itself possesses an elevated basal activity due to a spontaneous activation of receptors (*vide infra*). A class of drug that reverses such elevated basal effect is termed *inverse agonist*; these will be described in later discussions of antagonists.

It will be seen that the common currency of pharmacology in describing drug effect is the dose-response curve. Such curves are a function of two molecular properties of the drugs that produce them, namely, affinity and efficacy for a biological receptor.

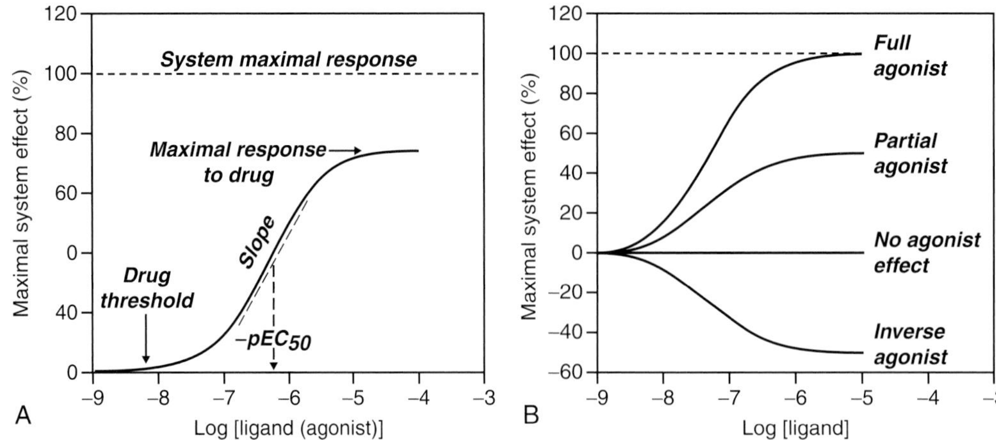

Figure 4.1 Dose-response curves. (A) Basic nomenclature for dose-response relationships. A given agonist may not produce the maximal response capability of the system. The potency of a given agonist is quantified by the location parameter along the concentration axis. For example, the pEC_{50} is the – logarithm of the molar concentration of the agonist that produces 50% of the maximal response to the agonist (not the system). (B) Classical ligand behaviors in functional systems. A ligand with positive efficacy can produce the system maximal response in well–coupled systems (if the ligand has high positive efficacy); under these circumstances it is referred to as a full agonist. If the maximal response to the ligand is below the system maximal response, it is referred to as a partial agonist. Ligands with no efficacy or such a low level of efficacy that the system cannot produce a visible response are antagonists. A ligand with negative efficacy (*vide infra*) can reduce the basal response if that basal response is elevated due to constitutive receptor activity.

As a prerequisite to a discussion of these properties, it is useful to describe the biological target, in this case the receptor.

4.3 RECEPTORS

One of the most important concepts to emerge from early pharmacological studies (1840 to 1940) is the concept of the biological receptor. Although the actual physical nature of receptors was not known, it was realized that they allowed cells to recognize drugs and read the chemical information encoded in them. Early concepts of receptors likened them to locks and drugs as keys (i.e., as stated by the biologist Paul Ehrlich, "...substances can only be anchored at any particular part of the organism if they fit into the molecule of the recipient complex like a piece of mosaic finds its place in a pattern..."). The main value of receptors was that they put order into the previously disordered world of physiology. For example, it is observed that the hormone epinephrine produces a wealth of dissimilar physiological responses such as bronchiole muscle relaxation; cardiac muscle positive inotropy, chronotropy, and lusitropy; melatonin synthesis; pancreatic, lacrimal and salivary gland secretion; decreased stomach motility; urinary bladder muscle relaxation; skeletal muscle tremor; and vascular relaxation.

The understanding of how such a vast array of biological responses could be mediated by a single molecule is difficult until it is realized that these processes are all mediated by the interaction of epinephrine with a single protein receptor, in this case the β-adrenoceptor. Thus, when this receptor is present on the surface of any given cell, it will respond to epinephrine and the nature of that response will be determined by the encoding of the receptor excitation produced by epinephrine to the cytosolic biochemical cascades controlling cellular function.

In a conceptual sense, the term receptor can refer to any single biological entity that responds to drugs (i.e., enzymes, ion channels, transport proteins, DNA, and structures in the nucleus). In terms of the mechanisms and thermodynamics of ligand binding described in this chapter, the model for the receptor will be a seven-transmembrane receptor, a protein residing on the cell membrane (half of the receptor faces out to the extracellular space and half into the cytoplasm) that is capable of recognizing chemicals such as hormones and neurotransmitters present in the extracellular space, and transmitting signals from these to the cell interior. This information is transmitted through changes in protein conformation; that is, the drug does not enter the cell nor does the receptor change the nature of the drug (as would an enzyme). With this biological target in mind, the molecular nature of ligand-receptor interaction can now be described mechanistically. The first process to be described is the binding of a drug to the receptor—the nature of ligand-affinity.

4.4 AFFINITY

A simple model of ligand binding, originally designed to describe the binding of chemicals to metal surfaces in the making of filaments for light bulbs, was published by the chemist Irving Langmuir; accordingly, it is referred to as the Langmuir adsorption isotherm and it still forms the basis for the measurement and quantification of drug affinity today. In Langmuir's model, a drug molecule has an intrinsic rate of onset (referred to as the *rate of condensation* by Langmuir) onto the target (in Langmuir's system, the target was the surface of metal but in the context of pharmacodynamics, the target is the binding pocket of a biologically relevant protein such as a receptor). This rate of onset (denoted k_1) is driven by changes in energy; the energy of the system containing the drug in the receptor binding pocket is lower than the energy of the system with the drug not bound in the pocket.

The drug also has an intrinsic *rate of evaporation* away from the target, which describes the change in energy when the molecule diffuses away from the surface. In pharmacological terms, this is referred to as the *rate of offset* of the drug away from the receptor (denoted k_2). When a drug is present in the compartment containing the receptor, then the concentration gradient controls the movement of drug molecules. The absence of drug in the receptor binding pocket drives the binding reaction toward drug binding to the receptor. As more drug binds, the bound drug will diffuse out of the binding pocket in accordance with its natural tendency to do so (defined by the energy changes dictated by the rate of offset). This leads to an equilibrium whereby the rate of drug leaving the binding pocket will equal the rate of drug approaching and entering the binding pocket.

The ratio of rates (namely k_2/k_1) determines the amount of drug bound to the receptor at any one instant and this becomes a measure of how well the drug binds to the receptor, that is, the affinity of the drug for the receptor. This ratio is referred to as the equilibrium dissociation constant (denoted K_{eq}). Langmuir's calculation was centered on calculation of the fraction of the total area of surface bound by the chemical and is denoted as ρ_A. Fraction of total area left free for further binding of new molecule to the surface is given by $1 - \rho_A$. The amount of drug (denoted $[A]$) bound to the surface is the product of the concentration of drug available for binding ($[A]$), the rate of onset (k_1), and the fraction of surface left free for further binding ($1 - \rho_A$):

$$\text{Rate of binding} = \partial[AR]/\partial t(+) = [A]k_1(1 - \rho_A) \quad (4.1)$$

Similarly, the amount of drug diffusing away (evaporating) from the surface is given by the amount bound (ρ_A) and the intrinsic rate of evaporation of offset k_2:

$$\text{Rate of diffusion off} = \partial[AR]/\partial t(-) = \rho_A k_2 \quad (4.2)$$

At equilibrium, the fractional amount diffusing toward the receptor is equal to the fractional amount diffusing away from the receptor:

$$[A]k_1(1 - \rho_A) = \rho_A k_2 \quad (4.3)$$

Defining K_{eq} as k_2/k_1, the following relationship for the fractional amount bound (ρ) known as the Langmuir adsorption isotherm is given as:

$$\rho_a = \frac{[A]}{[A] + K_{eq}} \quad (4.4)$$

When the concentration of the drug is equal to K_{eq}, then $\rho = 0.5$; that is, the K_{eq} is the concentration of drug that occupies 50% of the available receptor population. Therefore, the magnitude of K_{eq} is inversely proportional to the affinity of the drug for the receptor. For example, consider two drugs, one with $K_{eq} = 10^{-9}$ M and another with $K_{eq} = 10^{-7}$ M. The first drug occupies 50% of the receptors at a concentration 1/100 of that required by the second. Clearly the drug with $K_{eq} = 10^{-9}$ has a higher affinity for the receptor than the one with $K_{eq} = 10^{-7}$ M.

If a direct measure of the amount of bound ligand can be made (for instance, if the ligand is radioactive and the quantity of radioactive-ligand complex could be quantified), a direct measure of K_{eq} can be made; this can be accomplished with saturation binding experiments with radioactive ligands. A shortcoming of this approach is the fact that the affinity of only radioactive drugs can be obtained in this way. However, interference with the binding of a radioactive drug by any drug that binds to the same receptor can also yield a direct measure of the affinity of the nonradioactive drug (antagonism, to be described later).

4.5 EFFICACY

The second fundamental property of a ligand is efficacy. This is basically the result of ligand binding to the receptor. Specifically in cellular systems, it is defined as the change in behavior of the receptor toward its host (the cell) upon binding of the ligand. The most common setting for observing efficacy is in the effect of agonists on cellular systems. On a molecular scale, it is useful to consider how an agonist elicits a change in the receptor to cause cellular activation. Whereas enzymes bind their substrates in energetically constrained conformations to stretch bonds to a breaking point (or to create a new bond), receptors do not change their substrates, nor are they permanently altered by their interaction with drugs. Instead, an agonist activates the receptor when it binds and the activation ceases when the agonist diffuses away. Historically, it was thought that the binding of the drug deformed the receptor and produced an activated state through drug binding (protein conformational induction). However, such a mechanism is energetically extremely unfavorable.

A much more reasonable mechanism, in terms of energetics, is through protein conformational selection. In this scheme, drugs bind to a limited number of preexisting receptor conformations and stabilize those through binding (at the expense of other conformations—Le Chatelier's principle of an equilibrium responding to perturbation). Through selective affinity of the ligand for receptor active states, a bias in the collection of conformations results. If two conformations are interconvertible, then a ligand with higher affinity for one of the conformations will enrich it through selective binding. This can be shown as follows. Assume two receptor conformations R and R^* controlled by an equilibrium dissociation constant L where $L = [R^*]/[R]$:

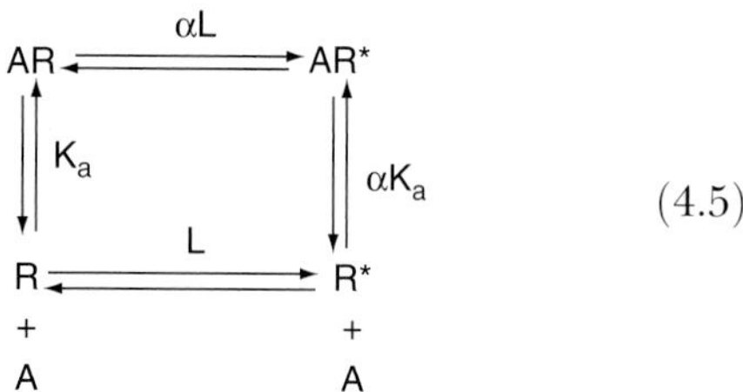

(4.5)

Consider a ligand A with an affinity (defined as the equilibrium association constant $K_a = k_1/k_2$) of K_a for receptor state R and αK_a for receptor state R^*, where the factor α denotes the differential affinity of the agonist for R^*; that is, $\alpha = 10$ denotes a 10-fold greater affinity of the ligand for the R^* state. The effect of α (selective affinity) on the ability of the ligand to alter the equilibrium between R and R^* can be calculated by examining the amount of R^* (both as R^* and AR^*) present in the system in the absence of A and in the presence of A. The equilibrium expression for $[R^*] + [AR^*])/[R_{tot}]$ where $[R_{tot}]$ is the total receptor concentration given by the conservation equation $[R_{tot}] = [R] + [AR] + [R^*] + [AR^*])$ is:

$$\rho = \frac{L(1 + \alpha[A]/K_A)}{[A]/K_A(1 + \alpha L) + 1 + L} \tag{4.6}$$

where K_A is the equilibrium dissociation constant of the agonist-receptor complex. In the absence of agonist ($[A] = 0$), $\rho_0 = L/(1 + L)$ while in the presence of a maximal concentration of ligand (saturating the receptors; $[A] \to \infty$) $\rho_\infty = (\alpha(1 + L))/(1 + \alpha L)$. Therefore, the effect of the ligand on the proportion of the R^* state is given by the ratio ρ_∞/ρ_0. This ratio is given by:

$$\frac{\rho_\infty}{\rho_0} = \frac{\alpha(1 + L)}{(1 + \alpha L)} \tag{4.7}$$

It can be seen from Equation 4.7 that if the ligand has an equal affinity for both the R and R^* states ($\alpha = 1$), then ρ_∞/ρ_0 will equal unity and no change in the proportion of R^* will result from maximal ligand binding. *However*, if $\alpha > 1$, then the presence of the conformationally selective ligand will cause the ratio ρ_∞/ρ_0 to be > 1 and the R^* state will be enriched by presence of the ligand. If the R^* state promotes physiological response, then ligand A will promote response and be an agonist. This defines binding as an active, not passive process. Specifically, if a ligand has selective affinity for a collection of protein conformations, it will actively change the make-up of that collection. It is this active property of ligands that can result in physiological cellular response (efficacy).

Ligand affinity and efficacy both emanate from the thermodynamic forces that promote association of the ligand with the receptor, thus they are related. However, they can also be dissociable properties that vary independently with changes in chemical structure. In fact, it is the fact that the affinity of a series of alkyltrimethylammonium compounds for muscarinic receptors had differing abilities to produce ileal smooth muscle contraction that led the Scottish pharmacologist R.P. Stephenson to postulate the second fundamental property of drugs (efficacy). Specifically, in Stephenson's system, it was reasoned that the compounds needed to have another intrinsic property to differentiate one from the other. It is useful to note the independence of affinity and efficacy on chemical structure for drug development as these scales can be manipulated separately *en route* to a defined therapeutic entity (as in the case of the discovery and synthesis of the important class of histamine receptor H2 antagonists for the treatment of peptic ulcer). In this instance, a chemical effort to enhance the affinity and eliminate the efficacy of the natural agonist histamine for the target H2 receptor resulted in the synthesis of cimetidine, a potent molecule with high affinity for the H2 receptor but no efficacy. This molecule competes with histamine to antagonize the production of stomach acid and thus promotes healing of ulcers.

Since Stephenson's theoretical revolution of receptor theory, a model of drug function has emerged that is based on experimentally observed relationships between receptor occupancy by a ligand and the production of pharmacological response. This scheme, called the operational model of drug action, has emerged as the preeminent method of quantifying relative efficacy in experimental systems. It is worth considering this model and the ramifications of its use in the drug discovery process.

Early receptor theory used the concept of efficacy as a multiplicative factor relating response and receptor occupancy; that is, response is a function of stimulus which itself is $= \rho_A \bullet e$ where ρ_A is receptor occupancy (Eq. 4.4) and efficacy (denoted e). It was also recognized that cells processed stimulus in myriad different ways to produce the observed response. This ambiguity was dealt with by the abstract notion that a monotonic but undefined function $f(S)$ converted stimulus to response. The undefined nature of this function was negated by equating equal responses in any given experiment to allow for cancellation of the response function; it is assumed that equal responses emanate from equal stimuli. A theoretical shortcoming of this theoretical approach is the fact that there is no experimental or physiological basis for the parameter "e". This shortcoming was removed by the introduction of the operational model.

The basis of the operational model is the experimental finding that the experimentally obtained relationship between agonist-induced response and agonist concentration resembles a model of enzyme function presented in 1913 by Louis Michaelis and Maude L. Menten. This model accounts for the fact that the kinetics of enzyme reactions differ significantly from the kinetics of conventional chemical reactions. It describes the reaction of a substrate with an enzyme as an equation of the form reaction velocity = (maximal velocity of the reaction x substrate concentration)/(concentration of substrate + a fitting constant K_m). The parameter K_m characterizes the tightness of the binding of the reaction between substrate and enzyme or the concentration at which the reaction rate is half the maximal value. It can be seen that the more active the substrate, the smaller will be the value of K_m. Comparison of this equation with Equation 4.4 shows that it is identical to the Langmuir adsorption isotherm relating binding of a chemical to a surface. Both of these models form the basis of drug receptor interaction, thus the kinetics involved are referred to as Michaelian or Langmuirian in form.

The operational model relates tissue response to a Michaelis-Menten type of equation of the form:

$$\text{Response} = \frac{[AR]E_{max}}{[AR] + K_E} \tag{4.8}$$

where $[AR]$ is the concentration of the amount of agonist-activated receptor, E_{max} is the maximal response that the system is able to produce under saturating stimulation (as the V_{max} in the Michaelis-Menten enzyme reaction), and K_E is the equilibrium dissociation constant of the activated receptor and response element (cellular machinery that responds to the activated receptor to generate cellular response) complex. In this sense, Equation 4.8 treats the cell as a comprehensive virtual enzyme utilizing the activated receptor as the substrate and cellular response as the product. In practice, the cascade of biochemical reactions initiated by activated receptor is a series of Michaelis-Menten-like reactions that can be modeled by a single mathematical function of the Michaelis-Menten form. For example, if the first reaction in the cascade is modeled by:

$$y_1 = \frac{x}{x + \beta_1} \tag{4.9}$$

and where the output y_1 becomes the input for a second function of the form:

$$y_2 = \frac{y_1}{y_1 + \beta_2} \tag{4.10}$$

a series of such functions can be generalized to the form:

$$y_n = \frac{x}{x(1 + \beta_n(1 + \beta_{n-1}(1 + \beta_{n-2}(1 + \beta_{n-3})..)..)\ldots) + (\beta_n \bullet ..\beta_1)} \tag{4.11}$$

which can be rewritten in the form of Equation 4.8 where $E_{max} = (1 + \beta_n (1 + \beta_{n-1}(1 + \beta_{n-2} (1 + \beta_{n-3})..)\ldots)..)^{-1}$ and $K_E = (\beta_n \ldots \bullet .. \beta_1)/(1 + \beta_n (1 + \beta_{n-1}(1 + \beta_{n-2} (1 + \beta_{n-3})..)\ldots)..)$. It can be seen that the product of a succession of reactions of the form of Equation 4.8 results in a general equation of the form of Equation 4.8.

The K_E is the concentration of AR complex that produces half maximal response (the K_m for the Michaelis-Menten model). Therefore, the magnitude of the K_E reflects the activating power of the agonist; that is, high efficacy agonists will have a lower K_E value than low efficacy agonists. The amount of $[AR]$ complex is given by the Langmuir adsorption isotherm for the fractional receptor occupancy of the agonist (ρ_A from equation 4.4) to yield $[AR]$ from $[AR] = \rho_A \bullet [R_t]$ where $[R_t]$ is the concentration of receptors. Combining Equations 4.4 and 4.8 leads to:

$$\text{Response} = \frac{[A]/K_A[R_t]/K_E}{[A]/K_A([R_t]/K_E + 1) + 1} \tag{4.12}$$

The model defines a parameter τ as $[R_t]/K_E$ to present the description of agonist response as:

$$\text{Response} = \frac{[A]/K_A \bullet \tau}{[A]/K_A \bullet (\tau + 1) + 1} \tag{4.13}$$

An important and versatile parameter in the operational equation is τ; this constant incorporates the intrinsic efficacy of the agonist (a property of the molecule) and elements describing the efficiency of the tissue as it converts agonist-derived stimulus into tissue response (receptor density and K_E, the constant relating receptor activation and cellular response). The magnitude of K_E is also unique for each tissue since it is an amalgam of the series of biochemical reactions unique to the cell.

Equation 4.13 predicts that there will be a sigmoidal relationship between agonist concentration and tissue response; this is what is observed in pharmacological systems so the theory predicts experimental observation. Another important aspect of the operational model is that it predicts a displacement of the receptor occupancy curve (defining binding of the agonist to the receptor population) and observed tissue response (Figure 4.2). The magnitude of the displacement is controlled by the receptor density, the efficiency of receptor coupling, and the intrinsic efficacy of the agonist. As noted in the previous discussion, this is τ.

The inset to Figure 4.2 shows a parabolic relationship between receptor occupancy and cellular response; this is characteristic of the amplification of biological systems in general. However, the actual steepness of this relationship is unique for every agonist; that is, for a low efficacy agonist, it will not be as skewed and for very low efficacy agonists, it can nearly be linear. For high efficacy agonists where the relationship is skewed, it can be seen that essentially a maximal cellular response can be obtained with a low level of receptor occupancy; this is a phenomenon referred to as *receptor reserve* or *spare receptors*.

The maximal response of most tissues to powerful natural agonists (neurotransmitters, hormones) is produced by partial activation of the total receptor density and the remaining receptors appear to be "spare" and in fact participate in making the tissue more or less sensitive to the agonist. For example, the ileum of guinea pigs produce maximal force of isometric contraction to the natural autacoid histamine by activation of only 3% of the available receptors. Therefore, in practical terms, 97% of the receptor population can be removed or inactivated with no diminution of the

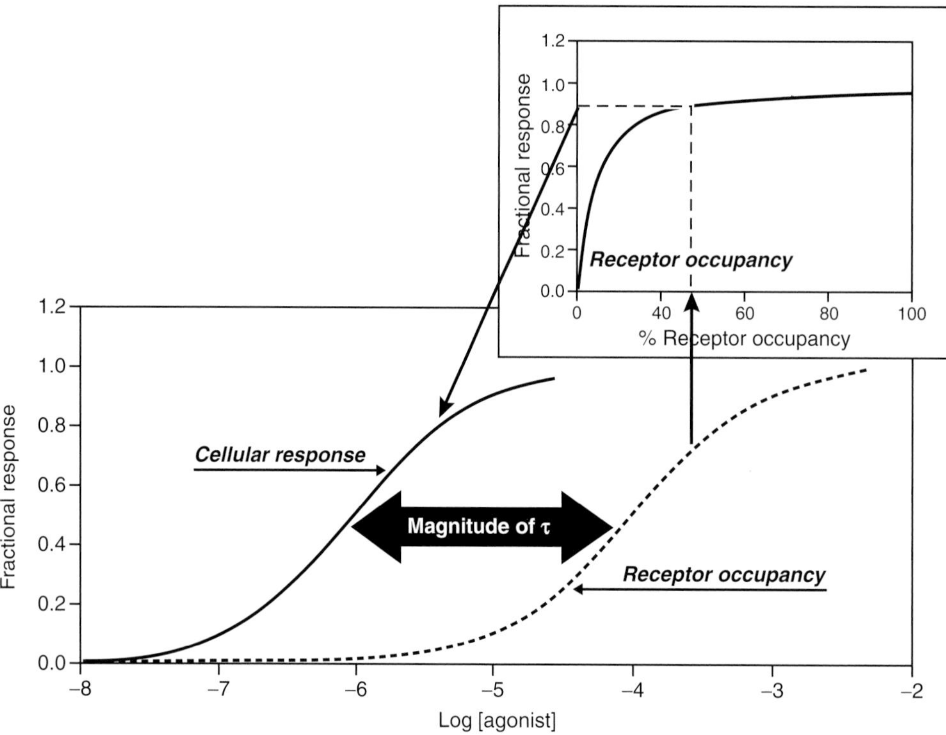

Figure 4.2 The effect of positive efficacy on displacement of receptor occupancy curves from response curves. A highly skewed relationship between receptor occupancy and tissue response can be produced by high efficacy of the ligand, a high number of receptors in the tissue, and an efficient coupling between receptors and cellular response mechanisms (value of τ in the operational model).

maximal response to histamine (albeit a loss in the sensitivity to histamine). The term receptor reserve has historically been associated with the tissue (it involves the number of receptors in a given tissue and the efficiency with which they are coupled to the stimulus-response machinery of the cell). However, the intrinsic efficacy of the agonist is intimately involved in the magnitude of receptor reserve. Thus, the magnitude of the receptor reserve for two different agonists will be different; the agonist with the higher efficacy will have a greater receptor reserve—one agonist's spare receptor is a weaker agonist's essential one.

An inspection of Equation 4.13 shows the relationship between cellular response and affinity. Specifically, changes in affinity can affect only the location parameter of the dose-response curve and not the maximal response. In contrast, the magnitude of τ can control both the maximal response to the agonist and the location parameter of the dose-response curve. However, the dependence of these dose-response curve parameters on affinity and efficacy are not continuous. If the agonist produces partial agonism, then efficacy controls only maximal response and affinity controls only location on the concentration axis. If the agonist produces full agonism, both affinity and efficacy control only the location parameter of the dose-response curve (since maximal response is fixed at the tissue maximum).

The major use of the operational model is the prediction of agonism in tissues. Specifically, the ratio of efficacies of two agonists (as ratios of τ values) is a tissue-independent measure of relative efficacy that can be measured in one test tissue and applied to all tissues. This is an important aspect of experimental pharmacology as drugs are almost always tested and developed in one type of system for use in another (i.e., the therapeutic one). Reliance on tissue-dependent measures of drug activity (i.e., pEC_{50}, maximal response) therefore would be capricious and difficult to apply to the therapeutic environment without a tool such as the operational model to negate the effects of tissue type.

4.6 ANTAGONISM

The previous discussion considers the effect of a single molecule on cellular function through a receptor. Another vast therapeutic application of drugs involves the use of one molecule to interfere or otherwise modify the effects of another molecule that produces a cellular effect (the latter usually being a naturally occurring agonist such as a hormone or neurotransmitter). Most commonly the interfering molecule is introduced therapeutically to block the effects of the agonist (antagonize response). It should be noted that a subset of such interactions may not block agonist effect but actually may potentiate agonist effect; this will be discussed later in this chapter. There are basically two molecular mechanisms of receptor antagonism. The first to be considered is orthosteric interaction whereby the antagonist physically precludes binding of the agonist to the active site of the receptor (steric inhibition). The second is where the antagonist binds to its own site on the receptor (separate from that of the endogenous agonist) to affect agonist response through a conformational change in the receptor.

4.6.1 Orthosteric Antagonism

The model for orthosteric receptor antagonism involves the binding of an agonist [A] to a receptor R and the antagonism of that binding by an antagonist [B]. The equation for the calculation of the agonist receptor occupancy at any time for a concentration of agonist A in the presence of a concentration of antagonist B is:

$$\rho_{AB} = ([A]/K_A/([A]/K_A + 1)) \bullet (1 - (\vartheta(1 - e^{-k_2\Phi t})) + \rho_B\, e^{-k_2\Phi t})) \qquad (4.14)$$

where:

$$([B]/K_B)/([B]/K_B + [A]/K_A + 1) \qquad (4.15)$$

and

$$([B]/K_B)/([B]/K_B + 1) \qquad (4.16)$$

$$\Phi = ([B]/K_B + [A]/K_A + 1)/([A]/K_A + 1) \qquad (4.17)$$

In practice, antagonism is measured by assessing the system sensitivity to the agonist (determination of a dose-response curve to the agonist), elimination of the agonist from the system with washing (drug-free medium), equilibration of the system with a concentration of antagonist for a sufficient time to allow an equilibrium to be attained between the antagonist and the free receptors, and then the reassessment of sensitivity of the system to the agonist in the presence of the antagonist. For the latter experimental procedure to be conducted under equilibrium conditions, there must be sufficient time for the agonist, antagonist, and receptors to come to proper equilibrium during the course of the experiment to determine the sensitivity of the system to agonist in the presence of the antagonist. The temporal requirements for equilibrium under these conditions demand that there must elapse sufficient time for the antagonist to dissociate from the receptors in accordance with mass action equilibria and for the agonist to reassociate with these receptors. There are experimental factors that control whether or not this condition can be met; these include the density of the receptors in the tissue, their efficiency of coupling, the efficacy of the agonist, the time available to measure agonist response in the presence of antagonist and the dissociation rate of the antagonist.

Figure 4.3 shows a schematic diagram of the system for orthosteric antagonism. Two temporal extremes will be considered first. Complete competitive equilibrium can be achieved when there is sufficient time for the antagonist, agonist, and receptors to come to correct equilibrium when agonist response is measured in the presence of the antagonist. In practical terms, this usually occurs when the dissociation rate of the antagonist is rapid such that the agonist can attain correct receptor occupancy. This kinetic extreme is modeled by Equation 4.14, where the time allowed for measurement of response is much greater than the dissociation rate of the antagonist (time/k_2 > 10). Under these circumstances, Equation 4.14 reduces to the equation for simple competitive antagonism:

$$\rho_A = \frac{[A]/K_A}{[A]/K_A + [B]/K_B + 1} \qquad (4.18)$$

A characteristic feature of Equation 4.18 is that the receptor occupancy by the agonist (ρ_A) will be complete ($\rho_A \rightarrow 1$) when $[A] \gg [B]$. In molecular terms, this is the condition whereby large excess concentrations of agonist will compete for antagonist, and receptor occupancy will essentially revert to complete occupancy by the agonist. This highlights a feature of competitive antagonism, namely that the receptor will be occupied by the ligand with the higher affinity or the one present at the highest concentration. Experimentally, this type of antagonism is characterized by parallel shifts to the right of the agonist dose-response curve with no diminution of the maximal response (Figure 4.3A).

The other temporal extreme is where there is a complete insufficiency of time to allow the antagonist to dissociate from the receptors during the period of measurement of the agonist response. This usually occurs in the testing of very slow offset antagonists (i.e., ones that essentially irreversibly occupy the receptors during the timecourse of agonist response measurement). Under these conditions, time/k_2 < 0.01 and Equation 4.14 reduces to the Gaddum equation for noncompetitive antagonism:

$$\rho_A = \frac{[A]/K_A}{[A]/K_A(1 + [B]/K_B) + [B]/K_B + 1} \qquad (4.19)$$

It can be seen from Equation 4.19 that the presence of the antagonist ($[B] \neq 0$) essentially precludes complete receptor occupancy by the agonist (ρ_A always <1 with nonzero values of [B]). Clearly if there is a receptor reserve for the agonist, then maximal response may still be obtained with a submaximal agonist receptor occupancy. Therefore, in cases where there is a receptor reserve for agonist, antagonism according to Equation 4.19 may not produce a depression of maximal response. However, there are a great many situations where antagonism according to Equation 4.19 will depress the maximal response. This type of antagonism, depicted in Figure 4.3B, is termed insurmountable or noncompetitive.

It can be seen from the previous discussion that the kinetics of antagonist offset can determine the behavior of the orthosteric antagonist. If the antagonist has a rapid offset, then the antagonism will be competitive with no diminution of agonist maximal response (termed surmountable; see Figure 4.3A). In contrast, if the antagonist produces persistent receptor binding and has a slow rate of offset from the receptor, then the antagonism could be noncompetitive with a depressed maximal response to the agonist (Figure 4.3B). It should be

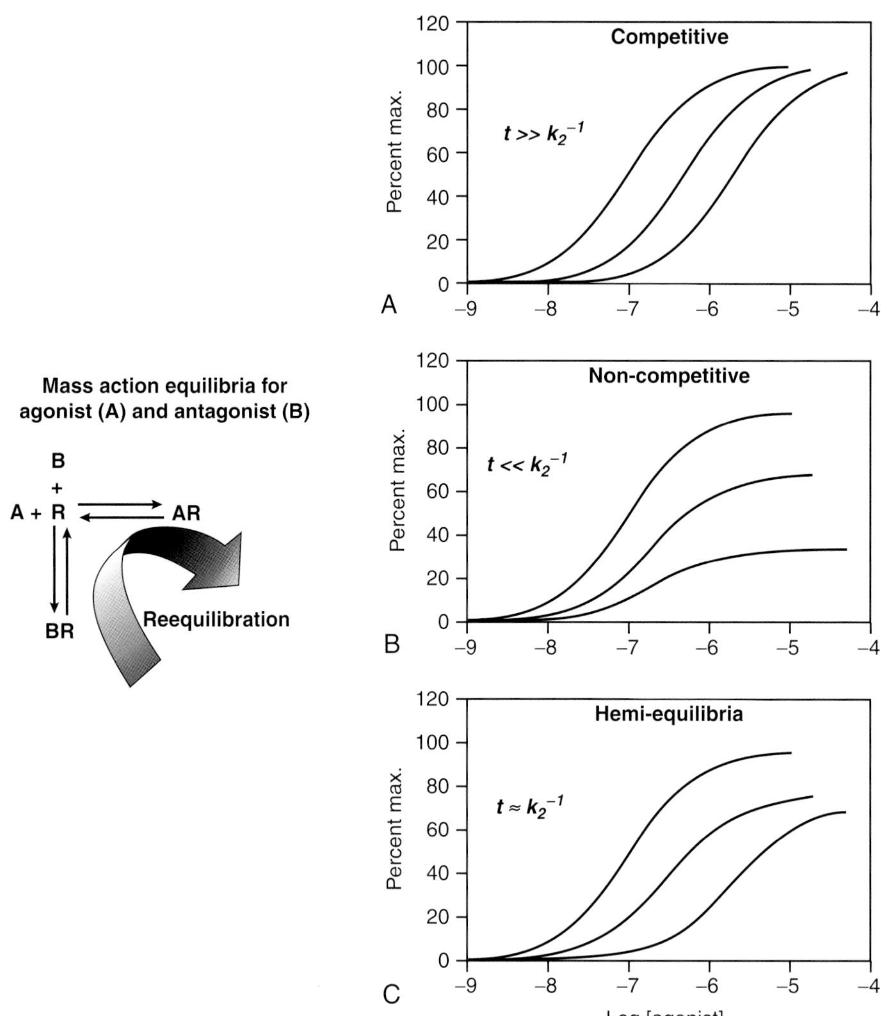

Figure 4.3 Orthosteric antagonist effect. Mass action equilibria between receptors, an agonist A, and an antagonist B is governed by the concentration of each ligand in the receptor compartment and the equilibrium dissociation constants of the respective ligand-receptor complexes. However, there must be time allowed for this proper equilibrium to be attained. When there is, dextral displacement of agonist occupancy curves with no diminution of maxima is observed (competitive antagonism, panel A). In contrast, if there is insufficient time allowed for reequilibration to occur, then insurmountable antagonism with depressed agonist maximal occupancy is observed (noncompetitive, panel B). In a midpoint region where a partial reequilibration can occur, then a hemi-equilibrium is observed, characterized by dextral displacement of the curves with some depression of maxima (panel C).

noted that the experimental system used to measure the antagonism is also important. For example, measurement systems that utilize rapid transient responses (such as intracellular calcium release) leave little time for agonist and antagonist to come to equilibrium with the receptors during collection of pharmacological response. These assays tend to show slow offset antagonists as noncompetitive. Since the temporal conditions *in vivo* are not known, it is difficult to predict whether noncompetitive antagonism seen in an *in vitro* test assay will translate into a noncompetitive antagonism in the therapeutic situation. For this reason, the labels of competitive and noncompetitive are not useful and are similar to agonist behaviors such as full and partial agonism. However, a persistent noncompetitive antagonism does predict a relevant degree of receptor target coverage in the *in vivo* therapeutic situation suggesting that this behavior, seen in a test system, may be a useful predictor of therapeutic value.

Between the extremes of time/k_2 < 0.1 and time/k_2 > 10 lies a variable kinetic behavior region known as *hemi-equilibria*. This may be described as cases where there is "almost enough time" for the agonist and antagonist to fully equilibrate with the receptor population. Under these circumstances, a mixture of behaviors is seen with a simple competitive antagonist-like behavior observed at low agonist receptor occupancies (parallel shift of the agonist dose-response curve and a noncompetitive depression of the maximal response seen at higher agonist receptor occupancies (Figure 4.3C).

4.6.2 Allosteric Modulation

The other major mechanism available for two drugs to interact at a single receptor is through allosteric modulation. In this mechanism, the allosteric modulator binds to its own site on the receptor to stabilize a unique allosteric conformation. The effect of such a ligand (referred to as an allosteric modulator, designated *B*) on the primary natural ligand is produced through a conformational change of the receptor, therefore the interaction between the ligands is not through steric hindrance but rather through the protein itself via a ternary complex of the endogenous ligand for the receptor (designated [*A*]), the allosteric modulator, and the receptor (designated *R*; see later):

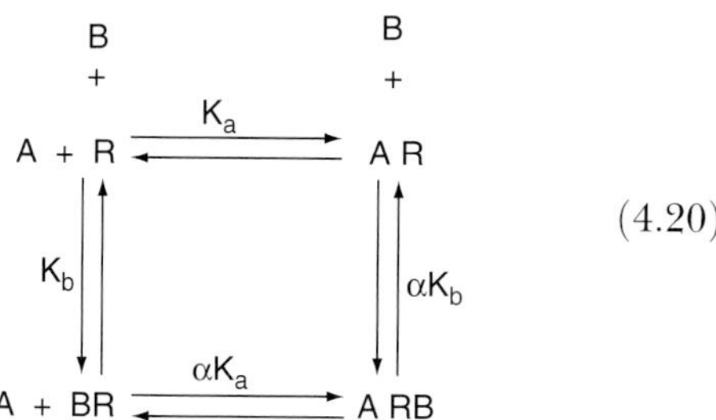

(4.20)

The effect of the modulator on the affinity of the receptor for ligand *A* is quantified by a factor α (designated the cooperativity constant); the affinities of ligands *A* and *B* for the receptor are K_a and K_b, respectively. Under these circumstances, the effect of an allosteric modulator on the binding of ligand *A* is given by:

$$\rho_A = \frac{[A]/K_A(1+\alpha[B]/K_B)}{[A]/K_A(1+\alpha[B]/K_B)+[B]/K_B+1} \qquad (4.21)$$

Equation 4.21 defines the changes in affinity of the receptor for *A* when the modulator *B* is bound; these can be positive (increase affinity when $\alpha > 1$) to yield potentiation of binding or negative (decrease affinity when $\alpha < 1$) to yield antagonism. It should be noted that, unlike orthosteric antagonism, binding is not precluded by a negative allosteric modulator. Instead, the affinity of the receptor is simply reset to a lower level. Since allosteric effect is mediated by binding of the modulator at a separate site, it is saturable; when the allosteric sites are completely bound by modulator, the effect reaches a maximal limit (Figure 4.4).

Also in contrast to orthosteric antagonism, allosteric modulation can have separate effects on agonist affinity and efficacy. This is the result of the fact that modulators essentially stabilize a new conformation of the receptor. Therefore, an extended model of allosteric modulation of receptors is required to accommodate allosteric effects on agonist efficacy. The model for this is an amalgam of the one shown in scheme 4.20 (with receptor occupancy given by Eq. 4.21) and the operational model for agonism (Eq. 4.13) to yield the following equation for response to agonist *A* in the presence of allosteric modulator *B*:

$$\text{Response} = \frac{[A]/K_A\tau(1+\alpha\xi[B]/K_B)E_{max}}{[A]/K_A(1+\alpha[B]/K_B+\tau(1+\alpha\xi[B]/K_B))+[B]/K_B+1} \qquad (4.22)$$

where K_A and K_B are the equilibrium dissociation constants of the agonist and antagonist receptor complexes, respectively, and E_{max} is the maximal response of the system. As with Equation 4.21, α refers to the multiple change in affinity for the agonist produced by the modulator. However,

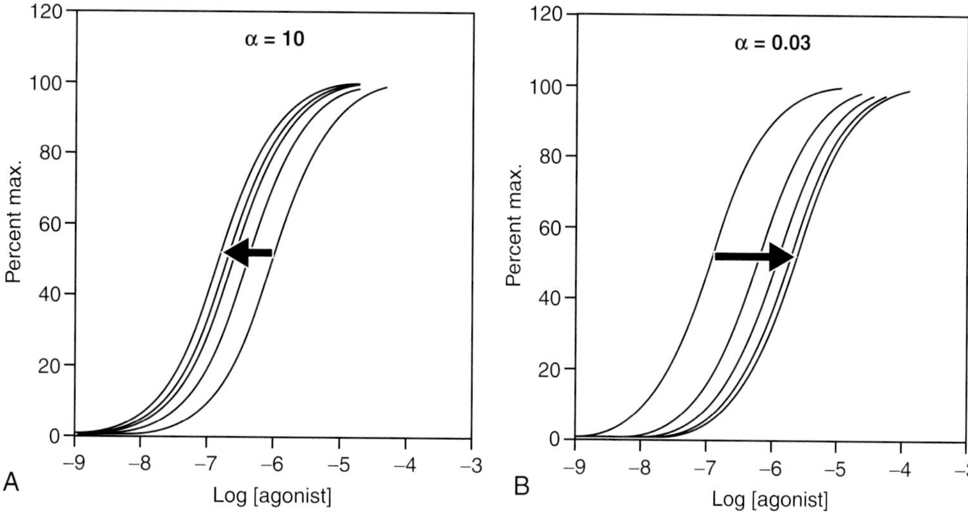

Figure 4.4 Allosteric effects on ligand affinity. The effects of an allosteric modulator on ligand affinity are shown (term α in Eq. 4.21). Positive modulation ($\alpha > 1$) produces shifts to the left of agonist occupancy curves until the allosteric effects stops with saturation of the allosteric binding site. Thus, a 10-fold shift to the left is observed for $\alpha = 10$ (panel A). Negative effects on affinity are produced when $\alpha < 1$ characterized by shifts to the right of the agonist occupancy curves ($\alpha = 0.03 =$ 30-fold shift to the right) (panel B).

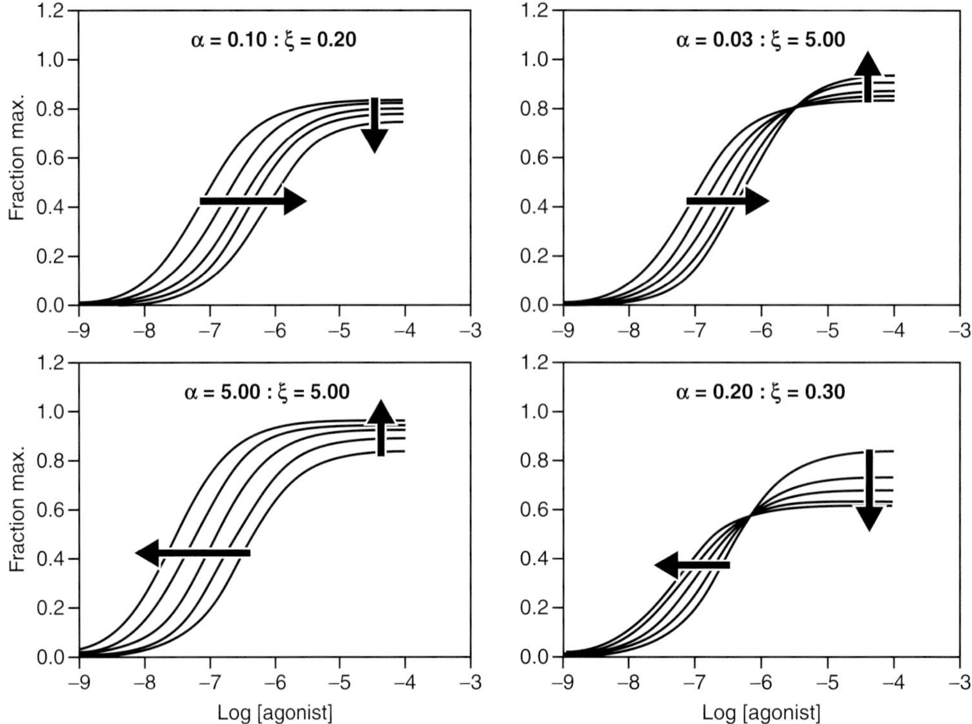

Figure 4.5 Allosteric effects on receptor function. Allosteric modulators may affect affinity (through the term α in Eq. 4.22) and efficacy through the term ξ (Eq. 4.22). Various combinations such as decreased affinity and efficacy (panel A), decreased affinity and increased efficacy (panel B), increased affinity and efficacy (panel C), and increased affinity with decreased efficacy (panel D) can result.

this model takes into account receptor function (as with Eq. 4.13, τ incorporates the efficacy of the agonist and the ability of the system to yield response). In this model, the agonist and modulator-bound receptor complex has the potential ability to signal, therefore ξ refers to the multiple in the efficacy of the agonist when the receptor is bound by a modulator ($\xi = \tau'/\tau$, where τ' is the efficacy of the agonist when the modulator is bound to the receptor). This permits the model to predict a range of effects on affinity and efficacy of the agonist (Figure 4.5).

One of the more interesting effects predicted by Equation 4.22 is for a modulator that increases the affinity but decreases the efficacy of an agonist. Since allosteric effects are reciprocal, this means that the agonist also increases the affinity of the receptor for the modulator. This leads to an interesting scenario whereby the antagonist modulation becomes more potent with higher levels of agonist; that is, the antagonism increases as the system is more highly driven. The reciprocal is also true whereby the affinity for the antagonist is low when there is no agonist present; this may lead to a reduction of side effects. One such modulator is ifenprodil for the NMDA receptor.

4.7 CONSTITUTIVE RECEPTOR ACTIVITY

The previous discussions have been confined to systems that essentially are quiescent until activated by an agonist (i.e., hormone, neurotransmitter). For these, activation (by a natural or synthetic agonist) can be described by the operational model (Equation 4.13), whereas interference with this process (antagonism) can be orthosteric (Equation 4.14) or allosteric (Equation 4.22). These models are general representations of pharmacological function and transcend actual molecular mechanism of receptor function; in this regard they are flexible and have the advantage of being generally applicable to most tissue systems. However, one pharmacological phenomenon that requires more mechanistic elaboration to be described is constitutive receptor activity. This is the occurrence of elevated basal response in a tissue due to spontaneous formation of receptor active states made in the absence of agonist. The only way to affect such activity is through the use of a class of molecule called an inverse agonist. To discuss constitutive activity and inverse agonism, the extended ternary complex receptor model must be considered.

4.8 EXTENDED TERNARY COMPLEX MODEL

A large family of therapeutically relevant membrane receptors is the seven-transmembrane receptor family, so named because of their structure. Conformational changes in this protein induced by intracellular and extracellular ligands permit information transfer from the outside to the inside of the cell. When these receptors become activated, they bind with other membrane-bound (i.e., *G*-protein) or cytosolic (i.e., *β*-arrestin) proteins. The model describing such a system was termed the ternary complex model for the complex of receptor, ligand, and *G*-protein. Subsequent demonstration that receptors can produce cell activation in the absence of agonist led to an extension of this model to what is now called the extended ternary complex model. This model describes the spontaneous formation of an active state receptor ($[R_a]$) from an inactive state receptor ($[R_i]$) according to an allosteric constant ($L = [R_a]/[R_i]$). The active state receptor can form a complex with *G*-protein ($[G]$) spontaneously to form R_aG or agonist activation can induce formation of a ternary complex AR_aG.

$$\begin{array}{ccccc} & & & G \searrow \gamma K_g & \\ AR_i & \overset{\alpha L}{\rightleftarrows} & ARa & \rightleftarrows & AR_aG \\ K_a \updownarrow & & \alpha K_a \updownarrow & & \updownarrow \alpha\gamma K_a \\ R_i & \overset{L}{\rightleftarrows} & Ra & \rightleftarrows & R_aG \\ & & & G \nearrow K_g & \end{array} \qquad (4.23)$$

The fraction ρ of *G*-protein activating species (producing response), namely $[R_aG]$ and $[AR_aG]$, as a fraction of the total number of receptor species $[R_{tot}]$, is given by:

$$\rho = \frac{L[G]/K_G(1 + \alpha\gamma[A]/K_A)}{[A]/K_A(1 + \alpha L(1 + \gamma[G]/K_G)) + L(1 + [G]/K_G) + 1} \qquad (4.24)$$

where the ligand is $[A]$ and K_A and K_G are the equilibrium dissociation constants of the ligand-receptor and G-protein–receptor complexes, respectively. As with the allosteric model, the term α refers to the multiple difference in affinity of the ligand for R_a over R_i. For instance, $\alpha = 10$ refers to the case where the ligand has a 10-fold greater affinity for R_a over R_i. Similarly, the term γ defines the multiple difference in affinity of the receptor for G-protein when the receptor is bound to the ligand; that is, $\gamma = 10$ means that the ligand bound receptor has a 10-fold greater affinity for the G-protein than the ligand unbound receptor. For this model, α and γ describe the ability of the ligand to selectively cause the receptor to couple to G-proteins, therefore they quantify the ligand efficacy.

As noted in Equation 4.7, selective binding of a ligand to a receptor species will bias the entire system toward selective production of that species; therefore, positive values for α and γ would produce an agonist. However, this model predicts a vectorial nature for efficacy as well, namely that it can be positive (as for agonists) but also negative. Thus selective affinity for the inactive receptor state ($\alpha, \gamma < 1$) will reverse receptor activation in systems where activation is present either through the presence of agonist or, notably, spontaneously (*vide infra*). This will be observed as inverse agonism, but only in systems that demonstrate constitutive receptor activity. The mechanistic detail of the extended ternary complex model can take into account the phenomenon of constitutive receptor activity. It can be seen from Equation 4.24 that even in the absence of ligand ($[A] = 0$), the fraction of receptor in the active state may be positive:

$$\text{Constitutive Activity} = \frac{L[G]/K_G}{L(1 + [G]/K_G) + 1} \qquad (4.25)$$

The most common experimental and pathological setting for constituive receptor activity is in cases of high membrane receptor density. The allosteric constant L dictates the ratio between spontaneous existence of active state and inactive state receptors ($L = [R_a]/[R_i]$); therefore, the larger the number of receptors, the larger the ambient number of active state receptors. At very high receptor levels, there will be sufficient active state receptors to produce an elevated basal response in the tissue; such systems then are considered to have pharmacologically relevant constitutive receptor activity. The dependence of constitutive activity on $[R_i]$ is given by

$$\frac{[R_aG]}{[G_{tot}]} = \frac{[R_i]}{[R_i] + (K_G/L)} \qquad (4.26)$$

where $[R_i]$ is the receptor density, L is the allosteric constant describing the propensity of the receptor to spontaneously adopt the active state, and K_G is the equilibrium dissociation constant for the activated receptor–*G*-protein complex. Constitutive activity is favored by a large value of L (low energy barrier to spontaneous formation of the active state) and/or a tight coupling between the receptor and the *G*-protein (low value for K_G). Figure 4.6A shows the appearance of constitutive receptor activity with rising levels of membrane receptor density. Figure 4.6B shows the effects of positive agonists and inverse agonists on the elevated basal response of a constitutively active system.

4.9 CONCLUSIONS

This chapter discusses ligand binding to receptors from the point of view of molecular mechanism and pharmacological consequences. Although the binding of a ligand to a protein generally can be described by a simple model of molecular binding to an inert surface (Langmuir adsorption isotherm), more complex binding models can confer texture on the system to allow binding to produce an effect. For instance, selective binding to one of two protein states can bias the total amounts of those two states; this can lead to tissue activation (agonism) or reversal of spontaneous activation of receptors (inverse agonism). An equilibrium between receptor states can also lead to spontaneous elevation of tissue response (constitutive receptor activity). The interpretation of receptor active states by cells leads to a further diversity in signaling, thereby

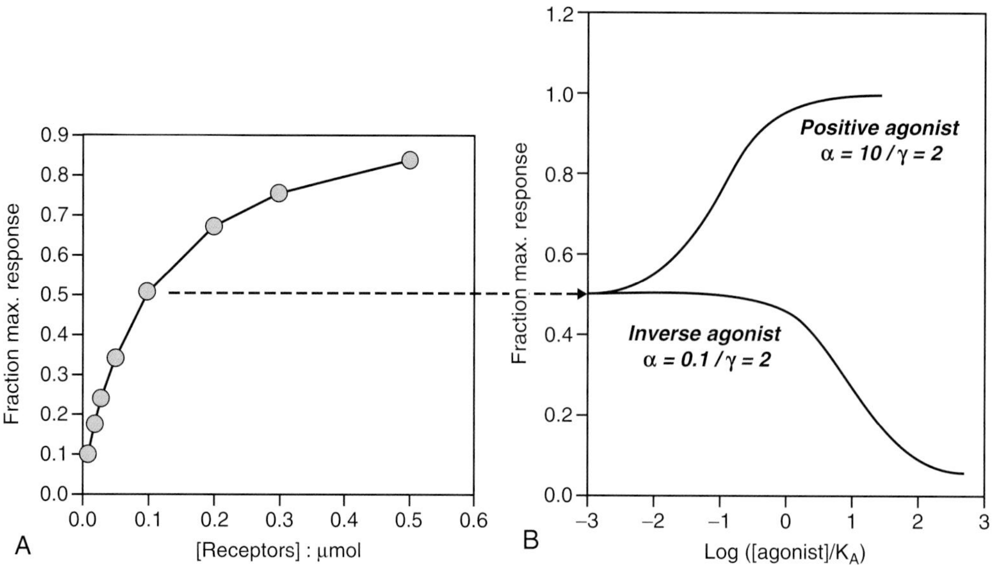

Figure 4.6 Constitutive activity and inverse agonism. (A) Constitutive activity as a function of receptor density according to Equation 4.26 ($K_G = 10^{-8}$ M, $L = 10^{-3}$). (B) Effects of a positive agonist ($\alpha = 10$, $\gamma = 2$, parameters for Eq. 4.24) and inverse agonist ($\alpha = 0.1$, $\gamma = 0.1$) in a constitutively active system.

illustrating the enormous flexibility in receptor-mediated information transfer. An understanding of the first step in this process (ligand binding) is useful in realizing the potential control of these systems for therapeutic advantage.

REVIEW QUESTIONS

1. Essentially, the affinity of a drug molecule can be thought of as a concentration. What is the usual concentration used to quantify affinity this and what does it mean in molecular terms?
2. The operational model equation uses a parameter tau to quantify efficacy. How exactly is tau defined and why is it useful in drug discovery?
3. What is meant by orthosteric antagonism? Allosteric antagonism? Which one produces a saturable effect and why?
4. A slow-onset, long-acting antagonist may produce noncompetitive antagonism in the FLIPR response system (rapid transient responses) but competitive (surmountable) effects in 24-hour assays like reporters. Why?
5. An experimental antagonist appears to increase in activity with increasing levels of agonism in the system. What mechanism could be responsible for such behavior?
6. Some antagonists depress basal responses but others do not. What type of system is required to observe such an effect and what is the molecular mechanism responsible for it (inverse agonism)?

REFERENCES

Black, J. W., & Leff, P. (1983). Operational models of pharmacological agonist. *Proceedings of the Royal Society of London [Biol], 220,* 141.

Burgen, A. S. V. (1981). Conformational changes and drug action. *Federal Proceedings, 40,* 2723–2728.

Kenakin, T. P. (2001). Inverse, protean, and ligand-selective agonism: Matters of receptor conformation. *The FASEB Journal, 15,* 598–611.

Kenakin, T. P. (2004). *A Pharmacology Primer: Theory, Application and Methods.* Academic Press/ Elsevier, Amsterdam, pp 1–324.

Kenakin, T. P. (2004). Principles: Receptor theory in pharmacology. *Trends in Pharmacological Sciences, 25,* 186–192.

Kew, J. N. C., Trube, G., Kemp, J. A. (1996). A novel mechanism of activity-dependent NMDA receptor antagonism describes the effect of ifenprodil in rat cultured cortical neurons. *Journal of Physiology,* 497.*3*: 761–772.

Rang, H. P. (2006). The receptor concept: Pharmacology's big idea. *British Journal of Pharmacology, 147,* S9.

Samama, P., Cotecchia, S., Costa, T., & Lefkowitz, R. J. (1993). A mutation-induced activated state of the β_2-adrenergic receptor: Extending the ternary complex model. *The Journal of Biological Chemistry, 268,* 4625–4636.

Stephenson, R. P. (1956). A modification of receptor theory. *British Journal of Pharmacology, 11,* 379–393.

Chapter

5

Hormesis and Pharmacology

Edward Calabrese

OUTLINE

5.1 INTRODUCTION

5.1.1 Pharmacology and the Dose Response

The historical foundations of the dose-response relationship in pharmacology were based principally on the classic research and publications of Alfred J. Clark and his contemporary and successor John Henry Gaddum. Based on extensive research on the quantitative actions of drugs such as acetylcholine and atropine, these authors concluded that combining drugs with specific receptor groups could be mathematically described by the same relationships employed in the Langmuir adsorption isotherm. This conclusion assumed that the responses of a tissue were directly proportional to its specific receptor groups as occupied by the drug, that the receptor occupation followed the law of mass action, and that drug molecules would have equal access to all receptor groups. This perspective became the dominant pharmacological dose-response paradigm for the remainder of the twentieth century.

Despite its dominant general intellectual "hold" on the field of pharmacology, this dose-response model of Clark & Gaddum has required growth, refinement, and correction over the past nearly 80 years. In fact, soon after the theoretical formulation by Clark in the 1930s it was recognized that adsorption equations other than Langmuir's would frequently fit the dose response data just as well, and that a maximal response may not require maximal receptor occupation. However, despite such early recognized limitations in this pharmacological model of the dose response, the

Langmuir equation became commonly adopted as well as the belief that the maximal response required the complete occupation of receptors by the agent.

Although this conceptual framework of the pharmacological dose response relationship has had a long history of qualitative predictive utility, it often provided less than satisfactory quantitative agreement with experimentally derived data as noted by Stephenson, then at the University of Edinburgh. During subsequent decades it was often reported that the observed dose-response relationship did not follow the predicted form. Some drugs, now called partial agonists, could stimulate tissues but could not produce the expected normal maximum response. Nor, as was pointed out by Paton of the University of Oxford, could the model of Clark and Gaddum account for the antagonism shown by partial agonists to more powerful agonists, tissue desensitization following exposure to highly specific stimulants (acetylcholine, histamine) as well as responses when a vigorous excitation is replaced quickly by competitive antagonism.

These examples of theory limitations and others led to modification in the receptor-based dose response concept during the middle decades of the twentieth century. Most notably was that of Ariens at the University of Nijmegan in The Netherlands, who proposed that the drug-receptor union may have varying effectiveness, which he called *intrinsic activity*, and which Stephenson referred to as *efficacy*. This efficacy or intrinsic activity concept became expressed in quantitative terms as the rate constant of the second step of a drug-receptor process that yielded the active form of the receptor.

Among the challenges affecting the receptor-based model of Clark and Gaddum, biphasic dose response curves, particularly those with a single active chemical group, present a significant problem for the occupation receptor theory. By 1957 Ariens and his colleagues had proposed that biphasic dose-response curves might occur if a drug interacted with two receptor systems. In fact, as early as 1906, Henry Dale noted that adrenaline can act at both excitatory and inhibitory receptors in the vasculature, leading Robert F. Furchgott, then Chair of Pharmacology at State University of New York/Downstate and later, Nobel Laureate, some 50 years later to propose that these receptors may occur on the same smooth muscle cell. However, it was not until the 1960s that numerous, yet isolated biphasic dose-response relationships began to be reported for drugs of pharmacological importance. Of significance was that these responses were accounted for by the presence of two opposing receptor populations. In a review of this literature Szabaldi, from the University of Manchester, noted that most of the sympathomimetic amines activate opposite receptors in smooth muscle preparations, with α type receptors being stimulating and β receptors being negative. Likewise, in the early 1980s, a number of researchers reported that histamine can activate both excitatory and inhibitory receptors with H_1 type excitatory receptors being stimulating and H_2 receptors being inhibitory.

During the 1970s it also became recognized that two opposing receptor populations to the same agonist were often present on the same neuron. This was shown to be the case in vertebrates for acetylcholine, dopamine, and 5-HT. Likewise, similar receptor strategies were reported in vertebrates for 5-HT, and histamine on sympathetic ganglion cells along with numerous other examples.

Based on this cumulative evidence Szabaldi developed a theoretical model to describe how agonists and antagonists act in pharmacological systems containing opposite acting receptors. He noted that this model was derived from the combination of "double agonists" and functional antagonism of Ariens. Double agonism was generally defined as a phenomenon when "a compound induces an effect by interaction with two different specific receptors, but by means of a common effect." Szabaldi determined that his model was a special case of double agonism when two receptors that are activated by the agonist mediate opposite effects. Further, if the two types of receptors are assumed to be functionally independent, the model for functional antagonism is employed; the quantitative features of the model are described by the algebraic sum of the induced effects produced by the activities of both receptors.

This model is very general and could account for a wide range of dose response relationships depending on assumed affinities and intrinsic activities. Of particular interest is that the model can account for hormetic-like biphasic dose response relationships. Over the next 30 years the number of examples of biphasic dose responses has greatly proliferated to include now up to nearly 40 receptor families affecting a range of biological endpoints that govern essential physiological and behavioral functions.

The model of Szabaldi has served as a theoretical and practical foundation that has been expanded upon by others. Based on research on α-lactalbums production by rat mammary gland explants, Quirk and Funder at Prince Henry's Hospital in Melbourne were able to account for biphasic dose responses even for highly specific glucocorticoids with binding to a single receptor. This was explained with a model of a single "turn-on" nuclear receptor site for glucocorticoid receptors and multiple, preemptive glucocorticoid regulatory refinements. This model is consistent with that of Jarv, at the University of Tartu in Estonia, that agonistic and antagonistic effects of ligands may be related to their binding in two separate sites of the same receptor molecule. Evidence supporting this model was initially published in 1980 by Jarv and his colleagues for the muscarinic acetylcholine receptor.

Although pharmacological evaluation of biphasic dose responses has dominated the literature from the 1970s to the present, it is important to note that there is both a convergence of concept and a reformulation of such perspectives in the area of toxicology and more broadly in systems biology. In 2004, Leuchenko at Johns Hopkins and several colleagues at the California Institute of Technology presented a framework for biphasic regulation that is conceptually similar to the model of Szabaldi and the work of Calabrese under the concept of hormesis. Four types of biphasic regulatory schemes were proposed, with the first two being quite similar to the one-receptor model of Quirk and Funder, and the one-agonist, two-receptor model of Szabaldi. However, the paper added a further dimension of progressive complexity.

The biphasic response in their third scheme or model (i.e., type III) results from signal transduction activities that are removed from the response element (ligand-receptor complex). In this situation, the biphasic nature of the response derives from the properties of the signal transducing components. The authors proposed a variety ways in which the biphasic dose response could occur depending on the type of properties of the response element (RE), molecular inputs, and complexity of the biochemical pathways.

The fourth model of biphasic regulation (type IV) requires two inputs to affect the response rather than one as in the preceding cases. This is seen in combinatorial inhibition when a molecule binds with two or more interacting molecules to form a single functional complex as is the case with scaffold proteins. A second type IV receptor involves two or more interactions between an activator and the activated molecules for full activation. Examples of both biphasic regulation with scaffold protein concentrations and distributive activators are seen in the MAPk cascades. A third category of type IV biphasic regulation acts via immediate enzymatic feedback from the activated molecule onto the activator molecule.

The authors speculated on the adaptive significance of biphasic regulatory strategies. Such responses provided tunable filtering of the magnitude of the incoming signal. They claim that each type of biphasic regulation can determine the maximum, sensitivity, and strength of the response. The composite of the four strategies may have broad biological significance at multiple levels including global and local domains.

Hormesis is a dose-response phenomenon characterized by a low-dose stimulation and a high-dose inhibition. This type of dose-response relationship may be described as an inverted U-shaped dose response or a J-shaped dose response (Figure 5.1). Whether the dose response is an inverted U- or J-shape is determined by the endpoint that is measured. For example, in the cases of growth, longevity, or cognition, the results would be plotted as an inverted U-shaped dose response. In the case of disease incidence such as cancer incidence, cardiovascular disease incidence, and other diseases, the results are typically plotted as J-shaped dose responses. However, regardless of whether the results are seen as inverted U- or J-shaped dose responses they fit into the descriptive framework of a hormetic dose-response. As will be demonstrated in this chapter, the hormetic dose response is highly generalizable, occurring across the broad spectrum of plant, microbiological, invertebrate, and vertebrate organisms and in *in-vitro* and *in-vivo* systems. It represents an adaptive response that is evolutionarily based, and needs to be evaluated within that context.

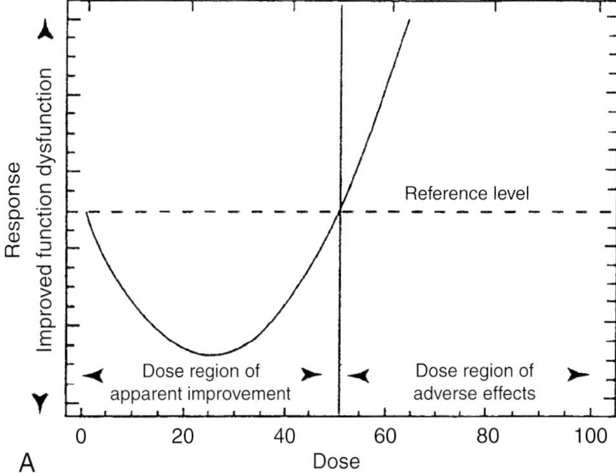

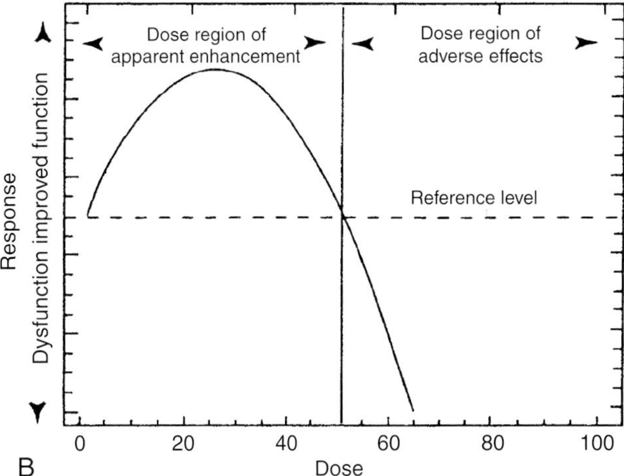

Figure 5.1 Hormetic dose responses: J- and inverted U-shaped. (Source: Davis and Svendsgaard, 1990)

5.1.2 Hormesis: Origin of Concept and Terminology

The term *hormesis* was first reported in the peer-reviewed journal literature in 1943 by Chester Southam and John Ehrlich, based on research assessing the effects of extracts from the Red Cedar tree on fungal metabolism. The term hormesis is believed, however, to have first appeared in the undergraduate thesis of Chester Southam, then a student at the University of South Dakota in 1941. A final draft of this thesis reveals that Southam originally used the term *toxicotrophism* to describe the inverted U-shaped dose response in the Red Cedar extract induced fungal growth response. However, this term was neatly crossed out with the term *hormesis* printed over it. (A copy of the original undergraduate thesis may be found at www.hormesissociety.org.) Thus, we don't know whether the term originated from Southam or Ehrlich. However, the concept of hormesis is generally is recognized as having been developed and nurtured in a substantial way first by Hugo Schulz, starting in the early 1880s at the University of Grieswald in Northern Germany. The initial observations of the hormetic dose response were made in experiments assessing the effects of various chemical disinfectants on yeast metabolism based on the measurement of liberated carbon dioxide. That low doses of toxic metals would stimulate the metabolism of yeasts was totally unexpected, forcing Schulz to replicate these initial and critical findings repeatedly as described in an autobiographical statement approximately 40 years later:

> *Since it could be foreseen that experiments on fermentation and putrescence in an institute of pathology would offer particularly good prospects for vigorous growth, I occupied myself as well as possible, on accordance with the state of our knowledge at the time, with this area. Sometimes when working with substances that needed to be examined for their effectiveness in comparison to the inducers of yeast fermentation, initially working together with my assistant, Gottfried Hoffmann, I found in formic acid and also in other substances the marvelous occurrence that if I got below their indifference point, i.e., if, for example, I worked with less formic acid than was required to order to halt the appearance of its anti-fermentive property, that all at once the carbon dioxide production became distinctly higher than the controls processed without the formic acid addition. I first thought, as is obvious, that there had been some kind of experimental or observation error. But the appearance of the overproduction continually repeated itself under the same conditions. First I did not know to deal with it. And in any event, at that time still did not realize that I had experimentally proved the first theorem of Arndt's fundamental law of biology.*

Despite Schulz's experimental awakening, perhaps the earliest discovery of the biphasic dose response was made some 30 years earlier by the renowned pathologist Rudolf Virchow at the University of Wurzburg, who observed an increased beating activity of ciliae of the tracheal epithelia of post mortem mucosa by sodium and potassium hydroxide at low concentrations and inhibition by higher concentrations. Even though Virchow incorporated this concept into his famous "cellular pathology" framework, as was recently pointed out by Dietrich Henscher, Schulz was the scientist who not only saw broad biological and medical significance in these findings but also devoted himself to this area, thereby making him the most substantive early developer of the hormesis concept.

The significance of Schulz for the hormetic dose-response relationship was unfortunately that of a two-edged sword. On the positive side his intuition suggested that this biphasic dose response was basic and may well be the most fundamental dose response relationship, thus having enormous generalizability. This belief suggested that his initial findings were of considerable importance to all areas of the biological/medical sciences interested in the dose-response relationship. Furthermore, Schulz thought that his findings provided the explanatory principle underlying the medical practice of homeopathy. This placed Schulz in the middle of the long-festering philosophical, medical, legal, and economic conflict between what is now called "traditional" medicine and homeopathy. In effect, Schulz sided with homeopathy, becoming a scientific hero of sorts to the German homeopathic community at that time, but also the object of scorn, ridicule, and criticism of the mainstream biomedical and clinical sciences soon after his discovery and continuing throughout his long career, and even down to the present time, some 75 years after his death.

5.1.3 Historical Marginalization of Hormesis

As a result of Schulz's decision to move the concept of hormesis into the traditional medicine-homeopathy dispute he unknowingly created the conditions within which his dose-response discovery (or rediscovery) would become marginalized, at best, by the biomedical community over the next century. Schulz became seen as carrying the scientific banner of homeopathy, and as such, became the object of criticism by powerful and extremely accomplished leaders of the pharmacological academic community such as Alfred J. Clarke, Professor of Pharmacology at Edinburgh University, still a revered name in academic pharmacology with graduate fellowships and a distinguished chair named in his honor at the University of Edinburgh. In a succession of journal articles and books, some of an extremely prestigious nature, Clark repeatedly highlighted the work of Schulz with criticism, disbelief, and derision; he also made strong efforts to portray homeopathy as monolithic "high dilutionists" in order to further ensure the marginalization of homeopathy and Schulz's ideas, when, in fact, that wing of the homeopathic movement constituted only a very small fraction of homeopathic practitioners. In his book entitled *The Mode of Action of Drugs on Cells*, Clark stated that "many pharmacologists have pointed out that it (Arndt-Schulz Law) expresses no general truth. It is interesting to note that no trace of evidence in support of such a law can be found in the majority of drugs." A further statement in the 1933 text by Clark noted that "evidence in favor of this law can easily be obtained from experimental errors." In addition, Clark singled out the work of Samuel Hanheman, the creator of homeopathy theory and practice, in an article dealing with "scientific quackery."

Since Clark was a founding member of the British Pharmacology Society in 1929 (www.bps.ac.uk/meetings/index.jsp), holder of the most prestigious academic Chair in Pharmacology in the United Kingdom, and possibly Europe, the author of major textbooks on pharmacology and toxicology, editorial board member of numerous leading journals in pharmacology, an advisor to numerous governmental panels and committees, he was professionally respected and highly influential. Furthermore, in the forward to the book, *Towards Understanding Receptors*, Robinson in 1981 referred to Clark's *Handbook of Experimental Pharmacology* as the "now classic monograph on *General Pharmacology*, a book that had great influence on a number of individuals." After Schulz died in 1931 there was not even symbolic opposition to the relentless chorus of criticism directed toward the hormetic concept; criticism that Clark's writings extended long after his untimely death in 1941. It is evident that Clark was no ordinary intellectual opponent, casting a long and understandably influential shadow upon the field that extended across disciplines, countries, and decades.

Of considerable further significance is that two of Clark's quantitatively focused colleagues, Chester Bliss and John Henry Gaddum, independently created the probit analysis model that was used to quantitatively characterize dose-response relationships, including responses at low doses. In this context a paper by Bliss included an appendix by the eminent biostatistician Ronald Fisher, himself perhaps the founder of modern biostatistics, which proposed the use of the maximum likelihood estimate to estimate threshold responses using the probit analysis model. Of profound future importance was that Fisher so constrained the model such that responses could only asymptotically approach the control value, never dipping below control values. Responses below controls were forced to be seen as background noise, never real effects. Such constraining of the dose response to always be above the control no matter how low the dose, effectively implied that hormetic effects were not real, but only manifestations of noise or random error.

These constraints were soon adopted by researchers in the U.S. NCI to model dose-response data for chemical carcinogens. The first instance of such constrained modeling of tumor incidence was published in the early 1940s by Bryan and Shimkin who, by following the guidance of Fisher, "ignored" below control responses in the low-dose zone, using the maximum likelihood estimate method where they applied the probit model even though response data clearly below control values were present. This intellectual framework of ignoring possible hormetic dose-responses was later adopted by regulatory agencies in the United States. and elsewhere as a standard procedure for assessing cancer risks at low doses, and remains so to the present.

The hormetic dose-response model was marginalized further in the hazard assessment process used by regulatory agencies, such as EPA and FDA. The goal of the hazard assessment is to obtain a no observed adverse effect level (NOAEL) (i.e., the highest dose that does not differ in a statistically significant manner from the control group), which can then be used in the risk assessment/management process to which are applied a host of uncertainty factors (UF) such as interspecies UF, inter-individual UF, less than lifetime exposure (LL Uncertainty Factor), and so on. Since the hazard assessment process assumes the existence of a threshold dose, only a few doses were believed necessary to estimate the NOAEL dose. Thus, toxicology has long been dominated by the hazard assessment process as imposed on the field by regulatory agencies largely due to their control over the dispersal of grant/contract monies to university scientists and their congressionally mandated risk-assessment decision-making authority. As a result of this regulatory agency dominance, toxicology became a high-dose, few-doses discipline. When the high-dose, few-doses framework is combined with a dose-response modeling procedure that constrains responses to be above the controls, it becomes nearly self-evident that the concept of hormesis would not only have become marginalized by modern toxicology but actually denied in theory, practice, and in regulations.

This goal of hormesis "concept" denial was the product of a strikingly successful strategy by pharmacologists led by Clark who were powerfully placed within the traditional medical establishment. In fact, the first generation of toxicologists in most governmental regulatory settings were educated and trained as pharmacologists in medical schools, and were successful in passing along their dose-response perspectives and biases not only to the newly created regulatory agencies that governed the testing of all drugs and chemicals but to new generations of pharmacologists, toxicologists, and all biomedically trained scientists down to the present time. So successful was this intellectual control of the dose response within toxicology and pharmacology that it was not until approximately 2000 that major toxicology texts introduced the term and concept of hormesis, and it was not until 2005 that the U.S. Society of Toxicology had a workshop specifically on hormesis at its 2005 annual Society meeting.

The concept of hormesis has been victimized, therefore, by the long conflict between traditional medicine and homeopathy, a battle in which homeopathy was vanquished. In the course of this conflict the concept of hormesis became collateral damage. The eliminating of the hormesis concept compelled the fields of pharmacology and toxicology to seek its replacement, and this role fell to the threshold model. As will be demonstrated in this chapter, the threshold dose-response model often fails to predict accurately the response of doses below the threshold. This central failing of the threshold dose response to predict low-dose effects accurately undermines the usefulness that pharmacology and toxicology should offer society, while being seen as a major flaw that has been missed and unappreciated by essentially the entire disciplines of pharmacology and toxicology since their inception.

The term hormesis, as noted earlier, was created by Chester Southam and John Ehrlich some 60 years after its initial experimental basis was uncovered by Schulz. Numerous publications generally supportive of the Schulz findings were subsequently published. Some of these investigations were designed to replicate and extend the findings of Schulz concerning the effects of toxic substance on yeast, and others utilized bacteria, fungi, and plant species with chemicals and/or radiation. Recognizing the controversial nature of the findings of Schulz, Ferdinande Hueppe, a famous microbiologist and protégé of Robert Koch, noted that even though Schulz had a close association with the homeopathic tradition this should not be a reason to reject his scientific findings, which were reproducible. August Bier, the renowned spinal surgeon who was nominated on numerous occasions for the Nobel Prize in medicine, also became a strong supporter of Schulz during his term as a Professor at the University of Greiswald. In fact, in 1931 Auguste Bier officially nominated Schulz for a Nobel Prize based upon the original research showing the low-dose stimulation of yeast in 1888.

Despite the strong identification of this concept with Schulz, numerous independent researchers such as Jensen commonly observed this dose-response relationship, often without any apparent knowledge that this biphasic dose-response was actually part of a controversial dose response concept of Schulz. Other investigators created a journal called *Cell Stimulation* based upon the Arndt-Schulz Law/hormesis concept. However, after what appeared to be a very successful initial six years, the publication was ceased in 1930 for reasons that are unclear.

The Arndt-Schulz Law, therefore, failed to thrive during the early decades of the twentieth century. The reasons for this failure are many. Although the intimidating presence of passionate and powerful opponents such as Clark were clearly critical factors in its demise, this law also failed because of inadequate leadership and organization, lack of understanding of its biological significance and experimental requirements and need for enhanced statistical power for assessing in low-dose treatments and a heightened need for replication. Numerous potential leaders who published papers on the hormesis concept never stepped forward on this issue or linked their findings to the scientific concepts embedded in the Arndt-Schulz Law. These included Benjamin Duggar, a notable researcher from the later 1890s to the early 1950s. Duggar, who first observed the hormetic phenomenon in the late 1890s as a graduate student in Germany, went on to have a very long, productive, and influential career, even being nominated for the Nobel Prize in 1950 following his discovery of the drug chlortetracycline (Aureomycin®), while working at the Lederle pharmaceutical company several years after his academic retirement at the age of 72 from the University of Wisconsin.

Perhaps the largest missed opportunity for influence was that Duggar had a close academic relationship with Alexander Hollaender, the creator of the Environmental Mutagen Society and director of the Oak Ridge National Laboratory from its creation in 1946 for nearly the next quarter-century. Charles Lipman, professor at the University of California and later Dean at that institution, published findings indicating that low levels of toxic metals enhanced plant growth. In fact, Lipman is believed to be the first scientist to present his data in a major litigation in support of the hormesis concept. Charles Edward Winslow, a very accomplished Yale University Professor, directed numerous graduate student dissertations in bacteriology with a strong focus on chemically induced biphasic dose responses from the mid 1910s until the early 1930s. Yet, Winslow, who was to become a major influence in the field as Editor-in-Chief of *Bacteriology* and the *American Journal of Public Health* until 1956, never communicated with Schulz and apparently never realized the public-health implications of the frequently reported hormetic responses by his stream of Ph.D. students. He never focused the attention of the public-health journal on the implications of hormetic dose-responses even though he observed these in his students' research for many years. Thus, although there were prestigious researchers whose findings were highly supportive of the hormetic concept, none stepped forward to either defend Schulz or challenge the traditional paradigm, or became fascinated with the inherent scientific questions raised by the hormesis concept or its implications as did Schulz. A notable possible exception to this general situation was August Bier, who himself became professionally damaged because of his support for Schulz despite his high standing within the scientific and medical communities.

The hormetic concept also failed to thrive because it was not well understood by its advocates and the scientific community in general. This lack of understanding was evident for most of the twentieth century. The most significant lack of insight relates to the quantitative dose response features, and that such dose-response features would originate via a direct stimulatory response or as an overcompensation response to a disruption in homeostasis (Figure 5.2). Numerous researchers had observed low-dose stimulatory responses following chemical or radiation exposures. This led to entrepreneurial attempts to exploit these observations for commercial benefit. This was typically true within the context of plant growth stimulation.

When experiments were conducted on the effects of plant stimulation, such as radiation, the results were often mixed as was the case with a massive research activity undertaken by the USDA. This study involved some 13 different agricultural research centers and 20 different commercial plant species. In this extraordinary undertaking, which tested the effects of radionucleides on plant growth/yield, the results were not generally supportive of the hormetic perspective. In effect this investigation was a type of death knell for the practical implementation of the hormetic concept into government-sponsored research programs. Even though the data did not support a hormetic interpretation, it must be emphasized that the research strategy and study design were amazingly inadequate to test the hormetic hypothesis, reflecting a lack of understanding by the organizers of this large study. No preliminary toxicity testing was conducted on any plant species; all species received the identical treatment, and only one concentration was employed in the study. Thus, it is hard to imagine that a poorer study could have been devised. Nonetheless, with the generally nonsupportive findings following such a massive effect, resources were no longer directed to this area.

5.1.4 Rebirth of Scientific Credibility and Centrality

Despite its experimental failings, medical opposition, linkage to homeopathy, difficulty to prove, and lack of understanding, scientists continued to publish a flow of papers throughout the decades of the twentieth century that were consistent with the hormesis hypothesis. During this first half of the twentieth century the hormesis concept became embodied in the terms Arndt-Schulz Law or Hueppe's Rule. However, in 1943 Chester Southam and John Ehrlich, apparently

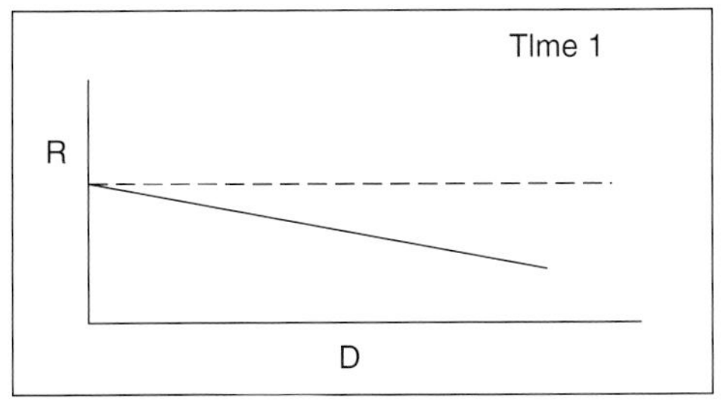

At Time 1 there is a dose dependent decrease, consistent with a toxic response.

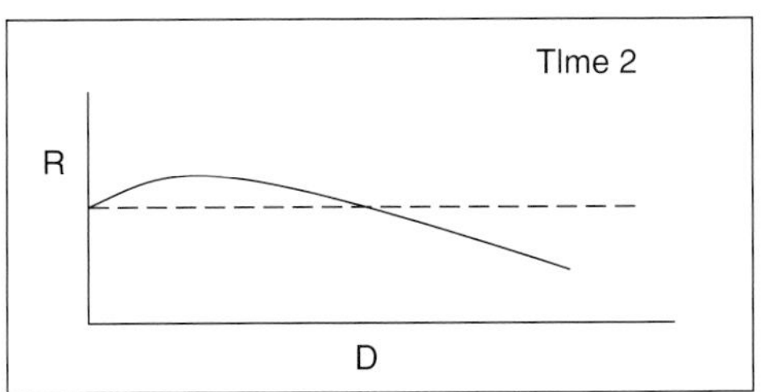

At Time 2 there is the start of a compensatory response, as is evident by the low stimulatory response within the low dose range.

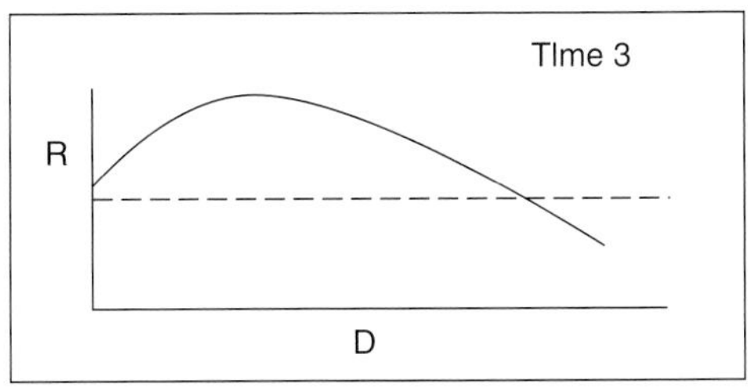

At Time 3 the compensatory response achieves its maximum increase over controls at the low dose. At high doses a complete compensatory response is not achieved. As time progresses the low dose stimulatory response may be expected to return to the control value.

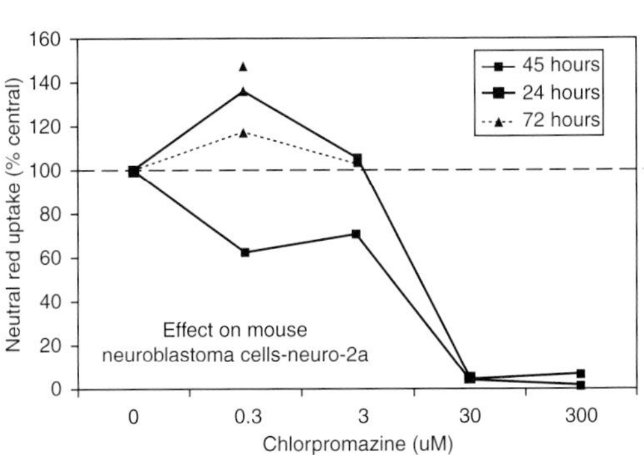

Example: Dose-time-response concerning the effects of chlorpromazine on neutral red uptake of mouse neuroblastoma cells. (Andres et al., 1999)

Figure 5.2 Overcompensation stimulation (hormesis) within a dose-time-response relationship. Response (R) on the vertical axis, dose (D) on the horizontal axis. (Source: Calabrese, 2005c)

unaware of the earlier terms, introduced the term hormesis (but apparently aware of bacterial studies, probably from Winslow's students) to describe a biphasic dose response, with a low-dose stimulation and high-dose inhibition. Despite its introduction in 1943 the term hormesis was not often cited until the 1990s following the publication of two books on hormesis by Thomas Luckey, several broad literature summaries, especially one in 1982 by Anthony Stebbing, a conference on radiation hormesis in 1985 (with the peer-reviewed proceedings published in 1987 in *Health Physics*), and a series of directed activities by BELLE and publications of Calabrese and Baldwin at the University of Massachusetts/Amherst. In fact, the term hormesis was cited in the Web of Science database only twice prior to 1982. By the end of 2006, hormesis/hormetic had been cited over 10,000 times in that database.

5.2 HORMESIS

5.2.1 Common Terms Used for Hormetic Dose Responses

Although now there are numerous articles citing hormesis in various scientific databases, there are numerous other terms that have been used to describe dose-response relationships with the same quantitative features of the hormetic dose response. These similar descriptive terms include Yerkes-Dodson Law, nonmonotonic dose-response, nonlinear dose response, J-shaped dose-response, U-shaped dose-response, biphasic dose-response, BELL-shaped dose-response, functional antagonism, hormologosis, overcompensation, rebound effect, bitonic, dual effect, bidirectional effect, bimodal effects, Arndt-Schulz Law, Hueppe's Rule, and subsidy gradient, among others. Thus, the hormetic concept was much more prevalent in the literature than the use of the hormetic term itself might suggest. In fact, it is not unreasonable to assume that for every literature citation using the term hormesis there may be 20 to 40 additional hormetic-like dose responses where authors have used a different descriptive term or perhaps where data, though reported, were not formally acknowledged in the results section of the papers nor mentioned in the discussion section or possibly mistaken as background variation and dismissed.

Of particular interest is that the specific description (i.e., terms used) for the hormetic dose response concept tends to be scientific subdiscipline-specific (Table 5.1). The use of different terms for the same dose-response phenomenon by numerous biological/biomedical subdisciplines has resulted from the normal and relentless evolution of biological subdisciplines becoming progressively more specialized. Although scientific specialization has yielded great benefits in terms of ever greater mechanistic insights, it also has resulted in progressively less communication between various scientific disciplines, even ones that have been historically closely aligned. As a result, each subdiscipline has created its own professional societies, journals, annual meetings, and academic-specific specialty departments. This typically leads to intellectual isolation, and conditions in which new terms are created with modified understandings and usages as the biological specialty interest evolves into a new subdiscipline. In the case of biphasic dose-response relationships there are now many subbiological disciplines, each with its own term and concept for what is argued here as most likely the same biological phenomenon. In this way each discipline has created its own term for the same or closely related concept, which this chapter calls hormesis. This procedure has undercut the capacity of the broader field of biology to recognize that the hormetic response is highly generalizable. Thus, due to the profound trend toward hyperscientific specialization, a basic and general biological principle has been missed.

Table 5.1 Hormetic-like Dose Responses with Differing Names by Different Scientific Disciplines

Scientific Disciplines	Descriptive Terms
Subsidy gradient	Ecology
U-shaped	Epidemiology
Yerkes-Dodson law	Behavioral psychology
Bell-shaped	Pharmacology
Nonmonotonic	Human toxicology/risk assessment
Functional antagonism	Pharmacology
J-shaped	Epidemiology
Adaptive response	Radiation biology
Biphasic dose response	Many disciplines
Arndt-Schulz law	Historical value only

5.2.2 Evidence Supporting Hormesis

In light of the fact that numerous terms have been employed to describe hormetic dose-responses and often investigators fail to recognize and acknowledge this effect in their published data, a hormetic database was created in order to systematically collect and assess hormetic dose-responses. The information collected has permitted an evaluation of the quantitative features of the hormetic dose-response relationship, but it has also revealed that hormetic dose-responses occur independent of biological model, endpoint measured, and chemical class. Based upon information contained in this database several dozen dose-response relationships were selected in order to demonstrate the occurrence of hormetic dose-responses across model, endpoint, and chemical class (Figure 5.3).

In addition to this database, a second database was created by Calabrese and Baldwin in order to estimate the frequency of hormesis in the toxicological and pharmacological literature using *a priori* entry and evaluative criteria. This second database was created based on the suggestion by Kenny Crump of Environ Corporation that a frequency expectation of hormesis in the toxicological literature was needed in order to evaluate its potential public health significance. Based on this second database a frequency of hormesis was estimated at approximately 40%. That is, for every 100 dose-responses satisfying the entry study design criteria, 40% satisfied the *a priori* evaluative criteria for hormesis. These data were then used to assess whether the traditional threshold model or the hormetic dose-response model was more frequent in the toxicological and pharmacological literature. In this head-to-head comparison the threshold model was observed to poorly predict below-threshold responses whereas the hormetic model was quite effective. These observations were subsequently supported in an evaluation of a U.S. NCI database evaluation of 57,000 dose responses of 2200 potential antitumor agents with a built-in replication feature.

This study demonstrated that the hormetic model was highly effective in estimating responses below the toxic threshold whereas the threshold model again failed to do so. This type of evidence suggests that the threshold model may have an inherent flaw that precludes accurate predictions of low-dose effects whereas the opposite appears to be the case for hormesis.

Despite the fact that the hormetic dose-response is very generalizable and has out-competed and shown the significant limitations of the threshold model, it is not possible at present to absolutely identify and prove hormesis. That is, hormesis is a dose-response phenomenon, not a specific effect. Judgments can be made about hormesis based on the strength of the study design, statistical power, magnitude of the response, reproducibility of the findings and whether the dose-response can be effectively deconstructed and reconstructed via the use of the synthetic agonists and antagonists.

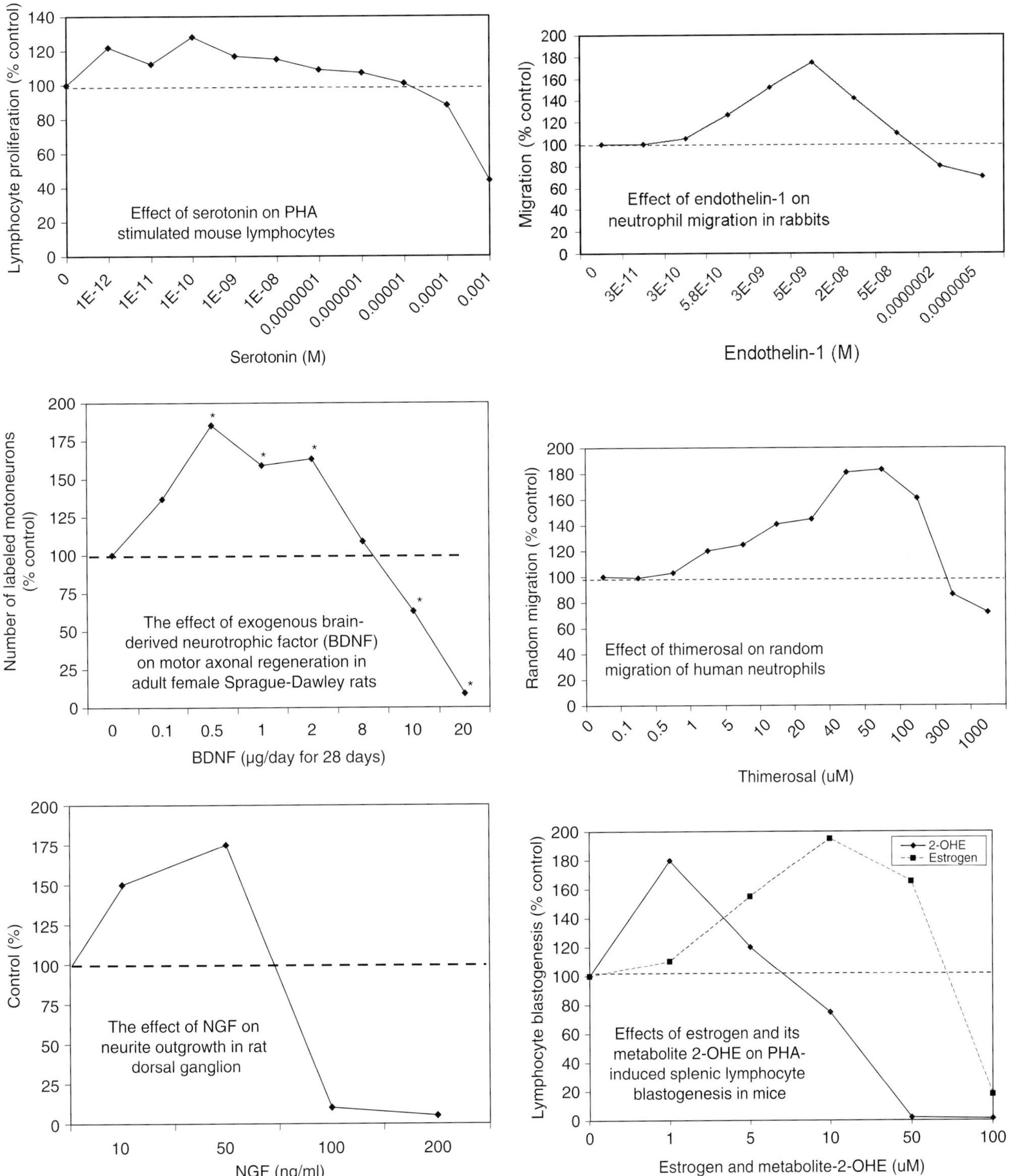

Figure 5.3 Representative biomedical hormetic dose responses.

(Continued)

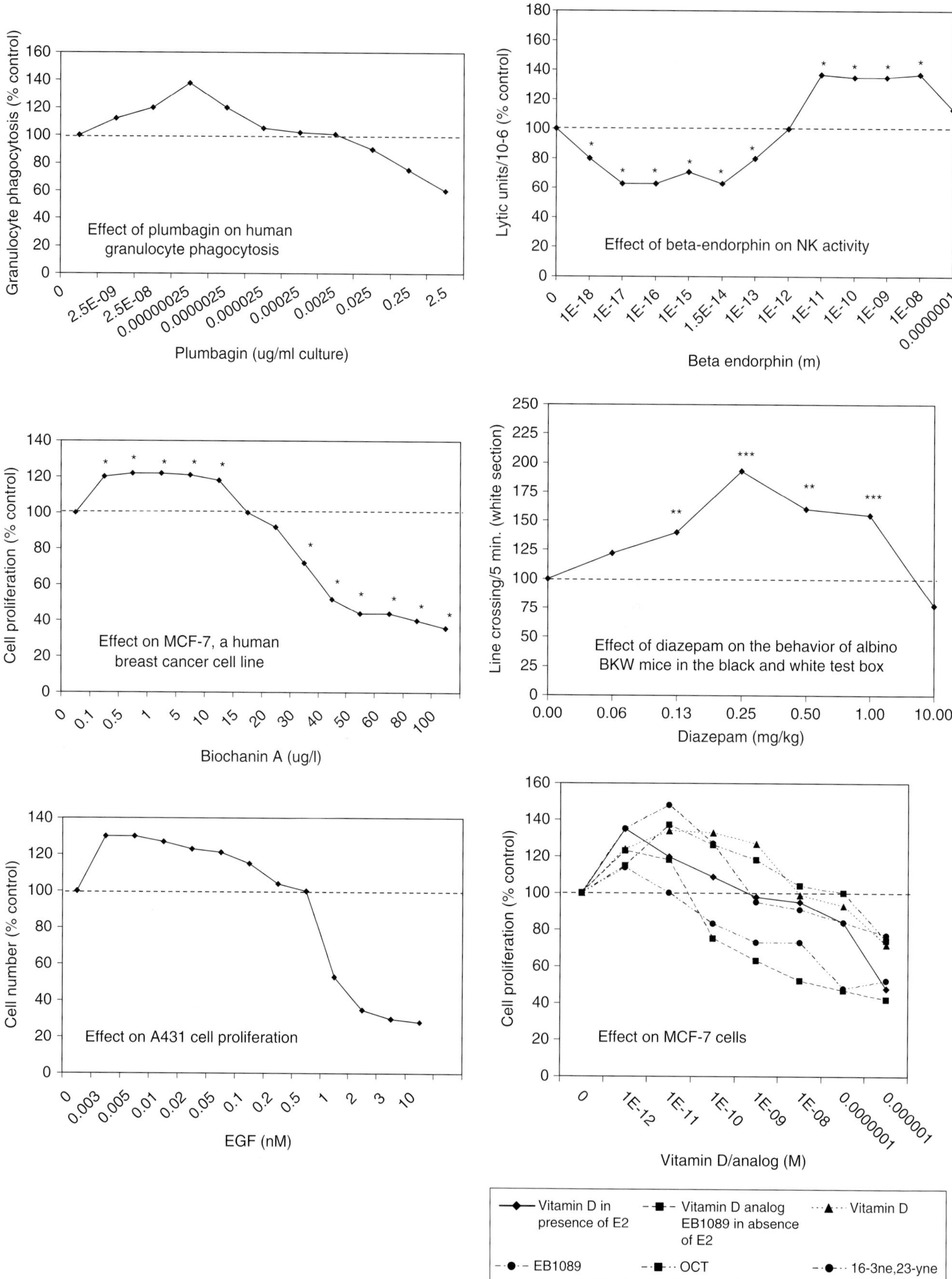

Figure 5.3, Cont'd.

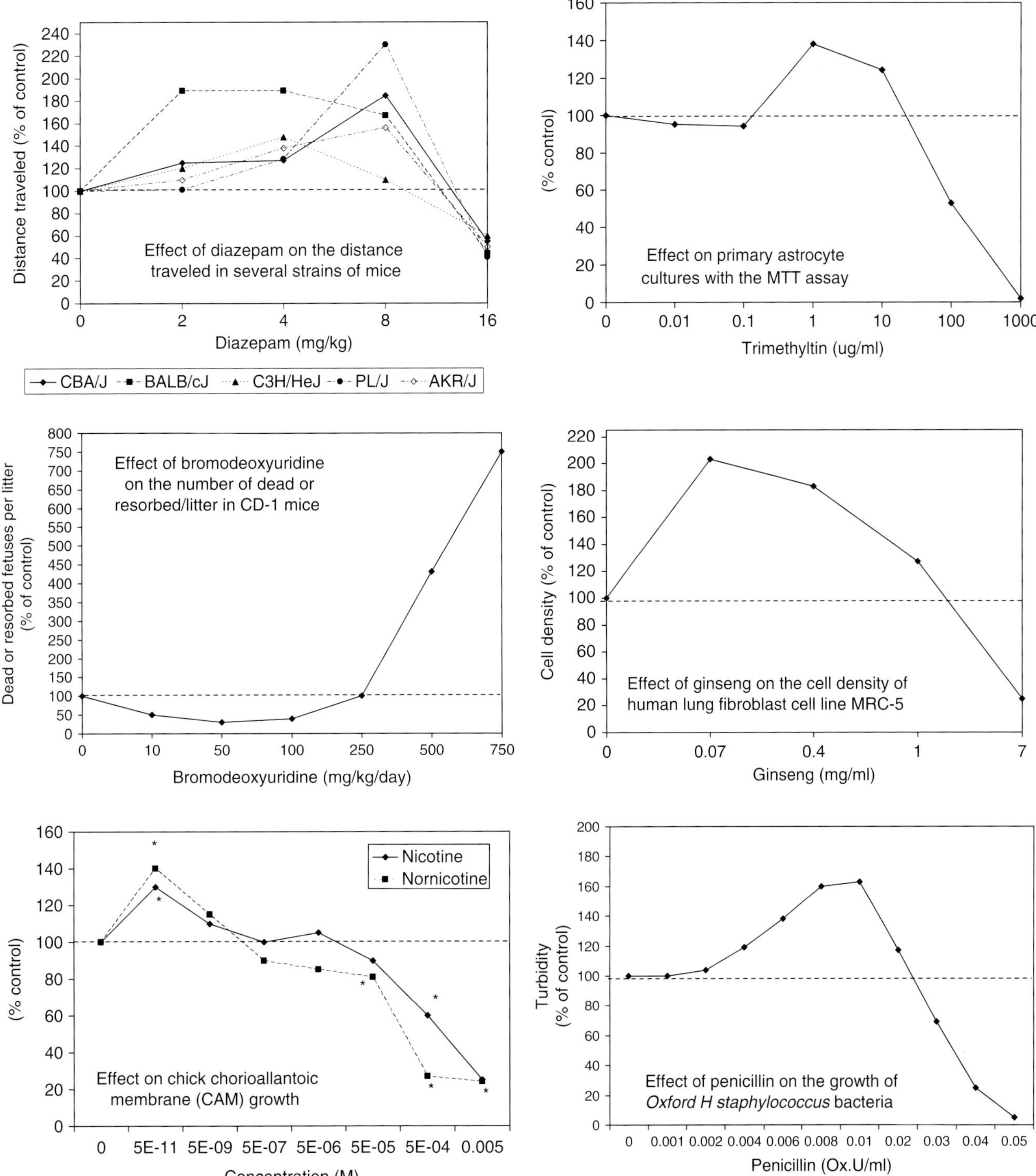

Figure 5.3, Cont'd.

(Continued)

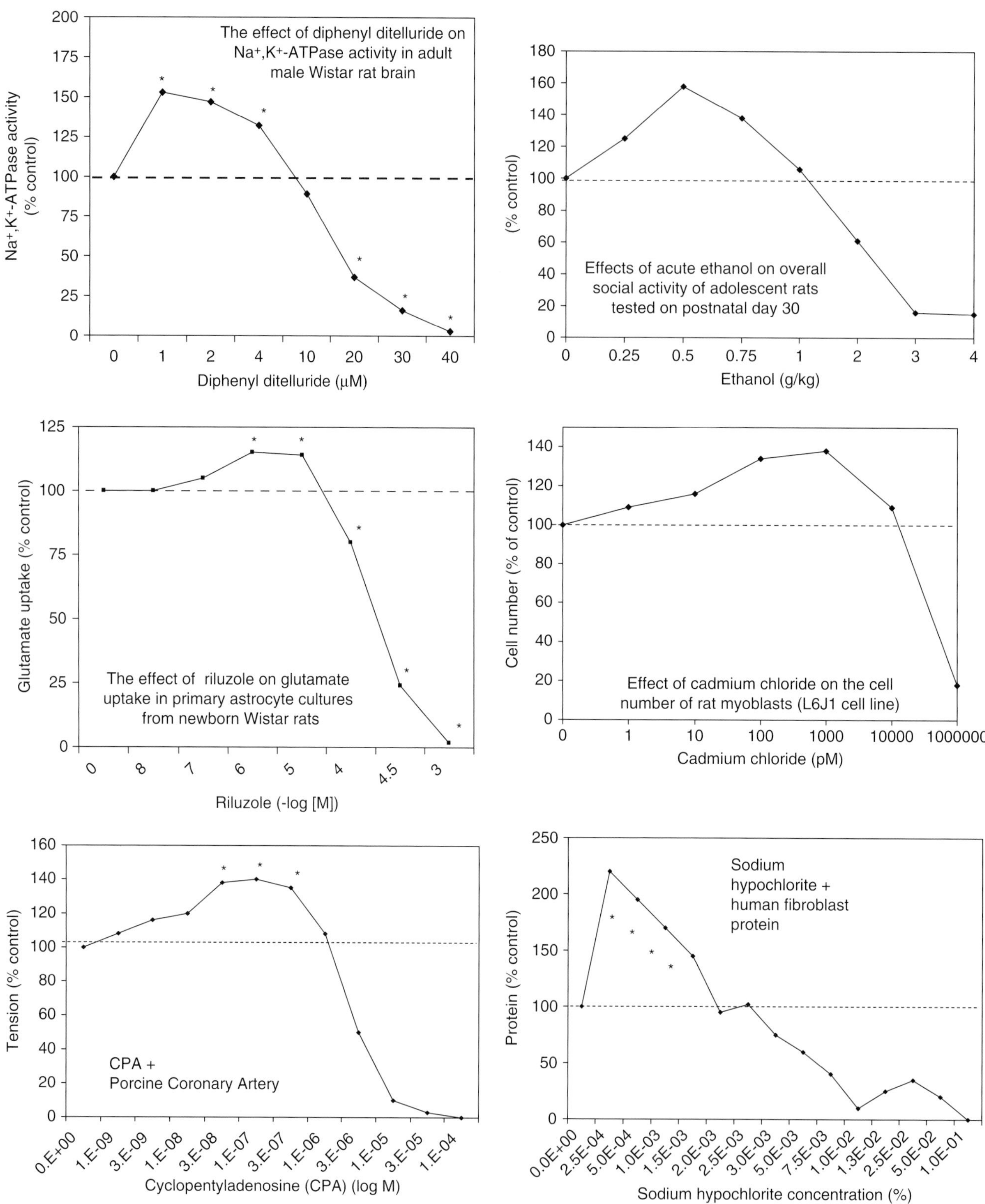

Figure 5.3, Cont'd.

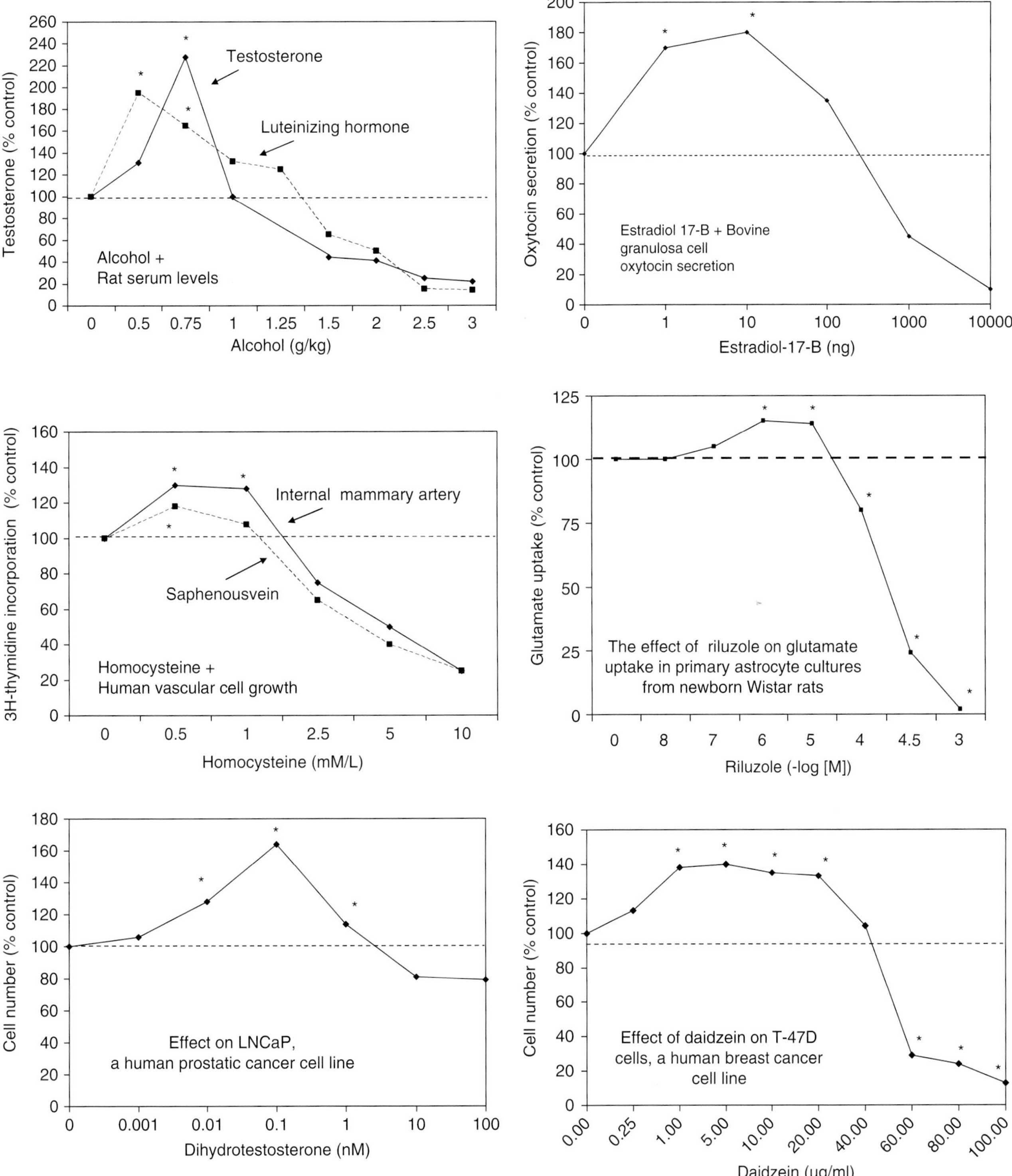

Figure 5.3, Cont'd.

(Continued)

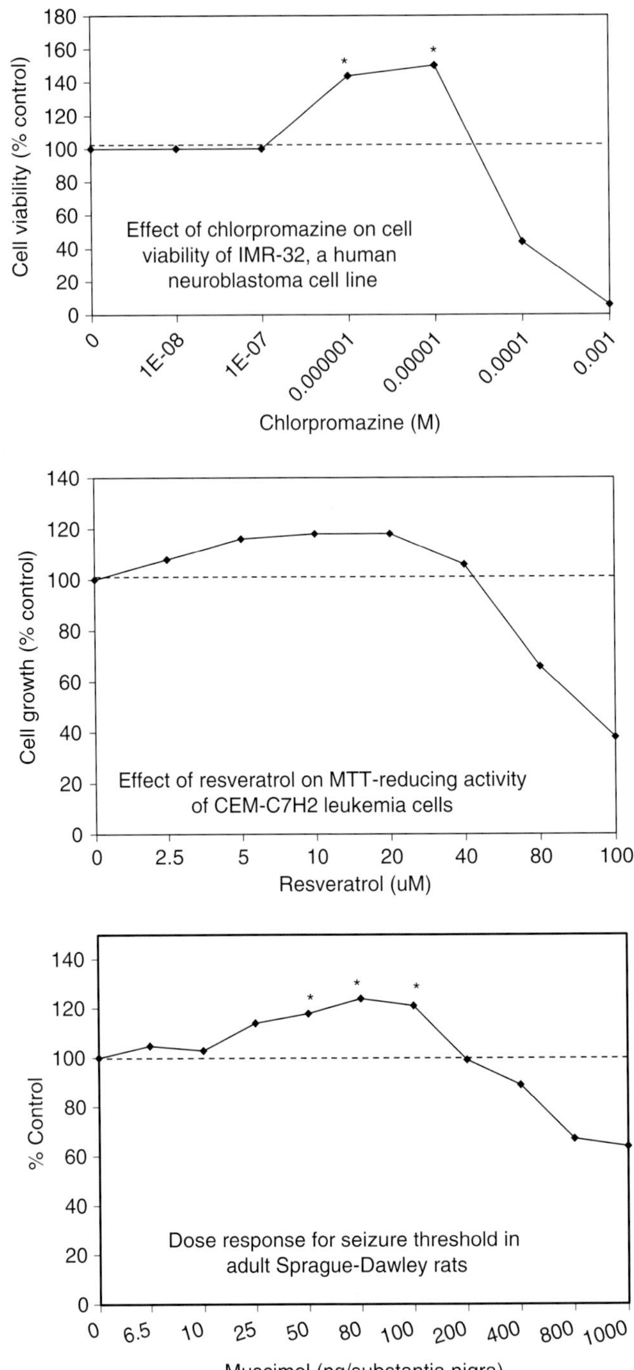

Figure 5.3, Cont'd.

5.2.3 Hormesis Characteristics

The hormesis database, as we just noted, has been created based upon *a priori* evaluative criteria. These criteria included requirements relating to study design, control group characteristics, magnitude/range of the stimulatory response, statistical significance, and reproducibility of the findings. Information from about 40 fields of interest are collected on each hormetic dose response. To date there are nearly 8000 examples of dose-response relationships displaying dose-response characteristics that satisfied the evaluative criteria for a hormetic response designation. Detailed evaluations of this database have revealed that hormetic dose responses are independent of biological model, endpoint measured, and chemical class/

physical stressor, thereby suggesting that hormesis is a highly generalizable phenomenon. Yet, as suggested earlier, the vast majority of dose-response relationships that display hormesis have been described with other terms, thereby masking the frequency of this phenomenon in the literature.

5.2.3.1 The Hormesis Stimulation: Direct or Compensatory Response to Damage?

Key questions are why is the hormetic dose-response modest, and what are its implications? Considerable evidence indicates that hormetic dose-responses represent a modest overcompensation to a disruption in homeostasis. This was observed initially over a century ago by Townsend and extended to other biological models and endpoints in the subsequent decades. This was particularly the case with the research of Branham, who not only replicated the earlier research of Schulz, but clarified the dose-time response relationship. Similar observations were made by Smith, who demonstrated that stimulation of mycelium growth was a reproducible phenomenon except that it occurred only following the UV-induced damage, with the subsequent stimulation representing the modest overcompensation response now called hormesis.

These observations were essential to the refinement of the hormetic concept since they led to the conclusion that the stimulatory response was not a direct one, but one made as a rebound-like effect in response to damage. Despite these validations of the Schulz findings and their capacity to be generalized, this conclusion, surprisingly, was thought to be a refutation of the Arndt-Schulz Law, and was argued as such by several highly regarded radiation health scientists in the first half of the twentieth century. Among the highly visible leaders of the intellectual opposition was Holzknecht, who had studied with the X-ray discovering Nobel laureate, Willhelm Conrad Roentgen, for three years, developed the first method for measuring X-rays, created the International Society of University Professors of Medical Radiology, and who became the first European professor of medical roentgenology. As a result of his high standing in the field, Holzknecht's views were broadly influential and adopted by numerous international leaders, including Shields Warren, a prestigious Harvard University professor and the first Director of the Division of Biology and Medicine of the U.S. Atomic Energy Commission. In fact, the highly influential Warren reached the critical conclusion that the "assumption that small doses of X-ray or radium radiation are stimulatory (the Arndt Schulz Law) is invalid. The slight evidences of proliferative activity offered as evidence by the proponents of this hypothesis are in fact only reparative responses to the injury that has been done."

Warren was on solid scientific grounds in recognizing that compensatory stimulation typically was observed following tissue damage. Data to support the existence of such reparative overcompensation stimulation following radiation-induced damage have been widely observed and reported as seen in the reports of Hektoen, head of Pathology at the University of Chicago and later director of the U.S. NCI, with respect to antibody production, and numerous others in the early and mid decades of the twentieth century. Thus, the rejection of the Arndt-Schulz Law by notable leaders in the field of radiation health, including Shields Warren, which was based on a conclusion that the stimulation was merely a manifestation of a response to damage rather than a direct stimulatory effect, was perhaps the critical scientific judgment of the twentieth century that led to the marginalizing of the hormesis concept.

This highly visible and vocal opposition to the Arndt-Schulz Law as seen in the writings of Warren, failed to note that the process being rejected was a fundamental feature of the toxicological dose-response curve as seen in plant and animal models. This was the case regardless of whether the damage was caused by chemical agents or radiation. The compensatory stimulation was recognized as being modest (i.e., 30–60% greater than control values) and consistently distanced from the traditional toxicological threshold with an overall dosage range of about 10- to 100-fold (Figure 5.4). These observations supported the conclusion that this response was most likely compensatory following some degree of damage.

These observations should not have lead to a refutation of the Arndt-Schulz Law but to a more refined understanding of its temporal features along with its implications for the quantitative features of the dose response. Yet instead of offering such a biological-based refinement that could account for the low dose stimulatory response, leaders in the field rejected the Arndt-Schulz Law and the hormesis concept and the fields of pharmacology, toxicology, and radiation health followed their lead.

Over the next nearly seven decades the most provocative aspect in the evolution of the concept of hormesis was that it was now most consistently accepted as an overcompensation response following an initial disruption in homeostasis. This accepted definition of hormesis is ironically the same concept that was rejected by leaders in the field in the early to mid decades of the twentieth century. Although Holzknecht, Warren, and their colleagues were quite correct in recognizing that a modest stimulation predictably follows a disruption in homeostasis, they did not anticipate its biological and societal significance. This contributed to the long-term intellectual suppression and marginalization of the concept. Somehow the findings of Schulz were rejected even though they had been repeatedly replicated.

The research of Anthony Stebbing at the Marine Biological Station in the late 1970s and early 1980s provided the theoretical integration of hormesis as being based in a compensatory dose-time response relationship. The Stebbing insights were expanded by Calabrese, who found substantial support for this interpretation in the biomedical literature.

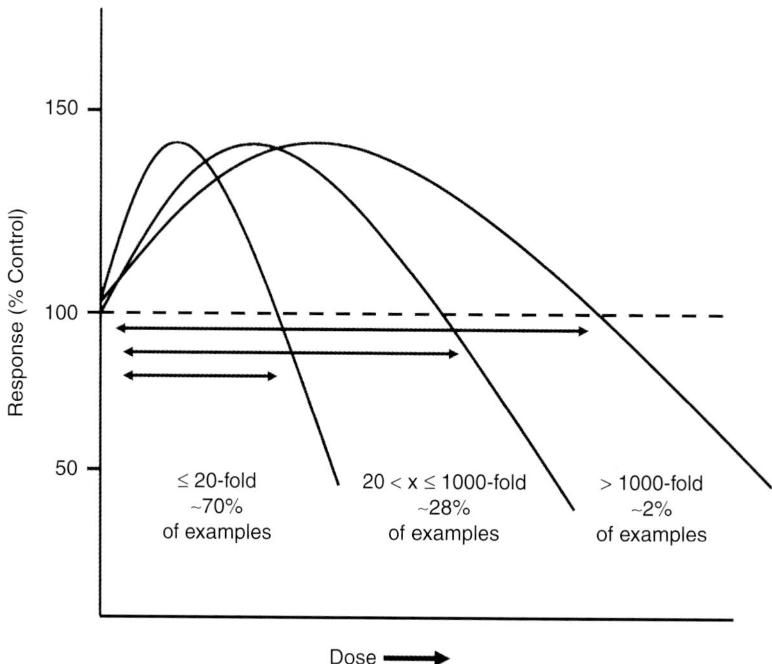

Figure 5.4 Stylized dose-response curves reflecting the relative distribution of stimulatory dose ranges. Note the maximum stimulatory response is usually 130–160% of the control value regardless of the width of the stimulatory dose range; the inverted U-shaped curve was used for illustrative purposes only, whereas examples in the hormesis database include both inverted U- and U-(J-)shaped curves depending upon the endpoint measured. (Source: Calabrese and Baldwin, 2003b)

5.2.3.2 Quantitative Features of the Hormetic Dose Response

Magnitude of Stimulatory Response The quantitative features of the hormetic dose-response have remarkable consistency. This is especially the case with respect to the maximum stimulatory response range, which is typically around 30 to 60% greater than the control. This relatively modest stimulatory response is the most consistent and distinctive feature of the hormetic dose-response. This modest magnitude of response provides significant challenges in the assessment of hormetic dose-responses as it becomes critical to distinguish a "true" hormetic response from random variation. It is therefore particularly important that hypotheses relating to hormesis have strong study designs, including special consideration for both the number and spacing of doses. Although there is no fixed operational number of doses, it is ideal to have sufficient doses that define the threshold and an adequate number of doses in the below-threshold zone in order to evaluate possible hormesis.

Hormesis may be missed by investigators where the low dose stimulatory response is not statistically significant. In such cases, numerous investigators may conclude that the nonstatistically significant modest low-dose response was due to background "noise" or random error. In these cases, the researchers may make a decision not to replicate the experiments using greater statistical power in the lower dosage range, a factor that may be necessary to pursue hypotheses relating to whether a hormetic response may exist in this experimental system. However, as often has been the case, investigators often wrongly substitute statistical analyses for professional judgment and experience, rather than using it to enlighten and contribute to such evaluative and decision-making processes.

Variability in Magnitude of the Stimulatory Response Even though there are highly consistent observations of a modest stimulatory response in the hormetic zone, this response can vary at times in a significant manner with an approximate 30-fold range (e.g., ~10–300%). The causes of this variation have generally been neither explored nor systematically evaluated. Possible reasons for this variability may include the following:

1. **Variability due to study design**. Numerous studies have shown that maximum compensatory responses to a disruption in homeostasis are highly dependent upon how many repeat measures are made after the exposure to the chemical/physical stressor agent. If multiple measurements are made over time, the stimulatory zone can be well characterized. However, the stimulatory response is often published for only a single time point. This lack of temporal characterization of response may, in fact, be the most significant factor accounting for what appears to be a widespread variation in the magnitude of the stimulatory response (Figure 5.2).

2. **Possible damage and response relationship**. There may be a relationship between the degree of damage and the magnitude of the rebound effects (or stimulatory response). This is a factor that has generally been ignored except for a few cases.
3. **Regulatory Dysfunction**. A relatively large stimulatory response (i.e., over twice the control value) may be a sign of metabolic dysregulation. That is, high stimulatory responses may be a biomarker of an inefficient allocation of repair resources.
4. **Inherent Biology Variation**. There may also be inherent differences in compensatory repair in different biological models, tissues, and cellular systems as might possibly occur in aged and diseased subjects.
5. **Law of Initiative Values**. This law, which was first developed by Joseph Wilder, states that the magnitude of a response to an experimental stimulus is related to the prestimulus level. Wilder argued that this framework described the effects of activating drugs such as adrenalin on various autonomic variables. Higher initial levels were observed to be associated with smaller increases in the activating stimulus.

The Ceiling Effect Concept It is both interesting and important to note that the field of pharmacology introduced the term *ceiling effect* principally since the early 1990s, although it was first used as far back as the 1940s. It describes a somewhat quantitatively vague idea that stimulatory responses can be limited and will eventually plateau. This concept has now become widely accepted and shown to occur for numerous pharmacological endpoints and has been reported in over 600 articles in the past decade. An examination of the ceiling effect literature suggests that in many instances the investigators, in fact, may have been describing the maximum stimulatory response of a hormetic dose-response without being aware of this possibility.

Width of the Hormetic Stimulation Another feature of the hormetic dose-response is width of the stimulatory response in the low-dose zone; that is, below the zero equivalent point or toxicological threshold. Of the many dose responses in the hormesis database, 60% have a stimulatory concentration range of less than a factor of 10, and about 2% have a stimulatory range more than 1000-fold. The reason for this variability in the width of the hormetic stimulatory zone is uncertain. It is likely that the predominance of the dose responses having a relative small stimulatory range may be related to the highly homogenous nature of the experimental organisms and rigid control of experimental systems. It would be expected that the stimulatory response range may increase if the population under study were more heterogeneous. The implications of a narrow or wide stimulatory dose zone associated with a therapeutic dose range will affect the dosing strategies and patient treatment plans.

5.2.3.3 Why the Hormetic Stimulation Is Modest

Compensatory Stimulation A basis for the modest stimulatory response may be found within the biological framework of hormesis as a compensatory response. When a tissue is damaged a repair or compensatory response is initiated. The reparative goal would be to reestablish the original homeostasis condition within a given period of time. An assessment of data within the hormesis database includes dose-response relationships with single time and with multiple time points. The dose-time response relationship permits an assessment of the actual dynamics of the dose response. At initial or early time periods after exposure usually only toxicity is observed in a dose-dependent fashion. Over time the organism/tissue responds to the damage with evidence of reparative processes. Eventually the tissue(s) and organism(s) show responses at low doses that modestly exceed control or baseline responses, whereas at higher doses the compensatory response usually is not able to return to the control value, a phenomenon commonly reported in herbicide research. The net result is the hormetic biphasic dose response with its distinctive characteristic features.

Natural selection provides one possible reason why the hormetic response is modest. Selection ought to favor organisms that repair damage in a timely or efficient fashion. Excessive overcompensation would probably be reflective of an inefficient utilization of resources that would mitigate against long-term survival. Thus, the hormetic stimulation would appear to be a resource allocation issue ensuring that repair occurs without waste of precious resources needed for other functions and survival. This is most likely a factor limiting the typical maximum hormetic response to less than twice (i.e., two-fold) that of control and a reason why the maximum responses are typically only about 30 to 60% greater than the control value (Figure 5.3).

The adaptive value of hormesis is seen in numerous observations demonstrating that the prior low dose stress response in the so-called hormetic response range also acts as a form of preconditioning that elicits protection against toxicity threats from subsequent toxic exposures. In this sense, the low dose hormetic response would confer a selective advantage to organisms that experienced an initial modest toxic exposure and in situations where the modest toxic exposure was followed by the more massive one; a situation that would be expected to occur in both nature and evolutionary history. It is important to emphasize that a characterization of the prior low-dose response (i.e., adaptation) tends to reveal an inverted U-shaped dose response, similar to the hormetic dose response.

As an adaptive response, the modest overcompensatory response is therefore an expected one, rather than an extremely large one (e.g., more than three times the control response). Although this toxicological explanation is consistent with natural selection evolutionary theory, especially with respect to optimal resource allocation expenditure for the organisms, it has very significant and practical implications for researchers, regulatory agencies, and pharmaceutical companies.

Direct Stimulation Despite the fact that a large number of studies support the overcompensation interpretation, most experiments (~75%) in the hormesis database have multiple doses but only a single time point, making it impossible to assess hormesis as an overcompensation stimulation phenomenon in these instances. Under such circumstances it is not possible to assess the role of repair processes in the hormetic dose response. To make the situation more complicated there are a number of studies with an adequate number of doses and repeated measurements that reveal that some hormetic dose-response relationships seem to develop subsequent to direct stimulatory effects with no evidence of initial toxicity or inhibitory responses that are subsequently followed by compensatory stimulatory responses. Nonetheless, these examples of directly stimulated responses have the same quantitative dose-response features as those arising on account of the compensatory responses discussed earlier. Even though both types of dose responses (as a result of overcompensation or direct stimulation) likely employ different mechanisms, the same general quantitative features of the dose-response relationship emerge. This suggests that dose response features over a wide enough range of exposures may be related to the inherent plasticity of the biological system. The reason for the limited stimulatory response capacity may also be related to an overall adaptive strategy for proper resource allocation.

5.2.4 Hormetic Mechanisms

Most mechanistic studies dealing with hormetic dose response relationships in the pharmacological field have focused on receptor mediation of the biphasic dose response. A common and highly documented means to account for hormetic dose responses has been by the use of single agonists that can differentially bind to two different receptor subtypes that lead to opposing acting pathways (e.g., muscle concentration and relaxation). This strategy has been used widely across different receptor systems regardless of cell type. Table 5.2 lists a large number of receptor systems that display biphasic dose response relationships, consistent with the quantitative features of the hormetic dose-response via the use of agonist-opposing receptor subtypes as noted earlier. The means by which a hormetic biphasic dose response may originate may be even more complex, involving receptor cross-talk features. However, regardless of the specific tactic employed, the quantitative features of the hormetic dose-response are similar.

5.2.4.1 Proximate Mechanisms

Since thousands of examples of hormesis-like biphasic dose-responses exist in highly diverse biological systems, it is likely that there is no single proximate mechanistic explanation. Since there are probably unique proximate mechanisms for each example of hormesis, could there still be a more general "mechanism," and if so, what type of mechanism could it be? In essence, this question is divided into whether the quantitative features of the hormetic dose response, more specifically, the modest stimulatory responses that occur independent of model, endpoint, and agent has originated independently in each species or is a common ancestral trait that has been highly conserved and is therefore broadly generalizable. If these were traits that evolved *de novo* independently for the same functional response, then a universal selective pressure would have had to occur. The alternative argument is that early in evolution the hormetic response was selected and conserved as life evolved from single cells to more complex levels of organization. If this were the case, then the hormetic dose response would be highly conserved and more basic than the plethora of reported proximate mechanisms for its final explanation.

Table 5.2 A Partial Listing of Receptor Systems Displaying Biphasic Dose-Response Relationships (Source: Calabrese and Baldwin, 2003b)

Adenosine	Neuropeptides[1]
Adrenoceptor	Nitric oxide
Bradykinin	N-methyl-D-aspartate (NMDA)
Cholecystokinin (CCK)	Opioid
Corticosterone	Platelet-derived growth factor
Dopamine	Prolactin
Endothelin	Prostaglandin
Epidermal growth factor	Somatostatin
Estrogen	Spermine
5-hydroxytryptamine (5-HT) (serotonin)	Testosterone
Human chorionic gonadotrophin	Transforming growth factor β
Muscarinic	Tumor necrosis factor α

[1]For example, substance P and vasopressin.

5.2.4.2 A Possible Common Mechanistic Strategy for Hormesis

Since the hormetic response is generalizable and exhibits a consistent quantitative magnitude across species, it can be viewed allometrically. Could allometric scaling of hormetic responses be linked to allometric genes that provide the underlying blue prints of organismal architectural design? This conceptual framework, which links hormesis to allometry, may be a means to understanding why such a broad range of dose responses using different proximate mechanisms (e.g., different receptors in different cells) appear quantitatively similar. It may be that the hormetic dose-response is a measure or expression of the plasticity of the biological system, and that this is a function of resource allocation. The proximate mechanisms that facilitate this response are cellular tactics acting in conformity to the more general strategy of adaptive response within the context of a coordinated system of resource conservation/allocation controlled by allometric gene clusters.

5.3 SELECTED ISSUES

5.3.1 Hormesis in Drug–Drug Interactions (DDIs) and Mixed Chemical Systems

The concept of drug–drug interactions (DDIs) is well established in pharmacology (see Chapter 12). So advanced has been the state of development that a variety of commercial products have long been used by pharmacies to assist patients in avoiding possible harmful effects from taking multiple drugs. Major reviews in the pharmacological literature concerning drug interactions were published as long as 40 years ago (also see Chapter 12). These influential publications summarized a considerable amount of information concerning DDIs, and also offered rational frameworks upon which new information could be added. They clearly highlighted the need for more systematic efforts to characterize DDIs, while affording a means to providing real-time information about DDIs in a real-life setting.

The need to gather and assess drug interaction information and to transfer this information to physicians and pharmacists experienced a major advance when the American Pharmaceutical Association (APhA) evaluated the best way to disseminate DDI information to practitioners. Their analysis identified the following key desirable features of DDI monographs:

- An assessment of the quality of the scientific literature reporting each DDI
- An assessment of the likelihood of occurrence and clinical significance of the DDI
- Provision of practical and specific recommendations concerning ways to avoid the harmful effects of a DDI

The APhA efforts culminated in a consensus document in 1971 called "Evaluations of Drug Interactions," the intent of which was to offer sufficient information to allow physicians and pharmacists to make "authoritative judgments" concerning specific drug interactions. This effort paved the way for the collection of DDI information into commercial electronic data bases.

The efforts to compile and characterize information about DDIs into databases was paralleled by similar activities in the area of environmental health sciences regarding exposures to chemical mixtures. The U.S. EPA initiated work on the creation of Guidelines for the Health Risk Assessment of Chemical Mixtures in January, 1984, issuing final guidelines on September 24, 1986. The major difference between the two approaches was that the pharmaceutically oriented strategy was intended to prevent adverse DDIs from occurring in patients, whereas the EPA goal was to assist federal and state agencies in predicting the potential for toxic interactions associated with exposure to complex chemical mixtures in drinking water and ambient air. That is, the EPA guidelines were oriented toward public safety, whereas the DDI databases were developed to minimize adverse drug reactions in patients on an individualized basis.

The entire orientation of the assessment of complex chemical exposures and DDIs in the domains of public health/environment and pharmacy/medicine, respectively, was to prevent adverse health effects. Neither of these efforts took account of the possibility of hormetic responses. However, hormetic dose-responses have been reported within the context of complex mixtures such as petroleum, tobacco smoke, waste water effluents, and in studies with well-defined chemical composition.

With respect to pharmacological investigations, hormetic dose response studies have been emphasized in the extensive research of John Flood and colleagues concerning memory enhancing drugs. In their research numerous drugs were assessed for their capacity to enhance memory, principally in mouse models. In essentially all cases the dose responses were U-shaped. That is, drugs displaying the U-shaped dose response had an optimal dose that maximized the memory response in the mice, with performance decreasing at lower and higher doses. These initial studies led Flood and colleagues to explore whether these memory active agents would interact with each other and further enhance the memory process. The follow-up interaction studies did, in fact, reveal greater than additive responses in most cases. The combined drug treatments did not increase the maximum memory response in mice beyond that induced by a single agent (ceiling effect). However, the amounts of combined drug needed to achieve the optimal response (i.e., ceiling effect) were markedly reduced in the interaction experiments. The research of Flood was novel, possibly representing the first systemic evaluation of DDIs and hormesis. The authors acknowledged that they were unable to increase the performance (beyond what is now called a ceiling effect), but emphasized that possible side effects could be reduced by the combined exposures since the total amount of drug now needed to achieve the maximum performance was markedly reduced.

The findings of Flood are striking and profoundly insightful. These studies indicate that the concept of drug interaction is different when dealing with a therapeutic outcome rather than toxicity. In the case of a therapeutic outcome such as memory we are concerned with a hormetic dose-response. These findings suggest that the magnitude of the hormetic response remains capped by the ceiling effect. Nevertheless, this ceiling effect can be achieved at lower doses of two drugs acting synergistically, opening the door to sustaining a benefit while reducing the risks. If this concept is broadly generalizable it has significant implications for toxicological and pharmacological theory, clinical medicine, and the pharmaceutical industry.

That drug or chemical interactions might be constrained by hormetic dose response relationships possessing ceiling effect limitations is a phenomenon that may extend to broad research areas and biology in general. For the pharmaceutical industry this suggests that limits in biological plasticity might constrain maximum responses of drug combinations to something less than two-fold as is seen in most hormetic dose-response curves.

Interaction studies have also been investigated in other pharmacological systems, including those dealing with opiate receptors and potential involvement with epileptic seizures using animal models. More specifically, morphine interacts in a synergistic manner with the opiate antagonist naltrexone to enhance the threshold of epileptic seizures in the mouse model. Of particular note is that the synergistic interaction was seen principally at the level of doses eliciting low percentage responses, an observation consistent with the observations by Flood and coworkers.

5.3.2 Epidemiological Considerations: Issue of Population Heterogeneity

If a population were comprised of multiple subgroups widely differing in susceptibility to a chemical agent this could have a significant effect on the assessment of a hormetic effect. Two factors to consider are the dose-response relationships of the individual population subgroups and their relative percentage within the total population. Figure 5.5 plots a theoretical dose response (e.g., cognition) for five different populations (numbers 1–5) studied. In this figure each population is comprised of the same five subpopulation groups, each of which has a unique susceptibility profile (see dose response below graph). Hypothetical dose response curves have been created for each subgroup. These subgroups have been combined to create five different populations (1–5), all with differing proportions of the same five subpopulations. The figure plots the dose-response curve for each population. It is important to note that a population may or may not show a hormetic dose-response based entirely upon the relative populations of the subpopulation groups comprising the population and their dose-response characteristics. In this example, only groups 2 and 3 show hormesis. However, the only difference among these populations is the relative proportion of the subpopulation group. Other comparisons could be made using different dose-response characteristics

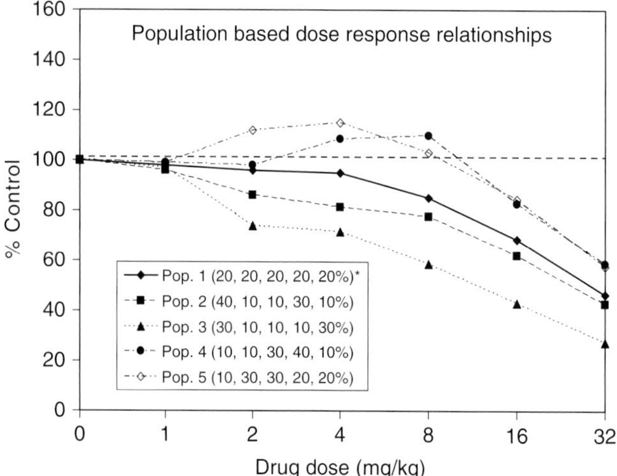

Hypothetic Dose (mg/kg)	Subpopulation 1	Subpopulation 2	Subpopulation 3	Subpopulation 4	Subpopulation 5
	Response % Control				
Control	100	100	100	100	100
1	90	100	100	100	100
2	60	120	100	100	100
4	40	105	140	110	80
8	20	80	120	145	60
16	5	70	95	132	40
32	2	55	60	95	20

*Population 1 is comprised of equal proportion (20%) of subgroups 1–5. See the relative proportions comprising the other populations (Populations 2–5). The numbers in the ( ) indicate the relative proportion of each subgroup comprising each population.

Figure 5.5 Population-based dose-response relationships in which each dose response is comprised of five distinct subpopulations (with unique dose-response relationships—hypothetical data not shown) in which a different proportion of the subpopulation (see legend) contributed to the total population dose response.

and populations subgroup proportionality assumptions, which could have resulted in other unique sets of population dose response curves. This exercise is of value since it indicates that population-based dose response evaluations (i.e., epidemiological assessment) if conducted in heterogenous populations, cannot always provide meaningful insight into the real nature of the dose response relationship, or insights into mechanism(s) responsible for the observed dose-response relationship.

5.3.3 Statistical Considerations

The statistical analysis of hormetic dose response relationships is amenable to a variety of strategies depending on the goals of the research team. The vast majority of experimental papers exhibiting hormetic dose response relationships have utilized analysis of variance methods in attempts to isolate doses that display statistically significant treatment related effects. However, over the past decade a number of other attempts have been made to model hormetic dose-response relationships. For example, in 1989 Brain and Cousens introduced low-dose stimulatory effects in dose-response modeling by modification of the four-parameter logistic function. Even though their publication was a groundbreaking effort, integrating the hormesis concept into mainstream biostatistical modeling, some of their procedures had limitations (e.g., requiring reparameterization) that restricted the model's range and application.

Other investigators have proposed the use of general linear model methods in which the dose variable is given in linear, quadratic, and under certain conditions higher-order polynomials. Use of such modeling has been criticized, since fitting a quadratic term to describe the hormetic effect requires several doses in the hormetic response zone, a condition that may often not be satisfied. In addition, this methodology has no parameter that directly simulates the magnitude of the hormetic effect. In light of these limitations Nina Cedergreen and her colleagues at the Royal Veterinary and Agricultural University in Denmark have recently proposed a new empirical model that can describe and test for hormetic responses in a broad range of dose response data, regardless of the slopes. Preliminary evaluation of the model indicated that it had a variety of advantages over previous modeling attempts such as the dose range over which it could detect hormetic responses and its handling of variability. Since the concept of hormesis is relatively new it is expected that statistical methods in this area will attract considerable attention with marked refinements.

5.4 ADAPTIVE RESPONSE, PRECONDITIONING AND AUTOPROTECTION: HOW THESE CONCEPTS RELATE TO HORMESIS

These three terms represent important concepts in the biomedical sciences. Each has its own origin and historical development and biological applications. Each has had an evolution that is unique and distinct from the other as they have tended to reside in different subsets of the biomedical research domain. However, all three are remarkably similar, if not identical, response phenomena. Historically, the concept of adaptive response originated from the initial findings of Leona Samson and John Cairns in 1977, which revealed that a prior low dose of a mutagen actually protected against the mutagenic effects of a subsequent and more massive dose of the same or different mutagens. This work was confirmed and considerably expanded over the next three decades and has become a central concept in chemical and radiation mutagenesis. The concept of autoprotection preceded that of adaptive response by almost a decade, and described situations in which a prior low dose of carbon tetrachloride protected against the capacity of a subsequent and more massive dose of this agent to cause toxicity and death. These findings have also been repeatedly confirmed and expanded to multiple organs and agents. The third concept is that of preconditioning, which was first reported in 1986 by Charles Murry and colleagues at Duke University who noted that a prior series of low ischemic challenges significantly reduced damage from a subsequent experimentally induced myocardial infarction in the dog model. As in the case of the other two concepts, preconditioning has been confirmed and generalized and is now a central feature in biomedical research.

Each of these concepts involves a limited prior exposure that leads to an enhanced capacity to protect the biological system against a subsequently more massive challenge. However, in each of these systems the adaptive-provoking doses have been shown to have an optimal range, and to display hormetic-like biphasic response relationships. These observations indicate that the biological phenomena of adaptive response, preconditioning, and autoprotection are all cases of hormesis, and further support the conclusion that hormesis is a central and highly generalizable concept in the biological and biomedical sciences.

5.5 IMPLEMENTING HORMESIS INTO PHARMACOLOGY AND TOXICOLOGY

The modest hormetic stimulation (i.e., ceiling effect) has profound significance for the fields of toxicology and pharmacology and the pharmaceutical industry. Regardless of the intended consequences of a new drug, the nature of the hormetic dose- response relationship strongly suggests that there are biological limits to the magnitude by which a drug can enhance a therapeutic outcome. In patient treatment this obviously has implications for efficacy as well as response expectations.

Hormesis should and can impact pharmacology in a variety of practical ways (Table 5.3), as described next.

5.5.1 Drug Discovery

The concept of hormesis should be formally considered in structure-activity-relationship (SAR) evaluation studies. If the low-dose stimulatory response is

Table 5.3 Overview of Biomedical Implications of Hormesis

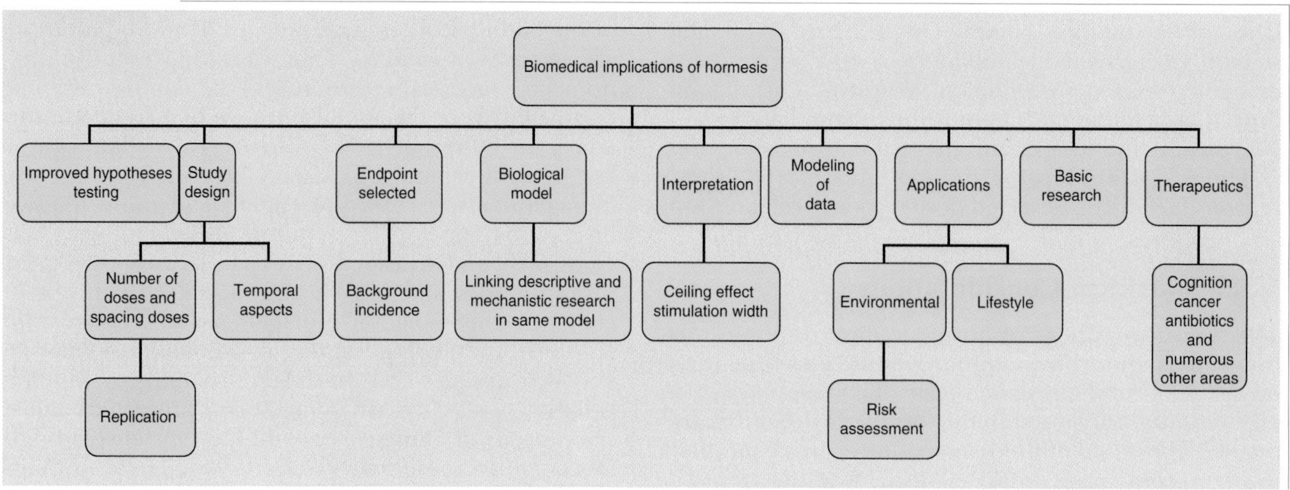

considered harmful to the patient and/or the general public, then the structural determinants contributing to that response should be identified and evaluated. Similarly, if the low-dose stimulation confers benefits to the patient or general public, then the relevant SAR features should be identified and retained. A growing number of researchers have explored the relationship of SAR and the hormetic dose-response relationship, using natural herbicides, natural fungicides, antidepressant and anxiolytic activities in animal models, and drug-enhancing cognitive responses. These papers are important since they suggest that the area of SAR can be applied with success to the assessment of hormetic dose-response relationships.

5.5.2 Drug Development

An important feature in drug development is the initial screening of candidate drugs. Although such screening methods can be quite variable, the concept of hormesis indicates that a critical factor in this process should be a cost-effective assessment of the dose-response continuum. The concept of agent screening can be significantly affected if it is assumed that the nature of the dose response is linear at low doses, follows a threshold, or is hormetic. This chapter has illustrated that hormetic dose-response relationships are common in toxicology and pharmacology and may be considered an expectation for many systems and endpoints. This suggests that preliminary screening activities need to have the capacity to identify and quantitate the hormetic dose-response relationship in early drug development so that candidate drugs are not lost or potential benefits unrecognized.

5.5.3 Selection of Animal Models of Human Disease

In the case of drug discovery and development, animal populations with a relatively high incidence of the target condition must be used. Subsequent drug treatments are designed to assess the extent to which they can palliate or cure the condition. The opposite strategy has been adopted in testing for chemical toxicity in animals. Animal models with a low spontaneous disease background are usually selected so that pathology doesn't confound observations of chemical toxicity. Otherwise an extraordinary sample size would be required. Unfortunately, minimizing background disease in animal populations virtually erases the opportunity to study hormesis, since little opportunity is left to improve function in already healthy animals.

5.5.4 Endpoint Selection

Although most endpoints are amenable to a hormesis evaluation, some commonly assessed endpoints are inherently problematic. For example, serum enzyme activities such as those routinely taken to assess liver toxicity, such as ALT and AST, would not be a means to study hormesis because any changes from normal, whether high or low, may be indicative of some underlying pathology. In order to assess whether liver changes would be reflective of a hormetic response it may be necessary to utilize an animal model with a high predisposition to liver disease or to create experimental conditions that would promote the early onset of liver disease.

5.5.5 Selection of Doses

It is essential that a broad dose response relationship be established. The initial goal should be to estimate the threshold response. This typically is achieved by high-end dosing to establish frank effect and lowest observed effect levels. Subsequent experimentation should be designed to explore possible subthreshold responses with the threshold as part of the frame of reference. In order to study subthreshold responses it is advisable to explore a 1000-fold dose range below the threshold, with semi-log dose spacing. This would involve the use of at least six doses below the established threshold.

5.5.6 Estimating the Threshold

The threshold may be estimated following a traditional EPA-based NOEL approach, which identifies the highest dose that does not differ from the control group in a statistically significant manner. This dose would be called the NOEL, and would serve as a quasi-estimate of the threshold. An alternative approach would employ the benchmark dose (BMD) methodology in which data are modeled to estimate a response that approaches the threshold response level.

5.5.7 Dose-Time-Effect

The hormetic dose-response can occur as an overcompensation to a disruption in homeostasis or as a direct stimulation. The incorporation of a repeated measures analysis component into the study design would be an essential element in both identifying and understanding dose-response relationships. Dose-time-effects relating to hormesis have typically been associated with the concept of a "rebound"/overcompensation effect with a robust supportive literature.

5.5.8 Clinical Relevance

The hormetic dose response model indicates that the maximum stimulatory response is modest, being best described as a ceiling effect with the maximum response occurring typically between 30 and 60% greater than control responses. The clinical implications of increases of this limited magnitude must be appreciated in order to determine the clinical effectiveness of pharmaceutical agents.

5.5.8.1 Drug–Drug Interactions Revisited

Multiple agents inducing hormetic dose response relationships display interactions that are equal to or greater than additive responses. However, a key feature of hormetic drug–drug interactions is that they would be expected to be constrained by the response ceiling effect. Thus, the resultant interactions likely would not increase the response beyond that imposed on the system by its inherent plasticity. The maximum interaction response therefore likely would be within two-fold of the control value. However, the doses of individual agents needed to achieve the effect could be profoundly lowered by the interaction.

5.5.9 Some Examples of Hormesis in Pharmacology

5.5.9.1 Diuretics, Bone Strength, and Hormesis

Epidemiological studies from several research teams have reported that long-term use of thiazide diuretics, such as hydrochlorothiazide (HCTZ), increase bone density and reduce hip fractures. These findings were consistent with numerous clinical observations that thiazides reduced urinary calcium resorption, which could lead to increased serum calcium levels and a reduction in serum parathyroid hormone (PTH) concentrations. These effects would be expected to minimize bone resorption. HCTZ has a direct inhibitory effect on bone resorption, and it also had a direct anabolic effect on human osteoblasts *in vitro* with the response conforming to a hormetic-like biphasic dose response with a maximum stimulation of about 60%. The recommended therapeutic drug dose of HCTZ in patients ranges from 12.5 to 100 mg, yielding serum concentrations up to 1 μM. The effective concentrations of HCTZ that elicit an anabolic effect on osteoblasts *in vitro* were between 0.1 and 1 μM, well within the clinically relevant serum HCTZ levels. Although still speculative, the *in vitro* hormetic anabolic effect may therefore be clinically relevant, and may contribute to the beneficial effect of HCTZ on bone mineral density and hip fracture rates.

5.5.9.2 Chemotherapeutic Antitumor Agents

The effects of numerous chemotherapeutic agents have been assessed for their capacity to inhibit the replication of various tumor cell types. Many of these investigations have led to the generally unexpected observations of biphasic dose-response relationships with a stimulatory response at low doses and inhibitory responses at higher doses consistent with the hormetic dose-response findings. Hormetic dose-responses were noted by Calabrese in more than 130 tumor cell lines from over 30 tissue types for over 120 different agents. The quantitative features of these dose response relationships were similar regardless of the tumor cell line or agent evaluated. This could have serious ramifications for the design of treatment cycles. For example, agents with long biological half-lives would be of particular concern due to persistence in the patient for several weeks in concentrations low enough to be dose stimulatory to tumors (e.g., suramin).

5.5.9.3 Minoxidil

Attempts to grow hair by chemical treatment have had a long history. However, in 1980, it was reported that minoxidil, a systemic antihypertensive agent, enhanced the growth of hair in patients. Over the next two decades minoxidil became the most widely employed drug to treat androgenic alopecia (AGA). The mechanism by which minoxidil enhances hair growth involves, at least to some extent, the restoration of normal keratinocyte proliferation via the regulation of calcium channels by its metabolite, minoxidil sulfate.

In more recent years there has been a focus on the direct effects of minoxidil on keratinocytes. However, such findings have not yielded a consistent and clear assessment of the effects of minoxidil due to the wide variety of cell sources, culture conditions, and different research methods employed. As a result of this lack of clarity an extensive and highly systematic study was conducted by Boyera and colleagues of the effects of minoxidil on human keratinocytes from different donors, different sources (i.e., interfollicular keratinocytes, follicular keratinocytes from microdissected hairs or plucked hairs), a diverse set of experimental conditions (e.g., high and low calcium medium, with or without serum, high or low epidermal growth factor content), using multiple but complementary endpoints to assess cellular proliferation (i.e., BrdU incorporation, mitochondrial dehydrogenase activity, lysosome content, protein content, lactate dehydrogenase release, and involucrin expression). The experiments revealed that regardless of the specific experimental condition assessed, minoxidil induced a biphasic concentration-response curve with stimulatory effects at low (i.e., micromolar) concentrations, and antiproliferative, pro-differentiative and partial cytotoxic effects at higher concentrations (i.e., millimolar).

This study is extraordinary due to the large number of experimental conditions tested, the number of endpoints, and the broad range of concentrations assessed. The overall consistency of the dose-response relationships that emerged adds considerable reliability to the findings. The dose-response relationship revealed that the amplitude of the stimulatory response was typically in the range of 15 to 30% greater than control with a stimulatory concentration range of approximately 10- to 100-fold. Despite the changes in experimental conditions and the use of multiple endpoints, the consistency in the quantitative features of the dose-response relationships is remarkably striking.

The relevance of the biphasic concentration response for the chemical use of minoxidil remains speculative. In general, the maximum plasma levels of minoxidil following systemic administration of hair growth-promoting doses is 0.775 μM, a value that consistently induces stimulatory cell proliferation responses *in vitro*. Thus, minoxidil treatment at low doses should maintain keratinocyte proliferation in pathological conditions such as AGA, while concomitantly retarding premature commitment to differentiative pathways. However, the authors noted that it is possible that minoxidil may accumulate in some compartments of the follicle, especially the hair shaft rich in keratins and melanins. Resultant millimolar concentrations of the drug could occur adjacent to the keratogenic zone, thereby favoring keratinocyte differentiation along with hair shaft thickening.

5.6 REMAINING ISSUES

5.6.1 Are Hormetic Effects Beneficial?

Hormesis is a dose-response phenomenon characterized by low-dose stimulation and high-dose inhibition. The determination of whether the hormetic stimulation is beneficial or not should be decoupled from a decision as to whether the response is hormetic or not. Hormetic effects themselves can be beneficial, neutral, or harmful depending on the specific circumstances. For example, a low-level exposure to an antibiotic may stimulate the growth of harmful bacteria that could be harmful to human patients yet theoretically beneficial to the bacteria. As a general concept, hormesis is an adaptive response that has been evolutionarily favored and is highly conserved. Therefore, it would be expected to confirm benefit to the species and individual. However, there can be situations in which adaptive responses may become maladaptive, and these need to be carefully evaluated.

5.6.2 Does Hormesis Impose a Cap on Drug-Induced Benefits or Performance Improvements?

Pharmaceuticals can be used to improve human and animal health in many ways. This may include the killing of harmful microorganisms and tumor cells or the enhancement of various types of performance in many complex biological systems or processes, including the immune system, hair growth, cognitive function, and others. However, the hormetic dose-responses have defined the plasticity of drug enhancing performance to be in the 30 to 60% range at maximum. These observations of hormetically-constrained performance limitations have important implications for setting appropriate levels of expectations in drug development and the clinic.

5.6.3 Statistical Significance and Hormesis

Hormetic dose responses often have been overlooked or dismissed incorrectly or prematurely because the low-dose stimulation may not have achieved statistical significance. Given the mild limits of enhancement of the (hormetic) stimulatory responses, the low-dose end of dose-response experiments should be sufficiently powered to affirm or deny the existence of hormesis.

5.6.4 Cell Culture and Hormesis

The extensive expansion of cell culture studies in the 1980s has had a major impact on the study of hormesis, because it has permitted the use of large numbers of doses to be evaluated with minimal costs. Since an evaluation of hormesis requires very powerful study designs with larger numbers of doses/concentrations and careful consideration of dose/concentration spacing, cell culture experiments have permitted detailed assessment of numerous hormetic hypotheses.

5.6.5 Drug Potency and Hormesis

One of the important features of the hormetic dose response is that agents of widely varying potencies exhibit similar quantitative features of the dose-response relationship. That is, more potent agents do not induce greater stimulatory responses though they elicit the stimulatory response at a lower dose.

5.6.6 Multiple Exposures to Hormetic Agents: Good or Bad?

The answer to this question is *maybe*. Evidence has shown that additive and greater than additive effects of these agents can occur when the exposures are sufficiently low and when responses are at or below the hormetic-imposed ceiling effect limit of about 30 to 60% above the control group. At higher doses the stimulatory effect quickly becomes less than additive, and at still higher doses inhibitory effects will occur.

5.6.7 Human Heterogeneity and Hormesis

There is considerable heterogeneity within the human population. In the case of hormetic dose-response relationships, the available evidence indicates that hormetic dose responses occur in subgroups with widely differing susceptibility. Although the quantitative features of the dose response for those with low and higher risks are similar, the hormetic response is shifted to the left in the more susceptible subgroups. On occasion, the hormetic dose response is not present in the more susceptible subgroup, suggesting that its absence may be a contributing factor to the increased susceptibility.

5.6.8 Will Multiple Effects Occur for the Same Treatment?

It is highly likely that pharmaceutical agents and toxic substances will induce multiple effects in different organ systems. It is also likely that each endpoint may display its own hormetic response with a unique dose-response relationship. Evidence for multiple hormetic dose-response relationships caused by the same agent for differing endpoints in different organs is not uncommon. This type of information is often hard to obtain since the findings are widely distributed in different biomedical subdisciplines and not integrated. In addition, most papers consider only endpoints related to a single organ system.

5.6.9 Are There Substances That Are Not Hormetic?

Factors affecting hormesis depend on the stressor agent and the biological system being stressed, challenged, or activated. Stebbing has long argued, and with considerable justification, that the organism is key and responds in a general fashion to a very broad range of stressor agents. However, it is also true that chemical specificity can be an important factor affecting the occurrence of hormetic dose-response relationships. Structure-activity relationship studies in the pharmaceutical domain have clearly demonstrated some of the structural determinants of hormetic dose responses. Both perspectives have validity and need to be integrated.

5.7 SUMMARY AND CONCLUSION

The hormetic dose-response relationship is not only the most fundamental dose-response relationship, but also a basic biological concept with extremely broad evolutionary, biomedical, and toxicological implications. The introduction of this concept into the central core of pharmacology and toxicology educational practices is both long overdue and essential for the development of these respective fields.

The history of the dose response in pharmacology is complex, having been shown to be one that has been strongly influenced by cultural norms, medical ideologies, economic competition, governmental influences, public health protectionist philosophy, and scientific studies and assessment. It has been the contention of this chapter that decisions concerning what is the most fundamental nature of the dose response have been dominated by factors other than the underlying science. Although there is strong documentation to support this conclusion, it can be hard to accept because it suggests that some of the very foundations of modern biomedical science have not been scientifically based.

This chapter describes how the scientific community has struggled with the dose-response concept, how it came to reject the hormesis perspective and ultimately settled on the threshold dose response model as a quasi-default model, guiding study designs and data assessment. In addition, this chapter has tried to challenge this perspective by presenting the dose response in a broader context and by permitting an evaluation of the entire dose response continuum including possible responses below and above the threshold dose. The data supporting the existence of the hormetic dose-response model is now not in question. However, it is still not yet agreed upon as to how general this concept is, and whether it could be considered a universal phenomenon and a missed general principle of biomedical sciences. Nonetheless, it is long overdue that textbooks in the field of pharmacology begin to incorporate the concept of hormesis as it is likely to have the capacity to transform study hypotheses, study designs, and the process of drug discovery, development, and clinical evaluation.

REVIEW QUESTIONS

1. What is the medical practice of homeopathy? How does it address the issue of dose response? Why would Hugo Schulz, the developer of the hormesis concept, have thought that he had discovered the underlying principal of homeopathy? Critically assess whether there is any scientific relationship between the concept of hormesis and homeopathy.
2. Proving that hormesis is not simply random error has long posed a significant challenge to the biomedical community. Is there a process that you can propose that would test that hormesis has occurred? What kind of certainty would be associated with this process?

3. Although it is claimed that hormesis is broadly generalizable and independent of animal model, endpoint measured, and chemical class, are there situations that exist in which hormesis cannot be effectively studied and assessed? If there are such situations, identify several and explain the underlying reasons why they cannot be assessed properly within an experimental setting.
4. Epidemiological research can have an important role in the public health assessment of drugs, chemical toxins, and radiation. Discuss the challenges that hormesis poses to the field of epidemiology as it attempts to better understand the nature of the dose response in the low-dose zone. For example, in the field of toxicology most biological models are very homogeneous, whereas in epidemiology, human populations are very heterogeneous.
5. Are biphasic dose-response relationships with similar quantitative features using different animal models, measuring widely differing endpoints and with highly diverse chemical agents, likely to be manifestations of the same biological concept? Discuss the pros and cons of this interpretation. Or should they all be treated as a specific phenomenon?
6. How could the concept of hormesis affect the process of drug discovery, drug development, and clinical trials?
7. How can clinicians utilize knowledge of the quantitative features of the hormetic dose-response in the treatment of patients?
8. Is the J-shaped dose response that is widely reported for alcohol consumption and various types of cardiovascular disease an example of hormesis? Why or why not? Explain.
9. Would you expect that the reason why some people are at higher or lower risk of experiencing drug side-effects is due to their lack of capacity to display a hormetic dose-response? Please explain.
10. Is hormesis a general principle in pharmacology or simply a paradoxical dose response that occurs in isolated situations? What is meant by paradoxical within the context of dose response? Would this characterization have relevance to the concept of hormesis?
11. How should the FDA address the question of hormesis in its data requirements and evaluation processes?
12. Should hormetic dose responses have to be demonstrated in each case or can it be assumed to occur if it is in fact far more common than the threshold response? Should there be a default dose response model? Why? Why not?

REFERENCES

Alexander, L. T. (1950). Radioactive materials as plant stimulants—Field results. *Agron J, 42*, 252–255.

Andres, M. I., Repetto, G., Sanz, P., & Repetto, M. (1999). Biochemical effects of chlorpromazine on mouse neuroblastoma cells. *Vet. Hum. Toxicol., 41*, 273–278.

Ariens, E. J. (1954). Affinity and intrinsic. *Archives Internationales de Pharmacodynamie, 99*, 175–187.

Ariens, E. J., & Degroot, W. M. (1954). Affinity and intrinsic-activity in the theory of competitive inhibition. 3. Homologous decamethonium-derivatives and succinyl-choline-esters. *Archives Internationales de Pharmacodynamie et de Therapie, 99*, 193–205.

Ariens, E. J., Van Rossum, J. M., & Simonis, A. M. (1957). Affinity, intrinsic activity and drug interactions. *Pharmacological Reviews, 9*, 218–236.

Ariens, E. J., Simonis, A. M., & Van Rossum, J. M. (1964a). Drug-receptor interaction: Interaction of one or more drugs with one receptor system. In E. J. Ariens (Ed.), *Molecular Pharmacology* (pp. 119–286).

Ariens, E. J., Simonis, A. M., & Van Rossum, J. M. (1964b). Drug-receptor interaction: Interaction of one or more drugs with different receptor systems. In E. J. Ariens (Ed.), *Molecular Pharmacology* (pp. 287–393). New York: Academic Press.

Barlow, R. B. (1994). Problems associated with the partiality of a partial agonist. *Trends in Pharmacological Sciences, 15*, 320.

Beck, B., Slayton, T. M., Calabrese, E. J., Baldwin, L. A., & Rudel, R. (2001). The use of toxicology in the regulatory process. In A. W. Hayes (Ed.), *Principles and Methods of Toxicology* (4th ed., pp. 23–75). Philadelphia: Taylor & Francis.

Bliss, C. I. (1935a). The comparison of dosage-mortality data. *The Annals of Applied Biology, 22*, 307–333.

Bliss, C. I. (1935b). The calculation of the dosage-mortality curve. *The Annals of Applied Biology, 22*, 134–167.

Brain, P., & Cousens, R. (1989). An equation to describe dose-responses where there is stimulation of growth at low doses. *Weed Res., 29*, 93–96.

Branham, S. E. (1929). The effects of certain chemical compounds upon the course of gas production by baker's yeast. *Journal of Bacteriology , 18*, 247–284.

Brenchley, W. E. (1914). *Inorganic Plant Poisons and Stimulants.* London: Cambridge University Press.

Bryan, W. R., & Shimkin, M. D. (1943). Quantitative analysis of dose-response data obtained with three carcinogenic hydrocarbons in strain C3H male mice. *Journal of the National Cancer Institute, 3*, 503–531.

Buchanan, R. E., & Fulmer, E. I. (1930). *Physiology and Biochemistry of Bacteria. Vol. II. Effects of Environment Upon Microorganisms.* Baltimore, MD: The Williams and Wilkins Company.

Calabrese, E. J. (2005a). Paradigm lost, paradigm found: The re-emergence of hormesis as a fundamental dose response model in the toxicological sciences. *Environmental Pollution, 138*, 378–411.

Calabrese, E. J. (2005b). Hormetic dose-response relationships in immunology: Occurrence, quantitative feature of the dose response, mechanistic foundations, and clinical implications. *Critical Reviews in Toxicology, 35*, 89–295.

Calabrese, E. J. (2005c). Cancer biology and hormesis: Human tumor cell lines commonly display hormetic (biphasic) dose responses. *Critical Reviews in Toxicology, 35*, 463–582.

Calabrese, E. J. (2005d). Historical blunders: How toxicology got the dose-response relationship half right. *Cellular and Molecular Biology, 51*, 643–654.

Calabrese, E. J. (2004a). Hormesis: From marginalization to mainstream. A case for hormesis as the default dose-response model in risk assessment. *Toxicology and Applied Pharmacology, 197*, 125–136.

Calabrese, E. J. (2003). Special issue: Hormesis: Environmental and biomedical perspectives—Introduction. *Critical Reviews in Toxicology, 33*(3–4), 213–214.

Calabrese, E. J. (2001). Overcompensation stimulation: A mechanism for hormetic effects. *Critical Reviews in Toxicology, 31*, 425–470.

Calabrese, E. J., & Baldwin, L. A. (2003a). Toxicology rethinks its central belief—Hormesis demands a reappraisal of the way risks are assessed. *Nature, 421*(6924), 691–692.

Calabrese, E. J., & Baldwin, L. A. (2003b). Hormesis: The dose-response revolution. *Annual Review of Pharmacology and Toxicology, 43*, 175–197.

Calabrese, E. J., & Baldwin, L. A. (2003c). Hormesis at the National Toxicology Program (NTP): Evidence of hormetic dose responses in NTP dose-range studies. *Nonlinearity Biol Toxicol Med, 1*, 455–467.

Calabrese, E. J., & Baldwin, L. A. (2003d). The hormetic dose response model is more common than the threshold model in toxicology. *Toxicological Sciences, 71*(2), 246–250.

Calabrese, E. J., & Baldwin, L. A. (2002). Defining hormesis. *Human & Experimental Toxicology, 21*, 91–97.

Calabrese, E. J., & Baldwin, L. A. (2001a). Hormesis: A generalizable and unifying hypothesis. *Critical Reviews in Toxicology, 31*, 353–424.

Calabrese, E. J., & Baldwin, L. A. (2001b). Hormesis: U-shaped dose-response and their centrality in toxicology. *Trends in Pharmacological Sciences, 22*(6), 285–291.

Calabrese, E. J., & Baldwin, L. A. (2001c). The frequency of U-shaped dose-responses in the toxicological literature. *Toxicological Sciences, 62*, 330–338.

Calabrese, E. J., & Baldwin, L. A. (2001d). Agonist concentration gradients as a generalizable regulatory implementation strategy. *Critical Reviews in Toxicology, 31,* 471–474.

Cedergreen, N., Ritz, C., and Streibig, J. C. (2005). Improved empirical models describing hormesis. *Env. Toxicol. Chem., 24,* 3166–3172.

Calabrese, E. J., & Baldwin, L. A. (1997). The dose determines the stimulation (and poison): Development of a chemical hormesis database. *Intern'tl. J. Toxicol., 16,* 545–559.

Calabrese, E. J., & Blain, R. (2005). The occurrence of hormetic dose responses in the toxicological literature, the hormesis database: an overview. *Toxicol. Appl. Pharmacol., 202*: 289–301.

Clark, A. J. (1926). *Applied Pharmacology* (1st ed., p. 430). London: J & A Churchill.

Clark, A. J. (1937). *Handbook of Experimental Pharmacology.* Berlin: Verlig Von Julius Springer.

Clark, A. J. (1933). *Mode of Action of Drugs on Cells.* London: Arnold.

Cokkinos, D. V. (2002). Preconditioning—A paradigm of yin and yang. *Hellenic Journal of Cardiology: HJC = Hellenike Kardiologike Epitheorese, 43,* 179–182.

Dale, H. H. (1906). On some physiological actions of ergot. *The Journal of Physiology (London), 34,* 163–206.

Davies, J. M. S., Lowry, C. V., & Davies, K. J. A. (1995). Transcient adaptation to oxidative stressing yeast. *Archives of Biochemistry and Biophysics, 317,* 1–6.

Davis, J. M., & Svensgaard, D. J. (1990). U-shaped dose-response curves - their occurrence and implications for risk assessment. *J. Toxicol. Env. Health, 30,* 71–83.

Duggar, B. M. (1948). Aureomycin—A product of the continuing search for new antibiotics. *Annals of the New York Academy of Sciences, 51,* 177.

Eaton, D. L., & Klaassen, C. D. (2003). Principles of toxicology, Chapter 2. In *Casarett & Doull's Essentials of Toxicology* (pp. 6–20).

Flood, J. F., Smith, G. E., & Cherkin, A. (1988). 2-drug combinations of memory enhancers—Effect of dose ratio upon potency and therapeutic window, in mice. *Life Sciences, 42,* 2145–2154.

Flood, J. F., Smith, G. E., & Cherkin, A. (1985). Memory enhancement—Supra-additive effect of subcutaneous cholinergic drug-combinations in mice. *Psychopharmacology, 86,* 61–67.

Flood, J. F., Smith, G. E., & Cherkin, A. (1983). Memory retention—Potentiation of cholinergic drug-combinations in mice. *Neurobiology of Aging, 4,* 37–43.

Furchgott, R. F. (1955). The pharmacology of vascular smooth muscle. *Pharmacological Reviews, 7,* 183–265.

Gaddum, J. H. (1936). The quantitiative effects of antagonistic drugs. *The Journal of Physiology, 89,* 79.

Gaddum, J. H. (1957). Theories of drug antagonism. *Pharmacological Reviews, 9,* 211–268.

Gaddum, J. H. (1933). Methods of biological assay depending on the quantal response. *Med Res Counc Ond Sp Rep Ser No 183,* London: H.M. Stationery Office.

Gaddum, J. H. (1962). The pharmacologists of Edinburgh. *Ann Rev, 2,* 1–10.

Garant, D. S., Xu, S. G., Sperber, E. F., & Moshe, S. L. (1995). Age-related differences in the effects of GABAA agonists microinjected into rat substantia nigra: Pro- and anticonvulsant actions. *Epilepsia, 36,* 960–965.

Heald, F. D. (1896). On the toxic effect of dilute solutions of acids and salts upon plants. *Bot Gaz, 22,* 125–153.

Hektoen, L. (1918). Further studies on the effects of roentgen ray on antibody-production. *The Journal of Infectious Diseases, 22,* 28–33.

Hektoen, L. (1920). Further observations on the effects of roentegenization and splenectomy on antibody production. *The Journal of Infectious Diseases, 27,* 23–30.

Henschler, D. (2006). The origin of hormesis: Historical background and driving forces. *Human & Experimental Toxicology, 25,* 347–351.

Honar, H., Riazi, K., Homayoun, H., Sadeghipour, H., Rashidi, N., Ebrahimkhani, M. R., et al. (2004). Ultra-low dose naltrexone potentiates the anti-convulsant effect of low dose morphine on clonic seizure. *Neuroscience, 129,* 733–742.

Hotchkiss, M. (1923). Studies on salt actions. VI. The stimulating and inhibitive effect of certain cations upon bacteria growth. *Journal of Bacteriology , 8,* 141–162.

Hussar, D. A. (1969). Mechanisms of drug interactions. *Journal of the American Pharmaceutical Association, 9,* 208.

Jarv, J. (1994). An alternative model for model-shaped concentration response curve. *Trends in Pharmacological Sciences, 15,* 321.

Jarv, J., Toomela, T., & Karelson, E. (1993). Dual effect of carbachol on muscarinic receptor. *Biochemistry and Molecular Biology International, 30,* 649–654.

Jensen, G. H. (1907). Toxic limits and stimulation effects of some salts and poisons on wheat. *Bot Gaz, 43,* 11–44.

Josephs, I. (1931). (Professor Doctor Fuido L. Ed.). Holzknecht. *Radiology, 17,* 1316–1318.

Kahlenberg, L., & True, R. H. (1896). On the toxic action of dissolved salts and their electrolytic dissociation. *Bot Gaz, 22,* 81–124.

Laughlin, R. B., Ng, J., & Guard, H. E. (1981). Hormesis—A response to low environmental concentrations of petroleum-hydrocarbons. *Science, 211,* 705–707.

Leuchenko, A., Bruck, J., & Sternberg, P. W. (2004). Regulatory modules that generate biphasic signal response in biological systems. *Systematic Biology, 1,* 139–148.

Lipman, C. B. (1909). Toxic and antagonistic effects of salts as related to ammonification by Bacillus Subtilis. *Bot Gaz, 48,* 105–125.

Lipman, C. B. (1915). Letter of C.B. Lipman concerning injuries by metals in the soil to the Selby Smelter Commission. In *Report of the Selby Ssmelter Commission.* Department of the Interior, Bureau of Mines, Bull. 98 (pp. 466–467). Washington Government Printing Office.

Luckey, T. D. (1980). *Ionizing Radiation and Hormesis.* Boca Raton, CRC Press.

Luckey, T. D. (1991). *Radiation Hormesis.* Boca Raton, CRC Press, Inc.

Middler, S., Pak, C. Y., Murad, F., & Bartter, F. C. (1973). Thiazide diuretics and calcium metabolism. *Metabolism: Clinical and Experimental, 22,* 139–146.

Miller, W. M., Green, C. A., & Kitchin, H. (1945). Biphasic action of penicillin and other sulphonamide similarity. *Nature, 1,* 210–211.

Murry, C. E., Jennings, R. B., & Reimer, K. A. (1986). Preconditioning with ischemia: A delay of lethal cell injury in ischemic myocardium. *Circulation, 75,* 1124–1136.

Mutscheller, A. (1925). Physical standards of protection against Roentgen ray dangers. *AJR. American Journal of Roentgenology, 13,* 65–69.

Oliva, A., Meepagala, K. M., Wedge, D. E., Harries, D., Hale, A. L., Aliotta, G., et al. (2003). Natural fungicides from *Ruta graveolens* L. leaves, including a new quinolone alkaloid. *Journal of Agricultural and Food Chemistry, 51,* 890–896.

Paton, W. D. M. (1961). A theory of drug action based on the rate of drug-receptor combinations. *Proceedings of the Royal Society of London, Series B, 154,* 21–69.

Paton, W. D. M., & Perry, W. C. M. (1953). The relationship between depolarization and block in the cat's superior cervical ganglion. *The Journal of Physiology, 119,* 43–57.

Quirk, S. J., & Funder, J. W. (1988). Steroid receptors, and the generation of closely coupled/biphasic dose response curves. *Journal of Steroid Biochemistry, 30,* 9–15.

Ray, W. A., Downey, W., Griffin, M. R., & Melton, L. J., III. (1989). Long-term use of thiazide diuretics and risk of hip fracture. *Lancet,* (I), 687–690.

Robison, G. A. (1981). Forward. In J. W. Lamble (Eds.), *Towards Understanding Receptors* (pp. v–x). New York: Elsevier/North-Holland.

Rovati, G. E., & Nicosia, S. (1994a). Lower efficacy: Interaction with an inhibitory receptor or partial agonism? *Trends in Pharmacological Sciences, 15,* 140–144.

Samson, L. & Cairns, J. (1977). A new pathway for DNA in *Escherichia coli. Nature, 267,* 281–283.

Salle, A. J. (1939). *Fundamental Principles of Bacteriology* (pp. 317–338). New York: McGraw-Hill Book Company, Inc.

Salsburg, D. (2001). *The Lady Tasting Tea. How Statistics Revolutionized Science in the Twentieth Century* (pp. 75–77). New York: W.H. Freeman and Company.

Schackell, L. F. (1925). The relation of dosage to effect. II. *The Journal of Pharmacology and Experimental Therapeutics, 25,* 275–288.

Schackell, L. F. (1923). Studies in protoplasm poisoning. I. Phenols. *The Journal of General Physiology, 5,* 783–805.

Schulz, H. (1888). *UBer Hefegifte. Pflugers Archiv. Fue die gesamte Physiologie des Menschen und der Tiere, 42,* 517–541.

Smith, E. C. (1935). Effects of ultra-violet radiation and temperature on Fusarium. II. Stimulation. *Bull Tor Bot Club, 62,* 151–164.

Smyth, H. F., Jr. (1967). Sufficient Challenge. *Food and Cosmetics Toxicology, 5,* 51–58.

Southam, C. M., & Erlich, J. (1943). Effects of extracts of western red-cedar heartwood on certain wood-decaying fungi in culture. *Phytopathology, 33,* 517–524.

Stebbing, A. R. D. (1982). Hormesis—The stimulation of growth by low levels of inhibitors. *Sci Tot Env, 22,* 213–234.

Stephenson, R. P. (1956). A modification of receptor theory. *British Journal of Pharmacology, 11*, 379–393.
Stolman, A. (1967). Combined action of drugs with toxicological implications. Part I. *Progress in Chemical Toxicology, 3*, 305–361.
Stolman, A. (1969). Combined action of drugs with toxicological implications. Part II. *Progress in Chemical Toxicology, 48*, 257–395.
Szabadi, E. (1977). A model of two functionally antagonistic receptor populations activated by the same agonist. *Journal of Theoretical Biology, 69*, 101–112.
Taliaferro, W. H., & Taliaferro, L. G. (1951). Effect of x-rays on immunity: A review. *Journal of Immunology (Baltimore, Md.: 1950), 66*, 181–212.
Van Ewijk, P. H., & Hoekstra, J. A. (1993). Calculation of the EC50 and its confidence interval when subtoxic stimulus is present. *Ecotoxicology and Environmental Safety, 23*, 25–32.
Verney, E. B., & Barcroft, J. (1941). A.J. Clark (Obituary). *Obituary Notices of Fellows of the Royal Society, 3*, 969.
Warren, S. (1945). The histopathology of radiation lesions. *Physiological Review, 25*, 225–238.
Wilder, J. (1931/1976). The "law of initial values," a neglected biological law and its significance for research and practice. Translated from *Zeitschrift fur die gesamte Neurologie und Psychiatrie 137*: 317–338. In S. W. Proges & M. G. H. Coles (Eds.), *Psychophysiology* (pp. 38–46). Stroudsburg, PA: Dowden, Hutchinson & Ross, Inc.
Wilder, J. (1967). *Stimulus and Response: The Law of Initial.* Value, 25. Bristol: Wright.
Winslow, C. E. A., & Dolloff, A. F. (1928). Relative importance of additive and antagonistic effects of cations upon bacterial viability. *Journal of Bacteriology, 15*, 67–92.
Zell-Stimulations-Forschungen. (1924–1930). Vol. 1–3. In M. Popoff & W. Gleisberg (Eds.). Berlin: Paul Pare.
Zimmerman, F. T., Burgemeister, B. B., & Putnam, T. J. (1948). The ceiling effect of glutamic acid upon intelligence in children and in adolescents. *The American Journal of Psychology, 104*, 593–599.

REFERENCES FOR FIGURE 5.3.

1. Bonnet, M., Lespinats, G., & Burtin, C. (1984). Histamine and serotonin suppression of lymphocyte response to phytohemagglutinin and allogeneic cells. *Cell. Immunol., 83*, 280–291.
2. Elferink, J. G. R., & De Koster, B. M. (1994). Endothelin-induced activation of neutrophil migration. *Biochem. Pharmacol., 48*(5), 865–871.
3. Boyd, J. G., & Gordon, T. (2002). A dose-dependent facilitation and inhibition of peripheral nerve regeneration by brain-derived neurotrophic factor. *European Journal of Neuroscience, 15*, 613–626.
4. Elferink, J. G. R., & DeKoster, B. M. (1998). The effect of thimerosal on neutrophil migration. A comparison with the effect on calcium mobilization and CD11B expression. *Biochem. Pharmacol., 55*(3), 305–312.
5. Conti, A. M., Fischer, S. J., Windebank, A. J. (1977). Inhibition of axonal growth from sensory neurons by excess nerve growth factor. *Ann. Neurol., 42*, 838–846.
6. Pfeifer, R. W., & Patterson, R. M. (1986). Modulation of lectin-stimulated lymphocyte agglutination and mitogenesis by estrogen metabolites: Effects on early events of lymphocyte activation. *Acrch. Toxicol., 58*, 157–164.
7. Wanger, H., Kreher, B., & Jurcic, K. (1988). In vitro stimulation of human granulocytes and lymphocytes by pico- and femtogram quantities of cytostatic agents. *Drug Res., 38*(1), 273–275.
8. Williamson, S. A., Knight, R. A., Lightman, S. L., and Hobbs, J. R. (1987). Differential effects of beta-endorphin fragments on human natural killing. *Brain, Behav. Immun., 1*, 329–335.
9. Hsu, J-T., Hung, H-C., Chen, C-J., Hsu, W-L., & Ying, C. (1999). Effects of the dietary phytoestrogen biochanin A on cell growth in the mammary carcinoma cell line MCF-7. *J. Nutr. Biochem., 10*, 510–517.
10. Costall, B., Jones, B. J., Kelly, M. E., Naylor, R. J., & Tomkins, D. M. (1989). Exploration of mice in a black and white test box: Validation as a model of anxiety. *Pharmacol. Biochem. Behav., 32*, 777–785.
11. Kawamoto, T., Sato, J. D., Jonathan, A. L., Polikoff, J., Sato, G.H., & Mendelsohn, J. (1983). Growth stimulation of A432 cells by epidermal growth factor: Identification of high-affinity receptors for epidermal growth factor by an anti-receptor monoclonal antibidy. *Proc. Nat. Acad Sci., 80*, 1337–1341.
12. Love-Schimenti, C. D., Gibson, F. C. D., Ratnam, A. V., & Bikle, D. D. (1996). Antiestrogen potentiation of antiproliferative effects of vitamin D3 analogues in breast cancer cells. *Cancer Res., 56*, 2789–2794.
13. Crabbe, J. C., Gallaher, E. J., Cross, S. J., & Belknap, J. K. (1998). Genetic Determinants of Sensitivity to Diazepam in Inbred Mice. *Behav. Neurosci., 112*(3), 668–667.
14. Cookson, M. R., Mead, C., Austwick, S. M., & Pentreath, V. W. (1995). Use of the MTT assay for estimating toxicity in primary astrocyte and C6 glioma cell cultures. *Toxic. In Vitro, 9*, 39–48.
15. Daston, G. P., Rogers, J. M., Versteeg, D. J., Sabourin, T. D., Baines, D., & Marsh, S. S. (1991). Interspecies Comparisons of A/D Ratios: A/D Ratios are not Constant Across Species. *Fund. Appl. Toxicol., 17*, 696–722.
16. Fulder, S. J. (1977). The Growth of Cultured Human Fibroblasts Treated with Hydrocortisone and Extracts of the Medicinal Plant Panax ginseng. *Exp. Geront., 12*, 125–131.
17. Ji, L., Melkonian, G., Riveles, K., & Talbot, P. (2002). Identification of pyridine compounds in cigarette smoke solution that inhibit growth of the chick chorioallantoic membrane. *Toxicol. Sci., 69*, 217–225.
18. Miller, W. M., Green, C. A., & Kitchin, H. (1945). Biphasic Action of Penicillin and Other Sulphonamide Similarity. *Nature, 1*(155), 210–211.
19. Borges, V. C., Rocha, J. B. T., & Nogueira, C. W. (2005). Effect of diphenyl diselenide, diphenyl ditelluride and ebselen on cerebral Na^+, K^+-ATPase activity in rats. *Toxicology, 215*, 191–197.
20. Varlinskaya, E. I., Spear, L. P., & Spear, N. (2001). Acute effects of ethanol on behavior of adolescent rats: Role of social context. *Alcoholism:Clin. Exper. Res., 25*(3), 377–385.
21. Frizzo, M. E., Dall'Onder, L. P., Dalcin, K. B., & Souza, D. O. (2004). Riluzole Enhances Glutamate Uptake in Rat Astrocyte Cultures. *Cell. Mol. Neurobiol., 24*(1), 123–128.
22. Von Zglinicki, T., Edwall, C., Ostlund, E., Lind, B., Nordberg, M., Ringertz, N. R., & Wroblewski, J. (1992). Very Low Cadmium Concentrations Stimulate DNA Synthesis and Cell Growth. *J. Cell Sci., 103*(4), 1073–1081.
23. Merkel, L. A., Lappe, R. W., Rivera, L. M., Cox, B. F., & Perrone, M. H. (1992). Demonstration of vasorelaxant activity with an A_1-selective adenosine agonist in porcine coronary artery: involvement of potassium channels. *J. Pharmacol. Exp. Ther., 260*, 437–443.
24. Hidalgo, E., & Dominquez, C. (2000). Growth-altering effects of sodium hypochlorite in cultured human dermal fibroblasts. *Life Sci., 67*, 1331–1344.
25. Cicero, T. J., & Badger, T. M. (1977). Effects of alcohol on the hypothalamic-pituitary-gonadal axis in the male rat. *J. Pharmacol. Exp. Ther., 201*, 427–433.
26. Voss, A.K., & Fortune, J.E. (1993). Estradiol-17-b has a biphasic effect on oxytocin secretion by bovine granulose cells. *Biol. Reprod., 48*, 1404–1409.
27. Tang, L., Mamotte, C.D.S., Van Bockxmeer, F.M., & Taylor, R.R. (1998). The effect of homocysteine on DNA synthesis in cultured human vascular smooth muscle. *Atherosclerosis, 136*, 169–173.
28. Frizzo, M.E., Dall'Onder, L.P., Dalcin, K.B., & Souza, D.O. (2004). Riluzole Enhances Glutamate Uptake in Rat Astrocyte Cultures. *Cell. Mol. Neurobiol., 24*(1), 123–128.
29. Lee, C., Sutkowski, D.M., Sensibar, J.A., Zelner, D., Kim, I., Amsel, I., Shaw, N., Prins, G.S., & Kozlowski, J.M. (1995). Regulation of proliferation and production of prostate-specific antigen in androgen-sensitive prostatic cancer cells, LNCaP, by dihydrotestosterone. *Endocrinology, 136*, 796–803.
30. Ying, C., Hsu, J-T, Hung, H-C, Lin, D-H, Chen, L-F.O., & Wang, L-K. (2002). Growth and cell cycle regulation by isoflavones in human breast carcinoma cells. *Reprod. Nutr. Dev., 42*, 55–64.
31. Abe, K., Sekizawa, T., & Kogure, K. (1986). Biphasic effects of chlorpromazine on cell viability in a neuroblastoma cell line. *Neurosci. Letters, 71*, 335–339.
32. Bernhard, D., Schwaiger, W., Crazzolara, R., Tinhofer, I., Kofler, R., & Csordas, A. (2003). Enhanced MTT-reducing activity under growth inhibition by resveratrol in CEM-C7H2 lymphocytic leukemia cells. *Cancer Letters, 195*, 193–199.
33. Garant, D.S., Xu, S.G., Sperber, E.F., & Moshe, S.L. (1995). Age-related differences in the effects of GABAA agonists microinjected into rat substantia nigra: pro- and anticonvulsant actions. *Epilepsia, 36*, 960–965.

Chapter

6 Signal Transduction and Second Messengers

Karen Lounsbury

OUTLINE

Central to the communication between cells is the process of signal transduction. Signal transduction is the mechanism by which cell surface receptors receive information from extracellular signals such as hormones and neurotransmitters, and amplify this information through the actions of second messengers. Second messengers in turn activate pathways intrinsic to processes such as protein secretion, cell differentiation, and cell division. Many pharmacological agents elicit their clinical activity and side effects through interactions with receptors and/or their downstream signaling targets. As our understanding of receptor signaling has progressed, intracellular signaling molecules have become a major target of drug discovery. This chapter will review the major receptor-mediated signaling pathways and will outline current and future therapeutic strategies to target these pathways.

6.1 RECEPTOR COMMUNICATION

Receptors are the primary sensors of the cell environment, but ligand binding alone is useless without signal transduction. The effect of a pharmacologic agent on the ability of receptors to couple to downstream signals thus defines whether it will increase (agonist) or decrease (antagonist) the physiologic activity of the receptor. Selective regulation of the magnitude, time-course, and spread of the signal allows a single ligand to transmit a complex set of physiological effects. Signal transduction by receptors can be broken into four major categories:

- Ion channels
- G protein-coupled receptors
- Receptor tyrosine kinases
- Intracellular receptors

6.1.1 Ion Channels

Ion channels can be regulated by receptors either directly (ligand-gated) or indirectly (second-messenger regulated) to modulate the passage of ions and other hydrophilic molecules across the plasma membrane. This regulated movement of ions can have effects on the membrane potential (i.e., K^+ efflux) as well as on downstream signaling pathways (i.e., Ca^{2+} influx). The specifics of this regulation will be covered in Chapter 7.

6.1.2 G-Protein-Coupled Receptors

G-protein-coupled receptors are the most abundant class of receptors and are responsible for regulating a multitude of physiologic processes including vision, muscle contraction, secretion, and neurotransmission. These receptors are inserted into the plasma membrane in a serpentine fashion that results in seven transmembrane domains. When a ligand binds to the active site of the receptor, a conformational change occurs within the intracellular domains resulting in the activation of a guanine nucleotide-binding protein (G-protein).

Prior to the knowledge that G-proteins existed, there was a great deal of information regarding the interactions of agonists and antagonists with receptor proteins present within cell membranes, but there was little understanding of how receptors communicated with their downstream targets. A tremendous amount of research from 1970 to 1990 revealed that there are three separate proteins necessary for signal transduction including the receptor (R), which recognizes external signals; the effector (E), which is responsible for the production of second messengers; and the G-protein (G), which is necessary for communication between the receptor and effector (Figure 6.1). The importance of this research on our understanding of cell signaling is evidenced by the Nobel Prize for Physiology or Medicine awarded to U.S. scientists Alfred Gilman and Martin Rodbell for their pioneering research in the discovery of G-proteins and the role of these proteins in signal transduction in cells.

G-proteins function as signal transducers through their cyclical regulation influenced primarily by receptors and guanyl nucleotides (Figure 6.2). G-proteins are heterotrimeric in structure, made up of an α subunit, which confers both catalytic activity and signaling function, and a βγ heterodimer subunit complex, which targets the G-protein to the appropriate membrane receptor and can also interact with downstream effectors. A G-protein is considered to be in an "inactive" state when its α subunit is bound to GDP and associated with its respective βγ subunit. When a receptor is coupled to a G-protein heterotrimer, it exhibits an increased affinity for its corresponding agonist. An agonist binding to the receptor induces activation of the G-protein by stimulating exchange of bound GDP for GTP on the α subunit, which promotes release of the βγ subunit. The free GTP-α and βγ subunits can functionally couple to their downstream effector molecules (i.e., Gs coupling to adenylyl cyclase). Because exchange of GTP for GDP is the limiting step, ligand-mediated receptor activation is the key activator of signaling by G-proteins.

The GTPase activity inherent to the α subunit hydrolyzes the bound GTP to GDP, resulting in a decreased affinity for effector and an increased affinity for βγ. The GTPase activity thus acts as a turnoff and recycling mechanism for the α subunit. The turnoff mechanism can be enhanced by G-protein interaction with specific regulator of G-protein signaling (RGS) isoforms, which act as both GTPase activating proteins and as antagonists of the interaction between α subunits and their receptors.

The use of G-proteins as a relay between receptor ligand binding and effector activation has important implications toward effectiveness of signaling. First, the time-course of the effect is not dependent on ligand binding, but instead on the length of second messenger activation. Thus, the relatively slow hydrolysis of GTP by the G-protein maintains the signal well after ligand has dissociated. Second, the dispersion of second messengers by G-protein coupling greatly increases the spatial effectiveness of the signaling throughout the cell. Together these mechanisms amplify the ligand-initiated signal to broadcast a programmed effect from a single source.

Heterotrimeric G-proteins can couple signals from over 1000 receptor subtypes, and their effector molecules include both ion channels and a variety of enzymes. There are 16 α, 5 β, and 14 γ genes, so a large number of subunits are produced, and they can combine in various ways. There are specific functions for both the α subunits and the βγ heterodimers. The α subunits can be divided into five families, Gs, Gi, Gt, Gq, and G12/13, each with a relatively characteristic set of effectors. A compilation of functions reported for specific receptor-G-protein coupling can be found in Table 6.1.

6.1.2.1 G-Protein-Coupled Second Messengers

Despite the diversity of receptor subtypes, there is a relatively small subset of G-protein-coupled second messengers that are the convergence point for multiple receptors. This convergence allows for a complicated

R ⇨ G ⇨ E ⇨ Second messengers

Input Transduction Output

Figure 6.1 Amplification of signals by second messengers.

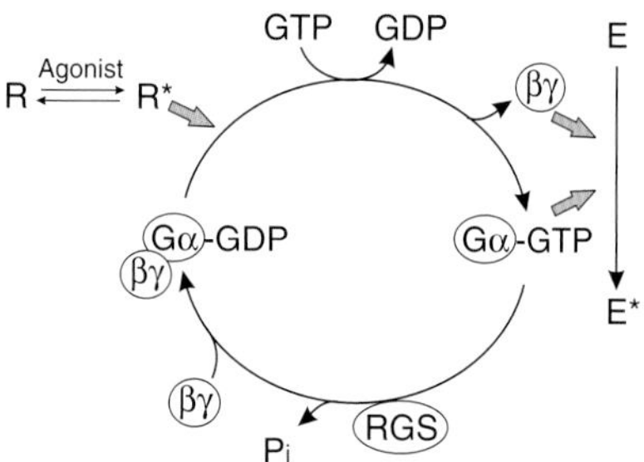

Figure 6.2 GTPase cycle of G protein activation.

Table 6.1 Heterotrimeric G protein Signaling Pathways

G protein	Receptors	Effectors
Gs	β-adrenergic amines, glucagon, histamine, serotonin	Adenylyl cyclase cAMP
Gi	α2-adrenergic amines, acetylcholine, opiods, serotonin	Adenylyl cyclase K+ channels
Golf	Odorants	Adenylyl cyclase
Go	Neurotransmitters(?)	Adenylyl cycase(?)
Gq	Acetylcholine, serotonin	Phospholipase C IP3, DAG, Ca2+
Gt	Photons (rhodopsin and color opsins)	cGMP phosphodiesterase cGMP

environment to be processed into a coordinated cellular effect. Following are the primary G-protein-coupled second messenger signaling pathways that have been characterized in mammalian cells.

Gs/Gi Coupling to Adenylyl Cyclase Receptor coupling through Gs or Gi results in a cascade of events that begins with the stimulation or inhibition of adenylyl cyclase activity (Figure 6.3). Adenylyl cyclase catalyzes the conversion of ATP to 3′,5′-cyclic AMP (cAMP), which mediates a multitude of hormonal responses including carbohydrate metabolism, ion homeostasis, heart contractility, and neuronal signaling. Many of these activities of cAMP have been attributed to the activation of cAMP-dependent protein kinase (PKA), a ubiquitous protein with multiple substrates for phosphorylation. The catalytic subunits of PKA are held inactive through their interaction with regulatory subunits. When cAMP binds to the regulatory subunits, the active catalytic subunits are released and are able to promote phosphorylation of proteins containing PKA consensus phosphorylation sites. The specificity of cAMP effects is thus dependent on the expression and proximity of kinase substrates.

Perpetuation of the PKA-mediated phosphorylation signal is regulated by specific and nonspecific phosphatases that catalyze the removal of phosphate from the PKA substrates. The termination of the cAMP signal is mediated by its degradation to 5′-AMP by cyclic nucleotide phosphodiesterases that are selective for cAMP or able to degrade both cAMP and cGMP. Competitive inhibition of phosphodiesterases is one mechanism by which the methylxanthines such as caffeine and theophylline exert their effects.

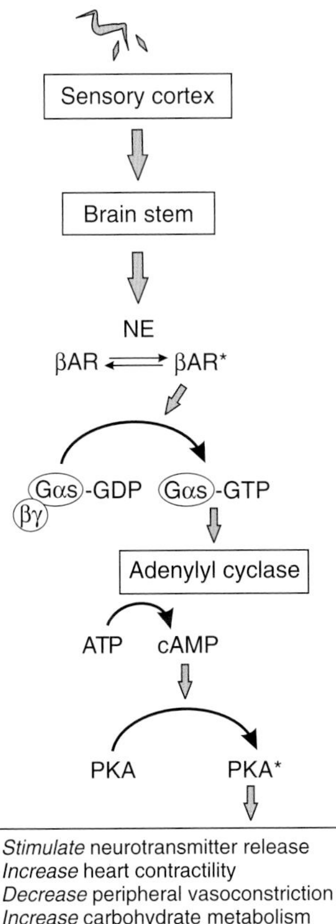

Figure 6.3 Signal amplification in the "fight-or-flight" response.

The G-proteins Gs and Gi are direct targets for bacterial toxins produced by V. cholerae and B. pertussis, respectively. Cholera toxin activates Gs independently of receptor activation causing increased activation of adenylyl cyclase and opening of ion channels in the epithelial lining of the colon. The increased flow of ions into the colon increases the osmotic transfer of water, resulting in diarrhea and often death due to dehydration. Pertussis toxin causes a modification of Gi, preventing it from interacting with its receptors or inhibiting adenylyl cyclase in the respiratory epithelium and phagocytotic immune cells. The resulting increase in adenylyl cyclase activity enhances cell invasion and inhibits phagocytotic functions. The clinical result is a pervasive cough, which has led to the reference to pertussis infection as whooping cough. Research leading to the identification of the mechanisms for these toxins was not only important clinically, but also fueled research to understand the receptor-G-protein-effector links.

Other G-proteins that are related to Gs and Gi include G_{olf} and Go. G_{olf} is structurally and functionally similar to Gs. G_{olf} was originally discovered in the olfactory neuroepithelium and striatum, but has subsequently been identified in several peripheral tissues as well. Like Gs, G_{olf} couples to activation of adenylyl cyclase. Although its role in the periphery has yet to be characterized, in the brain it is known to communicate odorant signals by coupling to olfactory receptors. Go has similar effector functions as Gi, including inhibition of adenylyl cyclase, but it is somewhat selectively expressed in the brain and heart. It is not clear why diversification to Go is advantageous, but new research suggests that Go is regulated by selective GTPase activating proteins that may fine-tune the response in a tissue-selective manner.

A classic example of the physiological effects mediated by the Gs/Gi-coupled signaling cascade is the "fight-or-flight" response (Figure 6.3). Beginning in the brain, the stressor signal (such as a loud noise or bright light) is relayed from the sensory cortex to the thalamus and brain stem. This signaling stimulates release of catecholamine neurotransmitters such as norepinephrine and dopamine in the locus ceruleus. The neurotransmitters bind to G-protein coupled receptors that activate adenylyl cyclase via Gs. The resulting production of cAMP enhances the catalytic activity of PKA. PKA then stimulates release of neurotransmitters that regulate neurons responsible for spontaneous "flight" responses. A prolonged stimulation of the locus ceruleus activates release of acetylcholine from the preganglionic neurons of the autonomic nervous system. Acetylcholine binds to nicotinic acetylcholine receptors in the adrenal medulla causing Na^+ influx, membrane depolarization, and release of epinephrine. Epinephrine has effects that are dependent on the array of receptors expressed on the membrane of target cells. Depending on the subtype, adrenergic receptors can couple to Gs, Gi, or Gq. Actions through β receptor/Gs coupling promote an increase in carbohydrate metabolism, heart contractility and lung action as well as dilation of blood vessels feeding the musculoskeletal system. Conversely, actions of epinephrine through α receptor coupling results in vasoconstriction of vessels feeding the gastrointestinal and renal systems. The result of these opposing actions of epinephrine allows the body to divert energy away from internal processes to the muscles for an optimal fight-or-flight response.

Gt Coupling to cGMP Phosphodiesterase In photoreceptor rod outer segments, light-activated rhodopsin activates transducin (Gt), which stimulates a cGMP-specific phosphodiesterase. This activation causes rapid degradation of cGMP resulting in the closure of cGMP-regulated sodium channels and membrane hyperpolarization. The resulting hyperpolarization reduces neurotransmitter release, thus the amount of neurotransmitter released is reduced in bright light and increases as light levels fall. The Gt signal is terminated following GTP hydrolysis. This chain of signaling events is called "the vertebrate phototransduction cascade" and is critical for rapidly adjusting the visual response to different light intensities.

Gq Coupling to Phosphoinositide Hydrolysis and Calcium Signaling Receptor coupling through Gq results in the activation of phospholipase C-β (PLC-β) (Figure 6.4). PLC-β enzymatically cleaves the membrane phospholipid phosphoatidylinositol-4,5-bisphopshate (PIP2) into diacylglycerol (DAG) and inositol trisphosphate (IP3). Both DAG and IP3 act as important second messengers. DAG remains in the membrane where it recruits and activates protein kinase C. IP3 stimulates the opening of IP3-mediated Ca^{2+} channels on intracellular organelles that store Ca^{2+} such as the endoplasmic reticulum. The release of Ca^{2+} into the cytoplasm regulates several signaling cascades including opening of ion channels and activation of Ca^{2+}/calmodulin-dependent kinases.

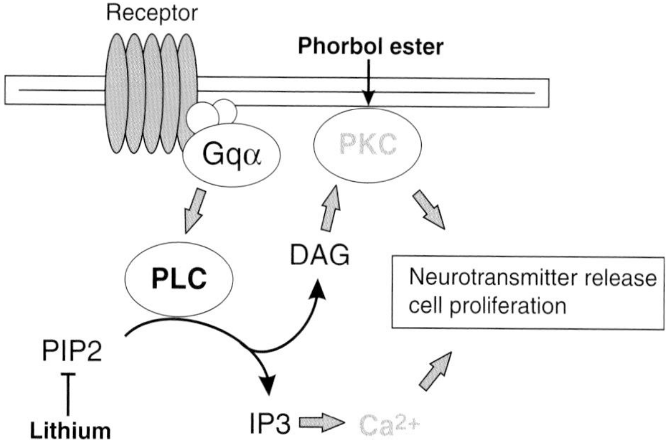

Figure 6.4 Gq signaling through phospholipase C (PLC).

The termination of signaling by Gq-generated second messengers is achieved by dephosphorylation of IP3 and deacylation of DAG. Removal of Ca^{2+} from the cytoplasm is achieved by Ca^{2+}-binding proteins and Ca^{2+}pumps. Ca^{2+} pumps in the plasma membrane remove Ca^{2+} from the cell whereas pumps in organellar membranes accumulate Ca^{2+} to replenish intracellular Ca^{2+} stores.

Because of its more complicated signaling cascade, Gq mediated signaling is more complex and cell-type specific. There are many isoforms of protein kinase C that have selective substrates and functions. In addition, different cell types express variable amounts of Ca^{2+}-mediated kinases and ion channels and Ca^{2+} can play a role in events ranging from cell contraction and secretion to gene expression and cell division.

Examples of exogenous agents that alter the Gq signaling pathway include phorbol esters, which mimic DAG to activate protein kinase C, and lithium, which blocks recycling of phosphoinositides. Phorbol esters are recognized as tumor promoters due to their ability to excessively activate protein kinase C-mediated signaling to upregulate cell growth. Conversely, lithium is used as a treatment for manic disorders because blocking the phosphoinositide signaling pathway prevents overactivity of signaling through excitatory amine neurotransmitter receptors in the brain such as dopamine and norepinephrine.

G12/G13 Coupling to Small GTPases G12 and G13 were discovered through their sequence homology to previously characterized G-proteins, and their functions are not yet completely known. Evidence thus far suggests that their main effectors are small GTPases. G12 reportedly interacts with the Ras GTPase, thus activating the MAP kinase cascade and cell proliferation (described later). It is not surprising then that G12 has been identified as a potential tumor-promoting oncogene. G13 couples to lysophosphatidic acid receptors and activates the small GTPase Rho. The Rho GTPase has several functions related to cytoskeleton rearrangements and signaling through protein kinases, thus G13 likely has an important role in cell motility.

Signaling by βγ Subunits Although initial reports were not readily accepted, it is now well established that the G-protein βγ subunit complex also has effector functions. Most cell types express multiple forms of β and γ subtypes, making individual assessments of physiologic function difficult. Although many functions have been attributed to selective βγ pairings, the best characterized functions are activating/inhibiting adenylyl cyclase, enhancing K^+ channel activity, and stimulating activity of phospholipase C-β. Like the G-protein α subunits, the effector activity is related to localization of targets, thus recruitment of scaffolding proteins that link protein regulators to membrane-bound enzymes is likely the most important role of the βγ complex. Although not directly targeted by pharmacologic agents, the loss of βγ subunits has been correlated to diseases including atherosclerosis, hypertension, and metabolic syndrome.

6.1.3 Receptor Tyrosine Kinases

Receptor tyrosine kinases (RTKs) mediate signaling by insulin and a variety of growth factors such as epidermal growth factor (EGF) and platelet-derived growth factor (PDGF). RTKs were discovered in 1980 and, because of their importance in the regulation of oncogenes and cell growth, there has been a flurry of progress in characterizing the mechanisms underlying their activity and regulation. Unlike G-protein-coupled receptors, RTKs are characterized by their intrinsic tyrosine kinase activity that becomes activated upon ligand binding. The majority of RTKs exist on the cell surface as monomers with a single transmembrane domain. When activated, these receptors dimerize and transfer phosphate to hydroxyl groups on tyrosines of target proteins within their vicinity (Figure 6.5). For most RTKs, autophosphorylation of the intracellular domain of the receptor is a key element to communication with second messengers.

The phosphorylated tyrosines on the RTK function as specific binding sites for proteins that contain SH2 (Src homology 2) domains. These proteins include enzymes such as phosphoinositide-3 kinase (PI3K) and phospholipase C (PLC) and adaptor proteins such as growth receptor binding protein-2 (Grb-2). The specificity of growth factor signaling is determined by the proximity of substrates that are directly phosphorylated by the receptor or that bind to adaptor proteins through SH2 domains. These proteins are often targeted to the receptor through specific scaffolding proteins that localize the appropriate targets to the receptor.

There are three primary mechanisms that have been identified for activation of effector proteins by RTKs as illustrated for PI3K signaling in Figure 6.5. The first mechanism involves recruitment of proteins to the membrane to mediate interactions with enzymes and lipid activators. The second mechanism is by mediating conformational change, which promotes activation; the third involves direct activation of enzyme activity by tyrosine phosphorylation. These three mechanisms work synchronously to accomplish localization, protein interaction, and enzyme activation.

6.1.3.1 Receptor Tyrosine Kinase-coupled Second Messengers

There has been rapid progress in multiple fields toward the understanding of signaling pathways activated by RTKs, and the picture that emerges is one that includes multiple signaling networks that modulate the flow of information to destinations in the membrane, cytoplasm, and nucleus. Described below are the RTK-coupled second messenger signaling networks that have been characterized in mammalian cells.

Ras/MAP Kinase Signaling Cascade All known RTKs stimulate activation of the small GTPase, Ras. Like heterotrimeric G-proteins, Ras activation requires exchange of GTP for GDP. Unlike heterotrimeric G proteins, Ras does not have a βγ subunit and has much less efficient intrinsic GTPase activity. For this reason, once activated by a GTP exchange factor, Ras remains active until it interacts with a GTPase activating protein (GAP). RTKs recruit the Ras GTP exchange factor, son-of-sevenless (SOS), via the SH2 and SH3 domains on the Grb-2 adaptor protein (Figure 6.6). Once at the membrane, SOS mediates exchange of GTP on Ras, thus stimulating its interaction and activation of downstream targets.

The downstream targets of Ras include both PI3K and the mitogen activated protein kinase (MAPK) cascade. Ras activates the first MAPK in the cascade, Raf kinase, which then stimulates MAP kinase (MEK) by phosphorylating a critical Ser residue in its activation domain. MEK then phosphorylates and activates the MAP kinase ERK (extracellular signal regulated kinase), which has functional targets in the plasma membrane, cytoplasm, and nucleus. MAP kinase signaling cascade is highly conserved throughout evolution and has an important role in the control of cell metabolism, cell division, and cell motility.

Termination of MAP kinase signaling can be accomplished by receptor downregulation, Ras interaction with its GAP, which catalyzes the hydrolysis of GTP on Ras, and by tyrosine and serine phosphatases that disrupt the kinase cascade. Gain of function mutations that

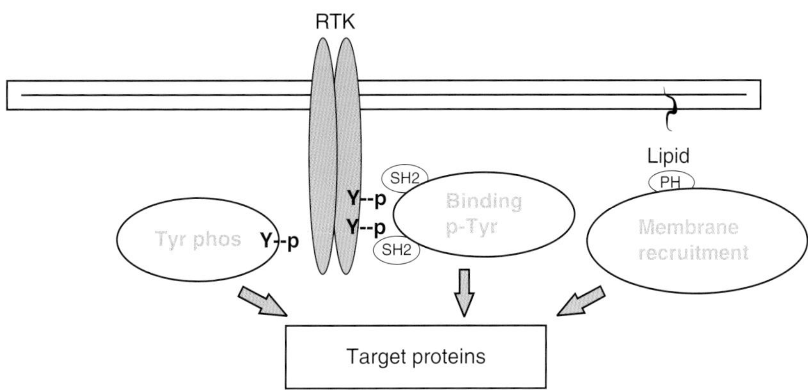

Figure 6.5 Growth factor signaling through receptor tyrosine kinases.

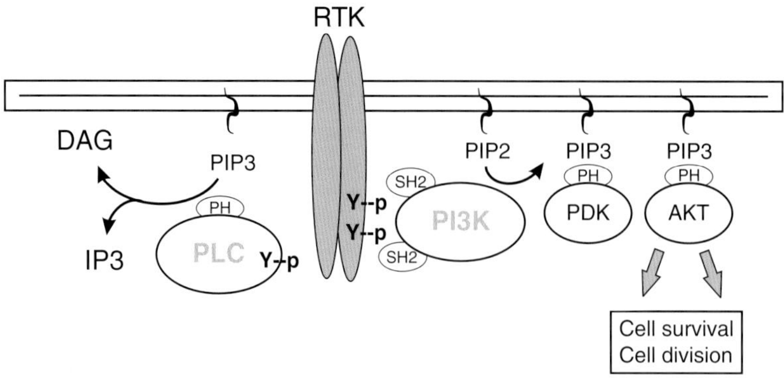

Figure 6.6 Ras/MAP kinase signaling cascade.

Table 6.2 Pipeline Targets of Growth Factor Signaling in Development

Drug/compound	Target	Mechanism	Clinical Phase
PTK/ZK	VEGFR	Tyr kinase inhib.	Phase I/II, colon, liver cancer
VandetanibZD6474	VEGFR, EGFR	Tyr kinase inhib.	Phase I/II, multiple studie
Axitinib/AG-013736	VEGFR, PDGFR	Tyr kinase inhib.	Phase I/II, multiple studie
Vatalanib/PTK787	VEGFR, PDGFR, c-Kit	Tyr kinase inhib.	Phase I/II, multiple studies
Lapatinib/GW572016	EGFR, ErbB2	Tyr kinase inhib.	Phase I/II, multiple studie
Dasatinib/BMS-354825	Src, Abl	Tyr kinase inhib.	Phase I/II, multiple studie
Nilotinib/AMN-107	**Abl**	**Tyr kinase inhib.**	**Phase III, Leukemia**
CP-751871	IGFR	Antibody	Phase II, combination therapy
Flavopiridol	Pan-cdk	Cell cycle Inhib.	Phase I/II, solid tumors
PD332991	Cdk4	Cell cycle Inhib.	Phase I/II Advanced cancer
PD0325901	MEK	Kinase inhibitor	Phase I/II Advanced cancer
ARRY-142886	MEK	Kinase inhibitor	Phase II, Melanoma
Sorafenib/BAY 43-9006	**RAF, VEGFR, PDGFR, c-Kit**	**Kinase inhibitor**	**Phase III, Kidney Cancer**

disrupt these termination signals can lead to uncontrolled cell growth that leads to many pathologies including inflammation, fibrosis, and cancer. These mutations are prevalent in leukemia, gastrointestinal, and gynecologic cancers and have also been linked to proliferative fibrotic diseases of the kidney, lung, and cardiovascular system.

Several anti-cancer agents, either approved or in development, target the kinase activity of RTKs and components of the MAP kinase cascade (Tables 6.2 and 6.3). The drug imatinib (Gleevec) was initially approved based on its inhibition of the tyrosine kinase activity of the intracellular RTK, Abl, which is associated with leukemia. Its dramatic success and relative selectivity for tumors has led to its further use as an RTK inhibitor in other cancers. Other successful anti-cancer agents that target RTKs in cancer include tamoxifen (Nolvadex) and trastuzumab (Herceptin), which target the estrogen receptor and ErbB2 RTKs, respectively, in breast cancer and bevacizumab (Avastin) that targets the VEGF RTK pathway in colon cancer. Drugs in the pipeline include multitargeted tyrosine kinase inhibitors and inhibitors of the Raf and MEK kinases. Newer methods of inhibiting these signaling pathways also are being developed that include selective knockout of RTK signaling

Table 6.3 Kinase Inhibitors Used Clinically

Drug	Target	Disease Indication
Small Molecules		
Imatinib (Gleevec)	Abl, PDGFR, c-Kit	Leukemia, GI Cancer
Gefitinib (Iressa)	EGFR	Lung Cancer
Erlotinib (Tarceva)	EGFR	Lung Cancer
Sorafenib (Nexavar)	VEGFR, PDGFR, c-Kit B-raf, Raf-1	Kidney
Sunitinib (Sutent)	VEGFR, PDGFR, c-Kit	
Biologics		
Trastuzumab (Herceptin)	ErbB2 (HER-2/neu)	Breast Cancer
Cetuximab (Erbitux)	EGFR	
Bevacizumab (Avastin)	VEGF	Colon, Pancreatic Cancer

components using gene silencing technology such as small interfering RNA (siRNA).

Phosphoinositol Metabolism RTKs stimulate phosphoinositol metabolism through their activation of phospholipase C-γ (PLC-γ) and phosphoinositide-3 kinase (PI3K) through binding of their SH2 domains to phospho-tyrosines on the receptor. Similar to Gq activation of PLC-β, activation of PLC-γ results in hydrolysis of PIP2 to form DAG and IP3, which promote PKC and Ca^{2+} signaling to their downstream cellular targets. Activated PI3K phosphorylates phosphoinositides to generate the second messengers, PI(3,4)P2 and PI(3,4,5)P3. PI(3,4,5)P3 induces membrane translocation of several proteins including soluble protein tyrosine kinases, protein kinase B (Akt), and nucleotide exchange factors for the small GTPases Arf and Rac. These proteins interact with the phosphoinositides through plextrin-homology domains (PH domains). These signaling proteins are important for the modulation of proteins that directly regulate cell survival by blocking apoptosis pathways (Figure 6.7).

Inactivation of these signaling pathways is mediated by phosphoinositide-specific phosphatases such as phosphatase and tensin homolog (PTEN). PTEN is a tumor suppressor protein that is mutated in several human cancers. Loss of PTEN results in unregulated cell survival, and thus aberrant cell growth.

6.1.4 Cytokine Receptors (Tyrosine Kinase-Associated Receptors)

Tyrosine kinase-associated receptors signal by recruiting activated cytosolic enzymes to the cell membrane. The resulting activation is similar to RTK signaling, but the kinase activity is not related directly to the receptor molecule. Classic examples of this type of receptor are cytokine receptors that modulate gene expression in immune cells as well as many other cell types. Cytokine receptors include receptors for interleukins, erythropoietin, and interferons.

When bound to ligand, these receptors dimerize and gain binding affinity for members of the Janus-kinase (JAK) family. This noncovalent binding increases the kinase activity of JAK, which sets into motion phosphorylation of multiple tyrosines on substrates including the receptor. Key substrates are the signal transducers and activators of transcription (STAT) proteins that dimerize via their phosphorylated tyrosines/SH2 interactions, and then translocate to the nucleus where they regulate gene transcription. The majority of identified gene targets are related to immune cell function. Overactivity of this pathway can lead to inflammatory disorders, whereas lack of pathway function results in immune suppression and susceptibility to infection.

The pathway is negatively regulated by protein tyrosine phosphatases and by feedback inhibition through STAT-mediated expression of suppressors of cytokine signaling (SOCs). Agonists for cytokine receptors are currently used to stimulate red blood cell maturation in anemia (erythropoietin) and to stimulate the immune system (interferons). The cascade nature of the cytokine pathway lends itself to future agents that specifically target components of the pathway.

6.1.5 Intracellular Receptors

Intracellular receptors require ligands that are membrane permeable and include receptors for steroid hormones, lipophilic vitamins, and small molecules such as nitric oxide and hydrogen peroxide. Members of the steroid hormone receptor family are structurally similar and exhibit similarities in their molecular mechanisms (Figure 6.8). In the absence of ligand, the receptor is retained in the cytoplasm by binding to heat shock protein 90 (HSP90), which conceals the receptor's nuclear localization signal. Following ligand binding, HSP90 is released and the receptor rapidly translocates to the nucleus. Steroid receptors

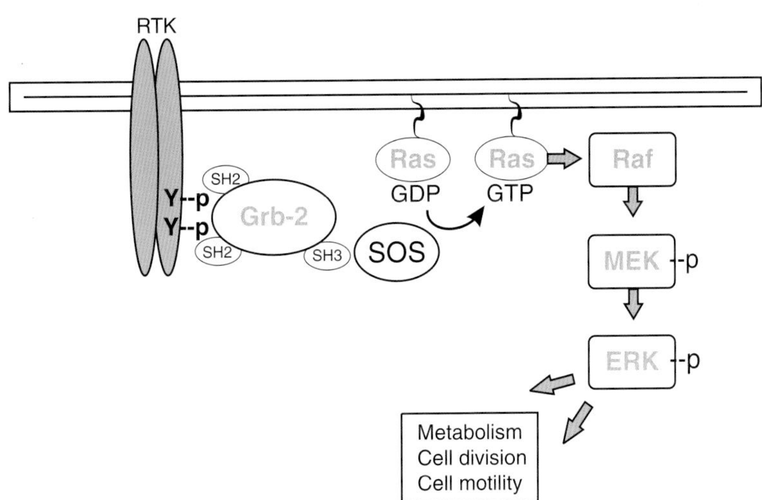

Figure 6.7 Phosphoinositide signaling by receptor tyrosine kinases.

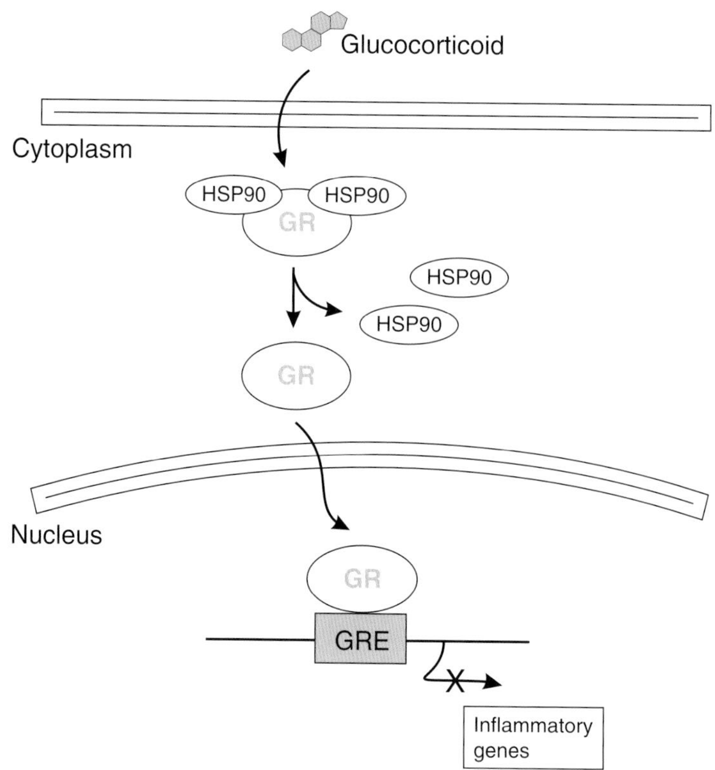

Figure 6.8 Glucocorticoid receptor signaling directly modulates gene transcription.

function as transcription factors, thus once in the nucleus they bind to specific steroid response elements on the DNA. These sequences are found in the regulatory region of genes, and binding by steroid receptors can either increase or decrease transcriptional activity of the gene. For example, glucocorticoids promote nuclear import of the glucocorticoid receptor, which results in an upregulation of anti-inflammatory genes and a downregulation of pro-inflammatory cytokines. Changes in gene transcription mediated by steroid receptors are relatively slow in onset yet result in long-term changes in gene expression. Thus pharmacologic agents that mimic steroid actions have a slow onset of effects, yet last a long time.

Nitric oxide is a small diffusible gas that has localized effects. Once inside the cell, NO activates soluble guanylyl cyclase, an enzyme that catalyzes the production of cGMP from GTP. The cGMP produced has the primary effect of activating cGMP-dependent protein kinase, which has a number of effects including smooth muscle cell relaxation. This mechanism of vasodilation is manipulated by a number of important vasodilating drugs that either mimic NO (such as nitroglycerin) or prevent degradation of cGMP (such as sildenefil).

6.1.6 Other Classes of Receptors

Although the majority of receptors fit into the classes described previously, there are some receptors that do not. Smaller classes of receptors include receptor tyrosine phosphatases that are found primarily in immune cells. These receptors can negate RTK signaling by catalyzing the removal of phosphate from tyrosines and can mediate immune suppression. Another small class of receptors has intrinsic serine/threonine kinase activity (transforming growth factor β receptor) and guanylyl cyclase activity (B-type natriuretic peptide receptor). A recombinant form of B-type natriuretic peptide (Nesiritide) is used in the treatment of heart failure to enhance vasodilation through the resulting increase in cGMP production as described for NO earlier.

6.2 RECEPTOR/SECOND MESSENGER CROSSTALK

Almost all second messenger signaling involves reversible phosphorylation, so it is easy to see how interactions between kinases across different second messenger systems can occur. Consensus sequences for phosphorylation can overlap leading to common substrates and, as demonstrated by the MAP kinase pathway, many kinases are themselves substrates for phosphorylation.

The phosphorylation modification lends itself to both signal amplification and to flexible regulation. Phosphorylation (-PO3) is a relatively dramatic modification in that it adds three negative charges to the protein, enough to significantly alter the three-dimensional conformation of the protein. The covalent phosphobond is also quite stable when compared to allosteric bond between receptor and ligand.

Although each signaling pathway has distinct "cassettes" of kinases and phosphatases, the downstream effects of second messenger pathways are not linear. Signal integration (crosstalk) occurs creating a complex network of communication between the different signaling pathways. Activation of G-protein-coupled receptors often results in transactivation of RTKs, and conversely signaling by RTKs can affect G-protein-coupled receptor activity. For example, activation of the angiotensin II receptor leads to activation of Gq, which couples to PLC-β activity. The resulting increase in Ca^{2+} and protein kinase C activity has direct effects on signaling components of the RTK pathway, namely, Ca^{2+}-mediated activation of the Raf kinase and protein kinase C phosphorylation of scaffolding proteins that enhance recruitment of the Ras GTP exchange factor, SOS. Conversely RTK signaling can lead to tyrosine phosphorylation of G-protein-coupled receptors and also has effects on the RGS proteins that stimulate GTPase activity. The overall result of a signal such as angiotensin II, therefore, is a combination of effects on multiple signaling pathways. These complicated effects make it more difficult to establish a single target for drug development, yet provide the potential for selectivity of pharmacological response depending on the cell environment and intracellular signaling networks.

6.3 SIGNAL TRANSDUCTION TARGETS FOR DRUG DISCOVERY

There has been an exhaustive quest to transfer the vast amount of information related to signal transduction that has been acquired over the last 60 years into specific molecularly targeted agents. Enzymology was the focus of drug discovery in the 1950s, which led to the development of many agents including the anticancer folate inhibitors and methotrexate. Both of these agents affect DNA synthesis, thus cells entering the cell cycle cannot undergo division and follow programmed cell death (apoptosis). Although relatively selective for rapidly dividing cells, the side-effects of these agents have significant morbidity including severe immune compromise.

With the advent of precise ligand binding studies and receptor cloning in the 1980s, many drugs were developed, or their mechanisms discovered, that act as agonists or antagonists of G-protein-coupled receptors. The disadvantage of many of these agents is the lack of specificity for receptor subtypes and the tendency to cause receptor downregulation and drug tolerance.

A better understanding of the genetics and cell signaling pathways involved in the regulation of cell division has led to molecular targets that are downstream of the receptor and are selective to second messenger pathways. Some current therapies, such as lithium to treat mania, had their mechanisms discovered long after they were used therapeutically. This modern approach to drug targets has especially benefited the cancer chemotherapy field. Several agents target signaling molecules such as tyrosine kinases and have shown efficacy in the treatment of a variety of cancers as described earlier (Table 6.3).

The future challenge of therapy targeted at signal transduction pathways entails both identifying the best targets and determining its overall effect on outcome. It is these two goals that have led to an increase in demand for clinical translational research. Patient-based research is necessary to reveal the effects of signal transduction crosstalk in a disease setting where both the targets and the outcome can be identified, measured, altered, and then correlated with prevention or progression of the disease state.

REVIEW QUESTIONS

1. What is the advantage of signaling by way of a receptor coupling to an enzyme?
2. How can a neurotransmitter elicit the opposite response in different cells? For example: epinephrine elicits heart muscle contraction and gastrointestinal smooth muscle relaxation.
3. What is the turn-off mechanism for Gq-mediated signaling?
4. If lithium blocks recycling of phosphoinositides, what receptor/G protein pathways will it affect?
5. What changes in the tyrosine kinase/Ras pathway could cause overactivity of the receptor pathway, possibly leading to unregulated cell division?
6. What is the leading target of newly approved anticancer drugs that act on the growth factor receptor/MAP kinase pathway?
7. The cytokine receptor signaling pathway in immune cells is referred to as the JAK/STAT pathway. How do JAK and STAT coordinately regulate the immune response?
8. How are steroid receptors regulated differently than plasma membrane receptors?
9. Explain the concept of transactivation between receptor signaling pathways. How does this affect individual signaling pathways?
10. What are the advantages and disadvantages of targeted therapies based on knowledge of signal transduction pathways?

REFERENCES AND FURTHER READING

Hubbard, K. B., & Hepler, J. R. (2006). Cell signalling diversity of the Gqalpha family of heterotrimeric G proteins. *Cell Signal, 18*(2), 135–150.

Many receptors for neurotransmitters and hormones rely upon members of the Gqalpha family of heterotrimeric G-proteins to exert their actions on target cells. Galpha subunits of the Gq class of G-proteins (Gqalpha, G11alpha, G14alpha, and G15/16alpha) directly link receptors to activation of PLC-beta isoforms, which in turn, stimulate inositol lipid (i.e., calcium/PKC) signaling. Although Gqalpha family members share a capacity to activate PLC-beta, they also differ markedly in their biochemical properties and tissue distribution that predicts functional diversity. Nevertheless, established models suggest that Gqalpha family members are functionally redundant and that their cellular responses are a result of PLC-beta activation and downstream calcium/PKC signaling. Growing evidence, however, indicates that Gqalpha, G11alpha, G14alpha and G15/16alpha are functionally diverse and that many of their cellular actions are independent of inositol lipid signalling. Recent findings show that

Gqalpha family members differ with regard to their linked receptors and downstream binding partners. Reported binding partners distinct from PLC-beta include novel candidate effector proteins, various regulatory proteins, and a growing list of scaffolding/adaptor proteins. Downstream of these signaling proteins, Gqalpha family members exhibit unexpected differences in the signaling pathways and the gene expression profiles they regulate. Finally, genetic studies using whole animal models demonstrate the importance of certain Gqalpha family members in cardiac, lung, brain, and platelet functions among other physiological processes. Taken together, these findings demonstrate that Gqalpha, G11alpha, G14alpha, and G15/16alpha regulate both overlapping and distinct signaling pathways, indicating that they are more functionally diverse than previously thought.

Milligan, G., & Kostenis, E. (2006). Heterotrimeric G-proteins: A short history. *British Journal of Pharmacology, 147* (Suppl. 1), S46–S55.

Some 865 genes in man encode G-protein-coupled receptors (GPCRs). The heterotrimeric guanine nucleotide-binding proteins (G-proteins) function to transduce signals from this vast panoply of receptors to effector systems including ion channels and enzymes that alter the rate of production, release or degradation of intracellular second messengers. However, it was not until the 1970s that the existence of such transducing proteins was even seriously suggested. Combinations of bacterial toxins that mediate their effects via covalent modification of the alpha-subunit of certain G-proteins and mutant cell lines that fail to generate cyclic AMP in response to agonists because they either fail to express or express a malfunctional G-protein allowed their identification and purification. Subsequent to initial cloning efforts, cloning by homology has defined the human G-proteins to derive from 35 genes, 16 encoding alpha-subunits, five beta and 14 gamma. All function as guanine nucleotide exchange on-off switches and are mechanistically similar to other proteins that are enzymic GTPases. Although not readily accepted initially, it is now well established that beta/gamma complexes mediate as least as many functions as the alpha-subunits. The generation of chimeras between different alpha-subunits defined the role of different sections of the primary/secondary sequence and crystal structures, and cocrystals with interacting proteins have given detailed understanding of their molecular structure and basis of function. Finally, further modifications of such chimeras have generated a range of G-protein alpha-subunits with greater promiscuity to interact across GPCR classes and initiated the use of such modified G-proteins in drug discovery programs.

Natarajan, K., & Berk, B. C. (2006). Crosstalk coregulation mechanisms of G protein-coupled receptors and receptor tyrosine kinases. *Methods in Molecular Biology, 332,* 51–77.

G-protein-coupled receptors (GPCRs) and receptor tyrosine kinases (RTKs) are transmembrane receptors that initiate intracellular signaling cascades in response to a diverse array of ligands. Recent studies have shown that signal transduction initiated by GPCRs and RTKs is not organized in distinct signaling cassettes, where receptor activation leads to cell division and gene transcription in a linear manner. In fact, signal integration and diversification arises from a complex network involving cross-communication between separate signaling units. Several different styles of crosstalk between GPCR- and RTK-initiated pathways exist, with GPCRs or components of GPCR-induced pathways being either upstream or downstream of RTKs. Activation of GPCRs sometimes results in a phenomenon known as transactivation of RTKs, which leads to the recruitment of scaffold proteins, such as Shc, Grb2, and SOS in addition to mitogen-activated protein kinase activation. In other cases, RTKs use different components of GPCR-mediated signaling, such as beta-arrestin, G protein-receptor kinases, and regulator of G-protein signaling to integrate signaling pathways. This chapter outlines some of the more common mechanisms used by both GPCRs and RTKs to initiate intracellular crosstalk, thereby creating a complex signaling network that is important to normal development.

Neer, E. J. (1995). Heterotrimeric G proteins: Organizers of transmembrane signals. *Cell, 80*(2), 249–257.

Neves, S. R., Ram, P. T., et al. (2002). G protein pathways. *Science, 296* (5573), 1636–1639.

The heterotrimeric guanine nucleotide-binding proteins (G-proteins) are signal transducers that communicate signals from many hormones, neurotransmitters, chemokines, and autocrine and paracrine factors. The extracellular signals are received by members of a large superfamily of receptors with seven membrane-spanning regions that activate the G-proteins, which route the signals to several distinct intracellular signaling pathways. These pathways interact with one another to form a network that regulates metabolic enzymes, ion channels, transporters, and other components of the cellular machinery controlling a broad range of cellular processes, including transcription, motility, contractility, and secretion. These cellular processes in turn regulate systemic functions such as embryonic development, gonadal development, learning and memory, and organismal homeostasis.

Schlessinger, J. (2000). Cell signaling by receptor tyrosine kinases. *Cell, 103*(2), 211–225.

Chapter

7 Drug Distribution

Patrick J. McNamara . Markos Leggas

OUTLINE

7.1 INTRODUCTION

Drug response, whether therapeutic or toxic, is dictated by drug concentration at sites of action located outside the site of drug administration. Thus, tissue distribution can often be a critical determinant of drug action, and is a complex process that involves drug transport across biological membranes into the blood, and distribution to sites of action or storage and eventually to sites of elimination.

7.1.1 Clinical Correlate: AIDS Pharmacotherapy Movement Across Biological Membranes

Successful treatment and control of HIV infection is now possible with treatments that combine different classes of drugs including reverse transcriptase inhibitors and protease inhibitors, among others. However, these drugs are completely ineffective against viral particles that find safe harbor in pharmacologically sequestered sites (e.g., the blood–brain barrier (BBB)) where drug concentrations are typically below the effective therapeutic range. Poor penetration into the brain is of concern clinically since the HIV virus may persist in the CNS where it acts as a reservoir for ongoing systemic infection. Another example where AIDS drug distribution is of importance is that of drug passage into breastmilk. HIV is present in breastmilk and can infect the nursing infant. This infection mechanism is a major issue in third-world countries where alternatives to breastfeeding are limited. Although extensive passage into breastmilk is generally thought to be an undesirable characteristic for most drugs, in third-world countries there may be a therapeutic advantage in treating HIV infected mothers with drugs that accumulate in breastmilk.

Drug distribution in such sites or “compartments” is a complex process that depends on the systemic circulation concentration and subsequent passage across single cell endothelial or epithelial membranes with specialized physical and molecular barrier functionality. For certain orally administered AIDS medications (e.g., zidovudine and didanosine), oral absorption is limited because of poor absorption from the GI tract, enzymatic biotransformation in the intestinal epithelium, or first-pass effects. For other AIDS drugs (e.g., protease inhibitors), oral absorption may be complete; however, drug distribution into the brain is limited by drug efflux proteins, which promiscuously interact and translocate lipophilic substrates back into blood as they diffuse into the BBB endothelium.

The goal of this chapter is to provide a context for understanding drug distribution into tissues and address those factors that play a major role in determining the rate and extent of drug distribution.

7.2 BIOLOGICAL MEMBRANES

In order to appreciate the role of biological membranes and tissue barriers as determinants of drug distribution, it is important to begin with an understanding of cell membranes.

7.2.1 Cell Membrane Properties

7.2.1.1 Lipid Bilayer

Biological cell membranes are composed largely of a phospholipid bilayer (Figure 7.1). These membranes are organized such that the nonpolar tail groups of the two bilayers associate with each other, and their respective polar head groups form the inner and outer surface of the membrane, respectively. Cholesterol is associated with the cell membrane where it increases the structural stability of the bilayer, especially in areas where multiple proteins interact with each other (e.g., lipid rafts) to perform specialized signaling functions. The physiochemical environment of the lipid bilayer provides an effective barrier to protect the cell from its environment and to maintain well-defined microenvironment conditions that are optimal for cellular function. The membrane is permeable to relatively small nonpolar substrates, but larger molecules as well as smaller charged molecules and ions have difficulty crossing the membrane. Transport of such molecules depends on selective permeability afforded to them by transmembrane transport proteins imbedded in the lipid bilayer.

7.2.1.2 Membrane Proteins

From a physiologic perspective, cells must control the entry of molecules and ions required for their nutritional and metabolic needs. They also must efficiently remove metabolic byproducts and prevent entry of harmful substances, except in the case of specialized cells (e.g., hepatocytes), which need to eliminate these substances from the body. Thus, to maintain homeostasis, cells have developed specialized transport mechanisms through the use of membrane proteins, which afford them exquisite control of the quantity, rate, and types of molecules that can permeate their cell membrane.

Proteins associated with membranes are classified as lipid anchored, peripheral, and integral. Many of the integral proteins facilitate communication between the intracellular and extracellular microenvironment by direct noncovalent interaction with peripheral proteins whereas others are primarily involved in transport. Here we expound on the latter process and the role of integral proteins in selectively controlling transport across cellular membranes.

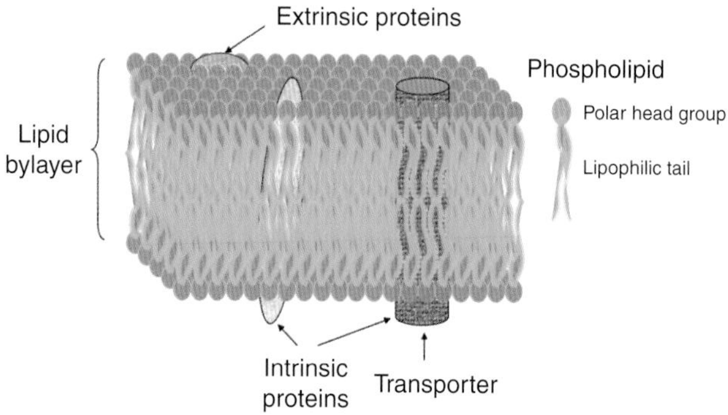

Figure 7.1 Lipid bilayer model.

Integral proteins are embedded in the membrane itself, to some degree, and are referred to as transmembrane proteins if they extend from one side of the membrane to the other. Typically these proteins have multiple domains or regions that are either primarily hydrophobic, if embedded in the lipid bilayer, or hydrophilic if localized in the extra- or intracellular environment. More complicated tertiary and quaternary protein domain structures allow for the formation of channels or pores where appropriate arrangement of hydrophilic and hydrophobic amino acids on the internal surface of each channel or pore dictates which molecules may enter or bind for subsequent translocation from one side of the membrane to the other. Based on this, some proteins exhibit considerable substrate specificity (e.g., GLUT1 a glucose transporter) whereas others appear much less specific (e.g., P-glycoprotein).

The transport mechanisms used by these proteins can be categorized based on use of energy. Channels and some types of carrier proteins function to carry substrates down a concentration gradient without the use of energy. Other carrier proteins require energy in the form of ATP to transport substrates against or up their concentration gradient.

Channel proteins allow substrate passage by forming an open space through the membrane. Channel opening or closing may be accomplished through a variety of mechanisms including changes in voltage gradients, secondary ligand binding, mechanical interaction via peripheral proteins, and chemical modification such as phosphorylation. Typically channel proteins display the highest substrate transfer rates since there is no need for binding or conformational changes other than the original opening of the channel. Also, in the case of ion transport, the formation of an electrochemical as well as a diffusion gradient leads to the most rapid transport process. Obviously, the substrate's physiochemical properties will dictate whether it will pass through the channel and further narrow the channel's substrate specificity. In contrast to channels, carrier proteins bind substrates weakly to a unique tertiary structural domain or "pocket" and translocate them by a conformational change. Once the substrate is released, the protein structure returns to its original more thermodynamically favorable conformation. Because of the need for this conformational change, release, and resetting of the protein's structure at each step, the transfer rates associated with carrier proteins are slower.

In contrast to the channel and carrier proteins described earlier, some carrier or transporter proteins utilize energy, in the form of ATP, either directly or indirectly to move substrates against their concentration gradient. In the case of carriers that use energy indirectly, also known as secondary active transporters, two transporters work in concert; one uses ATP and the other does not. Because of their capacity to move substrates against concentration gradients, transporters are of the greatest interest in terms of the movement of drugs across biological membranes. In general, these proteins function much like a carrier, but because they also require the binding and hydrolysis of ATP for the conformational changes and transport to occur, they transport substrates at the slowest rate.

7.2.1.3 Transporters

Transporters can greatly facilitate the passage of a drug from one side of a biological membrane to the other. Generally they are classified by their subcellular orientation (basolateral vs. apical), cellular direction of substrate flux (uptake vs. efflux transporters), energy source (primary vs. secondary energy source), or ability to move more than one substrate in more than one direction. The orientation of transporters is either apical or basolateral and these terms also are referred to as luminal or abluminal, respectively. There is a subtle difference in the assignment of subcellular orientation for a specific transporter depending on the cell type (i.e., epithelium or endothelium). In epithelial cells the basolateral membranes typically refer to the bottom and sides of the cell facing the basement membrane, whereas the apical side faces the lumen or cavity of the tissue, gland, or organ. Thus, basolateral transporters are in proximity to the capillary and venule networks and interact with substrates that have diffused through the basement membrane; hence, they control flux between the blood environment and the inside of the cell. Apical transporters regulate flux of substrates between the cell and the lumen of the tissue or organ (e.g., gastrointestinal track, bile duct, lung aveoli, etc.). In contrast to epithelial cells, the subcellular terminology is reversed in tight junction forming endothelial cells that constitute a blood–tissue barrier (e.g., blood–brain or blood–retinal barriers). Apically expressed transporters in endothelial cells control the flux of substrates between the lumen of the vessel (blood side) and the inside of the cell, whereas basolateral transporters control the flux between the tissue and the endothelium.

In terms of directional flux, uptake transporters dictate the movement of substrates into the cell (e.g., OATP family of transporters), whereas efflux transporters are largely responsible for the movement of drugs and their metabolites out of the cell (e.g., P-GP, BCRP, and MRP family of transporters). Transporters that depend on ATP hydrolysis are grouped into several families of ATP binding cassette proteins or ABC proteins. The energy of ATP hydrolysis causes a conformational change in the transporter, which allows for the translocation of the substrate from one side of the membrane to the other. Secondary energy transporters are driven by protein or ion gradients (e.g., Na^+). The translocation of the drug is driven by the movement of ion in the same direction (symporters) or in the opposite direction (antiporter) (Figure 7.2). A more appropriate term for these proteins is cotransporters since they can

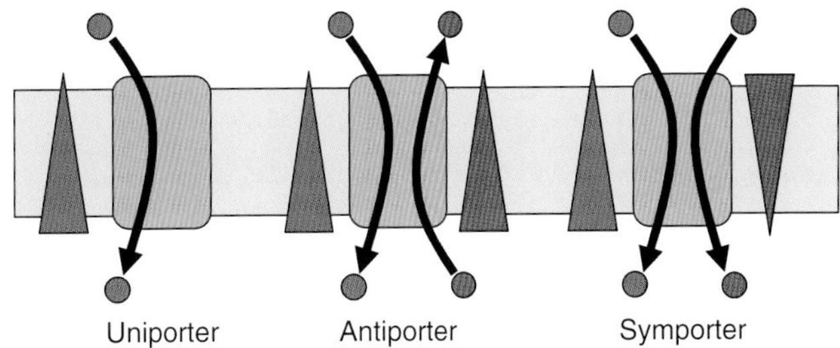

Figure 7.2 Functional models of membrane translocation by cotransporters. (Redrawn from Figure 15-2 in Lodish et al., 1995).

simultaneously transport two different solutes. A partial list of transporters implicated in cellular drug translocation is included in Table 7.1.

OAT/OCT Most solute transporters, including the members of the *SLC22*-family, share a predicted membrane topology with 12 transmembrane domains. This family comprises organic cation transporters (OCTs), as well as transporters for the zwitterion carnitine (OCTNs) and organic anion transporters (OATs).

Three polyspecific electrogenic cation transporters, OCT1, OCT2, and OCT3, have been identified. A number of properties are common to the OCT family: (1) all transport a variety of organic cations with different chemical structures; (2) all transport in an electrogenic manner, and their function is independent of Na^+, Cl^-, and H^+ ions; and (3) all are able to translocate cations across the plasma membrane in either direction. The OCTs vary somewhat in their tissue distribution with OCT1 largely expressed in the liver, OCT2 in the kidney, and OCT3 in a variety of tissues.

Other cation transporters of the SLC22 family appear to translocate the zwitterion carnitine together with Na^+ and/or organic cations (OCTN1 and OCTN2). OCTN1 appears to be an electroneutral H^+/organic cation antiporter that mediates efflux of organic cations from cells. OCTN2 is generally believed to function as a Na^+/carnitine cotransporter, but can also function as a polyspecific and Na^+-independent cation uniporter. Both OCTN1 and OCTN2 are expressed in a variety of tissues and can translocate a number of drugs.

A number of OATs function as dicarboxylate antiporters and are responsible for the movement of organic anions across cell membranes. OAT1 is expressed largely on the basolateral membrane of proximal tubule cells in the kidney and to a lesser degree in choroid plexus epithelium and brain neurons. OAT3 shares similar tissue distribution and subcellular orientation in the kidney and choroid plexus but is also expressed in brain capillary endothelial cells. By contrast, OAT2 has greater expression in the liver and OAT4 is expressed on the apical surface of renal tubules and serves as a reabsorptive pathway for organic anions.

Table 7.1 Characteristics of Transporters Involved in Drug Distribution

Gene Symbol	Alias	Substrates	Drugs	Tissue Expression	Ref
ABCB			*ATP-binding cassette, subfamily B (MDR/TAP)*		
ABCB1	MDR1	Neutral and organic cations	Doxorubicin, daunorubicin, vincristine, vinblastine, actinomycin-D, paclitaxel, docetaxel, etoposide, teniposide, bisantrene, homoharringtonine, imatinib	Intestine, liver, kidney, placenta, blood–brain barrier	Ito et al., 2005; Ambudkar et al., 2003
ABCC			*ATP-binding cassette, subfamily C (CFTR/MRP)*		
ABCC1	MRP1	Glutathione and other conjugates, organic anions, leukotriene C4	Doxorubicin, epirubicin, etoposide, vincristine, methotrexate	Ubiquitous	Ito et al., 2005; Ambudkar et al., 2003; Haimeur et al., 2004
ABCC2	MRP2	Glutathione and other conjugates, organic anions, leukotriene C4	Methotrexate, etoposide, doxorubicin, cisplatin, vincristine, mitoxantrone	Liver, kidney, intestine	Ito et al., 2005; Ambudkar et al., 2003; Haimeur et al., 2004
ABCC3	MRP3	Glucuronate and glutathione conjugates, bile acids	Etoposide, teniposide, methotrexate, cisplatin, vincristine, doxorubicin	Adrenals, intestine, kidneys, liver, pancreas	Ito et al., 2005; Ambudkar et al., 2003; Haimeur et al., 2004
ABCC4	MRP4	Nucleoside analogues, organic anions	Methotrexate, thiopurines	Ubiquitous	Ito et al., 2005; Ambudkar et al., 2003; Haimeur et al., 2004
ABCC5	MRP5	Nucleoside analogues, cyclic nucleotides, organic anions	6-Mercaptopurine, 6-thioguanine	Ubiquitous	Ito et al., 2005; Ambudkar et al., 2003; Haimeur et al., 2004
ABCC6	MRP6	Anionic cyclic pentapeptide		Liver, kidney	Ito et al., 2005; Ambudkar et al., 2003; Haimeur et al., 2004
ABCC10	MRP7	Glutathione conjugates, lipophilic anions		Liver	Ito et al., 2005; Ambudkar et al., 2003; Haimeur et al., 2004
ABCG			*ATP-binding cassette, subfamily G (WHITE)*		
ABCG2	BCRP	Endogenous compounds, sulfate conjugates, carcinogens	Doxorubicin, daunorubicin, mitoxantrone, topotecan, SN-38, nitrofurantoin, cimetidine	Placenta, intestine, mammary gland, liver	Ambudkar et al., 2003; Haimeur et al., 2004; Kusuhara and Sugiyama, 2006
SLC15			*Solute carrier family 15 (oligopeptide transporter)*		
SLC15A1	PEPT1	Di- and tripeptides	Valacylcovir, β-lactam antibiotics	Small intestine, kidney, liver	Biegel et al., 2006; Smith et al., 2004
SLC15A2	PEPT2	Di- and tripeptides	β-lactam antibiotics	Kidney, brain, lung, mammary gland	Biegel et al., 2006; Smith et al., 2004

SLC22			*Solute carrier family 22 (organic cation transporter)*		
SLC22A1	OCT1	Organic cations (e.g., TEA, MPP+, dopamine, tyramine)	Amantadine, memantine, metformin, acyclovir, azidoprocainamide, cimetidine, corticosteroids, quinidine, quinine, midazolam, verapamil	Liver	Dresser et al., 2001; Jonker and Schinkel, 2004; Koepsell et al., 2003
SLC22A2	OCT2	Organic cations (e.g., TEA, MPP+, choline, dopamine, tyramine)	Amantadine, memantine, cimetidine, debrisoquine, ganciclovir	Kidney, brain	Dresser et al., 2001; Jonker and Schinkel, 2004; Koepsell et al., 2003
SLC22A3	OCT3	Organic cations (e.g., TEA, MPP+, dopamine, tyramine, histamine, norepinephrine, serotonin)	Cimetidine, metformin	Liver, skeletal muscle, placenta, kidney, heart, lung, brain	Dresser et al., 2001; Jonker and Schinkel, 2004; Koepsell et al., 2003
SLC22A4	OCTN1	Organic cations	Quinidine, pyrilamine, verapamil, cephaloridin	Kidney, skeletal muscle, placenta, prostate, heart	Dresser et al., 2001; Jonker and Schinkel, 2004; Koepsell et al., 2003
SLC22A5	OCTN2	L Carnitine, organic cations	Cefepime, cefoselis	Skeletal muscle, kidney, prostate, lung, pancreas, heart, small intestine, adrenal gland, thyroid gland, liver,	Dresser et al., 2001; Jonker and Schinkel, 2004; Koepsell et al., 2003
SLC22A6	OAT1	Organic anions (e.g., PGE2, urate, uremic toxins)	PAH, NSAIDs, antiviral agents, MTX, OTA, β-lactam antibiotics, ACE inhibitors	Kidney, brain, placenta, eyes	Anzai et al., 2006; Sekine et al., 2006; Robertson and Rankin, 2006; You, 2004
SLC22A7	OAT2	Organic anions (e.g., PGE2, PGF2α)	Tetracycline, salicylate, acetylsalicylate	Liver, kidney	Anzai et al., 2006; Sekine et al., 2006; Robertson and Rankin, 2006; You, 2004
SLC22A8	OAT3	Organic anions (e.g., ES, cAMP, cGMP, E217βG, DHEAS, PGE2, PGF2α, OTA)	MTX, cimetidine	Kidney, skeletal muscle, brain, eyes, bone	Anzai et al., 2006; Sekine et al., 2006; Robertson and Rankin, 2006; You, 2004
SLC22A9	OAT4	Organic anions (ES, DHEAS, PGE2, PGF2α, OTA)	Tetracycline, MTX	Kidney, placenta	Anzai et al., 2006; Sekine et al., 2006; Robertson and Rankin, 2006; You, 2004
SLC28			*Solute carrier family 28 (sodium-coupled nucleoside transporter)*		
SLC28A1	CNT1	Pyrimidine nucleosides, adenosine	Zidovudine, lamivudine, zalcitabine, cytarabine	Liver, kidney, small intestine	Gray et al., 2004; Kong et al., 2004
SLC28A2	CNT2	Purine nucleosides, uridine	Didanosine, ribavirin	Kidney, liver, heart, brain, placenta, pancreas, skeletal muscle, colon, rectum, small intestine	Gray et al., 2004; Kong et al., 2004
SLC28A3	CNT3	Broadly selective for pyrimidines and purines	Cladrabine, gemcitabine, FdU, 5-fluorouridine, fludarabine, zebularine, AZT, ddC, ddI	Pancreas, trachea, bone marrow, mammary gland, intestine, lung, placenta, prostrate, testis, liver	Gray et al., 2004; Kong et al., 2004

Continued

Table 7.1 Characteristics of Transporters Involved in Drug Distribution—cont'd

Gene Symbol	Alias	Substrates	Drugs	Tissue Expression	Ref
SLC29		*Solute carrier family 29 (nucleoside transporters)*			
SLC29A1	ENT1	Pyrimidine and purine nucleosides	Cytarabine, gemcitabine	Ubiquitous	Kong et al., 2004; Baldwin et al., 2004
SLC29A2	ENT2	Pyrimidine and purine nucleosides, nucleobases	Cytarabine, gemcitabine, zalcitabine, zidovudine	Ubiquitous	Kong et al., 2004; Baldwin et al., 2004
SLC29A3	ENT3	Pyrimidine and purine nucleosides, nucleobases			Kong et al., 2004; Baldwin et al., 2004
SLCO		*Solute carrier organic anion transporter family*			
SLCO1A2	OATP-A, OATP	Bile salts, organic anions, hormone conjugates, eicosanoids	Saquinavir, methotrexate, fexofenadine, ouabain, indomethacin	Brain, kidney, liver, lung, small intestine	Hagenbuch and Meier, 2003, 2004; Ito et al., 2005
SLCO1B1	OATP-C, LST-1, OATP2	Bile salts, hormone conjugates, eicosanoids	Benzylpenicillin, pravastatin, fluvastatin, rifampin, methotrexate,	Liver	Hagenbuch and Meier, 2003, 2004; Ito et al., 2005; Konig et al., 2006
SLCO1B3	OATP8	Bile salts, organic anions	Digoxin, methotrexate, rifampin, paclitaxel	Liver, cancer cell lines	Hagenbuch and Meier, 2003, 2004; Ito et al., 2005; Konig et al., 2006
SLCO1C1	OATP-F	T4, rT3, BSP	Atorvastatin	Brain, testis (Leydig cells)	Hagenbuch and Meier, 2003, 2004; Ito et al., 2005
SLCO2A1	PGT	Eicosanoids		Ubiquitous	Hagenbuch and Meier, 2003, 2004; Ito et al., 2005
SLCO2B1	OATP-B, PGT	Bile salts, organic anions, hormone conjugates	Digoxin, benzylpenicillin, fexofenadine, fluvastatin	Liver, placenta, brain, heart, kidneys, intestine	Hagenbuch and Meier, 2003, 2004; Ito et al., 2005; Konig et al., 2006
SLCO3A1	OATP-D	E-3-S, prostaglandin	Benzylpenicillin	Ubiquitous	Hagenbuch and Meier, 2003, 2004; Ito et al., 2005
SLCO4A1	OATP-E	Taurocholate, T3, prostaglandin	Benzylpenicillin,	Ubiquitous	Hagenbuch and Meier, 2003, 2004; Ito et al., 2005
SLCO4C1	OATP-H	T3, T4	Digoxin, ouabine	Kidney	Hagenbuch and Meier, 2003, 2004; Ito et al., 2005
SLCO5A1	OATP-J				Hagenbuch and Meier, 2003, 2004; Ito et al., 2005
SLCO6A1	OATP-I. GST			Testis	Hagenbuch and Meier, 2003, 2004; Ito et al., 2005

OATPs Organic anion transporting polypeptides (OATP family) form a superfamily of sodium-independent transport systems that can flux a wide range of endogenous and exogenous organic compounds. As a family, these transporters have a wide tissue distribution. Many of these transporters serve an important role as uptake transporters in epithelial basolateral membranes, providing drug access from plasma into tissues including eliminating organs (i.e., kidney and liver). A growing body of evidence suggests this family of transporters is important in determining the disposition of a range of drugs. OATP1A2 (*SLCO1A2*) is located in the brain, kidney, liver, lung, and small intestine, and plays a role in the disposition of saquinavir, methotrexate, fexofenadine, ouabain, and indomethacin. OATP1B1 (*SLCO1B1*) and OATP1B3 (*SLCO1B3*) are generally associated with the liver and are involved in the hepatic uptake of benzylpenicillin, pravastatin, rifampin, and methotrexate.

P-Glycoprotein (P-GP) One of the most widely studied and clinically relevant drug transporters is P-GP (MDR or MDR1, which is the gene product of *ABCB1*). First associated with resistance of cancer cells to chemotherapeutic drugs, P-GP is now thought to play a central role in cellular, tissue, and systemic defense against drug or other xenobiotics exposure. P-GP has been identified in intestine, liver, kidney placenta and the blood–brain barrier. Doxorubicin, daunorubicin, vincristine, vinblastine, actinomycin-D, paclitaxel, docetaxel, etoposide, teniposide, bisantrene, imatinib, and many other drugs have been shown to be P-GP substrates. P-GP plays a distinct role in limiting the intestinal absorption and tissue distribution of drugs, while promoting their elimination into the bile and urine.

BCRP Another ABC family efflux drug transporter first associated with cancer cells and subsequently found to be very important in drug disposition is breast cancer resistance protein (BCRP (*ABCG2*)). Endogenous substrates for BCRP include sulfate conjugates, porphyrins, and potentially vitamins. Many anticancer drugs have also been identified as BCRP substrates including doxorubicin, daunorubicin, mitoxantrone, topotecan, SN-38, nitrofurantoin, and cimetidine. BCRP expression has been identified in intestine, liver, placenta, blood–brain barrier, the blood–cerebrospinal fluid barrier and the blood–mammary barrier. Like P-GP, BCRP appears to play a central role in reducing xenobiotic exposure by limiting absorption and distribution while enhancing the renal and hepatic elimination.

MRP Multiple drug resistance associated proteins (MRPs or *ABCC* family) are another important group of transporters. It is generally thought that these transporters are responsible for the cellular efflux of a number of drug metabolites (e.g., glutathione and other conjugates) once they have been formed intracellularly. The tissue distribution of MRP1 is wide spread and it appears critical in the disposition of doxorubicin, epirubicin, etoposide, vincristine, and methotrexate. By contrast, MRP2 is generally associated with organs of elimination (i.e., kidney, liver, and intestine). MRP2 has overlapping substrate profile with MRP1.

7.2.2 Tissue Barriers

The general principles described earlier for drug distribution into and out of cells can largely be applied to tissue barriers. Tissue barriers are made up of one or more cell types that collectively form a distinct boundary between one physiological environment (e.g., blood) and another (e.g., central nervous system). Typically these barriers protect the body or sensitive organs or tissues from exposure to substrates of the external environment including drugs. Several of these barriers will be discussed individually; however they have common features. The capillary beds in most systemic organs and particularly in the liver are thought to be "leaky" or fenestrated (i.e., the endothelial cells of the liver sinusoidal vascular bed do not form tight intercellular junctions). Substrates and nutrients from the blood can readily diffuse out of the blood and into the liver parenchymal cells very rapidly. For those tissues said to possess "barriers," cells tend to form tight intercellular junctions that limit rapid paracellular diffusion of proteins and polar compounds. These barriers may be composed of endothelial (e.g., blood–brain barrier) or epithelial cells (e.g., placental), or combinations of those cells working in concert to form a significant obstacle to drug passage into selective organs or tissues. In addition to tight junctions, many of these tissue barriers also appear to have a more differentiated cell type that gives rise to greater expression of transporters, which effectively limit or facilitate substrate passage across the membrane (Figure 7.3).

7.2.3 Flux Across Biological Membranes

Drug movement across barrier-forming biological membranes can generally be accomplished by three mechanisms (Figure 7.4). Typically paracellular passive diffusion occurs for ions and smaller drugs in those tissues that do not have tight junctions. In contrast, barrier forming membranes allow only molecules that are sufficiently hydrophobic to partition into the lipid bilayer of the plasma membrane and potentially diffuse to the other side of the cell. Carrier mediated transport is the most prevalent mechanism because it affords greater control as to the type and quantity of molecules that can be translocated. This mode may involve one or more transporters so that efficient vectorial transfer can occur, or just a single transporter that effluxes a substrate. In the latter case, the presence of a transporter on the side of

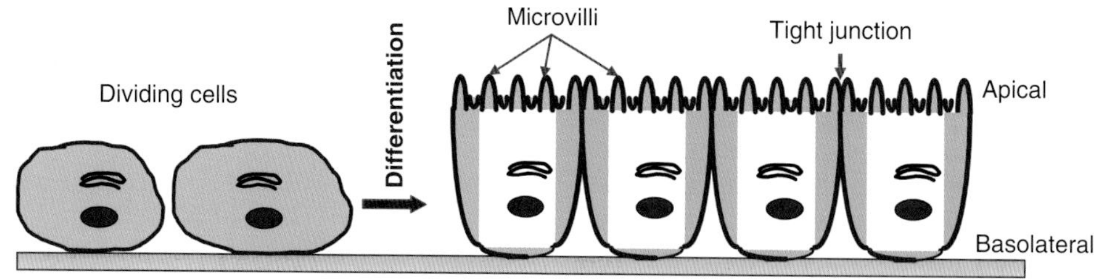

Figure 7.3 Model of cell differentiation on a basement membrane (or support structure) depicting polarization to reflect distinct apical and basolateral function. (Redrawn from Figure 6-9 in Lodish et al., 1995.)

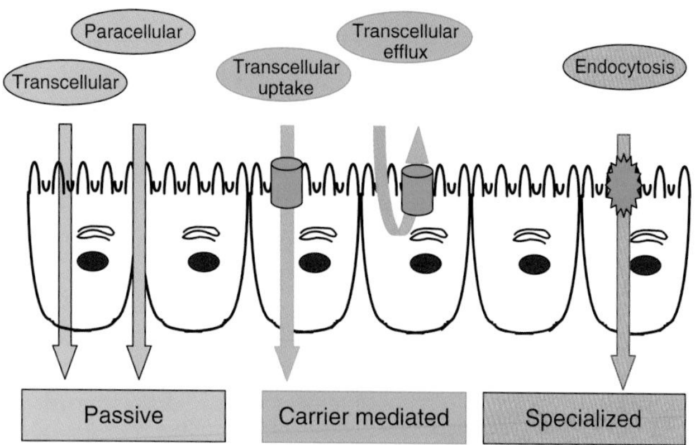

Figure 7.4 Mechanisms of drug flux across a polarized monolayer including passive diffusion, carrier mediated processes and specialized transport processes.

drug presentation could efflux drug back out of the cell by decreasing the intracellular (or in the case of P-GP, the intermembrane) drug concentration gradient. Drug transfer could also occur by specialized transport, which might include endocytosis. In this case, molecules may be transferred inside the cell while they are interacting with the membrane in a nonspecific fashion. However, the most efficient and controlled pathway involves molecules interacting with a cell surface receptor that subsequently triggers the formation of endocytic vesicles, which carry the receptor bound molecules into the cell where they are released for further use. This form of drug distribution is more likely for larger molecules and proteins and also has been used for the transport of drug delivery systems (e.g., liposomes or nanoparticles).

7.2.3.1 *Passive Diffusion*

Passive diffusion is a major process by which drugs cross cell membranes. Fick's law of diffusion is applied to drug transfer from outside the cell (C_o) to inside the cell (C_i) as viewed from the appearance of drug in the cell

$$F\left(\text{or}\,\frac{dC_i}{dt}\right) = \frac{DA(C_o - C_i)}{h} \tag{7.1}$$

where F is the mass transferred, D is the diffusion coefficient, A is the surface area of the membrane, $(C_o - C_i)$ is the drug concentration difference between outside and inside the cell, and h is the thickness of the membrane. If the outside drug concentration is maintained (Figure 7.5A), internal drug concentration accumulation driven by diffusion will eventually equilibrate with

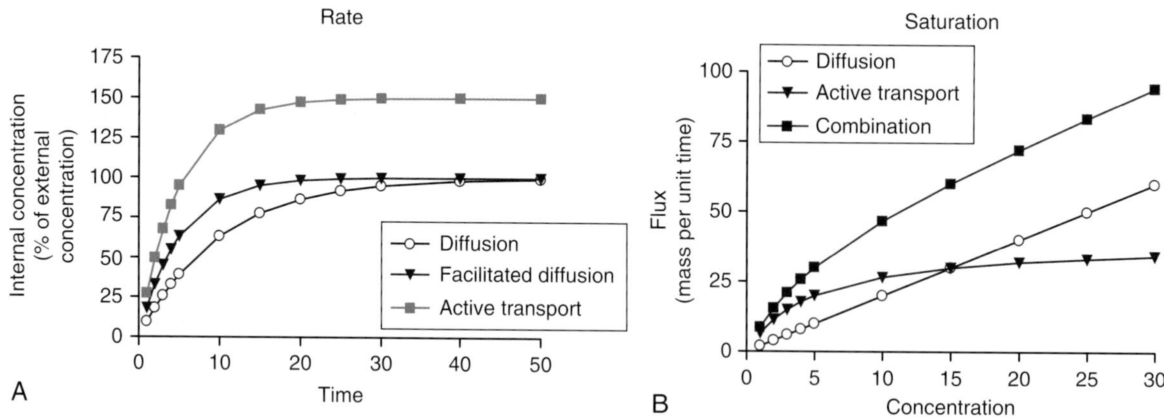

Figure 7.5 (A) Time course of internal drug concentration in a cell when exposed to a constant external concentration in which there is simple diffusion, facilitated diffusion, or active transport. (B) Drug flux as a function of drug concentration for diffusion, active transport, or a combination of both diffusion and active transport into a cell.

the external concentration. The flux rate is linear with respect to the external concentration; that is, the flux rate associated with diffusion is always proportional to drug concentration.

The relationship in Equation (7.1) forms a useful conceptual framework for assessing drug passage across a membrane (biological or other). Drug mass can be moved more quickly for those drugs with greater diffusivity (D) across thin (h) membranes with the greatest surface area (A). The diffusion coefficient is a measurement of how well a given molecule can diffuse in a particular medium. To cross a cell membrane the drug has to partition into the membrane and repartition out of the membrane into the cytoplasm on the other side.

Factors Influencing Passive Diffusion The cell bilayer, which is permeable to lipophilic molecules and favors their partitioning into the membrane, represents an important first step in flux across the membrane. In order to pass unassisted through the membrane, the drug must ultimately repartition out into the aqueous environment of the cytoplasm. Therefore, "good" drugs need a balance between hydrophilicity and lipophilicity. A very hydrophilic drug will have difficulty entering the cell whereas a drug that is too lipophilic may simply accumulate in the cell membrane. Figure 7.6 illustrates a pronounced correlation between lipophilicity and permeability across the blood–brain barrier for most drugs. Vinblastine and vincristine are exceptions to the correlation. Both are actively effluxed out of the brain by P-GP, hence lowering their apparent permeability.

A number of drug properties, in addition to lipophilicity, can influence passive diffusion. Many drugs possess ionizable functional groups, which give rise to two (or more) forms of the drug depending on the functional groups ionized (i.e., weak acids and weak bases), the pKa of the drug, and the pH of the environment surrounding the membrane. The charged form of the drug is thought to diffuse at a much slower rate

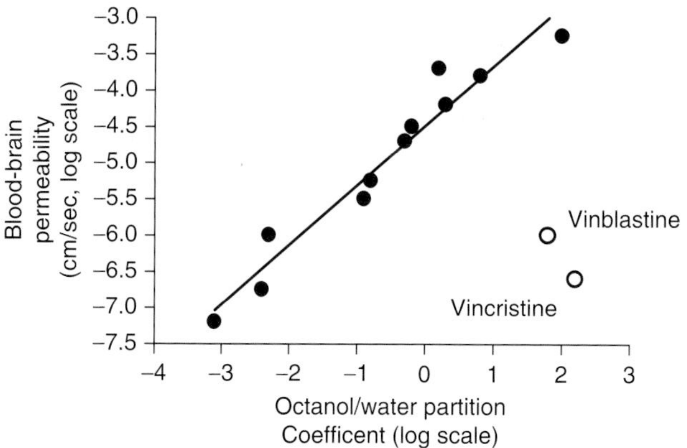

Figure 7.6 Influence of lipophilicity on the permeability of a number of drugs into the blood brain. (Adapted, in part, from Figure 4-4 in Rowland and Tozer, 2006; and from Grieg, 1989; and Grieg et al, 1990.)

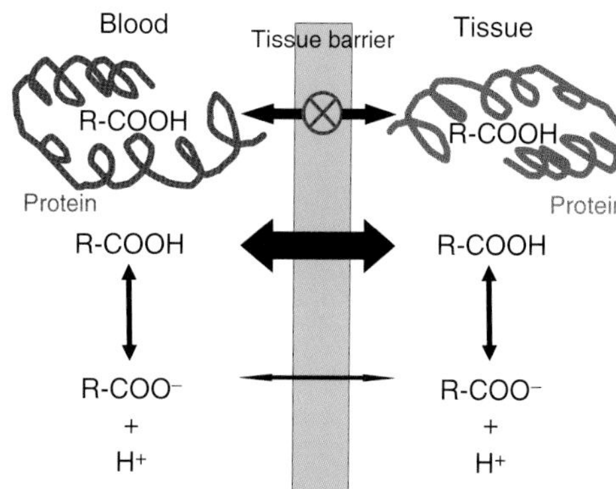

Figure 7.7 Schematic depicting the influence of ionization and protein binding on the passage of drugs across a biological membrane. The unionized, unbound form of the drug (R-COOH) is more readily translocated compared to the ionized (R-COO-) or bound drug.

(100-fold) than the unionized such that for general considerations, only unionized drug passes across the membrane (Figure 7.7). This practical assumption is widely applied. Molecular size also appears to be an important factor with the larger molecular radius of a drug slowing its diffusion across the membrane. In a similar fashion, drugs with greater hydrogen bonding potential are thought to be "stickier" as they pass through the membrane, slowing down this diffusion. With respect to drug passage from blood into tissues, binding to red blood cells or carrier proteins has also been shown to reduce the apparent diffusion of drug into cells or tissues by reducing the effective concentration gradient (e.g., unbound drug concentration). Conversely, drug plasma protein complexes are too large to readily diffuse across membranes (Figure 7.7).

7.2.3.2 Carrier Mediated Transport

Facilitated Diffusion A number of uptake transporters appear to exhibit facilitated diffusion with respect to their substrates (e.g., OCTs and ENTs). However, the most well-studied and often cited example of facilitated diffusion is the transport of glucose (i.e., GLUT or SLC2 transporter family). Facilitated diffusion involves a carrier protein, which aids the passage of a more hydrophilic solute across the membrane, but cannot work against the concentration gradient. For a drug transported into a cell by facilitated diffusion, the internal drug concentration accumulation will proceed at a faster rate than by simple diffusion; however, the internal concentration will equilibrate with the external concentration (Figure 7.5A). A key feature of a facilitated diffusion mediated process is that the flux rate associated with it can be saturated at higher drug concentrations (Figure 7.5B).

As applied to drug transfer from outside the cell (C_o) to inside the cell (C_i), the flux (F) of drug into the cell (via facilitated diffusion or active transport) can be described by the following equation:

$$F = \frac{T_{max}C_o}{(K_T + C_o)} \quad (7.2)$$

where T_{max} is the maximum flux rate, K_T is the dissociation constant, and C_o is the drug concentration outside the cell. The maximum flux rate is a function of the relative abundance of the transporter and the turnover rate of the substrate–transporter complex. The dissociation constant is inversely related to the binding affinity of the substrate for the transporter.

Active Transport Like facilitated diffusion, active transport involves a carrier protein, which aids the passage of a more hydrophilic solute across the membrane; however, an active transport process differs from facilitated diffusion in that it can transfer drugs against the concentration gradient. The difference in these two carrier mediated processes could be attributed to the difference in affinity for the two transporters in the cell. It is hypothesized that the affinity of the substrate for its facilitated carrier is the same when the complex is exposed externally and internally, resulting in no ability to accumulate drug. By contrast, the conformation of the substrate–transporter complex for active transport is thought to yield greater affinity on one side versus the other side of the membrane, resulting in the net flux of substrate in the direction of the lower affinity (either uptake or efflux across the membrane).

If the outside drug concentration is maintained (Figure 7.5A) internal drug concentration accumulation driven by an active transport process into the cell will eventually equilibrate at concentrations greater than the external concentration. Like facilitated diffusion, active transport mediated flux rate can be saturated at higher drug concentrations (Figure 7.5B).

For most drugs, flux into a cell (or across a tissue barrier) is a function of both diffusion (nonspecific, NS) and a carrier mediated process.

$$F = \frac{T_{max}C_o}{(K_T + C_o)} + NSC_o \quad (7.3)$$

The net effect of this combination would be drug flux across a membrane at a faster rate with low drug concentrations that slows to the flux of diffusion at higher concentrations. Drug concentration within the cell would be higher than external concentration for lower drug concentrations, but this difference would be minimized at concentrations well above the saturation concentration (i.e., K_T) for the uptake transporter.

Although this discussion was related to the active uptake into the cell (or flux across a membrane), many important transporters exist (e.g., P-GP, MRPs, BCRP) that exhibit active efflux transport. The same general mechanisms described above would hold however, the net flux would be in the opposite direction. A combination of passive diffusion into and active transport out of a cell would produce a drug flux that would appear at a slower rate for low drug concentrations, which eventually increase to that of diffusion at higher concentration. Drug within the cell would equilibrate at less than the external concentration for low drug concentrations, but this difference would be minimized at concentrations well above the saturation concentration (i.e., K_T) for the efflux transporter.

7.3 FACTORS INFLUENCING DRUG DISTRIBUTION

Most drugs leave the site of absorption, and distribute to sites of action and elimination by traveling in the blood. Distribution concepts need to consider the limitations of this physiological reality. For some drugs, the rate-limiting step in drug reaching the intracellular fluid is the time it takes the drug to reach the tissue, whereas for other drugs it is the passage out of the vascular space and into the tissue, which is rate limiting (Figure 7.8).

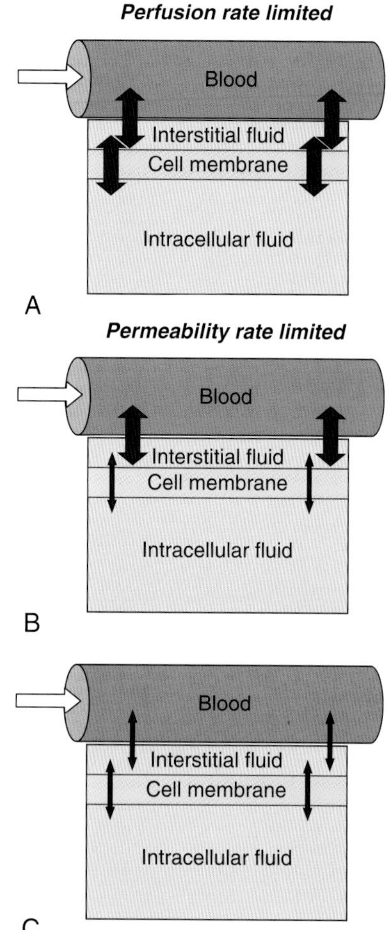

Figure 7.8 Model depicting perfusion rate limiting (A) and permeability limiting uptake in which the rate limited barrier is epithelium by itself (B) or in combination with the endothelium (C). (Redrawn from Figure 4-11 in Rowland and Tozer, 2006.)

7.3.1 Perfusion Rate

The perfusion rate of organs and tissues varies considerably (Table 7.2). The kidneys and liver are highly perfused, whereas bone and fat are perfused at much lower rates. Hence, for a drug that exhibits rapid permeability across cell membranes, the rate-limiting step is the blood flow carrying drug to the tissue (Figure 7.8A). A classic example of this scenario is thiopental. The distribution of thiopental out of the blood is very rapid and it first distributes into well-vascularized tissues, then muscle, and finally fat (Figure 7.9A). The loss of activity of this barbiturate is thought to arise in large part because of this redistribution phenomenon. This same pattern occurs with a number of other drugs and environmental contaminants that are very lipophilic.

Table 7.2 Blood Perfusion Rates for Various Organs and Tissues in an Adult Human (70kg) (Adapted from Table 5.2 in Rowland and Tozer, 2006.)

Organ	Perfusion Rate (ml/min)	% of Cardiac Output
Bone	250	5
Brain	700	14
Fat	200	4
Heart	300	4
Kidneys	1100	22
Liver	1350	27
Muscle	750	15
Skin	300	6

7.3.2 Permeability Rate

Although perfusion can limit the rate and extent of tissue penetration for some drugs, it is clear that permeability is a more significant barrier for distribution in most cases (Figure 7.9B). Relative to the rapid accumulation of thiopental the slower accumulation of barbital and salicylic acid in the CSF is thought to reflect the fact that their penetration is limited by something other than blood flow (i.e., permeability rate limited). For some tissues (i.e., muscle, kidneys, heart) the permeability barrier appears to be at the cell membrane (Figure 7.8B). In other tissues, such as the CNS, the barrier appears to be the capillary membrane (Figure 7.8C).

Many of the same factors which affect drug penetration into a cell can influence drug penetration into a tissue or organ. Although the general lipid membrane model (Figure 7.1) seems to convey similar permeability characteristics for most drugs, there are some properties of tissue barriers that limit the rate of drug penetration. Smaller hydrophilic drugs are able to pass through junctions between cells (paracellular pathway) in some tissues (Figure 7.4), whereas these same junctions in other tissues (e.g., GI tract, blood–brain barrier) are considered to be "tight," and drug passage is diminished between cells. The other property of tissue barriers is the relative abundance and orientation of transporters present. Most tissue barriers consist of well-differentiated cells that have different transporters expressed on basolateral and apical membranes. Such a difference in expression facilitates vectorial transport of substrates across a biological membrane. By contrast, P-GP expression in the GI tract and brain capillaries appears to limit drug penetration into the body or brain, respectively, by effluxing drug out of the membrane, thereby lowering intracellular concentration, which ultimately limits tissue accumulation. Drug properties (molecular size, lipophilicity, ionization, and protein binding) also play a crucial role in determining drug penetration across tissue barriers.

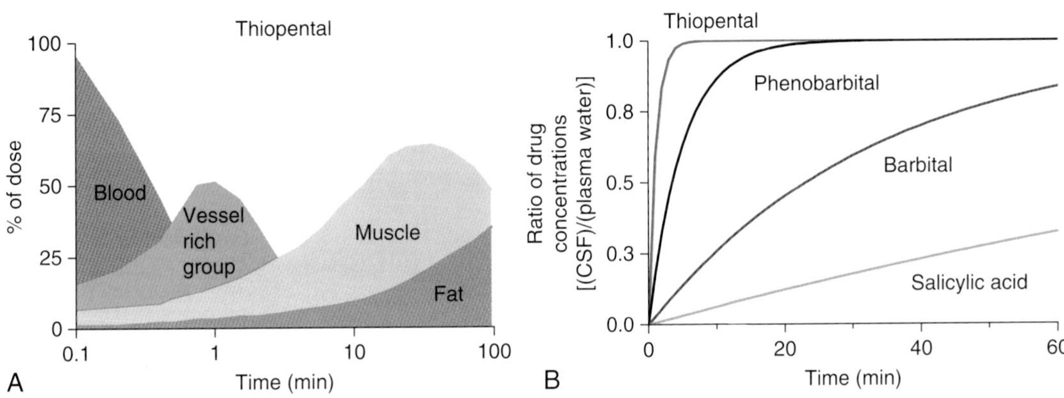

Figure 7.9 A. Illustrates the differences in perfusion rate on the proposed distribution and redistribution of thiopental. (Redrawn from http://www.cvm.okstate.edu/Courses/vmed5412/LECT006.htm) B. Drug equilibration in the cerebrospinal fluid with plasma water for various drugs in the dog (redrawn from Figure 5-11 in Rowland and Tozer, 2006, and Brodie et al., 1960. Plasma drug concentration was kept constant throughout the study. Thiopental displays perfusion limited distribution whereas the distribution of salicylic acid is permeability rate limited.

7.4 PHARMACOKINETIC/ PHARMACODYNAMIC DISTRIBUTION PROPERTIES

Both the rate and extent of drug distribution across tissue barriers can have a profound impact on pharmacokinetic and pharmacodynamic properties. The extent of drug distribution manifests itself locally as the tissue to plasma (or blood) concentration ratio. Collectively, the extent of distribution into all the tissues results in the apparent volume of distribution. Simply put, the pharmacokinetic parameter volume of distribution reflects the ratio of individual tissue to plasma drug concentration weighed for tissue volume. The rate of distribution (together with the extent of distribution) can influence the shape of the plasma versus time profile for a drug, which can give rise to differences in elimination half-life as well as onset and duration of action.

7.4.1 Tissue-to-Plasma (Blood) Ratio (T/P)

If it is assumed that only unbound, unionized drug can cross a tissue membrane by passive diffusion then the steady state drug concentration ratio of a tissue to plasma (T/P) is given by the following relationship

$$T/P = \frac{f_p^{un} f_p}{f_t^{un} f_t} K_F \qquad (7.4)$$

where f^{un} refers to the fraction unionized in plasma and tissue, f is the fraction unbound to proteins in the two spaces, and K_F a partitioning factor for drug in tissue fat.

Although some of the same factors influence the result, it is important to understand that this parameter is at steady state, hence the rate of permeability does not determine T/P. A highly permeable drug will cross the cell (tissue) membrane quickly, but will also leave quickly. Hence, the rate of distribution (or tissue equilibration) may be rapid for a more lipophilic drug, but the extent of distribution (reflected in T/P) may be no greater than a hydrophilic drug. The T/P ratio will be determined by factors such as ionization, due to pH differences in a tissue and blood, protein binding differences in tissue and blood, and partitioning into tissue fat.

7.4.2 Volume of Distribution

The volume of distribution reflects the relationship between the amount of drug in the body at steady state and plasma drug concentration. The volume of distribution is a mathematical concept, which does not necessarily reflect a physiological or "real" distribution space. This phenomenon can be illustrated by examining the volume of distribution for a number of drugs in Table 7.3. The volume of distribution of some drugs (e.g., chloroquine and digoxin) exceeds total body water (approximately 0.8 L/kg), whereas others (e.g., tolbutamide) are comparable to blood volume (0.08 L/kg).

Table 7.3 Apparent Volume of Distribution Values for a Number of Drugs (Data from Appendix Table A-II in Hardman et al., 2001)

Drug	Liters Per Kg
Chloroquine	150
Nortriptyline	30
Digoxin	7
Lidocaine	1.7
Theophylline	0.5
Tolbutamide	0.11

In a physiological sense, the volume of distribution can be conceptualized using the following relationship:

$$V_{ss} = V_p + \sum_{i=1}^{n} \left(\frac{T}{P}\right)_i V_i \qquad (7.5)$$

where V_p is the plasma volume, $(T/P)_i$ is the drug tissue-to-plasma concentration ratio in the ith tissue, and V_i is the volume of the ith tissue. The volume of distribution for chloroquine is so large because this lipophilic drug ($\log P = 4.7$) partitions into tissue fat; whereas digoxin ($\log P = 0.85$) large volume is attributed to its binding to muscle ATPases.

If the main factors controlling tissue distribution are differences between plasma and tissue binding then a derivative of Equation (7.5) can be written.

$$V_{ss} = V_p + \sum_{i=1}^{n} \left(\frac{f_p}{f_t}\right)_i V_i \qquad (7.6)$$

One clinically relevant observation that arises from this relationship is that the apparent volume of distribution for a drug is dependent upon the extent of plasma protein binding. Hence, drugs with more extensive plasma protein binding, like tolbutamide (95% bound), will have a lower volume of distribution than expected based on its lipophilicity ($\log P = 2.34$). This influence of plasma protein binding has been shown to contribute to the intersubject variability in the volume of distribution for a number of drugs (e.g., propranolol in liver disease).

7.4.3 Half-life ($t_{1/2}$)

Drug distribution can have a significant influence on elimination half-life. This influence is illustrated in Table 7.3. Glyburide and digoxin have comparable systemic clearances, but digoxin has a half-life, which is 10 times longer due to its more extensive distribution into tissues (larger V). Hence, the time course of digoxin is prolonged due to its extensive tissue distribution, not slow clearance. A similar situation can be found for montelukast and alprazolam (Table 7.4).

Table 7.4 Influence of Volume of Distribution (V) on Elimination Half-Life ($t_{1/2}$) for Selected Drugs with Similar Clearance Values (Cl) (Data from Appendix Table A-II in Hardman et al., 2001)

Drug	Cl [ml/(min*kg)]	V [L/kg]	$t_{1/2}$ [hr]
Glyburide	1.3	0.2	4
Digoxin	1.84	6	39
Montelukast	0.66	0.16	4
Alprazolam	0.74	0.72	12

7.5 SPECIFIC TISSUE BARRIERS

Although the general principles discussed here apply to all membranes, it is important to recognize that physiological (e.g., specific cell types, blood flow, and permeability) and molecular (e.g., uptake or efflux transporters) distinctions among tissue barriers can differentially affect drug distribution, which may be associated with efficacy or toxicity (Figure 7.10).

7.5.1 Blood–Brain Barrier and the Blood–Cerebrospinal Fluid Barrier

The blood–brain barrier (BBB) and the blood–cerebrospinal fluid barrier (BCB) at the choroid plexus are two major barriers between the CNS and blood (Figure 7.11). The BBB, however, has the most extensive surface area; approximately 1000 times that of the choroid plexus, which makes it the primary route for drug access to the brain. Furthermore, the high perfusion rate of the BBB allows lipophilic drug concentrations to equilibrate rapidly between the blood and brain.

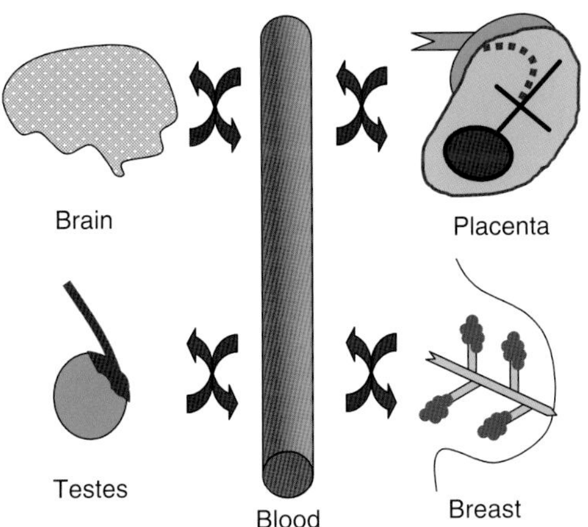

Figure 7.10 Select tissues for which a blood-tissue barrier is thought to be of importance in limiting drug distribution.

The BBB is comprised of microvascular endothelial cells, which unlike the systemic endothelium, are polarized and form tight junctions that impede paracellular flow and protect the brain by providing an effective barrier against the passage of many drugs. In addition, these cells exhibit low rates of endocytosis and limit nonspecific transcellular flux of potentially toxic substances. Transcellular passive diffusion across the BBB is generally restricted to small, unbound lipophilic drugs, but the BBB is also capable of macromolecular transcytosis through receptor mediated endocytosis. Although the endothelium presents the primary barrier, it appears that its physiological and molecular phenotype is maintained partially by adjacent astrocytes and pericytes (Figure 7.11A).

In contrast to the BBB, the endothelium of the choroid plexus is fenestrated, hence the true barrier for drug distribution across the choroid plexus is formed by a single continous layer of epithelial cells whose principal function is to control cerebral spinal fluid (CSF) homeostasis (Figure 7.11B). It also has tight paracellular junctions, but the flux of drugs across this barrier is much less extensive than the BBB due to its lower perfusion rate and smaller surface area.

The presence of these physical barriers allows for controlled transfer of nutrients and other substances into the brain through transporter mediated processes. There are a number of uptake transporters present at the BBB responsible for the flux of amino acids (System L, *SLC7A5*) and glucose (*GLUT1*) into the brain, which are critical for normal CNS function. The main drug efflux transporters located at the BBB include P-GP, BCRP, and MRP1 (*ABCC1*) (Figure 7.11C). Although endogenous physiological substrates of these transporters have not been identified in the brain, their function is considered primarily to be protecting the CNS from xenobiotics. Essentially, efflux transporters constitute a molecular barrier, which complements the physical endothelial barrier, and actively efflux drugs out of the brain. P-GP and BCRP have been shown to limit brain entry of a number of drugs, including HIV-1 protease inhibitors and anticancer agents. The choroid plexus barrier also has P-GP, BCRP and MRP1. In this case, P-GP expression appears to be subapical and may not contribute to efflux, whereas BCRP is expressed on the apical face of the epithelium and facilitates transfer of its substrates into the cerebrospinal fluid. In contrast, MRP1 and MRP4 are expressed in the basaloteral face of the epithelium and appear to impede entry of xenobiotics [PMID: 10675353; PMID: 15314169].

7.5.2 Placenta

The placenta is a complex membrane barrier system that separates the fetus from the mother and regulates the exchange of nutrients, gases, wastes, and

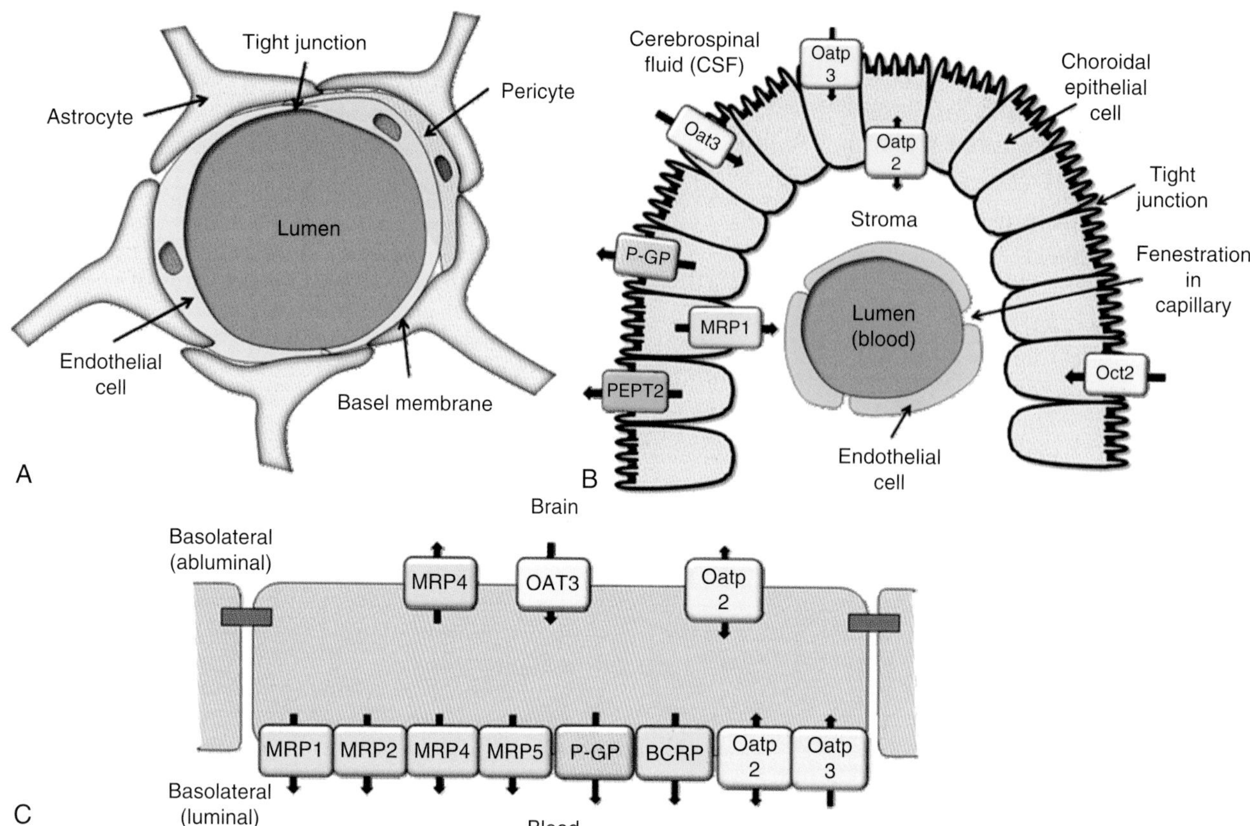

Figure 7.11 Schematic representation of the brain capillary (A), illustrating the interaction of capillary endothelial cells, pericytes, and astrocytes that result in tight junctions between endothelial cells, forming the blood–brain barrier (BBB) (redrawn from Figure 3 in Loscher and Potschka, 2005). The relationship between the choroid plexus and endothelial capillary is depicted in (B) (redrawn from Figure 6 in Loscher and Potschka, 2005). The capillary junctions are fenestrated and the barrier is thought to be the choroidal epithelial cells. A number of drug transporters have been identified in human and animals on this blood–cerebrospinal fluid (blood–CSF) barrier, including ABC transporters (P-GP and MRP1) as well as solute carriers (PEPT2, Oat3, Oatp2, Oatp3, and Oct3) (adapted from Kusuhara and Sugiyama, 2004). (C) represents the putative localization of drug transporters associated with the BBB (brain capillary endothelial cells), including ABC transporters (P-GP, BCRP, MRP1, MRP2, MRP4, and MRP5) as well as solute carriers (OAT3, Oatp2, Oatp3, as well as others) (adapted from Kusuhara and Sugiyama, 2005).

xenobiotics, including drugs. The placenta consists of the chorion frondosum (fetal tissue) and deciduas basali (maternal tissue) divided into functional units called cotyledons, which contains an effective barrier separating the maternal and fetal circulation. The barrier consists of the fetal capillary endothelia and the trophoblast, which contains the syncytiotrophoblast, a single-layered syncytium of polarized epithelial cells. Drug flux between mother and fetal blood includes their movement across the apical (toward maternal blood supply) and basolateral (toward fetal blood supply) membranes of the syncytiotrophoblast. The placenta is very well perfused and most lipophilic drugs can readily cross the placenta barrier by diffusion.

A number of transporters are present, which facilitate the transport of more hydrophilic nutrients, and some drugs. P-GP expression in the placenta is localized so that it effluxes drug back into the maternal circulation and limits fetal drug exposure to maternally adminstered drugs. This protective mechanism has been reported for a number of drugs including digoxin, saquinavir, and paxitaxel. Much like other barriers, BCRP also appears to be present in the placenta protecting the fetus from unwanted xenobiotics exposure. Members of the MRP and OATP family are also present in the placenta.

7.5.3 Mammary Gland

The mammary gland, like the placenta, is an important tissue for assessing risk exposure of the fetus or the newborn to maternal drugs. The mammary gland is comprised of large interconnecting alveoli, which produce milk. From there, the milk empties into collecting ducts that eventually empty into the sinuses beneath the areola, where it becomes available to the suckling infant. The functional unit for the milk production (and milk–blood barrier) in the mammary gland is a single layer of epithelial cells in the alveoli. These cells undergo extensive proliferation and are metabolically very active during lactation. Moreover, the mammary gland is very well perfused and the surface area is considerable. Hence, there is typically little lag time between the appearance of drug in milk relative to blood. There are exceptions to this generalization where certain drugs display a significant lag. Likewise, large milk producing ruminant animals are also likely to have a lag time in appearance due to the large milk volume resulting in slow equilibrium. To appreciate the factors influencing drug distribution into milk, it is important to note that milk pH is slightly lower (pH 7.2 in humans), trapping weak bases there is modest milk protein binding, and milk fat content is high. Highly lipophilic drugs may have large milk-to-serum ratios (M/S) due to extensive partitioning into milk.

A number of transporters have been reported to be expressed on the mammary epithelium (including glucose, amino acid transporters, and others). However, to date, only a handful of those have been shown to be important for drug transfer. BCRP appears to be an important transporter for drug transfer in the lactating mammary epithelium. Paradoxically, it is responsible for the accumulation of a number of drugs and toxins in this important nutritional fluid. The role of BCRP in drug accumulation into milk can be illustrated by examining the M/S of BCRP substrates in knockout mice (Table 7.5). Members of the OATP and MRP families also have been detected in human mammary epithelial cells. P-GP is not highly expressed in mammary epithelial cells and lactation appears to down regulate its mRNA levels.

Table 7.5 M to S from BCRP-/- Knockout Mice (van Herwaarden et al., 2005; Merino et al., 2005; Jonker et al., 2005; van Herwaarden and Schinkel, 2006)

	M/S		
	Wild-Type	**BCRP1-/-**	**Ratio**
Nitrofurantoin	45.7	0.6	76.2
PhIP	12.7	0.3	42.3
Cimetidine	13.6	2.2	6.2
Ciprofloxacin	4.44	2.19	2.0
Topotecan	6.75	0.8	8.4
Acylcovir	1.3	0.5	2.6
Folic Acid	0.023	0.021	1.1
Alfatoxin B1	0.7	0.18	3.9
IQ	0.95	0.28	3.4
Trp-P-1	1.15	0.43	2.7
DHEAS	0.15	0.13	1.2
DEHP	0.12	0.12	1.0

7.5.4 Testis

Developing germ cells are protected from xenobiotic exposure and immunological influences by a blood–testis barrier separating the seminiferous tubules from the blood. This barrier is created by the tight junction-forming Sertoli cells. Drugs must pass through Sertoli cells by either passive diffusion or active transport.

P-GP is highly expressed at the luminal surface of the capillary endothelial cells of testis capillaries where it appears to limit the exposure of the tissue to a number of substrates (e.g., ivermectin, vinblastine, and nelfinavir). The relatively high constitutive expression of MRP1 is cell-type specific and appears to play a role in the intercellular trafficking of steroids. The low expression level of BCRP and MRP2 in the blood–testis barrier suggests a functional role unlikely.

7.5.5 Intracellular Membranes

It is becoming increasingly more evident that the subcellular distribution of drugs is an important determinant of their toxicity. A number of anticancer and antiviral drugs exhibit significant mitochondrial toxicity that limits their clinical utility. The antiviral drug fialuridine with potent activity against hepatitis B virus produced severe toxicity in 7 of 15 patients in a phase II study, and this toxicity was not identified in preclinical studies. Unadkat and coworkers have demonstrated that the human equilibrative nucleoside transporter 1 (hENT1) is expressed on the mitochondrial membrane where it enhances the mitochondrial uptake and toxicity of fialuridine. Moreover, their data suggest that the lack of mitochondrial toxicity of this drug in rodents was due to the lack of mENT1 expression in the mitochondria. It is clear that transporters play an important role in the movement of drugs across intracellular membranes and thereby influence drug efficacy and toxicity.

7.6 SUMMARY

The goal of this chapter was to provide an understanding of the factors responsible for drug distribution into tissues. The physiochemical environment of the lipid bilayer (largely nonpolar) provides an effective barrier to protect the cell from its environment. Although relatively small nonpolar substrates can pass through the membrane, larger molecules as well as smaller charged molecules have difficulty crossing the membrane. The general principles described for drug distribution into and out of cells can be applied to tissue barriers as well. Typically, these tissue barriers protect the body or sensitive organs or tissues from exposure to substrates of the external environment, including drugs. Drug movement across biological membranes can be broadly categorized into three mechanisms including paracellular passive diffusion (ions and smaller drugs), transcellular transfer (sufficiently hydrophobic drugs), and carrier mediated transport involving one or more transporters. Drug distribution of larger molecular weight drugs or drug delivery systems into cells can occur by specialized transport, which might include endocytosis. Transporters can greatly facilitate the passage of a drug from one side of a biological membrane to another. A number of transporters (e.g., SLC22 family, OATPs) are involved in the active uptake into cells (or flux across a membrane), as well as important efflux transporters (e.g., P-GP, MRPs, BCRP) involved in the mechanism of active transport out of the cell or tissue barrier.

Drug properties including lipophilicity, the pKa of the drug, hydrogen bonding, and protein binding influence tissue distribution via passive diffusion. In addition to the drug properties, tissue characteristics also play a role, including the perfusion and capillary permeability of the tissue or organ as well as the specific transporter expression pattern at the tissue–blood barrier. A growing list of drugs appears to have their rate and extent of drug distribution into tissues linked to interactions with specific transporters. Unlike simple diffusion, these carrier mediated systems can be saturated and inhibited, which in turn may have clinical implications (drug interactions). Both the rate and extent of drug distribution across tissue barriers can have a profound impact on pharmacokinetic and pharmacodynamic properties (i.e., tissue-to-plasma concentration ratios, the apparent volume of distribution, the half-life and the time course of pharmacologic effect).

REFERENCES

Alcorn, J., et al. (2002). Transporter gene expression in lactating and nonlactating human mammary epithelial cells using real-time reverse transcription-polymerase chain reaction. *The Journal of Pharmacology and Experimental Therapeutics, 303*(2), 487–496.

Ambudkar, S. V., et al. (2003). P-glycoprotein: From genomics to mechanism. *Oncogene, 22*(47), 7468–7485.

Andiman, W. A. (2002). Transmission of HIV-1 from mother to infant. *Current Opinion in Pediatrics, 14*(1), 78–85.

Anzai, N., Kanai, Y., & Endou, H. (2006). Organic anion transporter family: Current knowledge. *Journal of Pharmacological Sciences, 100*(5), 411–426.

Bahn, A., et al. (2005). Murine renal organic anion transporters mOAT1 and mOAT3 facilitate the transport of neuroactive tryptophan metabolites. *American Journal of Physiology. Cell Physiology, 289*(5), C1075–C1084.

Baldwin, S. A., et al. (2004). The equilibrative nucleoside transporter family, SLC29. *Pflugers Archiv: European Journal of Physiology, 447*(5), 735–743.

Biegel, A., et al. (2006). The renal type H(+)/peptide symporter PEPT2: Structure-affinity relationships. *Amino Acids, 31*(2), 137–156.

Branch, R. A., James, J., & Read, A. E. (1976). A study of factors influencing drug disposition in chronic liver disease, using the model drug (+)-propranolol. *British Journal of Clinical Pharmacology, 3*(2), 243–249.

Breedveld, P., Beijnen, J. H., & Schellens, J. H. (2006). Use of P-glycoprotein and BCRP inhibitors to improve oral bioavailability and CNS penetration of anticancer drugs. *Trends in Pharmacological Sciences, 27*(1), 17–24.

Brodie, B. B., Kurz, H., & Schanker, L. S. (1960). The importance of dissociaton constant and lipid-solubility in influencing the passage of drugs into the cerebrospinal fluid. *The Journal of Pharmacology and Experimental Therapeutics, 130,* 20–25.

Dresser, M. J., Leabman, M. K., & Giacomini, K. M. (2001). Transporters involved in the elimination of drugs in the kidney: Organic anion transporters and organic cation transporters. *Journal of Pharmaceutical Sciences, 90*(4), 397–421.

Edwards, J. E., et al. (2005). Role of P-glycoprotein in distribution of nelfinavir across the blood-mammary tissue barrier and blood-brain barrier. *Antimicrobial Agents and Chemotherapy, 49*(4), 1626–1628.

Graff, C. L., & Pollack, G. M. (2004). Drug transport at the blood-brain barrier and the choroid plexus. *Current Drug Metabolism, 5*(1), 95–108.

Gray, J. H., Owen, R. P., & Giacomini, K. M. (2004). The concentrative nucleoside transporter family, SLC28. *Pflugers Archiv: European Journal of Physiology, 447*(5), 728–734.

Grieg, N. H. (1989). Drug Delivery to the Brain by Blood-Brain Barrier Circumvention and Drug Modification. In E. A. Neuwelt (Ed.), *Implications of the Blood-Brain Barrier and Its Manipulation.* New York: Plenum Medical Book Co.

Grieg, N. H., et al. (1990). Brain uptake and anticancer activities of vincristine and vinblastine are restricted by their low cerebrovascular permeability and binding to plasma constituents in rat. *Cancer Chemotherapy and Pharmacology, 26*(4), 263–268.

Hagenbuch, B., & Meier, P. J. (2003). The superfamily of organic anion transporting polypeptides. *Biochimica et Biophysica Acta, 1609*(1), 1–18.

Hagenbuch, B., & Meier, P. J. (2004). Organic anion transporting polypeptides of the OATP/ SLC21 family: phylogenetic classification as OATP/ SLCO superfamily, new nomenclature and molecular/functional properties. *Pflugers Archiv: European Journal of Physiology, 447*(5), 653–665.

Haimeur, A., et al. (2004). The MRP-related and BCRP/ABCG2 multidrug resistance proteins: Biology, substrate specificity and regulation. *Current Drug Metabolism, 5*(1), 21–53.

Hardman, J. G., Limbird, L. E., & Gilman, A. G. (2001). *Goodman and Gilman's The Pharmacological Basis of Therapeutics.* New York: McGraw-Hill.

Honkoop, P., et al. (1997). Mitochondrial injury. Lessons from the fialuridine trial. *Drug Safety: An International Journal of Medical Toxicology and Drug Experience, 17*(1), 1–7.

Ito, K., et al. (2005). Apical/basolateral surface expression of drug transporters and its role in vectorial drug transport. *Pharmaceutical Research, 22*(10), 1559–1577.

Jonker, J. W., & Schinkel, A. H. (2004). Pharmacological and physiological functions of the polyspecific organic cation transporters: OCT1, 2, and 3 (SLC22A1-3). *The Journal of Pharmacology and Experimental Therapeutics, 308*(1), 2–9.

Jonker, J. W., et al. (2005). The breast cancer resistance protein BCRP (ABCG2) concentrates drugs and carcinogenic xenotoxins into milk. *Nature Medicine, 11*(2), 127–129.

Kim, R., et al. (1998). The drug transporter P-glycoprotein limits oral absorption and brain entry of HIV-1 protease inhibitors. *The Journal of Clinical Investigation, 101*(2), 289–294.

Koepsell, H., Schmitt, B. M., & Gorboulev, V. (2003). Organic cation transporters. *Reviews of Physiology, Biochemistry and Pharmacology, 150,* 36–90.

Kolwankar, D., et al. (2005). Expression and function of ABCB1 and ABCG2 in human placental tissue. *Drug Metabolism and Disposition: The Biological Fate of Chemicals, 33*(4), 524–529.

Kong, W., Engel, K., & Wang, J. (2004). Mammalian nucleoside transporters. *Current Drug Metabolism, 5*(1), 63–84.

Konig, J., et al. (2006). Pharmacogenomics of human OATP transporters. *Naunyn-Schmiedeberg's Archives of Pharmacology, 372*(6), 432–443.

Kusuhara, H., & Sugiyama, Y. (2004). Efflux transport systems for organic anions and cations at the blood-CSF barrier. *Advanced Drug Delivery Reviews, 56*(12), 1741–1763.

Kusuhara, H., & Sugiyama, Y. (2005). Active efflux across the blood-brain barrier: Role of the solute carrier family. *NeuroRx, 2*(1), 73–85.

Kusuhara, H., & Sugiyama, Y. (2006). ATP-binding cassette, subfamily G (ABCG family). *Pflugers Arch.*

Lai, Y., Tse, C. M., & Unadkat, J. D. (2004). Mitochondrial expression of the human equilibrative nucleoside transporter 1 (hENT1) results in enhanced mitochondrial toxicity of antiviral drugs. *The Journal of Biological Chemistry, 279*(6), 4490–4497.

Lee, E. W., et al. (2006). Identification of the mitochondrial targeting signal of the human equilibrative nucleoside transporter 1 (hENT1): Implications for interspecies differences in mitochondrial toxicity of fialuridine. *The Journal of Biological Chemistry, 281*(24), 16700–16706.

Leslie, E. M., Deeley, R. G., & Cole, S. P. (2005). Multidrug resistance proteins: Role of P-glycoprotein, MRP1, MRP2, and BCRP (ABCG2) in tissue defense. *Toxicology and Applied Pharmacology, 204*(3), 216–237.

Lodish, H., et al. (1995). *Molecular Cell Biology* (3rd ed.). New York: W H Freeman and Company.

Loscher, W., & Potschka, H. (2005). Role of drug efflux transporters in the brain for drug disposition and treatment of brain diseases. *Progress in Neurobiology, 76*(1), 22–76.

Mao, Q., & Unadkat, J. D. (2005). Role of the breast cancer resistance protein (ABCG2) in drug transport. *The AAPS Journal, 7*(1), E118–133.

Mathias, A. A., Hitti, J., & Unadkat, J. D. (2005). P-glycoprotein and breast cancer resistance protein expression in human placentae of various gestational ages. *American Journal of Physiology. Regulatory, Integrative and Comparative Physiology, 289*(4), R963–R969.

Merino, G., et al. (2005). The breast cancer resistance protein (BCRP/ABCG2) affects pharmacokinetics, hepatobiliary excretion, and milk secretion of the antibiotic nitrofurantoin. *Molecular Pharmacology, 67*(5), 1758–1764.

Robertson, E. E., & Rankin, G. O. (2006). Human renal organic anion transporters: Characteristics and contributions to drug and drug metabolite excretion. *Pharmacology & Therapeutics, 109*(3), 399–412.

Rowland, M., & Tozer, T. N. (2006). *Introduction to pharmacokinetics and pharmacodynamics. The quantitative basis of drug therapy.* Philadelphia: Lippincott, Williams & Wilkins, p. 326.

Russell, L. (1977). Movement of spermatocytes from the basal to the adluminal compartment of the rat testis. *The American Journal of Anatomy, 148*(3), 313–328.

Scheepers, A., Joost, H. G., & Schurmann, A. (2004). The glucose transporter families SGLT and GLUT: Molecular basis of normal and aberrant function. *JPEN. Journal of Parenteral and Enteral Nutrition, 28*(5), 364–371.

Sekine, T., Miyazaki, H., & Endou, H. (2006). Molecular physiology of renal organic anion transporters. *American Journal of Physiology. Renal Physiology, 290*(2), F251–F261.

Sinko, P. J., et al. (1995). Oral absorption of anti-AIDS nucleoside analogues. 1. Intestinal transport of didanosine in rat and rabbit preparations. *Journal of Pharmaceutical Sciences, 84*(8), 959–965.

Sinko, P. J., et al. (1997). Oral absorption of anti-aids nucleoside analogues: 3. Regional absorption and in vivo permeability of 2′,3′-dideoxyinosine in an intestinal-vascular access port (IVAP) dog model. *Biopharmaceutics & Drug Disposition, 18*(8), 697–710.

Smith, D. E., Johanson, C. E., & Keep, R. F. (2004). Peptide and peptide analog transport systems at the blood-CSF barrier. *Advanced Drug Delivery Reviews, 56*(12), 1765–1791.

St-Pierre, M. V., et al. (2004). Temporal expression profiles of organic anion transport proteins in placenta and fetal liver of the rat. *American Journal of Physiology. Regulatory, Integrative and Comparative Physiology, 287*(6), R1505–R1516.

Strazielle, N., Khuth, S. T, & Ghersi-Egea, J. F. (2004). Detoxification systems, passive and specific transport for drugs at the blood-CSF barrier in normal and pathological situations. *Advanced Drug Delivery Reviews, 56*(12), 1717–1740.

Unadkat, J. D., Dahlin, A., & Vijay, S. (2004). Placental drug transporters. *Current Drug Metabolism, 5*(1), 125–131.

van Herwaarden, A. E., et al. (2005). Breast cancer resistance protein (Bcrp1/Abcg2) reduces systemic exposure of the dietary carcinogens aflatoxin B1, IQ and Trp-P-1 but also mediates their secretion into breast milk. *Carcinogenesis, 27*(1), 123–130.

van Herwaarden, A. E., & Schinkel, A. H. (2006). The function of breast cancer resistance protein in epithelial barriers, stem cells and milk secretion of drugs and xenotoxins. *Trends in Pharmacological Sciences, 27*(1), 10–16.

Wijnholds, J., et al. (2000). Multidrug resistance protein 1 protects the choroid plexus epithelium and contributes to the blood-cerebrospinal fluid barrier. *The Journal of Clinical Investigation, 105*(3), 279–285.

Wilson, J. T., et al. (1985). Pharmacokinetic pitfalls in the estimation of the breast milk/plasma ratio for drugs. *Annual Review of Pharmacology and Toxicology, 25*, 667–689.

You, G. (2004). The role of organic ion transporters in drug disposition: An update. *Current Drug Metabolism, 5*(1), 55–62.

Young, A. M., Allen, C. E., & Audus, K. L. (2003). Efflux transporters of the human placenta. *Advanced Drug Delivery Reviews, 55*(1), 125–132.

Zhuang, Y., et al. (2006). Topotecan central nervous system penetration is altered by a tyrosine kinase inhibitor. *Cancer Research, 66* (23), 11305–11313.

Chapter

8

Drug Metabolism

Kenneth Bachmann

OUTLINE

8.1 INTRODUCTION

8.1.1 Overview and History

The study of drug metabolism or biotransformation is vitally important to our understanding of the time course of drugs in the body, the structuring of dosage regimens, the pharmacology and toxicology of drug metabolites, and the interactions of multivalent drug combinations. Hydrophobicity is an important chemical characteristic of most drug molecules, because the probabilities of both good oral absorption and interactions with molecular targets tend to increase as hydrophobicity increases. Unfortunately, the probability of efficient renal or biliary excretion of drugs from the body diminishes as hydrophobicity increases. Thus, the metabolism or biotransformation of hydrophobic drug molecules to more hydrophilic molecules is a very important factor in the elimination of drugs from the body. Although the enzymes that mediate drug metabolism are found in many tissues, it is within the liver and the epithelial cells of the upper portion of the intestines where most drug metabolism occurs. For a drug that is subject to biotransformation, if it is administered by intravenous infusion, then the liver is likely to be the major site for biotransformation. On the other hand, it is possible that the same drug administered orally will be subject to biotransformation both in the intestine during absorption and in the liver as well. An overview of the relationship between intestinal and hepatic metabolism is shown in Figure 8.1.

The role of biotransformation on drug action was recognized as early as the mid-nineteenth century, however the scientific interest in drug metabolism grew exponentially after the discovery by Axelrod and Estabrook and coworkers that the liver red pigment described by Garfinkel and Klingenberg performed the function of hepatic drug-metabolizing oxido-reductases. The pigment was characterized as a cytochrome by Omura and Sato in the 1960s. The first human study of drug metabolism occurred in 1841 when Ure noted that hippuric acid could be isolated from the urine after the ingestion of benzoic acid, and the first metabolic interaction between drugs was reported by Hoffmann in 1877 who found that quinine could decrease the formation of hippuric acid from benzoic acid.

$$C_6H_5\text{–}C(=O)\text{–}OH \xrightarrow{HO\text{–}C(=O)\text{–}CH_2\text{–}NH_2} C_6H_5\text{–}C(=O)\text{–}NH\text{–}CH_2\text{–}CO_2H$$

Benzoic acid | Glycine | Hippuric acid

The preceding reaction is an example of a conjugation or synthetic reaction. Synthetic reactions constitute one of the two broad types of metabolic reactions that were initially classified by R. T. Williams in the middle of the twentieth century. Williams has been referred to as the founder of the field of drug metabolism. Some other mid-twentieth century scientists who are generally recognized as having advanced the field of drug metabolism in significant ways include Bernard B. Brodie, Sidney Udenfriend, James Gillette, Bert LaDu, and Julius Axelrod. Many of those who made major contributions to the field during the last half of the twentieth century took their training with Dr. Brodie at the National Institutes of Health.

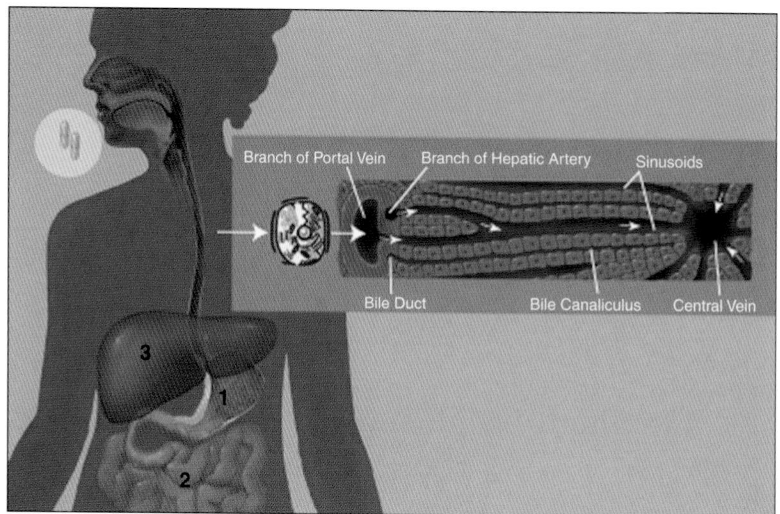

Figure 8.1 A drug taken orally first encounters the contents of the stomach (1). Dissolved drug will be principally absorbed from the small intestine (2). This process often exposes drug molecules to drug metabolizing enzymes within enterocytes (see #2 in the inset to the right). Drug molecules that traverse enterocytes intact will next be transported via the blood into the hepatic portal vein, and thus enter the sinusoids of the liver (3). The inset to the right shows the movement of drug molecules across the liver sinusoids from the hepatic portal vein (left) toward the central vein of the liver (right). As drug molecules move across the sinusoids they may be diffuse into or be transported into the hepatocytes where they can be biotransformed, transported into the bile cannaliculi, or transported back into the sinusoids. Once drug molecules and their metabolites enter the central vein (right side of inset), they gain access to the general circulation.

Williams proposed the dichotomous scheme of drug metabolism consisting of an initial phase (Phase I) that might possibly be followed by a second (Phase II). In Phase I a drug is either activated or inactivated by one of three types of irreversible chemical modifications or biotransformations, namely oxidation, reduction, or hydrolysis. Phase II was the synthetic phase, which Williams characterized as an additional inactivation step, though it is now understood that Phase II reactions can occur absent Phase I reactions, and that both Phase I and Phase II reactions can activate as well as inactivate drugs. Williams' dichotomy of metabolic reactions is still widely used today.

8.1.2 Biotransformation Pathways

Examples of how substrates might be biotransformed by either or both Phase I and/or II reactions are shown:

$$A \longrightarrow B$$

In this biotransformation B is the product of a Phase I reaction and is less active than A. An example would be the hydrolysis of the local anesthetic procaine (A) to *p*-aminobenzoic acid (B).

Procaine (H_2N–C_6H_4–C(=O)–O–CH_2–CH_2–NEt_2) → *p*-aminobenzoic acid (H_2N–C_6H_4–CO_2H)

$$A \longrightarrow C$$

In this reaction C is the product of a Phase I reaction and is more active than A. An example would be the hydroxylation of the urinary anti-infective, nalidixic acid (A), to hydroxynalidixic acid (C), which is about 16 times more potent as an anti-infective compared to nalidixic acid.

Nalidixic acid (Me, Et, CO_2H, O) → Hydroxynalidixic acid (HO–CH_2, Et, CO_2H, O)

$$A \longrightarrow B \longrightarrow Y$$

Here B is the product of a Phase I reaction and Y is the product of a Phase II reaction, and Y is less active than A. This occurs, for example, in the metabolism of the anticonvulsant drug, phenytoin. Phenytoin (A) is hydroxylated to an inactive metabolite, 5-(4′-hydroxyphenyl)-5-phenylhydantoin (4′-HPPH) (B), which is subsequently glucuronidated to 5-(4′-hydroxyphenyl)-5-phenylhydantoin (4′-HPPH) O-glucuronide (Y), an inactive metabolite and the most abundant form of phenytoin found in human urine of patients taking phenytoin.

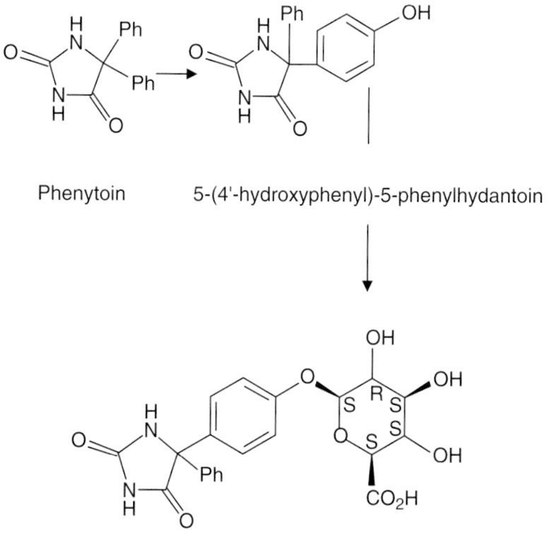

Phenytoin → 5-(4'-hydroxyphenyl)-5-phenylhydantoin → 4'-HPPH-O-glucuronide

A ⟶ B ⟶ Z

In this reaction B is the product of a Phase I reaction and Z is the product of a Phase II reaction, but the formation of Z actually increases the toxicity caused by the administration of A. For example the carcinogen, 2-acetylaminofluorene. (2-AAF) can be hydroxylated to N-hydroxy 2-acetylaminofluorene (B), which is also a carcinogen. Worse still, N-hydroxy-2-AAF can be glucuronidated (Z). However, the stable glucuronide metabolite (Z) can be excreted in bile and urine. Subsequently, the glucuronic acid portion of the molecule can be removed either enzymatically in the intestines or nonenzymatically in the kidneys regenerating N-hydroxy-2-AAF. Thus the glucuronide conjugate is, in essence, a vehicle for delivering sufficient quantities of N-hydroxy-2-AAF to the intestines (for transport to the liver as shown in Figure 8.1) and kidneys, ultimately facilitating AAF-induced liver and bladder cancer.

A ⟶ Y

In this reaction Y is the product of a Phase II reaction and is less active than A. A good example of this is the glucuronidation of the anxiolytic drug, lorazepam (A), which bears a hydroxyl group on C3. The C3 hydroxyl is glucuronidated, and the resulting glucuronide metabolite (Y) is devoid of anxiolytic activity. For lorazepam, then, the Phase II glucuronidation reaction in the liver is the major biotransformation step in the inactivation of the pharmacological activity of lorazepam.

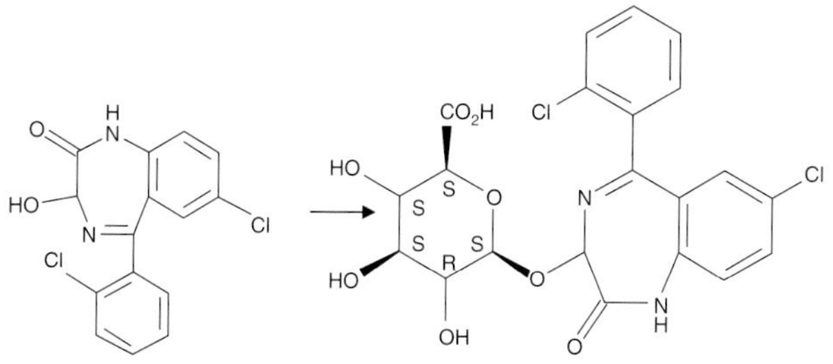

Lorazepam → Lorazepam glucuronide

A ⟶ Z

Here Z is again the product of a Phase II reaction, however Z is actually more active than A. An interesting example of this is the glucuronidation of morphine. Morphine (A) bears a hydroxyl group on C6, but when morphine is glucuronidated on the C6 hydroxyl to morphine-6-glucuronide (Z), the glucuronide conjugate is several times more active as an opiod agonist than morphine itself. However, the *in vivo* analgesic activity of this potent metabolite is limited by its poor penetration into the brain.

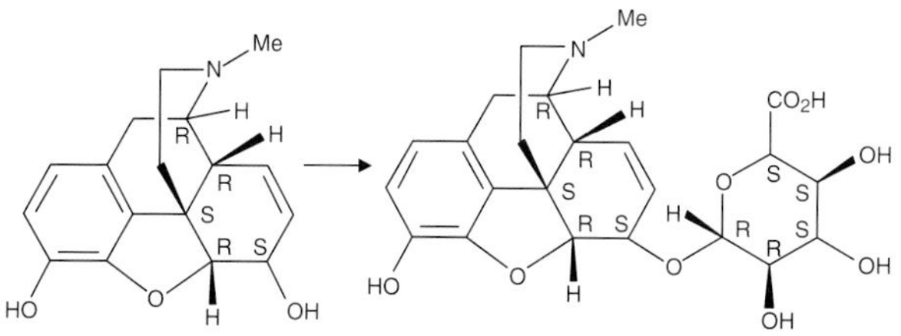

Morphine → Morphine 6-glucuronide

Examples of Phase I and Phase II reactions along with the types of enzymes that catalyze them are given in Tables 8.1 and 8.2.

The liver is the principal organ responsible for xenobiotic biotransformation, though some of the enzymes and biotransformations noted next occur in other tissues including the intestine, kidneys, placenta, lungs, and even the brain. A xenobiotic is a molecule that is foreign to the body, whereas an endobiotic is a molecule that is normally found in the body. Obviously, drugs are xenobiotics, though a few are human hormones or autocoids. Drugs with ester and amide bonds are subject to hydrolysis by esterase or amidase enzymes, respectively. A few drugs are subject to reductive reactions. Drug oxidations are among the most prominent type of biotransformation, and can encompass aliphatic or aromatic hydroxylations, N-oxidations, N-dealkylations, O-dealkylations, S-dealkylations, sulfoxidations, deaminations, or desulfurations. The Phase II (synthetic or conjugative) reactions include glucuronidation of hydroxyl functions, carboxyl functions, and amino groups; sulfonation of aromatic phenolic groups, alcohols, and amino groups; acetylation of aliphatic amines, aromatic amines, and hydrazino groups; glycine conjugation with carboxylic acid functions; glutathione conjugation with electrophiles; and methylation of aliphatic amines, N-containing heterocycles, phenols, and thiols. Selective examples of prominent key pathways are summarized in Table 8.1 (for Phase I biotransformations) and Table 8.2 (for Phase II biotransformations).

The wide array of enzyme families, subfamilies, and isoforms that mediates xenobiotic biotransformations serves as an important defense mechanism to protect the body against a dazzling variety of xenobiotic insults. Nebert (University of Cincinnati Medical Center) once drew a broad parallel between the immune system and the drug metabolizing enzymes, noting that both systems are adaptive and are capable of protecting the body against diverse molecular species.

Table 8.1 Phase I Biotransformations

Reaction Type	Biotransformation	Type of Enzyme	Representative Substrates
Hydrolysis			
Ester	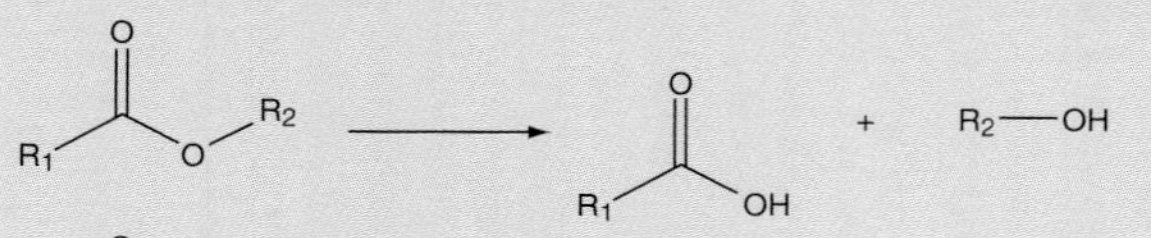	Esterase	Cocaine, esmolol, aspirin, enalapril, capecitabine, succinylcholine
Amide	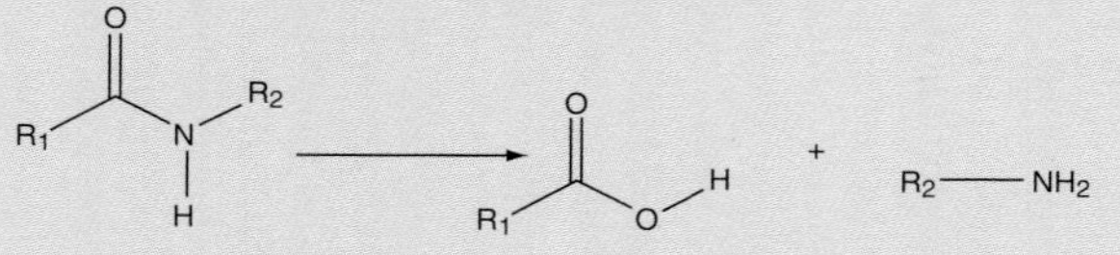	Amidase	Procainamide, loperamide, pyrazinamide, indapamide
Reduction			
Nitro reduction	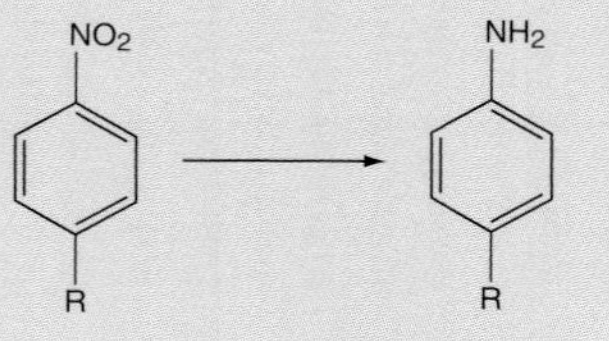	Cytochrome P450, cytochrome P450-reductase	Chloramphenicol
Hydration	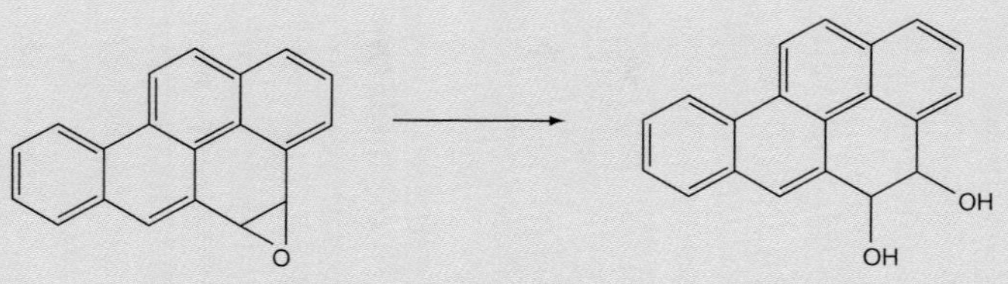	Epoxide hydrolase	Benzo[a]pyrene 4,5-epoxide (shown)
Oxidation			
Aromatic hydroxylation	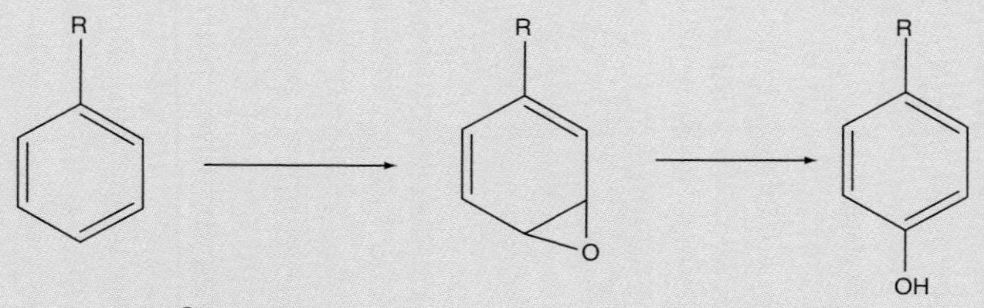	Mixed function oxidase (cytochromes P450)	Phenytoin, warfarin, midazolam, carvedilol
	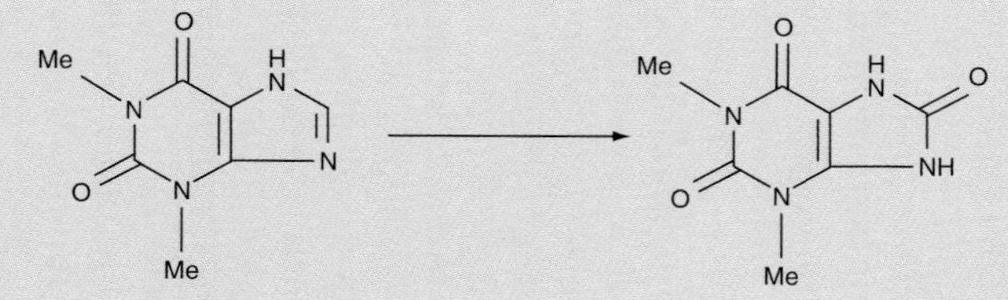	Xanthine oxidase	Caffeine, theophylline (shown)

Aliphatic hydroxylation	$R-CH_2CH_2CH_2-CH_3 \longrightarrow R-CH(OH)-CH_2CH_2-CH_3$	Mixed function oxidase (cytochromes P450)	Midazolam, cyclosporine, ibuprofen, valproic acid
O-dealkylation	$R-OCH_3 \longrightarrow R-OH + CH_2O$	Mixed function oxidase (cytochromes P450)	Dextromethorphan, codeine, fluvoxamine
N-dealkylation	$RNHCH_3 \longrightarrow RNH_2 + CH_2O$	Mixed function oxidase (cytochromes P450)	Fluoxetine, imipramine, diazepam, Flurazepam, olanzapine
N-oxidation	$R_1R_2NH \longrightarrow R_1R_2NOH$	Mixed function oxidase (cytochromes P450)	Acetaminophen, quinidine
S-oxidation	$R_1R_2S \longrightarrow R_1R_2S{=}O$	Mixed function oxidase (cytochromes P450)	S-omeprazole, cimetidine, thioridazine
Deamination	$R-CH(NH_2)-CH_3 \longrightarrow R-C(OH)(NH_2)-CH_3 \longrightarrow R-C(=O)-CH_3 + NH_3$	Mixed function oxidase (monoamine oxidase)	Amphetamine, epinephrine

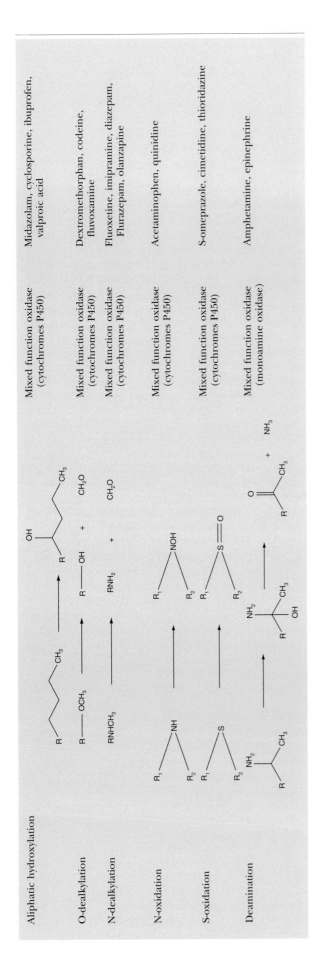

Table 8.2 Phase II Biotransformations

Reaction Type	Biotransformation	Enzyme	Representative Substrate
Glucuronidation	UDP-glucuronic acid + ROH → R-O-glucuronide + UDP	Glucuronosyl transferases	Acetaminophen, lorazepam, morphine, chloramphenicol
Acetylation	$SCoA{-}C(=O){-}CH_3$ + RNH_2 → $R{-}NH{-}C(=O){-}CH_3$ + CoA-SH	N-acetyltransferases	Isoniazid, procainamide
Sulfation	ROH + PAPS* → $R{-}OSO_3H$	Sulfotransferases	Acetaminophen
Glutathione conjugation	Glutathione + R-phenol → glutathione S-aryl conjugate → → $H_2C(S{-}C_6H_4{-}R){-}CH(NH_2){-}COOH$	Glutathione-S-transferases	Acetaminophen

*PAPS denotes 3′-phosphoadenosine-5′phosphosulfate

According to Josephy at the University of Guelph, Guengerich at Vanderbilt University, and Miners at Flinders University, the terminology that has been used to dichotomize drug metabolism into Phase I and Phase II reactions as originally described by Williams in the mid-twentieth century is dated, and should probably be supplanted by terminology that groups metabolic reactions into four simple categories. They have noted that fundamentally all drug metabolism falls into one of the following four categories:

- Oxidative reactions that are catalyzed by cytochromes P450 (CYPs), monamine oxidases (MAOs), peroxidases, xanthine oxidase (XO), or alcohol dehydrogenase
- Reductive reactions that typically involve either azo or nitro-reductions
- Conjugation reactions in which electrophilic adenosine-containing cofactors such as ATP, phosphoadenosine phosphosulfate (PAPS), acetylcoenzyme A (acetylCoA), uridine diphosphate glucuronic acid (UDPGA), or S-adenosylmethionine (SAM) react with nucleophilic groups such as –OH or $-NH_2$
- Nucleophilic trapping in which water, glutathione, or other nucleophiles react with electrophiles

8.2 DRUG METABOLIZING ENZYMES

Though in this chapter we will touch upon many of the drug-metabolizing enzymes, it has been estimated that about three-fourths of all currently marketed drugs are processed by the cytochrome P450 enzymes, and therefore the chapter will deal principally with those enzymes.

A tremendous amount of detailed information about the enzymatic biotransformation of xenobiotics has been discovered since the ground-breaking compendium of R. T. Williams in the mid-twentieth century. The wide-ranging findings encompass the genetic regulation of the drug-metabolizing enzymes, their cellular locale, their complete amino acid sequences, their polymorphisms, their crystal structures or deduced three-dimensional structures including the three-dimensional structures of their xenobiotic-binding domains, their preferred substrates and the molecular basis thereof, their enzyme kinetics, the kinetics and mechanisms of their inhibition, their allosteric regulation, the stoichiometry between enzymes, substrates, and cofactors, and the molecular mechanisms by which they biotransform substrates. Several journals are now published that focus principally on drug metabolism such as *Drug Metabolism and Disposition*, *Drug Metabolism Reviews*, *Current Drug Metabolism*, and *Xenobiotica*. A complete description of every drug metabolizing enzyme is beyond the scope of this chapter, however an attempt at summarizing important details of key drug-metabolizing enzymes follows, beginning with Phase I enzymes.

8.2.1 Esterases

8.2.1.1 Carboxylesterases

General Features Carboxylesterases (CES) catalyze the hydrolysis of xenobiotics with ester and amide functionalities (Table 8.1) yielding free acids as products. However, they are also capable of processing thioesters and carbamates as well. Substrates include drugs, carcinogens, and environmental toxins, and products may either be biologically less active or more active than the parent chemicals. CES are members of the serine esterase superfamily. Mammalian CES are products of a multigene family. A multigene family is a group of genes that have descended from a common ancestral gene and therefore have similar functions and similar DNA sequences.

The enzymes have molecular weights ranging from about 47 kDa (mouse and rhesus monkey) to 65 kDa (human), and can be found in liver, kidney, small intestine, heart, muscle, lung and other respiratory tissues, adipose tissue, CNS, and blood. Within the blood, CES have been found both in plasma as well as within leukocytes. Species differences in their presence in neuronal tissue and capillary endothelial cells of the CNS have led to some equivocation about their contribution to the blood–brain barrier. That is, the extent to which these enzymes might limit access of drugs into the brain by hydrolyzing them before they can diffuse from the blood into the brain isn't all that clear. CES are localized both in the cytosol, endoplasmic reticulum (ER), and in lysosomes.

Regulation Often, both endobiotics and xenobiotics can regulate the activities of drug-metabolizing enzymes. Decreases in enzyme activity can occur if a xenobiotic or endobiotic interacts with an enzyme to inhibit it. On the other hand, if a xenobiotic or endobiotic somehow stimulates the gene for an enzyme to increase its expression of the enzyme, then the enzyme is said to be induced. As discussed next and also in the chapter on drug interactions, many xenobiotics are capable of inducing the cytochrome P450 (CYP) enzymes. Hepatic CES appear to be partially regulated by pituitary hormones, though hormonal effects differ among CES isoforms. Many of the inducers of the cytochrome P450 enzymes (see later) have also been shown to induce microsomal CES. Examples include phenobarbital, polycyclic aromatic hydrocarbons, polychlorinated biphenyls, pregnenolone 16 α-carbonitrile (PCN), glucocorticoids, and the PPARα agonist, clofibrate. Although such xenobiotic regulation of the cytochromes P450 (CYPs) has been shown to alter dose requirements for drugs that are CYP substrates, the clinical consequences of xenobiotic-induced changes in the activity of microsomal CES may not be so profound.

Inhibition of CES activity, either hepatic microsomal or plasma CES activity, has been produced with disulfiram, chronic aspirin consumption, and nordihydroguaiaretic acid (NDGA). Here, too, the clinical consequences have not been shown to be as significant

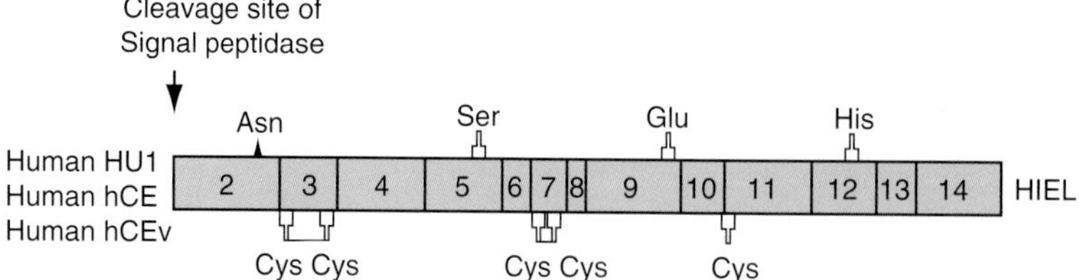

Figure 8.2 Deduced amino acid sequence for human liver CES. Trivial names of human CES are listed to the left. The disulfide bonds are Cys87-Cys 116 and Cys 274-Cys 285. (Modified from Annu. Rev. Pharmacol. Toxicol. 28:257–288, 1998, T. Satoh and M. Hosokawa.)

as the inhibition of CYP activity that can be elicited by the consumption of certain drugs and even some foods (see Chapter 12 on drug interactions).

Molecular Features and Pharmacogenetics Several conserved motifs occur across species and isoforms of the CES. Carboxy terminal tetrapeptides of either HIEL or HTEL seem to be important for the binding of human microsomal CES to the luminal side of the endoplasmic reticulum (ER). Some of the cysteines, the active site serine, and the histidine (Figure 8.2) are highly conserved, and mutations at these sites reduce CES activity. The human CES gene, localized on chromosome 16, is approximately 30 kb. Sequences on the 5′ flanking region of human liver CES may constitute binding sites for transcription factors such as GATA-1, NF-1, sterol regulatory element (SRE), and others. The deduced amino acid sequence for human liver CES isoforms is shown in Figure 8.2.

The active site for human liver carboxylesterase (hCE1) encompasses the three amino acids, serine, glutamic acid, and histidine as shown in Figure 8.3.

Sometimes the determination of enzyme crystal structures requires that a substrate be bound to the enzyme. The crystal structures of hCE1 in complex with homatropine, an anticholinergic drug, tacrine, a cholinesterase inhibitor, or naloxone, an opioid antagonist, have been

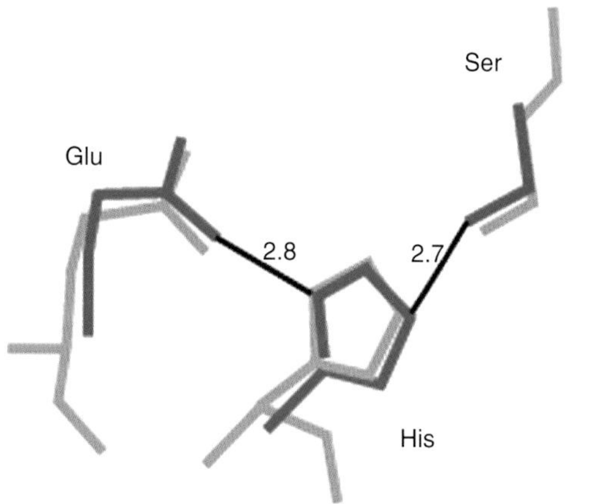

Figure 8.3 The key three active site amino acids, glutamic acid, serine, and histidine and their distances (nm) are shown for both hCE1 (green) and a bacterial carboxylesterase (gold). (Modified from Potter and Wadkins, Current Medicinal Chemistry volume 13, 2006; permission has been obtained from Potter.)

established (Figure 8.4). Depending upon the substrate that is bound, the enzyme-substrate complex contains either two trimers (homatropine or tacrine) or two tetramers (naloxone).

Since CES appear to play an important role in the activation of lipophilic ester prodrugs to pharmacologically active and more hydrophilic carboxylic acids or alcohols, there is increasing interest in their pharmacogenetics. The main idea here is to be able to identify those individuals with CES genotypes that will make them good candidates for responding to drugs that must be activated from a prodrug by CES. The CES are found in human liver, small intestine, kidney, lung, testes, heart, macrophages, monocytes, and even in the plasma. The human isoforms[1] are hCE1 and hCE2 (CES1 and CES2). Although many single nucleotide polymorphisms (SNPs) have been identified in the human CES2 gene encoding for hCE2, an enzyme that activates the anticancer drug irinotecan and plays a role in the inactivation of the local anesthetic agent procaine, only two SNPs have been definitively found to be responsible for reductions in the phenotypic activity of hCE2. Allele and haplotype frequencies in the CES2 gene are different between Europeans and Africans. Patients bearing these SNPs could be at risk of therapeutic failure when treated, for example, with irinotecan for cancer, since they would be incapable of activating the drug to its cytotoxic metabolite, 7-ethyl-10-hydroxycamptothecin (SN-38), which is three orders of magnitude more potent in its anticancer activity than its prodrug, irinotecan.

8.2.1.2 Cholinesterases

A common ancestral gene may have encoded CES, acetylcholinesterase (AChE), and thyroglobulin. Acetylcholinesterase and butyrylcholinesterase (BChE), like the CES enzymes, are members of the serine hydrolase superfamily. Cocaine (Table 8.1) is metabolized by hCE1, hCE2, and serum BChE. Though, as in the case of cocaine, there can be substrate overlap, each of these enzymes can also hydrolyze different substrates. There is noticeable sequence homology between them, particularly in the N-terminal half that includes the active serine site.

[1]An isoform is a protein that is similar though not identical to other proteins in its sequence and its function, but that is encoded by a different gene.

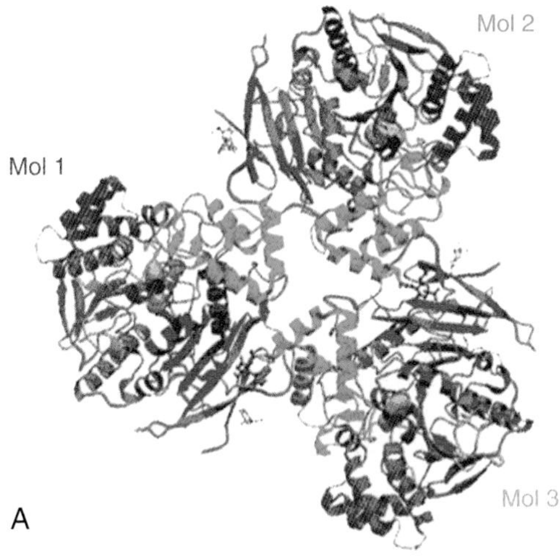

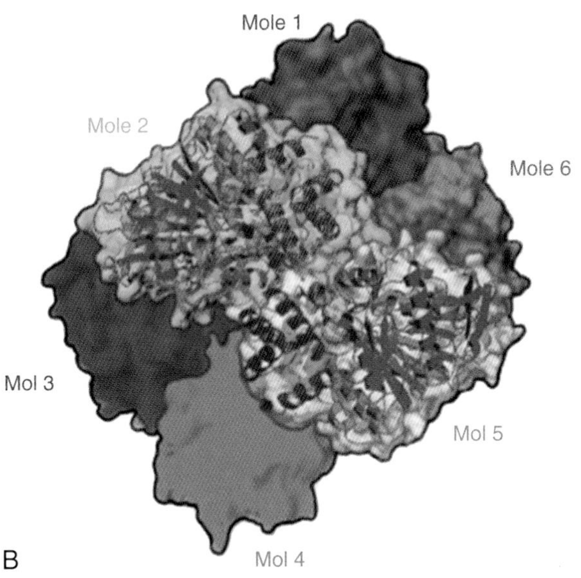

Figure 8.4 (A) "A trimer of hCE1 (MOL1, MOL2, and MOL3) complexed with tacrine viewed down the 3-fold axis of symmetry and into the catalytic gorge of the monomers. Catalytic domains, ab domains, and regulatory domains are in blue, green, and red respectively. Omega loops are in orange, the N-acetylglucosamines (NAG) are in cyan, and sialic acids are in dark green." (B) "A molecular surface representation of the hCE1 hexamer with a ribbon-representation of one pair of dimers within the hexamer superimposed. The hexamer is formed by the stacking of two trimers with active sites facing in." [Figure modified from Chemistry and Biology 10:341–249, 2003 by S. Bencharit et al; legend is quoted verbatim.

One of the earliest demonstrations of polymorphic metabolism was made by Kalow and colleagues at the University of Toronto. They were interested in examining why some patients appeared to be exquisitely sensitive to succinylcholine, a skeletal muscle relaxant that was widely used in anesthesia as an anesthetic adjunct. They found that BChE activity (then referred to as serum cholinesterase or pseudocholinesterase) was atypical in succinylcholine-sensitive individuals by virtue of a lower substrate affinity. They used an inhibitor of BChE, dibucaine, as a sort of probe to distinguish between individuals who possessed normal BChE activity and those who possessed atypical BChE activity. Dibucaine inhibited enzyme activity in the succinylcholine-sensitive patients (these would be those who possessed atypical BChE activity) by only 20%, compared to 80% inhibition of the "normal" esterase. In individuals who were heterozygous, dibucaine inhibition of the esterase was only 60%. Family studies revealed inheritance of a rare gene from both parents of individuals that were highly sensitive to succinylcholine, thereby giving rise to the expression of an atypical or variant form of BChE in plasma. Since the groundbreaking work of Kalow's group, other variants of this enzyme have been found, and the consequence of homozygously expressing these variants is an exaggerated response to the usual dose of succinylcholine, a substrate for the enzyme. That is, individuals expressing the atypical (variant) form of BChE, if treated with succinylcholine, could accidentally be recipients of relative succinylcholine overdoses capable of causing apnea or even suffocation. Other neuromuscular blocking agents that are used during anesthesia and that are also subject to hydrolysis by BChE are atracurium and mivacurium.

Currently in therapeutics, targeting the AChE for inhibition constitutes one treatment strategy for Alzheimer's disease, and those AChE inhibitors that are in use clinically as well as those still being developed, in fact, do show greater selectivity for inhibition of AChE compared to BChE. Inhibition of cholinesterases has other therapeutic purposes as well. Reversible cholinesterase inhibition with physostigmine is sometimes used to try and reverse some of the serious anticholinergic effects that occur with overdoses of tricyclic antidepressant drugs. On the other hand, dreaded nerve gases such as Tabun and Sarin are, in fact, irreversible inhibitors of the cholinesterases.

8.2.2 Epoxide Hydrolases

The epoxide hydrolases (EHs; EC3.3.2.3) hydrate simple epoxides to vicinal diols, and they hydrate arene oxides to trans-dihydrodiols (also see Table 8.1).

O
EH
OH
OH

Benzo[a]pyrene 4,5-epoxide → Benzo[a]pyrene-4,5-diol

These reactions tend to mitigate cellular damage arising from the oxidation of endobiotics or xenobiotics by oxidative enzymes (see oxido-reductases, later). The enzymatic oxidation of substrates can lead to the formation of epoxides that, absent detoxifying hydration by

EHs, are usually sufficiently reactive to cause protein and RNA adduction. This irreversible alteration of cellular macromolecules can result in cell damage, mutagenicity, or carcinogenicity.

There are several forms of EH that are immunologically and structurally distinct; some are localized in the cell cytoplasm, whereas others are found in the ER. We will address those EHs that are principally responsible for xenobiotic metabolism.

Cytosolic EH (MW~62 kDa) processes oxidation products of arachidonic acid and arachidonic acid metabolites, key autocoids in inflammatory and other processes, and also activates the linoleic acid oxide, leukotoxin, which is produced by leukocytes, to cytotoxic diols that appear to be the mediators of multiorgan failure and respiratory distress syndrome in some patients. With regard to xenobiotics, soluble EH also metabolizes trans-epoxide metabolites of xenobiotics.

Sequences of several mammalian soluble EHs have been published, and the human gene is approximately 45 kb with 19 exons. Cytoplasmic EH is inducible by PPARα agonists, including hypolipidemic agents such as clofibrate. Pathological and therapeutic consequences of inducing cytosolic EHs with PPARα agonists are unknown.

In humans a microsomal form of EH (mEH) is also found. mEH can catalyze trans-hydration of epoxides and arene oxides yielding reactive diol-epoxides. Xenobiotic substrates include carcinogenic polycyclic aromatic hydrocarbons (PAHs). Whereas diol-epoxide products tend to be highly reactive and carcinogenic or mutagenic, mEH can catalyze the detoxification of xenobiotics as well.

mEH has been found in human liver, lung, kidney, lymphocytes, epithelial cells, and ovary. The enzyme consists of a single polypeptide chain that is 455 amino acids in length with a molecular weight of approximately 52.96 kDa. Human mEH is encoded on a single gene, and the mEH gene (also known as HYL1) has been mapped to chromosome 1q42.1. Spielberg and colleagues (then in Toronto) suggested that individuals (including fetuses) expressing low levels of mEH appear to be at increased risk of "apparent" hypersensitivity reactions to aromatic anticonvulsant drugs that are oxidized to epoxide intermediates by the cytochrome P450 system (see later). The reactions range from fever and rash to eosinophilia and multiorgan failure, and have been reported to occur in about 1 in 5000 patients treated with such anticonvulsants as phenytoin, carbamazepine, and phenobarbital. Spielberg's work is supported by findings of Park at Liverpool University.

On the other hand, when Guenthner and colleagues evaluated the binding of anti-mEH monoclonal antibodies to liver samples biopsied from 21 different subjects they were unable to demonstrate structural epitope differences among them. The limitations, though, of their analysis preclude them from concluding that such differences, in fact, do not exist. Subsequently, others have evaluated phenotypic differences in mEH proteins with amino acid substitutions at positions 113 (Y/H) and 139 (H/R). The absence of significant phenotypic differences in these variants also raises questions about the clinical significance of mEH polymorphism. That is, the differences between rates of substrate metabolism by nonvariant forms of mEH and the variant forms may be no greater than the interindividual rates of metabolism that can be detected among individual nonvariant forms of mEH, anyway.

8.2.3 Oxido-Reductases

8.2.3.1 Mixed-Function Oxidases

Mixed function oxidases catalyze the oxidation of an extremely diverse array of lipophilic drug substrates as well as endobiotics such as steroid and thyroid hormones, fatty acids, and arachidonic acid metabolites. These oxidations have been broadly characterized as follows:

$$\mathrm{NADPH} + \mathrm{H}^+ + \mathrm{O}_2 + \mathrm{RH} \xrightarrow{\mathrm{MFO}} \mathrm{NADP}^+ + \mathrm{H}_2\mathrm{O} + \mathrm{ROH}$$

where MFO denotes mixed-function oxidase, RH is a generally lipophilic substrate, and ROH is a product (metabolite) that is more hydrophilic than the substrate. Electron equivalents are utilized in this reaction, and one of the atoms from the molecular oxygen is reduced to form water whereas the other is incorporated—sometimes transiently and sometimes permanently—into the metabolite.

8.2.3.2 Cytochromes P450

The most widely studied gene family of mixed-function oxidases and the one that participates more than any other in the oxidation of drugs is the cytochrome P450 family. The gene products or cytochrome P450 (CYP) enzymes are incredibly important in terms of the number of existing drugs that they process, their substrate specificity, polymorphism, and propensity to be determinants—often key determinants—in drug–drug interactions. Cytochrome P450 was initially observed as a liver pigment that, in the presence of carbon monoxide and dithionite, yielded an absorption peak at 450 nm. Upon fractionation of the liver the pigment was found to be concentrated in the microsomes. The term microsome, though commonly used, is a bit of a misnomer, because it implies the existence of a subcellular organelle called a microsome. In fact, there is no such organelle. Instead, microsomes are artifacts of cell preparation. They are actually pinched off portions of a cell's smooth endoplasmic reticulum (SER) that are formed during tissue homogenization. Frequently the so-called microsomal fraction of a tissue such as liver is acquired in order to study cytochrome P450 activity. To acquire the microsomal fraction, liver tissue is first homogenized. The homogenate is then centrifuged at a relatively slow speed, say 10,000 X g to remove cell debris, nuclei, and mitochondria. Then the supernatant is centrifuged at a high speed, about 100,000 X g. The pellet at the bottom is a rust-colored pellet consisting largely of microsomes (i.e., the SER). The microsomes are then harvested and resuspended to conduct experiments involving the CYP enzymes. The rust color of microsomes occurs because the major proteins are hemoproteins or iron-containing proteins, namely the CYPs.

The early characterization of a microsomal oxidase was based on observations of Garfinkel and Klingenberg near the middle of the twentieth century. Shortly thereafter, in 1962, Omura and Sato were credited with identifying the carbon-monoxide binding pigment as a hemoprotein that was designated as cytochrome P450 owing to its absorption peak at 450 nm in the presence of dithionate. Estabrook and colleagues, studying the role of this hemoprotein in bovine adrenal microsomal hydroxylation of steroids, established that cytochrome P450 was the terminal oxidase of bovine adrenal microsomal steroid C21 hydroxylase, and was responsible for the binding of substrates to the microsomal MFO system. Other key figures involved in purifying and establishing the role of P450 as the terminal element in microsomal (SER) electron transport were Lu and Coon. A schematic of electron transfer to cytochrome P450 is shown in Figure 8.5.

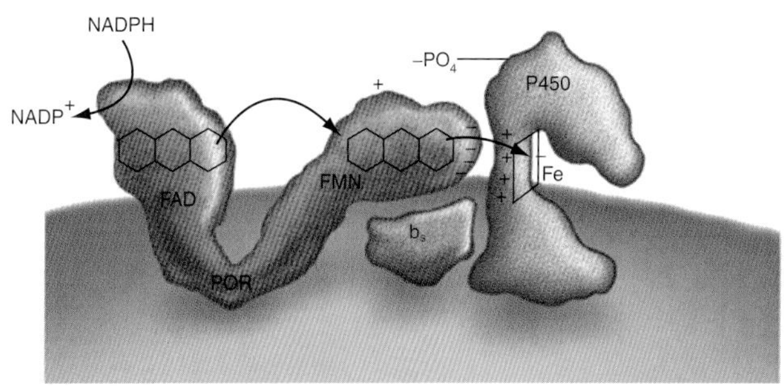

Figure 8.5 Schematic of electron transfer by microsomal P450 enzymes. NADPH interacts with cytochrome P450 oxido-reductase (POR), bound to the endoplasmic reticulum, and gives up a pair of electrons to the flavin adenine dinucleotide (FAD) moiety which elicits a conformational change, permitting the isoalloxazine rings of the FAD and flavin mononucleotide (FMN) moieties to come close together so that the electrons pass from the FAD to the FMN. Another conformational change returns the protein to its original orientation. The FMN domain of POR interacts with the redox partner binding site of the P450. Electrons from the FMN domain of POR reach the heme group to achieve catalysis. The interaction of POR and the P450 is coordinated by negatively charged acidic residues on the surface of the FMN domain of POR and positively charged basic residues in the redox partner binding site of the P450. Cytochrome b5 is also a source of electrons. (Figure and legend are modified from Endocrinology 146 (6):2544–2550, 2005 by Walter L. Miller.)

After a substrate binds to a cytochrome P450 isoform, it will acquire an oxygen atom. The sequence of events as stipulated by Guengerich at Vanderbilt is shown in Figure 8.6.

Notice that a prerequisite for substrate binding (step 1) is that the heme iron of cytochrome P450 must be at the +3 valency (ferric iron). Subsequent to binding an electron is transferred to P450 (step 2) via NADPH –P450 reductase (or POR as shown in Figure 8.5). This reduces the heme iron to ferrous iron, which is a prerequisite for the binding of molecular oxygen to the hemoprotein (step 3). A second electron, which may also arise from cytochrome b5 (step 4) and a proton (step 5) will lead to the formation of an

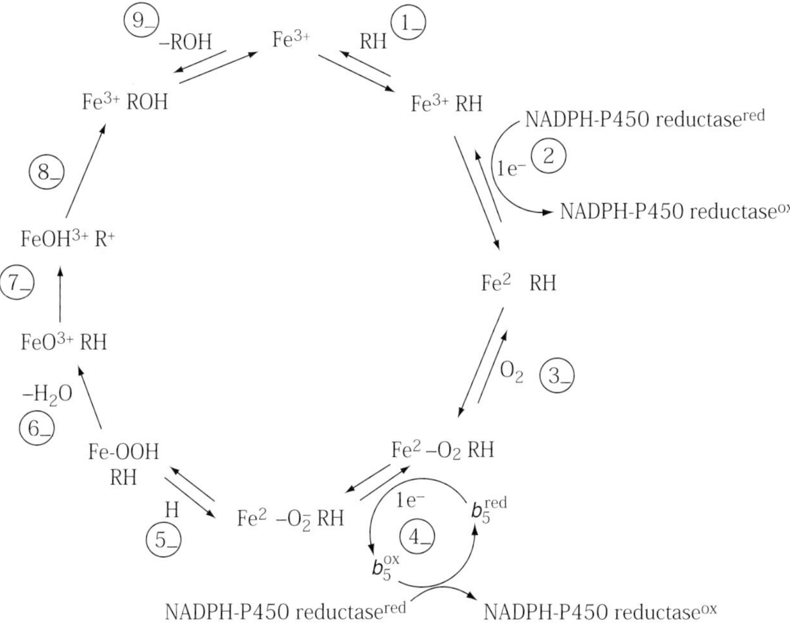

Figure 8.6 The sequential steps in substrate and molecular oxygen binding to cytochrome P450, and the subsequent oxidation of substrate. (Modified from F. P. Guengerich et al. Drug Metabolism and Disposition 26:1175–1178, 1998.)

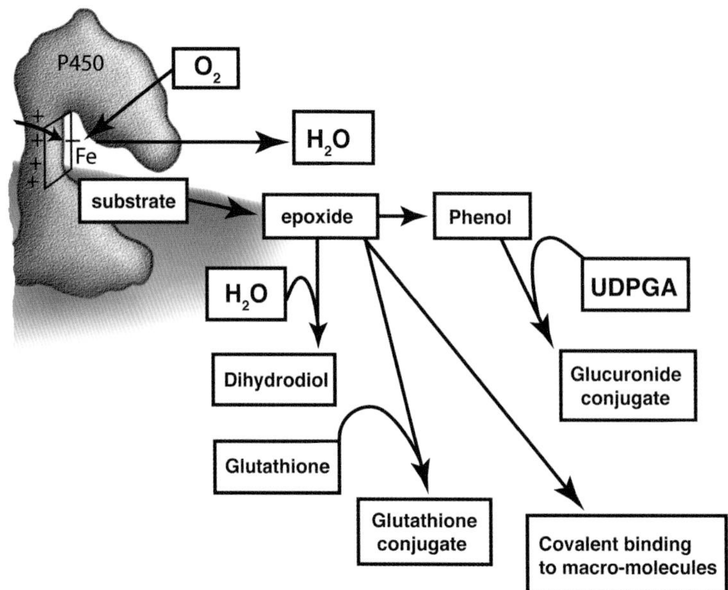

Figure 8.7 A schematic portrayal of aromatic substrate binding to P450 and substrate oxidation by P450. Note that an epoxide may form as an end-product or an intermediate. Also shown in the figure above are examples of post-oxidative steps including the hydration of an epoxide intermediate to a dihydrodiol, glutathione conjugation with the epoxide, conjugation of the phenol with UDPGA to yield a glucuronic acid conjugate. While these reactions are more likely to be detoxifying ones, the binding of a reactive epoxide intermediate to cell macromolecules leads to adverse outcomes.

FeOOH complex. The loss of water yields the $(FeO)^{3+}$ complex (step 6) that rearranges (step 7) and transfers an atom of oxygen to the complex-bound substrate (step 8). In the final step (step 9) the oxidized substrate is released, and the enzyme is regenerated.

If the substrate bears an aromatic ring, then the product may be a phenol arising through an expoxide intermediate as shown in Figure 8.7.

Tissue Distribution Though they are most densely distributed in the liver and the intestines, CYP enzymes that are responsible for xenobiotic metabolism are also found in the placenta, lung, lymphocytes, macrophages, kidney, and even the brain. Most of the cytochromes P450 that process xenobiotics are located within the endoplasmic reticulum. The membrane phospholipids to which the enzymes are anchored (see Figure 8.5) are important in the overall activity of the CYPs, and the relationship of P450 to the ER membrane is exemplified in Figure 8.5.

Structure Approximately 490 amino acids constitute the microsomal or SER Cytochrome P450 enzymes. David Lewis at the University of Surrey, among others, has shown the alignments for members of the CYP2 family, and indicated those sequences involved in membrane anchoring, alpha helical regions and substrate binding. Amino acid sequences of microsomal, mitochondrial, bacterial, and other CYPs are updated regularly online at http://drnelson.utmem.edu/CytochromeP450.html. Secondary structural segments of the bacterial enzyme, P-450_{CAM}, are shown in Figure 8.8. It was possible to study the details of the structure of P-450_{CAM} before most of the other P450

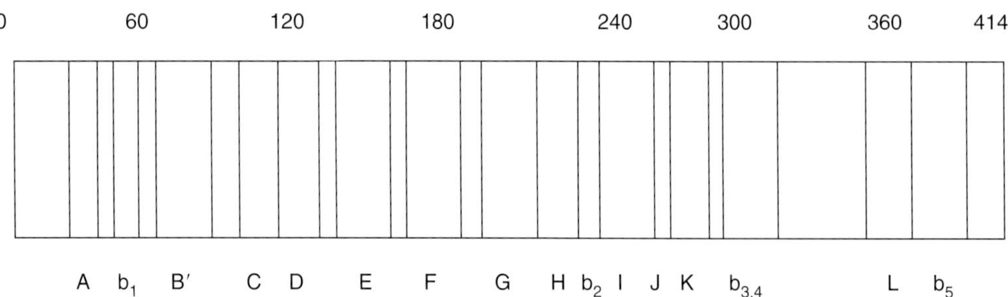

Figure 8.8 $P450_{CAM}$ secondary structural elements. Numbers above denote approximate residue numbers. Helical segments are represented by upper case letters, whereas lower case letters signify beta sheets. The heme thiolate which anchors the iron-containing and oxygen-binding heme moiety to the protein is near the start of the L helix. (Adapted from DFV Lewis and H. Moreels, J Computer Aided Molecular Design 6:235–252, 1992.)

enzymes, because unlike mammalian CYPs, P-450$_{CAM}$ is not membrane-bound, making crystallization less difficult. In Figure 8.8 the primary sequence of the enzyme is shown simply as a linear array of amino acids. Amino acid sequences appearing as helices (uppercase letters) or sheets (lowercase letters) are identified, and the width of each segment is a crude representation of the number of amino acids in each segment.

The X-ray crystal structure of the microsomal CYP2C5 is shown in Figure 8.9. As in Figure 8.8, the uppercase letters denote helices. Like the lowercase letters in Figure 8.8, the Greek symbols in Figure 8.9 denote beta sheets.

Topography No doubt the importance of phospholipids in the activity of the CYPs resides in their role as membrane lipids orienting CYP enzymes within the ER membrane. The hydrophobic region near the N-terminal end of the protein is the membrane-spanning domain and presumed to be an α-helix. The orientation of cytochrome P450 within the ER membrane has been depicted as in Figure 8.10.

The schematic shown in Figure 8.10 is a rather accurate portrayal of the orientation of cytochrome P450 in the ER membrane. Above the ER membrane it can be seen that the heme-containing portion of the CYP is oriented toward the cell cytoplasm, whereas the N-terminal end of the CYP is oriented toward the lumen of the SER. Compare Figure 8.10 with Figure 8.11, which is a homology model of rat cytochrome P450 2B1. Both models depict the major portion of the CYP protein presented to the cell cytoplasm while a helical portion of the protein anchors it to the SER membrane.

Conveniently, both NADPH cytochrome P450 oxidoreductase (POR) and cytochrome b5 are also anchored to the ER membrane by a single transmembrane helix. As shown in Figure 8.10, these proteins are oriented toward the cytoplasmic side of the ER membrane, and the portion of cytochrome P450 that interacts with these electron donors is also oriented toward the cytoplasmic side of the membrane.

Substrate Interactions with Cytochromes P450 Substrates for CYPs interact with the heme-thiolate, displacing the oxygen from the sixth coordination site. An example of this is shown in Figure 8.12, which portrays the

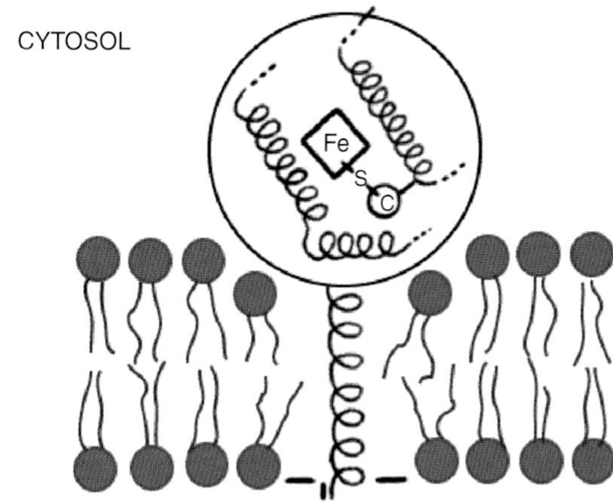

Figure 8.10 Orientation of cytochrome P450 within the ER membrane. The ligand-binding site is oriented toward the cytosol. An alpha-helical membrane spanning domain near the N-terminus anchors the enzyme to the ER membrane. (Modified from C. Brown and S. Black, J. Biol. Chem. 264 (8):4442–4449, 1989.)

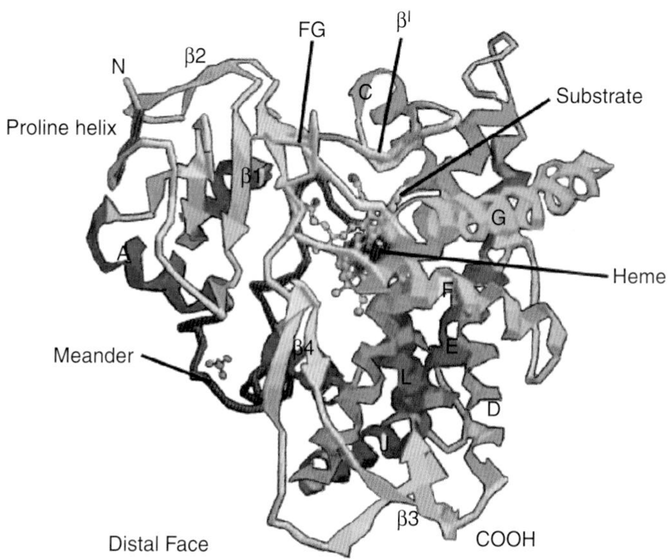

Figure 8.9 Ribbon representation of P450 2C5 crystal structure with several features labeled. (Modified from Williams, J. Cosme, V. Sridhar, E.F. Johnson, D.E. McRee, Journal of Inorganic Biochemistry 81 (2000) 183–190.)

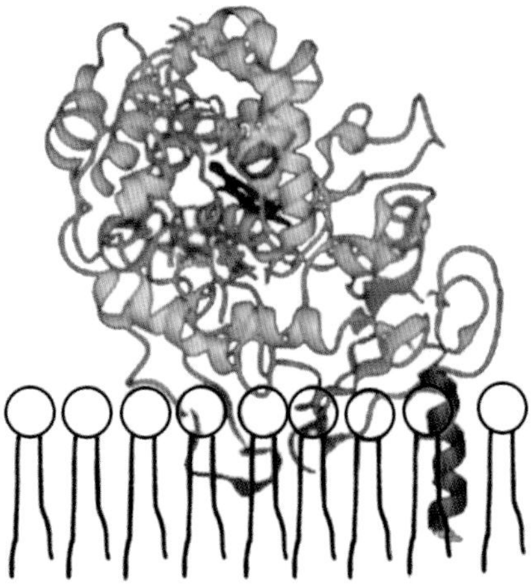

Figure 8.11 Homology model for rat P450 2B1. The proposed structure includes a hydrophobic membrane attachment domain and active sites which are consistent with the known substrate and inhibitor specificities of these P450s. (Modified from F.K. Friedman, http://home.ccr.cancer.gov/metabolism/friedman/fkfccr.htm)

binding and oxidation cycle as shown earlier in Figure 8.6, but delineates the changes in the planar orientation of the iron atom throughout the cycle.

In this schematic only the heme-thiolate portion of CYP is shown. The substrate need not necessarily bind directly to the heme.

Enzymology and Stoichiometry A depiction of the thermodynamic analysis of substrate, P450, and NADPH cytochrome P450 reductase interactions is shown in Figure 8.13.

Dr. Fred Guengerich at Vanderbilt University has published mechanistic schemata for cytochrome P450 involvement in an extensive array of both common and uncommon oxidative reactions and reductive reactions. Some of those are exhibited later in this chapter in a brief consideration of reductive reactions. Mechanisms for carbon hydroxylation, heteroatom oxygenation, N-dealkylation, O-dealkylation, alcohol oxidation, arene epoxidation, phenol formation, oxidation of olefins and acetylenes, reduction of nitro compounds, reductive dehalogenation, and azo reduction, to name a few, are provided.

Origin, Genetics, and Polymorphisms of Cytochromes P450 Though they are probably the most widely studied and the most prominent drug-metabolizing enzymes, how and when did the cytochromes P450 evolve? How are they named? And what are their similarities and dissimilarities?

After the recognition of the important role of the cytochromes P450 in drug oxidations dating back to the 1950s and 1960s, there was a relatively sharp scientific interest in these enzymes such that the rate of publication in the field appeared to outpace the rate of scientific publication generally in the biological sciences during the second half of the twentieth

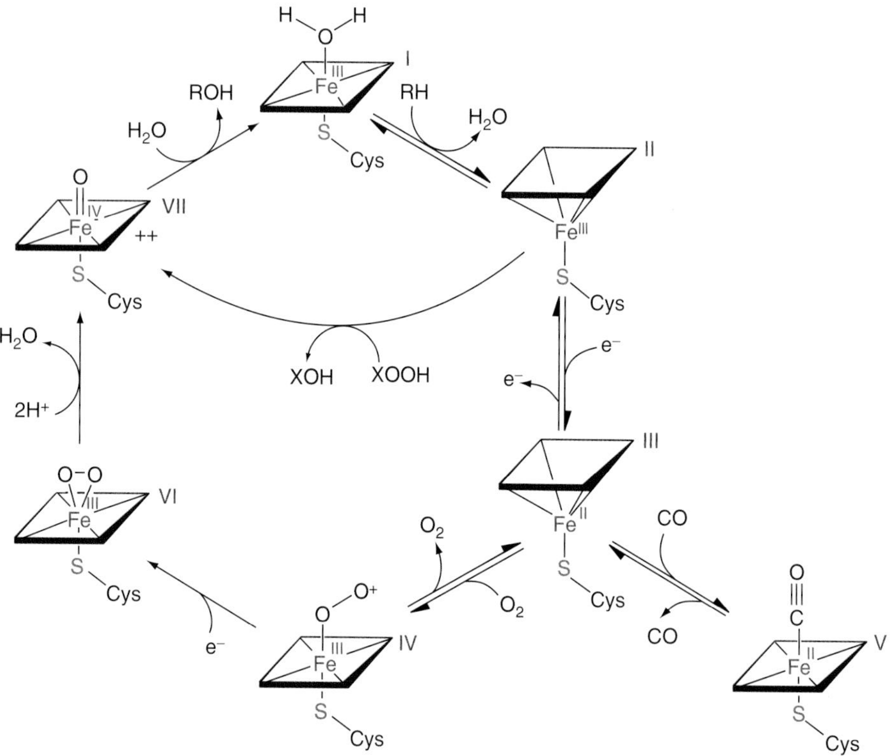

Figure 8.12 The most common reaction cycle for the interaction of xenobiotic substrates with microsomal cytochrome P450. In step I, the binding of substrate converts the iron complex from a low-spin ferric hexacoordinate to a high-spin ferric pentacoordinate in which the ferric iron is no longer in the plane of the heme.

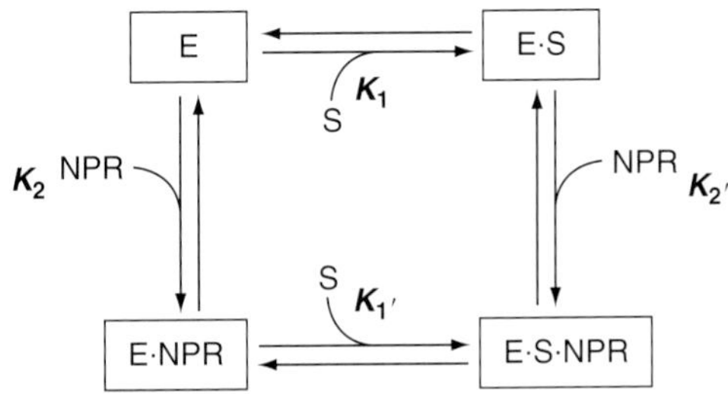

Figure 8.13 Interaction between cytochrome P450 (E), substrate (S), and NADPH cytochrome P450 reductase (NPR). (Modified from Shimada, Mernaugh, and Guengerich, Arch. Biochem. Biophys 435:307–216, 2005.)

century. Not surprisingly, as laboratories all over the world began to isolate and characterize these enzymes, they also assigned their own nomenclature to the enzymes. It became increasingly difficult to know whether enzymes discussed by one group of investigators were different from or identical to enzymes discussed by other groups of investigators. As molecular biological tools emerged in the 1980s still more cytochrome P450 enzymes could be expressed not only from liver but from other tissues as well. Finally, Daniel Nebert and other key investigators in the field organized the P450 Gene Superfamily Nomenclature Committee. The committee posts sequence alignments at its web site (http://drnelson.utmem.edu/CytochromeP450.html) along with bibliographic information.

It is thought that the original ancestral P450 gene arose approximately 3 billion years ago followed by rounds of expansion associated with gene and genome duplication. Though our interests here are in their role as xenobiotic processing enzymes, this gene superfamily likely originated to process endobiotics. There are hundreds of P450 gene families among animals, plants, and bacteria. The number of individual cytochrome P450 enzymes in animals number in the thousands. The current nomenclature is based on evolutionary relationships in primary amino acid sequence alignments of the enzymes. Thus, enzymes are assigned to the same family if they share at least 40% sequence identity. They are assigned to the same subfamily if they share greater than 55% amino acid sequence identity. There are at least 57 human P450 proteins. Happily, only 15 enzymes from three gene families are involved extensively in human drug metabolism. The enzyme families are identified by Arabic numbers after the prefix CYP, a shorthand reference to cytochrome P450. The three key cytochrome P450 or CYP families responsible for drug metabolism in humans are CYP1, CYP2, and CYP3. Subfamilies are denoted with uppercase letters (e.g., CYP1A). Individual enzymes are identified with the family designation, subfamily designation, and another Arabic numeral (e.g., CYP1A2). CYP genes are designated in italics (e.g., *CYP1A2*). The major CYP enzymes in human xenobiotic metabolism are listed in Table 8.3. Also shown are drugs that are known to inhibit CYP enzymes and drugs that increase CYP activity, typically by increasing the amount of enzyme in tissue (enzyme induction).

The lists of substrates, inhibitors, and inducers (see later sections on induction and inhibition for mechanisms and consequences of induction and inhibition) in Table 8.3 are highly abridged. Even so, it is easy to tell just by casual analysis that there is a considerable amount of nonselectivity in each of those areas. That is, some drugs are substrates for multiple CYPs. Some drugs are inhibitors of multiple CYPs. And some drugs such as rifampin can induce nearly every major human drug-metabolizing enzyme.

Pharmacogenetics is a term that is used frequently with reference to sequence variations in the alleles of individual CYP enzymes. Although exposure of individuals to a wide array of substances (including drugs and environmental chemicals) and/or conditions (such as infection and liver dysfunction) can alter the expression or activity of their CYP enzymes (these exposures have been characterized as host factors by Vesell at Hershey Medical Center), genetically based variation in the amino acid sequences of the CYP enzymes also has been shown to be responsible for significant interindividual variations in rates of drug metabolism. If a variant CYP gene—a gene other than the usual or most common or normal form (a.k.a. wild-type form) coding for a variant enzyme—occurs with a frequency of at least 1% in a population, the gene is said to be polymorphic. That means simply that within a population at least two forms of a CYP gene/enzyme exist: normal and variant. That portion of the population (at least 1%) bearing the variant CYP gene and expressing an abnormal form of the CYP enzyme *may* metabolize CYP substrates abnormally, though occasionally the expression of variant forms of CYP enzymes does *not* lead to unusual rates of substrate metabolism. Often, individuals who express a variant form of the enzyme metabolize drugs that are substrates for the enzyme much more slowly than normal. Even a single amino acid substitution engendered by a single nucleotide polymorphism (SNP) in a CYP gene may result in altered rates of drug metabolism.

Table 8.4 lists some of the allelic variants that are found among human CYP genes and includes the nomenclature and the actual nucleotide amino acid substitutions, the resultant abnormal phenotype, and an example of the clinical consequence.

In addition to the SNPs shown in Table 8.4, some alleles may be duplicated or multiplied even more, giving rise to higher than normal levels of enzymatic activity and ultra-rapid metabolic phenotypes. A good example of this is CYP2D6*2XN, where the N denotes the number of copies of active gene. The frequency of occurrence of CYP allelic variants among various ethnic and other subgroups continue to be characterized.

CYP2D6, CYP2C9, and CYP2C19 are among the most highly polymorphic of all CYP enzymes. Of these, the polymorphism of CYP2D6, which is responsible for the metabolism of ~25% of known drugs, has been studied most extensively. Three different research groups (Sjoqvist in Sweden, Smith in London, and Eichelbaum in Bonn) first described and characterized phenotypic and genotypic differences in the metabolism of substrates that were subsequently identified as CYP2D6 substrates.

Table 8.3 Role of CYPs in Human Drug Metabolism

P450	Percentage of Total Hepatic CYP Pool	Approximate Percentage of Drugs That are Substrates	Examples of Substrates	Examples of Inhibitors	Examples of Inducers
CYP1A2	15	~5	Fluvoxamine Caffeine Cyclobenzaprine Theophylline Thiothixene Olanzapine	Ciprofloxacin Fluvoxamine Ticlopidine	Halogenated biphenyls Polycyclic aromatic Hydrocarbons Omeprazole Rosiglitazone Phenylisothiocyanate
CYP2A6	<5	1–2	Acetaminophen Carbamazepine Cyclophosphamide Selegiline Flunitrazepam Nicotine	Clotrimazole Isoniazid Methoxypsoralen Valproic acid	Dexamethasone Phenobarbital Rifampin
CYP2B6	<5	1–2	Bupropion Carbamazepine Cyclophosphamide Selegiline Flunitrazepam Meperidine	Bupropion Selegiline Ethinylestradiol Phencyclidine Tamoxifen Ticlopidine	Clotrimazole Carbamazepine Phenobarbital Phenytoin Pioglitazone Rifampin Troglitazone Valproic acid Ritonavir
CYP2C8	<5	1–2	Disopyramide Amiodarone Clozapine Diclofenac Fluvastatin Nicardipine Paclitaxel Retinoic acid Rosiglitazone Torsemide Repaglinide	Amiodarone Celecoxib Felodipine Nicardipine Fluoxetine Ketoconazole Ritonavir Indinavir Troglitazone Zafirlukast Retinoic acid	Clotrimazole Phenobarbital Dexamethasone Gemfibrozil Rifampin Phenytoin Ritonavir
CYP2C9	20	10	Celecoxib Diclofenac Fluoxetine Fluvastatin Ibuprofen Irbesarten Naproxen Amitriptyline Phenytoin Tolbutamide Torsemide S-warfarin Rosiglitazone	Amiodarone Fluconazole Fluvoxamine Fluvastatin Isoniazid Sertraline Sulfaphenazole Trimethoprin Zafirlukast	Rifampin Clotrimazole Carbamazepine Hyperforin Phenobarbital Ritonavir
CYP2C19	<5	5	Amitriptyline S-mephenytoin Omeprazole Phenytoin Phenobarbital Propranolol Diazepam	Fluoxetine Fluvoxamine Ketoconazole Omeprazole Ticlopidine Topiramate	Carbamazepine Rifampin
CYP2D6	5	25	S-metoprolol Carvedilol Dextromethorphan Nortriptyline Propanolol Odansetron Chlorpromazine Codeine Flecainide Fluoxetine Haloperidol	Amiodarone Fluoxetine Methadone Celecoxib Doxorubicin	

Table 8.3 Role of CYPs in Human Drug Metabolism—Cont'd

P450	Percentage of Total Hepatic CYP Pool	Approximate Percentage of Drugs That are Substrates	Examples of Substrates	Examples of Inhibitors	Examples of Inducers
			Tamoxifen Thioridazine Venlafaxine		
CYP2E1	10	5	Acetaminophen Chlorzoxazone Enflurane Halothane Methoxyflurane Ethanol		Ethanol Isoniazid
CYP3A4 and CYP3A5	30	50	Alfentanyl Alprazolam Atorvastatin Cisapride Cyclosporine Diazepam Erythromycin Indinavir Lovastatin Midazolam Nifedipine Quinidine Ritonavir Saquinavir Simvastatin Triazolam Verapamil Zolpidem	Amprenavir Aprepitant Atazanavir Cimetidine Clarithromycin Cyclosporin Diltiazem Ethinylestradiol Erythromycin Fluconazole Itraconazole Ketoconazole Nefazodone Nelfinavir Ritonavir Saquinavir Telithromycin Troleandomycin Verapamil	Phenobarbital Carbamazepine Phenytoin Pioglitazone Rifampin St. John's wort Troglitazone

Table 8.4 Examples of Allelic Variations of Individual CYP Enzymes

Wild-type Allele†	Variant Allele	Nucleotide Substitution	Amino Acid Substitution	Phenotype	Clinical Consequence
CYP2A6*1	CYP2A6*2	1799T→A	L160H	No substrate metabolism	Nicotine is oxidized to cotinine by CYP2A6. Individuals with this genotype can more easily quit cigarettes
CYP2C9*1	CYP2C9*2	430C→T	$144C	Reduced rate of substrate metabolism	Significant increased risk of overanticoagulation during the initial dosing of warfarin
CYP2D6*1	CYP2D6*10	100C→T	P34Sl	Reduced rate of substrate metabolism	2–4 fold dose reductions required for imipramine, doxepin, nortriptyline, thioridazine, or haloperidol

†Phenotype of all wild-types is normal metabolism.

Early genotypic inferences were made on the basis of twin studies, but were subsequently confirmed more than a decade later in the laboratories of Meyers and Gonzalez. Today the known polymorphisms of CYP2D6 are maintained at the following web site: http://www.imm.ki.se/cypalleles/cyp2d6.htm.

Examples of the occurrence of variant *CYP2D6* alleles and their consequences are shown in Table 8.5.

A very interesting case control study about the pharmacogenetics of CYP1A2 was recently published in the Journal of the American Medical Association. It was reported that coffee drinkers who bear the *CYP1A2*1F* allele were at significantly greater risk of heart attack than coffee drinkers with the normal *CYP1A2*1* allele. Presumably the *CYP1A2*1F* subjects were slow metabolizers of caffeine.

An excellent discussion of cytochrome P450 pharmacogenetics was written by Haining and Yu (2003), and published in the book, *Drug Metabolizing Enzymes.* In their chapter, Haining and Yu discuss polymorphisms for virtually every important CYP isoform, paying special attention to CYP2C9 and CYP2D6.

Table 8.5 Human Polymorphic CYP2D6 Allelic Variants (Reproduced from Ingelman-Sundberg, 2005)

Major Variant Alleles	Mutation	Consequence	Allele Frequencies (%)			
			Caucasians	Asians	Black Africans	Ethiopians and Saudi Arabians
*CYP2D6*xn*	Gene duplication/ multiduplication	Increased enzyme activity	1–5	0–2	2	10–16
*CYP2D6*4*	Defective splicing	Inactive enzyme	12–21	1	2	1–4
*CYP2D6*5*	Gene deletion	No enzyme	2–7	6	4	1–3
*CYP2D6*10*	P34S, S486T	Unstable enzyme	1–2	51	6	3–9
*CYP2D6*17*	T107I, R296C, S486T	Altered affinity for substrates	0	0	20–35	3–9

In theory, knowledge of CYP genotypes should be useful in predicting individual phenotypes that will help in the selection of the most appropriate drug dosages for each person. Moreover, CYP genotyping is now commercialized for clinical application; that is, for predicting who might be candidates for high, normal, or low doses of certain drugs, or who might not be candidates for certain drugs at all. In 2006 the U.S. Food and Drug Administration approved Roche's AmpliChip genotyping device. This device, coupled with microarray instrumentation of Affymetrix, is currently available to assist physicians and other health care providers genotype a patient's CYP2D6 or CYP2C19 using a sample of blood. Once DNA is extracted from the blood sample it is applied to the AmpliChip and analyzed by the microarray instrumentation. The patient's CYP2D6 or CYP2C19 genotype then is reported to the physician to aid in decisions about dosing drugs that are processed by CYP2D6 or CYP2C19. The simplest example of this can be shown for CYP2C19. Suppose the normal allele is designated as *1 (*CYP2C19*1*), and the two variant alleles that can be expressed are *2 and *3, respectively. An individual could express one of the following combinations of two of these alleles: *1*1; *1*2; *1*3; *2*2; *2*3; or *3*3. From a single blood sample, the AmpliChip technology would determine which allelic combination of *CYP2C19* an individual possessed, and also whether or not a particular combination was likely to mean that the individual was a poor metabolizer of substrates for CYP2C19 (Table 8.3) or an extensive (i.e., normal) metabolizer of CYP2C19 substrates.

As it turns out, as long as an individual has one *1 allele, regardless of whichever other allele (s)he possesses, then (s)he will be an extensive (normal) metabolizer of CYP2C19 substrates. So, for example, if a patient's blood revealed by the AmpliChip technology that the patient's CYP2C19 enzymes, in fact, were expressed from *CYP2C19*2*3*, then the patient's physician would learn that the patient was a poor metabolizer of CYP2C19 substrates. If the patient required treatment with, say, phenytoin, it would be known from the outset that the safe and effective dose of phenytoin would likely be smaller than for most other patients.

However, in spite of the promise for individualizing drug therapy for substrates of CYP2C19 and CYP2D6, detecting correlations between single SNPs, diplotypes, or haplotypes of CYPs and phenotypic variations in drug metabolism will likely remain an important challenge in clinical pharmacology and drug metabolism for some time to come. Several issues that hamper establishing predictive correlations include:

- The growing number of genetic variants for each CYP that are continually being discovered
- The growing recognition that genomics is currently not a particularly good predictor of proteomics
- Lack of uniform agreement on the methods for clinically phenotyping CYP activities
- The relatively large sample sizes (i.e., populations) that must be simultaneously genotyped and phenotyped

An example of this problem was brought to light in a recent Japanese study conducted by Takata and colleagues who were interested in determining what types of correlations they could draw between CYP1A2*1F, CYP1A2*C genotypes, the CYP1A2*1K haplotype, and *in vivo* measures of CYP1A2 activity using theophylline and caffeine as probes. Even though they used a total of 350 Japanese patients and normal volunteers with phenotypic variations of 30-fold in patients and 70-fold in healthy volunteers, they concluded that those variations were not attributable to the two genotypes or the CYP1A2*K haplotype. The *post hoc* power analysis that they performed suggested that to establish any correlation between genotype and phenotype for CYP1A2 activity in their study they would have required more than 2000 subjects.

Phenotyping CYP Activity Certainly one of the difficulties in establishing correlations between drug metabolizing genotypes and phenotypes is rooted in the fact that the expression of many CYPs is either largely or at least partially regulated by environmental factors or host factors such as disease, exposure to chemicals (such as polycyclic aromatic hydrocarbons), and exposure to other drugs. With regard to disease, even the effects of liver disease on CYP activity depend upon both the specific CYP enzyme, and the extent of liver damage. This was demonstrated in humans with liver dysfunction by correlating Pugh scores with *in vivo* phenotyping measures by Robert Branch's group at the University of Pittsburgh and collaborators at the University of Florida, Gainesville. Their data suggested that CYP2C19 activity falls off rapidly even when hepatic function is not severely compromised. In contrast, CYP2E1 activity is sustained at near normal levels even during hepatic decompensation. CYP1A2 and CYP2D6 fall off slowly as hepatic function worsens.

To the extent, therefore, that the phenotypic expression of drug metabolizing enzyme activity is a function of such exposures, it would be useful to characterize the qualitative and quantitative impact of such exposures on the expression of drug metabolizing enzyme activity in humans. Phenotyping human drug-metabolizing enzyme activity is accomplished with both *in vitro* and *in vivo* experiments. The former experiments typically utilize human liver microsomes or heterologous expression systems engineered to express a single type of human drug-metabolizing enzyme. Probe substrates are added, and either the formation of metabolites or the disappearance of the substrate can be quantitated both in the absence and presence of other xenobiotics that are presumed to inhibit enzyme activity. Examples of probe substrates that have been used in *in vitro* phenotyping experiments are listed in Table 8.6.

Some commercially available phenotyping kits use an array of coumarin analogs designed to be relatively isozyme-specific substrates (probes) that are metabolized to products with easily measurable spectral characteristics. Other commercially available kits use microsomes from baculovirus-infected cells that overexpress individual human CYP isoforms and fluorescent substrates (Vivid® substrates) that can be incorporated into 1536 well formats. These simple systems do not readily lend themselves to the *in vitro* study of enzyme induction, however. The prediction of xenobiotic alteration of the expression of CYP activity *in vivo* from *in vitro* experiments will be discussed more completely in the chapter on drug–drug interactions.

The usual way in which *in vivo* phenotyping is done is to assess drug metabolizing enzyme activity both during and absent exposures (e.g. exposures to other drugs, chemicals, or diseases). *In vivo* drug-metabolizing activity of the enzymes of interest can be measured in one of several ways. One way is to measure the ratio of the concentration of an enzyme substrate to the concentration of one or more of its metabolites in a biological fluid (blood, urine, or saliva). Substrate selection must take account of the selectivity of its metabolism (e.g., the number of CYP enzymes that process the substrate) as well as the sites of metabolism (e.g., liver, intestines, or both). Often a particular metabolite of a probe is the product of the activity of a single CYP isoform, thus quantitating the formation of that metabolite provides adequate insight into the activity of a specific isoform. For example, although dextromethorphan is metabolized both by CYP3A4 and CYP2D6, it is only O-demethylated to dextrorphan by CYP2D6. Consequently the metabolic ratio (concentration of dextrorphan to dextromethrophan) after a single dose of dextromethorphan is an indication of the activity of hepatic CYP2D6 in humans.

Ideally, the substrate ought to be an endobiotic (e.g., cortisol) thereby obviating the necessity of administering a xenobiotic as an enzyme probe. However, the only accepted (and partially validated) endobiotic probe of a CYP enzyme is, in fact, cortisol. Its plasma or salivary levels in comparison to the levels of its metabolite, 6-hydroxycortisol, can be used to phenotype the activity of CYP3A4 in the liver. The generally accepted xenobiotic probes of human CYP activity are given in Table 8.7.

Some investigators favor the combined use of multiple CYP isoform probes in a single "cocktail" for the *in vivo* characterization of phenotypic activity of the major CYP enzymes in humans. In the "Pittsburgh cocktail" that is recommended by Richard Branch, Gary Matzke, and colleagues, caffeine, chlorzoxazone, dapsone, debrisoquin, and mephenytoin are used together for phenotyping CYP1A2, 2E1, 3A4, 2D6,

Table 8.6 Examples of Substrates (Probes) Used for *In Vitro* Phenotyping of CYP Activity

Cytochrome P450	Substrates Used as Probes for *In Vitro* Phenotyping
1A2	Ethoxyresorufin, phenacetin, caffeine, acetanilide, methoxyresorufin
2A6	Coumarin
2B6	S-mephenytoin, bupropion
2C8	Paclitaxel
2C9	S-warfarin, diclofenac, tolbutamide
2C19	S-mephenytoin
2D6	Bufuralol, dextromethorphan, metoprolol, debrisoquine, codeine
2E1	Chlorzoxazone, 4-nitrophenol, lauric acid
3A4	Midazolam, testosterone, nifedipine, felodipine, cyclosporine, terfenadine, erythromycin, simvastatin

Table 8.7 Xenobiotics Recommended for *In Vivo* Phenotyping of Human CYP Activities

Enzyme	Xenobiotic Probe
CYP1A2	Theophylline, caffeine*
CYP2C9	S-warfarin, tolbutamide*
CYP2C19	Mephenytoin*, omeprazole*
CYP2D6	Desipramine, debrisoquine*
CYP2E1	Chlorzoxazone*
CYP3A4	Midazolam†, buspirone, felodipine, simvastatin, lovastatin, atorvastatin*

*EUFEPS recommended probes. Probes unmarked with asterisk denote FDA-recommended probes.

†Oral midazolam plus intravenous erythromycin are recommended by EUFEPS for discriminating intestinal versus hepatic CYP3A4 activity.

and C19 activities, respectively. Joe Bertino Jr.'s group favors the combined use of caffeine, dextromethorphan, omeprazole, and midazolam for phenotyping the activities of CYP1A2, 2D6, C19, and 3A4, respectively. This drug combination has been referred to as the "Cooperstown cocktail." In order to use multiple CYP probes in single dose combinations as before, it is a requirement that none of the probes used in combination alter the metabolic ratios or clearances of any of the other probes. Both research groups have shown that to be true for the Pittsburgh and Cooperstown cocktails.

Quantitative Characterization of Drug Metabolizing Enzyme Activities This section is intended to outline the broad strategy for assessing drug metabolizing enzyme activities. For specific technical details, refer to classic techniques that have been described by G. Gordon Gibson and Paul Skett in their book, *Introduction to Drug Metabolism*, or an even older chapter written by Paul Mazel in the classic book, *Fundamentals of Drug Metabolism and Drug Disposition*, that was edited by Bert La Du, George Mandel, and E. Leong Way. Though originally published back in 1971 and no longer in press, the book is nevertheless still required reading for anyone with serious interests in the field. For more contemporary examples of the *in vitro* quantitation of drug metabolizing enzyme activities, sample any of the recent issues of *Drug Metabolism and Disposition, Journal of Pharmacology and Experimental Therapeutics, Current Drug Metabolism, Drug Metabolism Letters*, or *Xenobiotica* to name a few periodicals in which *in vitro* drug metabolism studies commonly are published.

Fundamentally, typical enzyme-substrate reactions can be characterized by the following expression:

$$E + S \underset{k_{-1}}{\overset{k_1}{\longleftrightarrow}} ES \xrightarrow{k_2} E + P \tag{8.1}$$

where E denotes the enzyme; S, the substrate; ES, the enzyme and substrate complex; and P, the product. Forward rate constants for the first and second steps are shown as k_1 and k_2, and the reverse rate constant for the first step is shown as k_{-1}.

Now, if the ES complex is in steady-state and substrate concentrations are saturating (i.e., occupy all enzyme active sites so that no enzyme molecules exist that are not occupied by substrate), then the rate of product formation will be maximal and its rate can be described by:

$$V_{max} = k_2[ES] \tag{8.2}$$

or

$$V_{max} = k_{cat} \times E \tag{8.3}$$

where k_{cat} is the enzyme catalytic constant in units of reciprocal time.

The Michaelis-Menten equation further describes the relationship between the initial rate of an enzyme-catalyzed reaction, v; the maximal rate of the reaction, V_{max}; the concentration of substrate, $[S]$; and the Michaelis-Menten constant, K_m. The K_m represents the substrate concentration required in order for $v = V_{max}/2$.

The Michaelis-Menten equation is as follows:

$$v = \frac{(V_{max} \times [S])}{(K_m + [S])} \tag{8.4}$$

If we were to plot a typical rate of enzyme-mediated product formation from a substrate as a function of substrate concentration, a plot such as the one shown in Figure 8.14 would typically describe the data.

Sometimes the data can be more readily visualized by transforming the data to linear graphics. This can be accomplished with a double-reciprocal or Lineweaver-Burke plot as shown in Figure 8.15.

The Lineweaver-Burke plot once provided a convenient method for estimating V_{max} with a discrete interpolated data point (note that $1/V_{max}$ is equivalent to the intercept at the ordinate), since in the direct plot (Figure 8.14), the plot of v versus $[S]$ asymptotically approaches a maximum. As it turns out, however, V_{max} can readily be estimated from the direct data (i.e., v versus $[S]$) using nonlinear regression.

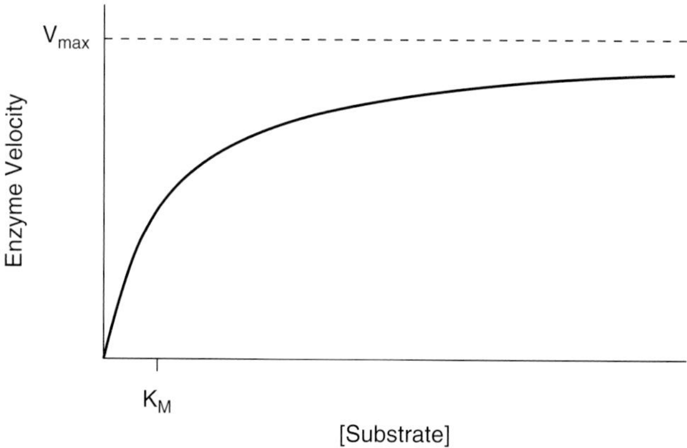

Figure 8.14 Plot of enzyme velocity, v, as a function of substrate concentrations, [S].

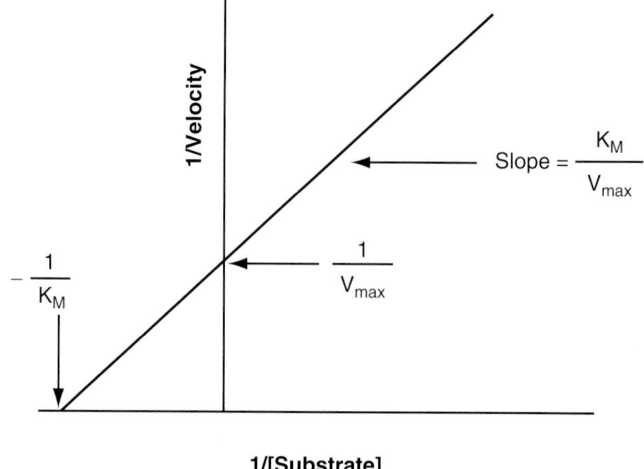

Figure 8.15 Lineweaver-Burke plot of enzyme kinetic data in which $1/v$ is plotted against $1/[S]$.

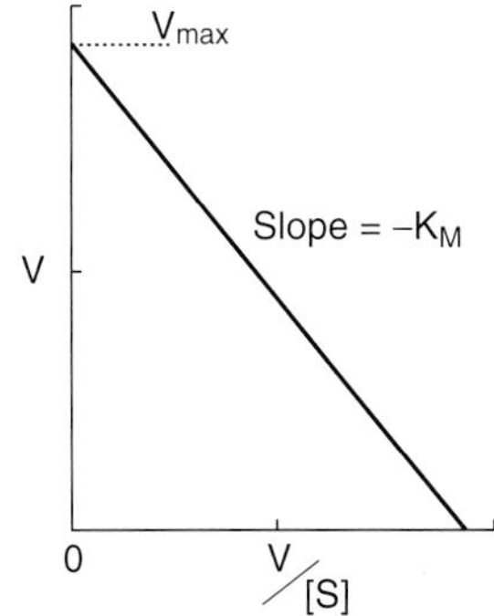

Figure 8.16 Eadie-Hofstee plot in which v is the enzyme reaction rate.

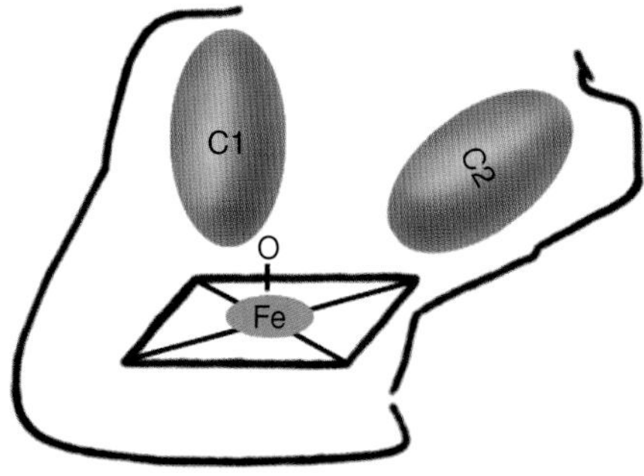

Figure 8.17 A hypothetical representation of two identical substrate molecules bound at the active site of a single enzyme.

The double-reciprocal plot spreads the data fairly unevenly, clustering data points near the origin. This data-weighting can give rise to errant estimates of the key Michaelis-Menten parameters, K_m and V_{max}.

Alternatively the data can be linearized in a plot of v versus $v/[S]$, known as an Eadie-Hofstee plot as shown in Figure 8.16.

The Eadie-Hofstee plot does a better job than the Lineweaver-Burke plot in evenly distributing the data points over the entire substrate concentration range, and can be a useful visual technique for ascertaining whether enzyme kinetics are typical (as shown) or atypical (see Figure 8.18, B and C). The Michaelis-Menten approach basically assumes that enzymes present a single binding site to each substrate. Estimates of V_{max} and K_m of drug substrates from *in vitro* experiments using either human hepatic microsomes or heterologous expression systems with human CYPs can permit the prediction of *in vivo* hepatic clearances of drugs. At substrate concentrations that are much smaller than K_m, the intrinsic hepatic clearance of the unbound drug $CL_{\text{int}_{unb}}$ will approximate the ratio of V_{max} to K_m as follows:

$$CL_{\text{int}_{unb}} = \frac{V_{max}}{K_m} \tag{8.5}$$

Scaling from an *in vitro* $CL_{\text{int}_{unb}}$ to an *in vivo* value is an easy matter in which scaling factors would include such things as the concentration of cytochrome P450 per mg of microsomal protein, the amount of microsomal protein per mg liver and the mass of an average liver.

It is now clear that many drug-metabolizing enzymes possess binding regions that can accommodate more than one substrate molecule as shown in Figure 8.17.

A homotropic effect occurs when the binding of one substrate molecule perturbs the rate of catalysis of a second molecule of the same substrate. It is possible for the homotropic effect to be either positive, that is, to give rise to an increased rate of catalysis (homotropic activation, positive cooperativity, or autoactivation), or a negative, that is, causing a decreased rate of catalysis (homotropic inactivation, negative cooperativity, or substrate inhibition). These circumstances cannot be adequately modeled by the simple Michaelis-Menten equation, and neither do direct plots of v versus $[S]$ appear hyperbolic nor do the Eadie-Hofstee plots appear linear, though changes in direct plots can be much more subtle than changes in the appearance of Eadie-Hofstee plots under these circumstances. Looking at A and B in Figure 8.18, the direct plots (hyperbolic in A and sigmoidal in B) may exhibit only subtle differences (i.e., the direct plots may not look very dissimilar). However, the Eadie-Hofstee plots (inset) clearly reveal the phenomenon of homotropic activation (B).

The inhibition of enzyme-mediated biotransformation of a drug substrate by a second drug will be discussed in a following section on enzyme regulation and in a subsequent chapter on drug–drug interactions as well.

In Silico Methods for Predicting Substrate Specificity Dr. David F. V. Lewis at the University of Surrey has examined the physical/chemical characteristics of CYP substrates as predictors of the preferred CYP isoform for their metabolism with a view toward predicting which isoforms would be most likely to participate in the processing of a new chemical entity (NCE) based on first principles. He has found predictors of enzyme selectivity in the molecular geometries of substrates. For example CYP1A2 substrates are likely to be planar molecules, basic, and have relatively small molecular weights. In contrast, CYP3A4 substrates are likely to be nonplanar (globular) with relatively large molecular weights. CYP2C9 substrates are likely to be acidic ($pKa \leq 5$), whereas CYP2D6 substrates are likely to be basic ($pKa \geq 12$). Using 3D molecular models of human CYPs constructed from a mammalian CYP2C5 crystallographic template, Lewis determined that overall substrate binding affinity to CYP enzymes was related to desolvation (or partitioning) energy, hydrogen bonding energy, π-π stacking interaction energy, loss of bond rotational energy, ion interaction energy, and loss of translational/rotational energy. Computing experimental binding energy (ΔG_{bind}) from the forementioned energies, Lewis found excellent correlations between ΔG_{bind} and reported K_m values (since $\Delta G = RT \ln K_m$) for nearly a total of 100 CYP substrates of 10 different CYP isoforms. For substrates of CYP2B6 a strong correlation (r = 0.980) existed between their

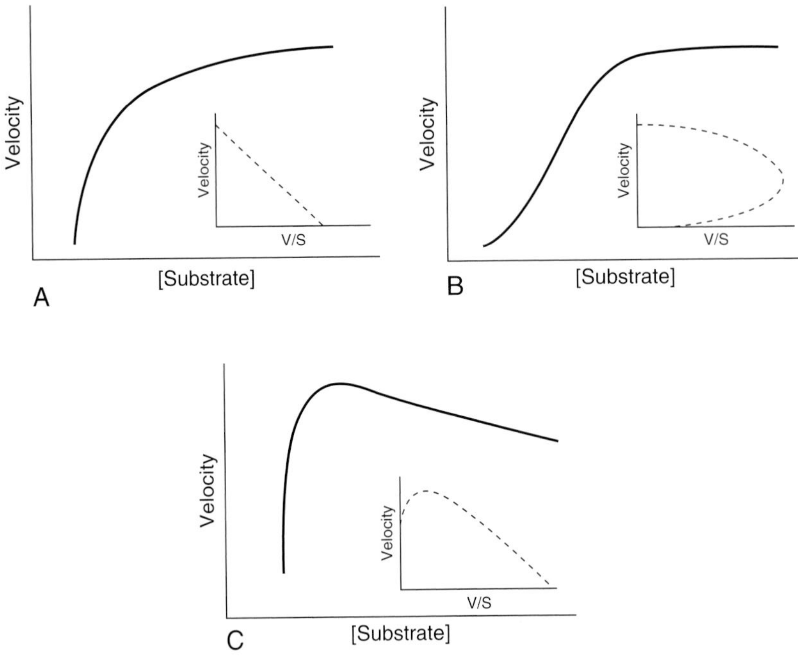

Figure 8.18 Representation of changes in deviations from Michaelis-Menten kinetics (A). Homotropic activation is depicted in B and substrate inhibition is shown in C. Inset curves denote Eadie-Hofstee plots for the same circumstances. (Modified from Atypical kinetic profiles in drug metabolism. J. Matthew Hutzler and Timothy S. Tracy, Drug Metabolism and Disposition 30:355-362, 2002.)

log*P* values and K_m values. For CYP3A4 substrates log*P* was also a key determinant of binding affinity, since ΔG_{bind} calculated as the sum of partitioning, hydrogen bond, π-π stacking, and loss of bond rotational energies, correlated highly (0.978) with an experimental ΔG_{bind} that was computed as $-RT$ ln *P*.

Empirical approaches to predicting which CYP isoforms are most likely to process a given substrate are data driven, dependent upon, for example, X-ray crystallographic analysis, sequence alignments, and site-directed mutagenesis, and include such things as homology modeling and molecular dynamics simulation. These computational approaches provide visual analyses. The accuracy of empirical approaches is highly dependent on the quality of the empirical data upon which models are structured. Empirical data that draws upon quantitative measures of the inhibition of a CYP enzyme by an array of inhibitory substances can be exhibited as three-dimensional models known as pharmacophores. Using this approach Sean Ekins has computed a pharmacophore model for inhibitors of CYP3A4 that is based on inhibition of midazolam 1′-hydroxylase that included three hydrophobes that were 5.2-8.8A from a hydrogen bond acceptor. Others (using different substrates and inhibitors) have similarly modeled pharmacophores for CYP3A4 inhibitors with three hydrophobes that were 4.2-7.1A from a hydrogen bond acceptor. A homology model of CYP3A4 based on CYP2C5 as the template is shown in Figure 8.19.

Several software programs are commercially available that predict metabolites from a 3D structure that can be entered through a graphical user input (GUI). These include TIMES®, META®, METEOR®, and MetabolExpert®. These predictive programs have been compared in terms of hardware requirements, input requirements, output formats, and explanations of reports (see Kulkarni, Zhu, and Blechinger, 2005).

Regulation of the CYP Enzymes

Increasing CYP Activity As alluded to earlier, the activity of CYP enzymes can be modulated by both genetic factors and environmental or host factors that include chemical (and drug) exposures, age, hormones, physical conditions (e.g., pregnancy), and disease states.

With old age, for example, comes a decrease in hepatic blood flow. If the rate of drug metabolism is so fast that the rate-limiting step in its metabolism is the rate at which the drug is delivered to the liver by liver blood flow, then the drug's metabolism is said to be *flow-limited*. Not surprisingly, the clearances of those drugs whose metabolism is flow-limited (e.g., propranolol) are significantly slower in the elderly. However, some investigators have also found decreased clearances for capacity-limited drugs in the elderly, too. A *capacity-limited* drug would be a drug whose rate of metabolism is limited, in fact, by the activity of the drug-metabolizing enzymes rather than the blood flow rate to the liver. This suggests that perhaps the activity of some drug-metabolizing enzymes actually can decline during old age. At the other end of the age continuum it has been well-established that many of the drug-metabolizing enzymes, especially Phase I enzymes, are absent prenatally, and become more prominent through the gestational period and postnatally. In contrast most Phase II enzymes can be detected by the second trimester.

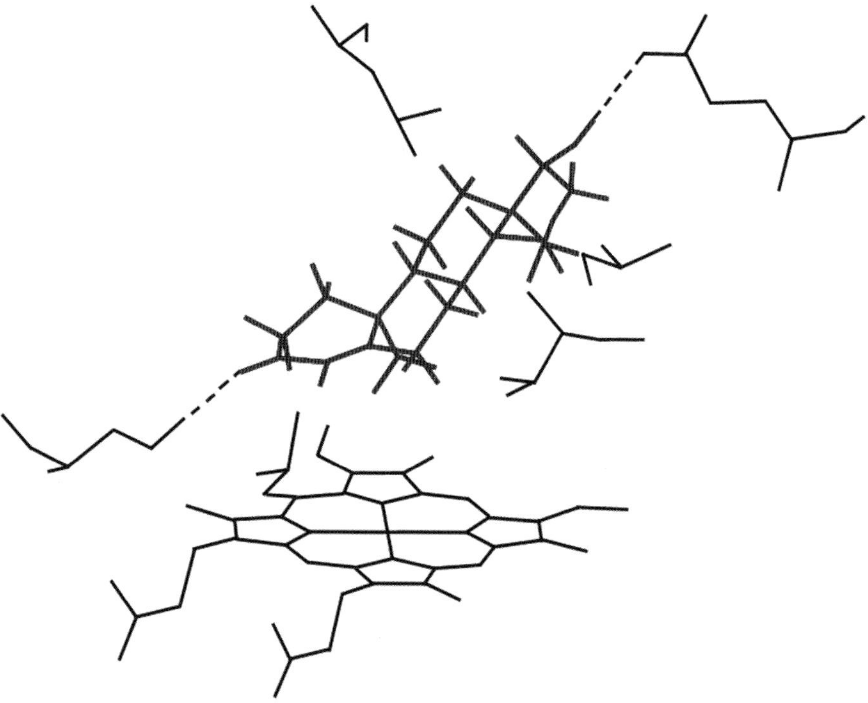

Figure 8.19 The substrate, testosterone, (in red) is shown within the active site of CYP3A4. Hydrogen bonds are dashed lines. The heme structure is shown in the bottom plane. (From DFV Lewis, Univ Surrey. Figure is Fig 6 from Xenobiotica 34:549–569, 2004.)

Although interindividual differences in CYP phenotype result from a wide array of variables it is at least worthwhile considering how other chemicals, particularly drugs, regulate CYP activities. Fundamentally, it is possible for one drug to either increase or decrease the activity of a CYP enzyme, thereby increasing or decreasing the metabolism of other substrates of that enzyme. Increases in the activity of a CYP enzyme are usually due to either the phenomenon of heterotropic activation (positive cooperativity) or enzyme induction. In the case of heterotropic activation, imagine that the two molecules depicted in Figure 8.16 are actually two different drug molecules (rather than two molecules of the same drug as shown). The binding of one of those molecules could increase the rate at which the enzyme processes the second molecule. A direct plot of v versus $[S]$ or an Eadie-Hofstee plot would be similar to the plots depicted in Figure 8.18B. However, it is more of a clinical concern if one drug actually increases the amount of enzyme that is expressed in a metabolizing tissue such as the small intestine or the liver, because a drug's disposition kinetics (e.g., clearance and half-life) will be more profoundly increased by increased enzyme expression than by heterotropic activation. That phenomenon (increased enzyme expression) is known as enzyme induction, and a great deal has been learned about the molecular features of enzyme induction since the pharmacological implications of the phenomenon were first reviewed in detail by Allan Conney in 1967.

It is now understood that nuclear receptors transduce the effects of most inducing agents on most of the inducible CYP enzymes. The identity of the aryl hydrocarbon (Ah) receptor, its activation by polycyclic aromatic hydrocarbons (PAHs), the subsequent translocation of the PAH-Ah receptor complex into the cell nucleus, and the subsequent increase in the transcription of *CYP1A1* resulting in increased cellular levels of its gene product, CYP1A1 was initially described by Daniel Nebert and colleagues (then at the NIH). Years later Evans and colleagues at the Salk Institute in La Jolla uncovered a similar role for another nuclear receptor, PXR or pregnane X receptor, in xenobiotic-induced increases in the expression of *CYP3A*. And another nuclear receptor, constitutive androstane receptor or CAR, has also been found to play a role in xenobiotic induction of some CYP enzymes. The primary structure of the PXR is shown schematically in Figure 8.20. Note that the PXR forms a heterodimer with the retinoid X receptor (RXR), and the DNA-binding domains (DBD) of the heterodimer bind to nucleotide sequences on regulated or target genes. These sequences are known as response elements. Additional details are provided in the figure legend.

A diagram of the binding of the PXR/RXR heterodimer to a response element, ER6, with the subsequent increased transcription of CYP3A4 protein is shown in Figure 8.21.

The hPXR structure is depicted in Figure 8.22.

The PXR is similar to other nuclear receptors. The arrow denotes that ligand entry occurs toward the back of the receptor. The small circle enscribes a flexible loop that may accommodate large ligands. The larger circle enscribes 70 residues that include two strands of

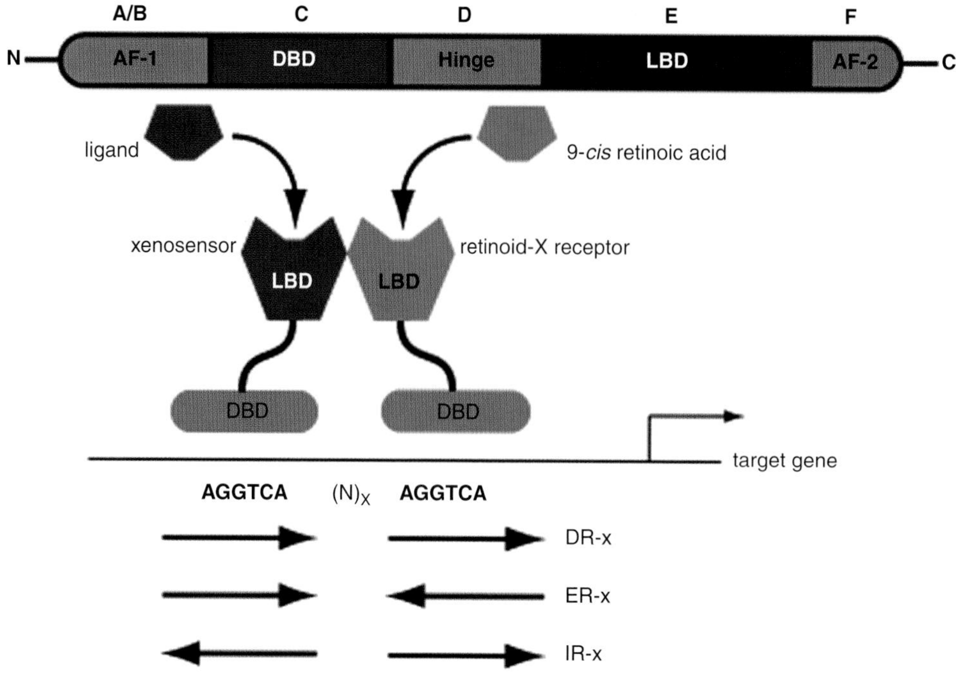

Figure 8.20 Upper part of the figure denotes the general structure of nuclear receptors consisting of four domains: an N-terminal region (denoted as AF-1), a DNA binding domain (DBD) with two zinc-finger motifs, a flexible hinge domain, a ligand binding domain (LBD), and terminal activation function domain (AF-2). The middle of the diagram portrays DNA binding of nuclear receptors. Here the xenobiotic-sensing nuclear receptors bind as heterodimers with the RXR to repeats of the nucleotide hexamer AGG/TTCA with variable spacing between (Nx). These response elements can be arranged either as direct repeats (DR), everted repeats (ER), or invertedrepeats (IR). (Figure is Fig 3 from Christoph Handschin and Urs A. Meyer. *Pharmacol Rev* 55:649–673, 2003.)

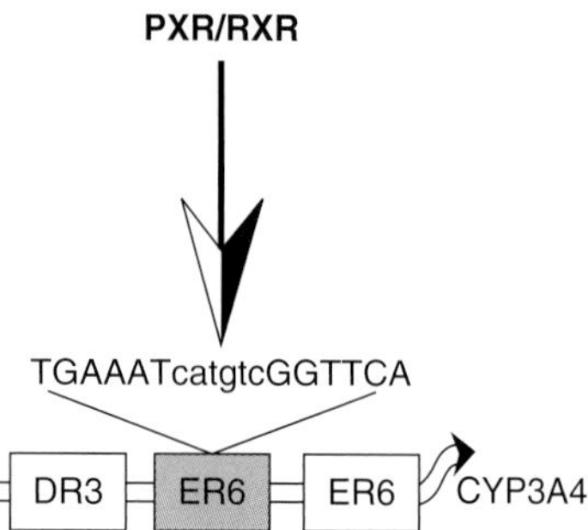

Figure 8.21 Binding of heterodimeric PXR/RXR toan ER6 response element of *CYP3A4*. The everted nucleotide sequences are shown with a spacer of six nucleotides between them. (From J.M. Pascussi et al./Biochimica et Biophysica Acta 1619 (2003) 243–253.)

ß sheets. A pharmacophore model of the human PXR, hPXR has been modeled showing three hydrophobic features and two hydrogen bond features (Figure 8.23.)

Some of the ligands that activate the PXR can activate the CAR, and conversely some CAR agonists are also PXR agonists. Moreover, some common response elements are shared by CYP3A genes and CYP2C genes, thus it is not surprising that some xenobiotics can promote transactivation of multiple CYPs.

A simple schematic depicting induction of the CYP2C and CYPA subfamilies is shown in Figure 8.24.

Though it would appear that most xenobiotic-induced increases in the cellular content of CYP enzymes are due to gene activation as shown earlier, there are examples of increased enzyme content that are due instead to enzyme stabilization. Although CYP2E1 ordinarily plays a minor role in the metabolism of ethanol, and CYP2E1 ordinarily accounts for only a very small percentage of the total CYP content in hepatocytes, the total amount of hepatic CYP2E1 can increase by as much as 10-fold in chronic alcoholics. However these increases have been ascribed to ethanol binding to CYP2E1 and stabilizing the enzyme (i.e., decreasing the enzyme's rate constant for degradation, k_{deg}, rather than increasing the rate of transcription of CYP2E1). These large increases in CYP2E1 content in the liver of alcoholics are responsible for CYP2E1 making a significant contribution to the metabolic elimination of alcohol in these individuals, and may also be partially responsible for the onset of alcohol-induced liver disease, since it can participate in the generation of reactive oxygen species (ROS).

Decreasing CYP Activity CYP activity, like that of any other enzyme, can also be decreased by endobiotics or xenobiotics. If, during drug metabolism, a substrate binds to a single active site, and that single site is also the binding site for another drug or inhibitor and the binding of the inhibitor can be reversed with high enough substrate concentrations, then the inhibition

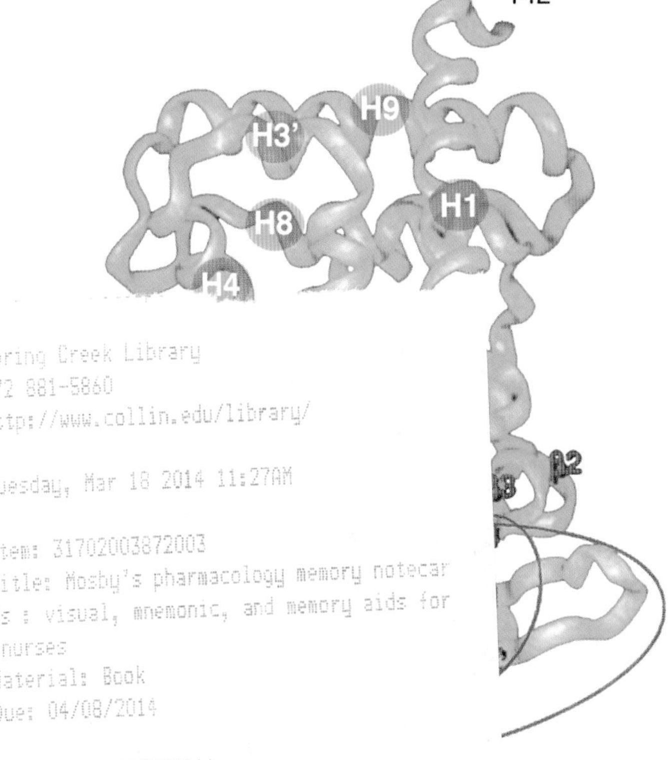

...ne human PXR. ...ca et Biophysica

...ances the V_{max} ... the inhibitor, ...hich is a bind- ...strate) will be ...f uninhibited

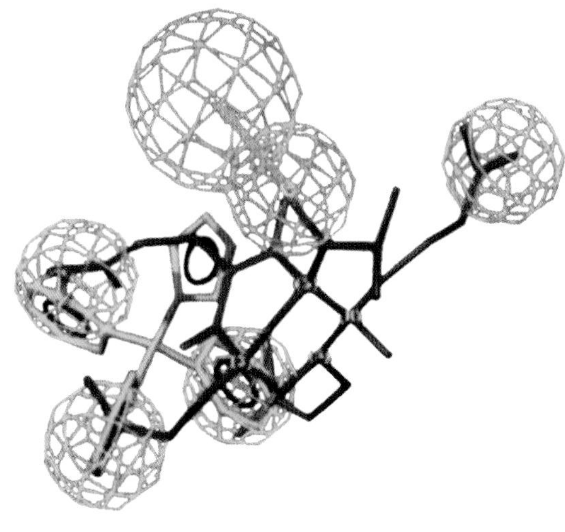

Figure 8.23 A pharmacophore model of hPXR. The blue features are hydrophobes, whereas the green denote hydrogen bond features. The red molecules is hyperforin, and the blue molecules is clotrimazole. (From *K. Bachmann et al./ Pharmacological Research 50 (2004) 237–246.*)

enzyme activity is shown on the left in Figure 8.25, whereas the Lineweaver-Burke plot to the right in would be an example of competitive inhibition.

Noncompetitive inhibition occurs if the inhibitor binds at a site that is distinct from the substrate-binding site, product formation is slowed, and the addition of large amounts of substrate cannot overcome the inhibition. Under these circumstances the V_{max} of the enzyme would be decreased, but the K_m should be unchanged. If a xenobiotic can bind to the enzyme-substrate complex only in the presence of substrate, and then slows the rate of product formation, then the inhibition is described

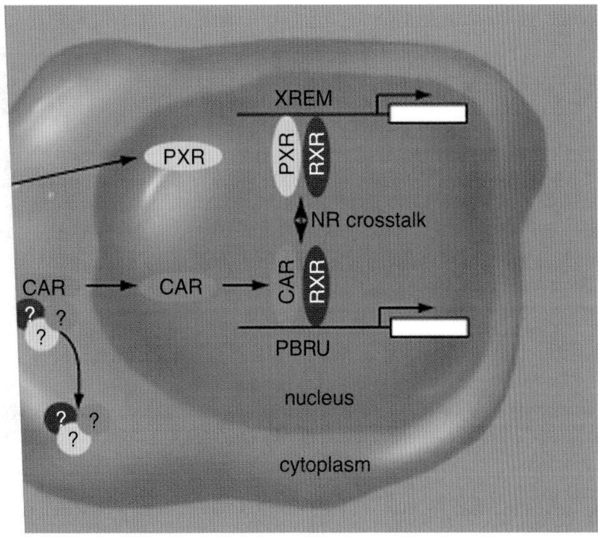

Figure 8.24 Activation of CYP genes by PXR and CAR. The question marks denote proteins that may have to be released from CAR in order for CAR to translocate into the cell nucleus. XREM, xenobiotic response enhancer module; PBRU, phenobarbital-responsive enhancer unit. (Modified from Christoph Handschin and Urs A. Meyer. *Pharmacol Rev* 55:649–673, 2003.)

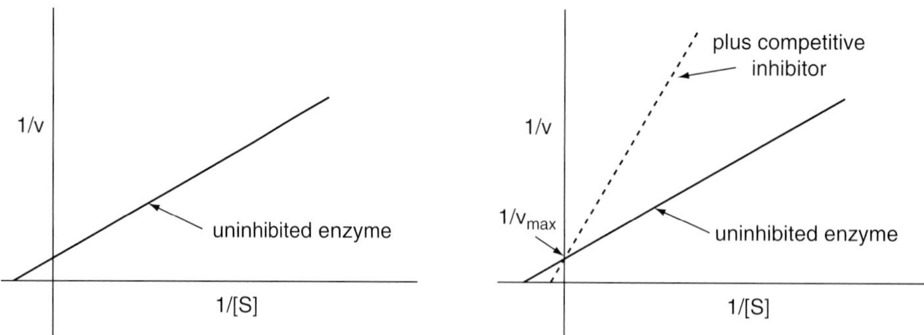

Figure 8.25 Lineweaver-Burke plots characterizing normal enzyme activity (left) and in the presence of a competitive inhibitor (upper curve, right panel).

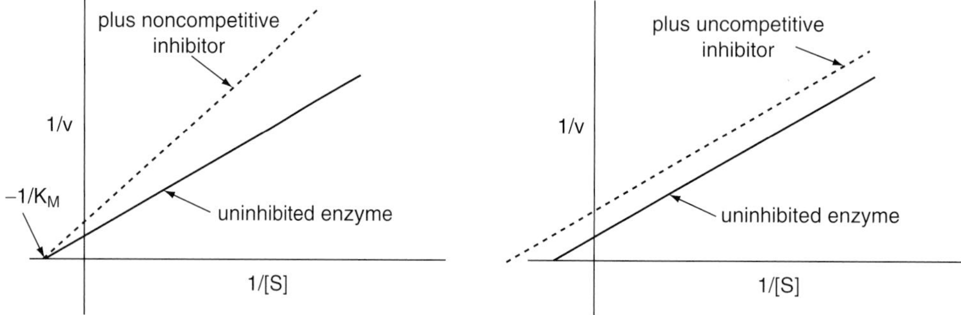

Figure 8.26 Non-competitive inhibition (left) and un-competitive inhibition (right). In both panels the lower curve denotes uninhibited enzyme activity.

as uncompetitive. In this case both Michaelis-Menten parameters, K_m and V_{max}, decrease.

Examples of noncompetitive and uncompetitive enzyme inhibition are portrayed in Figure 8.26.

The velocity equations for the reversible inhibitory reactions depicted in Figures 8.25 and 8.26 would be as follows:

For competitive inhibition,

$$v = \frac{V_{max} \times [S]}{K_m\left(1 + \frac{[I]}{K_i}\right) + [S]} \tag{8.6}$$

where all symbols are as defined in Equation (8.4), and K_i is the inhibitor constant, defined as the concentration of inhibitor required to decrease the V_{max} by 50%.

For noncompetitive inhibition,

$$v = \frac{V_{max} \times [S]}{K_m\left(1 + \frac{[I]}{K_i}\right) + [S]\left(1 + \frac{[I]}{K_i}\right)} \tag{8.7}$$

And for uncompetitive inhibition,

$$v = \frac{V_{max} \times [S]}{K_m + [S]\left(1 + \frac{[I]}{K_i}\right)} \tag{8.8}$$

Eadie-Hofstee plots for competitive and noncompetitive inhibition are portrayed in Figure 8.27. Notice that in the Eadie-Hofstee plots for a competitive inhibitor (left panel), the V_{max} (y-intercept) is not changed by any concentration of inhibitor $[I]$. The slope function denotes the K_m, and the steeper the slope, the higher the K_m and the poorer the binding of the substrate to the enzyme. In contrast, for a noncompetitive inhibitor the binding of the substrate is not affected by the inhibitor since the slopes are all comparable; however with increasing concentrations of inhibitor, the maximum rate of the reaction gets smaller (i.e., V_{max} decreases as shown in the right panel).

The cytochrome P450 enzymes, as mentioned, are now known to possess binding sites that may accommodate multiple substrate molecules or both substrate and inhibitor at the same time. Endobiotic or xenobiotic-mediated inhibition of a CYP in such a fashion would be characterized by negative cooperativity. Schematically, we could imagine a scenario similar to the one depicted in Figure 8.17, except that one of the molecules would be the substrate and the other an inhibitor. In this case the Eadie-Hofstee plot would no longer be linear as shown in Figure 8.27, but instead would appear as in Figure 8.28.

In addition to competitive, noncompetitive, and uncompetitive inhibition, reaction products may form that bind irreversibly or quasi-irreversibly to the enzyme and inactivate it. This type of phenomenon has been variously referred to as mechanism-based

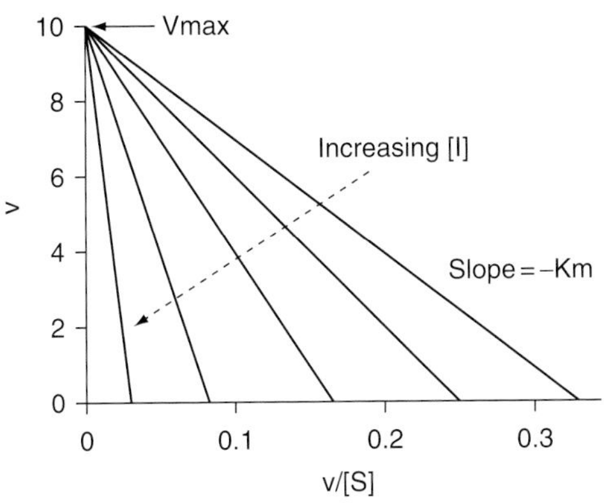

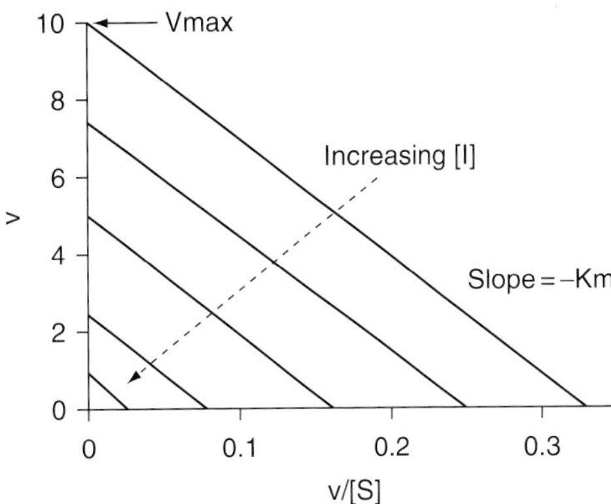

Figure 8.27 Eadie Hofstee plots of competitive (left) and non-competitive (allosteric) enzyme inhibition. (Modified from Houston et al. Chapter 7 Drug Metabolizing Enzymes Lee, Obach and Fisher, Eds, Fontis Media 2003.)

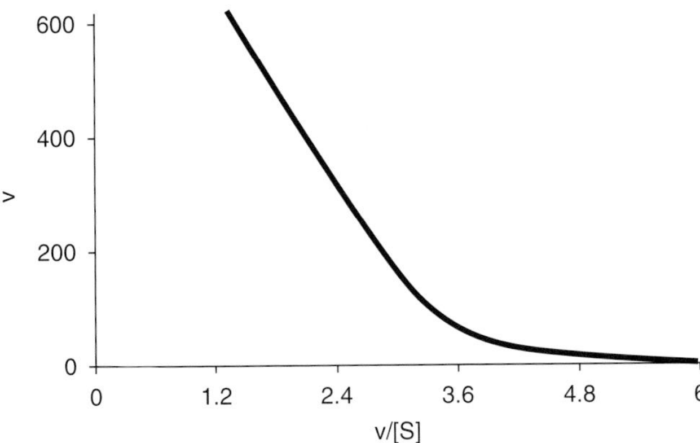

Figure 8.28 Simulated Eadie-Hofstee plot for negative cooperativity in the absence of enzyme inhibition, the plot would be linear (compare to competitive and non-competitive inhibition in Fig 8.27).

inhibition, metabolite-dependent inhibition, k_{cat} inhibition, and suicide inhibition. Metabolite-dependent inhibition can be modeled as:

$$E + I \underset{k_{-1}}{\overset{k_1}{\rightleftarrows}} EI \xrightarrow{k_2} EI' \xrightarrow{k_4} E_{inact} \quad (8.9)$$
$$EI' \xrightarrow{k_3} E + P$$

where E and E_{inact} denote the active and inactive forms of the enzyme, respectively; I represents the metabolite-dependent inhibitor; I' represents the active (inhibitory) metabolite; P, the product; and EI and EI' are enzyme-inhibitor complexes. The initial inactivation rate of the enzyme will be a function of the initial enzyme concentration, E_0 and the initial inactivation rate constant, k_{obs} as follows:

$$V_{inact} = k_{obs} \bullet E_0 \qquad (8.10)$$

and,

$$k_{obs} = k_{inact} \bullet \left(\frac{[I]_0}{K_{i,app} + [I]_0} \right) \qquad (8.11)$$

where

$$k_{inact} = k_2 \bullet k_4 / (k_2 + k_3 + k_4) \qquad (8.12)$$

The apparent inactivation rate constants of the enzyme, k_{obs}, can be estimated from a series of experiments in which each of several concentrations of inhibitor $[I]$ are used. For each $[I]$ the slope of enzyme activity versus preincubation time is measured. The array of k_{obs} values is then plotted against inhibitor concentrations $[I]$. The Ki_{app} is the $[I]$ that elicits a $k_{inact}/2$. Graphic representations of these experiments are shown in Figure 8.29.

Although relatively few drugs elicit covalent mechanism-based inhibition, the number of xenobiotic metabolites of CYP enzymes capable of causing metabolite-dependent enzyme inhibition is considerably larger than once thought. For that reason it makes some sense when screening drugs for their ability to inhibit CYP enzymes, to include preincubation periods long enough to permit the formation of inhibitory metabolites.

8.2.3.3 Oxidative Enzymes Other Than Cytochromes P450

Though the CYPs play the preeminent role in oxidative drug metabolism, collectively mediating the biotransformation of perhaps greater than 80% of all currently marketed drugs, there are also some other enzymes that mediate drug oxidations. Key non-CYP oxidative enzymes are listed in Table 8.8.

Monoamine Oxidases (MAO) There are two MAO isoforms, MAO A and MAO B, both of which are flavoenzymes that oxidize a wide array of neurotransmitter amines. However, they can also biotransform some xenobiotics. Both MAO isoforms consist of approximately 520 amino acid residues and share approximately 70% sequence identity. Their molecular weights are about 58K Daltons. Both isoforms are expressed in most tissues, though not necessarily in equivalent amounts. More MAO is found in liver and placenta, and least in the spleen. Actually MAO-B is

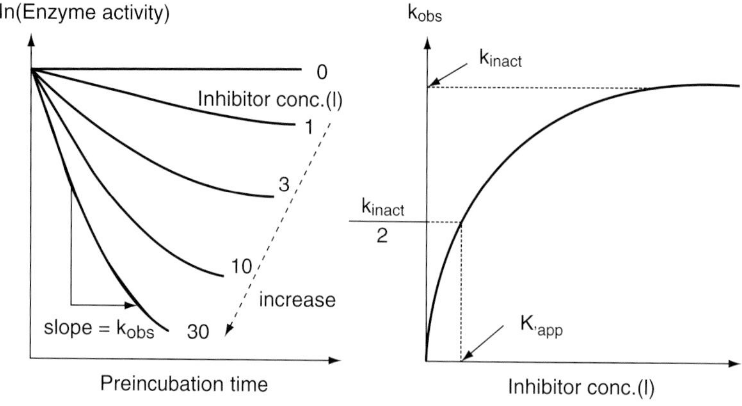

Figure 8.29 Estimation of k_{inact} and $K_{i,app}$ for mechanism-based inhibition. (From Sugiyama et al. Pharmacol Rev 50(3):387–411),

Table 8.8 Non-CYP Enzymes Capable of Mediating Drug Oxidations (Modified from Beedham, 1997)

Enzyme	Cofactors	Oxidation	Representative Type Substrate	Sample Substrate
Monoamine oxidase†	$FAD/0_2$	De-amination	Primary, secondary, and tertiary amines	Citalopram Triptans
Xanthine oxidase*	$NAD^+/0_2$ FAD	C-oxidation	Purines	6-mercaptopurine caffeine
Flavin monooxygenase	$NADPH/0_2$	N-oxidation	Secondary amines tertiary aliphatic amines	Desipramine Nicotine
Alcohol dehydrogenase	NAD^+	Alcohol oxidation	Primary alcohols	Ethanol
Aldehyde dehydrogenase	$NAD(P)^+$	Aldehyde oxidation	Aldehydes	Cyclophosphamide
Aldehyde oxidase*	O_2	Aldehyde oxidation	Aldehydes	Tolbutamide
		C-oxidation	N-heterocycles	Famciclovir

†MAOs are also enzymes that deaminate neurotransmitters such as norepinephrine and serotonin, and are also targets for monoamine oxidase inhibiting drugs that are used as antidepressant agents.
*Molybdenum-containing enzymes

not expressed at all in platelets. The two isoforms exhibit some differences in their substrate specificities. At least three different molecular mechanisms of amine oxidation have been described for MAO:

- A single electron transfer pathway
- A hydrogen atom transfer pathway
- A nucleophilic pathway

The crystal structure of MAO-B has been worked out, and indicates that the enzyme is a dimer that binds to membranes through a C-terminal transmembrane helix. The FAD moiety binds covalently to Cys397.

An important neurotoxin, MPTP, is activated to MPP^+ by MAO-B in the brain. The subsequent uptake of MPP^+ into the mitochondria of dopaminergic nerve terminals depletes the cells of ATP by inhibiting oxidative phosphorylation. MAOs are also therapeutic targets. Since these enzymes deaminate neurotransmitters such as norepinephrine and serotonin, their inhibition by monoamine oxidase inhibitors such as tranylcypromine is sometimes attempted with a view toward increasing central nervous system concentrations of norepinephrine and serotonin to ameliorate depressive illness.

Xanthine Oxidase (XO) XO is a homodimer consisting of two 150 Kdalton subunits. Like aldehyde oxidase and other molybdenum-containing enzymes XO catalyzes nucleophilic oxidations at electron-deficient carbons found within nitrogen-containing heterocyclic compounds. Like MAO, the highest levels of XO are found in the liver, though it has also been found in cardiac, pulmonary, and adipose tissue. Within those tissues XO appears to be localized in capillary endothelial cells. It has also been found in epithelial cells in lactating mammary glands. The mechanism by which XO mediates oxidation requires substrate binding to the molybdenum center with reducing

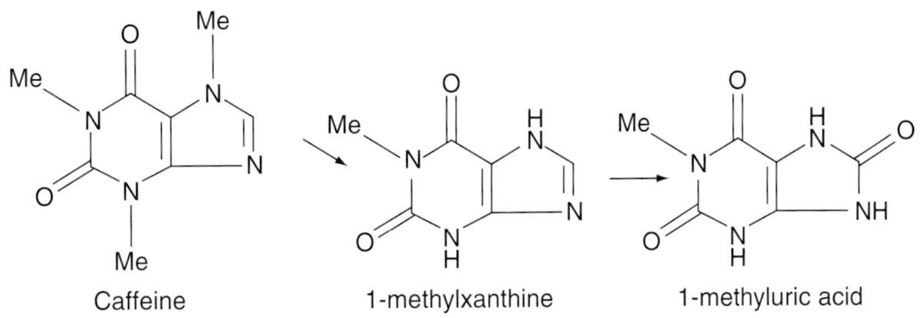

Figure 8.30 Oxidation of caffeine. The demethylation step is mediated by CYP, but the oxidation of C8 is mediated by XO (also shown in Table 8.1.)

equivalents introduced there subsequently shuttled to FAD. Purines are among the key substrates of XO, as shown for caffeine, in Figure 8.30.

The urinary ratio of 1-methyluric acid to 1-methylxanthine after a caffeine challenge can be used as a means to assess XO activity *in vivo.*

The oxidation of the endobiotic, hypoxanthine, to uric acid also requires XO, and can be inhibited by alloxanthine, an XO-mediated metabolite of allopurinol. Thus, allopurinol is, in essence, a pro-drug intended to inhibit XO in the treatment of hyperuricemia and gout. The oxidation of 6-mercaptopurine to thiouric acid is also mediated by XO. Folic acid and tetrahydrofolic acid are among the most potent inhibitors known for mammalian XO, exhibiting Ki values between 0.5 and 1.0 μM.

Aldehyde oxidases (AO) are also molybdenum-containing enzymes that, like XO, exist as homodimers of 300 Kdaltons. It is presumed that they behave mechanistically similarly to XO. Both AO and XO can mediate reductive reactions through the transfer of electrons from FADH2 to oxidized xenobiotic. For example, zonisamide can be reduced by AO to 2-sulfamoylacetylphenol.

Flavin Monoxygenases (FMO) These are FAD-containing enzymes that, like the CYPs, are localized in the endoplasmic reticulum (ER). FMOs are gene products of a gene family, and the isoforms are denoted simply by Arabic numerals, for example, FMO1, FMO2, and so on. These enzymes consist of approximately 530 amino acid residues, and have molecular masses of about 60 Kdaltons. In adult human liver FMO3 is most abundant, FMO5 is less abundant, and FMO1 is absent. FMO1 is expressed in brain, kidney, and fetal tissues. Though they appear to be subject to dietary and hormonal influences, not much is known about the influence of drugs on these enzymes (e.g. inhibition or induction).

The enzyme cycle for the FMOs (i.e., their catalytic mechanism), is not nearly as multifaceted as for the CYPs. Fundamentally, NADPH binds to FMO, thereby reducing FAD. Oxygen then binds to the NADP-FMO-$FAD_{reduced}$ complex to produce a hydroperoxyderivative that can be attacked by a nucleophilic S or N of the substrate. The distal peroxy oxygen is transferred to form the corresponding N-oxide or sulfoxide, and subsequent loss of water from the hydroxyflavin intermediate regenerates $FAD_{oxidized}$ as shown in Figure 8.31.

FMO substrates tend to be lipophilic nitrogen or sulfur-containing substances, and include numerous endobiotics and xenobiotics, particularly tertiary acyclic and cyclic amines, which are converted to stable N-oxides. Some examples include imipramine,

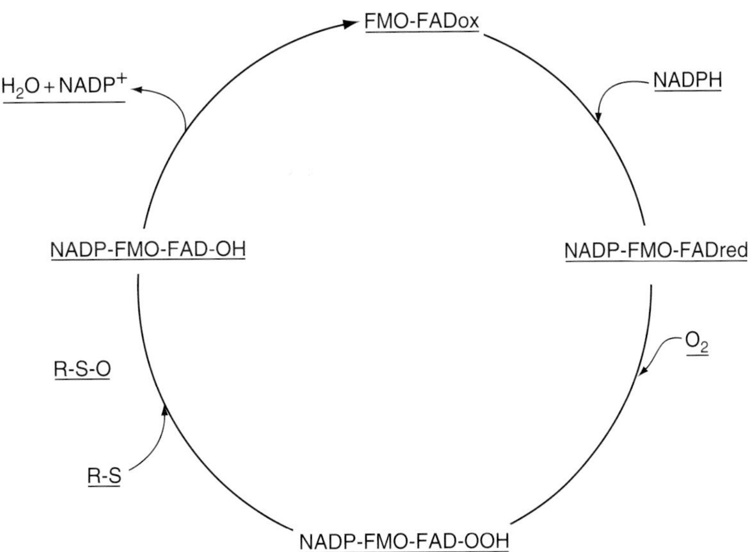

Figure 8.31 FMO catalytic cycle.

moclobemide, tamoxifen, xanomeline, and clozapine. S-oxygenation of thioethers is also mediated by FMOs, though sulfur-containing compounds in which the sulfur is adjacent to electron-withdrawing groups or heteroaromatic groups are generally poor FMO substrates. Methimazole, sulindac sulfide, and cimetidine appear to be subject to FMO-mediated S-oxygenation. In the United States, there currently are no good *in vivo* probes that are recommended for characterizing FMO3 activity in humans.

Several of the reactions catalyzed by enzymes listed in Table 8.8 are also catalyzed by CYPs. However, their role in providing complementary metabolic pathways when CYPs are inhibited, their regulation—both by induction and inhibition—their substrate selectivity, and their overall place in drug metabolism are issues that require greater exploration.

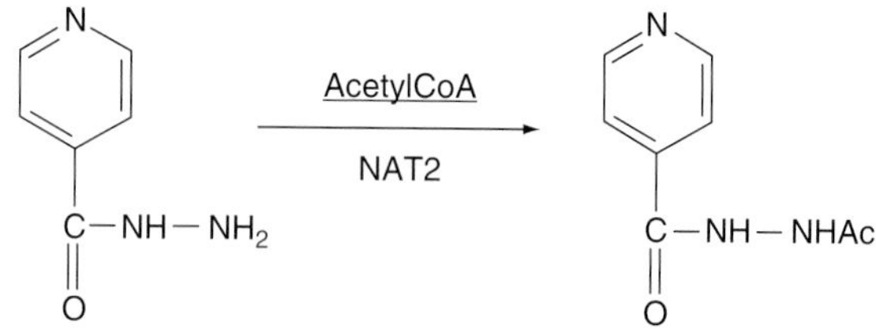

Figure 8.32 Acetylation of isoniazid by NAT2.

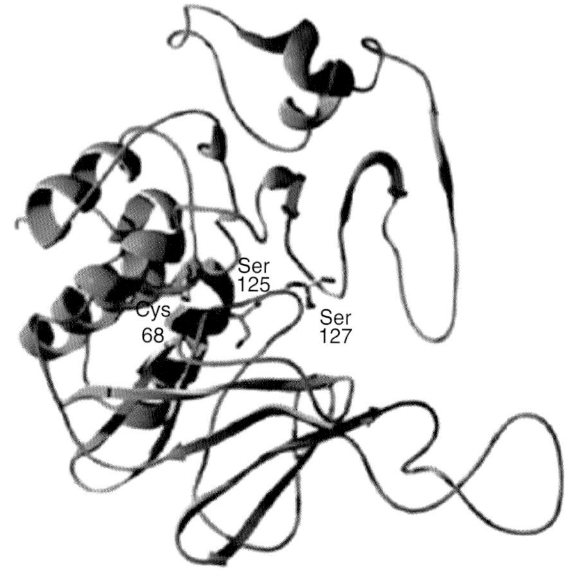

Figure 8.33 The presumed structure of human NAT2 shown below was constructed from the crystal structure of *Mycobacterium smegmatis* NAT using MODELLER. (Modified from Kawamura et al. Biochem Pharmacol 69:347–359, 2005.)

8.2.4 Phase II Enzymes

As stated much earlier in this chapter, the enzymes traditionally viewed as Phase II enzymes were those that often catalyzed the addition of functional groups such as acetate, sulfate, or glucuronate to molecular substituents such as hydroxyl functions that may have been enzymatically inserted by Phase I enzymes. Phase II enzymes also have often been thought of as conjugative enzymes, and the resultant metabolites often have significantly larger molecular weights than the parent molecules in addition to being more polar and hydrophilic. However, Phase II reactions can either be conjugation reactions, in which electrophilic adenosine-containing cofactors such as ATP, PAPS, acetylCoA, UDPGA, or SAM react with nucleophilic groups such as –OH or $-NH_2$, or they can be nucleophilic trapping reactions in which water, glutathione, or other nucleophiles react with electrophiles. Examples of Phase II reactions are shown in Table 8.2. In this chapter conjugation reactions involving PAPS, acetylCoA, and UDGA will be discussed followed by a discussion of nucleophilic trapping involving glutathione.

8.2.4.1 N-Acetyltransferases (NATs)

Arylamine N-acetyltransferases (NAT) are highly conserved in eukaryotes. These cytosolic enzymes transfer acetate from acetylCoA to primary amines, hydrazines, sulfonamides, and aromatic amines. They are 30 to 34 kDa in size. Humans express two functional NATs, NAT1 and NAT2. The genes for both isoforms encode 290 amino acids, and are found on chromosome 8. Their nucleotide sequences share 87% homology. These enzymes exhibit polymorphism, and allelic variation especially for NAT2 is associated with fast and slow acetylator phenotypes.

NAT2 detoxifies numerous drugs. The acetylation of isoniazid (INH) is shown in Figure 8.32. NAT2 is expressed mostly in the liver, intestinal epithelial cells, and colon. In contrast, NAT1 appears to metabolize fewer drug substrates even though it exhibits a more widespread tissue distribution. Para-aminobenzylglutamate (pABGlu) is thought to be the principal endobiotic substrate for NAT1.

An active Cys^{68} residue (Figure 8.33) participates in the transfer of acetate from acetylCoA onto arylamine substrates. Ser^{125} and Ser^{127} appear to be important determinants of substrate selectivity.

The discovery of polymorphic N-acetylation was linked to observations on the safety, metabolism, and pharmacokinetics of the antitubercular drug, isoniazid. When urinary excretion of isoniazid was evaluated in identical twins, fraternal twins, and unrelated subjects, the variability in its excretion depended upon genetic similarity. Ultimately, in a classic experiment by Evans and colleagues that measured the plasma isoniazid concentration in subjects who had taken a single 10 mg/kg dose of isoniazid, a clear polymorphic frequency distribution was revealed with an antimode of 2.5 ug/mL. Thus, two acetylator phenotypes were identified, and the slow acetylator phenotype had a frequency of 52%, and was an autosomal recessive trait. The slow acetylator phenotype, if treated with isoniazid (INH) is at increased risk of INH-induced arthralgias, neuropathy, and hepatotoxicity.

The slow acetylator phenotype for isoniazid is associated with a reduction in the amount of NAT 2, and occurs with a frequency of 50 to 60% in Caucasians; however, the frequency patterns can vary dramatically in different populations. NAT1 was originally thought to exhibit monomorphic metabolism, but has more recently been shown to exhibit polymorphisms in humans, too. Wild type alleles are *NAT1*4* and *NAT2*4*, respectively. As with the CYPs, it is not surprising that large numbers of SNPs have been discovered, and the up-to-date list of NAT alleles is maintained at http://www.louisville.edu/medschool/pharmacology/NAT.html.

Caffeine has been used to phenotype NAT2 using the urinary ratio of the caffeine metabolite, 5-acetylamino-6-formylamino-3-uracil (AFMU), or 5-acetyl-6-amino-3-uracil (AAMU), to various other caffeine metabolites (e.g., 1-methylxanthine (1X), 1-methylurate (1U)) or combinations of metabolites. Dapsone and sulfamethazine have also been used to phenotype NAT2.

The concordance of NAT2 genotypes and phenotypes has generally been disappointing, although a recent investigation in Chinese subjects suggests that NAT2 genotype may, in fact, predict phenotype. In any case, considerable efforts have been made to establish whether NAT2 genotypes bear associations with diseases, especially cancer. *NAT2* alleles associated with slow acetylator status appear to predict greater susceptibility to urinary bladder cancer, renal cell carcinoma, and pharyngeal cancer, whereas *NAT2* alleles associated with rapid acetylator status predict a higher risk of colorectal, lung, and laryngeal cancers. Environmental chemical exposures (e.g., heterocyclic amines in well-cooked meats or cigarette smoking) are codeterminants of risk.

8.2.4.2 Sulfotransferases (SULTs)

Enzymes mediating xenobiotic sulfonation are the sulfotransferase (SULT) enzymes. Most drugs, once sulfonated, become biologically less active and more water soluble, however xenobiotics such as N-hydroxy arylamines and N-hydroxy heterocyclic amines are actually activated by sulfotransferases to reactive electrophiles that can be mutagenic and/or carcinogenic. Cytosolic SULTs metabolize drugs and small endobiotics such as neurotransmitters (e.g., dopamine) and steroids including bile acids. The source of the sulfonyl group (SO_3^-) is adenosine 3′-phosphate 5′-phosphosulfate (PAPS). Both PAPS and substrate (ROH) bind to SULT yielding 3′-phosphoadenosine-5′-phosphate (PAP) plus R-OSO_3^-. In addition to hydroxyl functions, SULTs can sulfonate amino groups of arylamines.

Like the CYPs, SULTs comprise a superfamily of enzymes. Members of each family share at least 45% amino acid sequence identity, and members of each subfamily share at least 60% amino acid sequence identity. Table 8.9 displays the human SULT genes and their chromosome locations along with examples of some xenobiotic substrates.

SULT1A proteins are expressed in the liver, but also in extrahepatic tissues that are portals of entry of xenobiotics into the body including small and large intestine and the lungs. Its molecular weight is ca. 32 kDa. The sulfonation of acetaminophen is shown in Figure 8.34, and represents one of the major detoxification or inactivation pathways for acetaminophen. Another important inactivation pathway for acetaminophen is glucuronidation (see Section 8.2.4.3). If doses of acetaminophen are high enough, for example after an overdose, both of the aforementioned detoxification pathways can be saturated. Once that occurs, residual (i.e., nonsulfonated and nonglucuronidated) hepatic acetaminophen can be oxidized to a metabolite that can react with cellular macromolecules in the liver, causing hepatotoxicity.

In addition to sulfonating simple phenolic xenobiotics, SULT1A3 sulfonates endogenous catecholamines, and exhibits several nonsynonymous SNPs. It is much more highly expressed in fetal liver than in adult liver. SULTB1 is the major thyroid hormone sulfotransferase, and has been found in liver, small intestine, colon, and leukocytes. SULT1C2 is expressed in human fetal liver and spleen, and in adult kidney, stomach, and thyroid. SULT1E1 and SULT2A1 are expressed in the liver. SULT4A1 is found predominantly in the brain,

Table 8.9 Human *SULT* Genes and Examples of Human SULT Enzyme Xenobiotic Substrates

SULT	Chromosome	Xenobiotic Substrates
SULT1A1	16p11.2-12.1	Simple phenols, e.g., acetaminophen
SULT1A2	16p11.2-12.1	Simple phenols, e.g., p-nitrophenol
SULT1A3	16p11.2	Simple phenols, e.g., p-nitrophenol
SULT1B1	4q11-13	Simple phenols, e.g., 1-napthol
SULT1C2	2q11.2	Simple phenols, e.g., p-nitrophenol
SULT1C4	2q11.2	Simple phenols, e.g., p-nitrophenol
SULT1E1	4q13.1	17-ethinyl-estradiol, 2-hydroxyestradiol, 4-hydroxyestrone, tamoxifen
SULT2A1	19q13.3	Androgens, pregnenolone, bile acids, and carcinogens, e.g., 1-hydroxymethylpyrene
SULT2B1_v1	19q13.3	Pregnenolone
SULT2B1_v2	19q13.3	Cholesterol
SULT4A1	22q13.1-13.2	?

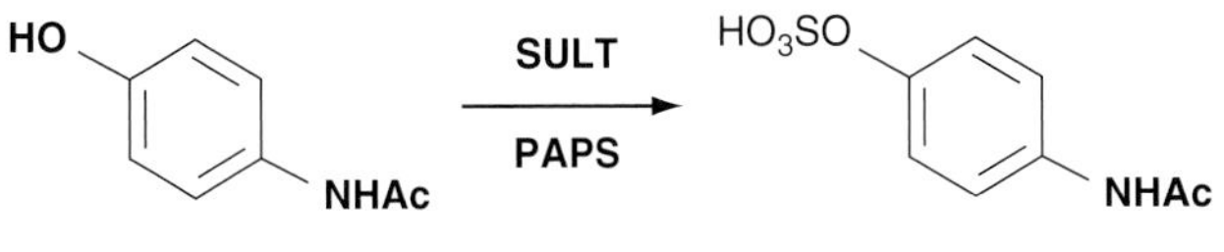

HO–C6H4–NHAc —(SULT, PAPS)→ HO_3SO–C6H4–NHAc

Figure 8.34 The sulfonation of acetaminophen.

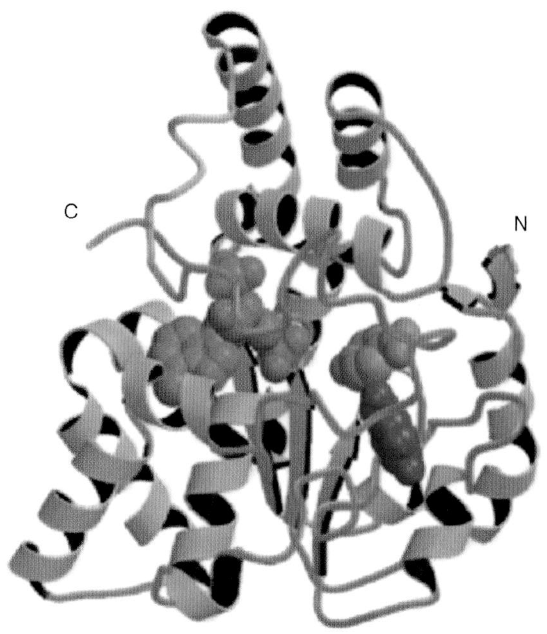

Figure 8.35 Crystal structure of cytosolic SULT1A1. PAPS is shown in purple, and the other two molecules are both *p*-nitrophenol. (Modified from N. Gamage et al. Toxicol. Sciences 90(1):5–22, 2006.)

and neither significant xenobiotic or endobiotic substrates have been identified yet.

The globular crystal structure of SULTs is shown in Figure 8.35.

ß sheets are involved in PAPS binding, and contain the key catalytic residues. The substrate binding site is an L-shaped hydrophobic pocket.

The regulation of SULTs is not particularly well understood. There is conflicting evidence as to whether CAR can induce SULTs. Similarly the effects of steroid hormones on SULTs varies depending upon cell lines. *SULT1A1* mRNA levels in primary human hepatocytes were unaffected by dexamethasone treatment, suggesting an absence of regulation by the glucocorticoid receptor (GR) and the PXR, although both the CAR and PXR have been found to be important regulators of *SULT*s in rodents. On the other hand SULT2A1 expression does appear to be regulated by PPAR in humans.

8.2.4.3 Glucuronidation

Glucuronidation of xenobiotics is an important way that many diverse organisms protect themselves against toxins, and the enzymes that detoxify xenobiotics by glucuronidation are the UDP-glucuronosyltransferases or UGTs. These are membrane-bound enzymes that transfer the glucuronic acid moiety from the uridine diphosphoglucuronic acid (UDPGlcA or UDPGA) to a nucleophilic functional group such as phenols and aliphatic alcohols, carboxylic acids, amines (including primary, secondary, or tertiary), sulfhydryl groups, and nucelophilic carbons. The addition of glucuronic acid to substrate molecules tends to increase their polarity and water solubility, and thus increases the extent of product excretion into bile, urine, or both. Increased biliary and urinary excretion of glucuronides is also attributable to their increased efflux by MRPs. Biliary secretion of glucuronide conjugates can be followed by intestinal hydrolysis of those conjugates by β-glucuronidases. The reabsorption of the parent drug and subsequent hepatic glucuronidation and intestinal hydrolysis by β-glucuronidases can lead to a pattern of entero-hepatic cycling, which can extend the half-life of the drug. In addition, the biological activity of the product (glucuronide conjugate), in most cases, is diminished or abolished. However, there are important examples of xenobiotic glucuronidation that elicit biologically active or toxic metabolites. For example morphine-6-glucuronide is a more potent opiod agonist than morphine itself.

UGTs play a significant role in Phase II detoxification of drugs in humans, and are reportedly responsible for more than one-third of all the Phase II metabolism of drugs. UGTs are also important enzymes in maintaining homeostasis of numerous endobiotics such as steroids, bilirubin, bile acids, and thyroid hormones.

As with other drug metabolizing enzymes, UGTs tend to be distributed in the endoplasmic reticulum (ER) of tissues that can be viewed as portals of entry into the body for xenobiotics (e.g., liver, epithelia of the nasal mucosa, GIT, skin, lungs, and placenta). However UGTs also are localized in brain, kidney, breast tissue, and prostate as well. Not surprisingly, the liver is the major site at which glucuronidation occurs. The distribution pattern of UGTs is broadly similar to that of the CYPs. Like the CYPs, the UGTs are a superfamily of enzymes. In humans there are three subfamilies known as UGT1A, UGT2B, and UGT2A (see later). Also like the CYPs, the UGT isoforms exhibit broad and overlapping substrate specificity.

UGTs consist of a 17-amino acid hydrophobic membrane-spanning domain that is near the C-terminus, and this sequence of amino acids anchors UGTs to the ER membrane. The greater portion of the protein, excluding the N-terminal signal peptide, is actually localized within the lumen of the ER cisternea. In contrast, the major portion of the CYPs is oriented to the cell cytoplasm (Figure 8.36). Thus, there is a close proximity between the products formed from CYP oxidation and UGTs, facilitating their Phase II metabolism by glucuronidation. Approximately 20 to 30 of the UGT terminal amino acids are oriented toward the cytoplasm. As with the CYPs, the activity of UGTs is dependent on the presence of phospholipids. The comparative orientations of CYPs and UGTs relative to the ER membrane, cell cytoplasm, and lumen of the ER is shown in Figure 8.36.

The molecular mechanism by which the glucuronic acid moiety is transferred to a nucleophilic substrate is depicted in Figure 8.37.

Although two *UGT* families encode multiple isoforms only the UGT1A, 2A, and 2B subfamilies play a prominent role in xenobiotic metabolism in humans. UGTs consist of ca. 530 amino acids and have molecular weights of 50 to 57 kDa. The substrate binding domain

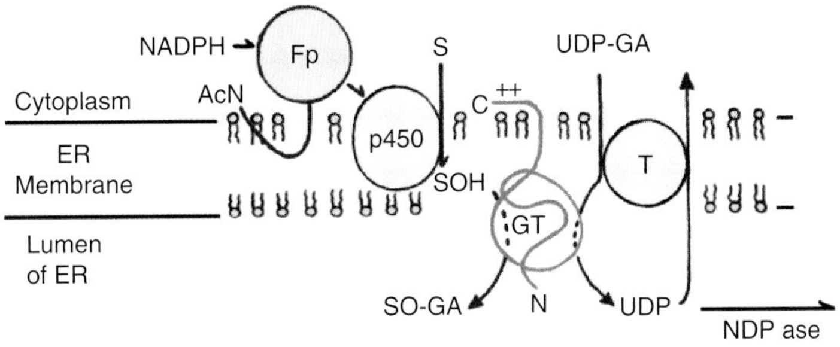

Figure 8.36 The topographical relationship between CYPs and UDGTs in the SER membrane. S denotes substrate, SOH denotes oxidized substrate, SO-GA refers to glucuronidated product. GT is UDGT, and T is a translocation protein for UDPGA. NDPase is nucleoside diphosphatase. ER is endoplasmic reticulum. (Modified from Iyanagi et al. J. Biol. Chem. 261:15607, 1986.)

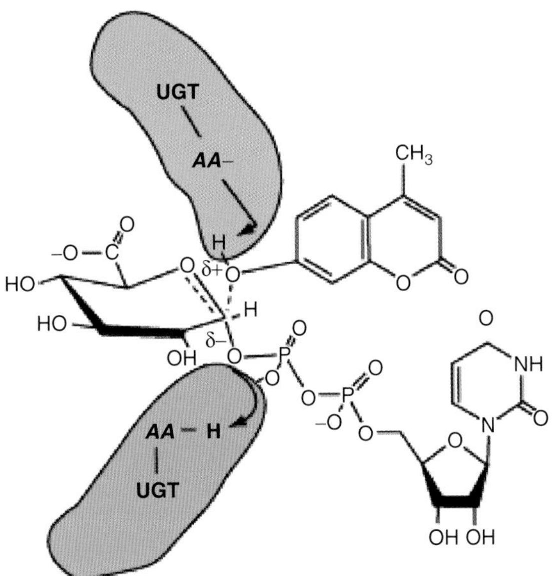

Figure 8.37 A general base involving aspartate-glutamate and histidyl residues deprotonates phenolic hydroxyls. UDP is the leaving group which is subsequently protonated by an acidic amino acid residue or a solvent molecule with proton exchange between basic and acidic catalytic amino acid residues. Notice that the C^1 atom of glucuronic acid begins with an alpha bond to the phosphate group of UDPGA, the final conjugate is in a β orientation. Modified from Radominska-Pandya et al. Drug Metabolism Reviews, 31(4), 817–899 (1999.). UDP; uridine diphosphate, UDPGA; uridine diphosphate glucuronic acid.

is near the N-terminal region of the proteins, whereas the cosubstrate-binding domain is nearer to the carboxy-terminus. The *UGT1* family arises from a single gene locus on chromosome 2q37. UGT2 genes are found on chromosome 4q13. *UGT* genes exhibit polymorphic forms, and of course there are polymorphic forms of the proteins. These polymorphisms have continued to be charted in human populations along with their clinical, physiological, and pathological consequences.

UGT1 isoforms, tissue locales, and prominent endogenous substrates are listed in Table 8.10.

Representative xenobiotic substrates for the major human UGT subfamilies are shown in Table 8.12.

Although it has been appreciated for some time that glucuronidation of both endo- and xenobiotics was a mechanism for either diminishing their biological activity and/or increasing their excretion via bile or urine, it has been only much more recently that biological activation was also a consequence of the glucuronidation of some chemicals. For example, the 3-O-glucuronide of lithocholic acid is highly cholestatic. Likewise, as alluded to before, the 6-O-glucuronide of morphine is a more potent opiod agonist than morphine, itself. Acylglucuronides of some NSAIDs are responsible for severe adverse effects including immunological reactions and hepatotoxicity. In some cases glucuronide conjugation of xenobiotics, although not altering their toxicity *per se*, nevertheless contributes to their carcinogenic effects. An interesting example of this is the glucuronidation of hydroxylamines such as N-hydroxy 2-acetylaminofluorene. 2-acetylaminofluorene (2-AAF) causes cancer of the liver and bladder in rats, and its N-hydroxylated metabolite is even more carcinogenic. We might think that the N-glucuronide of N-hydroxylamines might diminish the hepatotoxicity of

Table 8.10 UGT1 Isoforms and Their Tissue Localization and Endogenous Substrates (From Radominska-Pandya et al., 1999)

Isoform (Expression System)	Tissue Localization	Major Endogenous Substrates	Functional Group Glucuronidated[a]
UGT1A1 (V79, HK293)	Liver, gallbladder, intestine	Bilirubin	COOH
		Estriol	OH
		β-Estradiol	OH
		2-Hydroxyestriol	OH
		2-Hydroxyestrone	OH
		2-Hydroxyestradiol	OH
UGT1A3 (HK293)	Liver, gallbladder	2-Hydroxyestrone	OH
		2-Hydroxyestradiol	OH
		Estrone	3-OH
		5,6-Epoxy-atRA[b]	COOH
		4-OH-atRA[b]	COOH
		LA[b]	COOH
UGT1A4 (HK293)	Liver, gallbaldder, intestine	Androsterone	OH
		Epiandrosterone	OH
		5α-Androstane-3α,17β-diol	OH
		5β-Androstane-3α,11α,17β-triol	OH
		5α-Pregnan-3α,20α-diol	OH
		5α-Pregnan-3β,20β-diol	OH
		5-Pregnene-3β-ol-20-one	OH
		16α-Hydroxypregnenolone	OH
UGT1A5			
UGT1A6	Liver, gallbladder, stomach, intestine	None known	
UGT1A7	Stomach, intestine	None known	
UGT1A8 (HK293)	Intestine	Estrone	OH
		2-Hydroxyestrone	OH
		4-Hydroxyestrone	OH
		2-Hydroxyestradiol	OH
		4-Hydroxyestradiol	OH
		Dihydrotestosterone	OH
		5α-Androstane-3α,17β-diol	OH
UGT1A9 (V79)	Liver	Thyroxine	OH
		Reverse triiodothyronine	OH
UGT1A10 (HK293)	Gallbladder, stomach, intestine	2-Hydroxyestrone	OH
		4-Hydroxyestrone	OH
		Dihydrotestosterone	OH

[a]Exact positions for hydroxyl glucuronides are given when known.
[b]Abbreviations: LA, lithocholic acid; atRA, all *trans*-retinoic acid.

the precursor substances. However, it appears that the N-glucuronide is relatively stable, and can be excreted via the bile into the intestine, or can be excreted into the urine. In the acidic pH of the urine, the glucuronic acid is hydrolyzed, regenerating the hydroxylamine. In the intestine, bacterial ß-glucuronidases likewise can split the glucuronic acid molecule from the conjugate also regenerating hydroxylamine. The hydroxylamine can subsequently form DNA adducts in the liver, with epithelial cells in the bladder or the intestine.

Finally, there has been great interest in determining the relationships between UGT genetic variants and various pathological conditions. Here is a brief description of the key findings.

UGT1A1 is the UGT principally responsible for bilirubin glucuronidation. There are 60 rare mutations in the *UGT1A1* gene known to date, but only a few of them occur with a sufficient frequency ($\geq$ 1%) to represent polymorphisms.

The wild-type allele is *UGT1A1*1*. The most common variant allele is *UGT1A1*28*, and this variant is associated with a form of hyperbilirubinemia known as Gilbert's syndrome. This variant is expressed more in Caucasians (2–13%) and Africans (16–19%) than Asians (0–3%). Expression of the variant enzyme not only predicts increased risk of Gilbert's syndrome, but also a slower glucuronidation rate for acetaminophen and lorazepam. Perhaps even more importantly, the active form of irinotecan, an antineoplastic agent, is more toxic to patients with *UGT1A1*28*. Irinotecan is actually activated by CES to an active metabolite, SN-38 (or 7-ethyl-10-hydroxycamptothecin), which is highly toxic. SN-38, however, is glucuronidated by UGT1A1. Cancer patients with alterations in the promoter region of *UGT1A1*28* exhibited more irinotecan-induced toxicity.

An association with breast cancer was found in African-American women with low UGT activity alleles (e.g., *UGT1A1*28* and *UGT1A1*34*), though no

Table 8.11 UGT1 Isoforms and Their Tissue Localization and Endogenous Substrates (From Radominska-Pandya et al., 1999)

Isoform (Expression System)	Tissue Localization	Major Endogenous Substrates	Functional Group Glucuronidated[a]
UGT2B4 (V79)	Liver	HDCA[b]	6α-OH
UGT2B4 allele (COS7) (formerly 2B11)	Liver	Androsterone[c]	3-OH
		5α-Androstane-3α,17β-diol[c]	OH
		5β-Pregnan-11α,17β-diol-20-one[c]	OH
		5β-Pregnan-3α,11β,17α-triol-20-one[c]	
UGT2B7(Y) (HK293, COS-7)		4-Hydroxyestrone	4-OH
		4-Hydroxyestradiol	OH
		Androsterone	3-OH
		Epitestosterone	OH
		5β-Androstane-3α,17β-diol	OH
		5β-Pregnan-3α-ol-11,20-dione	3α-OH
		5β-Pregnan-11α-ol-3,20-dione	11α-OH
		HDCA	OH
		C20αβ[b]	3α-OH
		C20αβ	COOH
UFT2B7(H) (HK293, COS-1	Liver	Androsterone	3-OH
	Intestine	Epitestosterone	OH
	Kidney	4-Hydroxyestrone	OH
		2-Hydroxyestrone	OH
		4-Hydroxyestradiol	OH
		Estriol	17β-OH
		LA[b]	3α-OH
		HDCA	6α-OH
		C20αβ	3α-OH
		C20αβ	COOH
		C20ββ[b]	COOH
		atRA[b]	COOH
		5,6-epoxy-atRA	COOH
		4-OH-atRA	COOH
		4-OH-atRA[c]	4-OH
		Linoleic acid	COOH
		Linoleic acid 9,10-diol	9-OH, 10-OH
		Linoleic acid 12,13-diol	12-OH, 13-OH
		13-HODE[a]	13-OH, COOH
		13-Oxe-ODE[a]	COOH
UGT2B10 (COS-7)	Liver	None known	
UGT2B11 (HK293)	Prostate and LNCaP cells, liver, kidney, mammary gland, skin, adipose, adrenal gland	None known	
UGT2B15 (HK293)	Liver	Dihydrotestosterone	OH
	Prostate and LNCaP cells	5α-Androstane-3α,17β-diol	OH
		5α-Androstane-3α,11β,17β-triol	OH
	Breast		
	Skin		
UGT2B17 (HK293)	Prostate and LNCap cells	Testosterone[c]	17β-OH
		Dihydrotestosterone[c]	17β-OH
		Etiocholanone[c]	3α-OH
		Androsterone[c]	3α-OH
		5α-Androstane-3α,17β-diol[c]	17β-OH
		5α-Androstane-3α,11β,17β-triol[c]	OH
		5α-Androstane-3α,11α,17β-triol[c]	OH
		5α-Androstane-3α,17β-triol[c]	OH
		5α-Pregnane-3α,20α-diol[c]	OH

[a]Exact positions for hydroxyl glucuronides are given when known.

[b]Abbreviations: HDCA: hyodeoxycholic acid; C20αβ: 3α-hydroxyetianic acid; C20ββ: 3β-hydroxyetianic acid; LA: lithocholic acid; atRA: all *trans*-retinoic acid; atRAc: all *trans*-retinyl acetate; 13-HODE: 13-hydroxy-9,11-octadecadienoic acid; 13-Oxo-ODE: 13-oxo-9, 11-octadecadienoic acid; nd: not determined.

[c]A limit of sensitivity for glucuronidation assays of 15 pmol/mg/min was assumed. Values for enzymatic activity toward these substrates were well below this limit.

Table 8.12 Typical Xenobiotic Substrates for the UGT1A and 2B Subfamilies

Isoform	Tissues	Xenobiotic Substrates	Functional Group Glucuronidated
UGT1A1	Liver, gallbladder, intestine	Quercetin, naringenin, 1-naphthol	-OH
UGT1A3	Liver, gallbladder	2-aminoflurorene naringenin 4-methylumbelliferone	N -OH -OH
UGT1A4	Liver, gallbladder, intestine	Amitryptyline Imipramine Trifluoperazine	N N N
UGT1A6	Liver, gallbladder, stomach, intestine	Acetaminophen	-OH
UGT1A8	Intestine	Naringenin propafol	-OH -OH
UGT1A9	Liver	Acetaminophen 4-methylumbelliferone quercetin	-OH -OH -OH
UGT2B7	Liver	Morphine Naloxone Nalorphine Codeine Hydromorphone Buprenorphine	3-OH & 6-OH -OH -OH -OH -OH -OH
UGT2B15	Liver	Naringenin 4-methylumbelliferone	-OH -OH

increased risk for breast cancer was found among Caucasian women with low UGT activity alleles.

Although the *UGT1A6* genotype was not found to be a risk factor for colon adenoma, it was found to play a role in the chemopreventive effects of NSAIDs in colon adenoma. Americans with low activity genotypes of *UGT1A7*, namely **3* and **4*, were found to be more at risk of oropharyngeal cancer than those with high activity genotypes, *viz. UGT1A7*1* and **2*. The risks were greater still in African-Americans (vs. Caucasian Americans) and smokers (vs. nonsmokers). The combination of low-activity UGT1A7 and dietary heterocyclic amine exposure was associated with an increased risk of colon cancer.

Polymorphisms of UGT2B7 do not account for variability in the glucuronidation of substrates for this enzyme, such as morphine or epirubicin. However, UGT2B7 appears to be overexpressed in neoplastic mammary foci, and this overexpression may provide early protection in the early stages of breast cancer.

At present, it is not clear whether interindividual variability in rates of drug glucuronidation is more appropriately ascribed to genetic polymorphism or to host factors such as age, sex, disease, diet, or other environmental influences. However some genetic polymorphisms have been associated with hyperbilirubinemia and with some cancers.

Regulation of UGTs Multiple chemicals have been found to induce UGT activity in humans. Among them are the same substances that are agonists of the human PXR (e.g., rifampin, carbamazepine, phenytoin, and phenobarbital). In particular, hepatic UGT1A1 is most abundantly upregulated through PXR agonism, though heptic UGT1A6, 1A3, and 1A4 are less extensively upregulated by the PXR. In contrast none of the UGT2B isoforms appear to be upregulated by PXR.

With regard to UGT inhibition there appear to be two important considerations. First, glucuronidation can be inhibited by a decrease in the cellular content of the cosubstrate, UDPGA. Second, some xenobiotics can actually inhibit UGT activity. For example, gentamycin is a weak inhibitor of bilirubin and salicylamide glucuronidation. Novobiocin has also been demonstrated to slow bilirubin glucuronidation by competitively inhibiting substrate binding to the enzyme. Tertiary amines such as amitriptyline, imipramine, and chlorpromazine can potently inhibit the glucuronidation of steroids such as testosterone, androsterone, and estriol. Ketoprofen is a competitive inhibitor of UGT2B7 capable of slowing S-oxazepam glucuronidation.

8.2.4.4 Glutathione-S-Transferases (GSTs)

GSTs actually possess a variety of catalytic activities, however the activity of interest in this chapter is the catalysis of the conjugation of reduced glutathione with a wide array of electrophilic compounds. The general reaction is shown in Figure 8.38.

A common product resulting from glutathione conjugation is a mercapturic acid as shown in Figure 8.39. Mercapturic acids are excreted by the renal organic anion antiport system in the proximal tubular epithelia of the kidney.

Other catabolic products include sulfenic acids (R-SOH), S-glucuronides, S-methylconjugates, cysteine-S-conjugates, and more.

Not surprisingly, the several different human GSTs are products of distinct genes. The cytosolic GSTs are

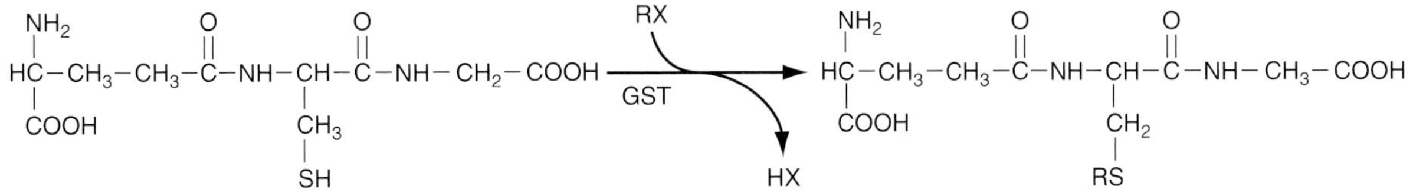

$$HC(NH_2)(COOH)-CH_3-CH_3-C(=O)-NH-CH(CH_3SH)-C(=O)-NH-CH_2-COOH \xrightarrow[GST]{RX} HC(NH_2)(COOH)-CH_3-CH_3-C(=O)-NH-CH(CH_2RS)-C(=O)-NH-CH_3-COOH + HX$$

Figure 8.38 Reduced glutathione (GSH) is shown on the left. GST catalyzes the reaction of GSH with an electrophilic substrate, RX, to yield a glutathione conjugate (right).

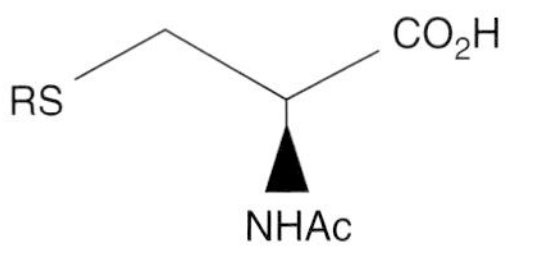

RS, CO_2H, NHAc

Figure 8.39 Mercapturic acid product of GST conjugation.

grouped into five families: alpha, A; mu, M; pi, P; theta, T; and zeta, Z; with subfamily members more than 40% amino acid sequence identity. There are additionally three membrane-associated (microsomal) GSTs that do not share sequence homology with the cytosolic GSTs. A three-dimensional image of dimerized rat liver GST is shown in Figure 8.40.

GSTs possess two binding sites; one for glutathione and another for substrate. Site-directed mutagenesis studies have shown that tyrosine 6 is vital for stabilizing the thiolate anion of glutathione, and that if substituted with another amino acid, GST activity can decline by 90%.

Subclasses of GSTs are denoted by Arabic numerals separated by a hyphen, and genetic variants thereof are further denoted with lowercase roman letters. Examples of human GSTs are given in Table 8.13, along with the tissues in which they have been found in the greatest density.

Though large numbers of pesticides and other toxic xenobiotics have been shown to be substrates for GSTs, relatively few drugs are biotransformed by GST. Among them are ethacrynic acid, doxorubicin, thiotepa,

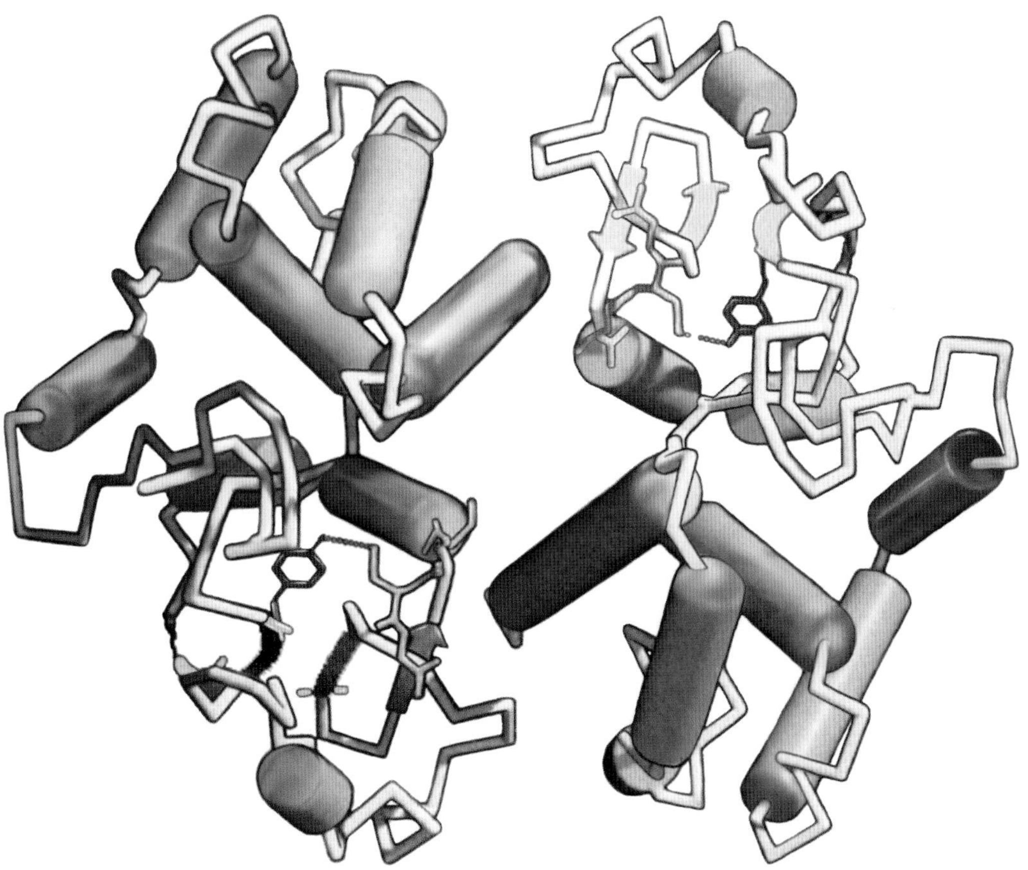

Figure 8.40 Drawing of Raster 3D images for the dimer of the asymmetric unit glutathione S-transferase 3-3 from rat liver and B strands are indicated by yellow arrows and α helices by blue barrels. Active site tyrosine is shown in red and GSH in purple. The spatial relationship between the two active sites in the dimer is shown. (Modified from Xinhua Ji, Pinghu Zhang, Richard Armstrong and Gary Gilliland Biochemistry 31:10169–10184, 1992.)

Table 8.13 Tissue Distribution of Several Human UGTs

GST	Tissues
GSTA1-2	Liver, kidney, testis
GSTM1a-1a	Liver, cerebrum, prostate, testis, skeletal muscle
GSTM3-3	Small intestine, cerebrum, testis
GSTT1-1	Liver, kidney, small intestine, cerebrum
GSTZ1-1	Liver

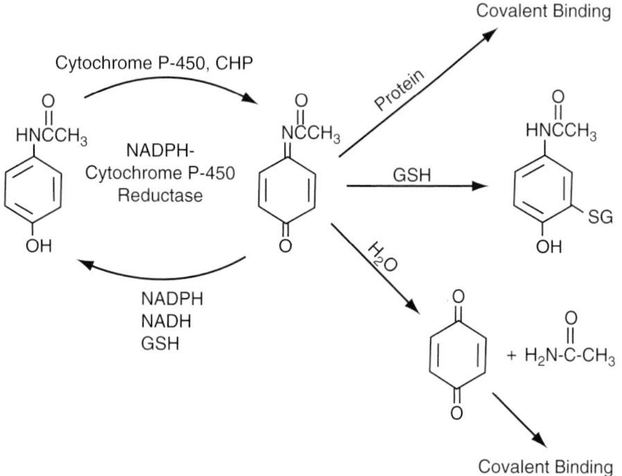

Figure 8.41 Formation of NAPQI by hepatic cytochrome P450 and subsequent detoxification by glutathione (GSH). (Modified from Dahlin et al. Proc Natl Acad Sci 81: pp 1331, 1984.)

nitroglycerin, menadione, cyclophosphamide, BCNU, busulfan, and chlorambucil. A reactive intermediate of acetaminophen, N-acetyl-p-benzoquinonimine (NAPQI), thought to be the acetaminophen metabolite responsible for acetaminophen-induced hepatotoxicity, is detoxified by glutathione conjugation as shown in Figure 8.41.

One of the more interesting features of glutathione and its conjugation with xenobiotics resides in the dichotomous outcomes of conjugation. The conjugates of the xenobiotic drugs listed earlier are either less toxic or inactive, however glutathione conjugates of geminal dihalomethanes (CH_2X_2) and vicinal dihaloalkanes ($X\text{-}CH_2CH_2\text{-}X$) are unstable and can lead to cytotoxicity. The precise organ toxicity of glutathione conjugates depends upon the cellular transport mechanisms and the activities and localization of enzymes such as β-lyase. Much of the pioneering work on glutathione-dependent toxicity was performed by M. W. Anders at the University of Rochester. An important issue related to glutathione cellular toxicity is that of GST polymorphism. In humans *GSTM1*, *GSTM3*, *GSTT1*, and *GSTP1* are all polymorphic. The GSTM1 null genotype has been linked in several studies to a slightly elevated risk for lung cancer and also emphysema in smokers. Similarly the *GSTM1* null genotype has been linked in several (though not all) studies to an increased risk in bladder cancer, again especially in smokers. There may also be an increased risk of stomach cancer among *GSTM1* null genotypes, though this association is less certain, perhaps owing to the small size of the studies conducted so far. Equivocal findings exist regarding the *GSTM1* null phenotype and risk of colon cancer. However a considerable risk has been found for esophageal and head and neck cancers, though no risk has been found for breast, cervical, oral, or liver cancers.

The *GSTT1*0* (homozygous null) phenotype occurs with a frequency of 12 to 24% in most Caucasians, 24% in African Americans, and 45 to 60% in Asians. In both Hispanics and African-Americans a combination of the *GSTT1* and *GSTM1* deletions has been associated with increased risks of brain astrocytoma and meningioma. The *GSTT1* deletion by itself has been implicated as a risk factor for myeloplastic diseases, colon cancer, basal cell carcinomas, and bladder cancer in nonsmokers. Finally, allelic variants of GSTP1, which encodes for the most abundant GST in many tissues, have been associated with testicular and bladder cancers as well as teratomas.

8.3 CONCLUSIONS AND KEY POINTS

A diverse array of drug metabolizing enzymes evolved in order to process endobiotics and to protect organisms from xenobiotic insults. These enzymes are distributed in many tissues, but are most prevalent within the liver, the major drug-metabolizing organ. In most cases the metabolites that form as a result of drug metabolism are more hydrophilic and water soluble than the parent molecules, and more readily excreted in the bile or urine. Not surprisingly, drugs and other xenobiotics can be chemically altered or biotransformed by many different kinds of reactions, depending on the chemical nature of the substrate. Thus esters and amides can be hydrolyzed. One of the most widely used drugs is aspirin, acetylsalicylic acid, and it is subject to hydrolysis as shown:

COOH, O–C(=O)–CH3 → CO2H, OH + CH_3COOH

Ester and amide hydrolytic reactions are mediated principally by carboxylesterases (CES), though other esterases play a role in the hydrolysis of a limited number of esters. Other key biotransformations include oxidations and conjugation reactions.

By far the most important oxidative enzymes are the cytochromes P450 (CYPs). These enzymes are hemoproteins found primarily in the smooth endoplasmic reticulum, and are most prevalent in the liver and the epithelial cells of the gastrointestinal tract. They mediate epoxidations and hydroxylations of aliphatic groups and aromatic rings, N and O dealkylations, and the addition of oxygen atoms to N and S atoms as well. They account for the biotransformation of the overwhelming majority of existing drugs. They also play a major role in the problem of drug–drug interactions (see Chapter 12), because they can be inhibited by other drugs and/or induced by other drugs. Xenobiotic inhibition of the CYPs results from the direct interaction of inhibitors with these enzymes, however induction most often results from transactivation involving the PXR nuclear receptor.

Other oxidative enzymes, though certainly important in the biotransformation of some drugs (e.g., xanthine oxidase contributes to the overall metabolism of substances such as caffeine and theophylline), are not responsible for the metabolism for very many drugs compared to the CYP enzymes.

Synthetic or Phase II biotransformations consist of either conjugation or nucleophilic trapping in which moieties such as acetate, sulfate, glucuronic acid (conjugations), or glutathione (nucleophilic trapping) are added to either preexisting functional groups or functional groups arising from oxidative biotransformations. The preeminent enzymes responsible for these reactions are the NATs, STs, UGTs, and GTTs. The NATs exhibit polymorphism, and the significance of this is quite clear for the drug, isoniazid. Isoniazid is an antitubercular drug, subject to acetylation by NAT2.

The acetylation of isoniazid by NAT2 occurs as shown:

$$\text{(pyridin-4-yl)}-C(=O)-NH-NH_2 \longrightarrow \text{(pyridin-4-yl)}-C(=O)-NH-N\text{-}OCH_2CH_3$$

Among Caucasians, approximately half are slow acetylators of isoniazid. These individuals:

- Exhibit somewhat longer plasma half lives (roughly 3–5 hrs compared to 1.5–2 hrs for the other half who are normal or rapid metabolizers)
- Are more likely to experience isoniazid-induced hepatoxicity
- Are more likely to experience isoniazid-induced neurotoxicity
- Are more likely to experience isoniazid-induced arthralagias

Synthetic or Phase II reactions, though generally conceded to further increase metabolite hydrophilicity and decrease biological activity, have been shown to occasionally increase the likelihood of toxicity rather than decrease it. This can occur if Phase II metabolites are stable enough to be transported to tissues or organs where they can be hydrolyzed to more biologically active compounds, or if the Phase II metabolites themselves are reactive enough to covalently bind to cell macromolecules.

Though best exemplified for the CYPs, individual drug metabolizing enzymes are isoforms of enzyme families. The individual enzymes within a family differ in their amino acid sequences, and the genes from which they are transcribed differ in their nucleic acid sequences. Therefore, distinct genetically based differences in enzyme expression and activity have been found. In some cases, most notably for CYP2C9, CYP2C19, and CYP2D6, definitive correlations have been found between the genotype of drug metabolizing enzymes and the activity (phenotype) of the enzyme. It is now possible to phenotype the activity of many drug-metabolizing enzymes in humans, particularly the CYPs. In most cases this requires the administration of probe drugs, however. It is also possible to evaluate the genotypes for some drug metabolizing enzymes. New polymorphisms are being discovered continuously, and genotype alone doesn't always predict phenotype. Nevertheless, the emerging strategies for assessing both genotype of drug-metabolizing enzymes and the phenotypic expression of their activity, for example using "cocktails" of probe drugs, is bringing the era of individualized drug dosing tantalizingly close. In fact, in addition to Amplichip technology discussed for CYP2C19 and CYP2D6, another technology has been made commercially available to identify colorectal cancer patients expressing a variant form of UGT1A1, thereby placing them at increased risk for severe adverse reactions to irinotecan.

In addition to genetic factors, drug metabolizing enzyme activity is, to a large extent, subject to environmental regulation. Environmental regulation can be elicited by changes in an individual's condition (i.e., pathology), by exposure to environmental chemicals such as polycyclic aromatic hydrocarbons, or by exposure to other drugs. Environmental chemicals and other drugs can inadvertently slow the metabolism of a particular drug substrate by inhibiting the enzyme(s) responsible for its biotransformation. The nature of that inhibition may be competitive, noncompetitive, or metabolite-dependent inhibition. Whether enzyme inhibition plays out in a clinically important way will depend upon such things as the Ki of the inhibitor for the enzyme(s) of interest, and also the concentration of the inhibitor in the vicinity of the enzyme(s) (see Chapter 12 for more details). Exposure to environmental chemicals (including other drugs) might also increase the expression of the key enzyme(s) associated with biotransformation of a specific drug of interest. This phenomenon is known as enzyme induction, and in most cases results from transactivation of the gene for the enzyme that is mediated by the activation of nuclear receptors such as PXR or CAR.

There are many examples of drug–drug interactions in which one drug (sometimes called a victim drug) is a substrate for a drug-metabolizing enzyme and another drug (sometimes called a perpetrator drug) can increase the amount of the enzyme responsible for the biotransformation of the victim drug. In this type of drug–drug interaction the perpetrator drug renders the victim drug less effective or ineffective, unless the dose of the victim drug is increased. A good example of this is the effect of the antitubercular and antistaphylococcal drug rifampin on the effectiveness of oral contraceptives that contain low doses of ethinyl estradiol. Ethinyl estradiol is oxidized by CYP3A4 in the liver. Rifampin, through PXR activation, can significantly increase the amount of CYP3A4 in the liver and cause the levels of ethinyl estradiol to become ineffective. The unintended outcome is the loss of the contraceptive effect.

Software has emerged and continues to be refined and developed for predicting the likely biotransformation pathways by which a drug is likely to be metabolized. In addition to the chemical structure, the molecular characteristics of a drug such as molecular size, planarity, K_m, and pKa can be used to predict which CYP isoforms are most likely to metabolize it. Such predictions can be confirmed with relatively simple *in vitro* tests using individual human CYPs that are expressed in heterologous expression systems. Additionally, the rates of organ (e.g., liver) clearance can be predicted from *in vitro* data in which either the rate of formation of metabolites is measured or the rate of consumption of the substrate drug is measured. From these measurements it becomes possible to predict whole organ and *in vivo* drug clearances in humans. In addition to heterologous expression systems, predictions of drug clearance can be made from *in vitro* experiments using human liver microsomes or human hepatocytes. However, careful attention must be paid to account for protein binding, nonspecific binding, and other parameters that will be different among different *in vitro* systems and between *in vitro* systems and the intact liver.

REVIEW QUESTIONS

1. What are the general types of Phase I reactions mediated by drug metabolizing enzymes? Name a key enzyme responsible for each general type of Phase I reaction.
2. What are the major types of synthetic (or Phase II) reactions? Identify the enzymes that mediate each type of synthetic reaction.
3. What are some features of cytochrome P450 enzymes that distinguish them from other Phase I enzymes?
4. What molecular events account for the ability of a drug such as rifampin to increase the expression of cytochrome P450 3A4?
5. What are the V_{max} and K_m for an enzyme-substrate interaction, and how would they change in the presence of a competitive inhibitor or a non-competitive inhibitor?
6. For which CYP enzymes is allelic variation most well characterized? How does this variation affect the drug metabolizing activity of these enzymes?
7. How would the phenotypic expression of CYPs be characterized in humans (individuals or subpopulations)?
8. Why doesn't CYP genotype always predict CYP phenotype?
9. What structural feature of CYP enzymes is responsible for oxygen binding to the enzymes?
10. Describe the sequence of events that must occur in order for a substrate to be oxidized by cytochrome P450.
11. What molecular events must occur in order for one drug to induce the metabolism by cytochrome P450 of another drug?
12. Explain the phenomenon of homotropic activation. How would this affect a plot of v versus [S]? How would this affect the Eadie-Hofstee plot?

REFERENCES

Books

Gibson, G., & Skett, P. (2001). *Introduction to Drug Metabolism* (3rd ed.). Cheltenham, UK: Nelson Thornes.

Ioannides, C. (Ed.). (1996). *Cytochromes P450: Metabolic and Toxicological Aspects.* Boca Raton, CRC Press.

Jeffery, E. H. (Ed.). (1993). *Human Drug Metabolism: From Molecular Biology to Man.* Boca Raton, CRC Press.

Knoefel, P. K. (Ed.). (1972). *Absorption Distribution, Transformation, and Excretion of Drugs.* Springfield IL: Charles C. Thomas.

LaDu, B. N., Mandel, G., & Way, E. L. (Eds.). (1971). *Fundamentals of Drug Metabolism and Drug Disposition.* Baltimore, Williams & Wilkins.

Lash, L. H. (Ed.). (2005). *Drug Metabolism and Transport: Molecular Methods and Mechanisms.* Totowa, Humana Press.

Lee, J., Obach, R. S., & Fisher, B. (Eds.). (2003). *Drug Metabolizing Enzymes: Cytochromes P450 and Other Enzymes in Drug Discovery and Development.* Lausanne, Switzerland: Fontis Media.

Levy, R. H., Thummel, K., Trager, W. F., Hansten, D., & Eichelbaum, M. (Eds.). (2000). *Metabolic Drug Interactions.* Philadelphia: Lippincott Williams & Wilkins.

Pratt, W., & Taylor, P. (Eds.). (1990). *Principles of Drug Action: The Basis of Pharmacology* (3rd ed.). New York: Churchill Livingstone.

Woolf, T. (Ed.). (1999). *Handbook of Drug Metabolism.* New York: Marcel Dekker, Inc.

Monographs, Review Articles, and Original Papers

Anders, M. W., Dekant, W., & Vamvakas, S. (1992). Glutathione-dependent toxicity. *Xenobiotica; The Fate of Foreign Compounds in Biological Systems, 22,* 1135–1145.

Anon. (2003). Enzyme kinetics. *The Biological Catalysts,* 1–20.

Bachmann, C., & Bickel, M. H. (1986). History of drug meteabolism: The first half of the 20th century. *Drug Metabolism Reviews, 16,* 185–253.

Bachmann, K. A., Ring, B. J., & Wrighton, S. A. (2003). Drug–drug interactions and the cytochromes P450. In J. S. Lee, R. S. Obach, & M. B. Fisher (Eds.), *Drug Metabolizing Enzymes: Cytochromes P450 and Other Enzymes in Drug Discovery and Development* (pp. 311–336). Lausanne, Switzerland: Fontis Media.

Bachmann, K., et al. (2004). *Pharmacological Research, 50,* 237–246.

Beedham, C. (1997). The role of non-P450 enzymes in drug oxidation. *Pharmacy World and Science, 1,* 255–263.

Bencharit, S., Morton, C. L., Hyatt, J. L., Kuhn, P., KDanks, M. K., Potter, P. M., et al. (2003). Crystal structure of human carboxylesterase 1 complexed with the alzheimer's drug tacrine:from binding promiscuity to selective inhibition. *Chemistry & Biology, 10,* 341–349.

Bencharit, S., Morton, C. L., Xue, Y., Potter, P. M., & Redinbo, M. (2003). Structural basis of heroin and cocaine metabolism by a promiscuous human drug-processing enzyme. *Nature Structural Biology, 10,* 349–356.

Black, S. D. (1992). Membrane topology of the mammalian P450 cytochromes. *The FASEB Journal: Official Publication of the Federation of American Societies for Experimental Biology, 6,* 680–685.

Bock, K. W. (1991). Roles of UDP-glucuronosyltransferases in chemical carcinogenesis. *Critical Reviews in Biochemistry and Molecular Biology, 26,* 129–150.

Brown, C. A., & Black, S. D. (1989). Membrane topology of mammalian cytochrome P-450 from liver endoplasmic reticulum: determination by trypsinolysis of Phenobarbital-treated microsomes. *The Journal of Biological Chemistry, 264*, 4442–4449.

Burchell, B., & Coughtrie, M. W. H. (1997). Genetic and environmental factors associated with variation of human xenobiotic glucuronidation and sulfation. *Environmental Health Perspectives, 105*(4), 739–747.

Caldwell, J. (2006). Drug metabolism and pharmacogenetics: The British contribution to fields of international significance. *British Journal of Pharmacology, 147*, S89–S99.

Chang, T. K. H., & Waxman, D. J. (2006). Synthetic drugs and natural products as modulators of constitutive androstane receptor (CAR) and pregnane X receptor (PXR). *Drug Metabolism Reviews, 38*, 51–73.

Chen, B., Zhang, W. X., & Cai, W. M. (2006). The influence of various genotypes on the metabolic activity of NAT2 in a Chinese population. *European Journal of Clinical Pharmacology, 62*, 355–359.

Clarke, S. E. (1998). In vitro assessment of human cytochrome P450. *Xenobiotica; The Fate of Foreign Compounds in Biological Systems, 38*, 1167–1202.

Commandeur, J. N. M., Stijntjes, G. J., & Vermeulen, N. P. E. (1995). Enzymes and transport systems involved in the formation and disposition of glutathione S-conjugates. *Pharmacological Reviews, 47*, 271m–330m.

Conney, A. H. (2003). Induction of drug-metabolizing enzymes: A path to the discovery of multiple cytochromes P450. *Annual Review of Pharmacology and Toxicology, 43*, 1–30.

Conti, A., & Bickel, M. H. (1977). History of drug metabolism: discoveries of the major pathways in the 19th century. *Drug Metabolism Reviews, 6*, 1–50.

Cornelis, M. C., El-Sohemy, A., Kabagambe, E. K., & Campos, H. (2006). Coffee, CYP1A2 genotype, and risk of myocardial infarction. *JAMA: The Journal of the American Medical Association, 295*, 1135–1141.

Cotreau, M. M., von Moltke, L. L., & Greenblatt, D. J. (2005). The influence of age and sex on the clearance of cytochrome P450 3A substrates. *Clinical Pharmacokinetics, 44*, 33–60.

Dahlin, D. C., Miwa, G. T., Lu, A. Y., & Nelson, S. D. (1984). N-acetyl-p-benzoquinone imine: a cytochrome P-450-mediated oxidation product of acetaminophen. *Proceedings of the National Academy of Sciences of the United States of America, 81*, 1327–1331.

Danielson, P. B. (2002). The cytochrome P450 superfamily: Biochemistry, evolution and drug metabolism in humans. *Current Drug Metabolism, 3*, 561–597.

De Graaf, C., Vermeulen, N. P. E., & Feenstra, K. A. (2005). Cytochrome P450 in silico: An integrative modeling approach. *Journal of Medicinal Chemistry, 48*, 2725–2755.

De Groot, M. J., & Vermeulen, N. P. E. (1997). Modeling the active sites of cytochrome P450s and glutathione s-transferases, two of the most important biotransformation enzymes. *Drug Metabolism Reviews, 29*, 747–799.

Eaton, D. L., & Bammler, T. K. (2000). Glutathione S-transferases. In R. H. Levy, K. E. Thummel, W. F. Trager, P. D. Hansten, & M. Eichelbaum (Eds.), *Metabolic Drug Interactions* (pp. 175–189). Philadelphia: Lippincott Williams and Wilkins.

Ekins, S., Degroot, M. J., & Jones, J. P. (2001). Pharmacophore and three-dimensional quantitative structure activity relationship methods for modeling cytochrome P450 active sites. *Drug Metabolism and Disposition: The biological fate of Chemicals, 29*, 936–944.

Ekins, S., Stresser, D. M., & Williams, J. A. (2003). In vitro and pharmacophore insights into CYP3A enzymes. *TIPS, 24*, 161–165.

Estabrook, R. W. (1996). Cytochrome P450: From a single protein to a fmily of proteins—with some personal reflections. In C. Ioannides (Ed.), *Cytochromes P450 Metabolic and Toxicological Aspects* (pp. 3–28). Boca Raton, CRC Press.

Fisher, M. B., Paine, M. F., Strelevitz, T. J., and Wrighton, S. A. (2001). The role of hepatic and extrahepatic UDP-glucuronosyltransferases in human drug metabolism. *Drug Metabolism Reviews, 33*, 273–297.

Fretland, A. J., & Omiecinski, C. J. (2000). Epoxide hydrolases: Biochemistry and molecular biology. *Chemico-Biological Interactions, 129*, 41–59.

Friedman, F. K. Accessed at http://home.ccr.cancer.gov/metabolism/friedman/fkfccr.htm

Gardner-Stephen, D., Heydel, J. M., Goyal Am Lu, Y., Xie, W., Lindblom, T., Mackenzie, P., et al. (2004). Human PXR variants and their differential effects on the regulation of human UDP-glucuronosyltransferase gene expression. *Drug Metabolism and Disposition: The biological fate of Chemicals, 32*, 340–347.

Gamage, N., Barnett, A., Hempel, N., Duggleby, R. G., Windmill, K. F., Martin, J. L., et al. (2006). Human sulfotransferases and their role in chemical metabolism. *Toxicological Sciences: An Official Journal of the Society of Toxicology, 90*, 5–22.

Gonzalez, F. J., Guengerich, F. P., Gunsalus, I. C., Johnson, E. F., Loper, J. C., Sato, R., et al. (1991). The P450 superfamily: Update on new sequences, gene mapping, and recommended nomenclature. *DNA and Cell Biology, 10*, 1–14.

Guengerich, F. P. (2001). Common and uncommon cytochrome P450 reactions. *Chemical Research in Toxicology, 14*, 612–650.

Guengerich, F. P. (2003). Cytochromes P450, drugs, and diseases. *Molecular Interventions, 3*, 194–204.

Guengerich, F. P., Hosea, N. A., Parikh, A., Bell-Parikh, L. C., Johnson, W. W., Gillam, E. M. J., et al. (1998). Twenty years of biochemistry of human P450s: Purification expression, mechanism and relevance to drugs. *Drug Metabolism and Disposition: The biological fate of Chemicals, 26*, 1175–1178.

Guillmette, C. (2003). Pharmacogenomics of human UDP-glucuronosyltransferase enzymes. *The Pharmacogenomics Journal, 3*, 136–158.

Handschin, C., & Meyer, U. A. (2003). Induction of drug metabolism: The role of nuclear receptors. *Pharmacological Reviews, 55*, 649–673.

Haining, R. L., & Yu, A. (2003). Cytochrome P450 pharmacogenetics. In J. S. Lee, R. S. Obach, & M. B. Fisher (Eds.), *Drug Metabolizing Enzymes: Cytochromes P450 and Other Enzymes in Drug Discovery and Development* (pp. 375–419). Lausanne, Switzerland: Fontis Media.

Hein, D. W., Doll, M. A., Fretland, A. J., Leff, M. A., Webb, S. J., Xiao, G. H., et al. (2000). Molecular genetics and epidemiology of the NAT1 and NAT2 acetylation polymorphisms. *Cancer Epidemiol Biomarkers & Prevention, 9*, 29–42.

Hollenberg, P. (1992). Mechanisms of cytochrome P450 and peroxidase-catalyzed xenobiotic metabolism. *The FASEB Journal: Official Publication of the Federation of American Societies for Experimental Biology, 6*, 686–694.

Houston, J. B., Kenworthy, K. E., & Galetin, A. (2003). Typical and atypical enzyme kinetics. In J. S. Lee, R. S. Obach, & M. B. Fisher (Eds.), *Drug Metabolizing Enzymes: Cytochromes P450 and Other Enzymes in Drug Discovery and Development* (pp. 211–254). Lausanne, Switzerland: Fontis Media.

Hutzler, J. M., & Tracy, T. S. (2002). Atypical profiles in drug metabolism reactions. *Drug Metabolism and Disposition: The biological fate of Chemicals, 30*, 355–362.

Ingelman-Sundberg, M. (2005). Genetic polymorphisms of cytochrome P450 2D6 (CYP2D6): Clinical consequences, evolutionary aspects and functional diversity. *The Pharmacogenomics Journal, 5*, 6–13.

Ito, K., Iwatsubo, T., Kanamitsu, S., Ueda, K., Suzuki, H., & Sugiyama, Y. (1998). Prediction of Pharmacokinetic Alterations Caused by Drug-Drug Interactions: Metabolic Interaction in the Liver. *Pharmacologial Reviews, 50*, 387–412.

Iyanagi, T., Haniu, M., Sogawa, K., Fujii-Kuriyama, Y., Watanabe, S., Shively, J. E., & Anan, K. F. (1986). Cloning and characterization of cDNA encoding 3-methylcholanthrene inducible rat mRNA for UDP-glucuronosyltransferase. *The Journal of Biological Chemistry, 261*, 15607–15614.

Jones, J. P., Mysinger, M., & Korzekwa, K. R. (2002). Computational models for cytochrome P450: A predictive electronic model for aromatic oxidation and hydrogen atom abstraction. *Drug Metabolism and Disposition: The biological fate of Chemicals, 30*, 7–12.

Josephy, D., Guegerich, F. P., & Miners, J. O. (2005). Phase I and Phase II drug metabolism: Terminology that we should phase out? *Drug Metabolism Reviews, 37*, 575–580.

Kawamura, A., Graham, J., Mushtaq, A., Tsifsoglou, S. A., Vath, G. M., Hanna, P. E., et al. (2005). Eukaryotic arylamine N-acetyltransferase: Investigation of substrate specificity by high throughput screening. *Biochemical Pharmacology, 69*, 347–359.

Klaassen, C. D., & Boles, J. W. (1997). The importance of 3′-phosphoadenosine 5′-phosphosulfate (PAPS) in the regulation of sulfation. *The FASEB Journal: Official Publication of the Federation of American Societies for Experimental Biology, 11*, 404–418.

Korzekwa, K. R., & Jones, J. P. (1993). Predicting the cytochrome P450 mediated metabolism of xenobiotics. *Pharmacogenetics, 3*, 1–18.

Koymans, L., Den Kelder, G. M., Te, J. M., & Vermeulen, N. P. E. (1993). Cytochromes P450: Their active-site structure and mechanism of oxidation. *Drug Metabolism Reviews, 25*, 325–387.

Kubo, T., Kim, S., Sai, K., Saito, Y., Nakajima, T., Matsumto, K., et al. (2005). Functional characterization of three naturally occurring single nucleotide polymorphisms in the *CES2* gene encoding carboxylesterase 2 (HCE-2). *Drug Metabolism and Disposition: The Biological Fate of Chemicals, 33*, 1482–1487.

Kirchheiner, J., Roots, I., Goldammer, M., Rosenkranz, B., & Brockmoller, J. (2005). Effect of genetic polymorphisms in cytochrome P450 (CYP) 2C9 and CYP2C8 on the pharmacokinetics of oral antidiabetic drugs. Clinical relevance. *Clinical Pharmacokinetics, 44*, 1209–1225.

Kulkarni, S. A., Zhu, J., & Blechinger, S. (2005). In silico techniques for the study and prediction of xenobiotic metabolism: a review. *Xenobiotica; The Fate of Foreign Compounds in Biological Systems, 35*, 955–973.

Lang, D., & Kalgutkar, A. S. (2003). Non-P450 mediated oxidative metabolism of xenobiotics. In J. S. Lee, R. S. Obach, & M. B. Fisher (Eds.), *Drug Metabolizing Enzymes: Cytochromes P450 and Other Enzymes in Drug Discovery and Development* (pp. 483–539). Lausanne, Switzerland: Fontis Media.

Laurenzana, E. M., Hassett, C., & Omiecinski, C. J. (1998). Post-transcriptional regulation of human microsomal epoxide hydrolase. *Pharmacogenetics, 8*, 157–167.

Lewis, D. F. V. (2000). On the recognition of mammalian microsomal cytochrome P450 substrates and their characteristics: towards the prediction of human P450 substrate specificity and metabolism. *Biochemical Pharmacology, 60*, 293–306.

Lewis, D. F. V. (2003). On the estimation of binding affinity (ΔG_{bind}) for human P450 substrates (Based on K_m and K_D values). *Current Drug Metabolism, 4*, 331–340.

Lewis, D. V. F., Ito, Y., & Goldfarb, P. S. (2006). Structural modeling of the human cytochromes P450. *Current Drug Metabolism, 13*, 2545–2652.

Lewis, D. V. F., & Moereels, H. (1992). The sequence homologies of cytochromes P450 and active-site geometries. *Journal of Computer-Aided Molecular Design, 6*, 235–252.

Lu, A. Y. H., Wang, R. W., & Lin, J. H. (2003). Cytochrome P450 in vitro reaction phenotyping: A re-evaluation of approaches used for P450 isoform identification. *Drug Metabolism and Disposition: The Biological Fate of Chemicals, 31*, 345–350.

Mackenzie, P. I., Miners, J. O., & McKinnon, R. A. (2000). Polymorphisms in UDP glucuronsyltransferase genes: functional consequences and clinical relevance. *Clinical Chemistry and Laboratory Medicine: CCLM/FESCC, 38*, 889–892.

McLean, A. J., & Le Couteur, D. G. (2004). Aging biology and geriatric clinical pharmacology. *Pharmacological Reviews, 56*, 163–184.

Meijer, J., & Depierre, J. W. (1988). Cytosolic epoxide hydrolase. *Chemico-Biological Interactions, 64*, 207–249.

Miller, W. L. (2004). P450 oxidoreductase deficiency: a new disorder of steroidogenesis with multiple clinical manifestations. *Trends in Endocrinology and Metabolism: TEM, 15*, 311–315.

Miller, W. L. (2005). Minireview: regulation of steroidogenesis by electron transfer. *Endocrinol, 146*, 2544–2550.

Murphy, P. J. (Ed.). (2005). *History of Xenobiotic Metabolism.* http://www.issx.org/hisjan.html, accessed July, 2005.

Nebert, D. W., Nelson, D. R., Coon, M. J., Estabrook, R. W., Feyereisen, R., Fuji-Kuriyama, Y. et al. (1991). The P450 superfamily: Update on new sequences, gene mapping, and recommended nomenclature. *DNA and Cell Biology, 10*, 1–14.

Nebert, D. W., Nelson, D. R., & Feyereisen, R. (1989). Evolution of the cytochrome P450 genes. *Xenobiotica; The Fate of Foreign Compounds in Biological Systems, 19*, 1149–1160.

Negishi, M., Pedersen, L. G., Petrotchenko, E., Shevstov, S., Gorokhov, A., Kakuta, Y., et al. (2001). Minireview: Structure and function of sulfotransfersases. *Archives of Biochemistry and Biophysics, 390*, 149–157.

Nelson, D. R., Koymans, L., Kamataki, T., Stegeman, J., Feyereisen, R., Waxman, D. J. et al. (1996). P450 superfamily: Update on new sequences gene mapping, accession numbers and nomenclature. *Pharmacogenetics, 6*, 1–42.

Omiecinski, C. J., Hassett, C., & Hosagrahara, V. (2000). Epoxide hydrolase—polymorphism and role in toxicology. *Toxicology letters, 112-113*, 365–370.

Pascussi, J. M., Gerbal-Chaloin, S., Drocourt, L., Maurel, P., Vilarem, M. J. (2003 Feb 17). The expression of CYP2B6, CYP2C9 and CYP3A4 genes: a tangle of networks of nuclear and steroid receptors. *Biochimica et Biophysica Acta, 1619(3)*, 243–253.

Pascussi, J. M., Dvorak, Z., Gerbal-Chaloin, S., Assenat, E., Drocourt, L., Maurel, P., et al. (2004). Regulation of xenobiotic detoxification by PXR, CAR, GR, VDR, and SHP receptors: Consequences in physiology. *HEP, 166*, 409–435.

Potter, P. M., & Wadkins, R. M. (2006). Carboxylesterases-detoxifying enzymes and targets for drug therapy. *Current Medicinal Chemistry, 13*, in press.

Radominska-Pandya, Anna., Czernik, Piotr., Little, Joanna., Battaglia, Eric., Mackenzie, Peter. (1999). Structural and Functional Studies of UDP-Glucuronosyl transferases. *Drug Metabolism Reviews, 31(4)*, 817–899.

Radominska-Pandya, A., Bratton, S., & Little, J. M. (2005). A historical overview of the heterologous expresson of UDP-glucuronosyltransferase isoforms over the past twenty years. *Current Drug Metabolism, 6*, 141–160.

Rushmore, T. H., & Pickett, C. B. (1993). Glutathione-S-transferases, structure, regulation and therapeutic implications. *The Journal of Biological Chemistry, 268*, 11475–11478.

Saini, S., Sonoda, J., Xu, L., Toma, D., Uppal, H., Mu, Y., et al. (2004). A novel constitutive androstane receptor-mediated and CYP3A-independent pathway of bile acid detoxification. *Molecular Pharmacology, 65*, 292–300.

Sato, T., & Hosokawa, M. (1995). Molecular aspects of carboxylesterase isoforms in comparison with other esterases. *Toxicology Letters, 82/83*, 439–445.

Satoh, T., & Hosokawa, M. (1998). The mammalian carboxylesterases: from molecules to functions. *Annual Review of Pharmacology and Toxicology, 38*, 257–288.

Schenkman, J. B. (2000). Cytochromes P450: Historical overview. In R. H. Levy, K. E. Thummel, W. F. Trager, P. D. Hansten, & M. Eichelbaum (Eds.), *Metabolic Drug Interactions* (pp. 51–60). Philadelphia: Lippincott Williams and Wilkins.

Shimada, T., Mernaugh, R. L., & Guengerich, F. P. (2005). Interactions of mammalian cytochrome P450, NADPH-cytochrome P450 reductase, and cytochrome b5 enzymes. *Archives of Biochemistry and Biophysics, 435*, 207–216.

Sonoda, J., Xie, W., Rosenfeld, J. M., Barwick, J. L., Guzelian, P. S., & Evans, R. M. (2002). Regulation of a xenobiotic sulfonation cascade by nuclear pregnane X receptor (PXR). *Proceedings of the National Academy of Sciences of the United States of America, 99*, 13801–13806.

Svensson, C. K., & Hein, D. W. (2005). Phenotypic and genotypic characterization of N-acetylation. In L. H. Lash (Ed.), *Drug Metabolism and Transport: Molecular Methods and Mechanisms* (pp. 173–196). Totowa, Humana Press.

Szklarz, G. D., & Halpert, J. R.. (1997). Molecular modeling of cytochrome P450 3A4. *Journal of Computer-Aided Molecular Design, 11*, 265–272.

Takata, K., Saruwatari, J., Nakada, N., Nakagawa, M., Fukuda, K., Tanaka, F., et al. (2006). Phenotype-genotype analysis of CYP1A2 in Japanese patients receiving oral theophylline therapy. *European Journal of Clinical Pharmacology, 62*, 23–28.

Tephly, T. R., & Green, M. D. (2000). UDP-glucuronosyltransferases. In R. H. Levy, K. E. Thummel, W. F. Trager, P. D. Hansten, & M. Eichelbaum (Eds.), *Metabolic Drug Interactions* (pp. 161–173). Philadelphia: Lippincott Williams and Wilkins.

Thummel, K. E., Kunze, K. L., & Shen, D. (2000). Metabolically-based drug-drug interactions: Principles and mechanisms. In R. H. Levy, K. E. Thummel, W. F. Trager, P. D. Hansten, & M. Eichelbaum (Eds.), *Metabolic Drug Interactions* (pp. 3–19). Philadelphia: Lippincott Williams and Wilkins.

Von Wachenfeldt, C., & Johnson, E. F. (1995). Structures of eukaryotic cytochrome P450 enzymes. In P. Ortiz de Montellano (Ed.), *Cytochrome P450: Structure, Mechanism, and Biochemistry* (2nd ed., pp. 183–223). New York: Plenum Press.

Waxman, D. J. (1999). P450 gene inductin by structurally diverse xenochemicals: Central role of nuclear receptors CAR, PXR, and PPAR. *Archives of Biochemistry and Biophysics, 369*, 11–23.

Weber, W. W., & Hein, D. W. (1985). N-acetylation pharmacogenetics. *Pharmacological Reviews, 37*, 25–79.

Wells, P. G., Mackenzie, P. I., Chowdhury, J. R., Guillemette, C., Gregory, P. A., Ishii, Y., et al. (2004). Glucuronidation and the UDP-glucuronosyltransferases in health and disease. *Drug Metabolism and Disposition: The Biological Fate of Chemicals, 32*, 281–290.

Williams, P. A., Cosme, J., Sridhar, V., Johnson, E. F., & McRee, D. E. (2000). Microsomal cytochrome P450 2C5: comparison to microbial P450s and unique features. *Journal of Inorganic Biochemistry, 81*, 183–190.

Williams, P. A., Cosme, J., Vinkovic, D. M., Ward, A., Angove, H. C., Day, P. J., et al. (2004). Crystal structures of human cytochrome P450 3A4 bound to metyrapone and progesterone. *Science, 305*, 683–686.

Williams, J. A., Johnson, K., Paulauskis, J., & Cook, J. (2006). So many studies, too few subjects: Establishing functional relevance of genetic polymorphisms on pharmacokinetics. *Journal of Clinical Pharmacology, 46*, 258–264.

Wu, M. H., Chen, P., Wu, X., Liu, W., Strom, S., Das, S., et al. (2004). Determination and analysis of single nucleotide polymorphisms and haplotype structure of the human carboxylesterase 2 gene. *Pharmacogenetics, 14*, 595–605.

Yoshinari, K., Petrotchenko, E. V., Pedersen, L. C., & Negishi, M. (2001). Crystal structure-based studies of cytosolic sulfotransferase. *Journal of Biochemical and Molecular Toxicology, 15*, 67–75.

Zhou, S., Chan, S. Y., Goh, B. C., Chan, E., Duan, W., Huang, M., et al. (2006). Mechanism based inhibition of cytochrome P4503A4 by therapeutic drugs. *Clinical Pharmacokinetics, 44*, 279–304.

Chapter

9

Drug Excretion

David R. Taft

OUTLINE

9.1 INTRODUCTION

Clearance is the most important determinant of drug disposition, as clearance dictates the amount of drug that must be administered to maintain therapeutic effectiveness. Consequently, alterations in drug clearance due to genetics, disease, or drug–drug interactions can result in poor therapeutic outcomes. Drug clearance consists of two general pathways: metabolism and excretion. In Chapter 8, Dr. Kenneth Bachmann provides an excellent overview of drug metabolism. The purpose of drug metabolism (or biotransformation) is to render lipophilic molecules more hydrophilic so that the body can more readily excrete them.

Excretion is the removal of waste substances from body fluids, substances that include drugs and their metabolites. Excretion predominantly occurs via urine formed in the kidneys; other routes of drug excretion from the body include bile, saliva, breast milk, and exhaled air. Drug excretion depends on transport across various organs and tissues in the body. Over the past decade, numerous drug transport proteins have been identified, and significant progress has been made in their cloning, functional expression, and characterization. Identification of the transporter(s) responsible for the excretion of a given compound allows for the elucidation of potential drug interactions (drug–drug, drug–disease). Furthermore, modulation of these transport systems can elicit changes in clearance and, consequently, drug activity.

This chapter provides a comprehensive summary of drug excretion. The chapter begins with an overview of membrane transporters in terms of classification, nomenclature, and organ expression. Next, various routes of drug excretion are detailed with regard to mechanisms and transport systems involved, and the factors affecting these processes. Renal and biliary excretion are emphasized because of their importance in drug disposition, however brief discussions of drug excretion by other organs and tissues are also provided. Following a section presenting emerging issues affecting the field of drug excretion, the chapter concludes with perspectives for the future in this important and ever-expanding field.

9.2 OVERVIEW OF MEMBRANE TRANSPORTERS INVOLVED IN DRUG EXCRETION

Membrane transporters perform a central function in drug excretion. Although Heinenman first proposed the phenomenon of drug transport in 1870, identification and characterization of membrane transporters continues to evolve. Transporter protein science is a rapidly emerging field, and numerous transporters have been identified in various regions of the body including the liver, gastrointestinal (GI) tract, and kidney. Together with the metabolizing enzymes (e.g., cytochrome P-450), membrane transporters form a primary defense mechanism against the potential toxic effects of xenobiotics.

The term *transporter* refers to a variety of membrane proteins with diverse functions and structures. Transporters can mediate either facilitated or active transport (Figure 9.1). Facilitated transport involves movement of drug across a membrane down an electrochemical gradient. Conversely, active transporters rely on energy-coupling mechanisms (e.g., ATP hydrolysis) to move drug. These transporters can also create ion/solute gradients across membranes (secondary active transport), which in turn drive uphill membrane transport of drugs.

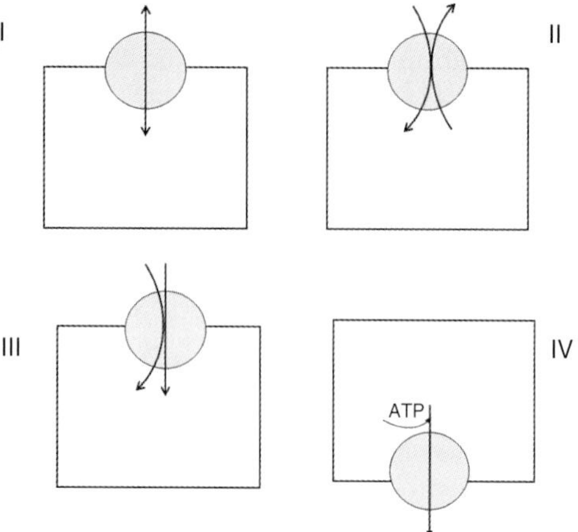

Figure 9.1 Mechanisms of drug transport (uptake and efflux) across cellular membranes. I. Facilitated transport proceeds along an electrochemical gradient (bidirectional). II. Ion exchange transport rives uphill transport of drug (antiport, secondary-active transport). Ion gradients are generated and maintained by ion pumps (ATPases). III. Ion coupled transport (symport, another secondary active transport system). IV. Primary active, ATP dependent transport. These transporters bind or hydrolyze ATP as a control gate to transport ions and drugs out of cells. Examples include ABC Transporters and ATPases. With kind permission from Springer Science +Business Media: Plugers Archiv: European Journal of Physiology, The ABCs of solute carriers: Physiological, pathological and therapeutic implications of human membrane transport proteins, volume 447, 2004, pp. 465–468, M.A. Hediger, M. Romero, J.B. Peng, A. Rolfs, H. Takanaga, & E.A. Bruford, Figure 1.

With the completion of the human genome project, the Human Genome Organization (HUGO) maintains a list of gene families, classified on the basis of amino acid sequence identity. In terms of drug excretion, two transporter gene families are of particular importance: ATP-binding cassette (ABC) transporters and solute carrier (SLC) transporters. These transporters are termed *polyspecific* because they transport compounds with diverse sizes and molecular structures. Each of these transporter families is discussed next.

9.2.1 ATP-Binding Cassette (ABC) Transport Family

The ATP-binding cassette (ABC) transporter superfamily consists of membrane-bound, ATP-driven transporters that pump drugs, drug metabolites, and endogenous metabolites out of cells. ABC transporters are classified based on amino acid sequence and phylogeny. At present there are 49 known human ABC family members belonging to seven different subfamilies. Transporters in this family include p-glycoprotein (P-gp), breast cancer resistant protein (BCRP), and the multidrug resistance protein (MRP) subfamily.

9.2.1.1 P-glycoprotein (Pgp, ABCB1)

Resistance of tumor cells to chemotherapeutic drugs is a major challenge in treating cancer. Multidrug resistance (MDR) is defined as decreased cellular sensitivity to a broad range of chemotherapeutic drugs. Pgp is an ATP-dependent drug efflux membrane transporter, thereby limiting intracellular drug uptake. A link between Pgp and MDR is well established. Overexpression of Pgp in cancer cells results in a poor clinical outcome of chemotherapy. A striking feature of Pgp is its broad substrate specificity, as Pgp is known to transport a large number of unrelated compounds. In addition to anticancer medications, substrates for Pgp include antibiotics, antivirals, immunosuppresants, and cardioactive drugs (Table 9.1).

The development of gene knock-out animal models has resulted in detailed characterization regarding the tissue distribution of the Pgp and its importance in pharmacology as a protective mechanism against potentially toxic compounds. Pgp is expressed in apical membranes of a number of organs and tissues including the intestine, liver, kidney, and brain. The importance of Pgp as a barrier to oral drug absorption and CNS distribution has been confirmed through studies comparing drug disposition in Pgp-deficient and wild-type mice. Likewise, its expression in proximal tubular epithelium of the kidney and canalicular membrane of the liver point to a role of Pgp in drug excretion.

Modulation of Pgp activity is considered a potential approach to reverse MDR and improve therapeutic outcomes in cancer patients. Initial clinical studies with Pgp inhibitors such as verapamil and cyclosporin showed modest success in reversing resistance in a small number of patients, but significant

Table 9.1 List of Clinically Relevant Substrates and Inhibitors of Pgp. Reprinted from European Journal of Pharmaceutical Sciences: Official Journal of the European Federation for Pharmaceutical Sciences, Volume 27, C.J. Endres, P. Hsiao, F.S. Chung, and J.D. Unadkat, The role of transporters in drug interactions, pp. 501–517, Copyright 2006, with permission from Elsevier.

Substrates		
Analgesics	**H_2-receptor Antagonists**	**Cardioactive Medications**
Asimadoline	Cimetidine	Verapamil
[D-Penicillamine 2,5]-enkephalin (DPDPE)	Ranitidine	Diltiazem
Anticancer agents	**Antigout agents**	**Digoxin**
Vincristine	Colchicine	Quinidine
Vinblastine	**Antidiarrheal agents**	**Antihypertensives**
Paclitaxel	Loperamide	Losartan
Doxorubicin	**Antiemetics**	Atovastatin
Daunorubicin	Domperidone	**Immunosuppressants**
Epirubicin	Ondansetron	Cyclosporin A
Bisantrene	**Antifungals**	FK506
Mitoxantrone	Ketoconazole	Tacrolimus
Etoposide	Itraconazole	**Corticosteroids**
Actinomycin D	**Antihistamines**	Dexamethasone
HIV protease inhibitors	Fexofenidine	Hydrocortisone
Saquinavir	Cetirizine	Corticosterone
Ritonavir	**Diagnostic agents**	Triamcinolone
Nelfinavir	Rhodamine 123	**Antibiotics**
Indinavir	Hoechst 33342	Erythromycin
Lopinavir	**β-Blockers**	Gramicidin D
Amprenavir	Talinolol	Valinomycin
Inhibitors		
First Generation	**Second Generation**	**Third Generation**
Verapamil	Dexverapamil	LY335979 (Zosuquidar)
Nicardipine	PSC833 (Valspodar)	XR9576 (Tariquidar)
Quinacrine	GF120918 (Elacridar)	R101933 (Laniquidar)
Cyclosporin A	VX-710 (Biricodar)	OC 144-093 (ONT-093)

side effects were observed with these therapeutically active medications. A number of second- and third-generation Pgp-inhibitors are in drug development (Table 9.1). These agents are specific inhibitors of Pgp; that is, they demonstrate inhibitory activity but are devoid of pharmacologic effects. Given the wide tissue distribution and broad substrate specificity of Pgp, inhibition of induction of Pgp may lead to significant drug–drug interactions, resulting in altered drug disposition.

9.2.1.2 Breast Cancer Resistance Protein (BCRP, ABCG2)

BCRP is a recently identified ABC transporter, originally identified by its ability to confer drug resistance that is independent of other ABC transporters including Pgp. Because it contains a single N-terminal ATP binding cassette, BCRP is referred to as a *half-transporter*. Nevertheless, BCRP is present in various tissues including the intestine, liver, kidney, brain, and placenta. Like Pgp, BCRP is localized on the luminal membrane, where it functions to extrude drugs from the cell.

The substrate specificity of BCRP shows considerable overlap with PGP and includes topotecan derivatives, anthracyclines (e.g., doxorubicin, mitoxantrone), etposide, and prazosin. Correspondingly, Pgp modulators such as GF120918 have been shown to also inhibit BCRP activity. Although the overall contribution of BCRP to drug disposition remains to be elucidated, this novel transporter may play an important role in protecting fetal exposure to harmful xenobiotics as well as mediate excretion of drugs into breast milk during lactation.

9.2.1.3 Multidrug Resistant Proteins (MRP, ABCC)

The ABCC family of ABC transporters includes nine drug transporters, referred to as multidrug resistance proteins (MRPs). Like Pgp and BCRP, MRPs have also demonstrated MDR to cancer cells. Nine MRP transporters have been identified. As detailed in Table 9.2,

Table 9.2 The MRP Transporter Subfamily: Tissue Localization and Substrate and Inhibitor Specificity. Reprinted from European Journal of Pharmaceutical Sciences: Official Journal of the European Federation for Pharmaceutical Sciences, Volume 27, C.J. Endres, P. Hsiao, F.S. Chung, and J.D. Unadkat, The role of transporters in drug interactions, pp. 501–517, Copyright 2006, with permission from Elsevier.

	Localization			
Transporter	**Tissue**	**Membrane**	**Substrates**	**Inhibitors**
MRP1 (ABCC1)	Ubiquitous	Basolateral	Methotrexate, GSH, doxorubicin, vincristine, estradiol-17-β-D-glucuronide	MK571, cyclosporine A, indomethacin, probenecid, sulfinpryazone, PSC933. LY475776
MRP2 (ABCC2)	Liver, kidney, intestine	Apical	Methotrexate, vinblastine, etoposide, 2,4-dinitrophenyl-S-glutathione	MK571, furosemide, indomethacin, benzbromarone
MRP3 (ABCC3)	Liver, kidney, intestine, bile ducts	Basolateral	Methotrexate, vincristine, estradiol-17-β-D-glucuronide	
MRP4 (ABCC4)	Prostate, lung, muscle, pancreas, bladder	Apical	Estradiol-17-β-D-glucuronide, cyclic nucleotide (cAMP, cGMP), GSH, PMEA	Probenecid, dipyridamole
MRP5 (ABCC5)	Ubiquitous	Basolateral	Cyclic nucleotide analogs, heavy metals (Cd), GSH, 6-mercaptopurine	Probenecid, sulfinpyrazone, zaprinast, trequinsin, sildenafil
MRP6 (ABCC6)	Liver, kidney	Basolateral	Enothelial receptor antagonist BQ-123, leukotiene C_4, 6-mercaptopurine	
MRP7 (ABCC7)	Colon, skin, testis		Leukotiene C_4, docetaxel, estradiol-17-β-D-glucuronide	MK571, cyclosporine A
MRP8 (ABCC8)	Liver, lung, kidney, fetal tissue		Cyclic nucleotides (cAMP, cGMP), 5-fluorouracil	
MRP9 (ABCC9)	Breast, testis, brain, skeletal muscle, ovary			

these proteins are organic-anion pumps, but differ in substrate specificity, tissue distribution, and cell membrane location (i.e., basolateral vs. apical). Despite some substrate overlap with Pgp, MRP substrates include conjugates (glutathione, glucuronide) and other organic anions. Consequently, MRP proteins play a crucial role in the export of conjugated drug metabolites out of cells.

The most widely studied MRP isoform is MRP2. MRP2 mediates the efflux of conjugated compounds across the apical membrane of the hepatocyte into the bile canaliculi. This protein transports glutathione, glucuronide, and sulfate conjugates into the bile. MRP2 is also expressed on the apical membrane kidney and intestine cells, contributing to renal secretion and gut excretion of drugs. In the liver, MRP2 is believed to be involved in the biliary excretion of conjugated bilirubin. Natural mutations in the MRP2 gene have been linked to Dubin-Johnson syndrome (inherited conjugated hyperbilrubinemia), a disorder in which patients exhibit impaired transfer of anionic conjugates into bile.

MRP3 is a basolateral transporter that is expressed in the liver, intestine, and kidney. This protein is believed to play a role in the movement of drugs from the cell to the blood. Under cholestatic conditions, MRP3 is upregulated in the liver, suggesting a role in the removal of toxic organic anions via sinusoidal efflux from the hepatocyte.

9.2.1.4 Bile Salt Exporter Pump (BSEP, ABCC11)

BSEP is localized to the canalicular membrane of liver cells, where it mediates transport of conjugated bile acids such as taurine-amidates and acyl-glucuronides. BSEP has also been shown to transport the drug pravastatin. Mutations in BSEP have been linked to cholestatic liver disease. Despite its limited role in drug transport, inhibition of BSEP may be a cause of drug-induced hepatotoxicity. For example, the diabetes drug troglitazone was withdrawn from the market because of numerous reports on troglitazone-associated liver toxicity. It is believed that the metabolite troglitazone sulfate, a compound shown to inhibit BSEP, accumulates in the liver, resulting in cholestasis.

9.2.2 Solute Carrier (SLC) Transport Family

A second important family of drug transport proteins are the solute carrier transporters (SLC). SLC proteins play important physiological roles in the transport of nutrients and drugs. SLCs function by one of several mechanisms including facilitated, ion-coupled, and ion-exchange transport. Within each of the 43 SLC subfamilies that have been identified, transporters have at least 20 to 25% amino acid sequence identity. Table 9.3 lists the SLC transport families that play

Table 9.3 Solute Carrier (SLC) Families Involved in Drug Disposition

Gene Code	Name	# Isoforms
SLC15	Proton Oligopeptide Cotransporter Family (PEPT)	4
SLC21	Organic Anion Transporter Family (OATP)	11
SLC22	Organic Cation/Anion Transporter Family (OCT, OAT)	18
SLC28	Concentrative Nucleoside Transporter Family (CNT)	3
SLC29	Equilibrative Nucleoside Transporter Family (ENT)	4

important roles in drug disposition. These families are discussed individually later.

9.2.2.1 *Organic Anion Transporter Family (OAT, SLC22A)*

The OAT family plays a key role in drug excretion by the kidney, although these proteins are expressed in other tissues including the liver and the brain. Table 9.4 summarizes the various OAT isoforms that have been identified.

In terms of drug disposition, OAT1 is the most important member of this transport family. Expressed mainly in the kidney tubule cell, OAT1 is a dicarboxylate exchange protein that is responsible for basolateral uptake of organic anions such as para-aminohippurate (PAH). OAT1 mediates the excretion of a diverse array of substrates, including environmental toxins. Substrates for this transporter include antibiotics, antiviral nucleoside analogs, and nonsteroidal anti-inflammatory medications. In fact, more than 100 medications and toxic compounds have been found to interact with OAT1.

OAT2 is expressed in the liver and kidney. OAT3 has a broader tissue distribution including the brain, liver, and kidney. Like OAT1, OAT3 has a broad substrate specificity, and OAT3 is thought to participate in renal drug excretion.

9.2.2.2 *Organic Anion Transporting Polypeptide Family (OATP, SLC21A)*

OATP is a family of membrane transporters that mediate uptake of endogenous substrates and drugs. Although certain OATP isoforms are selectively involved in hepatic uptake of hydrophobic anions, most OATPs are widely expressed in various physiological barriers in the body, including the intestine, kidney, brain (brain capillary endothelial cells and

Table 9.4 The OAT Transporter Family: Tissue Distribution, Localization and Substrate Specificity. Reprinted from American Journal of Physiology: Renal Physiology, Volume 290, T. Sekine, H. Miyasaki and H. Endou, Molecular physiology of renal organic anion transporters, pp. 251–261, Copyright 2006, with permission from the American Physiological Society.

Transporter	Tissue Distribution	Membrane Localization	Substrates	Inhibitors*
OAT1 (SLC22A6)	Kidney, brain, skeletal muscle, placenta	Basolateral	PAH, duretics, antivirals, ACE inhibitors, antibiotics, ochratoxin A, NSAIDs, antineoplastics, mycotoxins	Probenecid, ellagic acid
OAT2 (SLC22A7)	Kidney, liver	Basolateral sinusoidal	PAH, salicylate, methotrexate, 5-fluorouracil, loop diuretics, carbonic anhydrase inhibitors	Probenecid, bromosulphthalein, cephalosporins
OAT3 (SLC22A8)	Kidney, choroid plexus, skeletal muscle	Basolateral luminal	Estrone sulfate, H_2-antagonists, antivirals uremic toxins, methotrexate, β-lactam antibiotics, NSAIDs, pravastatin	Probenecid, bromosulphthalein, cholate, melatonin
OAT4 (SLC22A11)	Kidney, placenta	Apical basolateral	Estrone sulfate, PAH, ochrotoxin A, tetracycline, zidovudine, bbumetanide, ketoprofen	Probenecid, bromosulphothalein
URAT1 (SLC22A12)	Kidney	Apical	Urate	Probenecid, sulfinpyrazone, benzbromarone losartan loop diuretics
OAT5 (SLC22A19)	Kidney		Ochratoxin A	
OAT6 (SLC22A20)	Olfactory mucosa			

*Transport inhibition can also occur through competitive inhibition by substrates for the transporter.

Table 9.5 The OATP Transporter Family: Species and Tissue Distribution

Transporter	Species	Tissue Distribution
OATP2A1 (SLC21A2)	Human, rat	Ubiquitous
OATP1A2 (SLC21A3)	Human	Kidney, liver, brain
OATP1A3-v1 (OAT-K1, SLC21A4)	Rat	Kidney
OATP1A3-v3 (OAT-K2, SLC21A5)	Rat	Kidney
OATP1B1 (LST-1, SLC22A6)	Human	Liver
OATP1B3 (LST-2, SLC22A8)	Human	Liver
OATP2B1 (SLC21A9)	Human	Brain, heart, intestine, kidney, liver, intestine
OATP3A1 (SLC21A11)	Human, mouse	Ubiquitous
OATP4A1 (SLC21A12)	Human, mouse, rat	Ubiquitous
OATP1C1 (SLC21A14)	Human	Brain, testis
OATP4C1 (SLC21A20)	Human, rat	Kidney

choroid plexus), lungs, and placenta (Table 9.5). Unlike OATs, there are considerable species differences in OATPs between rats and humans. Consequently, the nomenclature of OATP transporters is quite complicated.

The importance of OATPs to drug disposition is still evolving and remains to be clarified, although a role in renal and hepatic transport as well as uptake across the blood–brain barrier has been demonstrated. Despite the designation, OATP substrates are not limited to organic anions, but also include cations as well as neutral and zwitterionic compounds. Among the drugs known to be transported by OATP are enalapril (ACE inhibitor) pravastatin (HMG-CoA reductase inhibitor), fexofenadine (H1-antagonist), and digoxin (cardiac glycoside).

9.2.2.3 Organic Cation Transporter Family: Organic Cation Transporters (OCT, SLC22A) and Multidrug and Toxic Compound Extrusion Transporters (MATE)

The transport of cationic compounds across cells of the kidney, liver, and brain is mediated by a combination of two distinct transport families: OCTs and MATEs. Accordingly, these transporters play important roles in drug excretion. Six OCT proteins have been identified. OCT1 (SLC22A1), OCT2 (SLC22A2), and OCT3 (SLC22A3) mediate bidirectional, electrogenic facilitated diffusion of a variety of cations, including a number of medications (Table 9.6). These transporters are expressed in many organs and tissues, including strong expression in the liver (OCT1) and kidney (OCT2).

Table 9.6 OCT Substrates

Amantadine
Antivirals (acyclovir, ganciclovir)
Choline
Cisplatin
H_2-antagonists (cimetidine, ranitidine)
Metformin
Nucleoside analogs (lamivudine, emtricitabine)
N-methylnicotinamide
Paraquat
Procaine
Quinine
Quinidine
Tetraethylammonium
Trimethoprim
Verapamil

At least three additional OCT proteins have been identified: OCTN1 (SLC22A4), OCTN2 (SLC22A5), and OCTN3. OCTN1 is an organic cation/proton exchange transporter with wide distribution in the body. OCTN2 is a sodium-dependent transporter involved in the cotransport of carnitine. These two proteins are expressed in the brush border membrane of the kidney, suggesting a role in renal drug secretion.

In addition to OCT transporters, several new proton-cation antiporters have been identified. They belong to members of the multidrug and toxic compound extrusion family (MATE) and include MATE1, MATE2-B, and MATE2-K. Recent data suggests that MATE1 and MATE2-K function together as a detoxication system, and are responsible for the final step in the excretion of metabolic waste and xenobiotic organic cations in the kidney and liver through electroneutral exchange of H+. Among the medications that have been shown to interact with these transporters are tetraethylammonium, cimetidine, metformin, creatinine, procainamide, cisplatin, and topotecan.

9.2.2.4 Nucleoside Transporter Families: Concentrative Nucleoside Transporters (CNT, SLC28) and Equilibrative Nucleoside Transporters (ENT, SLC29)

Nucleosides and nucleoside analogs are used in antiviral and anticancer drug therapy. These drugs generally are hydrophilic in nature and require specialized transport proteins to facilitate their uptake and/or release from the cell. Nucleoside transporters are thought to play a key role in the disposition and nucleosides and nucleoside analogs. There are two families of nucleoside transport proteins, concentrative nucleoside transporters (CNT) and equilibrative nucleoside transporters (ENT).

CNT are localized primarily in the luminal (brush border) membrane of renal epithelial cells. Three isoforms have been identified: CNT1 (SLC28A1), CNT2 (SLC28A2), and CNT3 (SLC28A3). CNTs are involved in unidirectional cellular uptake cotransport with sodium. These secondary active transporters mediate active uphill transport of nucleosides.

Equilibrative nucleoside transporters are expressed primarily on the basolateral membrane and act as bidirectional facilitated diffusion transporters (downhill flux of nucleosides). Four isoforms have been identified: ENT1 (SLC29A1), ENT2 (SLC29A2), ENT3 (SLC29A3), and ENT4 (SLC29A4). ENTs have broad substrate specificities and are expressed in the basolateral membrane of many tissues ENT1 and ENT2 are involved in renal drug excretion.

9.2.2.5 Oligopeptide Transporter Family (PEPT, SLC15)

Members of the oligopeptide transporter (PEPT) family are of interest in drug disposition. The most important of these is PEPT1 (SLC15A1), which is expressed in the brush border membrane of the intestinal cell and plays a role in peptide absorption in the small intestine. In addition to di- and tripeptides, this intestinal transport system also mediates the absorption of ACE inhibitors, β-lactam antibiotics, and anticancer agents. A second transporter, PEPT2 (SLC15A2), has been identified in the luminal membrane of the kidney, and is thought to mediate peptide and drug reabsorption.

9.3 RENAL DRUG EXCRETION

9.3.1 Functional Overview of the Kidney

In the body, the physiologic role of the kidneys involves regulation of fluid volume, mineral composition, and acidity. This is accomplished by controlling the excretion and reabsorption of water and electrolytes. The kidneys also regulate some organic nutrients and excrete metabolic waste products and some foreign chemicals.

The functional unit of the kidney is the nephron (Figure 9.2). A human kidney contains approximately one million nephrons. Each nephron is composed of an initial filtering component, called the renal corpuscle, and a renal tubule specialized for reabsorption and secretion of water, electrolytes, and other solutes. The renal corpuscle consists of a compact tuft of interconnected capillary loops called the glomerulus, and a balloon-like capsule, called Bowman's capsule, into which the glomerulus protrudes. The Bowman's capsule is found in the outer part of the kidney, the cortex. Essentially, the capsule is a sealed, expanded sac at the end of the tubule, the rest of which elongates into a twisted and looped tubule in which urine is formed.

The portion of the renal tubule nearest the Bowman's capsule, the proximal tubule, leads to the descending and ascending limbs of the loop of Henle. Henle's loop dips down from the cortex of the kidney into the deeper tissues of the medulla before looping back up into the cortex. Here, the tubule once again becomes convoluted, forming the distal tubule. The distal tubule ultimately dips back into the medulla, where it connects with a collecting tubule. The collecting tubules from neighboring nephrons terminate into a common duct, into which urine is collected.

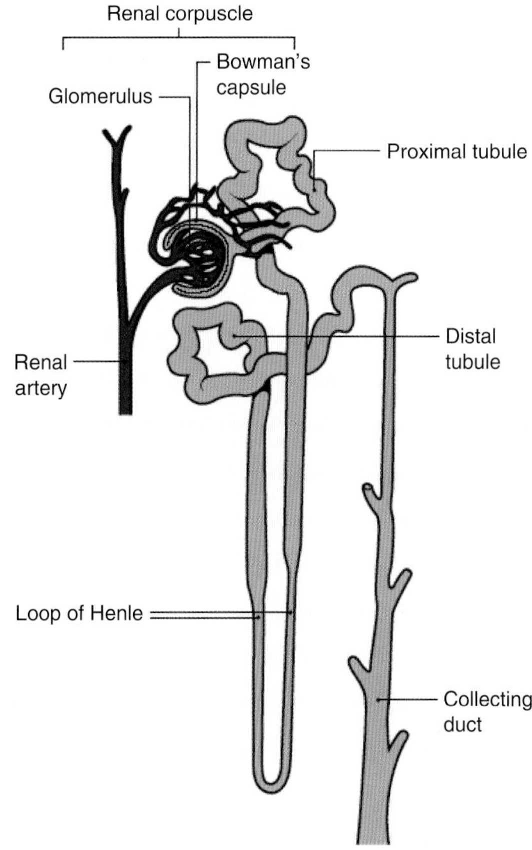

Figure 9.2 Structural overview of a nephron, the functional unit of the kidney. This figure was published in Anaesthesia and Intensive Care Medicine, Vol. 6, B.J. Pleurvy, Modes of drug elimination, pp. 277–279, Copyright Elsevier 2005.

Pharmacokinetic Primer 1 Calculating Renal Clearance

Drug excretion study design

Drug administered (example: IV bolus dose)

Both blood and urine collected for determined period of time post-dose

Blood is centrifuged → plasma. Plasma samples are assay for drug concentration.

Data is analyzed and area under the plasma concentration-time curve is measured

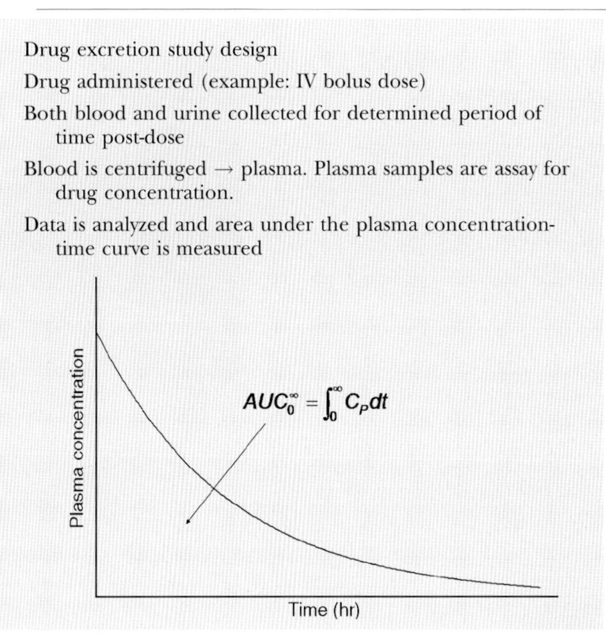

Continued

Pharmacokinetic Primer 1 Calculating Renal Clearance—Cont'd

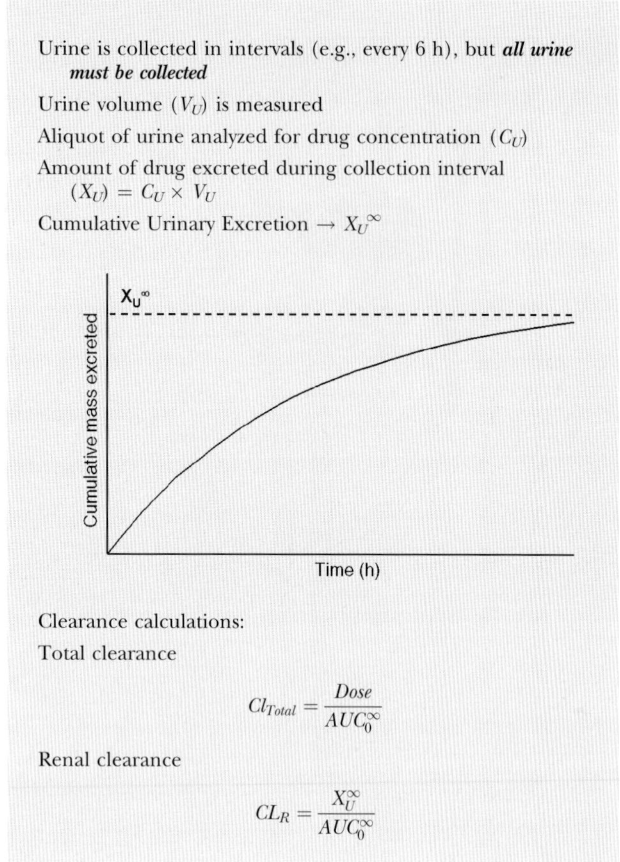

Urine is collected in intervals (e.g., every 6 h), but ***all urine must be collected***

Urine volume (V_U) is measured

Aliquot of urine analyzed for drug concentration (C_U)

Amount of drug excreted during collection interval (X_U) = $C_U \times V_U$

Cumulative Urinary Excretion → X_U^{∞}

Clearance calculations:

Total clearance

$$Cl_{Total} = \frac{Dose}{AUC_0^{\infty}}$$

Renal clearance

$$CL_R = \frac{X_U^{\infty}}{AUC_0^{\infty}}$$

9.3.2 Renal Drug Excretion

In addition to its role in water and electrolyte homeostasis, the kidney is the primary organ for excretion of drugs and their metabolites from the body. There are three basic processes involved in renal drug excretion: glomerular filtration, tubular secretion, and tubular reabsorption. The first two processes serve to extract drug from the blood into the urine. The last process, reabsorption, involves the movement of drug back into the blood. Thus, renal drug excretion reflects the relative contributions of these three mechanisms (Figure 9.3). The pharmacokinetic parameter that describes excretion by the kidney is renal clearance.

9.3.2.1 Glomerular Filtration

Urine formation begins with glomerular filtration, the bulk-flow of fluid from the glomerular capillaries into Bowman's capsule. The glomerular filtrate contents are essentially devoid of protein and cells, and contains most inorganic ions and low-molecular weight organic solutes (e.g., glucose) in virtually the same concentrations as in the plasma. The driving force for glomerular filtration is the hydrostatic pressure within the glomerular capillaries.

In humans, approximately 25% of renal plasma flow (450–600 ml/min) is filtered. Glomerular filtration rate (GFR), defined as the volume of filtrate formed per unit time, is commonly used to measure kidney function. GFR is measured as the clearance of a marker

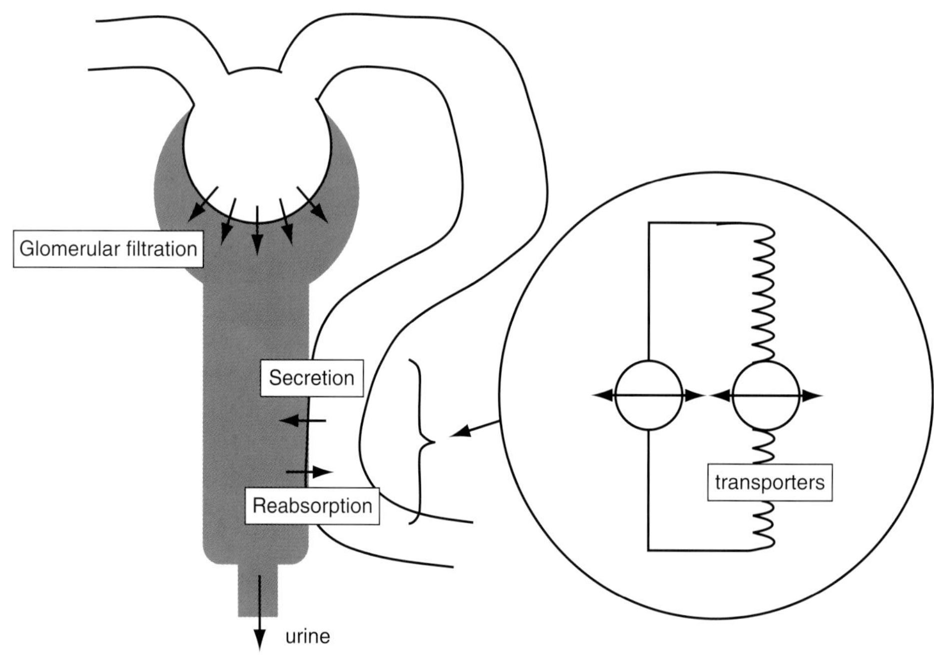

Figure 9.3 Schematic depiction of a nephron identifying mechanisms of drug excretion. Renal excretion involves glomerular filtration and secretion at the proximal tubules. Drug is returned to the systemic circulation via drug reabsorption. Reprinted from Annual Review of Pharmacology and Toxicology, Volume 45, Y. Shitara, H. Sato and Y. Sugiymama, Evaluation of drug-drug interaction in the hepatobiliary and renal transport of drugs, pp. 689–723, Copyright 2005, with permission from Annual Reviews.

substance that is entirely eliminated unchanged by the kidney, and excreted only by filtration (no tubular secretion or reabsorption). The two most commonly used markers are creatinine (an endogenous substance formed from muscle breakdown) and inulin (a polysaccharide molecule). In humans, normal GFR is 100–125 mL/min.

Two important factors governing drug filtration are molecular size and electrical charge. Small molecules (MW < 500) are filtered by the kidney. As molecular size increases, filterability becomes progressively smaller. Electrical charge is the second variable determining filterability of macromolecules. For any given size, negatively charged macromolecules are filtered to a lesser extent than neutral molecules. This is because the membrane surface of the renal tubule contains polyanions, which repeal negatively charged macromolecules during filtration.

Given these size and charge restrictions, glomerular filtration of large molecular weight, negatively charged molecules is negligible. This applies to plasma proteins such as albumin. Plasma protein binding is an important determinant of drug disposition and activity. Thus, assessment of plasma binding is routinely performed in drug development. The term commonly used to describe plasma binding is the fraction of drug unbound (f_U), the ratio of unbound and total plasma concentrations. For small drug molecules that undergo plasma protein binding, filtration by the kidney will be restricted to the unbound fraction of drug in the plasma, since protein-bound drug does not filter out of the glomerulus. Consequently, filtration clearance can be calculated as $[f_u \times GFR]$.

9.3.2.2 Tubular Secretion

Although most compounds that are renally eliminated undergo glomerular filtration, excretion via this mechanism can be relatively low, as in cases of extensive plasma binding. A second mechanism by which drug is extracted from the blood into the urine is proximal tubular secretion. Tubular secretion involves the translocation of drug from the plasma to the urine. Membrane-bound transporters are responsible for the movement of xenobiotics across the basolateral (blood → kidney) and luminal membranes (kidney → urine) of the kidney cell. Thus, tubular secretion contributes to the cellular accumulation and urinary excretion of many drugs, and is a contributing factor to the nephrotoxic effects of compounds such as antiviral agents and antibiotics. Additionally, these transporter systems are potential sites for significant drug–drug interactions *in vivo*. Identification and characterization of these transport systems has greatly enhanced understanding of renal drug transport, and of these systems (detailed in Section 9.3.3).

Physiologic factors affecting tubular secretion are renal plasma flow, plasma binding, and intrinsic clearance. Renal extraction ratio is defined as the ratio of renal clearance and renal plasma flow. The extraction ratio of a drug can be classified as restrictive or nonrestrictive. This classification is based upon the drug's relationship to binding by proteins in the plasma. Generally, the clearance of a high extraction compound is nonrestrictive; that is, the kidney is capable of extracting the entire amount of drug presented to it, regardless of the degree of protein binding. In this case, renal clearance approaches a maximum value, renal plasma flow. Hence, the elimination of a high extraction compound is sometimes referred to as perfusion rate-limited. An example is the organic anion, para-aminohippurate (PAH), which is used as a marker of renal plasma flow. The majority of excreted medications, however, are restrictively cleared, meaning that the drug excretion is limited to unbound drug in the plasma.

Pharmacokinetic Primer 2 Extraction Ratio Theory

Physiologic determinants of clearance include organ blood flow (Q), plasma protein binding (f_u), and intrinsic clearance (Cl_{INT}). Among the various physiologic models characterizing clearance, the most widely applied is the venous equilibration model. The venous equilibration model or "well-stirred" model assumes an eliminating organ is a single well-stirred compartment through which the concentration of unbound drug in the exiting blood is in equilibrium with the unbound drug within the organ. The model was originally used to characterize clearance by the liver, but was subsequently applied to renal excretion.

The venous equilibration model describes clearance as follows:

$$Cl = \frac{Q \times f_U \times Cl_{INT}}{Q + f_U \times Cl_{INT}}$$

In this model, Cl_{INT} is defined as the ability of the organ to remove drug in the absence of flow and binding restrictions. In terms of renal excretion, Cl_{INT} describes tubular secretion.

The extraction ratio is thus defined as the ratio of total drug clearance from an organ to the blood flow supplying that organ. Awareness of the extraction ratio of a drug and its classification as low ($E \leq 0.3$), intermediate ($0.3 < E < 0.7$), or high ($E \geq 0.7$) allows the prediction of the dependence of total organ clearance on the physiologic factors (Q, f_u, Cl_{INT}).

Extraction ratio can be classified as *restrictive* or *nonrestrictive*. This classification is based upon the drug's relationship to binding by proteins in the blood. Generally, the clearance of a high extraction compound is nonrestrictive; that is, the eliminating organ is capable of extracting the entire amount of drug presented to it regardless of the degree of protein binding. In these cases, the clearance approaches a maximum value, the blood flow to the organ ($Cl \approx Q$). Hence, the elimination of a high extraction compound is sometimes referred to as *perfusion rate-limited*.

Conversely, the opposite is observed for a compound with a low extraction ratio. The ability of the eliminating organ to remove drug depends on plasma binding and intrinsic organ clearance ($Cl \approx f_U \times Cl_{INT}$). Such compounds are referred to as restrictively cleared and elimination is dependent upon the free fraction of the drug in the blood.

9.3.2.3 Tubular Reabsorption

Whereas filtration and secretion systems in the kidney serve to eliminate drug from the blood into the urine, tubular reabsorption serves to counteract excretion from the blood. Active reabsorption occurs via the proximal tubule for many endogenous compounds (i.e., glucose, electrolytes), and advances in protein science indicate a role of renal transport systems in drug reabsorption by the kidney. Nevertheless, current data indicate that drug reabsorption is primarily a passive process. The primary driving force for passive reabsorption is the tubular reabsorption of water, which serves to concentrate the drug in urine with respect to plasma. It is the establishment of an electrochemical gradient that allows for back diffusion of drug molecules from tubular urine to blood. The degree of reabsorption is dependent upon physicochemical properties of the drug as well as physiologic variables.

Physicochemical properties that affect passive reabsorption include polarity, ionization state, and molecular weight. Small, nonionized, lipophilic molecules tend to be extensively reabsorbed. Physiologic variables that affect reabsorption include urine pH and urine flow rate. Generally, increasing the urine flow rate tends to decrease both the concentration gradient, contact time, and subsequently, the extent of reabsorption. Additionally, if the drug is weakly acidic or basic, perturbations in urine pH will influence reabsorption. In the case of weak acid such as aspirin, for example, alkalization of urine increasing drug ionization, resulting in reduced reabsorption and increased drug excretion.

Pharmacokinetic Primer 3 Characterization of Renal Excretion

The major processes involved in renal excretion are glomerular filtration, active tubular secretion, and passive reabsorption. Overall, renal excretion results from the net contributions of these three processes:

$$Cl_{Renal} = Cl_{Filtration} + Cl_{Secretion} - Cl_{Reabsorption}$$

Filtration clearance ($Cl_{Filtration}$) can be predicted from GFR and protein binding. Likewise, secretory clearance ($Cl_{secretion}$) is described by the venous equilibration model. However, it is difficult to accurately quantify the reabsorption of a drug. Thus, reabsorption in the kidney is best described in terms of the fraction of drug filtered and secreted that is reabsorbed (designated R), resulting in the following general equation describing renal clearance:

$$Cl_{Renal} = \left[f_U \times GFR + \left(\frac{Q \times f_U \times Cl_{INT}}{Q + f_U \times Cl_{INT}}\right)\right] \times (1 - R)$$

Knowledge of the extraction ratio of a particular compound allows the preceding to be simplified into more practical terms. Renal excretion drug interactions resulting from transport inhibition cause reductions in Cl_{INT}.

A particularly useful parameter for elucidating mechanisms of renal excretion is excretion ratio (*XR*). *XR* is simply renal clearance corrected for filtration clearance ($Cl_{Renal}/Cl_{Filtration}$):

$$XR = \frac{Cl_{Renal}}{f_U \times GFR} = \left[1 + \frac{Cl_{Secretion}}{f_U \times GFR}\right] \times (1 - R)$$

XR provides a general indication of the mechanism of elimination for the compound of interest, and is a reliable monitoring parameter for drug interaction assessment.

XR Value	Mechanism
XR = 1	Net Filtration
XR > 1	Net Secretion
XR < 1	Net Reabsorption

In general, it is difficult to accurately quantify drug reabsorption of a compound. A useful calculation to assess net excretion mechanisms is renal excretion ratio (XR). XR is calculated as the ratio of renal clearance and filtration clearance. Therefore, excretion ratio provides a general indication of the mechanism of elimination for the compound of interest. An XR greater than one is indicative of a net secretory process. Net reabsorption can be inferred when an XR value is less than one, and when renal clearance is dependent on urine flow rate or urine pH.

9.3.3 Membrane Transporters Involved in Renal Excretion

9.3.3.1 Tubular Transport of Organic Anions

The renal proximal tubule of the kidney contains several organic anion transport systems that secrete a wide array of exogenous compounds (Figure 9.4). At the basolateral membrane, OAT1 is the classic sodium-dependent organic anion transporter. This polyspecific protein mediates substrate uptake against an electrogenic gradient into the kidney cell in exchange for a dicarboxylate such as α-ketoglutarate. OAT1 substrates are amphiphilic and contain a negative charge. The prototypical substrate for OAT1 is PAH. Medications transported by OAT1 include antibiotics, antivirals, carbonic anydrase inhibitors, diuretics, and ochratoxin A (Table 9.7). OAT3 is a basolateral transporter similar to OAT1. Although there is some overlap of substrate specificity between both transporters, OAT3 transports sulfate- and glucuronide steroid conjugates. Both OAT1 and OAT3 are inhibited by probenecid.

At least two other transport systems mediate basolateral uptake of organic anions. OATP4C1 appears to play a role in digoxin excretion. Additionally, efflux of organic anions across the basolateral membrane has been proposed. This efflux system has been linked to members of the MRP transport family (MRP 6).

Once inside the tubular cell, there is a possibility of cytoplasmic binding or distribution into intracellular compartments. For example, the extensive renal accumulation of methazolamide in the kidney model was attributed to drug complexation with cytoplasmic carbonic anhydrase. Furthermore, biotransformation (most notably phase II metabolism) within the kidney cell is also possible. The role of intracellular distribution and metabolism on the renal disposition of organic anions requires further study.

Besides basolateral uptake, transepithelial transport and intracellular accumulation also depends on drug efflux across the apical brush border membrane. Although apical transport of organic anions is not completely understood, information is emerging regarding the translocation of organic anions across the luminal membrane into the urine. A number of transport pathways have been proposed for the luminal exit of acidic compounds, although the relative contribution of these mechanisms is species dependent. In rats, OATP1A3-v1 (OAT-K1) and OATP1A3-v3

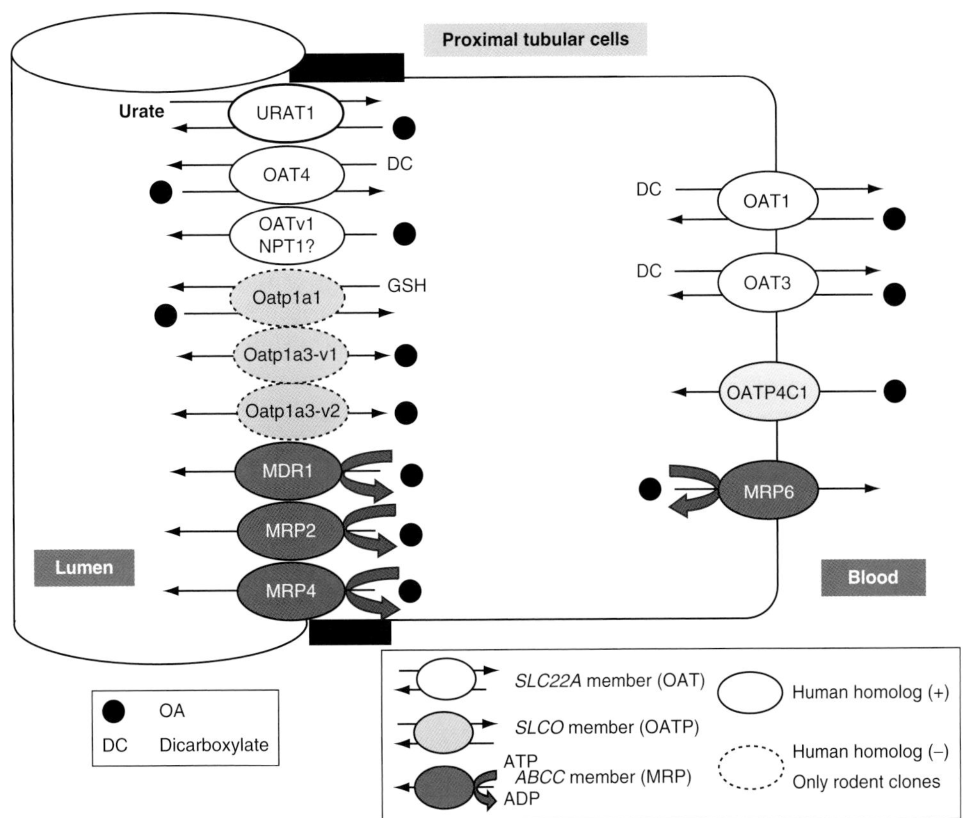

Figure 9.4 Organic anion (OA) transporters in proximal tubular cells. In the basolateral membrane, OAT1 and OAT3 mediate uptake of a wide range of relatively small and hydrophilic OAs from plasma. OATP4C1 is shown to transport digoxin. In the apical membrane, many OA transporters are identified. The role of URAT1 as an efflux transporter for various OAs into tubular lumen is suggested. In regard to the OATP members, large species differences are noted and their contribution to transepithelial transport of OA is still unclear. OATP1a3v1 and OATP1a3v2 could participate in tubular reabsorption and/or secretion of relatively hydrophobic anions such as bile acids, methotrexate, and PGE2. MRP2 and MRP4 extrude type II OAs from the cell into tubular lumen. MRP4 is shown to mediate the transport of PAH. OATv1 and its putative human ortholog NPT1 belong to the distinct transporter family (SLC17A). OATv1 would function as a voltage-driven OA transporter, which mediates efflux of OAs. Transporters whose human ortholog is not identified are depicted by dotted lines. Reprinted from American Journal of Physiology: Renal Physiology, Volume 290, T. Sekine, H. Miyasaki and H. Endou, Molecular physiology of renal organic anion transporters, pp. 251–261, Copyright 2006, with permission from the American Physiological Society.

Table 9.7 Substrates for OATs

Therapeutic Class	Examples
Carbonic anhydrase inhibitors	Acetazolamide, methazolamide
Cephalosporins	Cephalexin, ceftriaxone
Diuretics	Chlorothiazide, furosemide, bumetanide
HIV Inhibitors	Zidovudine, adefovir, cedofivir
NSAIDS	Salicylic acid, indomethacin flurbiprofen
Penicillins	Penicillin G
Sulfonamides	Sulfisoxazole
Miscellaneous	Ochratoxin A idoxyl sulfate PAH methotrexate tetracycline bile acids

(OAT-K2) are kidney-specific transporters that mediate facilitated transport. Two MRP isoforms, MRP2 and MRP4, are also expressed on the brush border membrane. MRP2 substrates include conjugated and unconjugated organic anions, methotrexate and PAH. MRP4 is a probenecid-sensitive transporter that has been linked to luminal transport of nucleoside analogs. Additionally, a member of the OAT family, OAT4, mediates bidirectional transport, although a role in substrate reabsorption by the kidney has been proposed.

Another transporter expressed in proximal tubule epithelial cells is URAT1. URAT1 is responsible for the reabsorption of urate in the kidney. Gout, an inflammatory disease, results from elevated body levels of uric acid. It is believed that an inherited deficiency in URAT1 expression is a causative factor in the disease. Treatment includes administration of uricosuric agents such a probenecid and sulfinpyrazone increase uric acid excretion through inhibition of URAT1.

9.3.3.2 Tubular Transport of Organic Cations

Renal excretion is a primary route of drug elimination for hydrophilic cationic drugs. Although hydrophobic compounds are also subject to filtration and renal secretion, these agents tend to be extensively reabsorbed by the kidney.

Organic cations are transported by the proximal tubule via a multistep process (Figure 9.5). At the basolateral membrane, transport proceeds by facilitated diffusion along an electrochemical gradient (driven by the inside-negative electrical potential difference) from the peritubular capillaries into the proximal tubular cells. The important transport carriers for basolateral uptake are thought to be OCT2 and OCT3, although a variant of OCT2 (OCT2A) has also been identified. It should be noted that OCT1 appears to be an important basolateral transporter in rats. Additionally, it appears that select cations such as TEA and cimetidine are substrates for OAT3, and this protein may also contribute to transport of cationic drugs from the plasma into the kidney cell.

Once inside the tubular cell, intracellular sequestration can result in extensive drug accumulation. This may involve drug binding to cytosolic proteins, or accumulation in vesicular compartments such as endosomes and lysosomes due to ion-trapping (these organelles have an acidic pH). The significance of intracellular sequestration on tubular transport of cationic drugs remains to be elucidated.

Luminal transport of cationic drugs across the brush border membrane into the urine mediated by proton-cation exchange proteins including OCTN1, MATE1, and MATE2-K. A Na^+-H^+ exchanger generates the proton gradient (intracellular > extracellular proton concentrations), with intracellular Na^+ levels maintained through Na^+-K^+-ATPase. Another transport system involved in efflux of organic cations is the MDR1/Pgp. Expressed on the brush border membrane the proximal tubule cell, P-gp, mediates efflux of a broad spectrum of cationic and hydrophobic drugs via an ATP-dependent mechanism.

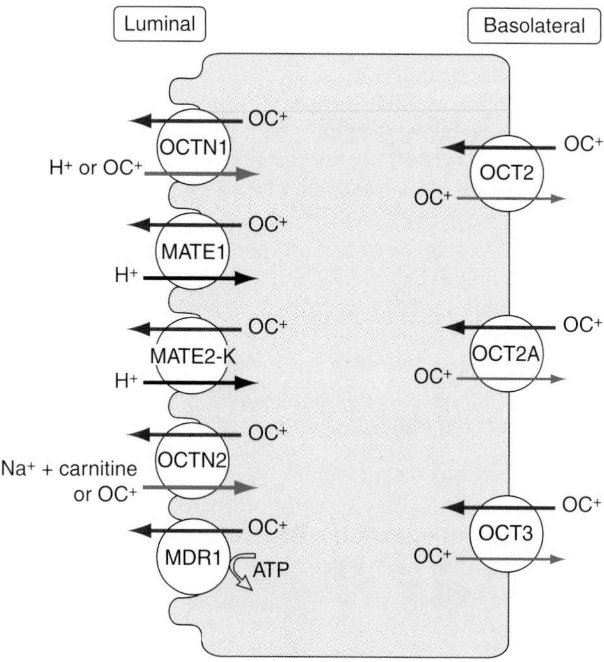

Figure 9.5 Organic cation transporters in plasma membranes of human renal proximal tubules. Red arrows indicate transport activities that are involved in cation secretion whereas green arrows indicate transport activities involved in cation reabsorption. MATE1 and MATE2-K are secondary active proton–cation antiporters. OCT2A is a splice variant of OCT2. The basolateral localization of OCT3 was observed in unpublished experiments. With kind permission from Springer Science+Business Media: Pharmaceutical Research, Polyspecific organic cation transporters: Structure, function, physiological roles, and biopharmaceutical implications, volume 24, 2006, pp.1227–1251, H. Koepsell, K. Lips and C. Volk, Figure 1.

9.3.3.3 Tubular Transport of Nucleosides and Nucleoside Analogs

As noted previously, nucleosides and nucleoside analogs are used to treat HIV infection as well as certain types of cancers (Table 9.8). Many of these drugs are readily excreted by the kidney. Consequently, renal tubular transport of these hydrophilic compounds involves various transport systems.

Nucleoside transporters are thought to play a key role in the renal disposition of nucleosides (Figure 9.6). There are two types of nucleoside transport processes: (1) concentrative nucleoside transporters (CNT1-CNT3) and (2) equilibrative nucleoside transporters (ENT1-ENT2). CNTs are localized primarily to the brush border membrane of renal epithelial cells and mediates active reabsorption of substrates into the cell by a sodium electrochemical gradient (Na^+ dependent secondary active transporters). ENTs are located primarily on the basolateral membrane, and function bidirectionally by facilitated diffusion (downhill flux of nucleosides), driven by substrate gradients. Accumulating evidence, however, suggests that ENTs may also be expressed at the brush border membrane, and therefore are involved in both secretion and reabsorption of nucleosides.

Presently, the role of nucleoside transporters on the pharmacokinetics of nucleoside drugs is poorly

Table 9.8 Nucleoside Analogs Used to Treat HIV Infection and Cancer

Anti-HIV Drugs	Anticancer Drugs
Aprictabine	Cytarabine
Azidothymidine	Clofarabine
Didanosine	Fludarabine
Emtricitabine	Gemcitabine
Lamivudine	Nelarabine
Stavudine	
Zalcitabine	

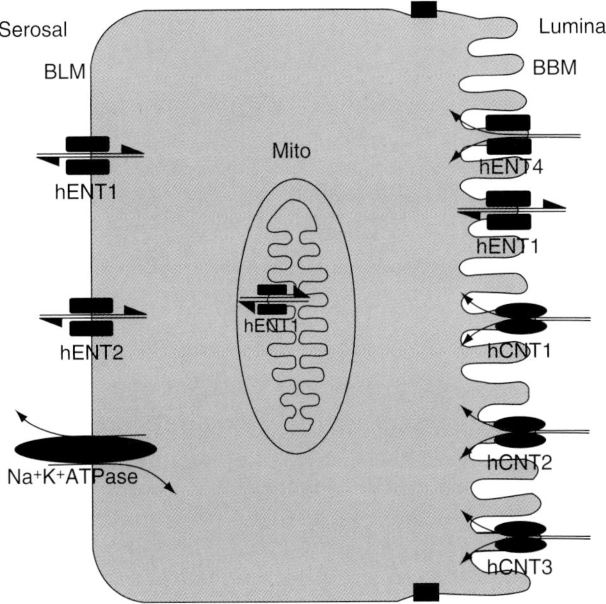

Figure 9.6 Nucleoside transporters in renal proximal tubule cells. Basolateral uptake proceeds by facilitated transport (bidirectional) via equilibrative nucleoside transporters (nENT1, hENT2). At the luminal membrane, concentrative nucleoside transporters (CNT1-3) mediate nucleoside reabsorption via cotransport with sodium. Additionally, a role of ENTs at the brush border membrane has been proposed. Reprinted from Biochemistry and Cell Biology, Volume 84, A.N. Elwi, V.L. Damaraju, S.A. Baldwin, S.D. Young, M.B. Sawyer, and C.E. Cass, Renal nucleoside transporters: Physiological and clinical implications, pp. 844–858, Copyright 2006, with permission from the NRC Research Press.

understood. However, nucleoside analogs have been shown to interact with polyspecific renal drug transporters including OCTs, OATs, MRPs, and Pgp. The renal excretion of several nucleosides (e.g., lamivudine, apricitabine emtricitabine) involves basolateral transport via a cimedtidine-sensitive transporter, OCT2. Likewise, azidothymidine is a substrate for OATs. MRP4, which has been found to mediate resistance to nucleoside antiviral and anticancer agents, is expressed in the brush border membrane of the proximal tubule, and may therefore play a role in the renal excretion of these agents.

9.3.4 Renal Drug Interactions

When two drugs are administered together, changes in pharmacokinetics and/or drug activity of one of both compounds can occur, resulting in a drug–drug interaction. Drug–drug interactions can involve various mechanisms of renal excretion. For example, reduced plasma binding (competitive or noncompetitive binding displacement) leads to increased filtration clearance of highly bound drugs. Alterations in urine pH can change the rate of passive drug reabsorption rate through manipulation of the plasma pH and/or urine pH, resulting in either an increased or decreased drug excretion renal elimination rate. This approach is used in cases of drug toxicity due to overdose as a means to increase drug excretion. However, the most important mechanism susceptible to renal drug interactions is alteration of tubular transport.

Due to the broad substrate specificity of the various renal transporters, it is not surprising that a number of competitive drug–drug interactions have been identified (Table 9.9). When two drugs compete for the same transporter, the renal clearance of one of the drugs is reduced, resulting in increased plasma exposure. In many cases, this can result in increased risk of toxicity. Examples in this category are inhibition of Pgp-mediated digoxin secretion by quinidine and inhibition of OAT-mediated methotrexate secretion by NSAIDS. On the other hand, secretory inhibition can also be an effective strategy to increase a drug's duration of action, as evidenced by the combined therapy of probenecid, a classic OAT inhibitor, and penicillin.

For several nephrotoxic medications (e.g., aminoglycosides, vancomycin), drug transport across tubular cells is a fundamental step in the onset of toxicity. Accordingly, the incidence of nephrotoxicity can be prevented by minimizing drug accumulation in the kidney. For example, cidofovir, a nucleoside analog used to treat cytomegalovirus retinitis, is correlated with high drug concentrations in kidney epithelial cells. Coadministration with probenecid has been shown to significantly lower the incidence of cidofovir nephrotoxicity in the clinical setting through inhibition of OAT1-mediated basolateral uptake.

Table 9.9 Drug–Drug Transporter Interactions in the Kidney

Transporter	Drug	Inhibitor	Result of Interaction
OAT	Penicillin	Probenecid	↑ duration of action of penicillin
	Methotrexate	NSAIDS	↑ plasma exposure of methotrexate leading to toxicity
	Cidofovir	Probenecid	↓ kidney accumulation and lower incidence of cidofovir nephrotoxicity
	Furosemide	Probenecid	↓ diuretic activity of furosemide
	Various	Uremic Toxins	↓ excretion of OAT substrates
OCT	Lamivudine	Trimethoprim	↑ plasma exposure of lamivudine
	Procainamide	Cimetidine	↑ procainamide toxicity
	Meformin	Cimetidine	↑ plasma exposure of metformin
Pgp	Digoxin	Quinidine	↑ digoxin plasma concentrations

9.3.5 Effects of Aging and Disease on Renal Drug Excretion

As people age, the kidneys progressively shrink (~10% ↓ per decade after age 20), and this is accompanied by decreased renal blood flow and GFR. Likewise, patients with hypertension, diabetes, and other diseases are at risk for developing chronic renal failure, a gradual and progressive loss of the ability of the kidneys to excrete wastes, concentrate urine, and conserve electrolytes.

For medications that are eliminated primarily by the kidney, dosage adjustments are sometimes required in patients with renal insufficiency secondary to disease or aging. This is a particular concern for those medications with a narrow therapeutic range (e.g., digoxin, vancomycin, aminoglycosides). The "intact nephron hypothesis" is based on the premise that, in patients with chronic renal failure, many of the nephrons are nonfunctional, but those that remain function normally. Therefore, the hypothesis implies that renal dysfunction results in parallel reductions in the three mechanisms of renal drug excretion (filtration, secretion, and reabsorption). This is the basis for GFR-based dosing of medications cleared primarily by the kidney. In other words, patients with reduced GFR are presumed to experience corresponding reductions in drug secretion and reabsorption.

Pharmacokinetic Primer 4 Methods to Estimate GFR

GFR is a standard measure of renal function and is critical in treating patients with renal dysfunction. Assessment of renal function is particularly important for drugs that are excreted primarily by the kidney, and have a narrow therapeutic range. Accordingly, modifications of drug dosing regimens are warranted in patients with renal impairment. Examples include aminoglycoside antibiotics, vancomycin, and digoxin.

The gold standard for measuring GFR is by monitoring the renal clearance of an ideal filtration marker, such as inulin, iothalamate, or iohexol. Renal clearance is calculated as follows:

$$Cl = \frac{UER}{C_{plasma}}$$

Direct assessment of GFR involves collection of urine for a prescribed period of time following drug administration (e.g., 24 hours). The urine volume is measured, and the concentration of marker in the urine is assayed. A plasma sample is also collected, typically at the midpoint of the collection period. Urinary excretion rate (*UER*) is estimated as urine flow rate (volume of urine collected divided by collection time) multiplied by urine concentration. Thus, clearance is estimated as follows:

$$Cl = \frac{UER \times C_{urine}}{C_{plasma}}$$

Although direct methods provide a more accurate measurement of GFR for a particular patient, these methods are time-consuming and require analytical methods that are not always readily available. As a result, GFR is routinely estimated based on the endogenous marker, creatinine clearance. Creatinine clearance is most commonly measured indirectly using any number of equations that have been developed based on a patient's measured serum creatinine (*SC*). These equations are based on patient characteristics such as age, gender, body weight, and height.

The most commonly applied formula is the Cockcroft-Gault equation (units: mL/min):

$$Cl_{creatinine} = \frac{(140 - Age) \times Wt}{72 \times SC}$$

The equation is multiplied by 0.85 for females.

The National Institute of Diabetes and Diseases of the Kidney (NIDDK) recommends the following equation:

$$Cl_{creatinine} = 186 \times (SC)^{-1.154} \times (Age)^{-0.203}$$

The equation is multiplied by 0.742 for females and by 1.210 for black patients. It estimates creatinine clearance as $mL/min/1.73m^2$.

However, questions have been raised regarding the accuracy of GFR-based dosing, for two general reasons. First, there is a concern that methods for calculating creatinine clearance, including nomgrams such as the Cockcroft-Gault equation, do not provide reliable GFR estimates in elderly patients, immunosupressed patients, and patients with HIV infection and rheumatoid arthritis. Second, the validity of the intact nephron hypothesis has been challenged, as it is unclear whether reductions in GFR are accompanied by similar reductions in other drug excretion mechanisms. In this regard, however, recent evidence does suggest that chronic renal failure does result in decreased expression of renal transporters (OCT2, OAT1), resulting in reduced drug secretion. Additionally, uremic toxins may directly alter renal drug excretion by inhibiting OAT transporter activity.

9.4 HEPATOBILIARY EXCRETION

Although the liver is commonly identified with its primary role of drug metabolism, one of the main functions of the liver is the formation of bile. Bile forms in the canaliculus between adjacent hepatocytes following active secretion bile acids and other components (phospholipids, bilirubin, cholesterol) across the canalicular membrane. These components are either synthesized by the liver or transported into the hepatocyte across the sinusoidal membrane. Bile acid secretion stimulates osmotic water flow across the canalicular membrane. The resulting bile drains into branches of intrahepatic bile ductules that converge to the common hepatic bile duct. In humans, 500 to 600 ml of bile is produced daily.

Beyond its physiologic role in the intestinal digestion of lipids and lipid-soluble vitamins, the bile also plays an important role in the excretion of xenobiotics, including drugs and their metabolites. This includes a diverse array of compounds, both polar and lipophilic, including, anions, cations, and neutral molecules. In humans, the molecular threshold is approximately 500 to 600, with renal excretion being the primary route of excretion for smaller molecules.

Hepatobiliary transport involves a series of pathways including drug uptake into the hepatocyte, intracellular translocation, biotransformation and egress into blood and/or bile (Figure 9.7). Accordingly,

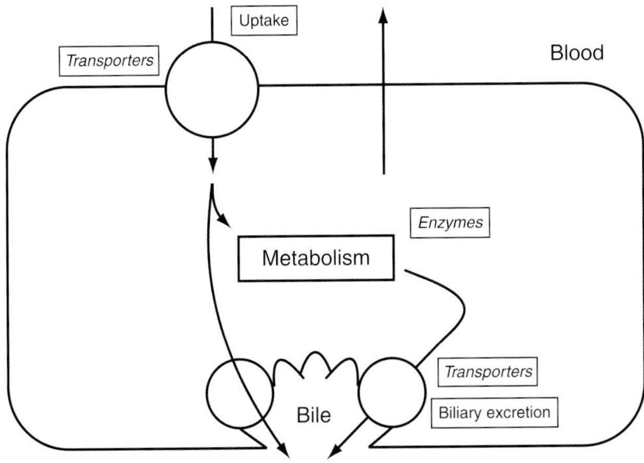

Figure 9.7 Diagram depicting mechanisms of hepatobiliary clearance. Drug can be taken up into hepatocytes via transporters and/or passive diffusion, followed by metabolism and/or biliary excretion. Mechanisms also exist for drug efflux across the sinusoidal membrane into the circulation. Reprinted from Annual Review of Pharmacology and Toxicology, Volume 45, Y. Shitara, H. Sato and Y. Sugiyama, Evaluation of drug-drug interaction in the hepatobiliary and renal transport of drugs, pp. 689–723, Copyright 2005, with permission from Annual Reviews.

membrane transporters play an important role in these processes of excretion, which are discussed next.

9.4.1 Drug Transport Across the Hepatocyte

Hepatic elimination involves a sequence of events involving drug uptake from the bloodstream, leading to intracellular metabolism and/or excretion. The liver has the capacity to efficiently extract protein-bound drugs from the circulation. These compounds have a high hepatic extraction ratio, defined as the rate of drug removal from the bloodstream by the liver relative to the rate of drug presentation to the liver (via the circulation). For those compounds with a high extraction ratio, clearance becomes limited by hepatic blood flow. Whereas these compounds tend to be rapidly metabolized, the first step in hepatic extraction is translocation of drug from the bloodstream into the hepatocyte. Accordingly, transport proteins in the sinusoidal (basolateral membrane) play a principal role in this process (Table 9.10).

Figure 9.8 provides a schematic representation of transport proteins that mediate sinusoidal uptake of drugs into the hepatocyte. Several members of the SLC family of proteins mediate bidirectional drug transport via a facilitative mechanism. The concentration gradient is created by the interplay of intracellular drug metabolism and drug efflux at the sinusoidal and canalicular membrane. Among the SLC transporters identified in Figure 9.8 is Na^+-taurocholate cotransporting polypeptide (NTCP, SLC10A1). Although NTCP is not directly involved in drug excretion to a significant extent, this is an important uptake system for bile salts from the bloodstream. NTCP has also been used to target anticancer drugs (cisplatin and chlorambucil) to the liver as bile acid derivatives.

Table 9.10 Human Hepatic Transport Proteins (Basolateral Transport)

Transporter	Substrates
NTCP	Bile acids, estrone-3-sulfate, bromosulphothalein
OATP1A2	Fexofenadine, bile acids, BQ-123
OATP1B1	HMG-CoA reductase inhibitors (atorvastatin, pravastatin); bile acids, bilirubin
OATP1B3	Bile acids, digoxin, rifampin; [D-penicillamine2,5]-enkephalin (DPDPE)
OATP2B1	Benzylpenicillin, estrone-3-sulfate, bromosulphothalein
OAT2	Prostaglandins, salicylate, tetracycline, zidovudine
OCT1	Tetraethylammonium, 1-methyl-4-phenylpyridinium (MPP^+)
MRP1	Anticancer agents (daunorubicin, doxorubicin, etoposide, vincristine
MRP3	Acetaminophen glucuronide, methotrexate
MRP4	Azidothymidine, methotrexate
MRP5	Cyclic nucleotides (cAMP, cGMP)
MRP6	BQ-123

Hepatic uptake of organic anions is mediated primarily by OATPs including OATP1B1 (LST1), OATP1B3 (LST2), and OATP2B1. These transporters have a broad substrate specificity. Besides organic anions, type II cations (bulky compounds with one or two charged groups in or near ring structures) and steroid molecules are taken up by the liver through OATP systems. Two additional SLC proteins involved in basolateral excretion by the liver are OAT2 and OCT1. OAT2 mediates sodium-independent transport of various anionic compounds including salicylate and methotrexate. OCT1 is involved in the bidirectional transport of small, type I organic cations such as tetraethylammonium and N-methylnicotinamide.

Pharmacokinetic Primer 5 Characterization of Hepatobiliary Excretion

Hepatic clearance is the net result of drug uptake into the hepatocyte, followed by metabolism and biliary excretion, with possible efflux of drug back into the circulation from the liver cell. Overall, hepatic clearance is traditionally described using the venous equilibration model:

$$Cl = \frac{Q \times f_U \times Cl_{INT}}{Q + f_U \times Cl_{INT}}$$

where Q is hepatic blood flow, f_U is the fraction of drug unbound in the circulation, and Cl_{INT} is intrinsic hepatic clearance. This parameter has been defined further to characterize the role of the individual processes of hepatobiliary transport and metabolism on clearance by the liver as follows:

$$Cl_{INT} = PS_{INFLUX} \times \frac{Cl_{H,INT}}{PS_{EFFLUX} + Cl_{H,INT}}$$

Continued

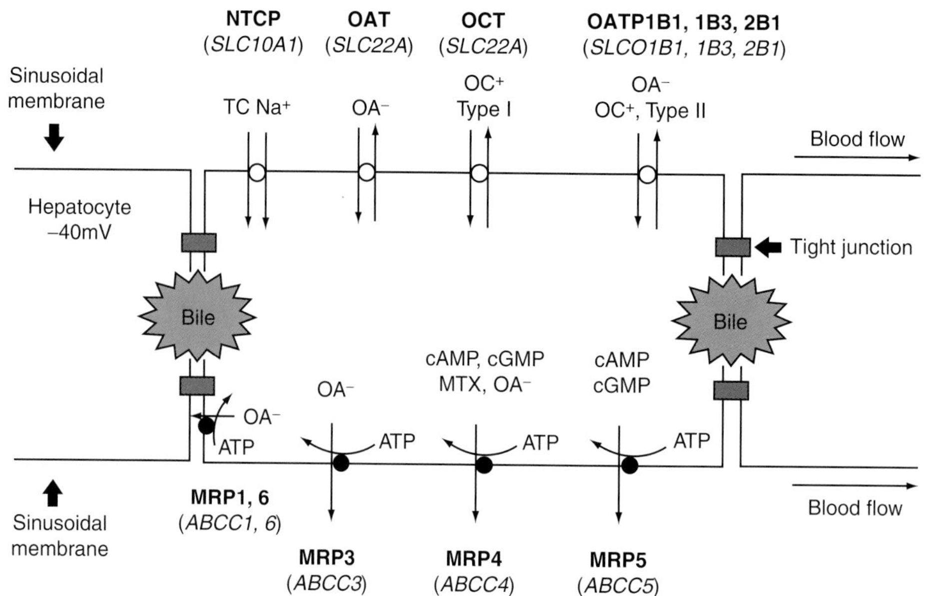

Figure 9.8 Substrate transport across sinusoidal membrane of hepatocytes. Blood flowing through the liver bathes hepatocytes and delivers solutes to the basolateral hepatic membrane for uptake. Important basolateral transport proteins (protein name is in bold type with gene symbol listed below) are depicted with arrows denoting the direction of transport and ATP-dependent transporters designated by •. For the OAT and OCT families, only mRNA have been detected in human liver. Typical substrates are listed including organic anions (OA–), organic cations (OC+), methotrexate (MTX) cyclic), adenosine 3′,5′cyclic monophosphate (cAMP) and guanosine 3',5'-cyclic monophosphate (cGMP). With kind permission from Springer Science+Business Media: Pharmaceutical Research, The complexities of hepatic drug transport: Current knowledge and emerging concepts, volume 21, 2004, pp. 719–735, P. Chandra and K.L.R. Brouwer, Figure 1.

Pharmacokinetic Primer 5 Characterization of Hepatobiliary Excretion—Cont'd

In this equation, PS_{INFLUX} and PS_{EFFLUX} are terms describing the membrane permeability of drug across the sinusoidal membrane of the hepatocyte for influx (blood → cytoplasm) and efflux (cytoplasm → blood). These processes are mediated by membrane transporters. $Cl_{H,INT}$ represents the intrinsic clearance for metabolism and biliary excretion of drug (also transporter-driven).

This equation can be simplified under the following conditions:

Sinusoidal efflux >>> intrinsic clearance ($PS_{EFFLUX} >>> Cl_{H,INT}$)

$$Cl_{INT} = PS_{INFLUX} \times \frac{Cl_{H,INT}}{PS_{EFFLUX}}$$

Sinusoidal efflux <<< intrinsic clearance ($Cl_{H<INT} >>> PS_{EFFLUX}$)

$$Cl_{INT} = PS_{INFLUX}$$

The implications are as follows.

Process	Role in Hepatic Clearance
Sinusoidal uptake	Always a determinant of net hepatic clearance (regardless of other mechanisms involved). Changes in sinusoidal uptake (e.g., due to transport inhibition) will affect overall hepatic clearance, even for drugs that are highly metabolized.
Metabolism	For highly metabolized drugs, this is a main route for hepatic elimination. Metabolism can be altered by enzyme inhibition and induction, and is highly variable due to factors such as environment and genetics.
Biliary excretion	Determinant of overall hepatic clearance, unless sinusoidal efflux is low ($Cl_{H,INT} >>> PS_{Efflux}$). When PS_{EFFLUX} is low, only a drastic reduction in biliary excretion (resulting from drug-mediated transport inhibition) will impact hepatic clearance.

In addition to SLC proteins, members of the MRP transport family play prominent roles in hepatic excretion of organic anions, including drugs and drug metabolites. MRPs are primarily involved in drug efflux from the hepatic cytosol to the bloodstream, and include MRP1, MRP3, MRP4, MRP5, and MRP6. It appears that, in addition to drug excretion, hepatic MRPs are important when biliary transport is impaired or blocked. Although expression of MRP1 is normally low in the liver, protein expression is induced during liver regeneration and under conditions of experimentally induced cholestasis (by endotoxin administration or bile-duct cannulation). Although MRP3 levels are also low under normal conditions, expression is induced by drugs such as phenobarbital. Additionally, MRP3 levels are increased in patients with genetic diseases caused by cases of MRP2 deficiency (e.g., Dubin-Johnson Syndrome). Under these conditions, upregulation of MRPs reduces bile acid levels in the hepatocyte by increasing efflux across the sinusoidal membrane into the blood.

9.4.2 Drug Distribution in the Hepatocyte

Following uptake across the basolateral membrane into the cytosol, drug disposition can proceed by one of several paths, most notably biotransformation. Additionally, drug and/or formed metabolites may be excreted across the canalicular membrane into bile (described later), or may be transported back into the circulation (sinusoidal membrane efflux) with subsequent renal excretion.

Besides the pathways noted earlier, the liver has the ability to sequester drugs and metabolites through various mechanisms. Although the importance of intrahepatic binding and distribution mechanisms to drug disposition has not been completely elucidated, several potential pathways are recognized. The cytosol of the hepatocyte can serve as a storage compartment, effectively decreasing the intracellular drug concentrations. Several cytosolic proteins including glutathione-s-transferase and fatty acid binding protein can complex organic anions. Hydrophobic anions and organic cations may undergo distribution to intracellular organelles such as lysosomes and endosomes. The acidic pH of these organelles facilitates cation accumulation via ionization. Mitochondria represent another potential drug distribution site, and this mechanism has been linked to toxicity associated with anticancer agents. Another intracellular site of cation accumulation is the cell nucleus, a mechanism that becomes significant when intracellular concentrations become high. This represents yet another potential mechanism for hepatic toxicity.

9.4.3 Drug Transport Across the Hepatic Canalicular Membrane

Biliary excretion of drug and metabolites involves one of several ATP-dependent transport proteins expressed on the canalicular membrane. These proteins are members of the ABC family of transporters (Table 9.11), and they mediate unidirectional (hepatic cytosol → bile) transport of substrates uphill against a large concentration gradient.

As illustrated in Figure 9.9, five transporters are known to participate in biliary excretion. The bile salt export pump, BSEP, has a limited role regarding drug excretion. However, this transporter is a potential site of drug interactions that can increase the risk of hepatotoxicity (see later). Among the drug transporters that have been identified, MRP2 (formerly known as cMOAT) mediates biliary excretion of a diverse number of substrates, including several drugs. As noted earlier, Dubin-Johnson syndrome is a type of hereditary hyperbilirubinemia resulting from absence of canalicular MRP2. To compensate for this deficiency, basolateral MRP3 expression is upregulated.

Besides MRP2, the other important canalicular transporter in terms of biliary drug excretion is MDR1 (Pgp). This widely studied transporter plays a major role in the excretion of numerous endogenous and exogenous compounds by the liver. Drug substrates for Pgp include anticancer agents, antivirals, cardiac medications, and opioid analgesics (Table 9.1). Another ABC transporter that may play an important role in biliary excretion is breast cancer resistance protein (BCRP).

Table 9.11 Human Canalicular Transport Proteins (Biliary Transport)

Transporter	Substrates
BSEP	Conjugated and unconjugated bile salts
MRP2	Quinolone antibiotics (grepafloxacin, lomefloxacin)
	β-lactam antibiotics (cefodizime, ceftriaxone)
	HMG CoA reductase Inhibitors (pravastatin)
	ACE inhibitors (temocaprilat)
	Methotrexate
	Campothecins (topotecan, irinotecan)
	Cisplatin
	Glucuronide, glutathione, and sulfate conjugates
MDR1 (Pgp)	See Table 9.1
MDR3	Phospholipids
BCRP	Daunorubicin, dauxorubicin, mitoxantrone

9.4.4 Enterohepatic Recycling

Enterohepatic recycling (EHR) is a feedback mechanism resulting from the combined roles of the liver and intestine. EHR begins with drug absorption across the intestine into the portal circulation, followed by uptake into the hepatocytes. Next, drug and or conjugated metabolites are secreted into the bile and returned to the intestine, where drug can be reabsorbed into the circulation, in some cases after deconjugation in the GI tract (Figure 9.10). As described previously, a number of drugs are secreted by the liver into bile, and are therefore capable of undergoing enterohepatic recycling. These include antibiotics, NSAIDS, hormones, opioids, digoxin, and warfarin.

Following extravascular dosing, drug absorption is generally more rapid than drug elimination. Thus, for drugs undergoing biliary excretion, EHR represents a secondary absorption phase for drug. From a pharmacokinetic perspective, therefore, EHR not only prolongs the elimination $t_{1/2}$, but may also produce multiple peaks in the plasma concentration-time profile of a drug.

Gut flora play an important role in EHR, as they produce various enzymes involved in the metabolism of drug conjugates that are secreted in the bile. Oral antibiotic therapy is thought to limit the efficacy of oral contraceptives. The mechanism of this interaction is interruption of EHR by eliminating gut flora responsible for enzymatic deconjugation of hormones. This makes females taking oral contraceptives susceptible to breakthrough bleeding or at increased risk of becoming pregnant.

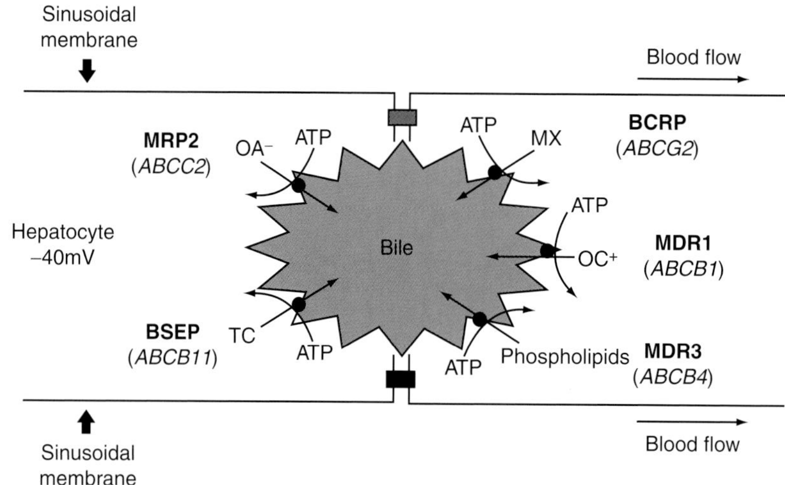

Figure 9.9 Human hepatic canalicular transport proteins. Important canalicular transport proteins are depicted with arrows denoting the direction of transport and ATP-dependent transporters designated by •. Typical substrates are listed (OA^-, organic anions; OC^+, organic cations; TC, taurocholate; MX, mitoxantrone). With kind permission from Springer Science +Business Media: Pharmaceutical Research, The complexities of hepatic drug transport: Current knowledge and emerging concepts, volume 21, 2004, pp. 719–735, P. Chandra and K.L.R. Brouwer, Figure 2.

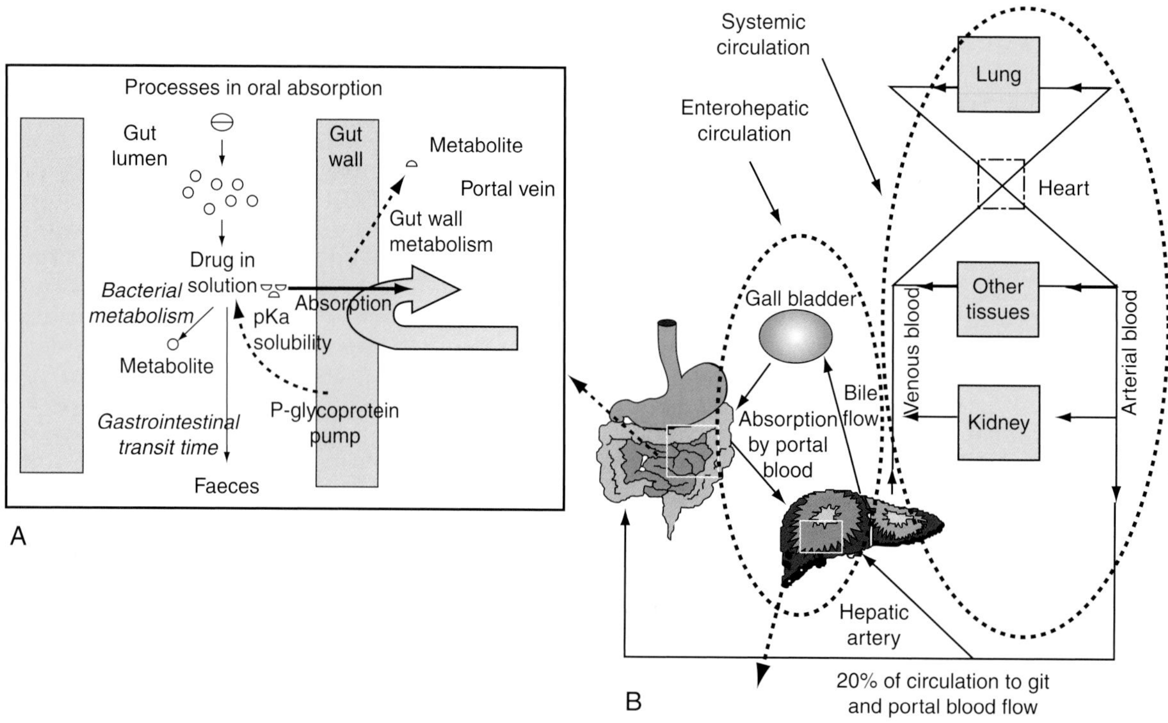

Figure 9.10 Schematic representation of enterohepatic recycling (B), and a detailed view of the factors affecting drug absorption from the intestine (A). Reprinted from Clinical Pharmacokinetics, Volume 41, M.S. Roberts, B.M. Magnusson, F.J. Burczynski, and M. Weiss, Enterohepatic circulation: Physiological, pharmacokinetic and clinical implications, pp. 751–790, Copyright 2002, with permission from Adis.

In cases of acute drug intoxications, activated charcoal is a commonly used treatment because of its ability to adsorb materials with a high capacity. Although timely single-dose administration is effective in preventing drug absorption of orally ingested drugs, repeated doses of activated charcoal have been shown to increase drug clearance, resulting in reduced plasma exposure of drug (Figure 9.11). This is the result of decreased enterohepatic recycling and increased drug exsorption from the intestine.

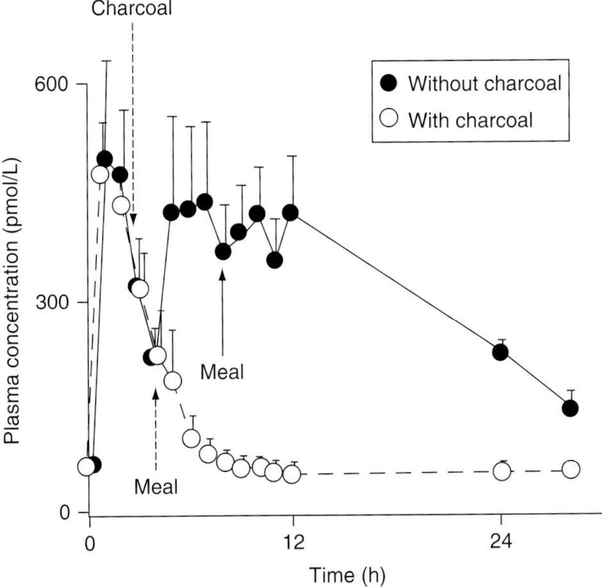

Figure 9.11 Inhibition of enterohepatic recycling of the hormone estriol by activated charcoal. Closed circles demonstrate how plasma levels show multiple peaks that are timed with meals (increased biliary transport; charcoal administration results in reduced plasma exposure and increased elimination). G.M. Heimer and D.E. Englund, 1986, Acta Endocrinologica, Vol. 113, pp. 93–95, (c) Society of the European Journal of Endocrinology (1986). Reproduced by permission.

9.4.5 Hepatobiliary Drug Interactions

Given its complexities with regard to the mechanisms and transport pathways involved, it is not surprising that hepatobiliary transport is a site for significant drug interactions (Table 9.12). These interactions can result from inhibition of sinusoidal drug transport, as demonstrated by the effects of OATP transport inhibition on the plasma exposure of HMG CoA Reductase inhibitors. Alternatively, biliary drug excretion can be attenuated by inhibition of canalicular membrane transporters, most notably Pgp and MRP2.

Although BSEP is not an important transporter of drugs, drug-inhibition of this transporter is a recognized mechanism for hepatotoxicity. Intracellular accumulation of cytotoxic bile salts subsequent to BSEP inhibition can produce cholestatic liver injury. The antidiabetic drug troglitazone was withdrawn from the U.S. market following reports of severe idiosyncratic hepatocellular injury, which was linked to inhibition of BSEP.

9.4.6 Disease Effects on Hepatobiliary Excretion

Both liver and kidney disease have been shown to affect hepatic clearance by reducing hepatic uptake, metabolism, and biliary excretion of drugs and their metabolites. In addition to altered drug metabolism, chronic liver disease alters through a number of mechanisms. Reduced plasma binding can affect the distribution and renal excretion of highly plasma bound medications (although these effects tend to offset one another). Hepatic blood flow is compromised, leading to reduced hepatic clearance of high extraction ratio medications such as propranolol and tissue plasminogen activator (t-PA). Likewise, portal shunting will decrease presystemic hepatic metabolism (i.e., first-pass effect), thereby increasing bioavailability. Liver disease also impairs transport systems on the sinusoidal and canalicular membrane of the hepatocyte. Consequently, for drugs primarily cleared by the liver, dosage reductions may be necessary in patients with liver disease.

Cholestasis is a condition characterized by impaired flow of bile, due to physical obstruction of the biliary tree or decreased bile secretion by the liver. Cholestasis produces alterations of enzyme activity in the liver (cytochrome P450) as well as altered transporter expression, with associated effects on drug clearance. As discussed previously, cholestasis can occur through inhibition of the canalicular membrane transporter, BSEP. In response to cholestasis, however, the liver has adaptive mechanisms to minimize cellular accumulation of toxic bile salts. These include upregulation of MRP3 to increase sinusoidal efflux, and downregulation of Na^+-taurocholate cotransporting polypeptide (NTCP), which mediates bile salt uptake from the blood to the liver.

For drugs that are primarily cleared by liver, there is a misconception that hepatic drug disposition will be unaffected by renal disease. Accumulating evidence has shown that deterioration of kidney function significantly reduces nonrenal clearance and alters the pharmacokinetics of some drugs that are predominantly metabolized or eliminated by liver through modulation

Table 9.12 Hepatobiliary Drug Interactions

Transporter	Drug	Inhibitor	Result of Interaction
Pgp	Mycophenolic Acid	Cyclosporin A	Reduced EHR resulting in ↓ systemic exposure
	Digoxin	Quinidine	↓ biliary excretion
	Ritonavir	Digoxin	↓ clearance following oral administration
OATP1B1	Cerivistatin	Gemfibrozil	5–6 fold ↑ in plasma AUC
	Rosuvastatin	Cyclosporin A	7 fold ↑ in plasma AUC
MRP2	SN-38 (metabolite of irinotecan	Probenecid	↓ biliary excretion, resulting in ↑ AUC
BSEP	—	Troglitazone Bosentan	Hepatotoxicity due to intracellular accumulation of bile salts

of biotransformation (Phase I, Phase II enzyme) and hepatobiliary transport. For example, OATP mediated drug uptake into the hepatocyte is impaired in renal failure, through reduced transporter expression and/or inhibition by uremic toxins.

9.5 OTHER ROUTES OF DRUG EXCRETION

9.5.1 Intestinal Exsorption

Oral dosing is the most important route for drug delivery. In the GI tract, the majority of drug absorption occurs in the small intestine. Bioavailability, defined as the fraction of an administered dose that reaches the systemic circulation, depends on a number of physicochemical (e.g., aqueous solubility, membrane permeability) and physiologic (e.g., degradation by intestinal enzymes) factors. Even though oral drug absorption was generally regarded as a passive process, research in transporter science has led to discovery of various drug transport systems in the GI tract that impact intestinal drug transport. The identification of these transporters not only accounts for the poor bioavailability of various lipophilic molecules, but they also represent formulation scientists with potential targets for systemic drug delivery (Figure 9.12).

In terms of intestinal drug transport, the most widely studied mechanism is Pgp. Based on the broad overlap in substrate and inhibitor specificities with Cytochrome P450 3A4 (the most important drug metabolizing exzyme), Pgp and CYP3A4 act as a concerted barrier to drug absorption in the GI tract. Indeed, a role of Pgp on the oral bioavailability has been demonstrated for a number of drugs through drug interaction studies (Table 9.13). Collectively, the results indicate that systemic exposure of Pgp substrates is increased following drug-induced transporter inhibition. In this regard, Pgp has been shown to limit oral absorption of several cancer agents (etoposide, paclitaxel, topotecan), and scientists believe that bioavailability can be improved by coadministration with Pgp inhibitors. Besides transport inhibition, induction of Pgp (resulting in increased expression), has a negative impact on oral drug absorption.

It is beyond the scope of this chapter to detail the role of intestinal transporters in drug absorption. However, it is worth noting that intestinal transport is bidirectional. In addition to allowing passage of drug molecules into the bloodstream through absorption, the GI tract is capable of extracting drugs from the

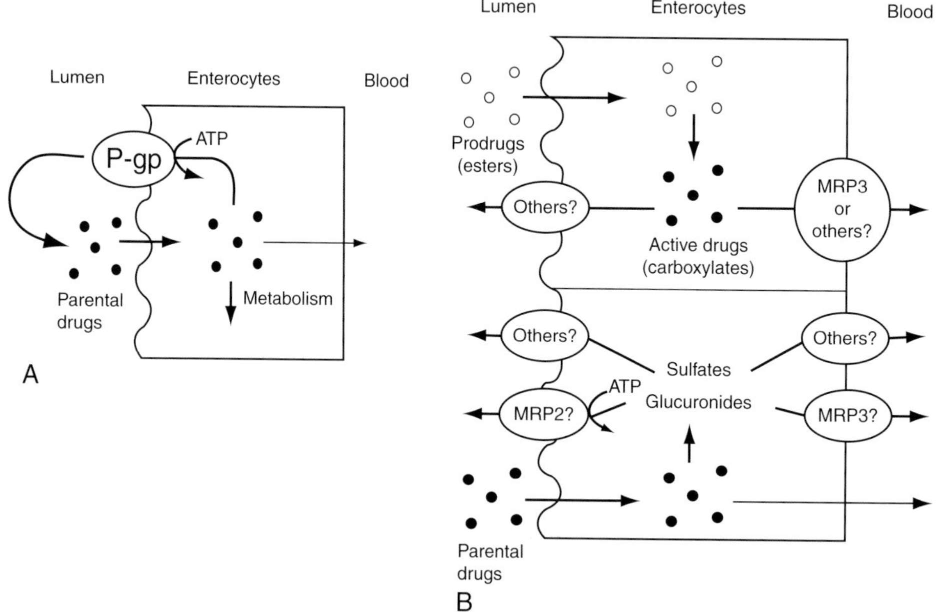

Figure 9.12 Schematic diagram illustrating the synergistic role of metabolic enzymes and efflux transporters. (A) Synergistic role of cytochrome P450 (CYP) 3A/3A4 and MDR1 P-glycoprotein (P-gp). After being taken up by enterocytes, some of the drug molecules are metabolized by CYP3A/3A4. Drug molecules that escaped metabolic conversion are eliminated from the cells into the lumen via P-gp. (B) Synergistic role of conjugative enzymes/carboxyesterases and efflux transporters for organic anions. After being taken up by enterocytes, some of the drug molecules are metabolized to form the glucuronide- and sulfated conjugates. Ester-type prodrugs are metabolized in enterocytes to form the active drugs (carboxylates). These conjugative metabolites and carboxylates are excreted from enterocytes via transporters for organic anions (such as multidrug resistance associated protein (MRP) 2 and 3, and other unidentified transporters). Reprinted from European Journal of Pharmaceutical Sciences: Official Journal of the European Federation for Pharmaceutical Sciences, Volume 12, H. Suzuki and Y. Sugiyama, Role of metabolic enzymes and efflux transporters in the absorption of drugs from the small intestine, pp. 3–12, Copyright 2000, with permission from Elsevier.

Table 9.13 Role of Pgp Modulation on Drug Exposure Following Oral Administration to Humans. Reprinted from Drug Metabolism and Pharmacokinetics, Volume 17, N. Mizuno and Y. Sugiyama, Drug transporters: Their role and importance in the selection and development of new drugs, pp. 93–108, Copyright 2002, with permission from the Japanese Society for the Study of Xenobiotics.

Pgp Inhibition	Inhibitor	Substrate	Effect
	Cyclosporine	Docetaxel*	↑ Oral bioavailability
		Paclitaxel*	
	Erythromycin	Cyclosporine*	↑ Cmax and AUC with no change in $t_{1/2}$ (suggests local effect on absorption)
		Fexofenadine	
		Talinolol	
		Saquinavir*	
	GF120918	Paclitaxel*	↑ Oral bioavailability
	Ketoconazole	Fexofenadine	↑ Cmax and AUC
		Saquinavir*	↑ AUC
	Valspodar	Digoxin	
Pgp Induction	**Inducer**	**Substrate**	**Effect**
	Rifampin	Digoxin	↓ Cmax and AUC with no change in $t_{1/2}$
		Fexofenadine	↓ Cmax and AUC
		Saquinavir	↓ Oral bioavailability
		Tacrolimus	↑ Intestinal Pgp expression,
	St Johns Wort	Digoxin	↓ Cmax and AUC

*Denotes compounds that are also substrates for CYP3A4, suggesting a dual role of Pgp and CYP on intestinal absorption.

circulation through intestinal exsorption. In this way, the intestine does represent yet another route from drug excretion in the body. The phenomenon of intestinal exsorption is not widely studied, and under normal conditions the intestine is not considered one of the primary organs for drug clearance, as are liver and kidney. However, in cases of acute drug toxicity, enterocapillary exsorption provides for a pathway for drug diffusion out of the bloodstream to increase systemic drug clearance, a process that is maximized by oral administration of activated charcoal. Additionally, preclinical studies have demonstrated a role of Pgp in intestinal exsorption of several drugs (digoxin, irinotecan) following IV dosing.

9.5.2 Drug Excretion into Breast Milk

The benefits of breast-feeding on the health and development of newborns are widely recognized, including reduced incidence of infections, diabetes, and sudden infant death syndrome. However, a mother's medication use during lactation increases the risk of infant drug exposure. Thus drug excretion into breast milk is important from a clinical and toxicological perspective. Although most drugs show minimal excretion into breast milk, adverse drug reactions in breast-fed babies have been attributed to antidepressants (fluoxetine, doxepine) and xanthines (caffeine, theophylline).

The potential impact of drug excretion into breast milk is greater for low molecular weight, lipophilic, cationic molecules with minimal plasma binding. These factors promote passive diffusion across the mammary gland. The acidic pH of milk favors retention of these compounds through ion-trapping; that is, a weakly basic molecule becomes ionized in the acidic pH, thereby restricting drug transfer back to the circulation. Evidence is also beginning to emerge regarding the role of transport systems in the mammary gland, although their identification and functional significance have not been elucidated.

9.5.3 Salivary Drug Excretion

Although saliva is considered a minimal route for drug excretion, it does have potential significance in the area of therapeutic drug monitoring (TDM). For medications with a narrow therapeutic range, plasma drug levels are used to assess clinical response. Obvious drawbacks to plasma monitoring include sample collection (invasive) and analysis. From a pharmacokinetic perspective, however, TDM typically involves measurement of total plasma concentrations of drug, whereas only unbound drug is available for distribution and activity.

Saliva is a possible alternative sampling fluid to plasma for therapeutic monitoring. A sample can be collected with minimal patient discomfort. Perhaps more importantly, saliva is protein-free, and saliva provides a measurement of the concentration of free (unbound) drug in the plasma (assuming distributional equilibrium). Saliva sampling has been proposed for therapeutic monitoring of anticonvulsant medications such as phenytoin and carbamazepine. It may also be beneficial in special patient populations such as children.

9.5.4 Other Routes of Drug Excretion

Although not widely reported in the scientific literature, other organs in the body are capable of drug excretion. The primary route of elimination of some inhalation anesthetics (e.g., isoflurane) is exhalation, a process that depends on cardiac output to the lung and alveolar ventilation. Given the current research focus on the pulmonary drug delivery, a better understanding of the role of pulmonary excretion of drug clearance is anticipated. Passive diffusion of lipophilic molecules across eccrine and lacrimal glands can result in drug excretion in sweat and tears, respectively. Likewise, sebaceous drug excretion is also possible. However, the overall contribution of these processes to drug excretion is considered minimal.

9.6 DRUG EXCRETION: ISSUES TO CONSIDER

9.6.1 Species Differences in Transporter Expression

Successful drug development requires application of preclinical data to predict clinical outcomes. Preclinical studies integrate physicochemical, pharmacokinetic, and toxicokinetic properties of a drug using a variety of experimental techniques at the molecular, cellular, organ, and whole animal level. Given the emergence of membrane transport systems as a fundamental determinant of drug excretion pathways, species differences in transporter expression and function impact the way in which preclinical data is collected and interpreted.

Rats are routinely the species of choice for preclinical drug disposition studies. Comparing rats and humans, not all membrane transporters are orthologous, meaning that amino acid sequences of transport proteins are among species. Transporters such as OATPs show significant differences between species (Table 9.5). Additionally, MRP2-mediated biliary excretion is much more efficient in rats. Although there is limited data available on species differences in transporters, this can have significant implications when interpreting data generated in preclinical studies.

It should also be pointed out that this chapter emphasized drug excretion in humans. As such, many of the figures and tables were based on transport mechanisms in man.

9.6.2 Gender Differences in Drug Excretion

The effect of gender on drug disposition and activity may have important clinical consequences. Differences in pharmacokinetics between males and females are attributed to biological differences between genders including body weight, body composition, and hormones. Moreover, sex-related differences in membrane transporter expression and activity are an underlying cause of these differences.

There are a vast number of drugs that undergo active secretion by the kidney. Therefore, disparities in renal excretion efficiency between males and females may result in gender differences in systemic exposure of narrow therapeutic range medications, and risks to nephrotoxic agents. As a consequence of reduced GFR, filtration clearance is lower in females. Moreover, research has shown differential expression of renal transporters between genders. Preclinical data demonstrate that renal OAT1 and OAT3 levels are increased in males, and female rats show increased expression of OAT2. Likewise, expression of OCT2 is increased in males, although there are no apparent differences in OCT3. Since it is unclear whether similar gender differences in transporter expression exist in humans, further studies are warranted in order to clarify the clinical importance of gender differences in renal excretion.

Studies conducted to date also point to gender-related differences in expression of Pgp and MDR2 in the canalicular membrane of hepatocyte, with higher expression in females compared to males. These differences, which appear to be regulated in part by sex hormones, may lead to differences in drug biliary excretion between genders.

9.6.3 Pharmacogenetics of Drug Excretion

Pharmacogenetics involves the impact of genetic variation on drug response. The link between genetically determined variation in drug metabolism enzymes (e.g., cytochrome p450, N-acetyltransferase) and intersubject differences in pharmacokinetics is well established. Likewise, there is an increasing awareness that differences in transporter expression can impact the efficacy and safety of pharmacotherapy.

In terms of drug excretion, recent discoveries point to genetic variations in the function of drug efflux transporters (ABC family) and cellular uptake transporters (SLC family). SNPs (single nucleotide polymorphisms) of these transport proteins are a potential source of interindividual variability in drug disposition and pharmacological response. For example, SNPs in Pgp, MRP2, or BCRP may lead to impaired biliary drug excretion. Likewise, genetic polymorphisms in OATPs, OATs, and OCTs can impact drug uptake across the hepatocyte (OATP) and renal epithelial cell, resulting in reduced hepatic and renal clearance.

9.6.4 Pharmacokinetics of Large Molecules

This chapter emphasized drug excretion mechanisms for small molecules, given that most medications fall into this category. It should be recognized, however, that peptide and protein therapeutics now constitute a substantial portion of the compounds under preclinical and clinical evaluation. Large molecule therapeutics represent promising approaches to treat a variety of diseases, but they also bring to light challenges to drug development scientists in terms of manufacturing drug delivery and bioanalysis. Additionally, large molecules have different pharmacokinetic profiles than conventional small molecule drugs. For example, peptide and protein drugs are cleared by the same catabolic pathways used to eliminate endogenous and dietary proteins. Although both the kidney and liver can metabolize proteins by hydrolysis, there is minimal clearance of protein therapeutics via conventional renal and biliary excretion mechanisms. You must recognize these differences when applying the principles and concepts presented in this chapter to large molecule therapeutics.

9.7 CONCLUSIONS AND FUTURE PERSPECTIVES

Pharmacokinetics, the mathematical characterization of drug disposition, is often referred to by the acronym ADME, which signifies the four key aspects of the body's handling of xenobiotics: absorption, distribution, metabolism, and excretion. It goes without saying, therefore, that excretion mechanisms in the kidney, liver, and other organs play a fundamental role in drug disposition. Since clearance is ultimately the link between the dose that a patient receives and the plasma level that is achieved, alterations in drug excretion due to disease, drug interactions, genetics, and other factors can have a direct impact on clinical outcomes. Consequently, effective drug therapy requires an understanding of the factors leading to intersubject variability in drug clearance.

The goal of this chapter was to highlight the major mechanisms involved in drug excretion. Our knowledge of drug movement across biological membranes has increased dramatically over the past decade, and this is only the beginning. Through advances in protein science, cellular uptake and efflux processes are being characterized at a molecular level. In the kidney for example, it was not very long ago that drug secretion was classified into two general systems for acids and bases, akin to our early view of cytochrome P450 being one enzyme. Following in the wake of the tremendous advances in the area of drug metabolism, the complexity of renal drug transport mechanisms has been brought to light over recent years, and our understanding of these processes continues to evolve. The same can be said for other organ systems such as the liver, intestinal tract, and CNS, and we have only scratched the surface in terms of our understanding in this area.

Looking forward, advances in molecular biology and genetic engineering will lead to further discoveries of how drugs and metabolites are transported by the kidney and liver. This will undoubtedly involve characterization of the substrate binding site of transport proteins and the mechanisms involved in transporter induction and inhibition. Furthermore, the role of genetic polymorphisms on individual transport systems will become better defined.

With regard to drug development, the availability of high-throughput screening tools for assessing transporter affinity will allow scientists to rapidly evaluate the role of individual transport systems on drug disposition *in vivo*. Having this information early on in the development process will positively impact drug candidate selection, and allow for development of safer and more efficacious drug therapies.

In the not too distant future, drug and dosage selection will be individualized based on a patient's genetic profile, which will be readily accessible by a physician at the point of care. This will not only involve selecting the appropriate therapy based on a patient's unique genome related to disease progression, but optimizing a dosing regimen based on the patient's genetic profile with regard to pharmacokinetics. Under this scenario of "personalized medicine," the risks to the patient in terms of ineffective therapy or likelihood for adverse effects will be minimized. In this regard, unraveling the mechanisms of drug excretion is an important endeavor, and progress in this area will undoubtedly play a pivotal role in optimizing therapeutic outcomes in the years to come.

REVIEW QUESTIONS

1. What are the two primary membrane transport families involved in drug excretion?
2. Describe the role of P-glycoprotein in multidrug resistance (MDR), including the potential therapeutic use of Pgp inhibitors to reverse MDR.
3. List and briefly describe three mechanisms of drug excretion by the kidney, including the factors affecting each of these processes.
4. What is the intact nephron hypothesis, and how does it apply to dosage determinations in patients with renal dysfunction?
5. List the main transport systems for drug transport across the basolateral and luminal membranes of the proximal tubule cell.
6. Characterize the general types of drug interactions originating through renal excretion mechanisms.
7. Explain the role of sinusoidal transport on hepatic clearance, and list the various transporters that mediate drug uptake into the hepatocyte.
8. Describe enterohepatic recycling in terms of the organs and mechanisms involved and the impact of enterohepatic recycling on pharmacokinetics.
9. Characterize the role of the transporter MRP3 as a protective mechanism during cholestasis.
10. How does inhibition of BSEP by medications potentially lead to hepatotoxicity?
11. Explain how renal disease affects hepatobiliary excretion.
12. Besides the renal and biliary excretion, what are other potential mechanisms of drug excretion?
13. Describe how pharmacogenomics will impact our understanding of drug excretion in the future, including its role on intersubject variability in patient response to drug therapy.

REFERENCES

Books

Gibson, G., & Skett, P. (2001). *Introduction to Drug Metabolism* (3rd ed.). Cheltenham, UK: Nelson Thornes.

Kwon, Y. (2001). *Handbook of Essential Pharmacokinetics, Pharmacodynamics and Drug Metabolism for Industrial Scientists*: Springer-Verlag.

Matern, S., Boyer, J. L., Keppler, D., & Meier-Abt, P. J. (Eds.). (2001). *Hepatobiliary Transport: From Bench to Bedside.* (Falk Symposium, Volume 121A). The Netherlands: Kluwer Academic Publishers, BV.

Rogge, M., & Taft, D. (Eds.). (2005). *Preclinical Drug Development*. Boca Raton, FL: Taylor and Francis.

Wang, B., You, G., & Morris, M. (2007). *Drug Transporters: Molecular Characterization and Role in Drug Disposition*. Hoboken: Wiley-Interscience.

Review Articles and Original Papers

Anzai, N., Kanai, Y., & Endou, H. (2006). Organic anion transporter family: Current knowledge. *Journal of Pharmacological Sciences, 100*, 411–426.

Ayrton, A., & Morgan, P. (2001). Role of transport proteins in drug absorption, distribution and excretion. *Xenobiotica; The Fate of Foreign Compounds in Biological Systems, 31*, 469–497.

Benet, L. Z., & Cummins, C. L. (2001). The drug efflux-metabolism alliance: Biochemical aspects. *Advanced Drug Delivery Reviews, 50*, S3–S11.

Bonate, P., Reith, K., & Weir, S. (1998). Drug interactions at the renal level: Implications for drug development. *Clinical Pharmacokinetics, 34*, 375–404.

Booth, C. L., Pollack, G. M., & Brouwer, K. L. R. (1996). Hepatobiliary disposition of valproic acid and valproate glucoronide: Use of a pharmacokinetic model to examine the rate-limiting steps and potential sites of drug interactions. *Hepatol, 23*, 771–780.

Borst, P., & Oude Elferink, R. (2002). Mammalian ABC transporters in health and disease. *Annual Review of Biochemistry, 71*, 537–592.

Brouwer, K. L. R., & Pollack, G. M. (2002). Pharmacogenomics: Is the right drug for the right patient sufficient? *Advanced Drug Delivery Reviews, 54*, 1243–1244.

Chandra, P., & Boiuwer, K. L. R. (2004). The complexities of hepatic drug transport: Current knowledge and emerging concepts. *Pharmaceutical Research, 21*, 719–735.

Chyka, P. A. (1995). Multiple-dose activated charcoal and enhancement of systemic drug clearance: Summary of studies in animals and human volunteers. *Journal of Toxicology. Clinical Toxicology, 33*, 399–405.

Dallas, S., Miller, D. S., & Bendayan, R. (2006). Multidrug resistance-associated proteins: Expression and function in the central nervous system. *Pharmacological Reviews, 58*, 140–161.

Dresser, M., Leabman, M. K., & Giacomini, K. M. (2001). Transporters involved in the elimination of drugs in the kidney: Organic anion transporters and organic cation transporters. *Journal of Pharmaceutical Sciences, 90*, 397–421.

Elwi, A. N., Damaraju, V. L., Baldwin, S. A., Young, J. D., Sawyer, M. B., & Cass, C. E. (2006). Renal nucleoside transporters: Physiological and clinical implications. *Biochemistry and Cell Biology = Biochimie et Biologie Cellulaire, 84*, 844–858.

Endres, C. J., Hsiao, P., Chung, F. S., and Unadkat, J. D. (2006). The role of transporters in drug interactions. *European Journal of Pharmaceutical Sciences: Official Journal of the European Federation for Pharmaceutical Sciences, 27*, 501–517.

Faber, K. N., Muller, M., & Jansen, P. L. M. (2003). Drug transport proteins in the liver. *Advanced Drug Delivery Reviews, 33*, 107–124.

Faber, K. N., Muller, M., & Jansen, P. L. M. (2003). Drug transport proteins in the liver. *Advanced Drug Delivery Reviews, 55*, 107–124.

Hediger, M. A., Romero, M. F., Peng, J. B., Rolfs, A., Takanaga, H., & Bruford, E. A. (2004). The ABCs of solute carriers: Physiological, pathological and therapeutic implications of human membrane transport proteins. *Pflugers Archiv: European Journal of Physiology, 447*, 465–468.

Heimer, G. M., & Englund, D. E. (1986). Enterohepatic recirculation of estriol: Inhibition by activated charcoal. *Acta Endocrinologica, 113*, 93–95.

Hood, E. (2003). Pharmacogenomics: The prominse of personalized medicine. *Environmental Health Perspectives, 111*, A581–A589.

Inui, K. I., Masuda, S., & Saito, H. (2000). Cellular and molecular aspects of drug transport in the kidney. *Kidney International, 58*, 944–958.

Ito, S., & Lee, A. (2003). Drug excretion into breast milk—overview. *Advanced Drug Delivery Reviews, 55*, 617–627.

Johnson, H. L., & Maibach, H. I. (1971). Drug excretion in human eccrine sweat. *The Journal of Investigative Dermatology, 56*, 182–188.

Kerb, H. (2006). Implications of genetic polymorphisms in drug transporters for pharmacotherapy. *Cancer Letters, 234*, 4–33.

Kivisto, K. T., & Niemi, M. (2006). Influence of drug transporter polymorphisms on pravastatin pharmacokinetics in humans. *Pharmaceutical Research, 24*, 239–247.

Koepsell, H., Lips, K., & Volk, C. (2006). Polyspecific organic cation transporters: Structure, function, physiological roles, and biopharmaceutical implications. *Pharmaceutical Research, 24*, 1227–1251.

Kushuhara, H., & Sugiyama, Y. (2002). Role of transporters in the tissue-selective distribution and elimination of drugs: Transporters in the liver, small intestine, brain and kidney. *Journal of Controlled Release: Official Journal of the Controlled Release Society, 78*, 43–54.

Kushuhara, H., Suzuki, H., & Sugiyama, Y. (1998). The role of P-glycoprotein and canalicular multispecific organic anion transporter in the hepatic excretion of drugs. *Journal of Pharmaceutical Sciences, 87*, 1025–1040.

Lam, Y. W. F., Banerji, S., Hatfield, C., & Talbert, R. L. (1997). Principles of drug administration in renal insufficiency. *Clinical Pharmacokinetics, 32*, 30–57.

Lin, J. H., & Yamazaki, M. (2003). Role of p-glycoprotein in pharmacokinetics: Clinical implications. *Clinical Pharmacokinetics, 42*, 59–98.

Liu, L., & Pang, K. S. (2005). The roles of transporters and enzymes in hepatic drug processing. *DMD, 33*, 1–9.

Mao, Q., & Unadkat, J. D. (2005). Role of the breast cancer resistance protein (abcg2) in drug transport. *The AAPS Journal, 7*, E118–E133.

Marzolini, C., Tirona, R. G., & Kim, R. B. (2004). Pharmacogenomics of the OATP and OAT families. *Pharmacogenomics, 5*, 273–282.

Masereeuw, R., & Russel, F. G. M. (2001). Mechanisms and clinical implications of renal drug excretion. *Drug Metabolism Reviews, 33*, 299–351.

Meijer, D. K. F., Smit, J. W., & Muller, M. (1997). Hepatobiliary elimination of cationic drugs: The role of P-glycoproteins and other ATP-dependent transporters. *Advanced Drug Delivery Reviews, 25*, 159–200.

Merino, G., van Herwaarden, A. E., Wagenaar, E., Jonker, J. W., & Schinkel, A. H. (2005). Sex-dependent expression and activity of the atp-binding cassette transporter breast cancer resistance protein (bcrp/abcg2) in liver. *Molecular Pharmacology, 67*, 1765–1771.

Mikkaichi, T., et al. (2004). The organic anion transporter (OATP) family. *Drug Metabolism and Pharmacokinetics, 1*, 171–179.

Mizuno, N., Niwa, T., Yotsumoto, Y., & Sugiyama, Y. (2003). Impact of drug transporter studies on drug discovery and development. *Pharmacological Reviews, 55*, 425–461.

Mizuno, N., & Sugiyama, Y. (2002). Drug trasnporters: Their role and importance in the selection and development of new drugs. *Drug Metabolism and Pharmacokinetics, 17*, 93–108.

Nakatani-Freshwater, T., Babayeva, M., Dontabhaktuni, A., & Taft, D. R. (2006). Effects of trimethoprim on the clearance of apricitabine, a deoxycytidine analog reverse transcriptase inhibitor, and Lamivudine in the isolated perfused rat kidney. *The Journal of Pharmacology and Experimental Therapeutics, 319*, 941–947.

Omote, H., Hiasa, M., Matsumoto, T., Otsuka, M., & Moriyama, Y. (2006). The MATE proteins as fundamental transporters of metabolic and xenobiotic organic cations. *Trends in Pharmacological Sciences, 27*, 587–593.

Otsuka, M., Matsumoto, T., Morimoto, R., Arioka, S., Omote, H., & Moriyama, Y. (2005). A human transporter protein that mediates the final excretion step for toxic organic cations. *PNAS, 102*, 17928–17928.

Oude Elferink, R. P. J., Meijer, D. K. F., Kuipers, F., Jansen, P. L. M., Groen, A. K., & Groothuis, G. M. M. (1995). Hepatobiliary secretion of organic compounds; Molecular mechanisms of membrane transport. *Biochimica et Biophysica Acta, 1241*, 215–268.

Pang, K. S., & Rowland, M. (1977). Hepatic clearance of drugs I: Theoretical considerations of a "well-stirred" model and a "parallel-tube" model. Influence of hepatic blood flow, plasma and blood cell binding, and the hepatocellular enzymatic activity on hepatic drug clearance. *Journal of Pharmacokinetics and Biopharmaceutics, 5*, 625–653.

Perri, D., Ito, S., Rowsell, V., & Shear, N. H. (2003). The kidney? The body's playground for drugs: An overview of renal drug handling with selected clinical correlates. *The Canadian Journal of Clinical Pharmacology = Journal Canadien de Pharmacologie Clinique, 10*, 17–23.

Pleuvy, B. J. (2005). Modes of drug elimination. *Anaesthesia and Intensive Care Medicine, 6*, 277–279.

Pritchard, J. B., & Miller, D. S. (1996). Renal secretion of organic anions and cations. *Kidney International, 49,* 1649–1654.

Pritchard, J. B., & Miller, D. S. (1997). Renal secretion of organic anions: A multistep process. *Advanced Drug Delivery Reviews, 25,* 231–242.

Rizwan, A. N., & Burckhardt, G. (2006). Organic anion transporters of the SLC22 family: Biopharmaceutical, physiological, and pathological roles. *Pharmaceutical Research,* 24, 1227–1251.

Roberts, M. S., Magnusson, B. M., Burczynski, F. J., & Weiss, M. (2002). Enterohepatic circulation: Physiological, pharmacokinetic and clinical implications. *Clinical Pharmacokinetics, 41,* 751–790.

Robertson, E. E., & Rankin, G. O. (2006). Human renal organic anion transporters: Characteristics and contributions to drug and drug metabolite excretion. *Pharmacology & Therapeutics, 109,* 399–412.

Sakaeda, T., Nakamura, T., & Okumura, K. (2003). Pharmacogenetics of MDR1 and its impact on the pharmacokinetics and pharmacodynamics of drugs. *Pharmacogenomics, 4,* 397–410.

Schinkel, A. H., & Jonker, J. W. (2003). Mammalian drug efflux transporters of the ATP binding cassette (ABC) family: An overview. *Advanced Drug Delivery Reviews, 55,* 3–29.

Sekine, T., Miyazaki, H., & Endou, H. (2006). Molecular physiology of renal organic anion transporters. *American Journal of Physiology. Renal Physiology, 290,* 251–261.

Shitara, Y., Horie, T., & Sugiyama, Y. (2006). Transporters as a determinant of drug clearance and tissue distribution. *European Journal of Pharmaceutical Sciences: Official Journal of the European Federation for Pharmaceutical Sciences, 27,* 425–446.

Shitara, Y., Sato, H., & Sugiyama, Y. (2005). Evaluation of drug-drug interaction in the hepatobiliary and renal transport of drugs. *Annual Review of Pharmacology and Toxicology, 45,* 689–723.

Statkevich, P., Fournier, D. J., & Sweeney, K. R. (1994). Characterization of methotrexate elimination and interaction with indomethacin and flurbiprofen in the isolated perfused rat kidney. *The Journal of Pharmacology and Experimental Therapeutics, 265,* 1118–1124.

Sun, H., Frassetto, L., & Benet, L. Z. (2006). Effects of renal failure on drug transport and metabolism. *Pharmacology & Therapeutics, 109,* 1–11.

Suzuki, H., & Sugiyama, Y. (2000). Role of metabolic enzymes and efflux transporters in the absorption of drugs from the small intestine. *European Journal of Pharmaceutical Sciences: Official Journal of the European Federation for Pharmaceutical Sciences, 12,* 3–12.

Sweeney, K. R., Hsyu, P. H., Statkevich, P., & Taft, D. R. (1995). Renal disposition and drug interaction screening of (-)-2′-deoxy-3′-thiacytidine (3TC) in the isolated perfused rat kidney. *Pharmaceutical Research, 12,* 1958–1963.

Sweet, D. H. (2005). Organic anion transporter (Slc22a) family members as mediators of toxicity. *Toxicology and Applied Pharmacology, 204*(3), 198–215.

Taft, D. R., Dontabhaktuni, A., Babayeva, M., Nakatani-Freshwater, T., & Savant, I. A. (2006). Application of the isolated perfused rat kidney model to assess gender effects on drug excretion. *Drug Development and Industrial Pharmacy, 32,* 919–928.

Tang, L., Persky, A. M., Hochhaus, G., & Meibohm, B. (2004). Pharmacokinetic aspects of biotechnology products. *Journal of Pharmaceutical Sciences, 93,* 2184–2204.

Tanihara, Y., Masuda, S., Sato, T., Katsura, T., Ogawa, O., & Inui, K. I. (2007). Substrate specificity of MATE1 and MATE2-K, human multidrug and toxin extrusions/H(+)-organic cation antiporters. Apr 13, 2007 (Epub ahead of print)

Tucker, G. I. (1984). Measurement of the renal clearance of drugs. *British Journal of Clinical Pharmacology, 12,* 761–770.

Wright, S. H., & Dantzler, W. H. (2004). Molecular and cellular physiology of renal organic cation and anion transport. *Physiological Reviews, 84,* 987–1049.

Zamek-Gliszczynski, M. J., Hoffmaster, K. A., Nezasa, K., Tallman, M. H., & Brouwer, K. L. R. (2006). Integration of hepatic drug transporters and phase II metabolizing enzymes: Mechanisms of hepatic excretion of sulfate, glucuronide, and glutathione metabolites. *European Journal of Pharmaceutical Sciences: Official Journal of the European Federation for Pharmaceutical Sciences, 27,* 447–486.

Zhou, F., & You, G. (2006). Molecular insights into the structure-function relationship of organic anion transporters OATs. *Pharmaceutical Research, 24,* 28–36.

Chapter

10

Pharmacokinetic Modeling

James P. Byers ▪ Jeffrey G. Sarver

OUTLINE

10.1 INTRODUCTION

Pharmacokinetics is a branch of pharmacology that employs mathematical models to describe what happens to a chemical substance within the body. The word *pharmacokinetics* combines the root word *kinetics*, which is the study of how things change with time, with the prefix *pharmaco*, which means pertaining to a pharmaceutical agent or drug. It follows then that pharmacokinetic (PK) models focus on how the concentration (or amount) of drug in the body changes with time. Changes in drug concentration with time depend on the relative rates of drug ADME processes (absorption, distribution, metabolism, and excretion) taking place in the body. PK models incorporate mathematical representations of the ADME processes to provide equations that relate drug concentrations versus time to biological parameters inherent in the ADME processes. PK models can then be applied in two different ways:

- Analyze measured drug concentration versus time data in order to evaluate the ADME biological parameters for the drug.
- Predict drug concentrations versus time based on estimated or previously measured ADME biological parameters for the drug.

The usefulness of PK models is ultimately derived from the fact that drug concentrations are indicative of the drug's duration and level of effect. A generalized view of the relationship between drug concentrations and drug effect is illustrated in Figure 10.1. Hence PK models are useful in deriving the biological parameters that control drug activity, as well as designing appropriate therapeutic dosing strategies. Drug concentrations in the target tissues (site of action) are most closely correlated with drug effects, but measuring or predicting target tissue concentrations is generally difficult if not impossible. Most drug concentration measurements, particularly those in humans, are made via whole blood, plasma (whole blood with cellular components removed), or serum (whole blood with cellular and clotting factors removed) samples. Plasma samples are most commonly used, so this chapter will use the general term *plasma concentration* (C_p) when referring to drug concentrations measured in the plasma, serum, or whole blood. Fortunately, plasma concentrations provide an adequate relationship with activity for a large majority of drugs, and PK models remain the primary means of designing and adjusting therapeutic dosing regimens.

Being a single chapter within a book describing a variety of pharmacology topics, there are limitations to the level of detail that can be provided in this chapter. As such, this chapter will describe the mathematical forms used in predicting concentrations and analyzing measured concentrations for the most common types

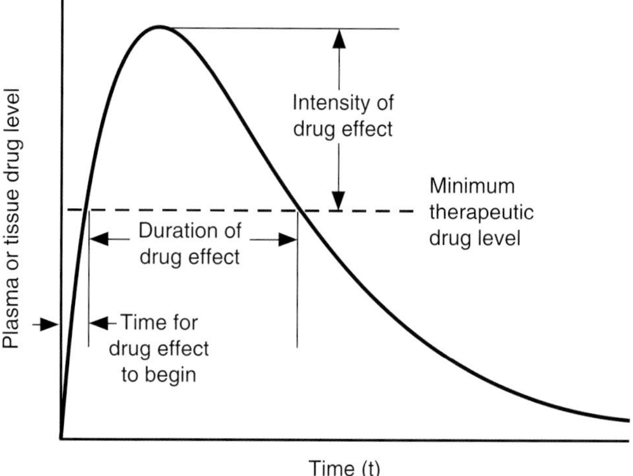

Figure 10.1 General relationship between drug concentration versus time and drug effect.

of PK models, but space does not allow for the inclusion of extensive application examples or problems. A number of textbooks devoted entirely to the topic of PK modeling are listed in the References, for readers needing more information. It should be further noted that while the discussions in this chapter take the substance under consideration to be a drug, the same equations and principles can be applied to many other types of chemical agent, such as toxins and environmental pollutants. The application of PK models to toxic substances is called *toxicokinetics*, and texts related to this application are also listed in the References.

10.1.1 Chapter Overview

This chapter is meant to provide readers with a basic understanding of the most commonly used types of PK models. It begins with a review of how the ADME processes, which have already been described in some detail in previous chapters, are defined and mathematically incorporated into PK modeling schemes. Equations are then developed for standard single and multiple compartment PK models as applied to a single delivery of drug by bolus intravenous injection (instantaneous absorption), intravenous infusion (zero-order absorption), and nonvascular routes such as oral, intramuscular, or subcutaneous drug delivery (first-order absorption). These models are then extended to the multiple dosing situations for each of these types of drug delivery. The principles behind other more advanced PK modeling concepts and approaches also are included at the end of this chapter.

10.1.2 Basic Pharmacokinetic Terms

A few basic terms must be defined before a meaningful discussion of PK models can take place. Figure 10.2 offers a schematic representation of some of the terms that will be used. The amount of drug delivered to the body is the *dose*. The means and location by which the drug is delivered to the body is the *route of administration*. Common routes of administration include intravenous (*IV*), oral ingestion (*po*), subcutaneous (*sc* or *sq*), and intramuscular (*IM*). The movement of drug molecules from the site of delivery to the systemic circulation is called *absorption*. For some routes of administration, a portion of the drug dose may never reach the systemic circulation. The fraction of the administered dose that reaches the systemic circulation is called the bioavailable fraction, or *bioavailability*.

Once absorbed into the systemic circulation, blood flow delivers the drug to the body tissues. In some cases, specific body tissues act as storage depots, with drug initially collecting in the tissues while plasma concentrations are high, then later being released back into the blood stream after plasma concentrations lower with time. This back and forth movement of a drug between circulating plasma and tissues (including the target tissue) is called *distribution*.

Pharmacodynamics is a term used to describe the relationship between drug concentrations (in the plasma or target tissue) and the resultant pharmacological effect. Enzymatic conversion of the drug molecule into a different chemical form is called *metabolism*, with the converted molecules labeled metabolites. *Excretion* is the process by which drug molecules or metabolites are discharged into body wastes, typically in the urine or feces. *Elimination* is a collective term for all processes that decrease the amount of drug in the body, which includes both metabolism and excretion. *Disposition* is the term for everything that happens to a drug in the body, so it represents the sum of all ADME processes.

10.1.3 Mathematics in Pharmacokinetics

Along with the basic PK terms in the previous section, some basic mathematical principles must also be reviewed in order to understand PK models. Although the equations in pharmacokinetics can sometimes seem overwhelming to the mathematically squeamish, it turns

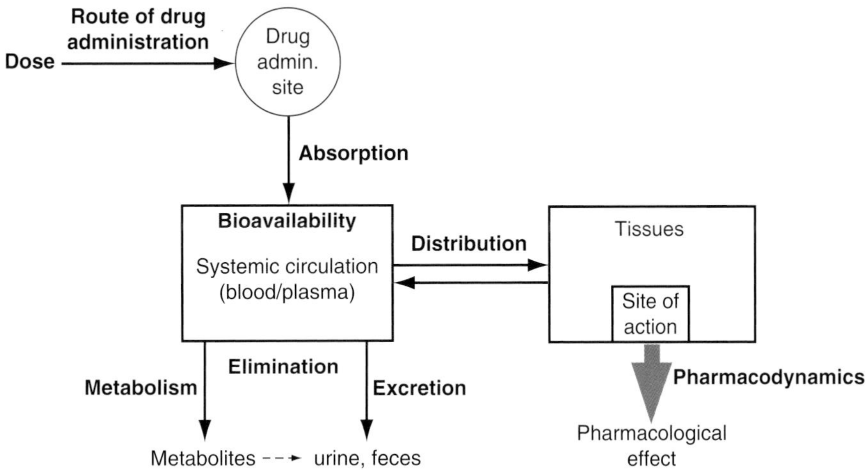

Figure 10.2 Simple schematic diagram illustrating common pharmacokinetic (PK) terms.

out that most of these equations involve only a few basic mathematical principles that show up repeatedly in different types of PK models. This section will review some of the mathematical principles that are encountered most frequently in pharmacokinetics.

10.1.3.1 Logarithms

A logarithm (typically abbreviated as log) is defined mathematically as the power (k) to which a base number (x) must be raised to produce a given product (y). This means that

$$\text{if } y = x^k \quad \text{then} \quad \log_x(y) = k \qquad (10.1)$$

where the subscript x after log indicates x is the base number used for the logarithm. Logarithms have a number of special properties, some of which are encountered frequently in PK modeling. First is that the logarithm of one always equals zero, no matter what value the base number (x) has:

$$\log_x(1) = 0 \qquad (10.2)$$

The second is that the logarithm of the product of two numbers is equal to the sum of the logarithm of the two numbers, so that

$$\log_x(y \cdot z) = \log_x(y) + \log_x(z) \qquad (10.3)$$

The logarithm of a number (z) raised to a power (k) follows the relation

$$\log_x(z^k) = k \cdot \log_x(z) \qquad (10.4)$$

The rules in Equations (10.3) and (10.4) can then be combined to give another useful relationship that will be encountered often:

$$\log_x(a \cdot z^k) = \log(a) + k \cdot \log_x(z) \qquad (10.5)$$

These are the logarithm properties that will be most pertinent to this chapter.

Although the base number (x) used in a logarithm can be any positive number, it turns out that only two different base numbers are commonly encountered in pharmacokinetics. The first, a logarithm using a base number of 10 ($\log_{10}$), is probably already familiar to many readers. It is used in many different disciplines, and can be written

$$\text{if } y = 10^k \quad \text{then} \quad \log_{10}(y) = k \qquad (10.6)$$

The second base number may not be as familiar to some readers, but it is actually encountered much more frequently in PK models as well as many other areas of mathematics. This base number is a natural constant called e, where e has an approximate value of 2.7182818, but the actual number of digits goes on forever without repeating. The logarithm with base e is called the natural logarithm, and often is written as ln, giving

$$\text{if } y = e^k \quad \text{then} \quad \log_e(y) = \ln(y) = k \qquad (10.7)$$

The constant e will be discussed further in the next section.

10.1.3.2 Exponential Function, Exponential Decay, and Half-Life

The exponential function can be defined as the constant e raised to some power, so that the exponential of k is simply e^k. The exponential function can also be defined as the inverse of the natural logarithm, which is essentially the same as rewriting Equation (10.7) in inverse order:

$$\text{if } \ln(y) = k \quad \text{then} \quad e^k = y \qquad (10.8)$$

Applying Equation (10.2) to the exponential function yields the useful fact that

$$\text{since } \ln(1) = 0 \quad \text{then} \quad e^0 = 1 \qquad (10.9)$$

An exponential decay is a special type of exponential function where time (t) appears in the exponent multiplied by a constant that is less than zero. A variable (z) undergoing exponential decay can be written in the general form

$$z = z_0 \cdot e^{-kt} \qquad (10.10)$$

where k is a positive constant (so $-k$ must then be a constant less than zero). The term z_0 is the initial value of the variable z (value at $t = 0$), which can be demonstrated by putting zero in for t

$$\text{at } t = 0 \quad z = z_0 \cdot e^{-k \cdot 0} = z_0 \cdot 1 = z_0 \qquad (10.11)$$

The general shape of the exponential decay for variable z is shown in Figure 10.3. The general form of exponential decay can be rewritten by taking the natural logarithm of both sides of Equation (10.10), which by the earlier logarithm relationships becomes

$$\ln(z) = \ln(z_0) - k \cdot t \qquad (10.12)$$

This equation shows $\ln(z)$ has a linear relationship versus time (t) of the form $y = b + mx$, where the dependent variable y is $\ln(z)$, the independent variable x is t, the intercept b equals $\ln(z_0)$, and the slope m equals $-k$. A plot of $\ln(z)$ versus time (t) yields a straight line as shown in Figure 10.4.

Variables undergoing exponential decay exhibit a special property, in that the value of the decaying variable always drops by half (50%) after a specific period

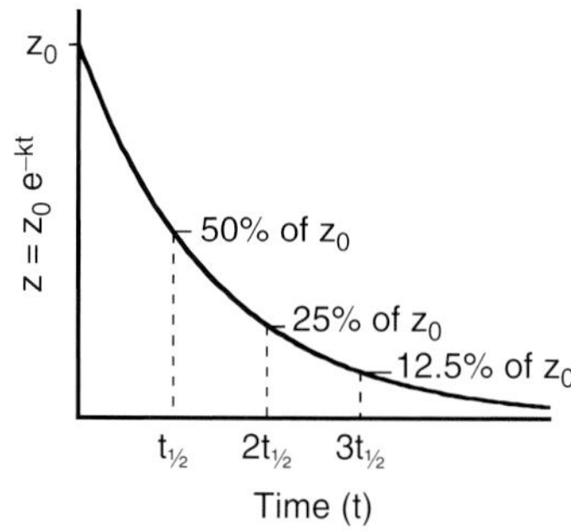

Figure 10.3 General shape of an exponential decay curve.

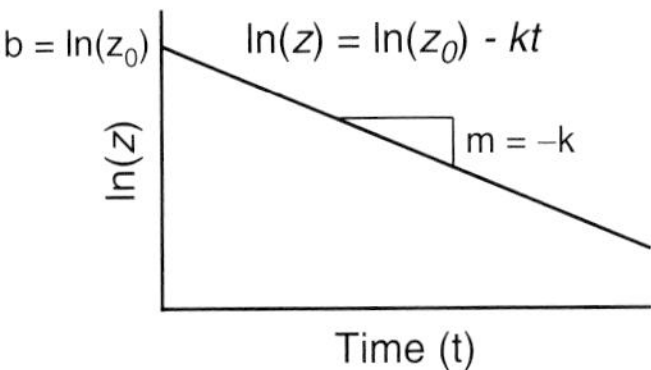

Figure 10.4 Linear relationship between the natural logarithm of an exponentially decaying variable (z) and time (t).

of time, called the half-life ($t_{1/2}$). The value of the half-life for an exponentially decaying variable such as z in Equation (10.10) can be related to the coefficient in the exponent (k) by the relation

$$t_{1/2} = \frac{\ln(2)}{k} \approx \frac{0.693}{k} \tag{10.13}$$

where the "approximately equal to" sign ($\approx$) is used because the actual value of ln(2) has an infinite number of nonrepeating digits. Since the value of the decaying variable decreases by 50% after each passage of a time interval equal to the half-life, the value of the variable is 50% of the initial value after one half-life, 25% (½ · ½) of the initial value after two-half-lives, 12.5% (½ · ½ · ½) of the initial value after three half-lives, and so on. Conversely, considering the amount the value has dropped from the initial value at time zero, there is a decrease of 50% after one half-life, 75% after two half-lives, 87.5% after three half-lives, and so on. The percent decrease versus the initial value can also be considered the amount of the decay process that has been completed. Table 10.1 lists the percent of initial value and percent of decay completed after different numbers of half-lives.

The decay process is often taken to be essentially finished after a certain number of half-lives. Different numbers of half-lives can be selected for this approximation, with five half-lives (~97% complete), seven half-lives (~99% complete), or 10 half-lives (~99.9% complete) being common estimates. In this chapter, an exponential decay process will be considered essentially complete after seven half-lives. In a related manner, an exponential decay term with a shorter half-life always becomes negligible compared to an exponential decay term with a longer half-life after a long enough period of time. From Equation (10.13) this yields

$$\text{for } k_1 > k_2 \quad B_1 \cdot e^{-k_1 \cdot t} < \\ < B_2 \cdot e^{-k_2 \cdot t} \quad \text{at large values of } t \tag{10.14}$$

where B_1 and B_2 are constants. This provides the useful relationship

$$\text{for } k_1 > k_2 \quad B_1 \cdot e^{-k_1 \cdot t} + B_2 \cdot e^{-k_2 \cdot t} \\ \approx B_2 \cdot e^{-k_2 \cdot t} \quad \text{at large values of } t \tag{10.15}$$

which will be utilized to simplify PK model equations under certain conditions.

Table 10.1 Percent of Initial Value and Percent Completion for an Exponential Decay Process

Time (t)	Percent of Initial Value	Percent Completion
$t_{1/2}$	50%	50%
$2 \cdot t_{1/2}$	25%	75%
$3 \cdot t_{1/2}$	12.5%	87.5%
$4 \cdot t_{1/2}$	6.25%	93.75%
$5 \cdot t_{1/2}$	3.125%	96.875%
$7 \cdot t_{1/2}$	0.781%	99.219%
$10 \cdot t_{1/2}$	0.098%	99.902%

10.1.3.3 Integration and Area Under the Curve

Many readers have probably had some exposure to calculus, which involves derivatives and integrals. Although both derivatives and integrals are used in developing PK models, this chapter will not go into detailed derivations of model equations, and you may be happy to learn that an extensive review of calculus is not forthcoming. This section will instead focus on the simple fact that the integral of a function $f(t)$ represents the area between the plot of the curve $y = f(t)$ and the horizontal axis represented by $y = 0$. This is illustrated in Figure 10.5. This area is called the area under the curve (AUC) in pharmacokinetics, which can then be written as

$$AUC = \int_0^\infty f(t)dt \tag{10.16}$$

As indicated earlier, exponential decay terms are the most commonly encountered functions in PK models. The integral of an exponential decay term such as that given in Equation (10.10) becomes

$$\int_0^\infty z_0 \cdot e^{-k \cdot t} dt = \frac{z_0}{k} \tag{10.17}$$

The integral of $f(t)$ between two time points t_n and t_{n+1} can also be approximated by the trapezoidal rule (illustrated in Figure 10.6) and can be written

$$\int_{t_n}^{t_{n+1}} f(t)dt \approx \frac{1}{2}\left[f(t_n) + f(t_{n+1})\right] \cdot \left(t_{n+1} - t_n\right) \tag{10.18}$$

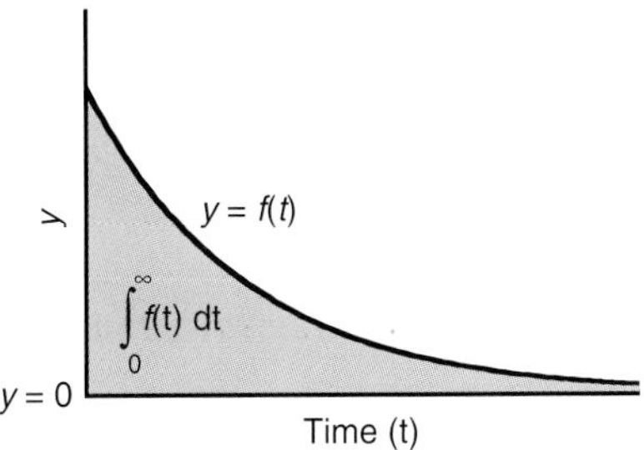

Figure 10.5 Graphical representation of the integral of the function $f(t)$ as the area under the curve.

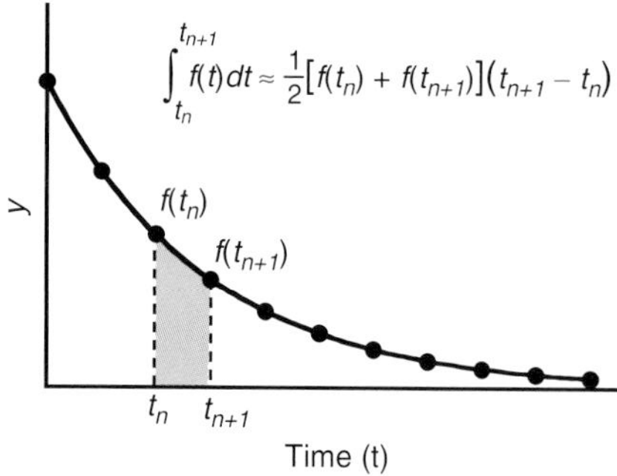

Figure 10.6 Graphical representation of the trapezoidal rule approximation for the integral of the function $f(t)$ between time points t_n and t_{n+1}.

Successive application of the trapezoidal rule to a series of points on the curve can be employed to estimate the total *AUC*. It will be shown later that the *AUC* has many important properties in PK models, so the calculation methods described here will become very useful.

10.2 CHEMICAL TRANSPORT

Before engaging in a detailed discussion of the PK modeling of ADME processes, it will be useful to discuss the basic mechanisms involved in the movement of chemicals from one location in the body to another. It will be shown that the physiochemical characteristics of the drug can have a large effect on this movement, particularly when it involves movement across a membrane or cellular barrier. In some cases, principles described in previous chapters for particular ADME processes will be discussed again here as they relate to other ADME processes (e.g., diffusion and active transport processes in Chapter 7 apply equally well to absorption and excretion processes) and PK model applications. Other aspects of chemical transport will be introduced that have not been thoroughly covered elsewhere in this book.

10.2.1 Passive Diffusion

The simplest form of molecular transport is passive diffusion. The driving force for passive diffusion is a concentration gradient. That is, a chemical in solution will move from an area of relatively high concentration to a region of lower concentration. Passive diffusion is the primary transport mechanism in many areas of the body where molecules must cross a membrane (outer surface of cell) or cellular barrier (layer of cells, such as in the capillary wall or intestinal wall) without the aid of specialized transporter proteins or fluid movement.

10.2.1.1 Passive Diffusion Transport Rate

The rate of passive diffusion transport across a membrane or cellular barrier is dependent on the concentration gradient as well as the characteristics of both the solute molecule and the barrier. The rate of transport (r_t) across the barrier can be written in the relatively simple form

$$r_t = PS\Delta C \tag{10.19}$$

where P is the barrier permeability (units of length per time), S is the surface area available for transport, and ΔC is the drug concentration difference across the barrier. The rate of transport, which has units of mass (or moles) per time, is then proportional to the permeability, surface area, and concentration gradient.

The relative magnitude of the surface area (S) is controlled largely by the geometry and physiology of the barrier that is being crossed. The capillary wall represents one of the most common barriers to diffusion transport in the body, as essentially all diffusion transport into and out of tissues occurs within a capillary bed. Maintaining capillary diameters as small as possible (generally about the same size as the diameter of a red blood cell) throughout the body effectively maximizes the capillary wall surface area available for transport, as the surface area per volume of a cylinder is inversely proportional to its diameter (hence smaller diameters give larger surface area). Some tissues exhibit specialized physiology to further enhance the surface area for transport. The cells lining the luminal (apical) side of the small intestinal wall offer an excellent example, where the cells have a highly invaginated surface structure that packs a large surface area into a small volume. The extra surface area effectively increases the rate at which nutrients (and drugs) are absorbed from the small intestines.

The concentration gradient across a barrier (ΔC) is determined largely by how rapidly molecules are transported away from the receiving side of the barrier. If the diffusing molecules build up on the receiving side, then the concentration gradient diminishes rapidly and diffusion quickly diminishes. If a high blood flow rate is maintained on the receiving side of a barrier, however, then molecules that cross the barrier are carried away rapidly, the concentration gradient remains large, and diffusion transport rates are kept high. The small intestine again offers an excellent example, as the high blood flow rate in the walls of the small intestine assure that nutrients (and drug molecules) diffusing across from the lumen are quickly carried away upon reaching the surrounding vasculature.

The permeability (P) of a solute molecule for a particular transport barrier depends on the thickness of the barrier, the types of the openings (if any) in the barrier, the size of the diffusing molecule, and in some cases the relative solubility of the molecule in the membrane lipid-bilayer. The thickness of the barrier affects the permeability since molecules must travel a longer distance in order to cross a thicker barrier. If the barrier has openings, such as fenestrations or gaps between cells, then molecules can often move more freely through the openings than through other parts of the barrier. Size of the solute molecule can affect the rate of transport across a barrier in several ways. First, larger molecules diffuse more slowly than smaller molecules due to hydrodynamic drag (friction between the molecule and the medium through which it is moving). Second, if the barrier contains openings of limited size, larger molecules have a harder time moving through the openings or can be completely excluded from the openings (e.g., drugs bound to large macroproteins such as albumin cannot fit through the openings in most barriers). If the barrier has no openings or the diffusing molecule is too large to fit through the openings, then passive transport across the barrier can occur only by molecular diffusion through the cell membrane lipid bilayer, which can be a much slower process.

Passive diffusion directly through the cell membrane highly depends on the solubility of the molecule in the lipid bilayer, which will be the focus of the next section. Some barriers in the body are specially modified to enhance or limit the transport of molecules through particular barriers. For example, relatively large gaps between cells in the small intestinal wall and fenestrations in kidney capillaries both increase the rate of transport across these barriers for many molecules. Conversely, capillaries in the central nervous system (CNS) have especially thick walls and extremely small gaps between cells, which limits the passage of molecules into the CNS and represents some of the factors responsible for the blood–brain barrier.

10.2.1.2 Diffusion through a Lipid Bilayer

When diffusion through the membrane lipid bilayer is the only option, solubility of the drug molecule in the lipid bilayer becomes very important. The extracellular and intracellular environments on each side of the membrane are aqueous in nature. Diffusion through the cellular membrane then constitutes movement from an aqueous environment, to a predominantly lipid environment within the membrane, and then to the aqueous environment on the other side of the membrane. Drug molecules with intermediate lipid solubility tend to be most effective at traversing the cell membrane. This is because drugs that are highly polar and lack solubility in a lipid-rich environment will not enter the membrane. Likewise, drugs that are extremely lipophilic easily dissolve in the lipid region of the membrane, but will not continue to diffuse through to the aqueous environment on the opposite side of the membrane.

A standard measure of lipid solubility is a physiochemical parameter called $\log P$. The $\log P$ of a solute is determined experimentally by adding the substance to a mixture of water and octanol. Water represents an aqueous, polar environment such as that surrounding each side of the lipid bilayer. Octanol represents a highly nonpolar solvent environment such as that found within the lipid bilayer. These two liquids are immiscible liquids, so they form a stable two-phase system much like an oil and water mixture. The solute is allowed to equilibrate between the two solvents, and the concentrations of the solute in both the octanol (C_O) and water (C_W) phases are measured. The $\log P$ is then given by the relationship:

$$\log P = \log_{10} K_{O/W} = \log_{10} \frac{C_O}{C_W} \tag{10.20}$$

where $K_{O/W}$ is the octanol/water equilibrium partition coefficient. A compound that has equal solubility in octanol and water has a $\log P$ equal to zero. Positive values of $\log P$ correspond to compounds that are more soluble in octanol than water and are lipophilic. Conversely, negative values of $\log P$ correspond to compounds that are more soluble in water than octanol and are more hydrophilic. As mentioned previously, it is generally the solute of intermediate lipophilicity and thus intermediate $\log P$ that can achieve the maximum rate of transport by diffusion through a lipid-bilayer membrane. It has been found that for many membranes and tissue barriers in the body, the $\log P$ that results in the maximum rate of diffusional transport is generally in the range of 2 to 3—that is, a solute that is 100 to 1000 times more soluble in octanol than water. Of course, the actual optimum value for diffusional transport will depend not only on the solute but also the nature of the membrane or barrier through which the molecule is being transported.

When the solute diffusing across a membrane barrier is a weak acid or base, the pH on either side of the membrane can have a profound effect on the rate of transport. This is because weak acids and bases can exist in either an ionized or neutral form, depending on the local pH. Given the nature of the phospholipid bilayer, transport by diffusion of the ionized forms of weak acids or bases across the bilayer is highly unfavorable, whereas neutral or uncharged forms more readily pass through the bilayer. This effect has already been described in Chapter 7, but it should be noted that this relationship is equally important in absorption and excretion processes. The relationship between charged and uncharged species for weak acid and bases is given by the following equations:

$$\text{Weak acid}: \quad HA \leftrightarrow A^- + H^+ \qquad \frac{[A^-]}{[HA]} = 10^{pH-pK_A} \tag{10.21}$$

$$\text{Weak base}: \quad RNH_3^+ \leftrightarrow RNH_2 + H^+ \qquad \frac{[RNH_2]}{[RNH_3^+]} = 10^{pH-pK_A} \tag{10.22}$$

For the weak acid, the neutral acid (HA) is favored when the local pH is less than the pK_A of the dissociation reaction. The converse is true for the weak base where the neutral species (RNH_2) is favored when the local pH is greater than the pK_A of its dissociation reaction. Hence an orally administered weak acid drug is more rapidly absorbed if its pK_A is above the pH 6.6 environment common in the duodenal region of the small intestine, maintaining a neutral form that more readily crosses the intestinal wall. Alternatively, an overdose of a weakly basic drug can be treated by acidifying the urine (e.g., by administering citric acid) in order to ionize the drug in the kidney tubules, which reduces the amount of drug reabsorbed in the tubules and hence increases urinary excretion.

10.2.2 Carrier Mediated Transport

Another means by which drug molecules traverse membrane barriers is by carrier mediated transport. This type of transport generally involves binding the substrate molecule to a specific binding site on a transmembrane protein that then transports the drug molecule to the other side of the membrane. Carrier mediated transport may be the only effective means by which some molecules are able to traverse membranes as they are either too large or too polar to effectively diffuse through the lipid bilayer. Some characteristics that are common to carrier mediated transporters are that they can be highly specific, they can be inhibited, and they are saturable. Substrate specificity may arise in situations where only a single or a narrow class of compounds may be able to properly bind to the transporter protein. However, there are transporter proteins that are able to bind to a wide variety of substrates. In these cases, the transporter is termed promiscuous. Inhibition of a transporter protein is possible for compounds that bind irreversibly to the protein, essentially rendering them useless for further transport. Saturable kinetics result from the fact that there are a limited number of carrier molecules located in the membrane, and once the substrate concentration reaches a level where all the carrier molecules are being utilized, further increases in the substrate concentration will have no further effect on the rate of transport across the membrane. The rate of transport (r_t) in this situation can generally be written in a Michaelis-Menten form:

$$r_t = \frac{V_{max,t} \cdot f_u C}{K_t + f_u C} \tag{10.23}$$

where $V_{max,t}$ is the maximum rate of facilitated transport in mass (or moles) per time, C is the substrate (drug) concentration in the region where the transporter picks up the solute, f_u is the unbound drug fraction (fraction of drug molecules that are not bound to macroproteins such as albumin), and K_t is the Michaelis-Menten transport constant representing the unbound substrate concentration at which the rate of transport is half the maximal rate. For many drugs, the unbound drug concentration ($f_u C$) is generally much lower than the value of K_t, in which case this equation can be simplified to

$$\text{for } f_u C << K_t, \quad r_t \approx \left(\frac{V_{max,t}}{K_t}\right) \cdot f_u C \tag{10.24}$$

Thus the rate of active transport is often proportional to the drug concentration, even when the transporter itself follows nonlinear Michaelis-Menten kinetics.

Carrier mediated transport can be further divided into two subclasses based on the means by which the carriers move the substrate molecule across the membrane. The first type of carrier mediated transport is called facilitated diffusion. In this case substrate molecules bind to the transporter but the driving force for their transport across the membrane is still a favorable chemical gradient. In the second type of carrier mediated transport, called active transport, substrate molecules are transported across the membrane against a chemical gradient (from a lower concentration region to a higher concentration region). Transport against a gradient is thermodynamically unfavorable and can be accomplished only by expending energy, generally supplied by the hydrolysis of ATP.

A comprehensive review of many important transporter molecules is provided in Chapter 7. It should be kept in mind that transporter proteins can affect absorption, excretion, and even metabolism processes as well as distribution. These transporters can also either enhance or reduce the rates of these processes, depending on which direction the transporters move the drug molecules. P-glycoprotein (Pgp) is a highly promiscuous efflux protein found at high levels in both the small intestinal wall and the blood–brain barrier. For drugs that are good substrates, Pgp can very effectively reduce intestinal absorption and prevent distribution to the CNS by binding drug molecules that have crossed the barrier and effluxing them back into the intestinal lumen or brain capillaries. Other transporter proteins are able to enhance intestinal absorption or CNS uptake for selected molecules. A variety of transporters are similarly present in the kidney tubules, most of which increase drug excretion by actively secreting certain types of molecules into the urine, but a few reduce excretion for selected types of molecules (e.g., sugars) by actively reabsorbing these molecules from the urine. Liver tissues are rich in transporters that enhance drug uptake, effectively increasing metabolic rates, as well as proteins that facilitate drug excretion into the bile.

10.2.3 Convective Transport

Convective transport occurs when solute molecules are carried along by fluid flow. The driving force for this type of transport is a pressure gradient that causes the fluid to flow from an area of high pressure to an area of low pressure. Convective transport can be much faster than passive diffusion or carrier-mediated transport, which is why the body generally relies on convective blood flow transport when molecules must be moved more than microscopic distances. Besides blood flow, convective transport also occurs by other types of fluid movement, such as in the lymphatic system and the kidney glomeruli. These latter cases are examples of convection by fluids being filtered across a cellular barrier.

10.2.3.1 Blood Flow Transport

Transport of drug molecules by flowing blood is an obvious example of convective transport. The heart pressurizes the blood causing it to flow through the pulmonary and systemic vasculature. The arterial portion of the systemic circulation delivers oxygen-rich blood, as well as any drug molecules dissolved in the blood, to the rest of the body. Drug molecules can enter the tissues via the capillary beds if the chemical gradient is favorable or there is an active transport system into the tissue. If the tissue already contains drug molecules from either previous distribution to the tissue or the tissue being a site of drug administration, then a chemical gradient or active transport in the opposite direction can cause drug molecules to move from the tissue into the blood, with venous blood flow then carrying the drug molecules back to the heart. The hepatic portal vein represents a specialized portion of the systemic circulation, where venous blood flow from the GI tract passes through the liver before returning to the heart. This allows the liver to remove and metabolize some of the drug molecules from the blood before they ever reach the heart or the rest of the body. This is known as hepatic (liver) first pass metabolism. In any of these cases, the transport rate (r_t) of drug via blood flow is given by

$$r_t = Q \cdot C_p \tag{10.25}$$

where Q is the plasma (or blood) flow rate in units of volume per time, and C_p is the concentration of drug in the plasma (or blood).

10.2.3.2 Filtration across a Cellular Barrier

Convection can also be important in transport across a cellular barrier. There are several examples in the body where pressure gradients are maintained on either side of a cellular barrier, causing transfer of fluid from the high pressure side of the barrier to the low pressure side. Two examples are shown in Figure 10.7. In the glomeruli of the kidney, the pressure in the Bowman's capsule space is lower than it is in the glomerular capillaries. Because of this, some of the fluid portion of the blood is filtered through the fenestrations in the glomerular capillaries into the Bowman's space. Also depicted in Figure 10.7 is what is known as Starling phenomena. The pressure of the blood near the arterial end of a capillary is greater than the surrounding tissue. This leads to the flow of fluid across the capillary wall into the tissue. Likewise, at the venous end of the capillary, the pressure of the blood is less than that in the tissue, leading to the fluid flow across the capillary wall back into the bloodstream. In each of these cases, the filtered fluid flow carries dissolved drug molecules across the cellular barrier.

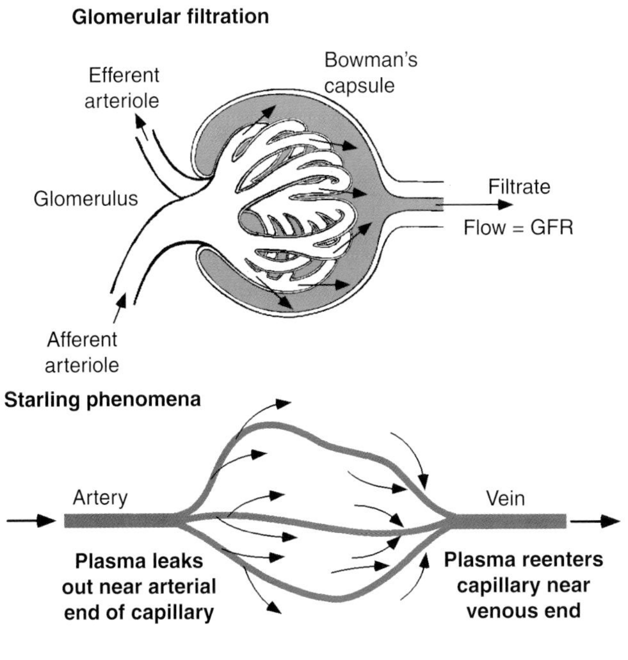

Figure 10.7 Examples of convective transport filtered through a cellular barrier, including glomerular filtration (top) and Starling phenomena (bottom).

Fluid flow does not generally occur through the cellular membranes themselves (transcellular transport), but rather through gaps or junctions between the cells (paracellular transport). This is the case in both of the previous examples. In the glomeruli and capillaries, liquid flows around the endothelial cells lining these conduits. The size of the gaps between the cells determines which solutes get through and those that cannot. In the glomeruli, molecules larger than about 60,000 molecular weight (MW) cannot make it through the openings. This excludes large macromolecules such as albumin from passing into the glomerular filtrate. Small molecules can readily move through these gaps unless they happen to be bound to macromolecules. The binding of drug molecules to protein macromolecules prevents the bound drug from moving through the gaps via convective transport. Thus the rate of convective transport (r_t) in the filtration case becomes

$$r_t = Q_{filt} \cdot f_u \cdot C_p \tag{10.26}$$

where Q_{filt} is the flow rate of the filtered fluid, f_u is the unbound drug fraction (fraction of drug molecules that are not bound to macroproteins such as albumin), and C_p is the total (unbound and bound) drug concentration in the plasma.

10.2.4 Perfusion versus Permeation Transport Limitations

Blood flow and membrane permeation are both important in PK processes. During absorption, drug molecules must permeate into the vasculature of the administration site (unless they are administered directly into a blood vessel, such as by IV injection), after which blood flow carries the drug away. Blood flow then delivers the drug to the vasculature within other tissues, from which the drug molecules must permeate from the blood vessel into the tissue during distribution. Similar blood flow delivery and permeation into tissues must occur in eliminating organs (such as the liver or kidneys) during metabolism and excretion. In each case, perfusion and permeation occur sequentially, and whichever process is slower controls the overall rate of drug transport. This can lead to two types of limiting situations, perfusion-limited and permeability-limited transport.

10.2.4.1 Perfusion-Limited Transport

In the perfusion-limited case, the permeation is relatively fast compared to perfusion of the tissue bed. This tends to occur when the barrier is thin or has many gaps, the drug has a low molecular weight and is near the optimal log*P* value, and the blood flow rate is not very high. Since permeation is relatively fast in this case, the plasma and the tissue on either side of the membrane barrier come into equilibrium in a very short period of time. It should be pointed out that at equilibrium, the concentration in the plasma and the tissue are not necessarily equal. At equilibrium, the plasma and tissue concentrations are related to one another by the relationship

$$K_T = \frac{C_T}{C_p} \quad (10.27)$$

where K_T is the equilibrium tissue partition coefficient. The reason the plasma and tissue concentrations can be different at equilibrium is that they each offer different environments, which may provide different levels of affinity or solubility for the drug molecule. When $K_T > 1$, the drug preferentially partitions into the tissue, as would be the case for a lipophillic drug in a tissue primarily composed of adipose. Conversely, $K_T < 1$ indicates preferential partitioning into the plasma, as would occur for a highly polar drug in adipose tissue. Figure 10.8 shows a situation where transport to or from the tissue is perfusion controlled. Drug is being delivered to the capillary bed at a rate equal to the product of the volumetric flow rate of plasma (Q) and the concentration of the drug in the arterial plasma (C_A):

$$\text{Drug Transport by Perfusion to Tissues} = Q\,C_A \quad (10.28)$$

Likewise, drug is removed from the tissue bed at a rate equal to the product of the volumetric flow rate of plasma and the concentration of the drug in the venous plasma (C_V):

$$\text{Drug Transport by Perfusion from Tissues} = Q\,C_V \quad (10.29)$$

Since the plasma and tissue reach equilibrium quickly, we can assume or approximate that the venous plasma is in equilibrium with the tissue, so from Equation (10.27) this becomes

$$C_V = \frac{C_T}{K_T} \quad (10.30)$$

The rate that drug is transported into or out of the tissue bed (r_t) is then equal to the difference between the rate of perfusion delivery and perfusion removal:

$$r_t = QC_A - QC_V = Q(C_A - C_V) = Q\left(C_A - \frac{C_T}{K_T}\right) \quad (10.31)$$

When written in this form, r_t is positive for net transport into the tissue (e.g., distribution to tissue), or negative for net transport out of the tissue (e.g., absorption from site of administration). This equation for perfusion-limited transport clearly shows that for this limiting case, transport between the blood and tissue is dependent solely on the rate of blood perfusion (Q) and not on the permeability (P) or surface area for transport (S) between the capillary lumen and tissue.

10.2.4.2 Permeability-Limited Transport

In permeability-limited transport, permeation across the membrane or cellular barrier is relatively slow compared to vascular perfusion. This tends to be the case where the membrane barrier is thick and tight, where there is relatively high blood flow, or when the drug molecule has difficulty crossing the barrier (log*P* very low or very high, or large molecular weight). Figure 10.9 illustrates schematically the permeability-limited case for drug transport into or out of a tissue. Since permeation is relatively slow, the plasma and the tissue on either side of the membrane barrier approach equilibrium conditions extremely slowly, and equilibrium will not be reached unless plasma drug levels hold steady for a very long time. It should be kept in mind that the concentration in the plasma and the tissue would not necessarily be equal even at

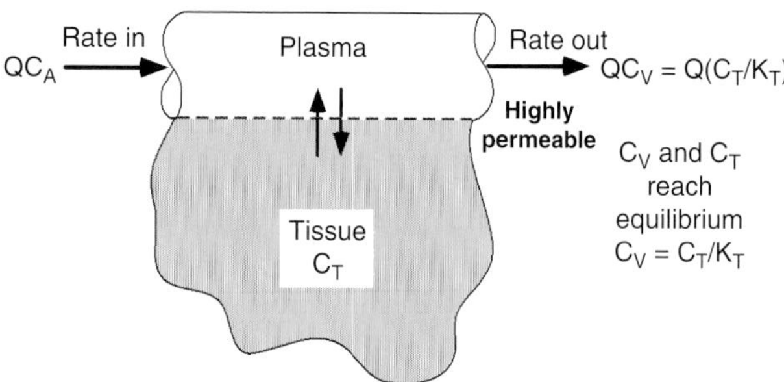

Figure 10.8 Perfusion-limited transport across the capillary wall allows the venous drug concentration (C_V) to reach equilibrium with the tissue drug concentration (C_T).

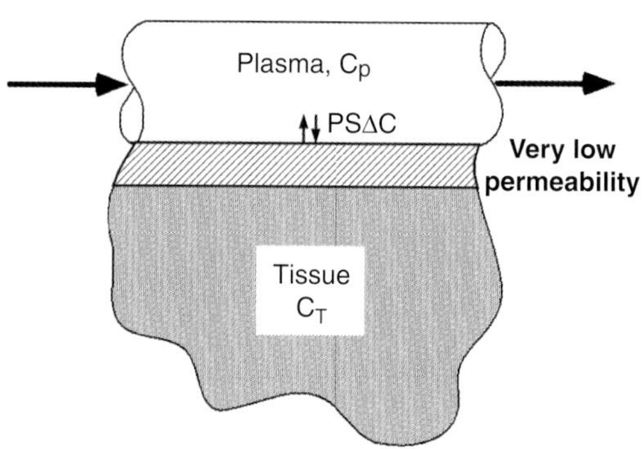

Figure 10.9 Permeability-limited transport across a low permeability capillary wall causes a slow approach to equilibrium between the plasma drug concentration (C_p) and tissue drug concentration (C_T).

equilibrium, but would be affected by the relative affinity and solubility of the drug in the plasma and the tissue. Thus the driving force for diffusion transport, ΔC, is not the difference between C_p and C_T, but is the difference between C_p and the plasma concentration that would be in equilibrium with C_T, which by the relationship in Equation (10.27) becomes

$$\Delta C = C_p - \frac{C_T}{K_T} \tag{10.32}$$

The rate of drug transport into or out of the tissue bed (r_t) is then given by combining Equations (10.19) and (10.32), which yields

$$r_t = PS \cdot \left(C_p - \frac{C_T}{K_T}\right) \tag{10.33}$$

where this equation is again written in a form where r_t is positive for net transport into the tissue (e.g., distribution to tissue) and negative for net transport out of the tissue (e.g., absorption from site of administration). As shown by this equation, the rate of transport in the permeability-limited case is dependent on the permeability and surface area of the transport barrier but is not dependent on the blood flow rate to the tissue. Hence changes in blood flow rate have little or no effect unless the flow drops so low that transport is no longer permeation-limited.

10.3 ABSORPTION

Absorption is the process by which a drug makes its way into the body, or more precisely, into the systemic circulation. Depending on the route of administration, there can be many obstacles that prevent some or even all of the drug molecules from reaching the systemic circulation. The route of administration can also have a large effect on the rate of drug absorption. A discussion of the many different routes of administration used for drug delivery has already been provided in Chapter 2. This section will focus on the factors that affect the extent and rate of drug absorption for common routes of drug administration, and the typical PK modeling approaches employed for drug absorption processes.

10.3.1 Extent of Absorption: Bioavailability

Unless a drug is administered directly to the site of therapeutic activity, drug molecules must reach the systemic circulation in order to be distributed to other tissues and produce the desired effect. For example, one of the most common routes of drug administration is via oral ingestion. However, the act of swallowing and having the drug present within the lumen of the GI tract does not constitute absorption. In order for an orally administered drug to elicit any effect (provided that the action is not along the GI tract itself), it has to pass through the stomach (where it may undergo some level of chemical degradation by acid hydrolysis) into the small intestines (where it may undergo some level of chemical, bacterial, or enzymatic degradation, or may have poor dissolution or solubility), cross the intestinal wall (where it may again undergo some level of enzymatic degradation, and may also be subject to active transport back into the intestinal lumen by P-glycoprotein or other transporters present at high levels in the intestinal wall) into the surrounding vasculature, after which it is carried by the portal vein to the liver (where it may undergo some level of enzymatic degradation, called hepatic first-pass metabolism since it occurs during the first pass of the drug through the liver), and then to the pulmonary circulation (where it can undergo some level of enzymatic degradation in the lungs), before finally reaching the systemic circulation and getting delivered to the rest of the body. Any fraction of the orally administered compound that is degraded along the GI tract, does not cross the intestinal wall (passing out of the body in fecal wastes), or undergoes metabolism prior to entering the systemic circulation, never becomes available to the rest of the body and hence is not bioavailable. Drugs delivered by other routes of extravascular administration (any route that does not deliver the drug directly into a blood vessel) can similarly undergo breakdown or other types of loss prior to reaching the systemic circulation. The advantages and disadvantages of different administration routes, and formulation methods employed to overcome some of these potential absorption problems, are discussed in detail in Chapter 2.

The fraction of the delivered drug dose that does successfully reach the systemic circulation is called the bioavailable fraction or bioavailability (F) of the drug. The total amount of drug that is absorbed into the systemic circulation ($A_{abs,tot}$) is then given simply by the product of the bioavailability (F) and dose (D) of the drug, or

$$A_{abs,tot} = FD \tag{10.34}$$

Bioavailability can range in value from 0 to 1 (or 0–100%), where a bioavailability of 0 (or 0%) corresponds to no drug molecules reaching the systemic circulation, and a bioavailability of 1 (or 100%) corresponds to the entire administered dose reaching the systemic circulation. Drugs that are administered directly to the systemic circulation via IV or intra-arterial injection are considered to have a bioavailability of 100%. Drugs delivered via extravascular routes of administration (oral, subcutaneous, intramuscular, nasal, inhaled, sublingual, transdermal, etc.) may have a bioavailability anywhere in the range of 0 to 100%. Most marketed drugs have a reasonably high bioavailability ($F > 50\%$) for any recommended extravascular routes of delivery, as a lower bioavailability would reduce their effectiveness, and tends to be associated with higher interpatient variability in bioavailability. Marketed drugs that do end up having a lower than desired bioavailability are generally administered exclusively by intravenous injection or infusion to avoid potential bioavailability problems.

10.3.2 Rate of Absorption

The mathematical description of the absorption rate can be quite complex, depending on the level of detail included in the mathematical analysis. However, the goal here, as it is for most PK modeling, is to keep the mathematics as simple as possible while maintaining sufficient details to adequately describe the process. It turns out that the absorption rate for most drug delivery routes can be accurately approximated as either instantaneous, zero-order, or first-order absorption. The meaning and application of each of these types of absorption is described in the following sections.

10.3.2.1 Instantaneous Absorption Rate

In order for absorption to be truly instantaneous, it would be necessary for the total amount of drug being absorbed (FD) to enter the systemic circulation in the instant after drug administration. This would essentially require an infinitely high rate of absorption over an infinitely short period of time. This is obviously impossible in the real world, but a close approximation occurs if the drug enters the systemic circulation at a very high rate over a very short period of time, such as illustrated in Figure 10.10. The best example of instantaneous absorption in actual practice is a bolus IV injection, in which the entire dose is injected into a vein over a brief period of time (typically several seconds). Since the drug directly enters the systemic circulation, absorption is complete as soon as the injection has been made, and the absorption process is as close to instantaneous as possible. Note that in the case of bolus IV injection, all of the drug enters the systemic circulation and hence the bioavailability (F) is 100%.

Other drug delivery situations that do not closely mimic true instantaneous absorption can still be approximated by this absorption model, as long as the absorption process occurs much more quickly than all other processes. For example, an orally ingested drug for which absorption is essentially complete after one or two hours could be approximated as instantaneous absorption if the distribution, metabolism, and excretion processes all take several days to approach completion. Note that even if an extravascular drug delivery can be treated as instantaneous absorption, the bioavailability (F) can still range from 0 to 100%. Specific criteria for when the instantaneous absorption approximation can be used will be provided later in this chapter after the necessary modeling concepts have been introduced.

10.3.2.2 Zero-Order Absorption Rate

The second type of absorption model that is commonly applied is zero-order absorption. Zero-order refers to the case where the absorption rate (r_{abs}) is taken to be proportional to the amount of drug remaining to be absorbed (A_{rem}) raised to the zero power, or

$$r_{abs} = k_0 A_{rem}^0 = k_0 \tag{10.35}$$

where k_0 is a zero-order rate constant with units of mass (or moles) per time. Since any number raised to the zero power is one, the rate of absorption is then constant and equal to k_0. The real-world drug delivery method that most closely approximates zero-order absorption is an intravenous (iv) infusion, in which drug is delivered at a steady rate directly into the systemic circulation. Infusions are typically delivered over some fixed time-period, which for most PK modeling purposes is taken to start at time zero ($t = 0$) and continue unchanged until some later time T ($t = T$). The absorption rate versus time can then be written mathematically as

$$\begin{aligned} r_{abs} &= 0 \quad \text{for } t < 0 \quad \text{and} \quad t > T \\ r_{abs} &= k_0 \quad \text{for } 0 < t < T \end{aligned} \tag{10.36}$$

which is illustrated graphically in Figure 10.11. Other drug administration methods that can be approximated by zero-order absorption include implantable or transdermal controlled release systems and intramuscular depot injections, all of which provide a reasonably steady rate of drug delivery over some period of time.

10.3.2.3 First-Order Absorption Rate

First-order absorption is the final approach that will be considered. Analogous to the zero-order absorption case, first-order absorption refers to the fact that the absorption rate (r_{abs}) is taken to be proportional to the amount of drug remaining to be absorbed (A_{rem}) raised to the first power (or power of one), giving

$$r_{abs} = k_a A_{rem}^1 = k_a A_{rem} \tag{10.37}$$

where k_a is a first-order absorption rate constant with units of 1/time or time^{-1}. Since any number raised to

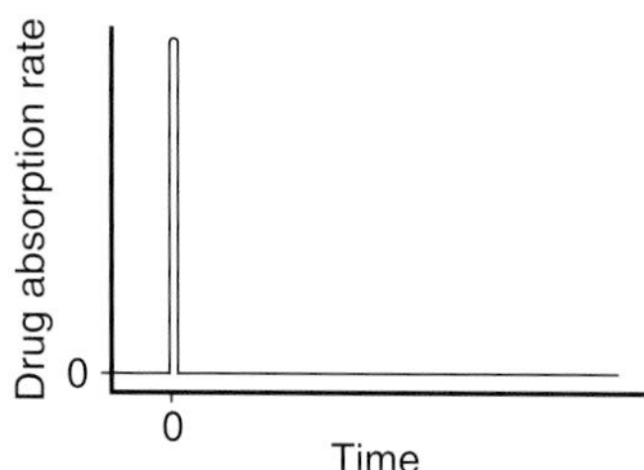

Figure 10.10 Graphical representation of an approximately instantaneous absorption rate.

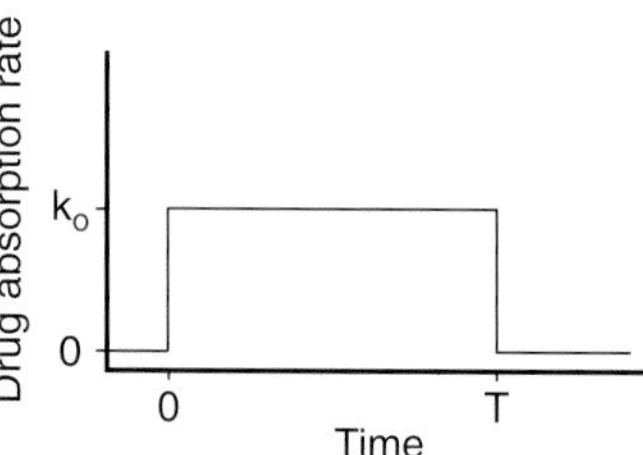

Figure 10.11 Graphical representation of a steady or zero-order absorption rate.

the power of one is itself, the rate of absorption is then proportional to the amount of drug remaining to be absorbed, with a proportionality constant of k_a. First-order absorption can also be said to follow "linear kinetics," since the absorption rate (r_{abs}) is a linear function of the amount of drug remaining to be absorbed (A_{rem}), with a slope of k_a and an intercept of zero.

First-order absorption often provides a realistic approximation for many types of extravascular drug delivery, including oral ingestion, subcutaneous injection, and intramuscular injection (when not used as a depot mode). The reason this is true can be demonstrated by several reasonable approximations. First, it is realistic to expect that the concentration of drug at the site of administration is much higher than the drug concentration in the plasma entering the site while absorption occurs. Second, it is reasonable to expect that the concentration of drug at the administration site is proportional to the amount of drug that remains to be absorbed (A_{rem}) at the administration site. Applying these reasonable approximations to either the perfusion-limited absorption case or the permeability-limited absorption case provides the same results, that the absorption rate should approximately equal A_{rem} multiplied by a constant no matter which type of transport limitation controls the absorption process. It can be demonstrated by similar logic that the absorption rate is also approximately proportional to A_{rem} when active transport dominates the absorption process as long as the unbound drug concentration at the site of administration is much less than the Michaelis-Menten constant K_t. Thus it is reasonable to expect that a first-order absorption model should be useful in modeling the absorption rate for most extravascular routes of drug administration (we encourage you to verify these findings on your own).

The relationship for first-order absorption in Equation (10.37) can be converted into a differential mass balance equation that can be solved (again, you are encouraged to try this on your own) to give

$$A_{rem} = FD \cdot e^{-k_a t} \tag{10.38}$$

and subsequently

$$r_{abs} = k_a FD \cdot e^{-k_a t} \tag{10.39}$$

For first-order absorption, the absorption rate then starts at a maximum value of $k_a FD$ at time zero ($t = 0$), after which it decreases with time by an exponential decay, as illustrated graphically in Figure 10.12. It can

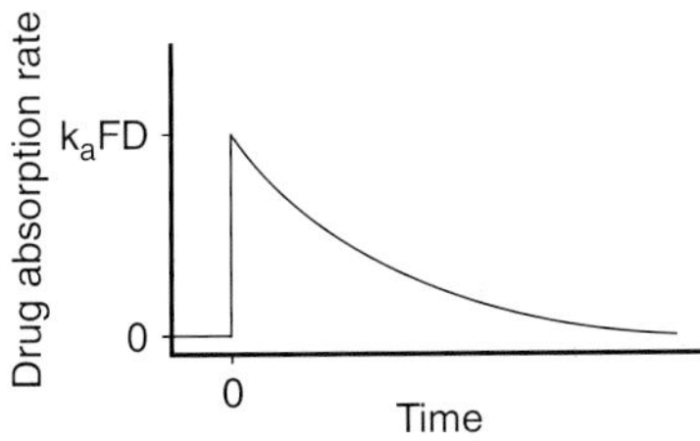

Figure 10.12 Graphical representation of a first-order absorption rate.

be shown from the earlier discussion of exponential decay processes that the absorption half-life is then

$$t_{1/2,abs} = \frac{\ln(2)}{k_a} \approx \frac{0.693}{k_a} \tag{10.40}$$

Thus for a first-order absorption rate, the absorption process is 50% complete after a single absorption half-life, 75% complete after two absorption half-lives, and about 99% complete (or essentially finished) after seven absorption half-lives. It should be kept in mind that these absorption half-life relationships apply only to first-order absorption processes.

10.4 DISTRIBUTION

The distribution process involves the movement of drug molecules between the systemic circulation and other tissues. Note that distribution is a two-way process that includes movement of drug from plasma to tissues as well as from tissues to plasma. In either case, drug transport occurs between capillaries and the surrounding tissue. The distribution process typically follows a three-stage process, illustrated sequentially in Figures 10.13, 10.14, and 10.15. The initial stage of distribution (Figure 10.13) starts when the drug first gets absorbed into the systemic circulation. At this stage, there is little or no drug present in the tissues,

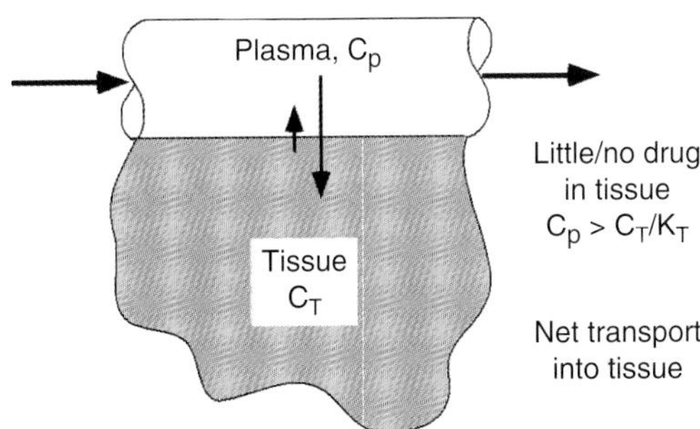

Figure 10.13 Graphical representation of the initial distribution stage when there is little or no drug present in the tissues and the net transport of drug is from plasma to tissue.

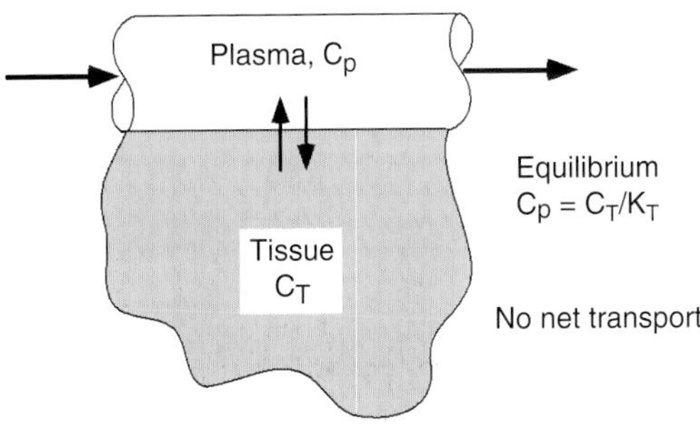

Figure 10.14 Graphical representation of the equilibrium distribution stage when there is no net transport of drug between plasma and tissue.

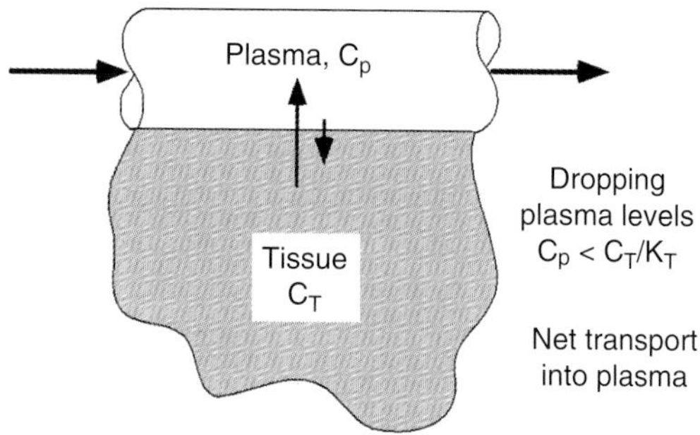

Figure 10.15 Graphical representation of the terminal distribution stage when plasma concentrations drop below tissue levels and the net transport of drug is from tissue to plasma.

and hence the movement of drug molecules is predominantly from plasma into the tissues. After a sufficient period of time, the plasma and tissues reach a distributional equilibrium or steady-state stage (Figure 10.14), where the rate of transport into the tissues equals the transport rate back into the plasma, and hence there is no net movement of drug molecules. At later times after absorption is complete and no new drug molecules are entering the circulation, plasma concentrations typically begin to drop more rapidly than tissue concentrations. Tissues then serve as drug storage reservoirs during this terminal redistribution stage (Figure 10.15), with the predominant direction of drug transport being from tissues back into the plasma.

Since the target site of a drug is rarely at the site of administration or in the systemic circulation, delivery of the drug to the target tissue by the distribution process is often a critical determinant of the drug's effectiveness. Many of the physiochemical and physiological factors involved in the distribution process have been discussed previously in Section 10.2 or in Chapter 7. This section will focus on the means by which the distribution process is incorporated and represented in PK models. This involves mathematical terms to represent both the extent of distribution and the rate of distribution transport.

10.4.1 Extent of Distribution

There are two types of parameters that can be employed to represent the extent of distribution in PK models. The first is a tissue partition coefficient (K_T), and the second is a volume of distribution (V). The definition of each of these parameters is provided in the following sections.

10.4.1.1 Tissue Partition Coefficient

The extent of drug distribution into particular tissues is related primarily to the relative concentration of drug molecules in the plasma versus tissue under equilibrium conditions. As mentioned previously in Section 10.2.4.1, plasma and tissue concentrations are generally not equal, even when they are in equilibrium with each other. This is because each offers a unique environment with different levels of affinity or solubility for the drug molecules. As mentioned in Chapter 7, the primary factors affecting differences in drug partitioning between tissue and plasma include the relative levels of protein binding, drug ionization, and inherent drug solubility. The first two factors are important because only drug molecules that are neutral (uncharged) and not bound to macroproteins can cross the capillary wall barrier under normal conditions. As a consequence, it is really the concentration of unbound, neutral drug molecules that come to equilibrium. The final term, the inherent drug solubility, is a consequence of solute/solvent interactions. Many tissues, particularly adipose and brain tissues, have a highly nonpolar nature, which provides a much higher solubility for lipophillic drug molecules than the mostly aqueous plasma. Conversely, polar molecules are much more soluble in the aqueous plasma environment. Combining each of these factors gives the following general relationship for the ratio of tissue versus plasma drug concentrations at equilibrium

$$\frac{C_T}{C_p} = K_T = \frac{f_{n,p}}{f_{n,T}} \cdot \frac{f_{u,p}}{f_{u,T}} \cdot \frac{C_{sol,T}}{C_{sol,p}} \tag{10.41}$$

where K_T is the overall equilibrium tissue-partition coefficient, f_n represents the fraction of neutral drug molecules in the plasma (p) and tissue (T) environments, f_u represents the unbound drug fraction (fraction of drug not bound to protein macromolecules) in each environment, and C_{sol} represents the inherent solubility of neutral, unbound drug in each environment. Note that if the tissue environment is predominantly lipid in nature (e.g., adipose tissue), then the ratio of the inherent solubilities can be taken to be similar to the octanol/water partition coefficient ($K_{o/w}$) and can be estimated from the drug's log$P$. Alternatively, the relative inherent solubilities can be related to $K_{o/w}$ and the lipid or fat content within the tissue. Note that K_T can generally be considered a constant for a given drug in a given tissue, but there are situations that can alter the partition coefficient and hence change the extent of tissue distribution for a given drug. One possibility would be if the pH of a tissue changes such as during tissue hypoxia, which could affect drug ionization and hence drug partitioning into tissues in certain disease states. Another situation that can cause clinical complications is the presence of a second drug or endogenous molecule that displaces the drug of interest from its normal protein binding site. This can dramatically change the distribution of the drug to the target tissue and hence could be the source of an important drug–drug interaction.

10.4.1.2 Volume of Distribution

Another PK parameter related to the extent of drug distribution is called the volume of distribution. The volume of distribution (V) is defined as the apparent volume in which the current amount of drug in the body (A_{body}) must be dispersed in order to give the current plasma concentration (C_p), which can be written

$$C_p = \frac{A_{body}}{V} \quad \text{or alternatively} \quad V = \frac{A_{body}}{C_p} \qquad (10.42)$$

The volume of distribution is a mathematical or theoretical concept, which does not generally represent a specific physiological volume within the body for most drugs, such as the plasma volume or extracellular fluid volume. In fact, many drugs, particularly highly lipophillic drugs, can have volumes of distribution that are many magnitudes higher than the entire volume of the body (e.g., chloroquine has a typical volume of distribution of about 150 L/kg, which ends up being more than two orders of magnitude larger than the actual volume of the body). The explanation for this disparity is that tissues with relatively large partition coefficients ($K_T >> 1$) dissolve a much greater amount of drug than would a similar volume of plasma. This disparity is explained further in Chapter 7, where it is also shown that the level of plasma protein binding can dramatically affect the apparent volume of distribution.

It should also be noted that different types of volumes of distribution can be defined for different types of PK models and in some cases for different time points during the distribution process. For a single compartment model, which will be the first type of PK model covered in this chapter, there is only a single volume of distribution (V) that never changes with time. For a multicompartment model, the volume of distribution is initially equal to the volume associated with just one particular compartment (V_1), then becomes equal to a larger volume (V_{ss}) at distributional steady-state as in Figure 10.14, and finally becomes equal to an even larger volume (V_{AUC}) at longer times as portrayed in Figure 10.15. All these seemingly difficult concepts will become much clearer after some of the actual PK models have been introduced.

10.4.2 Distribution Transport Rate

The distribution transport rate (r_{dist}) is a measure of how quickly drug molecules are exchanged between the plasma and the tissues. A rapid distribution transport rate causes the plasma and tissues to come quickly into equilibrium with each other, whereas a slower rate will cause a prolonged approach to equilibrium. As with the rate of absorption, different types of PK modeling approaches can be employed to approximate distribution rates. In the case of distribution there are essentially two types of models, instantaneous distribution and first-order distribution. The difference between the two types of models is in the number of compartments used to represent the drug disposition in the body.

10.4.2.1 Instantaneous Distribution Rate

Instantaneous distribution is represented by considering the body as a single compartment. This type of PK model can have parameters associated with how fast drug reaches the systemic circulation by absorption and how quickly drug is removed from the body by elimination, but there are no parameters to represent the time it takes for distribution because the plasma and tissues are assumed to instantly reach distributional equilibrium. As with instantaneous absorption, true instantaneous distribution is obviously physically impossible, as convective transport by blood flow and permeation of the capillary wall into tissues obviously takes some finite period of time. However, instantaneous distribution is a reasonable approximation when the time it takes for all tissues with significant drug concentrations to reach equilibrium with the plasma is substantially shorter than the time it takes for the elimination and absorption processes (unless absorption is essentially instantaneous as well). Note that the rate of transport to tissues that never reach particularly high concentrations of the drug do not have to be fast, as they play little or no role in determining the changes in plasma concentrations. Thus if distribution is primarily to tissues that have high blood perfusion rates (e.g., kidneys, liver, brain, muscle) and/or the drug has a high permeability across the capillary wall (e.g., small molecule near optimum log$P$, or extensive active transport mechanisms), then the assumption of approximately instantaneous distribution can be very reasonable. It also turns out that the instantaneous distribution (one-compartment) model involves much simpler mathematical equations. Thus it is not uncommon for this simplified model to be employed for ease of use, even if it does not give a particularly satisfactory approximation of the actual PK processes.

10.4.2.2 First-Order Distribution Rate

Analogous to first-order absorption, first-order distribution indicates that the rate of distribution (r_{dist}) from one location to another is proportional to the amount of drug remaining to be distributed (A_{rem}) raised to the power of one. This could be written for distribution in a manner analogous to first-order absorption (Section 10.3.2.3) in the form

$$r_{dist} = k_{dist} A_{rem}^1 = k_{dist} A_{rem} \qquad (10.43)$$

where k_{dist} is a distribution rate constant with units of per time or time^{-1}. As shown in Figures 10.13 through 10.15, however, distribution is by its very nature a bidirectional process. In order to account for this, PK models consider distribution to occur from one region (or compartment) to another region (or a second compartment), as well as simultaneously back in the opposite direction. This is illustrated in Figure 10.16.

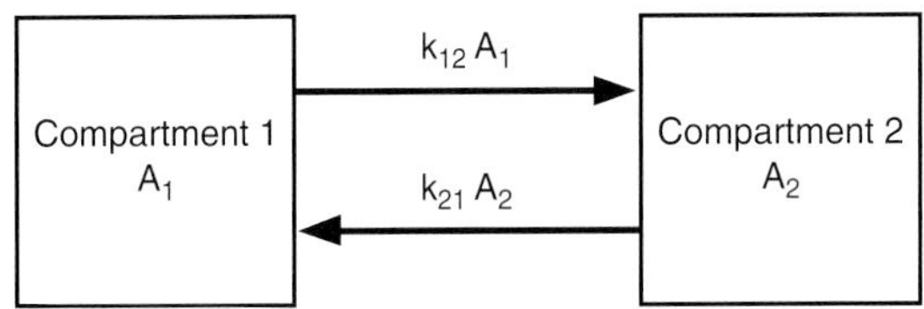

Figure 10.16 Graphical representation of the rates of distribution between two compartments.

By convention, compartment 1 is taken to include the systemic circulation, and compartment 2 represents the tissue or tissues that are exchanging drug molecules with the circulation. The amount of drug remaining in compartment 1 is labeled A_1, and the amount remaining in compartment 2 is A_2. The rate constant for distribution from 1→2 is labeled k_{12}, and the rate constant for distribution from 2→1 is k_{21}. The rate of distribution from 1→2 can then be written as

$$r_{dist,1\rightarrow 2} = k_{12}A_1 \quad (10.44)$$

and the distribution from 2→1 becomes

$$r_{dist,2\rightarrow 1} = k_{21}A_2 \quad (10.45)$$

All these conventional notation terms are illustrated in Figure 10.16. The overall net rate of distribution (taken as positive for net distribution from 1→2) can finally be expressed as

$$r_{dist,net,1\rightarrow 2} = k_{12}A_1 - k_{21}A_2 \quad (10.46)$$

It should be noted that as in absorption, first-order distribution represents linear kinetics, as the net rate of distribution is a linear function of the amount of drug remaining in compartment 1(A_1) and the amount of drug remaining in compartment 2(A_2). Also as in the absorption case, a half-life of distribution ($t_{½,dist}$) can be defined in terms of the distribution rate constants. However, because distribution occurs in more than one direction, and due to other model complications that will be explained later, the distribution half-life cannot be written as a simple function of k_{12} and k_{21}. It turns out that the distribution half-life is defined in terms of a "hybrid" rate constant (λ_1) by the equation

$$t_{½,dist} = \frac{\ln(2)}{\lambda_1} \approx \frac{0.693}{\lambda_1} \quad (10.47)$$

where this hybrid rate constant will be defined later as a relatively complex function of k_{12}, k_{21}, and another rate constant that has not been covered yet.

10.5 ELIMINATION (METABOLISM AND EXCRETION)

Metabolism and excretion, the final two ADME processes, both represent methods of drug elimination. Metabolism removes drug molecules from the body by converting them into different chemical forms, called metabolites. Excretion removes drug molecules from the body by discharging them into body wastes. Although the physiological basis for these two types of elimination are quite different, it turns out that the general PK modeling schemes employed for each are very similar. This section will first describe the important physiological considerations related to metabolism and excretion processes. The general modeling approaches and parameters used to describe elimination in PK models will then be provided.

10.5.1 Metabolism

Metabolism is the process by which drug molecules are converted into a different chemical form, typically by enzymatic reactions. The incredibly wide array of enzymes found in various tissues in the body are summarized in great detail in Chapter 8. The most notable class of enzymes are the cytochrome P450 (CYP) enzymes, which are responsible for the Phase I biotransformation of a very large percentage of marketed drug compounds. The liver has by far the highest levels of CYP enzymes in the body, although the GI tract, lungs, and to some extent the skin also have significant levels of CYP enzymes. It is interesting to note that any xenobiotic agent entering the body typically encounters one or more of these CYP-expressing tissues before any possible exposure to the rest of the body. Thus CYP enzymes serve as gatekeepers to protect the body against foreign chemical invaders entering via dermal absorption (skin), air-borne exposure (lungs), and oral ingestion (GI tract and liver first-pass metabolism), providing a means for the potentially toxic xenobiotics to be modified into less dangerous or more readily excretable forms before reaching other tissues. Besides the CYP enzymes, many other Phase I and Phase II enzymes are located throughout the body and play important roles in the metabolism of certain drugs and other xenobiotics. It is well recognized, however, that the liver is by far the most important site of metabolism in the body, being rich in CYP, other Phase I, and many Phase II enzymes. Thus although PK models incorporate metabolic processes from all tissues in the body, the liver is typically the primary focus of attention.

It should also be noted that although metabolism usually decreases the toxicity as well as activity of most drugs and xenobiotic agents, this is not always the case. For certain chemicals, a process called bioactivation can occur in which one or more of the metabolites are more active or more toxic than the parent compound. Acetaminophen, one of the most commonly taken drugs on the market, has a metabolite that can be extremely toxic to liver tissues at high concentrations. The levels of this metabolite are normally too low to cause problems, but if a person takes a high dose of acetaminophen, such as ingesting several types of cold or flu medicines that each contain their own dose of acetaminophen, then it can cause severe health complications.

Bioactivation can also cause a drug metabolite to be more therapeutically active than the parent drug molecule. For example, both codeine and morphine are converted into morphine-glucuronide metabolites, which are more effective at relieving pain than either of the parent drugs. When a drug molecule is specifically designed to become more active after metabolic bioactivation, it is typically called a *prodrug*. A prodrug approach is commonly used when the active form of a drug has poor bioavailability, either because it is poorly absorbed or degraded before reaching the systemic circulation. In these cases, the medication can be delivered as a prodrug that is readily absorbed and resists degradation. Once the prodrug reaches the liver or systemic circulation, enzymes convert it to the active form to yield the desired beneficial activity. Many ACE inhibitors, such as enalapril and quinapril, are delivered as oral prodrugs, which then get converted to their active forms by carboxylesterase enzymes in the liver.

10.5.1.1 Michaelis-Menten Enzyme Kinetics

Nearly all enzymes follow what is known as Michaelis-Menten kinetics, which was encountered in Section 10.2.2 for carrier-mediated transport processes. The Michaelis-Menten equation for the rate of metabolism (r_{met}) can be written as

$$r_{met} = \frac{V_{max,m} \cdot f_u C}{K_m + f_u C} \tag{10.48}$$

where $V_{max,m}$ is the maximum rate of metabolism in mass (or moles) per time, C is the drug concentration in the vicinity of the enzyme, f_u is the unbound drug fraction (fraction of drug molecules that are not bound to macroproteins such as albumin), and K_m is the Michaelis-Menten metabolism constant representing the unbound drug concentration at which the rate of metabolism is half of the maximal rate. As in the carrier-mediated transport case, the unbound drug concentration ($f_u C$) is generally much lower than the value of K_m, in which case this equation can be simplified to

$$\text{for } f_u C << K_m, \quad r_{met} \approx \left(\frac{V_{max,m}}{K_m}\right) \cdot f_u C \tag{10.49}$$

Thus the rate of metabolism is generally proportional to the drug concentration, even when the enzyme itself follows nonlinear Michaelis-Menten kinetics.

10.5.1.2 Metabolic Clearance and Hepatic Clearance

The clearance (CL) is a PK term that is typically defined as "the volume of plasma from which drug is completely removed per unit time." This definition may be useful in some strict technical sense, but for most people it is much more informative to say that the clearance (CL) relates the plasma drug concentration (C_p) to the overall elimination rate (r_{elim}) by the equation

$$r_{elim} = CL \cdot C_p \tag{10.50}$$

where CL has units of volume per time (like a flow rate). Clearance terms can be defined for specific types of elimination or for elimination in a particular organ or tissue, such as metabolic clearance (CL_{met}) or hepatic clearance (CL_H), so that the rate of metabolism (r_{met}) becomes

$$r_{met} = CL_{met} \cdot C_p \tag{10.51}$$

and the rate of hepatic metabolism ($r_{met,H}$) is

$$r_{met,H} = CL_H \cdot C_p \tag{10.52}$$

Hepatic metabolism can be considered to occur by a two-stage process, in which drug must first be delivered by convective blood flow transport to the liver, after which the enzymes in the liver convert the drug molecules to one or more metabolites. The hepatic clearance can then be written in a general form that accounts for both of these processes as

$$CL_H = \frac{Q_H f_u CL_{u,int}}{Q_H + f_u CL_{u,int}} \tag{10.53}$$

where Q_H is the hepatic plasma or blood flow rate (about 800 ml/min for plasma or 1.5 L/min for blood in humans), f_u is the unbound fraction of drug, and $CL_{u,int}$ is the intrinsic rate of enzyme activity for unbound drug molecules. The value of $CL_{u,int}$ can often be estimated from *in vitro* experiments with isolated liver cells or purified enzymes. The hepatic perfusion and enzymatic processes occur in series, and like the perfusion-limited and permeability-limited cases in chemical transport, hepatic metabolism can be limited by the slower of the two processes to give either perfusion-limited or enzyme-limited metabolic rates. For perfusion-limited hepatic metabolism, the enzymatic activity is sufficiently high to convert all the drug molecules entering the liver into metabolites, so that the hepatic metabolic rate is limited by the blood flow delivery of drug to the liver. The hepatic clearance for the perfusion-limited case is then

$$CL_H \approx Q_H \quad \text{when} \quad Q_H << f_u CL_{u,int} \tag{10.54}$$

Conversely, if the enzymatic activity is so low that only a small fraction of the drug entering the liver is metabolized, then the hepatic metabolic rate is enzyme-limited. The hepatic clearance for the enzyme-limited case becomes

$$CL_{H,enz} \approx f_u CL_{u,int} \quad \text{when} \quad f_u CL_{u,int} << Q_H \tag{10.55}$$

One fact that can be observed from this limiting-case analysis is that no matter how much intrinsic enzyme activity is present in the liver, the hepatic clearance (CL_H) can never be greater than the hepatic blood flow rate (Q_H).

10.5.1.3 First-Order Rate of Metabolism

As with previous first-order rate equations for absorption and distribution, a first-order equation for the metabolic rate (r_{met}) can be written

$$r_{met} = k_{met} \cdot A^1_{rem} = k_{met} \cdot A_{rem} \tag{10.56}$$

where k_{met} is a first-order metabolic rate constant, and A_{rem} is the amount of drug that remains. This equation can alternatively be written in terms of the metabolic clearance (CL_{met}) as

$$r_{met} = CL_{met} \cdot C_p \tag{10.57}$$

where CL_{met} is taken to be a constant for first-order metabolism and C_p is the plasma concentration of the drug. Note once again that first-order metabolism can be said to follow linear kinetics since the rate of metabolism is a linear function of the amount of drug remaining (with a slope of k_{met}) or the plasma concentration (with a slope of CL_{met}). The metabolic rates for most drugs do follow first-order or linear kinetics, which can be explained by the fact that the unbound drug concentration (f_uC) is generally much lower than the value of the Michaelis-Menten constant K_m. As indicated in Equation (10.49), this situation leads to the metabolic rate being approximately equal to some constant value multiplied by the plasma drug concentration, or alternatively by the amount of drug remaining. Cases where this approximation of first-order metabolism cannot be made will be discussed in Section 10.15.8.

10.5.2 Excretion

Excretion is defined as the discharge of drug molecules into any body waste that then leaves the body. Thus excretion in theory could include discharge into urine via the kidneys, feces via bile from the liver, exhaled air via the lungs, or sweat via the skin. For most drugs, however, the primary routes of excretion are into the urine via the kidneys or into bile/feces via the liver. Excretion into the urine is most common for water-soluble molecules, so many polar drugs with low log$P$ values are excreted unchanged directly into the urine. Lipophillic nonpolar drugs must generally undergo metabolism to more polar forms before being excreted into the urine. Drug molecules that are larger (MW > 500), lipophillic (log$P$ > 2), or glucuronide or glutathione conjugated are more likely to be excreted via the liver into the bile. Drugs excreted into bile end up in the intestines, where some of the drug molecules can be reabsorbed and thus recycled back into the systemic circulation. This is called the enterohepatic cycle, which can prolong the time that some drugs remain in the body. An analogous type of reabsorption can occur in the kidney tubules, which will be discussed in greater detail in the next section.

10.5.2.1 Excretion Clearance and Renal Clearance

As shown in Section 10.5.1.2, clearance terms can be defined for specific types of elimination or for elimination in a particular organ or tissue. Thus the rate of excretion (r_{excr}) is related to the excretion clearance (CL_{excr}) by

$$r_{excr} = CL_{excr} \cdot C_p \tag{10.58}$$

The renal (or urinary) excretion rate ($r_{excr,R}$) is similarly related to the renal clearance (CL_R):

$$r_{excr,R} = CL_R \cdot C_p \tag{10.59}$$

The renal excretion process has already been described in some detail in Chapter 9. Briefly, renal excretion is considered to occur in three distinct stages. The first stage is glomerular filtration, where about 20% of the plasma entering the kidney is filtered through the glomeruli as previously illustrated in Figure 10.7. This filtered plasma flow rate is called the glomerular filtration rate (GFR or Q_{GFR}) and averages about 100 to 125 ml/min in humans. Unbound drug is transported through the glomerular wall along with the filtered plasma. The filtered plasma continues to flow through the kidney tubule, while the blood leaving the glomeruli flows through the efferent arteriole. The tubule and efferent arteriole are kept in close proximity for intermolecular transport for quite a while after filtration. During this transit period, active transport proteins move selected molecules (including some drug molecules) from the arteriole blood into the tubule. This process is called tubular secretion, and has the effect of increasing the excretion of the transported molecules relative to that achieved by glomerular filtration alone. Conversely, molecules can also be reabsorbed from the tubule back into the arteriole blood, which generally occurs strictly by passive diffusion except for a few select types of molecules such as sugars. This process is called tubular reabsorption, and it has the effect of decreasing the excretion of reabsorbed molecules relative to that of glomerular filtration alone. Thus the overall renal excretion rate ($r_{excr,R}$) can be expressed as

$$r_{excr,R} = r_{glomerular\ filtration} + r_{tubular\ secretion} - r_{tubular\ reabsorption} \tag{10.60}$$

The rate of excretion due to glomerular filtration can be written directly from Equation (10.26) as

$$r_{glomerular\ filtration} = Q_{GFR} \cdot f_u \cdot C_p \tag{10.61}$$

where Q_{GFR} is the rate of plasma filtration flow through the glomeruli. The tubular secretion rate can be expected to be written as a Michaelis-Menten rate equation similar to that in Equation (10.23), whereas the rate of tubular reabsorption can be expressed as passive diffusion similar to that in Equation (10.19). Rather than trying to actually write these rates in strict equation forms, it is more common to compare the renal clearance (CL_R) to the value expected for glomerular filtration alone. The renal clearance due to filtration alone ($CL_{R,filt}$) becomes

$$CL_{R,filt} = f_u \cdot Q_{GFR} \tag{10.62}$$

If tubular secretion is significant for a given drug, then

$$CL_R > f_u \cdot Q_{GFR} \quad \text{for significant tubular secretion} \tag{10.63}$$

Conversely, if tubular reabsorption is significant for a given drug, then

$$CL_R < f_u \cdot Q_{GFR} \quad \text{for significant tubular reabsorption} \tag{10.64}$$

The experimental determination of renal clearance is relatively straightforward since urine and plasma can both be sampled and analyzed. The premise is that urine is collected over some time interval ($t_1 \rightarrow t_2$), and a plasma sample is drawn at the midpoint of the time interval. The amount of drug in the urine sample

(A_{urine}) and the midpoint plasma sample drug concentration ($C_{p,mid}$) are then measured by some analytical technique. The urinary or renal excretion rate ($r_{excr,R}$) for the collected urine sample is then given by

$$r_{excr,R} = \frac{A_{urine}}{t_2 - t_1} \tag{10.65}$$

The renal clearance (CL_R) can then be calculated from Equation (10.59) as

$$CL_R = \frac{C_p}{r_{excr,R}} = \frac{C_{p,mid}}{\left(\frac{A_{urine}}{t_2 - t_1}\right)} \tag{10.66}$$

The measured value of CL_R can then be compared to $f_u \cdot Q_{GFR}$ to determine whether tubule secretion or tubule reabsorption play significant roles in the urinary excretion of the drug.

10.5.2.2 First-Order Rate of Excretion

As with previous first-order rate equations, a first-order equation for the excretion rate (r_{excr}) can be written as

$$r_{excr} = k_{excr} \cdot A_{rem}^1 = k_{excr} \cdot A_{rem} \tag{10.67}$$

where k_{excr} is a first-order excretion rate constant, and A_{rem} is the amount of drug that remains. This equation can alternatively be written in terms of the excretion clearance (CL_{excr}) as

$$r_{excr} = CL_{excr} \cdot C_p \tag{10.68}$$

where CL_{excr} is taken to be a constant for first-order excretion and C_p is the plasma concentration of the drug. Note once again that first-order excretion can be said to follow linear kinetics since the rate of excretion is a linear function of the amount of drug remaining (with a slope of k_{excr}) or the plasma concentration (with a slope of CL_{excr}). The excretion rates for most drugs do follow first-order or linear kinetics, since the only potential source of saturable or nonlinear kinetics is the active secretion process in the renal tubules or into bile.

10.5.3 Pharmacokinetic Elimination Models

Since drug elimination can occur by metabolism or excretion, the overall elimination rate (r_{elim}) of a drug then becomes the sum of the metabolic rate (r_{met}) and the excretion rate (r_{excr})

$$r_{elim} = r_{met} + r_{excr} \tag{10.69}$$

These rate equations can be expressed in terms of clearance values, or they can be expressed in terms of first-order rate equations if the rates follow linear kinetics. Several other useful PK parameters are defined based on these elimination rate equations in the following sections.

10.5.3.1 Overall Elimination Clearance

The overall clearance (CL) has been defined in Section 10.5.1.2 as a parameter that relates the plasma drug concentration (C_p) to the overall elimination rate (r_{elim}) by the equation

$$r_{met} = CL \cdot C_p \tag{10.70}$$

where CL has units of volume per time (like a flow rate). Similar clearance terms and rate equations have also been defined for metabolism and excretion:

$$r_{met} = CL_{met} \cdot C_p \tag{10.71}$$

$$r_{excr} = CL_{excr} \cdot C_p \tag{10.72}$$

Combining these equations with Equation (10.69) gives the relationship

$$CL = CL_{met} + CL_{excr} \tag{10.73}$$

By a similar type of reasoning, it could be shown that the total clearance can also be written as the sum of metabolic and excretion clearances for each organ or tissue where metabolism or excretion of a drug takes place. For example, the overall clearance for a drug that undergoes hepatic metabolism as well as renal and bile excretion would become

$$CL = CL_H + CL_R + CL_{bile} \tag{10.74}$$

Additional clearance terms would be added to this sum as needed to account for the involvement of additional organs or tissues in drug elimination.

10.5.3.2 Overall First-Order Elimination Rate Constant

If the elimination rate, metabolic rate, and excretion rate all follow first-order (or linear) kinetics, then the overall first-order elimination rate constant (k) can be written as

$$r_{elim} = k \cdot A_{rem} \tag{10.75}$$

and the first-order rate constant for metabolism and excretion can be combined by

$$k = k_{met} + k_{excr} \tag{10.76}$$

Similarly, the overall elimination rate constant can also be written as the sum of metabolic and excretion rate constants for each organ or tissue where metabolism or excretion of a drug takes place. For the previous example in Equation (10.74), where a drug that undergoes hepatic metabolism as well as renal and bile excretion, the overall rate constant becomes

$$k = k_H + k_R + k_{bile} \tag{10.77}$$

Again, additional rate constants would be added to this sum as needed to account for the involvement of additional organs or tissues in drug elimination. Equations (10.70) and (10.75) can also be combined with the definition of the volume of distribution (V) in Equation (10.42) to give the relationship between the overall clearance (CL) and overall elimination rate constant (k) as

$$CL = V \cdot k \tag{10.78}$$

Note that this equation can be used only when elimination follows first-order (linear) kinetics, which will be the assumption for all the standard equations presented in this chapter.

10.5.3.3 Elimination Half-Life

The elimination half-life ($t_{½,elim}$) can be defined in the same way as was done previously for absorption and distribution by the equation

$$t_{½,elim} = \frac{\ln(2)}{k} \approx \frac{0.693}{k} \qquad (10.79)$$

This equation can then be combined with Equation (10.78) to give the relationship between clearance (CL) and the elimination half-life as

$$t_{½,elim} = \frac{V \cdot \ln(2)}{CL} \approx \frac{0.693 \cdot V}{CL} \qquad (10.80)$$

As with previous half-lives, this indicates that elimination is 50% complete after one elimination half-life, 75% complete after two elimination half-lives, and about 99% complete after seven elimination half-lives. Since elimination represents the final removal of drug molecules from the body, the elimination half-life also serves as the determining factor of how much of the originally absorbed drug remains in the body, so that 50% of the absorbed drug remains after one elimination half-life, 25% remains after two elimination half-lives, and only about 1% remains after seven elimination half-lives. The elimination half-life is the half-life value reported in drug handbooks as an indication of how long a drug remains active in the body.

10.5.3.4 Fraction of Drug Eliminated by Different Routes of Metabolism or Excretion

The fraction of absorbed drug eliminated by a particular route of metabolism or excretion ($f_{absD,route}$) can be represented by the ratio of the amount of drug eliminated by the route ($A_{elim,route}$) and the overall absorbed dose (FD) by the ratio

$$f_{absD,route} = \frac{A_{elim,route}}{FD} \qquad (10.81)$$

It turns out that the fraction in this equation is related to the clearance associated with this elimination route (CL_{route}) relative to the overall clearance (CL), or the rate constant for this route (k_{route}) relative to the overall elimination rate constant (k), as given by

$$f_{absD,route} = \frac{A_{elim,route}}{FD} = \frac{CL_{route}}{CL} = \frac{k_{route}}{k} \qquad (10.82)$$

Thus the fraction of absorbed drug that undergoes hepatic metabolism becomes

$$f_{absD,H} = \frac{A_{met,H}}{FD} = \frac{CL_H}{CL} = \frac{k_H}{k} \qquad (10.83)$$

and the fraction of absorbed drug that undergoes renal excretion into the urine as unchanged drug molecule (rather than as metabolites) becomes

$$f_{absD,unch,urine} = \frac{A_{unch,urine}}{FD} = \frac{CL_R}{CL} = \frac{k_R}{k} \qquad (10.84)$$

These terms can be rewritten as fractions of total drug dose eliminated by a given route ($f_{totD,route}$ or simply f_{route}) by accounting for the bioavailability (F), so that for a particular route

$$f_{route} = \frac{A_{elim,route}}{D} = F \cdot f_{absD,route} = F \cdot \left(\frac{CL_{route}}{CL}\right) = F \cdot \left(\frac{k_{route}}{k}\right) \qquad (10.85)$$

This can then be applied to hepatic metabolism to give

$$f_H = \frac{A_{met,H}}{D} = F \cdot \left(\frac{CL_H}{CL}\right) = F \cdot \left(\frac{k_H}{k}\right) \qquad (10.86)$$

For renal excretion of unchanged drug into urine, this becomes

$$f_{unch,urine} = \frac{A_{unch,urine}}{D} = F \cdot \left(\frac{CL_R}{CL}\right) = F \cdot \left(\frac{k_R}{k}\right) \qquad (10.87)$$

This last parameter, fraction of drug dose excreted unchanged in the urine, is often reported in drug handbooks and PK literature as a useful indication of where the drug ends up after removal from the body. If the amount of drug is measured in a series of urine samples, this relationship can also be used to evaluate some of the PK parameters discussed previously.

These calculations can be taken one step further to provide the actual amount of drug eliminated by a particular route. The amount of drug eliminated by hepatic metabolism becomes

$$A_{met,H} = FD \cdot \left(\frac{CL_H}{CL}\right) = FD \cdot \left(\frac{k_H}{k}\right) \qquad (10.88)$$

The amount of drug excreted unchanged in the urine is then

$$A_{unch,urine} = FD \cdot \left(\frac{CL_R}{CL}\right) = FD \cdot \left(\frac{k_R}{k}\right) \qquad (10.89)$$

The last equation once again tends to be the most useful, as the total amount of unchanged drug in the urine can be accurately measured by collecting repeated urine samples until drug is no longer detected in the urine. The total amount of drug measured in the urine samples then represents $A_{unch,urine}$. This measurement can be employed to validate the appropriateness of the PK model being used, or it can be employed to estimate the values of other PK parameters such as the bioavailability (F) or the renal clearance (CL_R).

10.6 ORGANIZATION OF SINGLE-DOSE PHARMACOKINETIC MODEL INFORMATION

The following sections will each describe one of the commonly used single-dose PK modeling approaches. To help make these sections easy to follow, and to make it easy to find information when used as a reference, each PK model section will be structured in a similar manner.

The opening discussion for each model will list general information about the model. This will include the common names for the model, drug dosing situations that are best represented by the model, and a brief outline of other topics that will be covered for the model.

10.6.1 Model Assumptions

All PK models involve several assumptions that allow the amazingly complex interactions between drug molecules and body systems to be simplified into a series of solvable equations. This section will describe the assumptions that are made or are inherent in each PK model. The implications of each assumption regarding application to real-world ADME processes will also be described. When the same assumption is applied to more than one model, it will be described in detail for the first model, with subsequent descriptions of the same assumption then simply referring back to the earlier description.

10.6.2 Setup and Solution of Mass Balance Equations

All PK models are derived by writing the governing mass balance equations for the model and then solving these equations mathematically. Mass balance equations are written in the general form

$$\frac{d}{dt}(\text{Amount of Drug}) = [\text{Rate of Drug In}] - [\text{Rate of Drug Out}] \quad (10.90)$$

where the term on the left-hand side of the equation represents the rate of change of the amount of drug in a given compartment, and the terms on the right represent the difference between the rates at which drug molecules enter and exit the compartment. There is always one mass balance equation for each compartment included in the model. The step-by-step derivation of the solution of these governing mass balance equations is not provided in this chapter. The equations are included, however, because they do allow readers to better understand how the resulting model equations arise, and they provide inquisitive readers with the information needed to derive the model equations on their own.

10.6.3 Plasma Concentration versus Time Relationships

The equations for plasma concentration versus time will be described in this section. Since half-life values are often used to understand how plasma concentrations vary with time, equations will also be given for all half-life relationships included in the model under consideration. The effect of each of the models' basic parameters on the shape of plasma concentration versus time will be discussed mathematically and shown graphically. Application of the model equations in predicting plasma concentrations will also be explained.

10.6.4 Estimating Model Parameters from Measured Plasma Concentration Data

The previous section explained how to estimate plasma concentrations based on known PK parameters for a drug; this section provides the methods for estimating the PK parameters of a drug based on experimental plasma measurements. The data analysis methods for each model have some steps in common, but each also contains calculations specific to the given model.

10.6.5 Special Cases of the Pharmacokinetic Model

Many of the models described in this chapter can have special case situations. One type of special situation occurs when a complex model can be reduced to a simplified model under certain circumstances. For these types of cases, the conditions under which the simplified model can be used are explained fully. Any modifications of the model equations that must be made to apply them to these cases will also be provided. A second type of special case involves modification of the standard model in order to properly represent a particular type of nonstandard circumstances. As in the first case, all necessary modifications to the model equations or data analysis will be explained fully.

10.7 ONE-COMPARTMENT BOLUS IV INJECTION (INSTANTANEOUS ABSORPTION) MODEL

The one-compartment bolus IV injection model is mathematically the simplest of all PK models. Drug is delivered directly into the systemic circulation by a rapid injection over a very short period of time. Thus the bolus IV injection offers a near perfect example of an instantaneous absorption process. Representation of the body as a single compartment implies that the distribution process is essentially instantaneous as well. The exact meaning of the assumptions inherent in this model are described in the next section. Model equations are then introduced that allow the prediction of plasma concentrations for drugs with known PK parameters, or the estimation of PK parameters from measured plasma concentrations. Situations in which the one-compartment instantaneous absorption model can be used to reasonably approximate other types of drug delivery are described later in Section 10.7.5.

10.7.1 Model Assumptions

The standard one-compartment bolus IV (or instantaneous absorption) model makes three inherent assumptions about the ADME processes that occur after drug delivery. The specific nature and implications of each of these assumptions are described in this section.

10.7.1.1 Instantaneous Absorption

As in all instantaneous absorption models, the entire absorbed dose of drug is taken to enter the systemic circulation instantly at time zero ($t = 0$). This provides an excellent approximation of the rapid drug delivery directly into the systemic circulation provided by a bolus IV injection, which truly occurs over a very short period of time (typically several seconds). However, this assumption does not actually require a strict interpretation of the word instantaneous. Even if an absorption process takes a substantial period of time (minutes or hours), it can still be approximated as instantaneous as long as absorption occurs quickly relative to other ADME processes. Thus, other routes of drug delivery besides a bolus IV injection can be approximated by instantaneous absorption if the time it takes for the absorption process to be essentially complete is very small compared to the half-life of elimination. The equations throughout most of this section are written specifically for a bolus IV injection, but modifications that can be employed to apply the equations to other drug delivery methods are described in Section 10.7.5.

10.7.1.2 Instantaneous Distribution

As in all standard one-compartment PK models, the body is represented by a single compartment, with plasma and tissue drug concentrations taken to reach equilibrium instantly. Drug distribution can never truly be instantaneous, as it cannot occur faster than the perfusion and permeation transport to the tissues. However, instantaneous distribution provides a reasonable approximation as long as all the tissues that eventually receive significant levels of drug approach equilibrium with plasma in a time period that is small compared to the elimination half-life. Many drug molecules are not accurately represented by a one-compartment instantaneous distribution model. In spite of this shortcoming, one-compartment models are often used, even when they do not apply well to the drug at hand. This is because the one-compartment model offers much simpler mathematics than multicompartment models, and the one-compartment approximation is often close enough for many drug modeling purposes (e.g., dosage adjustment or estimating drug accumulation during multiple dosing treatment). The assumption of instantaneous distribution also implies that the volume of distribution (V) for the body is a constant.

10.7.1.3 First-Order (Linear) Elimination Kinetics

As in all PK models described in this chapter, the rate of drug elimination is taken to follow first-order (or linear) elimination kinetics. Thus the rate of elimination is proportional to the amount of drug remaining to be eliminated. As discussed previously, this is often a reasonable approximation as most drug concentrations in the body are much less than the Michaelis-Menten K_m value of enzymes and transporter proteins.

10.7.2 Setup and Solution of Mass Balance Equations

A separate mass balance equation is written in the form of Section 10.6.2 for each compartment included in the model. Since this is a one-compartment model, only one mass balance equation is used. The amount of drug in the compartment is equal to the total amount of drug in the body (A_{body}). The absorbed dose of drug is given generally by multiplying the total dose (D) by the bioavailability (F). Since the bioavailability for an intravenous injection (F_{iv}) is by definition equal to 100% (or 1.0), the amount of drug absorbed for a bolus IV injection becomes equal to simply the injected dose (D_{iv}). From the instantaneous absorption assumption, the entire dose of drug (D_{iv}) enters the body instantly at time zero, which will be used as an initial condition for the mass balance equation. No additional drug enters the body compartment after time zero, so the rate of drug entering the compartment in the general mass balance equation is zero. The elimination rate is equal to the amount of drug remaining in the compartment (A_{body}) multiplied by an elimination rate constant (k). A schematic representation of this one-compartment bolus IV model is provided in Figure 10.17. The mass balance equation then becomes simply

$$\frac{dA_{body}}{dt} = -kA_{body} \quad \text{with} \quad A_{body} = D_{iv} \quad \text{at} \quad t = 0 \tag{10.91}$$

The differential equation provided by the mass balance can be solved to give

$$A_{body} = D_{iv}e^{-kt} \tag{10.92}$$

Note that derivations of the mass balance differential equation solutions are not being provided in this chapter, but if you are interested, you are encouraged

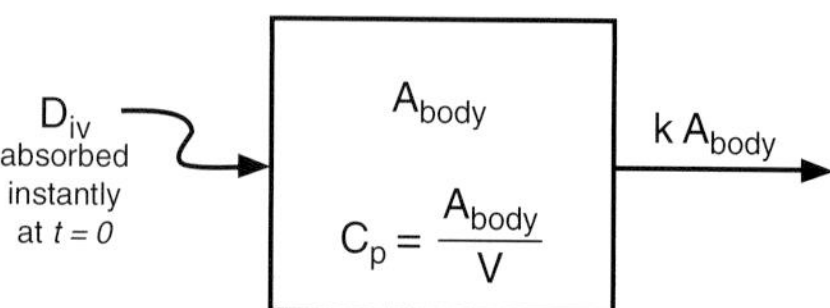

Figure 10.17 Schematic representation of the one-compartment model for a bolus IV injection.

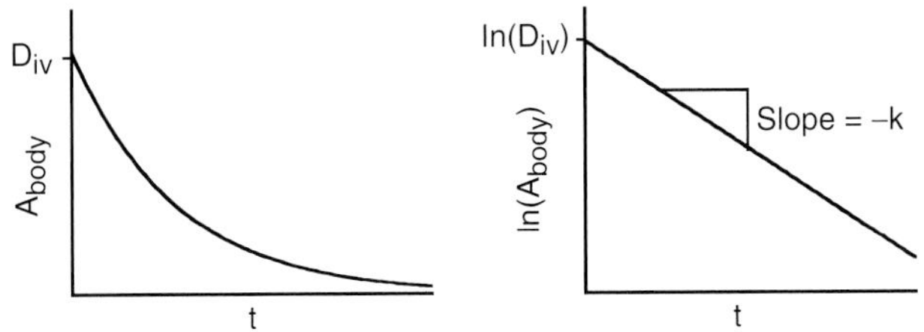

Figure 10.18 Graphical representation of the amount of drug in the body (A_{body}) versus time (t) and ln(A_{body}) versus t for a one-compartment PK model of a bolus IV injection.

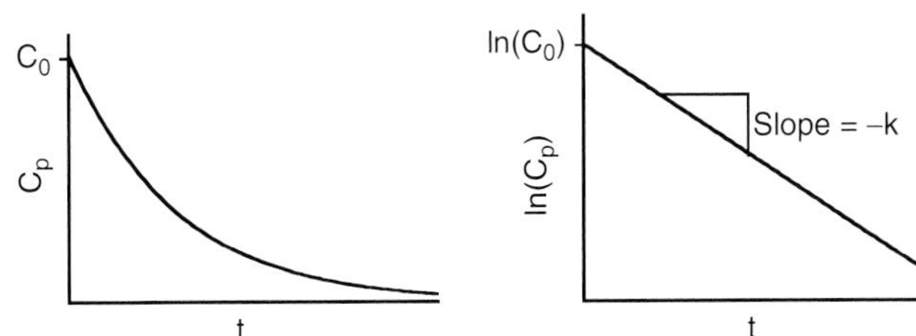

Figure 10.19 Graphical representation of the plasma concentration (C_p) versus time (t) and ln(C_p) versus t for a one-compartment PK model of a bolus IV injection.

to verify these solutions on your own. Taking the natural logarithm of both sides of this equation yields a log-linear form of the equation

$$\ln(A_{body}) = \ln(D_{iv}) - kt \tag{10.93}$$

where $\ln(A_{body})$ is the dependent linear variable (y), t is the independent linear variable (x), $\ln(D_{iv})$ is the linear intercept (b), and $-k$ is the linear slope (m). Graphical representations of the exponential Equation (10.92) and the log-linear Equation (10.93) are provided in Figure 10.18.

10.7.3 Plasma Concentration versus Time Relationships

The plasma concentration of drug (C_p) can be related to the amount of drug in the body (A_{body}) by the volume of distribution (V), as in the equation

$$C_p = \frac{A_{body}}{V} \tag{10.94}$$

Dividing both sides of Equation (10.92) by V then gives

$$C_p = \left(\frac{D_{iv}}{V}\right) \cdot e^{-kt} = C_0 \cdot e^{-kt} \tag{10.95}$$

where the initial plasma concentration (C_0) can then be written

$$C_0 = \frac{D_{iv}}{V} \tag{10.96}$$

Taking the natural logarithm of both sides of Equation (10.95) then gives the log-linear form

$$\ln(C_p) = \ln(C_0) - kt \tag{10.97}$$

Graphical representations of C_p and $\ln(C_p)$ versus t are provided in Figure 10.19.

10.7.3.1 Elimination Half-Life

The elimination half-life ($t_{½,elim}$) for the plasma concentration (C_p), which is the same as for the amount of drug in the body (A_{body}), can then be defined as

$$t_{½,elim} = \frac{\ln(2)}{k} \approx \frac{0.693}{k} \tag{10.98}$$

This equation can also be rearranged to

$$k = \frac{\ln(2)}{t_{½,elim}} \approx \frac{0.693}{t_{½,elim}} \tag{10.99}$$

which allows the elimination rate constant (k) to be calculated for a reported elimination half-life ($t_{½,elim}$) found in a drug handbook or research article. As explained previously, the elimination process is 50% complete after one $t_{½,elim}$, 75% complete after two $t_{½,elim}$, and about 99% complete after seven $t_{½,elim}$. Conversely, the plasma concentration is 50% of the initial value after one $t_{½,elim}$, 25% of the initial value after two $t_{½,elim}$, and about 1% of the initial value after seven $t_{½,elim}$. See Table 10.1 for more details.

10.7.3.2 Effect of Basic Model Parameters on the Plasma Concentration versus Time Curve

The effects of different model parameters on the plasma concentration versus time relationship can be demonstrated by mathematical analysis of the previous equations, or by graphical representation of a change in one or more of the variables. Equation (10.95) indicates that the plasma concentration (C_p) is proportional to the dose (D_{iv}) and inversely proportional to the volume of distribution (V). Thus an increase in D_{iv} or a decrease in V both yield an equivalent increase in C_p, as illustrated in Figure 10.20. Note that the general shape of the curve, or more specifically the slope of the line for $\ln(C_p)$ versus t, is not a function of D_{iv} or V. Equations (10.98) and (10.99) show that the

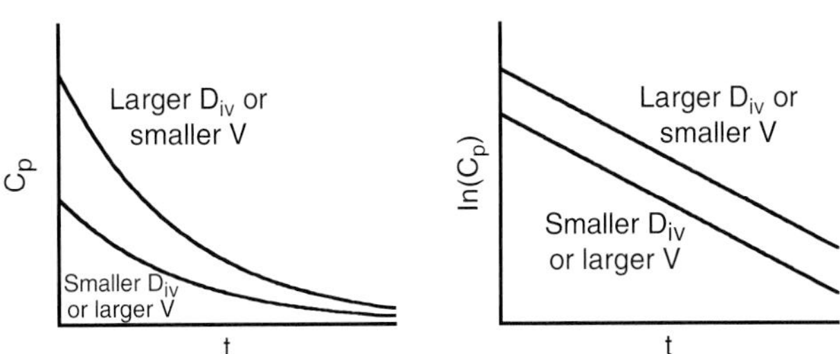

Figure 10.20 Graphical illustration of how plasma concentration (C_p) and ln(C_p) versus t change with an increase or decrease in the dose (D_{iv}) or volume of distribution (V).

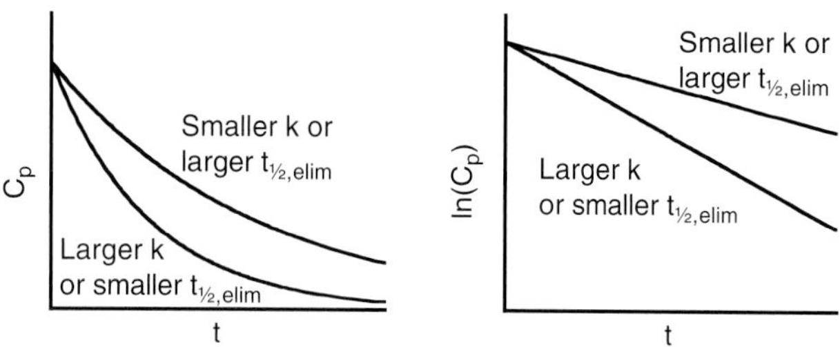

Figure 10.21 Graphical illustration of how plasma concentration (C_p) and ln(C_p) versus t change with an increase or decrease in the elimination rate constant (k) or elimination half-life ($t_{½,elim}$).

elimination rate constant (k) and the elimination half-life ($t_{½,elim}$) are inversely related to each other, so that an increase in one is equivalent to a decrease in the other. It can then be shown that an increase in k or a decrease in $t_{½,elim}$ do not affect the initial plasma concentration (C_0) in Figure 10.21, but they do make the plasma concentrations drop off more rapidly with time (a steeper or more negative slope in the log-linear plot).

10.7.3.3 Estimating Plasma Drug Concentrations

Average values for the volume of distribution (V) and elimination half-life ($t_{½,elim}$) for many drugs can be found in drug handbooks, pharmacology textbooks, or in PK research articles (which can be searched online). Once the values of these parameters have been obtained, the plasma concentration for the drug can be estimated for any time after bolus IV injection of a known drug dose by simply substituting the appropriate values for D_{iv}, V, k, and the desired time (t) into the previous model equations. Alternatively, Equation (10.95) can be solved for t to give

$$t = \frac{-\ln\left(\frac{C_p}{C_0}\right)}{k} \tag{10.100}$$

This equation can be used to calculate the time at which the plasma concentration (C_p) reaches a particular value.

10.7.4 Estimating Model Parameters from Measured Plasma Concentration Data

PK models can be employed in two distinct modes. The previous section described using known PK parameters from the literature to estimate plasma concentrations. This section explains how to use measured plasma concentration data to estimate the model parameters for the one-compartment bolus IV model.

Plasma samples for PK analysis by a one-compartment bolus IV model are typically collected at 5 to 12 time points after drug administration. The time interval between samples generally starts out small for early samples and increases for later samples. The drug concentration in each sample is then measured by some type of analytical chemistry technique.

10.7.4.1 Linear Regression of ln(C_p) versus t

The first step of nearly every PK data analysis procedure is to calculate the natural logarithm of each of the measured plasma concentration values. The values of ln(C_p) are then plotted versus the time (t) of sample collection. If the plot shows a series of points falling near a straight line, then the data can be well represented by the one-compartment bolus IV model. Early or late data points that do not fall on the line created by other points can be indicative of plasma sample analysis problems, or could indicate that the one-compartment bolus IV model is not the best PK model for the data, as indicated in Figure 10.22.

Once it has been verified that the data can be properly fit to a one-compartment bolus IV model, a linear regression analysis is performed on the data, with time (t) entered as the independent (x) data, and ln(C_p) entered as the dependent (y) data. Linear regression analysis can be performed on calculators that handle two-variable statistics, or using spreadsheet, graphing, or statistical analysis software on a computer. The analysis should provide values for the intercept (b) and the slope (m) that provide the best possible fit to the measured data in the form $y = b + mx$, as illustrated in Figure 10.23. The linear regression analysis also often provides a value called the correlation coefficient (r),

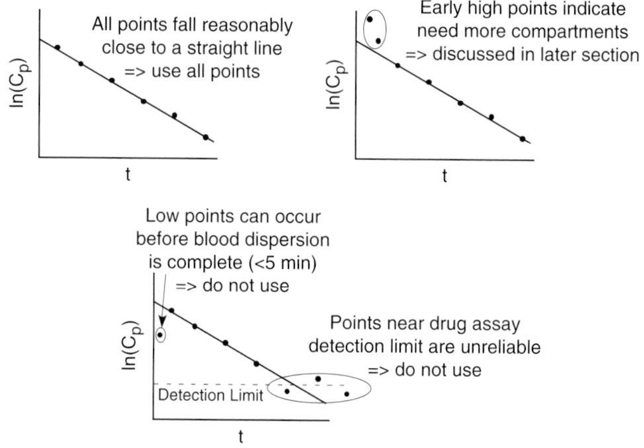

Figure 10.22 The graph of ln(C_p) versus time (t) should be inspected to evaluate whether the selected PK model is appropriate and determine if any points might be unreliable.

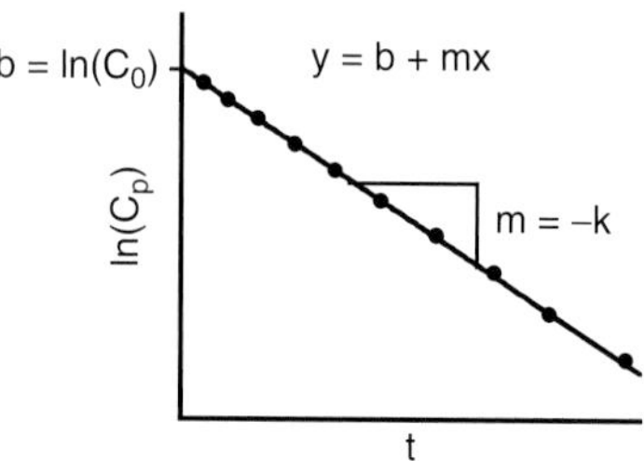

Figure 10.23 Analysis of measured plasma concentration (C_p) data by linear regression of ln(C_p) versus time (t).

which indicates how well the data is fit to a straight line. Data that falls very close to a straight line typically has a correlation coefficient near +1 or −1, with the sign of the value indicating whether the slope (m) is positive (+) or negative (−). The correlation can also be represented by the square of the correlation coefficient (r^2), in which case a good fit is indicated by values near +1. As a rough rule of thumb, data is fit reasonably well by a PK model if r is between −0.99 and −1 (r and the slope are always negative in this model) or r^2 is greater than about 0.98 in value. The intercept (b) from this fitted linear equation represents the best value for $\ln(C_0)$, from which C_0 can be calculated as

$$C_0 = e^b \tag{10.101}$$

The fitted slope (m) similarly represents the best value for $-k$, so that

$$k = -m \tag{10.102}$$

The elimination half-life ($t_{½,elim}$) can be calculated from k by Equation (10.98). The volume of distribution (V) can be calculated from the fitted value of C_0 by rearranging Equation (10.96) to give

$$V = \frac{D_{iv}}{C_0} \tag{10.103}$$

The overall elimination clearance (CL) for the one-compartment bolus IV model, discussed previously in Section 10.5.3.1, can then be calculated as

$$CL = Vk \tag{10.104}$$

Thus all the basic model parameters for the one-compartment bolus IV model can be determined from a single linear regression analysis of measured plasma concentration data.

10.7.4.2 Area under the Curve (AUC) Calculations

The area under the plasma concentration versus time curve, also called the area under the curve (AUC), ends up being an extremely useful parameter in PK models. It can be used as a means of evaluating the volume of distribution (V) and total elimination clearance (CL), it can provide a measure of the bioavailability (F) for extravascular drug delivery (see Section 10.9.4.4), and it provides a means to test the assumption of first-order linear elimination kinetics (as will be described in Section 10.15.8). As shown previously in Section 10.1.3.3, the AUC can be represented graphically as the area between the plasma concentration versus time curve and the horizontal axis, illustrated in Figure 10.24, or it can be written mathematically as

$$AUC = \int_0^{\infty} C_p \, dt \tag{10.105}$$

As indicated earlier, exponential decay terms are the most commonly encountered functions in PK models. Substituting the relationship for C_p versus t in Equation (10.95) gives the resulting equation forms

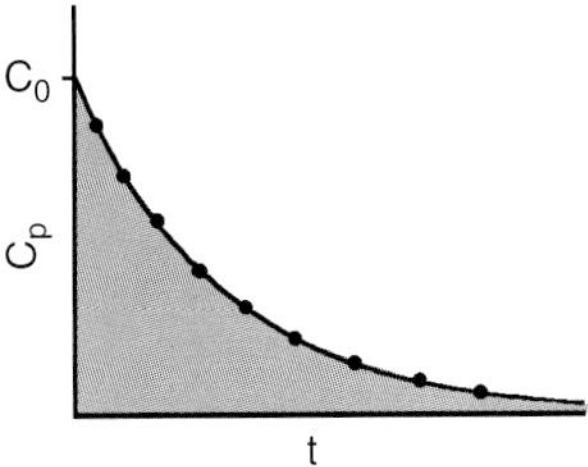

Figure 10.24 The shaded region represents the area under the plasma concentration versus time curve, known as the area under the curve (AUC).

$$AUC = \int_0^{\infty} C_0 \cdot e^{-k \cdot t} \, dt = \frac{C_0}{k} = \frac{D_{iv}}{Vk} = \frac{D_{iv}}{CL} \tag{10.106}$$

The simplest way to calculate AUC from measured plasma concentration data is to perform the linear regression analysis of $\ln(C_p)$ versus t as in the previous section, then substitute the values of C_0 and k derived from the intercept and slope into the equation

$$AUC = \frac{C_0}{k} \tag{10.107}$$

An alternative approach involves applying the trapezoidal rule to sequential pairs of measured plasma concentration values, as illustrated in Figure 10.25. From the general trapezoidal rule in Equation (10.18), the AUC of the left-most slice in Figure 10.25, representing the AUC for $t = 0 \rightarrow t_1$ or $AUC(0 \rightarrow t_1)$, becomes

$$AUC(0 \rightarrow t_1) \approx \frac{1}{2}\left[C_0 + C_1\right] \cdot t_1 \tag{10.108}$$

where C_0 is the estimate of the initial concentration from the linear regression analysis in the previous section, and C_1 is the plasma concentration measured at t_1. The AUC of each of the successive slices from t_1 up to t_f can then be estimated by applying the trapezoidal rule to each successive set of plasma concentration measurements. The general equation for these successive calculations for two successive plasma concentration measurements C_n and C_{n+1} made at t_n and t_{n+1} becomes

$$AUC(t_n \rightarrow t_{n+1}) \approx \frac{1}{2}\left[C_n + C_{n+1}\right] \cdot \left(t_{n+1} - t_n\right) \tag{10.109}$$

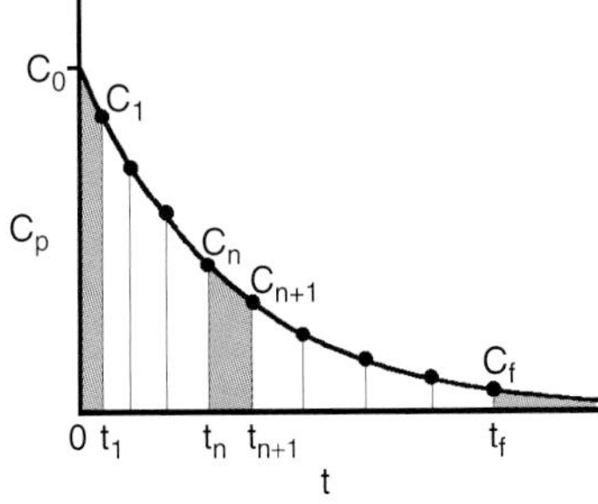

Figure 10.25 Graphical illustration of the application of the trapezoidal rule to numerically estimate the AUC.

Finally, the area under the curve for the final segment from t_f to an infinite time, called the tail of the curve, is given by the equation

$$AUC(t_f \to \infty) = AUC(tail) = \frac{C_f}{k} \tag{10.110}$$

Adding the AUC contribution from each slice in Figure 10.25 as estimated by these equations then yields an estimate for the total AUC. The value of AUC estimated from either of the described methods can then be used as an alternative means of evaluating the volume of distribution (V) and the overall elimination clearance (CL) by rearranging the relations in Equation (10.106) to give

$$V = \frac{D_{iv}}{k \cdot AUC} \tag{10.111}$$

$$CL = \frac{D_{iv}}{AUC} \tag{10.112}$$

For one-compartment models, these equations yield essentially the same values of V and CL as those estimated from the linear regression analysis of $\ln(C_p)$ versus t. It will be seen later that for two-compartment models, however, these equations can provide a more universal estimate of overall clearance and an entirely different type of distribution volume.

10.7.5 Special Cases of the One-Compartment Bolus IV (Instantaneous Absorption) Model

There are several special case situations in which the one-compartment bolus IV model can be applied as a reasonable approximation for administration routes other than bolus IV injection, or for drugs that do not quickly reach distributional equilibrium. The means by which the one-compartment bolus IV model can be employed in these situations are described here.

10.7.5.1 One-Compartment Zero-Order Drug Absorption with Short Duration of Drug Delivery

The one-compartment model for steady (zero-order) drug delivery will be covered in Section 10.8. For this type of model, drug is absorbed into the systemic circulation at a consistent or steady rate ($F \cdot k_0$) over some delivery period (T). Examples of this type of drug delivery include IV infusion as well as transdermal, implantable, or intramuscular controlled release systems. The general PK model for this situation is somewhat more complicated than the one-compartment instantaneous absorption case, as one type of PK equation must be used during the drug delivery period ($0 \leq t \leq T$), whereas a different equation is used after the drug delivery has stopped ($t > T$). It turns out that if the drug delivery duration (T) is much shorter than the elimination half-life ($t_{½,elim}$), then plasma concentrations are nearly the same as for the bolus IV injection case. The exact criteria for when this approximation can be used with reasonable accuracy will be covered in Section 10.8.5.3. For cases where this simplification applies, however, the one-compartment bolus IV equations can be used by simply replacing D_{iv} with $F \cdot k_0 \cdot T$.

10.7.5.2 One-Compartment First-Order Drug Absorption with Rapid Absorption

The one-compartment model with first-order absorption of drug will be covered in Section 10.9. For this type of model, the rate at which drug is absorbed into the systemic circulation is proportional to the amount of drug remaining to be absorbed (see Section 10.3.2.3 for details). Most types of extravascular drug delivery, including oral ingestion and subcutaneous injection, can be approximated by first-order absorption. The PK model for one-compartment first-order absorption is somewhat more complicated than the one-compartment instantaneous absorption case, as it involves two exponential terms rather than just one. It turns out that if the first-order absorption process is essentially completed at a time that is much shorter than the elimination half-life ($t_{½,elim}$), then plasma concentrations are nearly the same as for the bolus IV injection case. The exact criteria for when this approximation can be used with reasonable accuracy will be discussed in Section 10.9.5.3. When this simplification applies, the one-compartment bolus IV equations can be used by simply replacing D_{iv} with FD_{ev}, where D_{ev} represents the total dose delivered by the extravascular route.

10.7.5.3 Two-Compartment Instantaneous Drug Absorption Simplification

The two-compartment instantaneous absorption model will be covered in Section 10.10. Plasma concentrations of an instantaneously absorbed drug that follows two-compartment kinetics will yield early high points on the $\ln(C_p)$ versus t plot, as illustrated in Figure 10.22. The PK model for this situation is somewhat more complicated than the one-compartment instantaneous absorption case, as it involves two exponential terms rather than just one. It turns out that if the early high points are only slightly above the line formed by the rest of the data, then the one-compartment model provides a reasonable approximation to the actual plasma concentration. As mentioned previously, the simpler one-compartment model is actually used quite often even when it does not apply particularly well to a given drug (e.g., the early points are substantially above the line). This is because a one-compartment model is substantially easier to use, and because the difference between the models is generally only significant at times shortly after drug delivery. When this simplification is used, the one-compartment bolus IV equations can be employed without modification for a bolus IV injection, or with the modifications listed in Sections 10.7.5.1 and 10.7.5.2 for other routes of delivery.

10.8 ONE-COMPARTMENT IV INFUSION (ZERO-ORDER ABSORPTION) MODEL

Zero-order absorption occurs when drug enters the systemic circulation at a constant rate. An IV infusion, in which a drug solution is delivered directly into the systemic circulation at a steady flow rate, represents an idealized zero-order absorption case. Because of this, standard zero-order absorption models are typically called IV infusion models and are designed specifically for the IV infusion case. This particular section deals with the one-compartment IV infusion model, so as in the previous one-compartment bolus IV model, the body is modeled as a single compartment with the implication that the distribution process is essentially instantaneous. As with the other standard models, the exact meaning of the assumptions inherent in this model are described next. Model equations then are introduced that allow the prediction of plasma concentrations for drugs with known PK parameters, or the estimation of PK parameters from measured plasma concentrations. Modification of the one-compartment IV infusion (zero-order absorption) model to approximate other types of steady drug delivery are described in Section 10.8.5.

10.8.1 Model Assumptions

The standard one-compartment IV infusion (or zero-order absorption) model makes three inherent assumptions about the ADME processes that occur during and after drug delivery:

- Zero-order absorption
- Instantaneous distribution
- First-order (linear) elimination kinetics

The specific nature and implications of each of these assumptions are described next.

10.8.1.1 Zero-Order Absorption

As in all zero-order absorption models, the rate at which drug enters the systemic circulation is taken to be perfectly constant over a fixed period of time (from t equal 0 to T). This is an excellent approximation of the steady delivery of drug directly into the systemic circulation provided by an IV infusion. This assumption also offers a close approximation to other types of drug delivery that provide a reasonably steady release of drug into some region of the body. For example, the rate of drug absorption into the systemic circulation from a dermal patch can vary during the day as the body experiences variations in external temperature that alter the perfusion rate of the skin region where drug absorption occurs. The equations throughout most of this section are written specifically for an IV infusion, but modifications that can be employed to apply the equations to other drug delivery methods are described at the end of this section.

10.8.1.2 Instantaneous Distribution

This assumption is the same for all one-compartment models. See Section 10.7.1.2 for the details regarding this assumption.

10.8.1.3 First-Order (Linear) Elimination Kinetics

This assumption is the same for all PK models described in this chapter. See Section 10.7.1.3 for the details regarding this assumption.

10.8.2 Setup and Solution of Mass Balance Equations

A separate mass balance equation is written in the form of Section 10.6.2 for each compartment included in the model. For most PK models, this would imply that only a single mass balance equation would be needed. An IV infusion has an unusual discontinuity, however, in that drug is delivered into the systemic circulation at a steady rate over a fixed period of time ($0 \leq t \leq T$), after which the rate of drug delivery immediately drops to zero ($t > T$). In order to accommodate this discontinuity in drug delivery, separate mass balance equations must be written for the time period during infusion and the time period after infusion stops.

During either of these time periods, the amount of drug in the compartment is equal to the total amount of drug in the body (A_{body}). The elimination rate during each of these time periods is also given by the same relationship, as the amount of drug remaining in the compartment (A_{body}) multiplied by an elimination rate constant (k). The only process that changes during the two different time periods is the rate at which drug is absorbed. During drug infusion ($0 \leq t \leq T$), drug is delivered intravenously at a constant rate ($k_{0,iv}$). The rate of absorption is then given by multiplying the drug delivery rate by the bioavailability (F_{iv}), giving a drug absorption rate of $F_{iv} \cdot k_{0,iv}$. Since an IV infusion delivers drug directly into the systemic circulation, F_{iv} is by definition equal to 100% (or 1.0), and the rate of drug absorption simply equals the drug infusion rate ($k_{0,iv}$). For the post-infusion period ($t > T$), drug infusion is stopped completely and the rate of drug absorption is zero. A schematic representation of this one-compartment bolus IV model is provided in Figure 10.26.

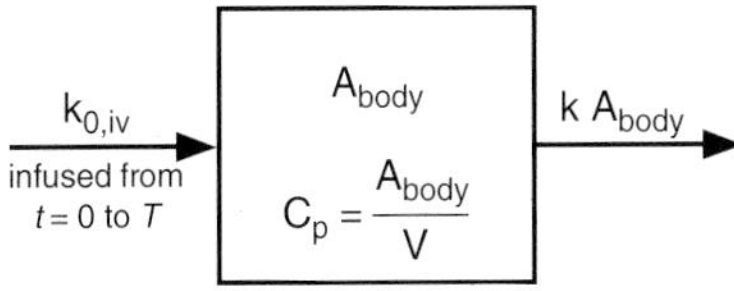

Figure 10.26 Schematic representation of a one-compartment IV infusion model.

The mass balance equation for the infusion period ($0 \le t \le T$) becomes

$$\frac{dA_{body}}{dt} = k_{0,iv} - kA_{body} \quad \text{for} \quad 0 \le t \le T \qquad (10.113)$$

Solution of this differential mass balance equation provides the following relationship for the amount of drug in the body (A_{body}) as a function of time during the infusion period:

$$A_{body} = \frac{k_{0,iv}}{k}(1 - e^{-k \cdot t}) \quad \text{for} \quad 0 \le t \le T \qquad (10.114)$$

The maximum amount of drug in the body ($A_{body,max}$) is equal to the amount of drug in the body at the exact instant when the infusion is stopped ($t = T$), which can be labeled A_T (A_{body} at $t = T$) and can be evaluated as

$$A_{body,max} = A_T = \frac{k_{0,iv}}{k}(1 - e^{-k \cdot t}) \qquad (10.115)$$

The mass balance equation for the post-infusion period (t > T), when there is no drug absorption, can be written

$$\frac{dA_{body}}{dt} = -kA_{body} \quad \text{for} \quad t > T \qquad (10.116)$$

which can then be solved to give

$$A_{body} = \frac{k_{0,iv}}{k}(1 - e^{-k \cdot T}) \cdot e^{-k(t-T)} = A_T \cdot e^{-k(t-T)} \quad \text{for} \quad t > T \qquad (10.117)$$

Taking the natural logarithm of both sides of this equation yields a log-linear form of the equation

$$\ln(A_{body}) = \ln(A_T) - k(t - T) \quad \text{for} \quad t > T \quad (10.118)$$

where $\ln(A_{body})$ is the dependent linear variable (y), $t - T$ is the independent linear variable (x), $\ln(A_T)$ is the linear intercept (b), and $-k$ is the linear slope (m). It is also possible to rearrange the variables in this equation to provide an alternative log-linear form

$$\ln(A_{body}) = [\ln(A_T) + kT] - kt \quad \text{for} \quad t > T \quad (10.119)$$

where $\ln(A_{body})$ is still the dependent linear variable (y), and $-k$ is still the linear slope (m), but t rather than $t - T$ is now the independent linear variable (x), and $\ln(A_T) + kT$ is now the linear intercept (b). Thus $\ln(A_{body})$ is a linear function of t and $t - T$ during the post-infusion period ($t > T$). Graphs of A_{body} and $\ln(A_{body})$ versus t for both the infusion period and the post-infusion period are provided in Figure 10.27.

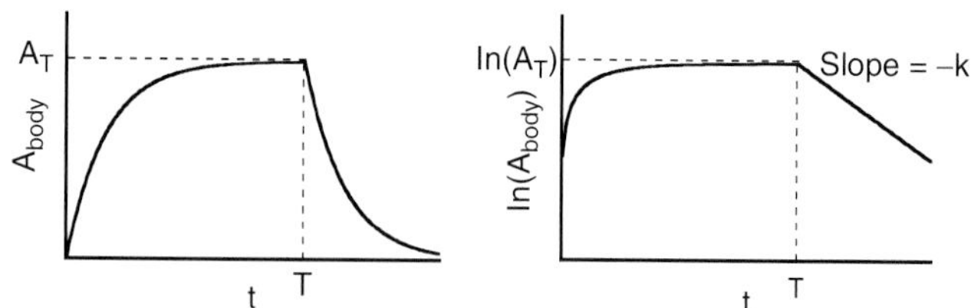

Figure 10.27 Graphical representation of the amount of drug in the body (A_{body}) versus time (t) and $\ln(A_{body})$ versus t for a one-compartment PK model of an IV infusion.

10.8.3 Plasma Concentration versus Time Relationships

As indicated numerous times previously, the plasma concentration of drug (C_p) is given by dividing the amount of drug in the body (A_{body}) by volume of distribution (V). The plasma concentrations during the IV infusion period can then be written directly from Equation (10.115) as

$$C_p = \frac{k_{0,iv}}{kV}(1 - e^{-k \cdot t}) \quad \text{for} \quad 0 \le t \le T \qquad (10.120)$$

The maximum plasma concentration, which is the concentration at time T (or C_T), becomes

$$C_{p,max} = C_T = \frac{k_{0,iv}}{kV}(1 - e^{-k \cdot t}) \qquad (10.121)$$

The plasma concentration for the postinfusion period can be shown from Equation (10.117) to be

$$C_p = \frac{k_{0,iv}}{kV}(1 - e^{-k \cdot t}) \cdot e^{-k(t-T)} = C_T \cdot e^{-k(t-T)} \quad \text{for} \quad t > T \qquad (10.122)$$

As with $\ln(A_{body})$, taking the natural logarithm of this equation provides two alternative log-linear forms for $\ln(C_p)$

$$\ln(C_p) = \ln(C_T) - k(t - T) \quad \text{for} \quad t > T \qquad (10.123)$$

where $\ln(C_p)$ is the dependent linear variable (y), $t - T$ is the independent linear variable (x), $\ln(C_T)$ is the linear intercept (b), and $-k$ is the linear slope (m), or

$$\ln(C_p) = [\ln(C_T) + kT] - kt \quad \text{for} \quad t > T \qquad (10.124)$$

where $\ln(C_p)$ is still the dependent linear variable (y), and $-k$ is still the linear slope (m), but t rather than $t - T$ is now the independent linear variable (x), and $\ln(C_T) + kT$ is now the linear intercept (b). Graphs of C_p and $\ln(C_p)$ versus t for both the infusion period and the postinfusion period are provided in Figure 10.28.

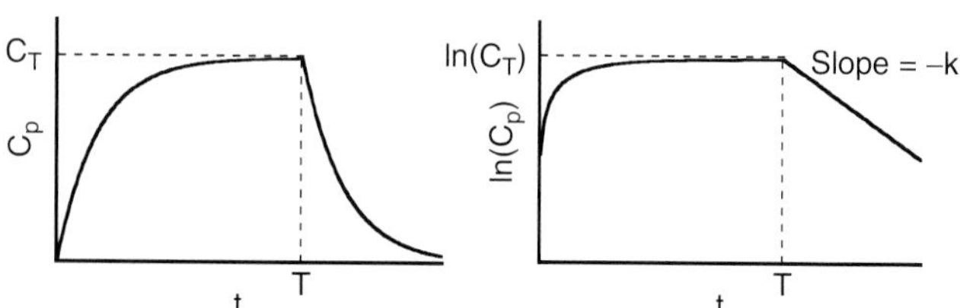

Figure 10.28 Graphical representation of the plasma concentration (C_p) versus time (t) and $\ln(C_p)$ versus t for a one-compartment PK model of an IV infusion.

10.8.3.1 Steady-State Conditions for IV Infusion (Zero-Order Absorption) Drug Delivery

The shape of the plasma concentration versus time curve during the infusion period can be altered dramatically by the duration of the infusion period. For a short infusion period (small T), plasma concentrations rise quickly throughout the infusion period. This is illustrated by the left graph in Figure 10.29. For a prolonged infusion period (large T), the plasma concentration initially rises quickly, but after a longer period of time the plasma concentration begins to level off at a particular concentration. This is illustrated by the right graph in Figure 10.29. The concentration levels off as the body approaches a condition known as steady-state, with the plasma concentration then approaching a steady-state concentration (C_{ss}). Steady-state occurs when the rate of drug entering the body exactly equals the rate at which drug is being eliminated. Since there is no net gain or loss of drug in the body at steady-state, the plasma concentration does not rise or fall. The drug absorption rate during the infusion period is known to be $k_{0,iv}$, and the elimination rate at any time can be written in terms of the overall clearance (CL) multiplied by the plasma concentration. Since the absorption rate and elimination rate are equal at steady-state, and the plasma concentration at steady-state is C_{ss}, it can then be written

$$k_{0,iv} = CL \cdot C_{ss} \quad \text{at steady-state} \tag{10.125}$$

which can be solved for the steady-state concentration to give

$$C_{ss} = \frac{k_{0,iv}}{CL} = \frac{k_{0,iv}}{k \cdot V} \tag{10.126}$$

This relationship can be used to rewrite Equation (10.120) for the plasma concentration during the infusion period in terms of the approach to steady-state conditions

$$C_p = C_{ss}(1 - e^{-k \cdot t}) \quad \text{for} \quad 0 \leq t \leq T \tag{10.127}$$

Thus the approach to steady-state follows a negative exponential decay, which essentially amounts to an upside-down exponential decay as can be seen in the right graph of Figure 10.29.

10.8.3.2 Elimination Half-Life

It should first be pointed out that the elimination rate constant (k) and the elimination half-life ($t_{½,elim}$) for a given drug in a given person (or animal) is not changed by the route of administration. Hence the values of k and $t_{½,elim}$ are the same for an IV infusion as they are for a bolus IV injection (or any other drug delivery method). Hence the relationship between these parameters remains the same as for a bolus IV injection

$$t_{½,\text{elim}} = \frac{\ln(2)}{k} \approx \frac{0.693}{k} \tag{10.128}$$

$$k = \frac{\ln(2)}{t_{½,elim}} \approx \frac{0.693}{t_{½,elim}} \tag{10.129}$$

Equation (10.122) indicates that the plasma concentration decays exponentially as soon as the infusion stops. This means that the plasma concentration (C_p) is 50% of the maximum value (C_T) at one $t_{½,elim}$ after infusion stops, 25% of C_T at two $t_{½,elim}$ after infusion stops, and about 1% of C_T at seven $t_{½,elim}$ after the infusion stops. Since the approach to steady-state during the infusion period follows an inverse exponential process, the plasma concentration (C_p) is 50% of the steady-state concentration (C_{ss}) after infusion for one $t_{½,elim}$, 75% of C_{ss} after infusion for two $t_{½,elim}$, and about 99% of C_{ss} after infusion for seven $t_{½,elim}$.

10.8.3.3 Effect of Basic Model Parameters on the Plasma Concentration versus Time Curve

The effects of different model parameters on the plasma concentration versus time relationship can be demonstrated by mathematical analysis of the previous equations, or by graphical representation of a change in one or more of the variables. Equations (10.120) and (10.122) indicate the plasma concentration (C_p) is proportional to the dosing rate ($k_{0,iv}$) and inversely proportional to the volume of distribution (V). Thus an increase in $k_{0,iv}$ or a decrease in V both yield an equivalent increase in C_p, as illustrated in Figure 10.30. Note that the general shape of the curve, including the slope of the line for $\ln(C_p)$ versus t during the post exposure period, is not a function of $k_{0,iv}$ or V. The elimination rate constant (k) and the elimination half-life ($t_{½,elim}$) are inversely related to each other, so an increase in one is equivalent to a decrease in the other. Changes in k or $t_{½,elim}$ have several important

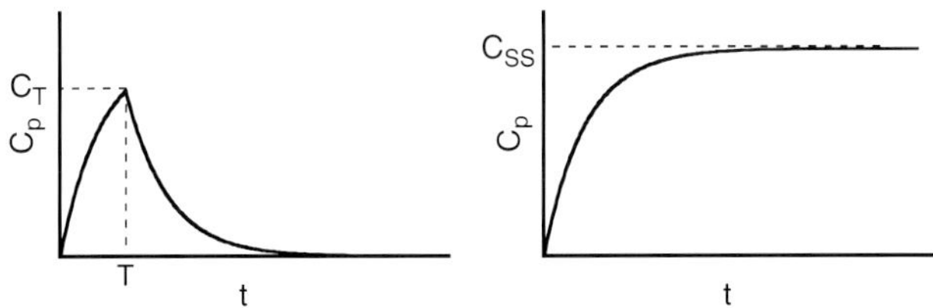

Figure 10.29 Graphical representation of the plasma concentration (C_p) versus time (t) for a relatively short infusion period (left) and a prolonged infusion period (right).

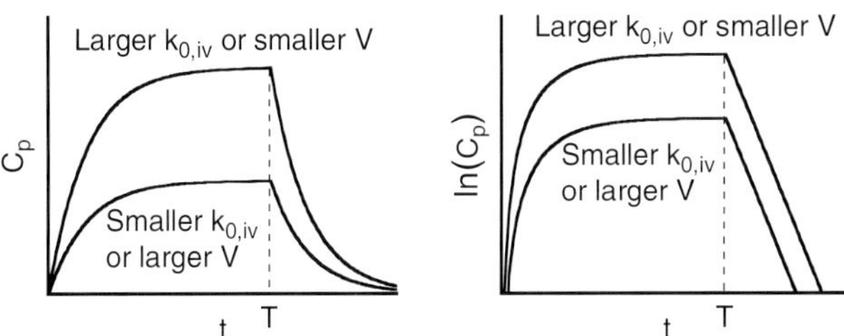

Figure 10.30 Graphical illustration of how plasma concentration (C_p) and $\ln(C_p)$ versus t change with an increase or decrease in the dosing rate (k_0,iv) or volume of distribution (V).

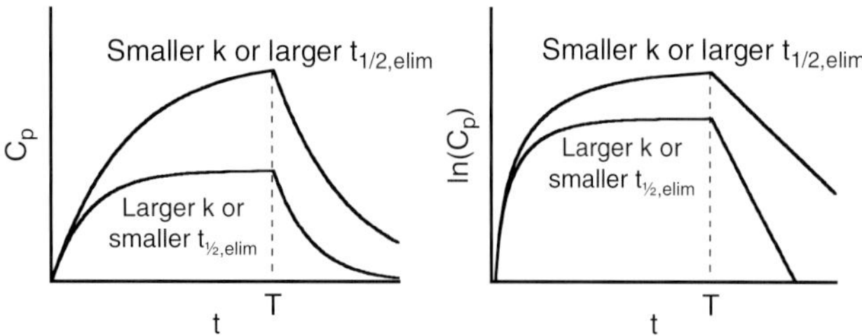

Figure 10.31 Graphical illustration of how plasma concentration (C_p) and $\ln(C_p)$ versus t change with an increase or decrease in the elimination rate constant (k) or elimination half-life ($t_{½,elim}$).

effects on the shape of C_p versus t, as illustrated in Figure 10.31. First, as in the bolus IV case, an increase in k or decrease in $t_{½,elim}$ causes plasma concentrations to drop-off more rapidly with time during the postinfusion period (a steeper or more negative slope in the log-linear plot). Second, an increase in k or decrease in $t_{½,elim}$ results in more drug being eliminated during the infusion period and hence lower plasma concentrations. Last, an increase in k or decrease in $t_{½,elim}$ causes the plasma concentrations to approach steady-state more quickly and more completely during the infusion period.

10.8.3.4 Estimating Plasma Drug Concentrations

Average values for the volume of distribution (V) and elimination half-life ($t_{½,elim}$) for many drugs can be found in drug handbooks, pharmacology textbooks, or in PK research articles (which can be searched online). Once the values of these parameters have been obtained, the plasma concentration for the drug can be estimated for any time during the infusion period or the postinfusion period by simply substituting the appropriate values for $k_{0,iv}$, V, k, T, and the desired time (t) into the previous model equations. Alternatively, the model equations can be solved for the time at which a particular plasma concentration will be reached during either the infusion period or the postinfusion period. For the infusion period, the time after the start of infusion to reach a particular plasma concentration (C_p) becomes

$$t = \frac{-\ln\left(1 - \dfrac{kVC_p}{k_0}\right)}{k} \quad \text{for} \quad 0 \leq t \leq T \qquad (10.130)$$

For the postinfusion period, the time after the end of infusion to reach a particular plasma concentration (C_p) is given by

$$t - T = \frac{-\ln\left(\dfrac{C_p}{C_T}\right)}{k} \qquad (10.131)$$

Note the maximum plasma concentration reached during an infusion is C_T, so entering a plasma concentration (C_p) value greater than C_T into either of these equations gives an irrational result.

10.8.4 Estimating Model Parameters from Measured Plasma Concentration Data

Plasma samples for PK analysis by a one-compartment IV infusion model can be collected either during the infusion period and/or during the postinfusion period. However, plasma samples from the postexposure period are easier to analyze by standard PK methods. PK parameters can be estimated from plasma concentration data collected during the infusion period only if the infusion is continued long enough ($T \geq 7 \cdot t_{½,elim}$) to provide a reasonable estimate for the steady-state plasma concentration (C_{ss}).

10.8.4.1 Linear Regression of Postinfusion Data

Analysis of postinfusion data for a one-compartment IV infusion model is nearly identical to the analysis of plasma concentrations in the one-compartment bolus IV model. The first step is to calculate the natural logarithm of each of the measured postinfusion plasma concentration values. If the concentration (C_T) is measured at $t = T$, then this value can be included in the postinfusion analysis as well. The values of ln (C_p) are plotted versus the time after infusion stopped ($t - T$) for each sample. If the plot shows a series of points falling near a straight line, then the data can be represented by the one-compartment IV infusion model. Just as in the bolus IV case, early high points above the line formed by most of the data indicate the one-compartment model is not the best PK model for the data, and erratic late data points could mean the values are unreliable, as illustrated in Figure 10.32.

Once it has been verified that the data fall approximately on a straight line, a linear regression analysis is performed on the data, with the time after infusion stops ($t - T$) entered as the independent (x) variable values, and $\ln(C_p)$ entered as the dependent (y) variable values. A graphical representation of this analysis is illustrated in Figure 10.33. The regression correlation (r or r^2) should always be recorded along with the best fit values of the intercept (b) and slope (m) for any linear regression analysis. The fitted slope (m) represents the best value for $-k$, so that

$$k = -m \qquad (10.132)$$

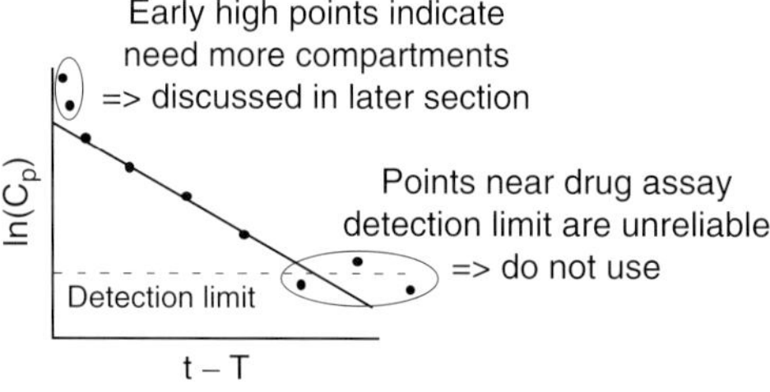

Figure 10.32 Check the graph of $\ln(C_p)$ versus time after infusion stops ($t - T$) for post-infusion data for unreliable measurements and to verify the PK model is appropriate.

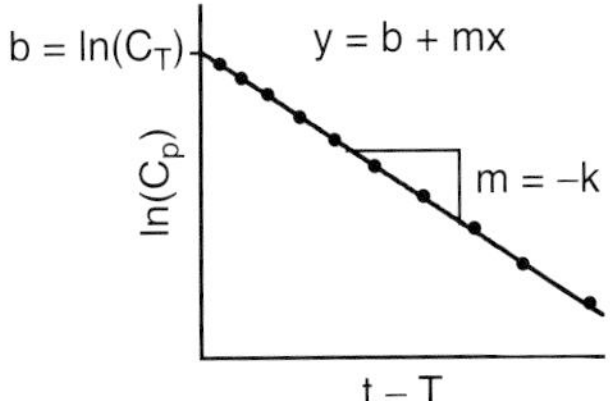

Figure 10.33 Analysis of measured post-infusion plasma concentration (C_p) data by linear regression of $\ln(C_p)$ versus time after infusion stops ($t - T$).

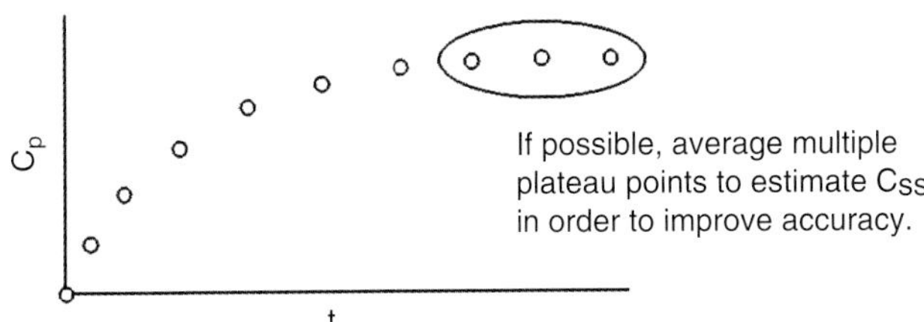

Figure 10.34 Analysis of measured infusion period plasma concentration (C_p) data requires an estimate for the steady-state plasma concentration (C_{ss}).

The fitted intercept (b) represents the best value for ln (C_T), from which C_T can be calculated as

$$C_T = e^b \tag{10.133}$$

The elimination half-life ($t_{½,elim}$) can be calculated from k by Equation (10.128). The volume of distribution (V) can be calculated from the fitted value of C_T by rearranging Equation (10.121) to

$$V = \frac{k_{0,iv}}{kC_T}(1 - e^{-k \cdot T}) \tag{10.134}$$

The overall elimination clearance (CL) can then be calculated as

$$CL = Vk \tag{10.135}$$

Thus all model parameters for the one-compartment IV infusion model can be determined from a single linear regression analysis of measured postinfusion plasma concentration data.

10.8.4.2 Linear Regression of Infusion Period Data

The basic PK parameters for a one-compartment IV infusion model can also be determined from infusion period plasma concentration data. This analysis requires an estimate of the steady-state concentration (C_{ss}), however, so plasma concentration measurements must be made for infusion times up to about $7 \cdot t_{½,elim}$ in order to perform this analysis. The mathematical basis for this analysis comes from Equation (10.127), which can be rearranged to become

$$C_{ss} - C_p = C_{ss}e^{-k \cdot t} \quad \text{for} \quad 0 \leq t \leq T \tag{10.136}$$

Taking the natural logarithm of both sides of this equation gives the log-linear form

$$\ln(C_{ss} - C_p) = \ln(C_{ss}) - kt \quad \text{for} \quad 0 \leq t \leq T \tag{10.137}$$

Thus measured plasma concentration data from the infusion period can be used in a linear regression analysis if the data is converted to the form $\ln(C_{ss} - C_p)$. The first step of the analysis is to estimate the value of C_{ss}, preferably by averaging the values of several measured plateau plasma concentrations as illustrated in Figure 10.34. The next step is then to calculate the values of $\ln(C_{ss} - C_p)$ for each of the remaining plasma concentrations (the measurements used to determine C_{ss} cannot be reused in this step). A plot of the ln ($C_{ss} - C_p$) values versus the infusion time (t) should be made to check for model appropriateness and unusable points, as illustrated in Figure 10.35. Once it has been verified that the data fall approximately on a straight line, a linear regression analysis is performed on the data, with the infusion time (t) entered as the independent (x) data, and $\ln(C_{ss} - C_p)$ entered as the dependent (y) data. A graphical representation of this analysis is illustrated in Figure 10.36. The fitted slope (m) represents the best value for $-k$, so that

$$k = -m \tag{10.138}$$

The fitted intercept (b) can be used to calculated the fitted value for C_{ss}:

$$C_{ss} = e^b \tag{10.139}$$

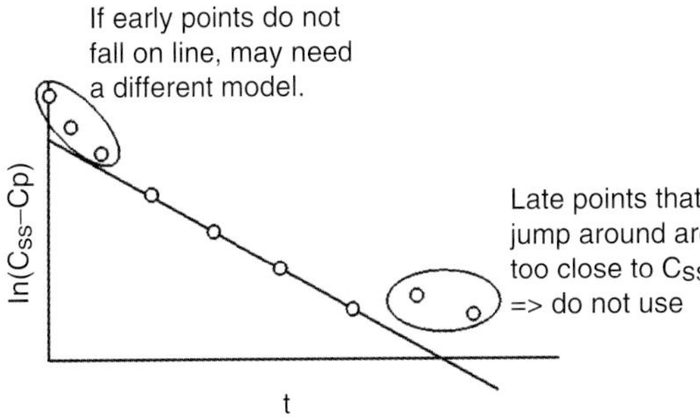

Figure 10.35 Check the graph of $\ln(C_{ss} - C_p)$ versus infusion time (t) for infusion period data for unreliable measurements and to verify the PK model is appropriate.

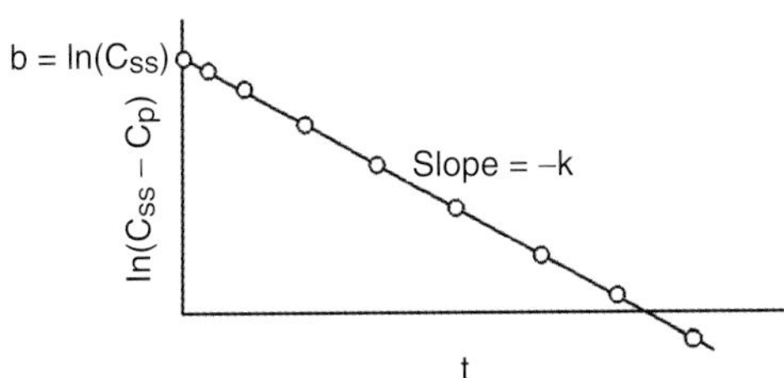

Figure 10.36 Analysis of measured infusion period plasma concentration (C_p) data by linear regression of $\ln(C_{ss} - C_p)$ versus infusion time (t).

which should closely match the estimated C_{ss} value from the first step of the data analysis. The elimination half-life ($t_{½,elim}$) can be calculated from k by Equation (10.128). The volume of distribution (V) can be calculated from C_{ss} by rearranging Equation (10.121) to give

$$V = \frac{k_{0,iv}}{k \cdot C_{ss}} \tag{10.140}$$

The overall elimination clearance (CL) for the one-compartment IV infusion model can then be calculated as

$$CL = Vk \tag{10.141}$$

Thus all the basic model parameters for the one-compartment IV infusion model can be determined from a linear regression analysis of measured infusion period plasma concentration data as long as an estimate of the steady-state plasma concentration can be made.

10.8.4.3 Area Under the Curve (AUC) Calculations

As discussed previously, the area under the plasma concentration versus time curve (AUC) can be very useful in determining the bioavailability of a drug and other PK parameters. The AUC for the one-compartment IV infusion model is represented graphically as the shaded area in Figure 10.37. The value of AUC for this model can be calculated directly by the equation

$$AUC = \frac{k_{0,iv}T}{Vk} = \frac{k_{0,iv}T}{Cl} \tag{10.142}$$

but this equation is useful only if all the PK parameters in this equation are already known. Note that since the product in the numerator ($k_{0,iv}T$) is exactly equal to the total IV infused dose (D_{iv}), this equation is in fact identical to the two terms on the right of Equation (10.106).

The AUC can alternatively be estimated by applying the trapezoidal rule to sequential pairs of measured plasma concentration values, as illustrated in Figure 10.38. Calculation of the slice of AUC between time zero and the first plasma measurement, $AUC\ (0 \rightarrow t_1)$, is different from the bolus IV case since the initial concentration (C_0) is zero, giving

$$AUC(0 \rightarrow t_1) \approx \frac{1}{2}\left(C_1 \cdot t_1\right) \tag{10.143}$$

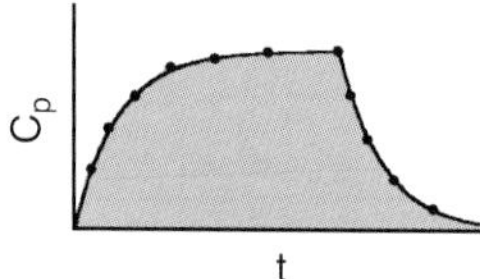

Figure 10.37 The shaded region represents the area under the plasma concentration versus time curve (AUC) for an IV infusion.

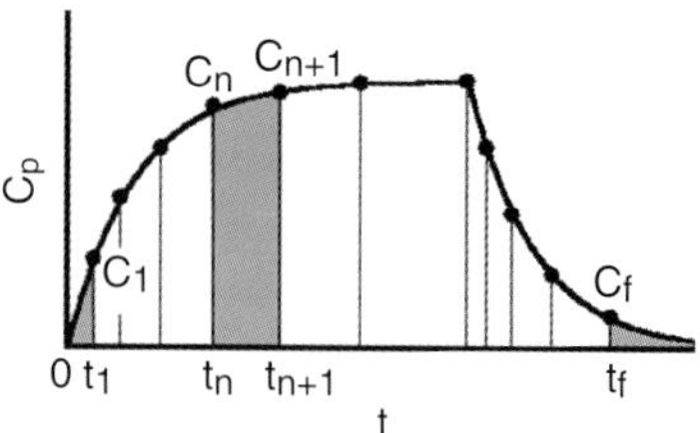

Figure 10.38 Graphical illustration of the application of the trapezoidal rule to numerically estimate the AUC for IV infusion data.

where C_1 is the plasma concentration measured at t_1. The AUC of each of the successive slices from t_1 up to t_f can then be estimated by applying the trapezoidal rule to successive sets of plasma concentration measurements. The general equation for successive plasma concentration measurements C_n and C_{n+1} made at t_n and t_{n+1} is the same as for the bolus IV case:

$$AUC(t_n \rightarrow t_{n+1}) \approx \frac{1}{2}\left[C_n + C_{n+1}\right] \cdot \left(t_{n+1} - t_n\right) \tag{10.144}$$

The AUC for the final segment from t_f to an infinite time is also the same as the bolus IV case:

$$AUC(t_f \rightarrow \infty) = AUC(tail) = \frac{C_f}{k} \tag{10.145}$$

Adding the AUC contribution from each slice in Figure 10.38 as estimated by these equations then yields an estimate for the total AUC. The value of AUC estimated from this calculation can then be used as an alternative means of evaluating the volume of distribution (V) and the overall elimination clearance (CL) by

$$V = \frac{k_{0,iv}T}{k \cdot AUC} = \frac{D_{iv}}{k \cdot AUC} \tag{10.146}$$

$$CL = \frac{k_{0,iv}T}{AUC} = \frac{D_{iv}}{AUC} \tag{10.147}$$

As with the one-compartment bolus IV model, these equations yield essentially the same values of V and CL as those estimated from the linear regression analyses of the previous sections for a one-compartment model. Comparison to Equations (10.111) and (10.112) shows that these equations are essentially identical to those for the bolus IV case, providing an initial glimpse of the universal nature of these AUC relationships.

10.8.5 Special Cases of the One-Compartment IV Infusion (Zero-Order Absorption) Model

Three special cases are considered for the one-compartment zero-order absorption model. First is the extension of the IV infusion equations to cover steady extravascular drug delivery. Second is the use of the one-compartment zero-order absorption model to approximate the plasma concentrations of drugs that follow two-compartment kinetics. The last case considered is the identification of conditions when a zero-order drug delivery over a short duration can be modeled as an instantaneous absorption process.

10.8.5.1 Zero-Order Extravascular Drug Delivery

A number of controlled drug release approaches deliver drug at a steady rate into an extravascular region of the body. Examples include transdermal patches, implantable pumps, and intramuscular depot injections. This situation is very similar to an IV infusion, except that a portion of the drug can be broken down or metabolized prior to reaching the systemic circulation. The fraction of delivered drug that reaches the systemic circulation is the bioavailability (F). The one-compartment IV infusion model equations can be applied to the steady extravascular drug delivery case by simply replacing the IV infusion rate ($k_{0,iv}$) with the extravascular drug delivery rate multiplied by the appropriate extravascular bioavailability, or $F \cdot k_{0,ev}$.

10.8.5.2 Two-Compartment Zero-Order Drug Absorption Simplification

The two-compartment IV infusion (zero-order absorption) model will be covered in Section 10.11. Plasma concentrations for steady absorption of a drug that follows two-compartment kinetics will yield a somewhat sharper rise during the drug delivery period, and early high points on the $\ln(C_p)$ versus $t-T$ plot of the post-absorption period. The PK model for this situation is more complicated than the one-compartment zero-order absorption case. It turns out that if the early high points during the postabsorption period are only slightly above the line formed by the rest of the data, then the one-compartment model provides a reasonable approximation to the actual plasma concentration. As mentioned several times previously, the simpler one-compartment model is used quite often even when it does not apply particularly well to a given drug. When this simplification is used for an IV infusion, the one-compartment IV infusion equations can be employed without modification. For the extravascular delivery case, the modifications listed in Section 10.8.5.1 are used.

10.8.5.3 One-Compartment Zero-Order Drug Absorption with Short Duration of Drug Delivery

It was previously discussed in Section 10.7.5.1 that under certain circumstances, a zero-order drug delivery process of short duration can be approximated as an instantaneous absorption process. The conditions under which this approximation gives reasonable results can be investigated mathematically using model simulations. These simulations are made by keeping the total absorbed dose ($FD = F \cdot k_0 \cdot T$) the same in each simulation. As illustrated in Figure 10.39, the instantaneous absorption model provides a reasonable approximation when $T \leq t_{½,elim}$. This criteria can be employed as a general rule of thumb, although the acceptable amount of difference between the models will depend on the required level of accuracy for a given application. When this approximation is used, the intravenous dose (D_{iv}) should be replaced by the total absorbed dose ($F \cdot k_0 \cdot T$) in the one-compartment bolus IV model equations.

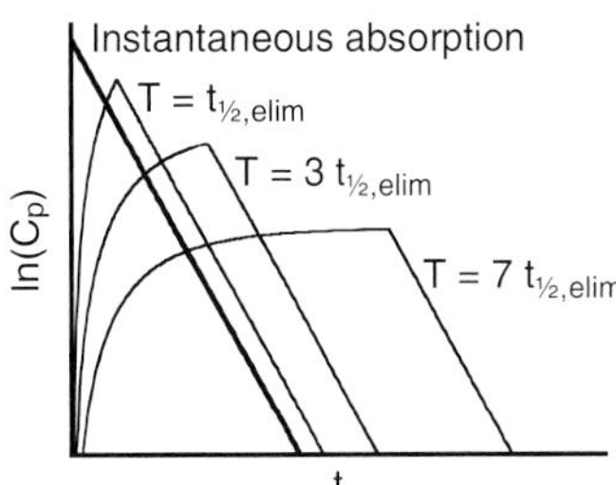

Figure 10.39 Graphical illustration of how closely a one-compartment instantaneous absorption model approximates one-compartment zero-order absorption plasma concentrations for different values of T relative to $t_{½,elim}$.

10.9 ONE-COMPARTMENT FIRST-ORDER ABSORPTION MODEL

First-order absorption occurs when drug enters the systemic circulation at a rate that is proportional to the amount of drug remaining to be absorbed at the site of administration. This is a very reasonable approximation for most routes of extravascular drug delivery, including oral ingestion and most injections into an administration site other than a blood vessel (with the only common exception being an intramuscular depot injection). This model is used most often for oral ingestion so it is sometimes called the one-compartment oral absorption model, but the equations in this section apply equally well to all extravascular routes. This section will provide the first example of a method of residual analysis of plasma concentrations. Similar residual methods will be employed for all types of two-compartment models in later sections. Evaluation of the bioavailability will also be discussed for the first time. Thus this section will introduce several new topics that are important for many other PK modeling situations.

10.9.1 Model Assumptions

The standard one-compartment first-order absorption model makes three inherent assumptions about the ADME processes that occur during and after drug delivery. The specific nature and implications of each of these assumptions are described in this section.

10.9.1.1 First-Order Absorption

As in all first-order absorption models, the rate at which drug enters the systemic circulation is taken to be proportional to the amount of drug remaining to be absorbed at the administration site. The rate of absorption is then highest immediately after drug administration at time zero, after which the absorption rate decays exponentially with time. As discussed in Section 10.3.2.3, this provides a very good approximation to the absorption rate for most routes of extravascular drug delivery, including oral ingestion and most injections not made into a blood vessel (with the only common exception being an intramuscular depot injection).

10.9.1.2 Instantaneous Distribution

This assumption is the same for all one-compartment models. See Section 10.7.1.2 for the details regarding this assumption.

10.9.1.3 First-Order (Linear) Elimination Kinetics

This assumption is the same for all PK models described in this chapter. See Section 10.7.1.3 for the details regarding this assumption.

10.9.2 Setup and Solution of Mass Balance Equations

A separate mass balance equation is written in the form of Section 10.6.2 for each compartment in the model. Since this is a one-compartment model, only one mass balance equation is needed. The amount of drug in the compartment is equal to the total amount of drug in the body (A_{body}). The rate of drug absorption is given by Section 10.3.2.3 to be a function of a first-order absorption rate constant (k_a), the bioavailability (F), and the administered dose (D). The elimination rate is equal to the amount of drug remaining in the compartment (A_{body}) multiplied by an elimination rate constant (k). A schematic representation of this one-compartment bolus IV model is provided in Figure 10.40. The mass balance equation then becomes

$$\frac{dA_{body}}{dt} = k_a FD \cdot e^{-k_a \cdot t} - kA_{body} \qquad (10.148)$$

The differential equation provided by this mass balance can be solved (with a little effort) to give

$$A_{body} = FD \cdot \left(\frac{k_a}{k_a - k}\right)(e^{-k \cdot t} - e^{-k_a \cdot t}) \qquad (10.149)$$

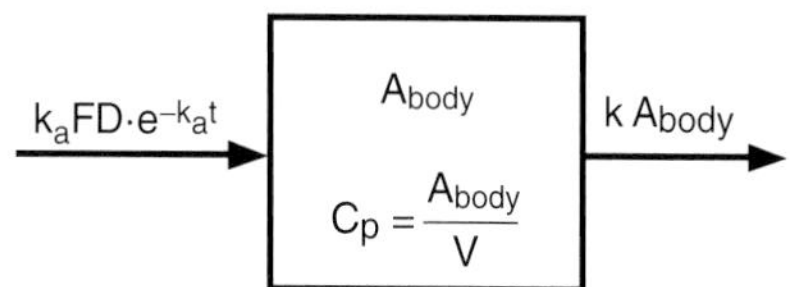

Figure 10.40 Schematic representation of the one-compartment model for first-order absorption.

This equation contains two exponential terms, so it does not follow a simple exponential decay. However, the fact that $k_a > k$ (except for a very rare special case situation discussed later) can be used to simplify the relationship for large values of time (t) to give

$$A_{body} \approx FD \cdot \left(\frac{k_a}{k_a - k}\right) \cdot e^{-k \cdot t} \quad \text{for large } t \qquad (10.150)$$

Taking the natural logarithm of both sides of this simplified equation yields the log-linear form

$$\ln(A_{body}) \approx \ln\left[FD \cdot \left(\frac{k_a}{k_a - k}\right)\right] - kt \quad \text{for large } t \qquad (10.151)$$

where $\ln(A_{body})$ is the dependent linear variable (y), t is the independent linear variable (x), $-k$ is the linear slope (m), and the natural logarithm of the term in square brackets is the linear intercept (b). This line that is formed at large t is called the terminal line. Graphical representations of Equations (10.149) and (10.151) are provided in Figure 10.41, with the terminal line clearly visible for large t in the log-linear graph.

10.9.3 Plasma Concentration versus Time Relationships

The plasma concentration of drug (C_p) is given by dividing the amount of drug in the body (A_{body}) by volume of distribution (V), yielding

$$C_p = \frac{FD}{V}\left(\frac{k_a}{k_a - k}\right)(e^{-k \cdot t} - e^{-k_a \cdot t}) = B_1(e^{-k \cdot t} - e^{-k_a \cdot t})$$
$$= B_1 e^{-k \cdot t} - B_1 e^{-k_a \cdot t} \qquad (10.152)$$

where the constant B_1 is defined as

$$B_1 = \frac{FD}{V}\left(\frac{k_a}{k_a - k}\right) \qquad (10.153)$$

in order to make it easier to write the equations. This equation can again be simplified for large values of time (t) by using the fact that $k_a > k$, which gives

$$C_p \approx B_1 \cdot e^{-k \cdot t} \quad \text{for large } t \qquad (10.154)$$

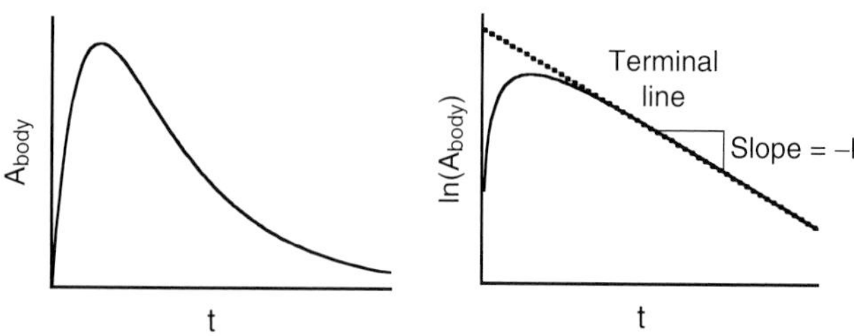

Figure 10.41 Graphical representation of the amount of drug in the body (A_{body}) versus time (t) and $\ln(A_{body})$ versus t for a one-compartment first-order absorption PK model.

This equation can then be written in a log-linear form as

$$\ln(C_p) \approx \ln(B_1) - kt \quad \text{for large } t \tag{10.155}$$

where $\ln(C_p)$ is the dependent linear variable (y), ln (B_1) is the linear intercept (b), t is the independent linear variable (x), and $-k$ is the linear slope (m). This relationship once again yields a terminal line at large t. Graphs of C_p and $\ln(C_p)$ versus t are provided in Figure 10.42. The plasma concentration reaches a maximum at a time (t_{max}) that can be related to k_a and k by the equation

$$t_{max} = \frac{\ln\left(\frac{k_a}{k}\right)}{k_a - k} \tag{10.156}$$

The maximum plasma concentration (C_{max}) is then given by substituting t_{max} in for t in Equation (10.152).

10.9.3.1 Absorption and Elimination Phases

The one-compartment first-order absorption plasma concentration versus time curve in Figure 10.43 shows a characteristic early rising period followed by a declining concentration period. The transition from concentration rise to concentration decline occurs at t_{max}. Concentrations rise for $t < t_{max}$ because the rate of drug absorption is greater than the rate of drug elimination. The absorption process can be said to dominate during the rising period, and hence the rising period is called the absorption phase. Conversely, concentrations decline for $t > t_{max}$ because the rate of drug elimination is larger than the rate of drug absorption for this time period. Hence elimination dominates during this later stage, which is then called the elimination phase. The concentration at $t = t_{max}$ is neither rising nor falling because the absorption rate and elimination rate are exactly equal to each other at this one point in time.

10.9.3.2 Absorption and Elimination Half-Lives

It should be pointed out first that the elimination rate constant (k) and the elimination half-life ($t_{½,elim}$) for a given drug in a given person (or animal) is not changed by the route of administration. Hence the values of k and $t_{½,elim}$ are the same for first-order absorption as they are for instantaneous or zero-order absorption (or any other drug delivery method). The relationship between the elimination parameters remains the same as given previously:

$$t_{½,elim} = \frac{\ln(2)}{k} \approx \frac{0.693}{k} \tag{10.157}$$

or rearranging,

$$k = \frac{\ln(2)}{t_{½,elim}} \approx \frac{0.693}{t_{½,elim}} \tag{10.158}$$

An absorption half-life cannot be defined for instantaneous or zero-order absorption, but for first-order absorption it becomes

$$t_{½,abs} = \frac{\ln(2)}{k_a} \approx \frac{0.693}{k_a} \tag{10.159}$$

or again by rearranging

$$k_a = \frac{\ln(2)}{t_{½,abs}} \approx \frac{0.693}{t_{½,abs}} \tag{10.160}$$

It was illustrated previously in Figures 10.41 and 10.42 that a terminal line forms at large values of time when $e^{-k_a \cdot t}$ becomes negligible compared to $e^{-k \cdot t}$. The exponential term with k_a in the exponent is associated with the absorption process. The absorption process is 50% complete after one $t_{½,abs}$, 75% complete after two $t_{½,abs}$, and about 99% complete after seven $t_{½,abs}$. So as an approximate rule of thumb, the absorption exponential generally becomes negligible and $\ln(C_p)$ values fall on a terminal line when $t > 7 \cdot t_{½,abs}$.

10.9.3.3 Effect of Basic Model Parameters on the Plasma Concentration versus Time Curve

The effects of different model parameters on the plasma concentration versus time relationship can be demonstrated by mathematical analysis of the previous equations, or by graphical representation of a change in one or more of the variables. Equation (10.152) indicates the plasma concentration (C_p) is proportional to the absorbed dose (FD) and inversely proportional to the volume of distribution (V). Thus an increase in FD or a decrease in V both yield an

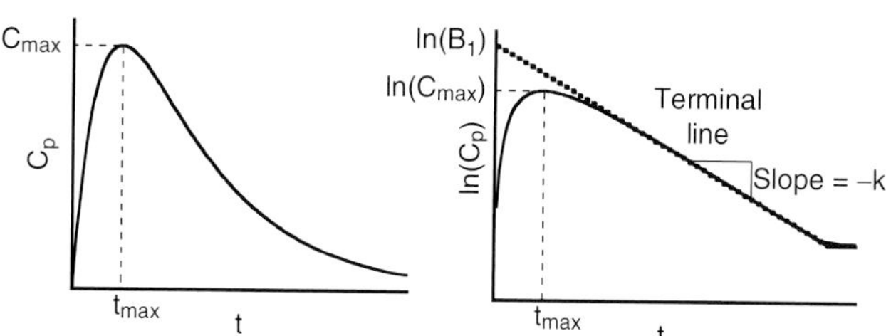

Figure 10.42 Graphical representation of the plasma concentration (C_p) versus time (t) and $\ln(C_p)$ versus t for a one-compartment first-order absorption PK model.

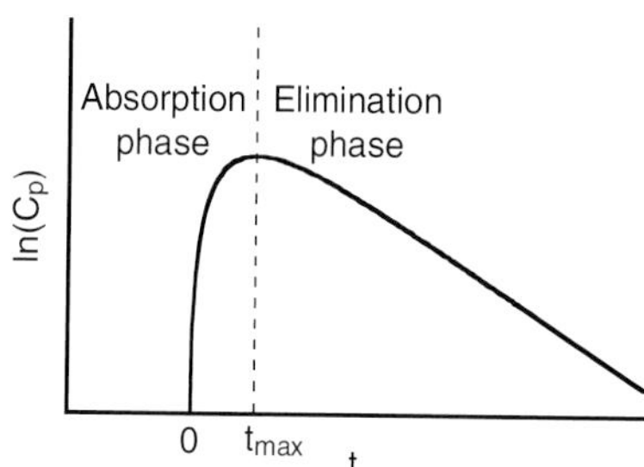

Figure 10.43 Graphical representation of the absorption phase (rising concentration) and elimination phase (falling concentration) for a one-compartment first-order absorption model.

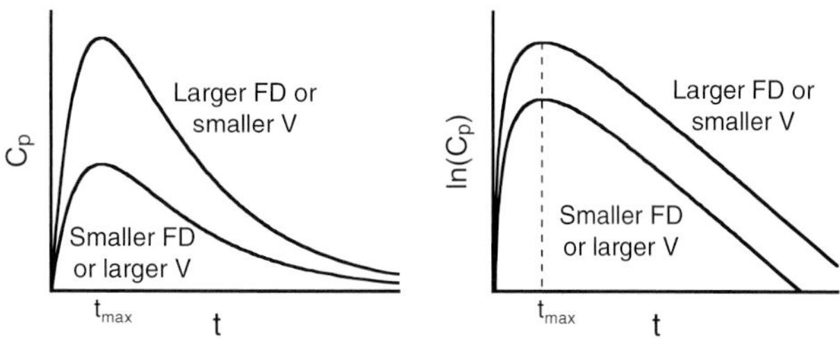

Figure 10.44 Graphical illustration of how plasma concentration (C_p) and $\ln(C_p)$ versus t change with an increase or decrease in the absorbed dose (FD) or volume of distribution (V).

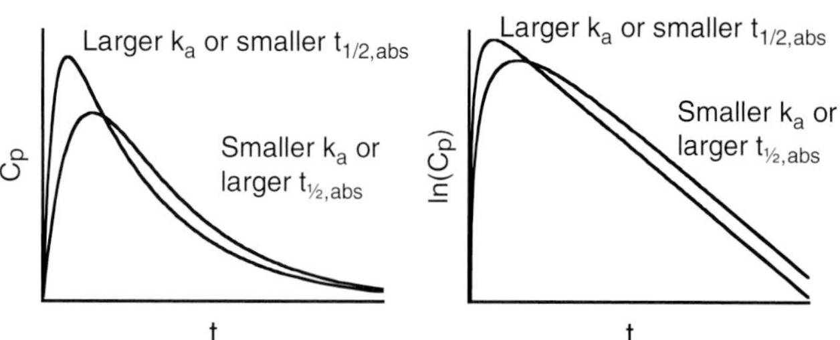

Figure 10.46 Graphical illustration of how plasma concentration (C_p) and $\ln(C_p)$ versus t change with an increase or decrease in the absorption rate constant (k_a) or absorption half-life ($t_{½,abs}$).

equivalent increase in C_p, as illustrated in Figure 10.44. Note that the general shape of the curve, including the value of t_{max} and the slope of the terminal line, are not a function of FD or V. The elimination rate constant (k) and the elimination half-life ($t_{½,elim}$) are inversely related to each other, so that an increase in one is equivalent to a decrease in the other. An increase in k or decrease in $t_{½,elim}$ causes concentrations to be lower at all times (since elimination is higher at all times), decreases the time for maximum concentration, and causes the terminal line slope to be more negative or to drop-off more rapidly with time, as illustrated in Figure 10.45. The values of k_a and $t_{½,abs}$ are similarly inversely related to each other, with an increase in k_a or decrease in $t_{½,elim}$ causing plasma concentrations to rise more rapidly during the absorption phase, maximum concentration to be reached earlier, and the terminal line to form earlier, but not affecting the slope of the terminal line. This relationship is illustrated in Figure 10.46.

10.9.3.4 Estimating Plasma Drug Concentrations

Average values for the volume of distribution (V), elimination half-life ($t_{½,elim}$), and bioavailability (F) for many drugs can be found in drug handbooks, pharmacology textbooks, or in PK research articles (which can be searched online). Values for the absorption rate constant or absorption half-life can sometimes be found in research articles, but many articles and most handbooks instead provide an estimate of t_{max} and C_{max}. It turns out that a crude estimate for

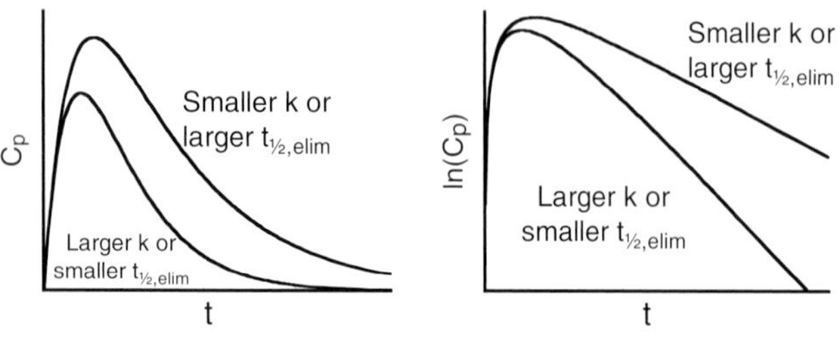

Figure 10.45 Graphical illustration of how plasma concentration (C_p) and $\ln(C_p)$ versus t change with an increase or decrease in the elimination rate constant (k) or elimination half-life ($t_{½,elim}$).

the absorption rate constant (k_a) can be determined from t_{max} with a little effort. The method involves a trial-and-error process where the value of k (calculated from the reported elimination half-life) and a guessed value for k_a are substituted into Equation (10.156) to determine a calculated value for t_{max}. If the calculated t_{max} does not closely match the literature value of t_{max}, then the process is repeated using a different guess for k_a. When the calculated t_{max} does finally closely match the reported value, then the guessed value of k_a is a crude but reasonable estimate of the actual absorption rate constant.

Once the values of these parameters have been obtained, the plasma concentration for the drug can be estimated for any time after drug administration by simply substituting the appropriate values for FD, V, k, k_a, and the desired time (t) into the previous model equations. Unlike the previous models, the time at which the plasma concentration reaches a given value cannot be solved directly for all time points. This is because the concentration equation contains two exponential curves, which under normal circumstances can only be solved by a trial-and-error technique (guess t, calculate C_p, continue until t gives the desired C_p). An exception occurs for plasma concentration (C_p) values at long times after drug administration, in which case the desired concentration is located on the terminal line. For this special case, plasma concentrations can be represented by the simplified terminal line equation, which can be solved directly for time to give

$$t = \frac{-\ln\left(\frac{C_p}{B_1}\right)}{k} \quad \text{for large } t \qquad (10.161)$$

As a general rule of thumb, this equation can be used to estimate t as long as $t > 7 \cdot t_{½,abs}$.

10.9.4 Estimating Model Parameters from Measured Plasma Concentration Data

Estimation of one-compartment first-order absorption parameters from measured plasma samples ends up being a bit more complicated and laborious than the previous models, but the methods are still relatively straightforward. Proper parameter evaluation ideally requires at least three to five plasma samples be collected during the absorption phase, and five to seven samples be collected during the elimination phase. Two stages of linear regression analysis are required to evaluate most of the parameters, and additional plasma concentration results from IV delivery of the same drug are required to fully evaluate all model parameters.

10.9.4.1 Linear Regression of Terminal Line Plasma Concentration Data

Elimination parameters are determined by linear regression analysis of the measured plasma concentration data falling on the terminal line. As always, the first step is to calculate the natural logarithm of each of the measured plasma concentration values. The values of $\ln(C_p)$ are then plotted versus time (t). If the plot shows later points falling near a straight terminal line with no early points above the terminal line, then the data can be well represented by the one-compartment first-order absorption model. As with previous one-compartment models, early high points above the terminal line indicate that the one-compartment model is not the best PK model for the data, and erratic late data points could mean the values are unreliable, as illustrated in Figure 10.47.

Once the data points located on the terminal line have been identified, a linear regression analysis is performed on the terminal line data. The time (t) is entered as the independent (x) data, and $\ln(C_p)$ is entered as the dependent (y) data. A graphical representation of this analysis is illustrated in Figure 10.48. The regression correlation (r *or* r^2) should always be recorded along with the best fit values of the intercept (b) and slope (m) for any linear regression analysis. The fitted slope (m) represents the best value for $-k$, so that

$$k = -m \tag{10.162}$$

The fitted intercept (b) represents the best value for $\ln(B_1)$, from which B_1 can be calculated as

$$B_1 = e^b \tag{10.163}$$

The elimination half-life ($t_{½,elim}$) can be calculated from k by Equation (10.157). These then represent all the parameters that can be evaluated from the terminal line data.

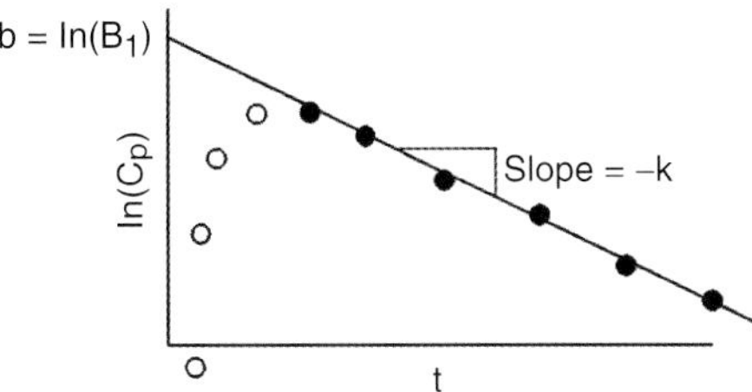

Figure 10.48 Linear regression analysis of $\ln(C_p)$ versus time for measured plasma concentrations falling on the terminal line.

10.9.4.2 Method of Residuals Analysis of Absorption Phase Plasma Concentration Data

The next step is to analyze the early measured plasma concentration values that were not used in the terminal line analysis. This is accomplished by a calculation scheme called the method of residuals. The values obtained from these residual calculations will then be analyzed by linear regression to get the absorption-related model parameters. The residual represents the difference between the value of the terminal line at a given value of time (t) and the actual measured concentration at the same value of t. A graphical representation of the residual values is provided in Figure 10.49, and the residual (R) is calculated for each data point not employed in the previous terminal line analysis by the equation

$$R = B_1 \cdot e^{-k \cdot t} - C_p \tag{10.164}$$

where C_p is the plasma concentration measurement for a plasma sample collected at time t. If the measured plasma concentrations follow the relationship in Equation (10.152), then the residual values should follow the relationship

$$\begin{aligned} R &= B_1 \cdot e^{-k \cdot t} - C_p \\ &= B_1 \cdot e^{-k \cdot t} - (B_1 \cdot e^{-k \cdot t} - B_1 \cdot e^{-k_a \cdot t}) \\ &= B_1 \cdot e^{-k_a \cdot t} \end{aligned} \tag{10.165}$$

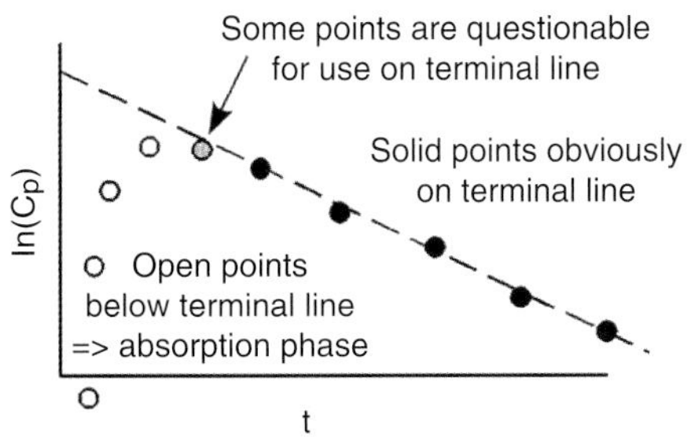

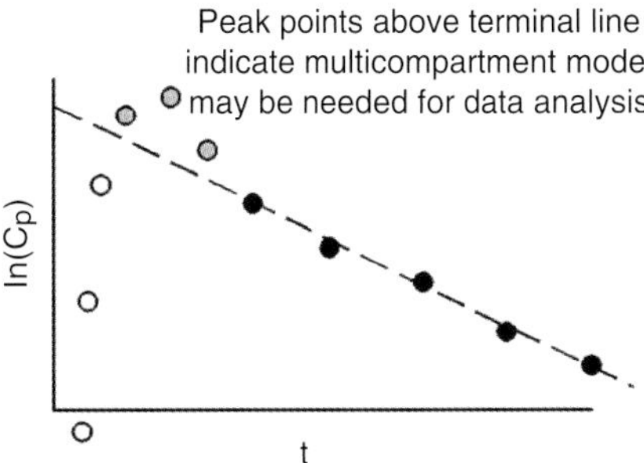

Figure 10.47 Check the graph of $\ln(C_p)$ versus t verify the one-compartment first-order absorption PK model is appropriate, and identify values falling on the terminal line.

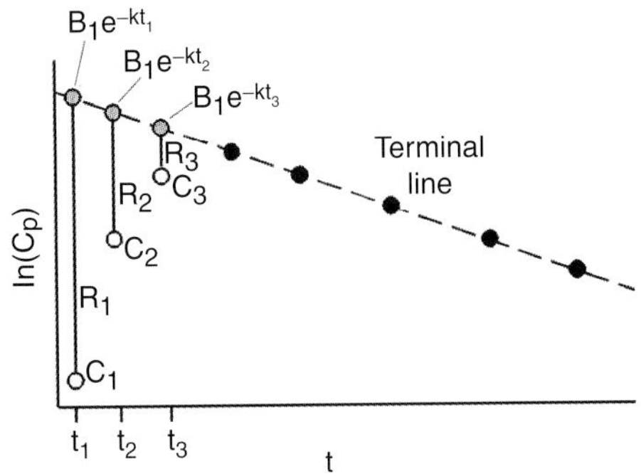

Figure 10.49 Calculation of residuals (R) from plasma concentration (C_p) data and fitted terminal line parameters.

Taking the natural logarithm of the left and right terms gives the log-linear form

$$\ln(R) = \ln(B_1) - k_a t \tag{10.166}$$

Thus a plot of $\ln(R)$ versus t should then give a series of points falling on a straight line, as in Figure 10.50. A linear regression analysis is then performed on the residual values, with time (t) entered as the independent (x) data, and $\ln(R)$ is entered as the dependent (y) data. The fitted slope (m_R) represents the best value for $-k_a$, so that

$$k_a = -m_R \tag{10.167}$$

The fitted intercept (b_R) represents $\ln(B_1)$, from which B_1 can be calculated as

$$B_1 = e^{b_R} \tag{10.168}$$

Note that the value of B_1 was already calculated from the $\ln(C_p)$ versus t terminal line analysis, and this newly calculated value should be very similar to the previous value. The value of the absorption half-life ($t_{½,abs}$) can then be calculated from Equation (10.159).

The terminal line analysis and the method of residuals analysis then provide values of k, $t_{½,elim}$, k_a, $t_{½,abs}$, and B_1. The model parameters that remain to be evaluated include the bioavailability (F), the volume of distribution (V), and the overall clearance (CL). However, the information derived thus far from the data cannot be used to solve explicitly for any of these three variables. The best that can be accomplished at this stage is values for the apparent distribution volume ($V_{app} = V/F$) and the apparent clearance ($CL_{app} = CL/F$) by the equations

$$V_{app} = \frac{V}{F} = \frac{D}{B_1}\left(\frac{k_a}{k_a - k}\right) \tag{10.169}$$

$$CL_{app} = \frac{CL}{F} = \frac{kV}{F} = k \cdot V_{app} \tag{10.170}$$

It turns out there is no way to evaluate the individual parameters V, CL, and F without measured plasma concentrations for the same drug delivered by IV. This analysis will be described shortly.

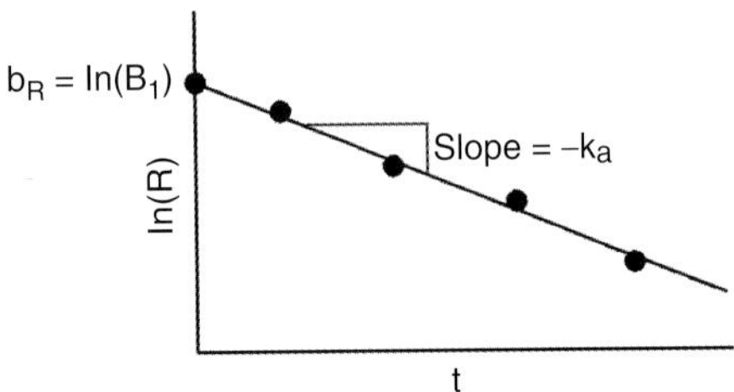

Figure 10.50 Linear regression analysis of calculated residuals for the absorption phase.

10.9.4.3 Area under the Curve (AUC) Calculations

First-order absorption processes end up being one of the cases where AUC values are needed in order to fully evaluate all model parameters. The AUC for the one-compartment first-order absorption model is represented graphically as the shaded area in Figure 10.51. The value of AUC for this model can be calculated directly by the equation

$$AUC = \frac{B_1}{k} - \frac{B_1}{k_a} \tag{10.171}$$

The AUC can alternatively be estimated by applying the trapezoidal rule to sequential pairs of measured plasma concentration values. Calculation of the slice of AUC between time zero and the first plasma measurement, $AUC(0 \rightarrow t_1)$, is the same as the zero-order absorption case since the initial concentration (C_0) of both is zero, giving

$$AUC(0 \rightarrow t_1) \approx \frac{1}{2}\left(C_1 \cdot t_1\right) \tag{10.172}$$

where C_1 is the plasma concentration measured at t_1. The AUC of each of the successive slices from t_1 up to t_f can then be estimated by applying the trapezoidal rule to each successive set of plasma concentration measurements. The general equation for these successive calculations for two successive plasma concentration measurements C_n and C_{n+1} made at t_n and t_{n+1} is the same as for each previous case:

$$AUC(t_n \rightarrow t_{n+1}) \approx \frac{1}{2}\left[C_n + C_{n+1}\right] \cdot \left(t_{n+1} - t_n\right) \tag{10.173}$$

Finally, the area under the curve for the final segment from t_f to an infinite time, called the tail of the curve, is also the same as the previous cases

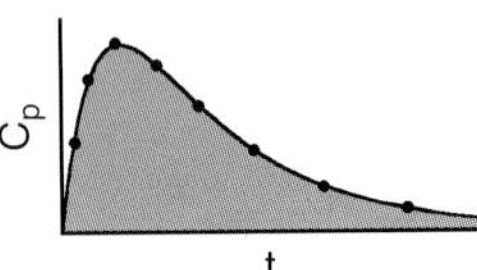

Figure 10.51 The shaded region represents the area under the plasma concentration versus time curve (AUC) for a one-compartment first-order absorption model.

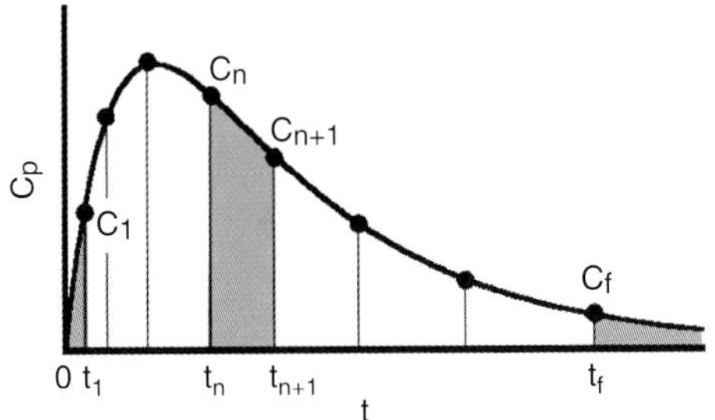

Figure 10.52 Graphical illustration of the application of the trapezoidal rule to numerically estimate the *AUC* for first-order absorption data.

$$AUC(t_f \rightarrow \infty) = AUC(tail) = \frac{C_f}{k} \tag{10.174}$$

Adding the *AUC* contribution from each slice in Figure 10.52 then yields an estimate for the total *AUC*. The value of *AUC* can be related to the distribution volume (V) and the overall clearance (CL) by the general relationship

$$AUC = \frac{FD}{k \cdot V} = \frac{FD}{CL} \tag{10.175}$$

As in the method of residuals analysis, the bioavailability (F), distribution volume (V), and overall clearance (CL) cannot be independently solved, but can only be written as the apparent values

$$V_{app} = \frac{V}{F} = \frac{D}{k \cdot AUC} \tag{10.176}$$

$$CL_{app} = \frac{CL}{F} = \frac{D}{AUC} \tag{10.177}$$

Thus once again the complete evaluation of model parameters cannot be determined from first-order plasma concentration measurements alone. Additional information is needed from intravenous drug delivery, as described in the next section.

10.9.4.4 Bioavailability Calculations

As discussed previously, the area under the plasma concentration versus time curve (*AUC*) can be very useful in determining the bioavailability of a drug and other PK parameters. The ratio of bioavailability values (F_1/F_2) for a drug delivered by two different routes is called the relative bioavailability. The relative bioavailability can be determined from the dose (D_1 and D_2) and *AUC* values (AUC_1 and AUC_2) of each route by the relationship

$$\frac{F_1}{F_2} = \frac{AUC_1 \cdot D_2}{AUC_2 \cdot D_1} \tag{10.178}$$

This relationship can be useful when comparing the relative bioavailability of two different formulations of the same drug (e.g., original versus generic forms) or when comparing two extravascular delivery routes for the same drug (e.g., oral versus intramuscular). If one route is extravascular (oral, subcutaneous, intramuscular, etc.) and the second is intravascular (*iv*), then the *iv* bioavailability (F_{iv}) is known to be 100% and the extravascular bioavailability (F_{ev}) can be determined directly as

$$F_{ev} = \frac{AUC_{ev} \cdot D_{iv}}{AUC_{iv} \cdot D_{ev}} \tag{10.179}$$

Thus comparison to *iv* measurements provides the absolute bioavailability. Once the bioavailability of a first-order absorption process is determined, the distribution volume (V) and clearance (CL) can be calculated from Equations (10.169) and (10.170) as

$$V = \frac{FD}{B_1}\left(\frac{k_a}{k_a - k}\right) \tag{10.180}$$

$$CL = kV \tag{10.181}$$

or by Equations (10.176) and (10.177) to give

$$V = \frac{FD}{k \cdot AUC} \tag{10.182}$$

$$CL = \frac{FD}{AUC} \tag{10.183}$$

Thus combining plasma concentration measurements from first-order absorption drug delivery and intravenous drug delivery allows the determination of all PK model parameters.

10.9.5 Special Cases of the One-Compartment First-Order Absorption Model

Three special cases are considered for the one-compartment first-order absorption model. First is a relatively rare situation known as a flip-flop situation. Second is the use of the one-compartment first-order absorption model to approximate the plasma concentrations of drugs that follow two-compartment kinetics. The last case considered is the identification of conditions when first-order drug delivery with rapid absorption can be modeled as an instantaneous absorption process.

10.9.5.1 Flip-Flop First-Order Absorption

For a small number of slowly absorbed drugs, a rare situation can occur under certain conditions in which the elimination rate constant (k) actually becomes larger than the absorption rate constant (k_a). This unusual situation with $k > k_a$ is called a flip-flop first-order absorption case. As counterintuitive as it may seem, it turns out that there is no way to differentiate the flip-flop situation ($k > k_a$) from the normal situation ($k_a > k$) based solely on first-order absorption plasma concentration data. The values of k_a and k merely swap with each other in the model equations, and the general shape of the plots in this section end up looking essentially the same. The only reliable way to identify a flip-flop situation is to collect plasma concentration data for an IV injection and compare the terminal line slope to that of the first-order absorption data. The slope for IV injection is known to be the elimination rate constant (k). Thus if the terminal line slopes of the IV and first-order absorption data are similar, then the drug follows normal kinetics. If the terminal line slope of the first-order absorption data is much less than that for IV, however, the drug follows flip-flop kinetics for the conditions under study. These situations are illustrated in Figure 10.53. In order to use the normal first-order absorption equations for the flip-flop case, we must swap k and k_a in each equation.

10.9.5.2 Two-Compartment First-Order Drug Absorption Simplification

The two-compartment first-order absorption model will be covered in Section 10.12. First-order absorption of a drug that follows two-compartment kinetics yields plasma concentrations near the peak concentration that are above the terminal line, as illustrated in Figure 10.47. The PK model for two-compartment first-order absorption is more complicated than the one-compartment first-order absorption case. It turns out that if the peak area high points are only slightly above the terminal line, then the one-compartment model provides a reasonable approximation to the actual plasma concentrations. As mentioned several times previously, the simpler one-compartment model is often used even when it does not apply particularly well to a given drug. When this simplification is used for first-order absorption, the one-compartment first-order absorption equations can be employed without modification.

10.9.5.3 One-Compartment First-Order Drug Absorption with Rapid Absorption

It was previously discussed in Section 10.7.5.2 that under certain circumstances, a first-order drug delivery process with rapid absorption rates can be approximated as an instantaneous absorption process. The conditions under which this approximation gives reasonable results can be investigated mathematically using model simulations. These simulations are made by varying the value of the absorption rate constant (k_a) relative to a fixed elimination rate constant (k). As illustrated in Figure 10.54, the instantaneous absorption model provides a reasonable approximation when $k_a \geq 7 \cdot k$, which can be expressed equivalently as $7 \cdot t_{½,abs} \leq t_{½,elim}$. These criteria can be employed as a general rule of thumb, although the acceptable amount of difference between the models will depend on the required level of accuracy for a given application. When this approximation is used, the intravenous dose (D_{iv}) should be replaced by the total absorbed dose (FD) in the one-compartment bolus IV model equations.

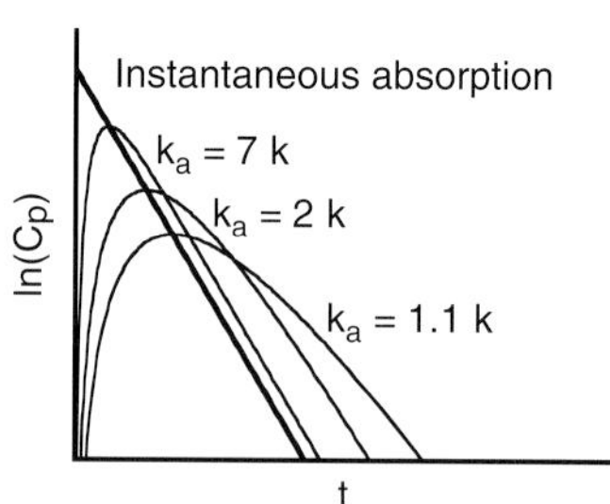

Figure 10.54 Graphical illustration of how closely a one-compartment instantaneous absorption model approximates one-compartment first-order absorption plasma concentrations for different values of *ka* relative to *k*.

10.10 TWO-COMPARTMENT BOLUS IV INJECTION (INSTANTANEOUS ABSORPTION) MODEL

The two-compartment bolus IV injection model is somewhat more mathematically complex than the one-compartment bolus IV injection model. As in the one-compartment model, drug is delivered directly into the systemic circulation by a rapid injection over a very short period of time. However, the body is now represented by two compartments, called compartment 1 and compartment 2. The systemic circulation is always included in compartment 1, commonly called the central compartment, which additionally contains any tissues that come to instantaneous (or rapid) equilibrium with the systemic circulation. The tissues in compartment 2, commonly called the tissue compartment, take substantially more time to reach equilibrium with the circulation. Two-compartment models also have an additional complexity that two different types of rate constants must be defined. "Micro" rate

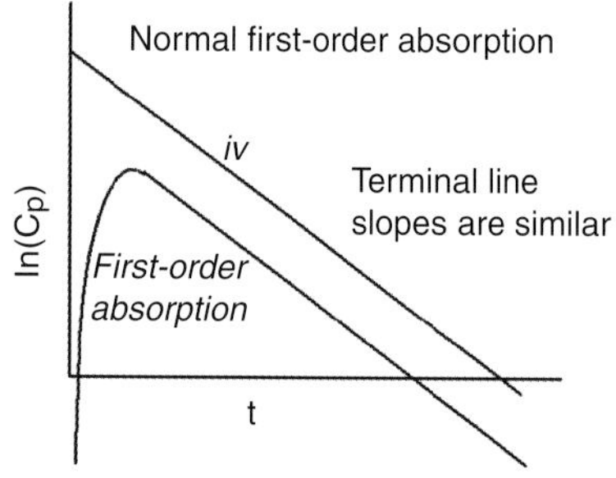

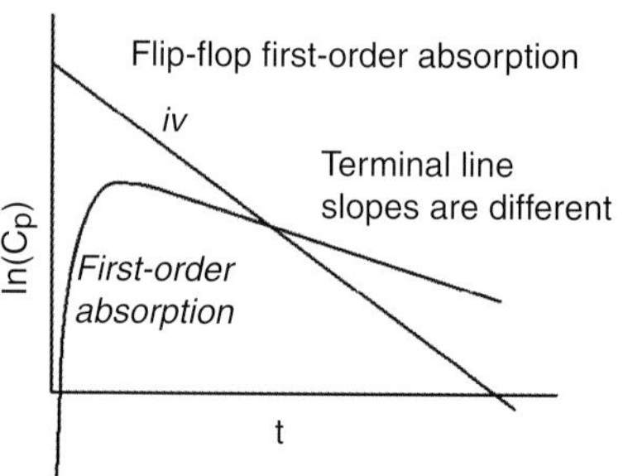

Figure 10.53 Graphical illustration of plasma concentrations for IV delivery versus first-order absorption for the normal and flip-flop situations.

constants are used in the mass balance equations, and the solution of these equations requires the definition of "hybrid" rate constants that are functions of the micro rate constants. As usual, this section will provide a summary of the model equations, plasma concentration analysis techniques, and special cases of the model.

10.10.1 Model Assumptions

The addition of a second compartment increases the number of inherent assumptions in the model to five. The specific nature and implications of each of these assumptions are described in this section.

10.10.1.1 Instantaneous Absorption

This assumption is the same for all instantaneous absorption models. See Section 10.7.1.1 for the details regarding this assumption.

10.10.1.2 Instantaneous Distribution throughout the Central Compartment

As in all compartmental models with more than one compartment, the central compartment (compartment 1) always contains the systemic circulation, and additionally contains all tissues that can be taken to reach equilibrium instantly with the systemic circulation. Drug distribution can never truly be instantaneous, as it cannot occur faster than the perfusion and permeation transport to the tissues. However, instantaneous distribution to the tissues in compartment 1 provides a reasonable approximation as long as these tissues approach equilibrium with plasma in a time period that is small compared to the elimination half-life. The assumption of instantaneous distribution throughout the central compartment also implies that the volume of distribution of this compartment (V_1) is a constant.

10.10.1.3 Approach to Equilibrium is Similar throughout the Tissue Compartment

As in all two-compartment models, the tissue compartment (compartment 2) contains tissues that take a significant period of time to reach equilibrium with the systemic circulation. The tissues in this compartment do not reach equilibrium with the systemic circulation quickly, however it is inherently assumed that they all approach equilibrium after a similar period of time. This doesn't mean that they all must approach equilibrium in an identical manner, merely that the approach to equilibrium is similar for all of the tissues in this compartment.

10.10.1.4 First-Order (Linear) Distribution Kinetics between Compartments

As in all standard two-compartment models, the rate of drug distribution transport between the two compartments is taken to follow first-order or linear kinetics. This means that the rate of drug transport from compartment 1 to compartment 2 is proportional to the amount of drug in compartment 1. Similarly, the rate of drug transport from compartment 2 to compartment 1 is proportional to the amount of drug in compartment 2. This assumption is generally reasonable as long as active transport molecules are not involved in the distribution process. If active transport is involved, then the assumption is still reasonable as long as the drug concentration is lower than the transporter Michaelis-Menten K_t constant in the vicinity of the transporter molecules.

10.10.1.5 First-Order (Linear) Elimination Kinetics

This assumption is essentially the same for all PK models described in this chapter. See Section 10.7.1.3 for the details regarding this assumption. For the standard two-compartment model, elimination is assumed to occur only from compartment 1.

10.10.2 Setup and Solution of Mass Balance Equations

A separate mass balance equation is written in the form of Section 10.6.2 for each compartment in the model. Since this is a two-compartment model, two mass balance equations are used. Variables A_1 and A_2 represent the amount of drug in compartment 1 and compartment 2, respectively. The total amount of drug in the body (A_{body}) is equal to the sum of A_1 and A_2. The absorbed dose of drug, generally written FD, can be simplified by the fact that F is 100% (or 1.0) for IV delivery, so the amount of drug absorbed for a bolus IV injection becomes simply the injected IV dose (D_{iv}). From the instantaneous absorption assumption, the entire dose of drug (D_{iv}) enters the systemic circulation in compartment 1 instantly at time zero, which will be used as an initial condition for the mass balance equation. No additional drug enters after time zero, so the rate of drug entering either compartment in the general mass balance equations is zero. Distribution between the compartments follows first-order kinetics, with the distribution rate of drug from compartment 1 to 2 equal to the micro distribution rate constant k_{12} multiplied by the amount of drug in compartment 1 (A_1), and the distribution rate from compartment 2 to 1 is given by the product of the micro distribution rate constant k_{21} and the amount of drug in compartment 2 (A_2).

Elimination occurs only from compartment 1 in the standard model form, with the elimination rate equal to the amount of drug remaining in compartment 1 (A_1) multiplied by a micro elimination rate constant (k_{10}). A schematic representation of this standard two-compartment bolus IV model is provided in Figure 10.55. The mass balance equation for compartment 1 is then

$$\frac{dA_1}{dt} = k_{21} \cdot A_2 - k_{12} \cdot A_1 - k_{10} \cdot A_1 \quad \text{with} \quad A_1 = D_{iv} \quad \text{at} \quad t = 0 \tag{10.184}$$

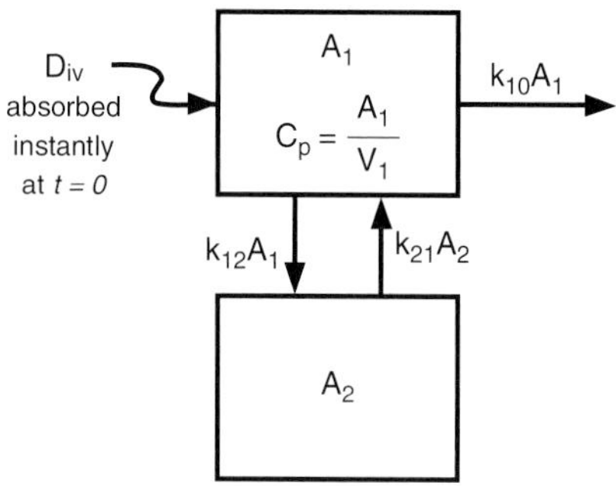

Figure 10.55 Schematic representation of the two-compartment bolus IV injection model.

and the mass balance equation for compartment 2 is

$$\frac{dA_2}{dt} = k_{12} \cdot A_1 - k_{21} \cdot A_2 \quad \text{with} \quad A_2 = 0 \quad \text{at} \quad t = 0 \tag{10.185}$$

Solving these two equations is substantially more involved than any of the previous one-compartment model equations, but with some mathematical manipulation the solution for A_1 and A_2 can be written in terms of the hybrid rate constants λ_1 and λ_2 as

$$A_1 = D_{iv}\left[\left(\frac{\lambda_1 - k_{21}}{\lambda_1 - \lambda_2}\right) \cdot e^{-\lambda_1 \cdot t} + \left(\frac{k_{21} - \lambda_2}{\lambda_1 - \lambda_2}\right) \cdot e^{-\lambda_2 \cdot t}\right] \tag{10.186}$$

$$A_2 = D_{iv}\left(\frac{k_{12}}{\lambda_1 - \lambda_2}\right)\left[e^{-\lambda_2 \cdot t} - e^{-\lambda_1 \cdot t}\right] \tag{10.187}$$

The hybrid rate constants are defined by the three relationships

$$\lambda_1 + \lambda_2 = k_{12} + k_{21} + k_{10} \tag{10.188}$$

$$\lambda_1 \cdot \lambda_2 = k_{21} \cdot k_{10} \tag{10.189}$$

$$\lambda_1 > \lambda_2 \tag{10.190}$$

which can be solved using a little more mathematical manipulation to give

$$\lambda_1 = \frac{1}{2}\left[(k_{12} + k_{21} + k_{10}) + \sqrt{(k_{12} + k_{21} + k_{10})^2 - 4 \cdot k_{21} \cdot k_{10}}\right] \tag{10.191}$$

$$\lambda_2 = \frac{1}{2}\left[(k_{12} + k_{21} + k_{10}) - \sqrt{(k_{12} + k_{21} + k_{10})^2 - 4 \cdot k_{21} \cdot k_{10}}\right] \tag{10.192}$$

Since $\lambda_1 > \lambda_2$, Equations (10.186) and (10.187) can be simplified for large time values to become

$$A_1 \approx D_{iv}\left(\frac{k_{21} - \lambda_2}{\lambda_1 - \lambda_2}\right) \cdot e^{-\lambda_2 \cdot t} \quad \text{for large } t \tag{10.193}$$

$$A_2 \approx D_{iv}\left(\frac{k_{12}}{\lambda_1 - \lambda_2}\right) \cdot e^{-\lambda_2 \cdot t} \quad \text{for large } t \tag{10.194}$$

Taking the natural logarithm of both sides yields a log-linear form for each of these equations at large time values

$$\ln(A_1) \approx \ln\left[D_{iv}\left(\frac{k_{21} - \lambda_2}{\lambda_1 - \lambda_2}\right)\right] - \lambda_2 \cdot t \quad \text{for large } t \tag{10.195}$$

$$\ln(A_2) \approx \ln\left[D_{iv}\left(\frac{k_{12}}{\lambda_1 - \lambda_2}\right)\right] - \lambda_2 \cdot t \quad \text{for large } t \tag{10.196}$$

Thus plots of $\ln(A_1)$ and $\ln(A_2)$ versus time should both have terminal line regions with a slope of $-\lambda_2$. Graphical representations of A_1 and $\ln(A_1)$ versus time are provided in Figure 10.56, and A_2 and $\ln(A_2)$ versus time are provided in Figure 10.57. The relative magnitudes of A_1 and A_2 depend on the tissue partition coefficients of the tissues included in compartment 2. Thus A_2 values could be lower than A_1 values at all times, or the A_2 values could rise above the A_1 values as the curves approach their terminal line regions.

10.10.3 Plasma Concentration versus Time Relationships

The plasma concentration of drug (C_p) can be related to the amount of drug in compartment 1 (A_1) by distribution volume of compartment 1 (V_1), as in the equation

$$C_p = \frac{A_1}{V_1} \tag{10.197}$$

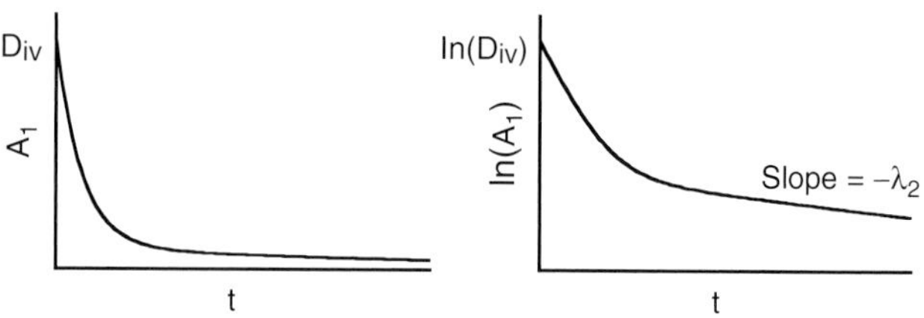

Figure 10.56 Graphical representation of the amount of drug in compartment 1 (A_1) versus time (t) and $\ln(A_1)$ versus t for a two-compartment bolus IV injection model.

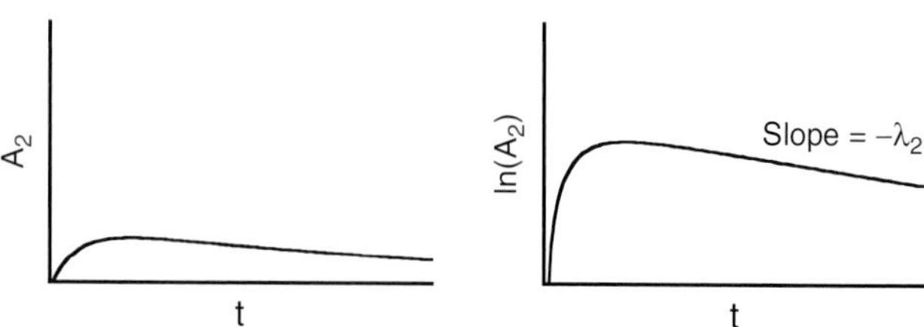

Figure 10.57 Graphical representation of the amount of drug in compartment 2 (A_2) versus time (t) and $\ln(A_2)$ versus t for a two-compartment bolus IV injection model.

Dividing both sides of Equation (10.186) by V_1 then gives

$$C_p = \frac{D_{iv}}{V_1}\left[\left(\frac{\lambda_1 - k_{21}}{\lambda_1 - \lambda_2}\right)\cdot e^{-\lambda_1 \cdot t} + \left(\frac{k_{21} - \lambda_2}{\lambda_1 - \lambda_2}\right)\cdot e^{-\lambda_2 \cdot t}\right] \quad (10.198)$$

It becomes easier to write this equation by defining the constants B_1 and B_2 as

$$B_1 = \frac{D_{iv}}{V_1}\left(\frac{\lambda_1 - k_{21}}{\lambda_1 - \lambda_2}\right) \quad (10.199)$$

$$B_2 = \frac{D_{iv}}{V_1}\left(\frac{k_{21} - \lambda_2}{\lambda_1 - \lambda_2}\right) \quad (10.200)$$

so that Equation (10.198) can be rewritten

$$C_p = B_1 \cdot e^{-\lambda_1 \cdot t} + B_2 \cdot e^{-\lambda_2 \cdot t} \quad (10.201)$$

It turns out that the initial plasma concentration (C_0) can be written

$$C_0 = \frac{D_{iv}}{V_1} = B_1 + B_2 \quad (10.202)$$

Since $\lambda_1 > \lambda_2$, Equation (10.201) can be simplified for large values of time as

$$C_p \approx B_2 \cdot e^{-\lambda_2 \cdot t} \quad \text{for large } t \quad (10.203)$$

Taking the natural logarithm of both sides of this equation then gives the log-linear form for the terminal line

$$\ln(C_p) \approx \ln(B_2) - \lambda_2 \cdot t \quad \text{for large } t \quad (10.204)$$

Graphical representations of the plasma concentration (C_p) and $\ln(C_p)$ versus time (t) are provided in Figure 10.58.

10.10.3.1 Distribution and Elimination Phases

The two-compartment bolus IV injection plasma concentration versus time curve in Figure 10.58 shows a characteristic early rapidly declining period followed by a more slowly declining terminal line concentration period. The early rapid decline is due to distribution to the tissue compartment, and hence this early period is called the distribution phase. Conversely, the slower decline at later times is due to drug elimination, and hence this later period is called the elimination phase. The distribution and elimination phases are illustrated in Figure 10.59.

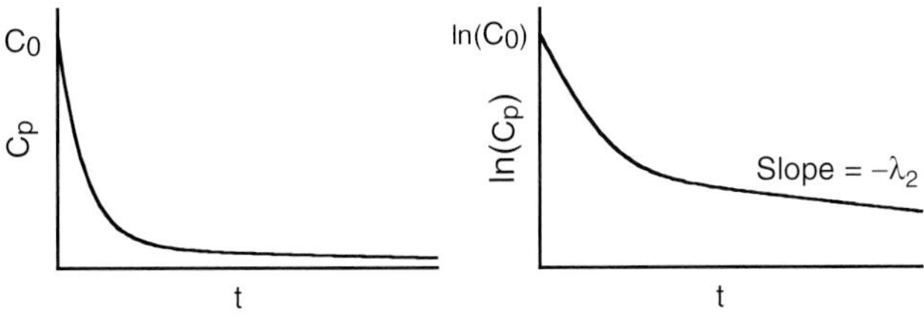

Figure 10.58 Graphical representation of the plasma concentration (C_p) versus time (t) and $\ln(C_p)$ versus t for a two-compartment bolus IV injection model.

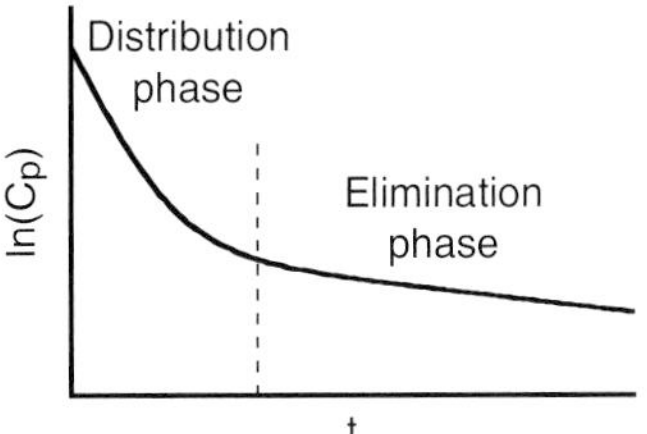

Figure 10.59 Graphical representation of the distribution phase (rapidly declining concentration) and elimination phase (slowly declining concentration) for a two-compartment bolus IV model.

10.10.3.2 Distribution and Elimination Half-Lives

The plasma concentration versus time relationship in Equation (10.198) contains two exponential decay terms. The first exponential decay term contains the larger hybrid rate constant (λ_1), which dominates at early times during the distribution phase. Hence λ_1 is called the hybrid distribution rate constant. The second exponential decay term contains the smaller hybrid rate constant (λ_2), which dominates at later times during the elimination phase. The slope of the terminal line is equal to $-\lambda_2$ rather than the negative value of the micro elimination rate constant ($-k_{10}$), and hence λ_2 is called the hybrid elimination rate constant. The relationships for the two-compartment elimination half-life are then written in terms of λ_2 as

$$t_{1/2,\text{elim}} = \frac{\ln(2)}{\lambda_2} \approx \frac{0.693}{\lambda_2} \quad (10.205)$$

$$\lambda_2 = \frac{\ln(2)}{t_{1/2,elim}} \approx \frac{0.693}{t_{1/2,elim}} \quad (10.206)$$

The distribution half-life are defined in terms of λ_1

$$t_{1/2,dist} = \frac{\ln(2)}{\lambda_1} \approx \frac{0.693}{\lambda_1} \quad (10.207)$$

$$\lambda_1 = \frac{\ln(2)}{t_{1/2,dist}} \approx \frac{0.693}{t_{1/2,dist}} \quad (10.208)$$

As illustrated earlier, a terminal line forms at large time values when $e^{-\lambda_1 \cdot t}$ becomes negligible compared to $e^{-\lambda_2 \cdot t}$. The exponential term with λ_1 in the exponent is associated with the distribution process. Hence the distribution process is 50% complete after one $t_{1/2,dist}$, 75% complete after two $t_{1/2,dist}$, and about 99% complete after seven $t_{1/2,dist}$. So as an approximate rule of thumb, the distribution exponential generally becomes negligible and $\ln(C_p)$ values fall on the terminal line when $t > 7 \cdot t_{1/2,dist}$.

10.10.3.3 *Effect of Basic Model Parameters on the Plasma Concentration versus Time Curve*

The effects of different model parameters on the plasma concentration versus time relationship can be demonstrated by mathematical analysis of the previous equations, or by graphical representation of a change in one or more of the variables. Equation (10.198) indicates the plasma concentration (C_p) is proportional to the bolus IV dose (D_{iv}) and inversely proportional to the compartment 1 distribution volume (V_1). Thus an increase in D_{iv} or a decrease in V_1 both yield an equivalent increase in C_p, as illustrated in Figure 10.60. Note that the general shape of the curve, including the slope of the terminal line, is not a function of D_{iv} or V_1. The hybrid elimination rate constant (λ_2) and the elimination half-life ($t_{½,elim}$) are inversely related to each other, so that an increase in one is equivalent to a decrease in the other. An increase in λ_2 or decrease in $t_{½,elim}$ causes concentrations to be lower at all times (since elimination is higher at all times), and causes the terminal line slope to be more negative or drop off more rapidly with time, as illustrated in Figure 10.61. The values of λ_1 and $t_{½,dist}$ are similarly inversely related to each other, with an increase in λ_1 or decrease in $t_{½,dist}$ causing plasma concentrations to drop more rapidly during the distribution phase and causing the terminal line to form earlier, but not affecting the slope of the terminal line. This relationship is illustrated in Figure 10.62.

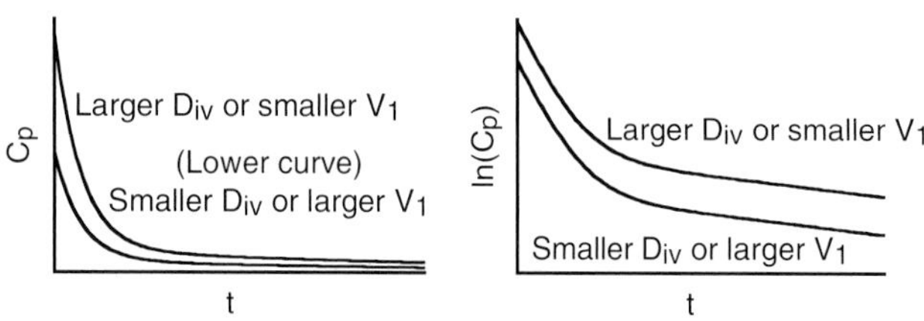

Figure 10.60 Illustration of how plasma concentration (C_p) and ln(C_p) versus *t* change with an increase or decrease in the bolus IV dose (D_{iv}) or compartment 1 distribution volume (V_1).

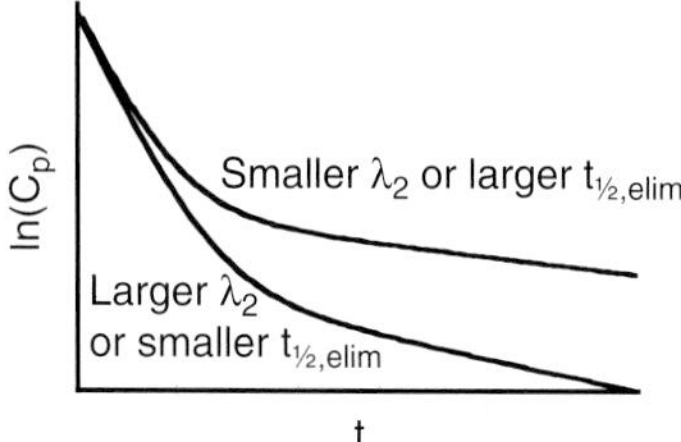

Figure 10.61 Illustration of how ln(C_p) versus *t* changes with an increase or decrease in the hybrid elimination rate constant (λ_2) or elimination half-life ($t_{½,elim}$).

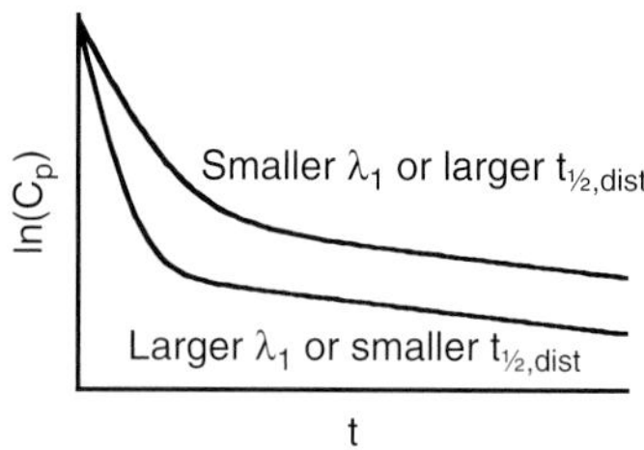

Figure 10.62 Illustration of how ln(C_p) versus *t* changes with an increase or decrease in the hybrid distribution rate constant (λ_1) or distribution half-life ($t_{1/2,dist}$).

10.10.3.4 *Estimating Plasma Drug Concentrations*

Average values for the elimination half-life ($t_{½,elim}$), and bioavailability (F) for many drugs can be found in drug handbooks, pharmacology textbooks, or PK research articles (which can be searched online). Values for the central compartment distribution volume (V_1) and the distribution half-life ($t_{½,dist}$) can typically only be found in research articles. Once the values of these parameters have been obtained, the plasma concentration for the drug can be estimated for any time after drug administration by simply substituting the appropriate parameter values and desired time (t) into the previous model equations. Unlike some of the previous models, the time at which the plasma concentration reaches a given value cannot be solved directly for all time points. This is because the concentration equation contains two exponential curves, which under normal circumstances can be solved only by a trial-and-error technique (guess t, calculate C_p, continue until t gives the desired C_p). An exception occurs for plasma concentration (C_p) values at long times after drug administration, in which case the desired concentration is located on the terminal line. For this special case, plasma concentrations can be represented by the simplified terminal equation, which can be solved directly for time to give

$$t = \frac{-\ln\left(\frac{C_p}{B_2}\right)}{\lambda_2} \quad \text{for large } t \tag{10.209}$$

As a general rule of thumb, this equation can be used to estimate t as long as $t > 7 \cdot t_{½,dist}$.

10.10.4 Estimating Model Parameters from Measured Plasma Concentration Data

Estimation of two-compartment bolus IV (instantaneous absorption) parameters from measured plasma samples ends up being quite similar to the one-compartment first-order absorption case. Proper parameter evaluation ideally requires at least three to five plasma samples be collected during the distribution phase, and five to seven samples be collected during the elimination phase. As in the one-compartment first-order absorption case, two stages of linear regression analysis are required to evaluate the parameters. The first stage involves analysis of measured plasma concentration data, and the second analysis is performed on calculated residual values.

10.10.4.1 Linear Regression of Terminal Line Plasma Concentration Data

Elimination parameters are determined by linear regression analysis of the measured plasma concentration data falling on the terminal line. As always, the first step is to calculate the natural logarithm of each of the measured plasma concentration values. The values of $\ln(C_p)$ are then plotted versus time (t). The plot should show later points falling on a terminal line with early points above the terminal line. Once the data points located on the terminal line have been identified, a linear regression analysis is performed on the terminal line data. The time (t) is entered as the independent (x) data, and $\ln(C_p)$ is entered as the dependent (y) data. A graphical representation of this analysis is illustrated in Figure 10.63. The regression correlation (r *or* r^2) should always be recorded along with the best-fit values of the intercept (b) and slope (m) for any linear regression analysis. The fitted slope (m) represents the best value for $-\lambda_2$, so that

$$\lambda_2 = -m \tag{10.210}$$

The fitted intercept (b) represents the best value for $\ln(B_2)$, from which B_2 can be calculated as

$$B_2 = e^b \tag{10.211}$$

The elimination half-life ($t_{½,elim}$) can be calculated from λ_2 by Equation (10.205). These then represent all the parameters that can be evaluated from the terminal line data.

10.10.4.2 Method of Residuals Analysis of Distribution Phase Plasma Concentration Data

The next step is to analyze the early measured plasma concentration values that were not used in the terminal line analysis. As in the one-compartment first-order absorption case, this is accomplished by the method of residuals calculations. The residual represents the difference between the value of the terminal line at a given value of time (t) and the actual measured concentration at the same value of t. Unlike the absorption phase points, which were below the terminal line, the distribution phase points are above the terminal line. The residual (R) values for the distribution phase are then calculated for each data point not employed in the previous terminal line analysis by the equation

$$R = C_p - B_2 \cdot e^{-\lambda_2 \cdot t} \tag{10.212}$$

A graphical representation of the residual value calculation is provided in Figure 10.64. If the measured plasma concentrations follow the relationship in Equation (10.201), then the residual values should follow the relationship

$$\begin{aligned} R &= C_p - B_2 \cdot e^{-\lambda_2 \cdot t} \\ &= (B_1 \cdot e^{-\lambda_1 \cdot t} + B_2 \cdot e^{-\lambda_2 \cdot t}) - B_2 \cdot e^{-\lambda_2 \cdot t} = B_1 \cdot e^{-\lambda_1 \cdot t} \end{aligned} \tag{10.213}$$

Taking the natural logarithm of the left and right terms gives the log-linear form

$$\ln(R) = \ln(B_1) - \lambda_1 \cdot t \tag{10.214}$$

Thus a plot of $\ln(R)$ versus t should then give a series of points falling on a straight line, as in Figure 10.65. A linear regression analysis is then performed on the residual values, with time (t) entered as the independent (x) data, and $\ln(R)$ is entered as the dependent (y) data.

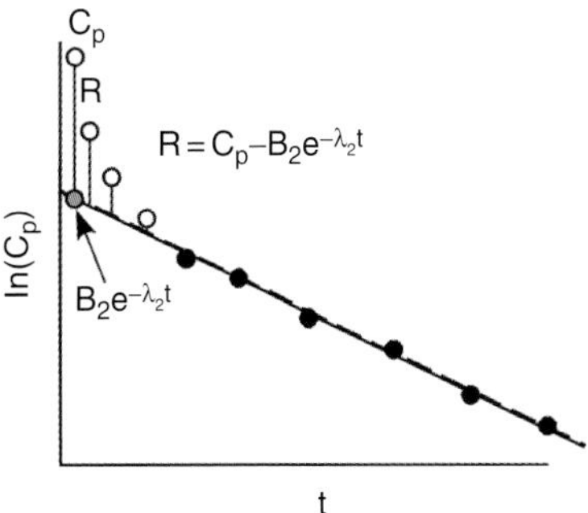

Figure 10.64 Calculation of residuals (R) from the fitted terminal line parameters and plasma concentration (C_p) data not used in terminal line analysis.

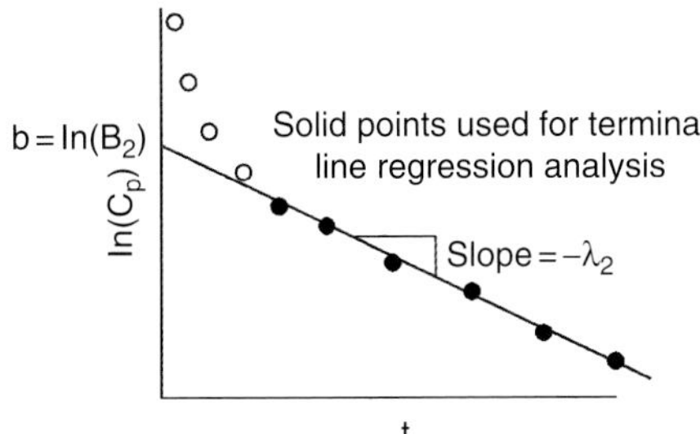

Figure 10.63 Linear regression analysis of $\ln(C_p)$ versus time for measured plasma concentrations falling on the terminal line.

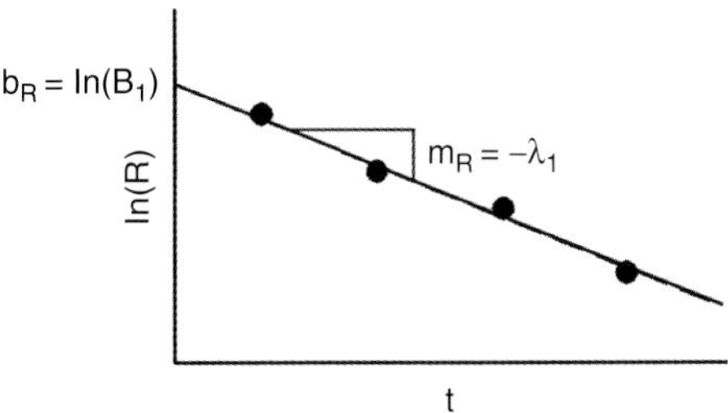

Figure 10.65 Linear regression analysis of calculated residuals for the distribution phase.

The fitted slope (m_R) represents the best value for $-\lambda_1$, so that

$$\lambda_1 = -m_R \tag{10.215}$$

The fitted intercept (b_R) represents $\ln(B_1)$, from which B_1 can be calculated as

$$B_1 = e^{b_R} \tag{10.216}$$

The value of the distribution half-life ($t_{½,dist}$) can then be calculated from Equation (10.207).

The values of B_1, λ_1, B_2, and λ_2 from the terminal line analysis and the method of residuals analysis can then be used to evaluate all the remaining model parameters that have been defined earlier in this section. The micro rate constants are given by the equations

$$k_{21} = \frac{B_1\lambda_2 + B_2\lambda_1}{B_1 + B_2} \tag{10.217}$$

$$k_{10} = \frac{\lambda_1\lambda_2}{k_{21}} \tag{10.218}$$

$$k_{12} = \lambda_1 + \lambda_2 - k_{21} - k_{10} \tag{10.219}$$

The central compartment distribution volume (V_1) can be evaluated by rearranging Equation (10.202) to give

$$V_1 = \frac{D}{C_0} = \frac{D}{B_1 + B_2} \tag{10.220}$$

The overall clearance (CL) is given simply by

$$CL = V_1 \cdot k_{10} \tag{10.221}$$

These then represent all the parameters that have been introduced so far for the two-compartment bolus IV (instantaneous absorption) model. Several additional parameters will be introduced in the following sections.

10.10.4.3 Area under the Curve (AUC) Calculations

The *AUC* of a two-compartment model can be used to define a new type of distribution volume, and as usual provides an alternate means to determine the overall clearance. The value of *AUC* for the two-compartment bolus IV model can be calculated directly by the equation

$$AUC = \frac{B_1}{\lambda_1} + \frac{B_2}{\lambda_1} \tag{10.222}$$

The *AUC* can alternatively be estimated by applying the trapezoidal rule to sequential pairs of measured plasma concentration values. Calculation of the slice of *AUC* between time zero and the first plasma measurement, $AUC(0 \rightarrow t_1)$, is the same as for the one-compartment bolus IV model case:

$$AUC(0 \rightarrow t_1) \approx \frac{1}{2}\left[C_0 + C_1\right] \cdot t_1 \tag{10.223}$$

where C_1 is the plasma concentration measured at t_1, and $C_0 = B_1 + B_2$. The *AUC* of each of the successive slices from t_1 up to t_f can then be estimated by applying the trapezoidal rule to each successive set of plasma concentration measurements. The general equation for these successive calculations for two successive plasma concentration measurements C_n and C_{n+1} made at t_n and t_{n+1} is the same for all PK models:

$$AUC(t_n \rightarrow t_{n+1}) \approx \frac{1}{2}\left[C_n + C_{n+1}\right] \cdot \left(t_{n+1} - t_n\right) \tag{10.224}$$

The area under the curve for the final segment from t_f to an infinite time, called the tail of the curve, is again similar to the one-compartment bolus IV model except that k is replaced by λ_2:

$$AUC(t_f \rightarrow \infty) = AUC(tail) = \frac{C_f}{\lambda_2} \tag{10.225}$$

Adding the *AUC* contribution from each slice as estimated by these equations then yields an estimate for the total *AUC*. The value of *AUC* from either of the described calculation methods can be related to the distribution volume of compartment 1 (V_1) and the overall clearance (CL) by the general relationship

$$AUC = \frac{D_{iv}}{V_1 \cdot k_{10}} = \frac{D_{iv}}{CL} \tag{10.226}$$

This yields alternative equations to evaluate V_1 and CL from the *AUC* that should yield nearly identical results to Equations (10.220) and (10.221)

$$V_1 = \frac{D_{iv}}{k_{10} \cdot AUC} \tag{10.227}$$

$$CL = \frac{D_{iv}}{AUC} \tag{10.228}$$

It turns out that another type of distribution volume, called V_{AUC}, can also be defined in terms of the area under the curve by the equation

$$V_{AUC} = \frac{D_{iv}}{\lambda_2 \cdot AUC} \tag{10.229}$$

which in turn provides yet another equation for overall clearance

$$CL = V_{AUC} \cdot \lambda_2 \tag{10.230}$$

Although the clearance (CL) defined in Equation (10.230) is the same as that in Equations (10.228) and (10.221), V_{AUC} is not the same as V_1. A discussion of the different distribution volume terms that can be defined for a two-compartment model is provided in the next section.

10.10.4.4 Distribution Volume Terms for a Two-Compartment Model

The general definition of the distribution volume (V) was previously given in Section 10.4.1.2 as

$$C_p = \frac{A_{body}}{V} \quad \text{or alternatively} \quad V = \frac{A_{body}}{C_p} \tag{10.231}$$

For a one-compartment PK model, the value of V is constant at all times and hence only a single distribution volume is defined. The volume of distribution for a two-compartment model changes with time, however, and hence several different types of distribution volumes are commonly defined for these models. The first distribution volume term is defined for time zero ($t = 0$). At time zero, $A_{body} = D_{iv}$ and $C_p = C_0$. These time zero values can be substituted into Equation (10.231) and combined with Equation (10.202) to show that $V = V_1$ at time zero. Another common distribution volume term is defined for the time when distributional steady-state occurs, as illustrated in Figure 10.14. There is no net transport of drug between compartments 1 and 2 at steady-state, as the transport rates in each direction are exactly equal. At the time when this occurs, a steady-state distribution volume (V_{ss}) can be defined by the equation

$$V_{ss} = V_1 \cdot \left(\frac{k_{21} + k_{12}}{k_{21}} \right) \qquad (10.232)$$

A final distribution volume is commonly defined for large time values, when redistribution of drug from compartment 2 to compartment 1 predominates, as illustrated in Figure 10.15. It turns out that the distribution volume under these conditions is equal to V_{AUC}, as defined earlier. In general, if the distribution volume changes with time, it always gets larger as time progresses. Thus it becomes universally true that $V_1 < V_{ss} < V_{AUC}$ for any two-compartment PK model.

10.10.5 Special Cases of the Two-Compartment Bolus IV (Instantaneous Absorption) Model

There are several common special case situations in which the two-compartment bolus IV model can be applied as a reasonable approximation for administration routes other than bolus IV injection. The means by which the two-compartment bolus IV model can be employed in these situations is described in this section. The criteria under which a drug following two-compartment instantaneous absorption can be approximated by a one-compartment instantaneous absorption model are also provided.

10.10.5.1 Two-Compartment Zero-Order Drug Absorption with Short Duration of Drug Delivery

As shown previously for the one-compartment case, the two-compartment model for steady (zero-order) drug delivery can be approximated by a two-compartment instantaneous absorption model as long as the drug delivery period (T) is relatively short compared to the elimination half-life ($t_{½,elim}$). As a general rule, the instantaneous model can be employed with reasonable accuracy as when $T \leq t_{½,elim}$. For cases where this simplification applies, the two-compartment bolus IV model equations can be used by simply replacing D_{iv} with $F \cdot k_0 \cdot T$.

10.10.5.2 Two-Compartment First-Order Drug Absorption with Rapid Absorption

Again similar to the one-compartment case, two-compartment first-order absorption of drug can be approximated by the two-compartment instantaneous absorption model as long as the absorption phase is completed at a very short time relative to the elimination half-life ($t_{½,elim}$). As a general rule of thumb, the instantaneous model can be employed with reasonable accuracy when $7 \cdot t_{½,abs} < t_{½,elim}$. When this simplification applies, the two-compartment bolus IV equations can be used by simply replacing D_{iv} with FD_{ev}, where D_{ev} represents the total dose delivered by the extravascular route.

10.10.5.3 Approximation of Two-Compartment Drug by One-Compartment Model

The two-compartment instantaneous absorption model is significantly more complex and harder to work with than the one-compartment instantaneous absorption model. Thus the one-compartment model is often used when it provides a reasonable approximation to the two-compartment values. In fact, the one-compartment model is often used even when a drug is known to significantly deviate from single compartment kinetics. Model simulations can be employed to evaluate under what conditions the one-compartment approximation is reasonable, and how much deviation occurs between the models under less ideal conditions.

Deviation between the one- and two-compartment instantaneous absorption models is related primarily to the relative values of the two-compartment constants B_1 and B_2 defined earlier. When $B_1 = 0$, the two-compartment model is identical to the one-compartment model. As the value of B1 becomes higher relative to the value of B2, the two-compartment model deviates more and more from the one-compartment model. Most marketed drugs have a B_1 value of zero up to about $50 \cdot B_2$. Figure 10.66 illustrates the model deviation at relative values of B_1 from zero (no deviation) up to $30 \cdot B_2$. Note that even with $B_1 = 30 \cdot B_2$, the deviation is only significant at early times and quickly dwindles to an insignificant difference. Thus it is not surprising that the one-compartment model is often used even for large values of B_1.

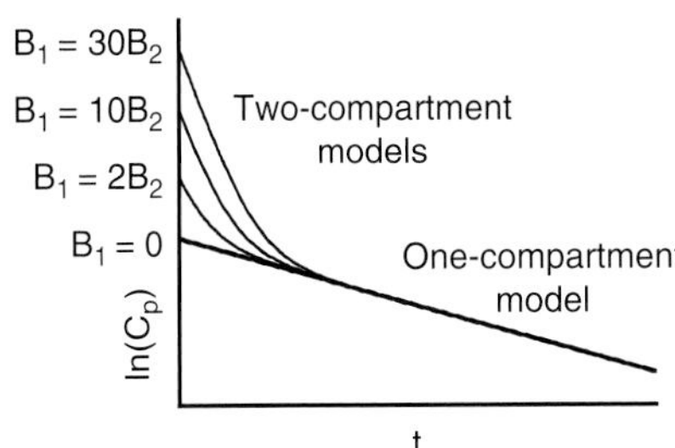

Figure 10.66 Approximation of a drug following two-compartment kinetics by a one-compartment bolus IV (instantaneous absorption) model.

As a general rule of thumb, however, typically it is recommended that the one-compartment model can be employed with reasonable accuracy for $B_1 \leq 2 \cdot B_2$. When this simplification is used, the one-compartment bolus IV equations in Section 10.7 can be used without modification for a bolus IV injection, or with the modifications listed in Sections 10.10.5.1 and 10.10.5.2 for other routes of delivery.

10.11 TWO-COMPARTMENT IV INFUSION (ZERO-ORDER ABSORPTION) MODEL

The two-compartment model scheme is applied to the steady delivery of drug into the systemic circulation (zero-order absorption) in this section. The only difference between the instantaneous absorption and zero-order absorption two-compartment models is in the type of drug absorption. Thus all descriptions of what is included in each compartment, the use of micro and hybrid rate constants, and the different types of distribution volumes are identical to the two-compartment bolus IV model values. As was done previously for zero-order absorption, the model equations are written specifically for the case of IV infusion, with modifications for other types of zero-order absorption described in Section 10.11.5.

10.11.1 Model Assumptions

The use of a two-compartment model with zero-order absorption results in five inherent model assumptions. The specific nature and implications of each of these assumptions are described in this section.

10.11.1.1 Zero-Order Absorption

This assumption is the same for all zero-order absorption models. See Section 10.8.1.1 for the details regarding this assumption.

10.11.1.2 Instantaneous Distribution throughout the Central Compartment

This assumption is the same for all compartmental models with more than one compartment. See Section 10.10.1.2 for the details regarding this assumption.

10.11.1.3 Approach to Equilibrium is Similar throughout the Tissue Compartment

This assumption is the same for all two-compartment models. See Section 10.10.1.3 for the details regarding this assumption.

10.11.1.4 First-Order (Linear) Distribution Kinetics between Compartments

This assumption is the same for all two-compartment models. See Section 10.10.1.4 for the details regarding this assumption.

10.11.1.5 First-Order (Linear) Elimination Kinetics

This assumption is essentially the same for all PK models described in this chapter. See Section 10.7.1.3 for the details regarding this assumption. For the standard two-compartment model, elimination is assumed to occur only from compartment 1.

10.11.2 Setup and Solution of Mass Balance Equations

A separate mass balance equation is written in the form of Section 10.6.2 for each compartment included in the model. Variables A_1 and A_2 represent the amount of drug in compartment 1 and compartment 2, respectively. Distribution and elimination rates can be written in terms of micro rate constants and first-order rate equations exactly as described for the two-compartment bolus IV model. As mentioned in Section 10.8, an IV infusion has an unusual discontinuity in that drug is delivered into the systemic circulation (directly into compartment 1) at a constant rate ($k_{0,iv}$) over a fixed period of time ($0 \leq t \leq T$), after which the rate of drug delivery drops to zero ($t > T$). A schematic representation of the standard two-compartment IV infusion model is provided in Figure 10.67. In order to accommodate this discontinuity in drug delivery, two mass balance equations must be written for compartment 1, one for the time period during infusion and the other for the time period after infusion stops. The mass balance equation for compartment 1 during the infusion period ($0 \leq t \leq T$) becomes

$$\frac{dA_1}{dt} = k_{0,iv} + k_{21} \cdot A_2 - k_{12} \cdot A_1 - k_{10} \cdot A_1 \quad \text{for} \quad 0 \leq t \leq T \tag{10.233}$$

The mass balance equation for compartment 1 during the postinfusion period ($t > T$) is

$$\frac{dA_1}{dt} = k_{21} \cdot A_2 - k_{12} \cdot A_1 - k_{10} \cdot A_1 \quad \text{for} \quad t > T \tag{10.234}$$

The mass balance equation for compartment 2 remains the same for both time periods:

$$\frac{dA_2}{dt} = k_{12} \cdot A_1 - k_{21} \cdot A_2 \quad \text{for} \quad t \geq 0 \tag{10.235}$$

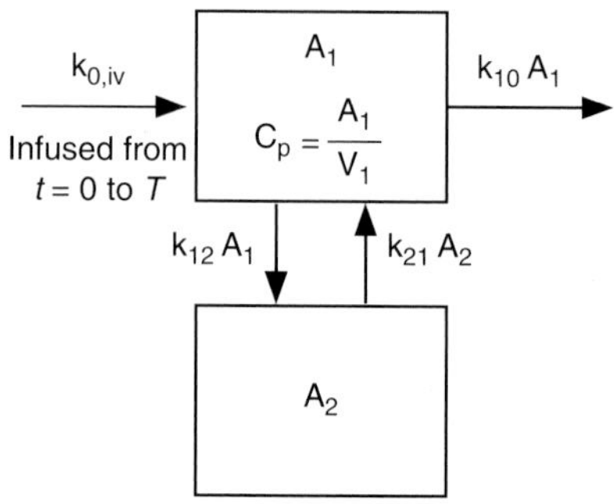

Figure 10.67 Schematic representation of the two-compartment IV infusion model.

Solution of these differential mass balance equations provides the following relationships for A_1 during the infusion period (for $0 \le t \le T$)

$$A_1 = \frac{k_{0,iv}(\lambda_1 - k_{21})}{\lambda_1(\lambda_1 - \lambda_2)}(1 - e^{-\lambda_1 \cdot t}) + \frac{k_{0,iv}(k_{21} - \lambda_2)}{\lambda_2(\lambda_1 - \lambda_2)}(1 - e^{-\lambda_2 \cdot t}) \quad (10.236)$$

and during the postinfusion period (for $t > T$):

$$A_1 = \left[\frac{k_{0,iv}(\lambda_1 - k_{21})(1 - e^{-\lambda_1 \cdot T})}{\lambda_1(\lambda_1 - \lambda_2)}\right] \cdot e^{-\lambda_1 \cdot (t-T)} + \left[\frac{k_{0,iv}(k_{21} - \lambda_2)(1 - e^{-\lambda_2 \cdot T})}{\lambda_2(\lambda_1 - \lambda_2)}\right] \cdot e^{-\lambda_2 \cdot (t-T)} \quad (10.237)$$

The hybrid rate constants used in these equations can be defined in terms of the micro rate constants exactly as previously listed for the bolus IV two-compartment model:

$$\lambda_1 = \frac{1}{2}\left[(k_{12} + k_{21} + k_{10}) + \sqrt{(k_{12} + k_{21} + k_{10})^2 - 4 \cdot k_{21} \cdot k_{10}}\right] \quad (10.238)$$

$$\lambda_2 = \frac{1}{2}\left[(k_{12} + k_{21} + k_{10}) - \sqrt{(k_{12} + k_{21} + k_{10})^2 - 4 \cdot k_{21} \cdot k_{10}}\right] \quad (10.239)$$

These relationships are utilized next to develop equations for plasma concentration versus time.

10.11.3 Plasma Concentration versus Time Relationships

The plasma drug concentration (C_p) is given by dividing the amount of drug in compartment 1 (A_1) by the distribution volume of compartment 1 (V_1). This yields the following equations for the infusion period (for $0 \le t \le T$):

$$C_p = \left(\frac{B_1}{1 - e^{-\lambda_1 \cdot T}}\right)(1 - e^{-\lambda_1 \cdot t}) + \left(\frac{B_2}{1 - e^{-\lambda_2 \cdot T}}\right)(1 - e^{-\lambda_2 \cdot t}) \quad (10.240)$$

and the postinfusion period (for $t > T$):

$$C_p = B_1 \cdot e^{-\lambda_1 \cdot (t-T)} + B_2 \cdot e^{-\lambda_2 \cdot (t-T)} \quad (10.241)$$

where the constants B_1 and B_2 are defined for the IV infusion model as

$$B_1 = \frac{k_{0,iv}(\lambda_1 - k_{21})(1 - e^{-\lambda_1 \cdot T})}{V_1\lambda_1(\lambda_1 - \lambda_2)} \quad (10.242)$$

$$B_2 = \frac{k_{0,iv}(k_{21} - \lambda_2)(1 - e^{-\lambda_2 \cdot T})}{V_1\lambda_2(\lambda_1 - \lambda_2)} \quad (10.243)$$

The plasma concentration at the end of infusion (C_T), which is also C_{max}, is given simply by

$$C_T = B_1 + B_2 \quad (10.244)$$

If the infusion lasts a long time, the plasma concentration approaches the steady-state concentration (C_{ss}), where the rate of elimination exactly equals the infusion rate, which gives

$$C_{ss} = \frac{k_{0,iv}}{CL} = \frac{k_{0,iv}}{V_1 \cdot k_{10}} = \frac{k_{0,iv}}{V_{AUC} \cdot \lambda_2} \quad (10.245)$$

Since $\lambda_1 > \lambda_2$, Equation (10.241) can be simplified for longer values of time after infusion stops as

$$C_p \approx B_2 \cdot e^{-\lambda_2 \cdot (t-T)} \quad \text{for large } t - T \quad (10.246)$$

taking the natural logarithm of both sides gives the log-linear form for the terminal line

$$\ln(C_p) \approx \ln(B_2) - \lambda_2 \cdot (t - T) \quad \text{for large } t - T \quad (10.247)$$

Note that the plasma concentration equation during the postinfusion period has the same form as the two-compartment bolus IV model (Section 10.10.3), except that the time after infusion stops ($t - T$) is substituted for (t). Graphical representations of the plasma concentration (C_p) and $\ln(C_p)$ versus time (t) for the two-compartment IV infusion model are provided in Figure 10.68.

10.11.3.1 Distribution and Elimination Phases during the Postinfusion Period

The postinfusion plasma concentration versus time curve in Figure 10.68 shows a characteristic early rapidly declining period followed by a more slowly declining terminal line period. The early rapid decline is due to distribution to the tissue compartment, and hence this early period is called the distribution phase. Conversely, the slower decline at later times is due to drug elimination, and hence this later period is called the elimination phase. The distribution and elimination phases are graphically illustrated in Figure 10.69.

10.11.3.2 Distribution and Elimination Half-Lives

The postinfusion plasma concentration versus time relationship in Equation (10.241) contains two exponential decay terms. The first exponential decay term contains the larger hybrid rate constant (λ_1), which dominates during the distribution phase. Hence λ_1 is called the hybrid distribution rate constant. The second exponential decay term contains the smaller hybrid rate

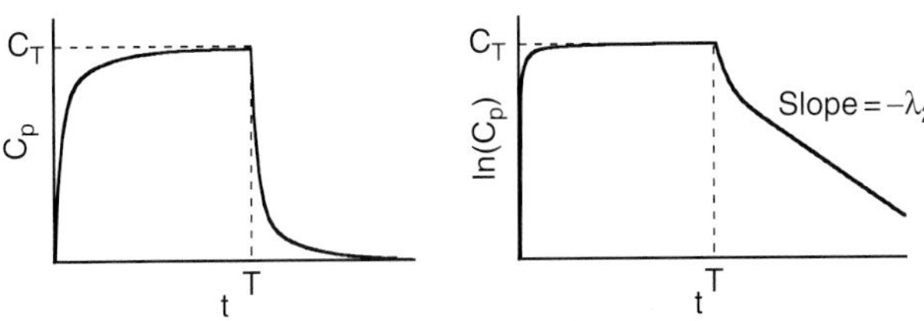

Figure 10.68 Graphical representation of the plasma concentration (C_p) versus time (t) and $\ln(C_p)$ versus t for a two-compartment IV infusion model.

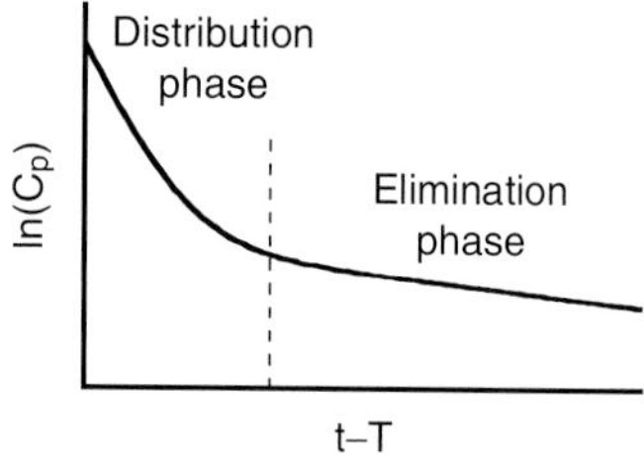

Figure 10.69 Graphical representation of the distribution phase (rapidly declining concentration) and elimination phase (slowly declining concentration) during the post-infusion period for a two-compartment IV infusion model.

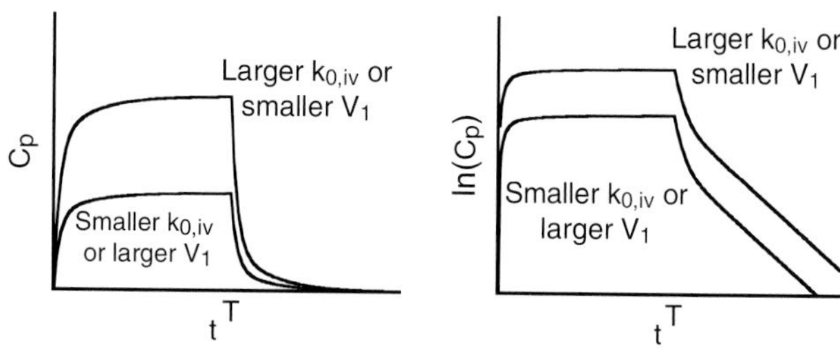

Figure 10.70 Illustration of how plasma concentration (C_p) and ln(C_p) versus t change with an increase or decrease in the IV dosing rate (k_0,iv) or compartment 1 distribution volume (V_1).

constant (λ_2), which dominates during the elimination phase. The slope of the terminal line is equal to $-\lambda_2$, and hence λ_2 is called the hybrid elimination rate constant. The relationship for the two-compartment elimination half-life is then written in terms of λ_2 as

$$t_{½,elim} = \frac{\ln(2)}{\lambda_2} \approx \frac{0.693}{\lambda_2} \tag{10.248}$$

or rearranging

$$\lambda_2 = \frac{\ln(2)}{t_{½,elim}} \approx \frac{0.693}{t_{½,elim}} \tag{10.249}$$

The distribution half-life is then defined in terms of λ_1 to give

$$t_{½,dist} = \frac{\ln(2)}{\lambda_1} \approx \frac{0.693}{\lambda_1} \tag{10.250}$$

or again by rearranging

$$\lambda_1 = \frac{\ln(2)}{t_{½,dist}} \approx \frac{0.693}{t_{½,dist}} \tag{10.251}$$

As illustrated earlier, a terminal line forms at long times when $e^{-\lambda_1 \cdot t}$ becomes negligible compared to $e^{\lambda_2 \cdot t}$. The exponential term with λ_1 in the exponent is associated with the distribution process. Hence the distribution process is 50% complete after one $t_{½,dist}$, 75% complete after two $t_{½,dist}$, and about 99% complete after seven $t_{½,dist}$. So as an approximate rule of thumb, the distribution exponential term generally becomes negligible and $\ln(C_p)$ values fall on the terminal line when $t - T > 7 \cdot t_{½,dist}$.

10.11.3.3 Effect of Basic Model Parameters on the Plasma Concentration versus Time Curve

The effects of different model parameters on the plasma concentration versus time relationship can be demonstrated by mathematical analysis of the previous equations, or by graphical representation of a change in one or more of the variables. The model equations indicate the plasma concentration (C_p) is proportional to the intravenous dosing rate ($k_{0,iv}$) and inversely proportional to the compartment 1 distribution volume (V_1). Thus an increase in $k_{0,iv}$ or a decrease in V_1 both yield an equivalent increase in C_p, as illustrated in Figure 10.70. Note that the general shape of the curve, including the slope of the terminal line, is not a function of $k_{0,iv}$ or V_1. The hybrid elimination rate constant (λ_2) and the elimination half-life ($t_{½,elim}$) are inversely related to each other, so that an increase in one is equivalent to a decrease in the other. An increase in λ_2 or decrease in $t_{½,elim}$ causes concentrations to be lower at all times (since elimination is higher at all times), and causes the terminal line slope to be more negative or to drop off more rapidly with time, as illustrated in Figure 10.71. The values of λ_1 and $t_{½,dist}$ are similarly inversely related to each other, with an increase in λ_1 or decrease in $t_{½,dist}$ causing plasma concentrations to drop more rapidly during the distribution phase and causing the terminal line to form earlier, but not affecting the slope of the terminal line. This relationship is illustrated in Figure 10.72.

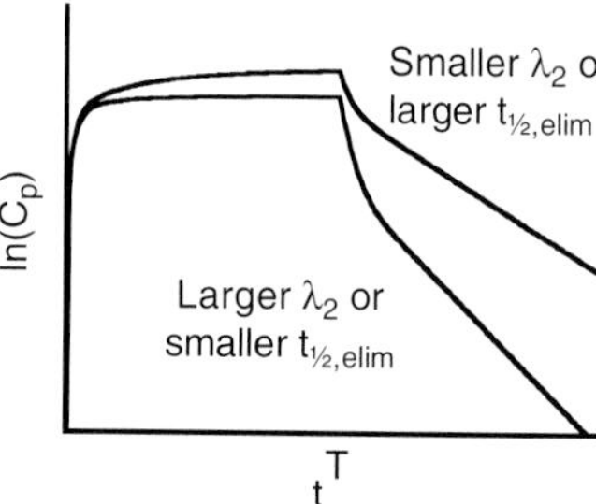

Figure 10.71 Illustration of how ln(C_p) versus t changes with an increase or decrease in the hybrid elimination rate constant (λ_2) or elimination half-life ($t_{½,elim}$).

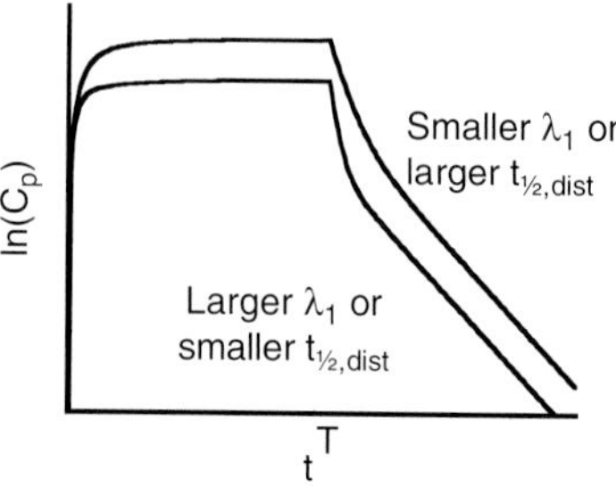

Figure 10.72 Illustration of how ln(C_p) versus t changes with an increase or decrease in the hybrid distribution rate constant (λ_1) or distribution half-life ($t_{½,dist}$).

10.11.3.4 Estimating Plasma Drug Concentrations

Average values for the elimination half-life ($t_{½,elim}$), and bioavailability (F) for many drugs can be found in drug handbooks, pharmacology textbooks, or in PK research articles (which can be searched online). Values for the central compartment distribution volume (V_1) and the distribution half-life ($t_{½,dist}$) can typically be found only in research articles. Once values of these parameters have been obtained, the plasma drug concentration can be estimated for any time after drug administration by substituting the appropriate parameter values and desired time (t) into the previous model equations. The time at which the plasma concentration reaches a given value cannot be solved directly for all time points. This is because the concentration equation during both the infusion period and postinfusion period contain two exponential terms, so that in general these equations can be solved for time only by a trial-and-error technique (guess t, calculate C_p, continue until t gives the desired C_p). An exception occurs for plasma concentration (C_p) values at long times after infusion stops, in which case C_p is located on the terminal line. For this special case, plasma concentrations can be represented by the simplified terminal line equation, which can be solved directly for time to give

$$t - T = \frac{-\ln\left(\frac{C_p}{B_2}\right)}{\lambda_2} \quad \text{for large } (t - T) \qquad (10.252)$$

As a general rule of thumb, this equation can be used to estimate t as long as $t - T > 7 \cdot t_{½,dist}$.

10.11.4 Estimating Model Parameters from Measured Plasma Concentration Data

Standard linear regression and method of residual analyses of two-compartment IV infusion (zero-order absorption) data is limited to samples collected during the postinfusion period. Plasma concentrations during the infusion period do not lend themselves to a linear analysis for a two-compartment model. Estimation of parameters from measured postinfusion plasma samples is quite similar to the two-compartment bolus IV (instantaneous absorption) case. Proper parameter evaluation ideally requires at least three to five plasma samples be collected during the distribution phase, and five to seven samples be collected during the elimination phase. Area under the curve (AUC) calculations can also be used in evaluating some of the model parameters.

10.11.4.1 Linear Regression of Postinfusion Terminal Line Plasma Concentration Data

Elimination parameters are determined by linear regression analysis of the measured postinfusion plasma concentration data falling on the terminal line. The analysis technique is mathematically and graphically identical to the analysis of two-compartment bolus IV data, except that the time after infusion stops ($t - T$) is used in place of the time (t), and the concentration at the end of infusion (C_T) is used in place of the initial concentration (C_0). As always, the first step is to calculate the natural logarithm of each of the measured plasma concentration values. The values of $\ln(C_p)$ are then plotted versus time after infusion stops ($t - T$). The plot should show later points falling on a terminal line with early points above the terminal line. Once the data points located on the terminal line have been identified, a linear regression analysis is performed on the terminal line data. The values of $\ln(C_p)$ are entered as the dependent variable (y) data time, and ($t - T$) values are entered as the independent variable (x) data. A graphical representation of this analysis is illustrated in Figure 10.73. The regression correlation (r or r^2) should always be recorded along with the best fit values of the intercept (b) and slope (m) for any linear regression analysis. The fitted slope (m) represents the best value for $-\lambda_2$, so that

$$\lambda_2 = -m \qquad (10.253)$$

The fitted intercept (b) represents the best value for $\ln(B_2)$, from which B_2 can be calculated as

$$B_2 = e^b \qquad (10.254)$$

The elimination half-life ($t_{½,elim}$) can be calculated from λ_2 by Equation (10.248). These then represent all the parameters that can be evaluated from the terminal line data.

10.11.4.2 Method of Residuals Analysis of Distribution Phase Plasma Concentration Data

The next step is to analyze the early measured plasma concentration values that were not used in the terminal line analysis. As in several previous models, this is accomplished by the method of residuals calculations. The residual values represent the difference between the value of the terminal line at a given value of time after infusion stops ($t - T$) and the actual measured concentration at the same value of $t - T$. The residual (R) values for the distribution phase are then

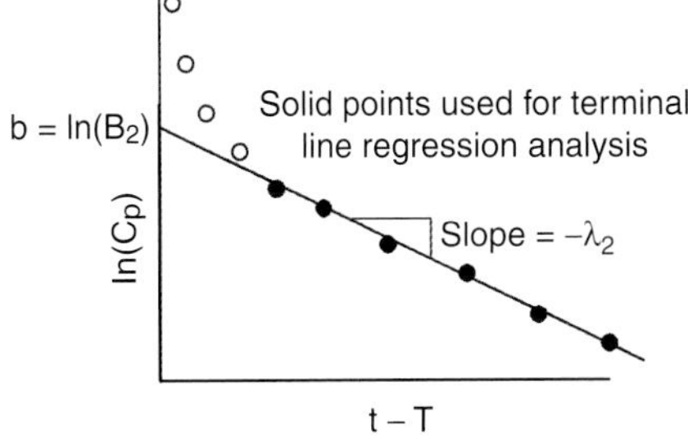

Figure 10.73 Linear regression analysis of $\ln(C_p)$ versus time after infusion stops ($t - T$) for measured plasma concentrations falling on the terminal line.

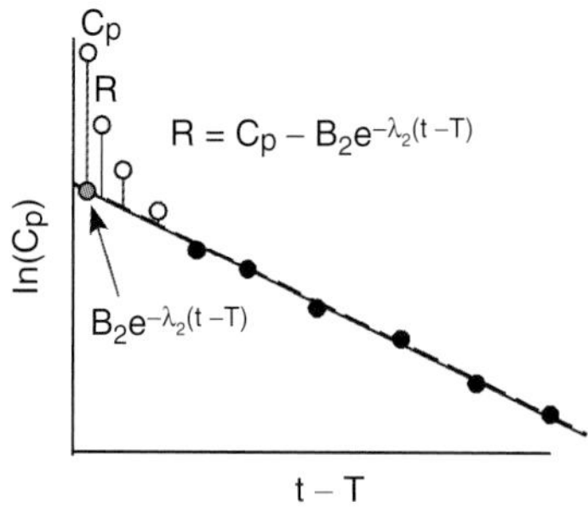

Figure 10.74 Calculation of residuals (R) from the fitted terminal line parameters and plasma concentration (C_p) data not used in terminal line analysis.

calculated for each data point not employed in the previous terminal line analysis by the equation

$$R = C_p - B_2 \cdot e^{-\lambda_2 \cdot (t-T)} \tag{10.255}$$

A graphical representation of the residual value calculation is provided in Figure 10.74. If the measured plasma concentrations follow the relationship in Equation (10.241), then the residual values should follow the relationship

$$\begin{aligned} R &= \left(B_1 \cdot e^{-\lambda_1 \cdot (t-T)} + B_2 \cdot e^{-\lambda_2 \cdot (t-T)}\right) - B_2 \cdot e^{-\lambda_2 \cdot (t-T)} \\ &= B_1 \cdot e^{-\lambda_1 \cdot (t-T)} \end{aligned} \tag{10.256}$$

Taking the natural logarithm of the left and right terms gives the log-linear form

$$\ln(R) = \ln(B_1) - \lambda_1 \cdot (t-T) \tag{10.257}$$

Thus a plot of $\ln(R)$ versus $t-T$ should then give a series of points falling on a straight line, as in Figure 10.75. A linear regression analysis is then performed on the residual values, with time after infusion stops ($t-T$) entered as the independent (x) data, and $\ln(R)$ is entered as the dependent (y) data. The fitted slope (m_R) represents the best value for $-\lambda_1$, so that

$$\lambda_1 = -m_R \tag{10.258}$$

The fitted intercept (b_R) represents $\ln(B_1)$, from which B_1 can be calculated as

$$B_1 = e^{b_R} \tag{10.259}$$

The value of the distribution half-life ($t_{½,dist}$) can then be calculated from Equation (10.250).

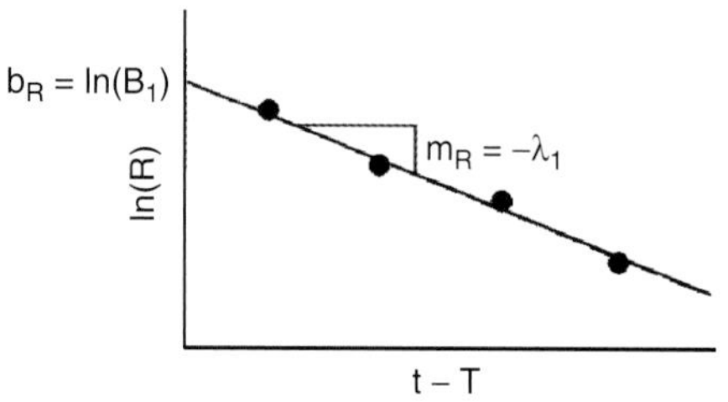

Figure 10.75 Linear regression analysis of calculated residuals for the distribution phase.

The values of B_1, λ_1, B_2, and λ_2 from the terminal line analysis and the method of residuals analysis can then be used to evaluate all remaining model parameters. The micro rate constants for the IV infusion (zero-order absorption) model are given by the equations

$$k_{21} = \frac{\left(\dfrac{B_1\lambda_1\lambda_2}{1-e^{-\lambda_1 T}} + \dfrac{B_2\lambda_1\lambda_2}{1-e^{-\lambda_2 T}}\right)}{\left(\dfrac{B_1\lambda_1}{1-e^{-\lambda_1 T}} + \dfrac{B_2\lambda_2}{1-e^{-\lambda_2 T}}\right)} \tag{10.260}$$

$$k_{10} = \frac{\lambda_1\lambda_2}{k_{21}} \tag{10.261}$$

$$k_{12} = \lambda_1 + \lambda_2 - k_{21} - k_{10} \tag{10.262}$$

The various distribution volume terms and overall clearance can be evaluated by

$$V_1 = \frac{k_{0,iv}}{\left(\dfrac{B_1\lambda_1}{1-e^{-\lambda_1 T}} + \dfrac{B_2\lambda_2}{1-e^{-\lambda_2 T}}\right)} \tag{10.263}$$

$$V_{ss} = V_1 \cdot \left(\frac{k_{21}+k_{12}}{k_{21}}\right) \tag{10.264}$$

$$V_{AUC} = V_1 \cdot \left(\frac{k_{10}}{\lambda_2}\right) \tag{10.265}$$

$$CL = V_1 \cdot k_{10} = V_{AUC} \cdot \lambda_2 \tag{10.266}$$

This gives values for all two-compartment IV infusion (zero-order absorption) model parameters.

10.11.4.3 Area under the Curve (AUC) Calculations

The value of AUC for the two-compartment IV infusion (zero-order absorption) model can be calculated directly by the equation

$$AUC = \frac{k_{0,iv}T}{CL} \tag{10.267}$$

but this equation is useful only if the clearance (CL) is already known. Note that since the product in the numerator ($k_{0,iv}$T) is exactly equal to the total IV infused dose (D_{iv}), or more generally the total absorbed dose (FD), this equation is in fact identical to the universal form

$$AUC = \frac{FD}{CL} \tag{10.268}$$

The AUC can alternatively be estimated by applying the trapezoidal rule to sequential pairs of measured plasma concentration values. Calculation of the slice of AUC between time zero and the first plasma measurement, $AUC(0 \rightarrow t_1)$, is the same as the one-compartment IV infusion since the initial concentration (C_0) is still zero, giving

$$AUC(0 \rightarrow t_1) \approx \frac{1}{2}(C_1 \cdot t_1) \tag{10.269}$$

where C_1 is the plasma concentration measured at t_1. The AUC of each of the successive slices from t_1 up to t_f can then be estimated by applying the trapezoidal rule to each successive set of plasma concentration measurements. The general equation for these successive calculations for two successive plasma concentration measurements C_n and C_{n+1} made at t_n and t_{n+1} is the same for all models

$$AUC(t_n \rightarrow t_{n+1}) \approx \frac{1}{2}\left[C_n + C_{n+1}\right] \cdot \left(t_{n+1} - t_n\right) \quad (10.270)$$

Finally, the area under the curve for the final segment from t_f to an infinite time, called the tail of the curve, is also the same as the two-compartment bolus IV case

$$AUC(t_f \rightarrow \infty) = AUC(tail) = \frac{C_f}{\lambda_2} \quad (10.271)$$

Adding the *AUC* contribution from these equations then yields an estimate for the total *AUC*. The value of *AUC* estimated from this calculation can then be used as an alternative means of evaluating the V_{AUC} and the clearance (CL) by

$$V_{AUC} = \frac{k_{0,iv} T}{\lambda_2 \cdot AUC} = \frac{D_{iv}}{\lambda_2 \cdot AUC} \quad (10.272)$$

$$CL = \frac{k_{0,iv} T}{AUC} = \frac{D_{iv}}{AUC} \quad (10.273)$$

In general, *AUC* calculations are not often used for IV infusion (zero-order absorption) unless the value is being compared to extravascular drug delivery for bioavailability calculations.

10.11.5 Special Cases of the Two-Compartment IV Infusion (Zero-Order Absorption) Model

There are several common special case situations for the two-compartment IV infusion model. One is a case where this model can be applied as a reasonable approximation for other routes of drug delivery. The other two are cases in which plasma concentrations can be reasonably approximated by a less complex model.

10.11.5.1 Zero-Order Extravascular Drug Delivery

A number of controlled drug release approaches deliver drug at a steady rate into an extravascular region of the body. Examples of this type of drug delivery include transdermal patches, implantable pumps, and intramuscular depot injections. This situation is very similar to an IV infusion, except that a portion of the drug can be broken down or metabolized prior to reaching the systemic circulation. The fraction of the delivered drug that reaches the systemic circulation is given by the bioavailability (F). The two-compartment IV infusion model equations in this section can be readily applied to the steady extravascular drug delivery case by simply replacing the IV infusion rate ($k_{0,iv}$) with the extravascular drug delivery rate multiplied by the appropriate extravascular bioavailability, or $F \cdot k_{0,ev}$.

10.11.5.2 One-Compartment Zero-Order Drug Absorption with Short Duration of Drug Delivery

As described in Section 10.8.5.3, under certain circumstances a zero-order drug delivery process of short duration can be approximated as an instantaneous absorption process. In general, the instantaneous absorption model provides a reasonable approximation when $T \leq t_{½,elim}$. This criteria can be employed as a general rule of thumb, although the acceptable amount of difference between the models will depend on the required level of accuracy for a given application. When this approximation is used, the intravenous dose (D_{iv}) should be replaced by the total absorbed dose ($F \cdot k_0 \cdot T$) in the bolus IV model equations.

10.11.5.3 Approximation of Two-Compartment Drug by One-Compartment Model

The two-compartment zero-order absorption model is more complex and harder to work with than the one-compartment zero-order absorption model. Thus the one-compartment model is often used when it provides a reasonable approximation to the two-compartment values. In fact, the one-compartment model is often used even when a drug is known to significantly deviate from single compartment kinetics. Just as in the case of the two-compartment bolus IV injection model in Section 10.10.5.3, as a general rule of thumb the one-compartment model can be employed with reasonable accuracy as long as $B_1 \leq 2 \cdot B_2$. When this simplification is used, the one-compartment IV infusion equations in Section 10.8 can be used without modification for an IV infusion, or with the modifications listed in Section 10.11.5.1 for steady extravascular delivery.

10.12 TWO-COMPARTMENT FIRST-ORDER ABSORPTION MODEL

First-order absorption occurs when drug enters the systemic circulation at a rate that is proportional to the amount of drug remaining to be absorbed at the site of administration. This is a very reasonable approximation for most routes of extravascular drug delivery, including oral ingestion and most injections into an administration site other than a blood vessel (with the only common exception being an intramuscular depot injection). This model is used most often for oral ingestion so it is sometimes called the two-compartment oral absorption model, but the equations apply equally well to all extravascular routes. Data analysis for two-compartment first-order absorption requires an extra stage of method of residuals calculations compared to the other two-compartment models. As with one-compartment first-order absorption, evaluation of the bioavailability will require comparison to IV drug delivery data. Thus the data analysis in this section will be the most complex of all the standard models discussed in this chapter.

10.12.1 Model Assumptions

The standard two-compartment first-order absorption model makes five inherent assumptions about the ADME processes that occur during and after drug delivery. The specific nature and implications of each of these assumptions are described in this section.

10.12.1.1 First-Order Absorption

This assumption is the same for all first-order absorption models. See Section 10.9.1.1 for the details regarding this assumption.

10.12.1.2 Instantaneous Distribution throughout the Central Compartment

This assumption is the same for all compartmental models with more than one compartment. See Section 10.10.1.2 for the details regarding this assumption.

10.12.1.3 Approach to Equilibrium is Similar throughout the Tissue Compartment

This assumption is the same for all two-compartment models. See Section 10.10.1.3 for the details regarding this assumption.

10.12.1.4 First-Order (Linear) Distribution Kinetics between Compartments

This assumption is the same for all two-compartment models. See Section 10.10.1.4 for the details regarding this assumption.

10.12.1.5 First-Order (Linear) Elimination Kinetics

This assumption is essentially the same for all PK models described in this chapter. See Section 10.7.1.3 for the details regarding this assumption. For the standard two-compartment model, elimination is assumed to occur only from compartment 1.

10.12.2 Setup and Solution of Mass Balance Equations

Separate mass balance equations are written in the form of Section 10.6.2 for each of the two compartments. Variables A_1 and A_2 represent the amount of drug in compartment 1 and compartment 2, respectively, and the total amount of drug in the body (A_{body}) is given by the sum of A_1 and A_2. The rate of drug absorption is a function of a first-order absorption rate constant (k_a), the bioavailability (F), and the administered dose (D). Distribution between the compartments follows first-order kinetics as described previously. Elimination occurs only from compartment 1 in the standard model form, with the elimination rate equal to the amount of drug remaining in compartment 1 (A_1) multiplied by a micro elimination rate constant (k_{10}). A schematic representation of this standard two-compartment first-order absorption model is provided in Figure 10.76. The mass balance equations for each compartment are then

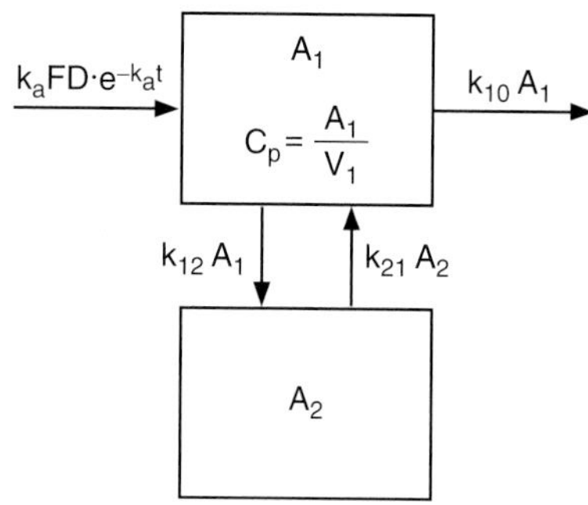

Figure 10.76 Schematic representation of the two-compartment first-order absorption model.

$$\frac{dA_1}{dt} = k_a FD \cdot e^{-k_a t} + k_{21} \cdot A_2 - k_{12} \cdot A_1 - k_{10} \cdot A_1 \quad (10.274)$$

$$\frac{dA_2}{dt} = k_{12} \cdot A_1 - k_{21} \cdot A_2 \quad (10.275)$$

Solving these two equations is substantially more involved than any of the previous PK model equations, but with some straightforward mathematical manipulations the solutions for A_1 and A_2 can be written in terms of the hybrid rate constants λ_1 and λ_2 as

$$A_1 = k_a FD \cdot \left[\frac{(\lambda_1 - k_{21}) \cdot e^{-\lambda_1 \cdot t}}{(\lambda_1 - \lambda_2)(k_a - \lambda_1)} + \frac{(k_{21} - \lambda_2) \cdot e^{-\lambda_2 \cdot t}}{(\lambda_1 - \lambda_2)(k_a - \lambda_2)} + \frac{(k_{21} - k_a) \cdot e^{-k_a \cdot t}}{(k_a - \lambda_1)(k_a - \lambda_2)} \right] \quad (10.276)$$

$$A_2 = k_a k_{21} FD \cdot \left[\frac{-e^{-\lambda_1 \cdot t}}{(\lambda_1 - \lambda_2)(k_a - \lambda_1)} + \frac{e^{-\lambda_2 \cdot t}}{(\lambda_1 - \lambda_2)(k_a - \lambda_2)} + \frac{e^{-k_a \cdot t}}{(k_a - \lambda_1)(k_a - \lambda_2)} \right] \quad (10.277)$$

The hybrid rate constants are defined as in the previous two-compartment models by

$$\lambda_1 + \lambda_2 = k_{12} + k_{21} + k_{10} \quad (10.278)$$

$$\lambda_1 \cdot \lambda_2 = k_{21} \cdot k_{10} \quad (10.279)$$

$$\lambda_1 > \lambda_2 \quad (10.280)$$

which can be solved to yield

$$\lambda_1 = \frac{1}{2} \left[(k_{12} + k_{21} + k_{10}) + \sqrt{(k_{12} + k_{21} + k_{10})^2 - 4 \cdot k_{21} \cdot k_{10}} \right] \quad (10.281)$$

$$\lambda_2 = \frac{1}{2}\left[(k_{12} + k_{21} + k_{10}) - \sqrt{(k_{12} + k_{21} + k_{10})^2 - 4 \cdot k_{21} \cdot k_{10}}\right] \quad (10.282)$$

It should be noted that the absorption rate constant (k_a) is taken to be greater than either of the hybrid rate constants. Hence $k_a > \lambda_1 > \lambda_2$, so the previous equations for A_1 and A_2 can be simplified for large time values to become

$$A_1 = \left[\frac{k_a FD \cdot (k_{21} - \lambda_2)}{(\lambda_1 - \lambda_2)(k_a - \lambda_2)}\right] \cdot e^{-\lambda_2 \cdot t} \quad \text{for large } t \quad (10.283)$$

$$A_2 = \left[\frac{k_a k_{21} FD}{(\lambda_1 - \lambda_2)(k_a - \lambda_2)}\right] \cdot e^{-\lambda_2 \cdot t} \quad \text{for large } t \quad (10.284)$$

Taking the natural logarithm of both sides yields a log-linear form for each of these equations:

$$\ln(A_1) \approx \ln\left[\frac{k_a FD \cdot (k_{21} - \lambda_2)}{(\lambda_1 - \lambda_2)(k_a - \lambda_2)}\right] - \lambda_2 \cdot t \quad \text{for large } t \quad (10.285)$$

$$\ln(A_2) \approx \ln\left[\frac{k_a k_{21} FD}{(\lambda_1 - \lambda_2)(k_a - \lambda_2)}\right] - \lambda_2 \cdot t \quad \text{for large } t \quad (10.286)$$

Thus plots of $\ln(A_1)$ and $\ln(A_2)$ versus time should both have terminal line regions with a slope of $-\lambda_2$. Graphical representations of A_1 and $\ln(A_1)$ versus time are provided in Figure 10.77, and A_2 and $\ln(A_2)$ versus time are provided in Figure 10.78. The relative magnitudes of A_1 and A_2 depend on the tissue partition coefficient (K_T) values of the tissues included in compartment 2. Thus A_2 values could be lower than A_1 values at all times, or the A_2 values could rise above the A_1 values as the curves approach their terminal line regions.

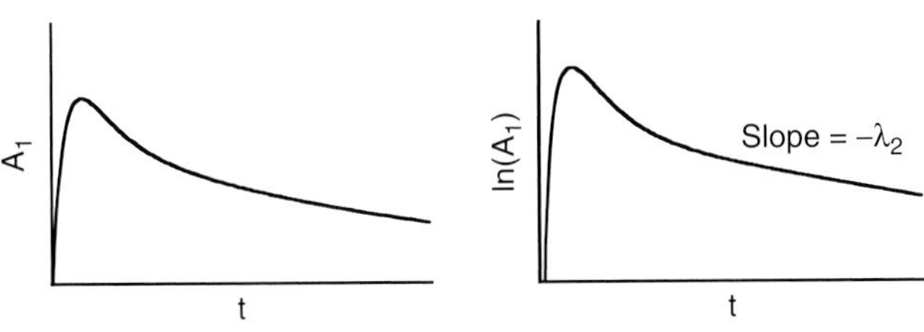

Figure 10.77 Graphical representation of the amount of drug in compartment 1 (A_1) versus time (t) and $\ln(A_1)$ versus t for a two-compartment first-order absorption model.

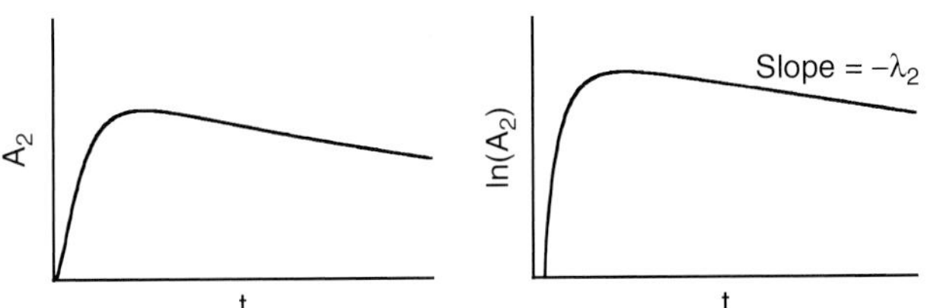

Figure 10.78 Graphical representation of the amount of drug in compartment 2 (A_2) versus time (t) and $\ln(A_2)$ versus t for a two-compartment first-order absorption model.

10.12.3 Plasma Concentration versus Time Relationships

The plasma concentration of drug (C_p) is given by dividing the amount of drug in compartment 1 (A_1) by distribution volume of compartment 1 (V_1), which yields

$$C_p = B_1 \cdot e^{-\lambda_1 \cdot t} + B_2 \cdot e^{-\lambda_2 \cdot t} + B_3 \cdot e^{-k_a \cdot t} \quad (10.287)$$

where the constants B_1, B_2, and B_3 are defined as

$$B_1 = \frac{k_a FD \cdot (\lambda_1 - k_{21})}{V_1(\lambda_1 - \lambda_2)(k_a - \lambda_1)} \quad (10.288)$$

$$B_2 = \frac{k_a FD \cdot (k_{21} - \lambda_2)}{V_1(\lambda_1 - \lambda_2)(k_a - \lambda_2)} \quad (10.289)$$

$$B_3 = \frac{k_a FD \cdot (k_{21} - k_a)}{V_1(k_a - \lambda_1)(k_a - \lambda_2)} \quad (10.290)$$

It turns out that B_3 is negative ($B_3 < 0$) and can be related to B_1 and B_2 by the relation

$$B_3 = -(B_1 + B_2) \quad (10.291)$$

Since $k_a > \lambda_1 > \lambda_2$, the plasma concentration versus time equation can be simplified for longer values of time as

$$C_p \approx B_2 \cdot e^{-\lambda_2 \cdot t} \quad \text{for large } t \quad (10.292)$$

Taking the natural logarithm of both sides gives the log-linear form for the terminal line:

$$\ln(C_p) \approx \ln(B_2) - \lambda_2 \cdot t \quad \text{for large } t \quad (10.293)$$

Graphical representations of the plasma concentration (C_p) and $\ln(C_p)$ versus time (t) are provided in Figure 10.79.

Unlike the one-compartment first-order absorption model, the time (t_{max}) of the maximum plasma concentration (C_{max}) cannot be written in a solved equation form. Thus determination of t_{max} and C_{max} for this model requires a trial-and-error approach in which a time (t) is guessed and the plasma concentration (C_p) is calculated repeatedly until the C_{max} and t_{max} are identified.

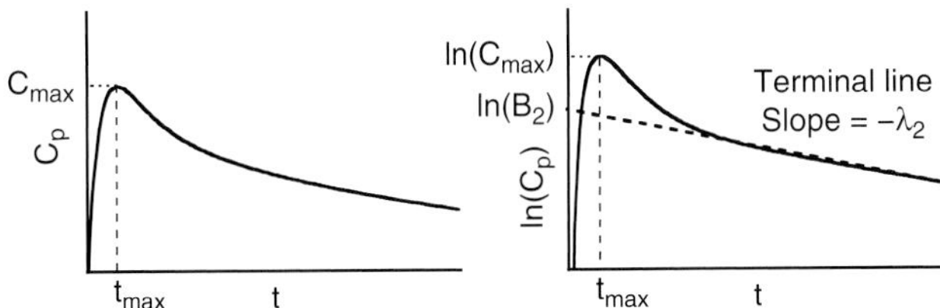

Figure 10.79 Graphical representation of the plasma concentration (C_p) versus time (t) and $\ln(C_p)$ versus t for a two-compartment first-order absorption model.

10.12.3.1 Absorption, Distribution, and Elimination Phases

The two-compartment first-order absorption plasma concentration versus time curve in Figure 10.79 displays a characteristic early rapid rise, which transitions into a rapidly declining period immediately after t_{max}, subsequently followed by a more slowly declining terminal line concentration period at later times. The early rise is due to absorption from the drug administration site, and hence this period is labeled the absorption phase. The rapid decline after t_{max} is caused by distribution to the tissue compartment, and hence is called the distribution phase. The slower decline at later times is due to drug elimination, and hence this later period becomes the elimination phase. The absorption, distribution, and elimination phases are graphically illustrated in Figure 10.80.

10.12.3.2 Absorption, Distribution, and Elimination Half-Lives

The plasma concentration versus time equation for the two-compartment first-order absorption model contains three exponential decay terms, and three corresponding phases in Figure 10.80. The first exponential decay term contains the larger hybrid rate constant (λ_1), which dominates just after t_{max} during the distribution phase. Hence λ_1 is called the hybrid distribution rate constant. The second exponential decay term contains the smaller hybrid rate constant (λ_2), which dominates at later times during the elimination phase. The third exponential decay curve contains k_a and dominates the early rising absorption phase. The two-compartment elimination half-life is then written in terms of λ_2 as

$$t_{½,elim} = \frac{\ln(2)}{\lambda_2} \approx \frac{0.693}{\lambda_2} \tag{10.294}$$

$$\lambda_2 = \frac{\ln(2)}{t_{½,elim}} \approx \frac{0.693}{t_{½,elim}} \tag{10.295}$$

The distribution half-life is defined in terms of λ_1 to give

$$t_{½,dist} = \frac{\ln(2)}{\lambda_1} \approx \frac{0.693}{\lambda_1} \tag{10.296}$$

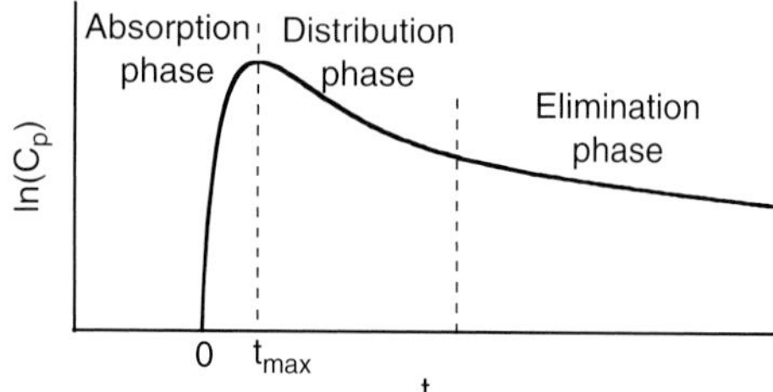

Figure 10.80 Graphical representation of the absorption phase (rapidly rising concentration), distribution phase (rapidly declining concentration after t_{max}), and elimination phase (slowly declining concentration) for a two-compartment first-order absorption model.

$$\lambda_1 = \frac{\ln(2)}{t_{½,dist}} \approx \frac{0.693}{t_{½,dist}} \tag{10.297}$$

Finally, an absorption half-life can be defined for first-order absorption in terms of k_a yielding

$$t_{½,abs} = \frac{\ln(2)}{k_a} \approx \frac{0.693}{k_a} \tag{10.298}$$

$$k_a = \frac{\ln(2)}{t_{½,abs}} \approx \frac{0.693}{t_{½,abs}} \tag{10.299}$$

Remembering that $k_a > \lambda_1 > \lambda_2$, it can readily be shown that $t_{½,abs} < t_{½,dist} < t_{½,elim}$. Hence the absorption process is completed before the distribution or elimination processes, and absorption is 50% complete after one $t_{½,abs}$, 75% complete after two $t_{½,abs}$, and is essentially (about 99%) complete after seven $t_{½,abs}$. The distribution processes is similarly 50% complete after one $t_{½,dist}$, 75% complete after two $t_{½,dist}$, and is essentially (about 99%) complete after seven $t_{½,dist}$. The terminal line forms at long times when $e^{-\lambda_1 \cdot t}$ and $e^{-k_a \cdot t}$ become negligible compared to $e^{-\lambda_2 \cdot t}$. As a general rule of thumb, the $\ln(C_p)$ values fall on the terminal line when $t > 7 \cdot t_{½,dist}$.

10.12.3.3 Effect of Basic Model Parameters on the Plasma Concentration versus Time Curve

As with all previous models, the effects of different model parameters on the plasma concentration versus time relationship can be demonstrated by mathematical analysis of the previous equations, or by graphical representation of a change in one or more of the variables. The plasma concentration (C_p) is proportional to the absorbed dose (*FD*) and inversely proportional to the compartment 1 distribution volume (V_1). Thus an increase in *FD* or a decrease in V_1 both yield an equivalent increase in C_p, as illustrated in Figure 10.81. Note that the general shape of the curve, including the time of maximum concentration and slope of the distribution phase and the terminal line, is not a function of *FD* or V_1. The hybrid elimination rate constant (λ_2) and the elimination half-life ($t_{½,elim}$) are inversely related to each other, so that an increase in one is equivalent to a decrease in the other. An increase in λ_2 or decrease in $t_{½,elim}$ causes concentrations to be lower at all times (since elimination is higher at all times), which causes the maximum concentration to occur slightly earlier, and causes the terminal line

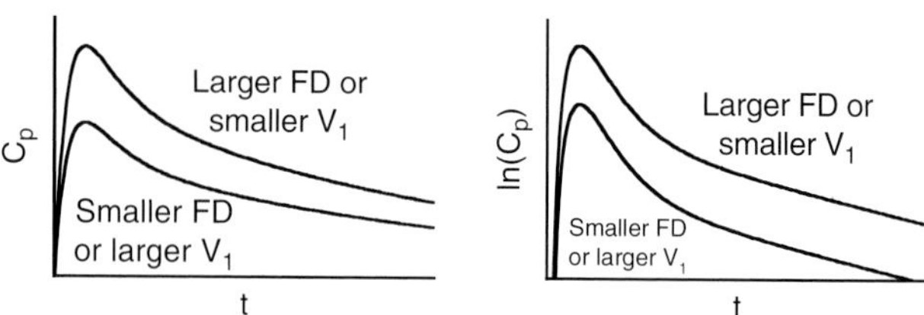

Figure 10.81 Illustration of how plasma concentration (C_p) and $\ln(C_p)$ versus *t* change with an increase or decrease in the absorbed dose (*FD*) or compartment 1 distribution volume (V_1).

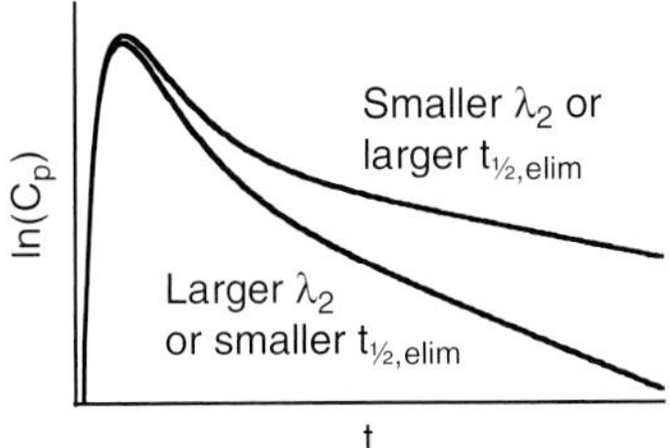

Figure 10.82 Illustration of how plasma concentration (C_p) and $\ln(C_p)$ versus t change with an increase or decrease in the hybrid elimination rate constant (λ_2) or elimination half-life ($t_{1/2,elim}$).

slope to be more negative or to drop off more rapidly with time, as illustrated in Figure 10.82. The values of λ_1 and $t_{1/2,dist}$ are similarly inversely related to each other, with an increase in λ_1 or decrease in $t_{1/2,dist}$ causing plasma concentrations to drop more rapidly during the distribution phase, making the maximum concentration occur earlier, and causing the terminal line to form earlier, but not affecting the slope of the terminal line. This relationship is illustrated in Figure 10.83. The values of k_a and $t_{1/2,abs}$ are also inversely related to each other, with an increase in k_a or decrease in $t_{1/2,abs}$ causing plasma concentrations to rise more rapidly during the absorption phase, and maximum concentration to be reached earlier, but not affecting the slope of the distribution phase or the terminal line. This relationship is illustrated in Figure 10.84.

10.12.3.4 Estimating Plasma Drug Concentrations

Average values for the elimination half-life ($t_{1/2,elim}$), and bioavailability (F) for many drugs can be found in drug handbooks, pharmacology textbooks, or in PK research articles (which can be searched online). Values for the central compartment distribution volume (V_1), distribution half-life ($t_{1/2,dist}$), and absorption rate constant (k_a) or half-life ($t_{1/2,abs}$) can typically be found only in research articles. Once the values of these parameters have been obtained, the plasma concentration for the drug can be estimated for any time after drug administration by simply substituting the appropriate parameter values and desired time (t) into

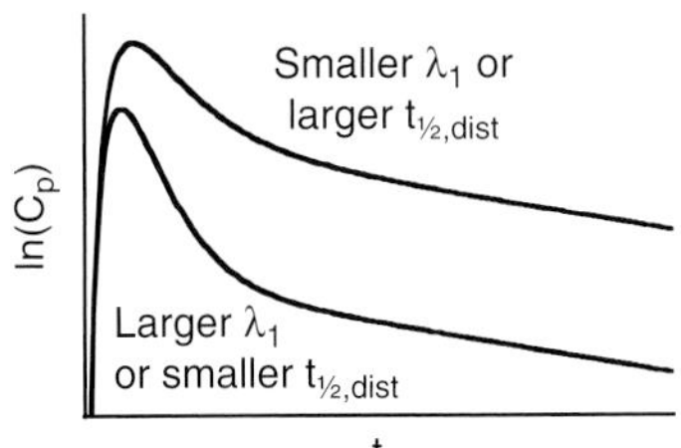

Figure 10.83 Illustration of how plasma concentration (C_p) and $\ln(C_p)$ versus t change with an increase or decrease in the hybrid distribution rate constant (λ_1) or distribution half-life ($t_{1/2,dist}$).

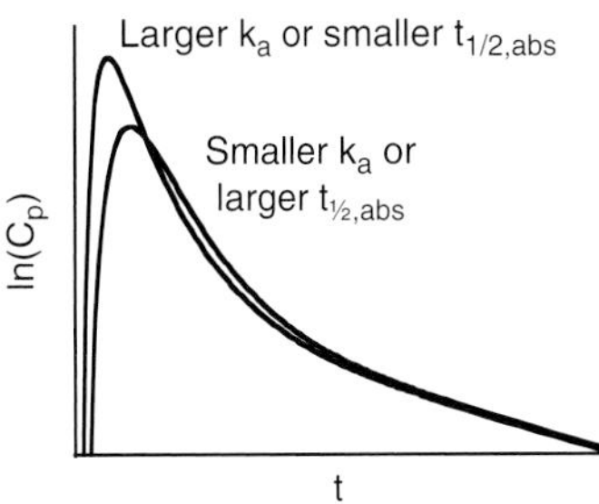

Figure 10.84 Graphical illustration of how plasma concentration (C_p) and $\ln(C_p)$ versus t change with an increase or decrease in the absorption rate constant (k_a) or absorption half-life ($t_{1/2,abs}$).

the previous model equations. As with all two-compartment models, the time at which the plasma concentration reaches a given value cannot be solved directly for all time points. This is because the concentration equation contains three exponential curves, which under normal circumstances can be solved only by a trial-and-error technique (guess t, calculate C_p, continue until t gives the desired C_p). An exception occurs for plasma concentration (C_p) values at long enough times that the desired concentration is located on the terminal line. For this special case, the time at which a particular plasma concentration is reached is given by

$$t = \frac{-\ln\left(\frac{C_p}{B_2}\right)}{\lambda_2} \quad \text{for large } t \qquad (10.300)$$

As a general rule of thumb, this equation can be used to estimate t as long as $t > 7 \cdot t_{1/2,dist}$.

10.12.4 Estimating Model Parameters from Measured Plasma Concentration Data

Estimation of two-compartment first-order absorption parameters from measured plasma samples ends up being more complicated and laborious than all previous models, but the methods are still relatively straightforward. Proper parameter evaluation ideally requires at least three to five plasma samples collected during the absorption phase, and three to five plasma samples collected during the distribution phase, and five to seven samples collected during the elimination phase. After the linear regression analysis of the $\ln(C_p)$ versus t terminal line, two stages of method of residuals calculations and fitting are required to evaluate all the rate constants. Additional plasma concentration results from IV delivery of the same drug are then required to fully evaluate the remaining model parameters.

10.12.4.1 Linear Regression of Terminal Line Plasma Concentration Data

Elimination parameters are determined by linear regression analysis of the measured plasma concentration data falling on the terminal line. As always, the first step is to

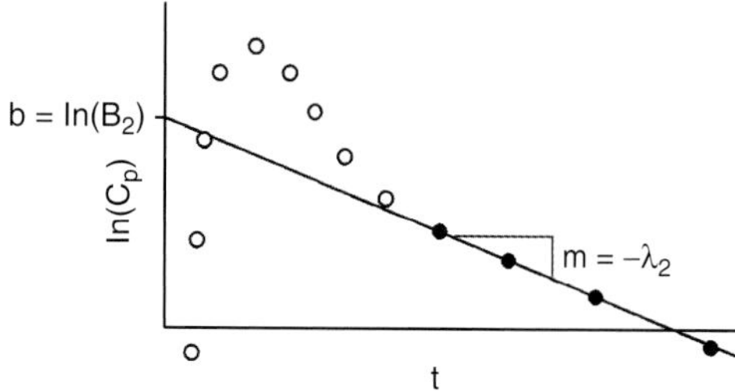

Figure 10.85 Check the graph of $ln(C_p)$ versus t to identify values falling on the terminal line, then perform a linear regression analysis on the terminal line values.

calculate the natural logarithm of each of the measured plasma concentrations. The values of $\ln(C_p)$ are then plotted versus time (t) to determine the points falling on the terminal line. A linear regression analysis is then performed on the terminal line data, with time (t) entered as the independent (x) data values, and $\ln(C_p)$ entered as the dependent (y) data values. A graphical representation of this analysis is shown in Figure 10.85. The regression correlation (r or r^2) should be recorded along with the best fit values of the intercept (b) and slope (m) for any linear regression analysis. The fitted slope (m) for the terminal line represents the best value for $-\lambda_2$, so that

$$\lambda_2 = -m \tag{10.301}$$

The fitted intercept (b) represents the best value for $\ln(B_2)$, from which B_2 can be calculated as

$$B_2 = e^b \tag{10.302}$$

The elimination half-life ($t_{½,elim}$) can be calculated from λ_2 by Equation (10.294). These then represent all the parameters that can be evaluated from the terminal line data.

10.12.4.2 Method of Residuals Analysis of Absorption and Distribution Phase Data

The next step is to analyze the early measured plasma concentration values that were not used in the terminal line analysis. In order to determine both the absorption and distribution parameters, two stages of method of residuals analysis must be performed on this data. The first set of residuals (R_1) represent the difference between the value of the terminal line at a given time (t) and the actual concentration measured at that time. A graphical representation of the first residuals is provided in Figure 10.86, and the first residual (R_1) is calculated for each data point not employed in the previous terminal line analysis by the equation

$$R_1 = C_p - B_2 \cdot e^{-\lambda_2 \cdot t} \tag{10.303}$$

where C_p is the plasma concentration measurement for a plasma sample collected at time t. If the measured plasma concentrations follow the relationship in Equation (10.287), then the first residual values should follow the relationship

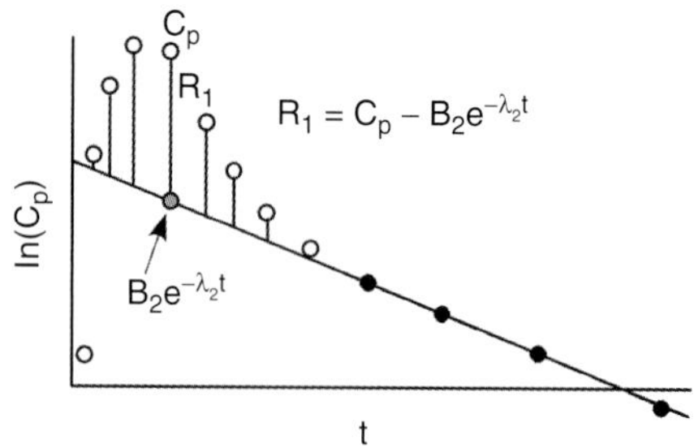

Figure 10.86 Calculation of first residuals (R_1) from plasma concentration (C_p) data and fitted terminal elimination line parameters.

$$\begin{aligned} R_1 &= (B_1 \cdot e^{-\lambda_1 \cdot t} + B_2 \cdot e^{-\lambda_2 \cdot t} + B_3 \cdot e^{-k_a \cdot t}) - B_2 \cdot e^{-\lambda_2 \cdot t} \\ &= B_1 \cdot e^{-\lambda_1 \cdot t} + B_3 \cdot e^{-k_a \cdot t} \end{aligned} \tag{10.304}$$

Since $k_a > \lambda_1$, at long time (generally $t > 7 \cdot t_{½,abs}$), this equation can be simplified to

$$R_1 \approx B_1 \cdot e^{-\lambda_1 \cdot t} \quad \text{for large } t \tag{10.305}$$

Taking the natural logarithm of the left and right terms gives the log-linear form

$$\ln(R_1) = \ln(B_1) - \lambda_2 \cdot t \quad \text{for large } t \tag{10.306}$$

Thus a plot of $\ln(R_1)$ versus t should give a series of later points falling on a new terminal line, as in Figure 10.87. A linear regression analysis is then performed on the first residual values falling on this new terminal line, with time (t) entered as the independent (x) data values, and $\ln(R_1)$ entered as the dependent (y) data values. The fitted slope (m_{R1}) represents the best value for $-\lambda_1$, so that

$$\lambda_1 = -m_{R1} \tag{10.307}$$

The fitted intercept (b_{R1}) represents $\ln(B_1)$, from which B_1 can be calculated as

$$B_1 = e^{b_{R1}} \tag{10.308}$$

The value of the distribution half-life ($t_{½,dist}$) can then be calculated from Equation (10.296).

Determination of the absorption parameters then requires a second stage of method of residuals analysis.

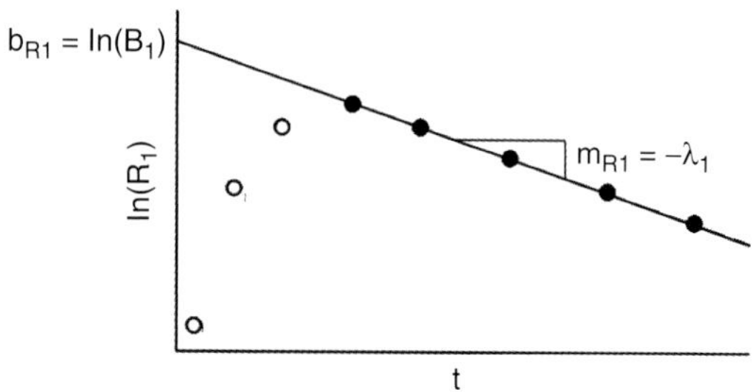

Figure 10.87 Linear regression analysis of the calculated first residuals falling on a new terminal distribution line to determine the distribution phase model parameters.

The second residual (R_2) values are calculated from the first residual (R_1) values that were not used in the first residual terminal line regression. Second residuals are calculated by the equation

$$R_2 = B_1 \cdot e^{-\lambda_1 \cdot t} - R_1 \quad (10.309)$$

which is represented graphically in Figure 10.88. If the first residuals are represented by Equation (10.303), then the second residuals are theoretically given by the equation

$$R_2 = B_1 \cdot e^{-\lambda_1 \cdot t} - (B_1 \cdot e^{-\lambda_1 \cdot t} + B_3 \cdot e^{-k_a \cdot t}) = -B_3 \cdot e^{-k_a \cdot t} \quad (10.310)$$

Taking the natural logarithm of this equation provides the log-linear form

$$\ln(R_2) = \ln(-B_3) - k_a \cdot t \quad (10.311)$$

Thus a plot of $\ln(R_2)$ versus t should give a series of points falling on a straight line, as in Figure 10.89. A linear regression analysis is then performed on the second residual values, with time (t) entered as the independent (x) data values, and $\ln(R_2)$ entered as the dependent (y) data values. The fitted slope (m_{R2}) represents the best value for $-k_a$, so that

$$k_a = -m_{R2} \quad (10.312)$$

The fitted intercept (b_{R1}) represents $\ln(-B_3)$, from which B_3 can be calculated as

$$B_3 = -e^{b_{R2}} \quad (10.313)$$

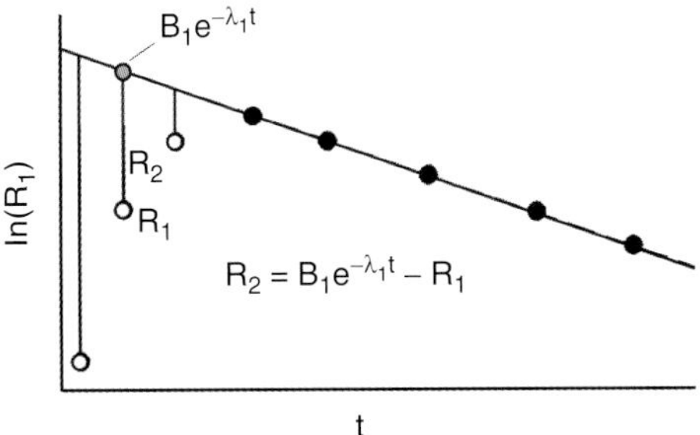

Figure 10.88 Calculation of second residuals (R_2) from the first residual values (R_1) and the fitted distribution phase parameters.

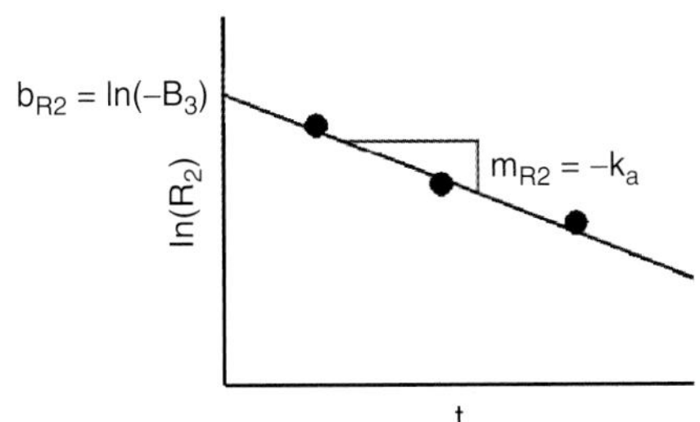

Figure 10.89 Linear regression analysis of the calculated second residuals to determine the absorption phase model parameters.

The value of the absorption half-life ($t_{½,abs}$) can then be calculated from Equation (10.298).

The remaining model parameters still to be determined include the overall clearance (CL) and the two-compartment distribution volumes (V_1, V_{ss}, V_{AUC}). As in the one-compartment first-order absorption model, these remaining model parameters cannot be calculated until the bioavailability (F) has been evaluated. This will require AUC calculations and a comparison to IV drug delivery results, as described in the next two sections.

10.12.4.3 Area under the Curve (AUC) Calculations

First-order absorption processes require AUC values in order to fully evaluate all model parameters. The AUC for the two-compartment first-order absorption model can be calculated using the method of residuals parameters by the simple equation

$$AUC = \frac{B_1}{\lambda_1} + \frac{B_2}{\lambda_2} + \frac{B_3}{k_a} \quad (10.314)$$

The AUC can alternatively be estimated by applying the trapezoidal rule to sequential pairs of measured plasma concentration values. Calculation of the slice of AUC between time zero and the first plasma measurement, $AUC(0 \rightarrow t_1)$, is the same as the zero-order absorption case since the initial concentration (C_0) of both is zero, giving

$$AUC(0 \rightarrow t_1) \approx \frac{1}{2}\left(C_1 \cdot t_1\right) \quad (10.315)$$

where C_1 is the plasma concentration measured at t_1. The AUC of each of the successive measurement time from t_1 up to t_f can then be estimated by applying the trapezoidal rule to each successive set of plasma concentration measurements. The general equation for these successive calculations for two successive plasma concentration measurements C_n and C_{n+1} made at t_n and t_{n+1} is the same as for each previous case

$$AUC(t_n \rightarrow t_{n+1}) \approx \frac{1}{2}\left[C_n + C_{n+1}\right] \cdot \left(t_{n+1} - t_n\right) \quad (10.316)$$

Finally, the area under the curve for the final segment from t_f to an infinite time becomes

$$AUC(t_f \rightarrow \infty) = AUC(tail) = \frac{C_f}{k} \quad (10.317)$$

Adding the AUC contribution from each successive time interval then yields an estimate for the total AUC. The value of AUC can be related to the overall clearance (CL) or to volume of distribution and rate constants by the general relationship

$$AUC = \frac{FD}{CL} = \frac{FD}{V_1 \cdot k_{10}} = \frac{FD}{V_{AUC} \cdot \lambda_2} \quad (10.318)$$

CL, V_1, and V_{AUC} cannot be evaluated by this relationship unless the bioavailability (F) is known.

10.12.4.4 *Bioavailability Calculations*

Evaluation of the bioavailability for a drug following two-compartment kinetics is identical to the methods employed for the one-compartment first-order absorption model. The ratio of bioavailability values (F_1/F_2) for a drug delivered by two different routes is called the relative bioavailability. The relative bioavailability can be determined from the dose (D_1 and D_2) and AUC values (AUC_1 and AUC_2) of each route by the relationship

$$\frac{F_1}{F_2} = \frac{AUC_1 \cdot D_2}{AUC_2 \cdot D_1} \tag{10.319}$$

This relationship is useful when comparing the relative bioavailability of different formulations of the same drug (e.g., original versus generic forms) or when comparing two extravascular routes for the same drug (e.g., oral versus intramuscular). If one route is extravascular (oral, subcutaneous, intramuscular, etc.) and the second is IV, then the IV bioavailability (F_{iv}) is known to be 100% and the extravascular bioavailability (F_{ev}) can be determined directly as

$$F_{ev} = \frac{AUC_{ev} \cdot D_{iv}}{AUC_{iv} \cdot D_{ev}} \tag{10.320}$$

Thus comparison to IV measurements provides the absolute bioavailability. Once the bioavailability is determined, the distribution volumes and clearance (CL) can be calculated by

$$V_1 = \frac{FD}{k_{10} \cdot AUC} \tag{10.321}$$

$$V_{ss} = V_1 \cdot \left(\frac{k_{21} + k_{12}}{k_{21}}\right) \tag{10.322}$$

$$V_{AUC} = \frac{FD}{\lambda_2 \cdot AUC} \tag{10.323}$$

$$CL = \frac{FD}{AUC} = V_1 \cdot k_{10} = V_{AUC} \cdot \lambda_2 \tag{10.324}$$

Thus combining plasma concentration measurements from first-order absorption drug delivery and intravenous drug delivery allows the determination of all PK model parameters.

10.12.5 Special Cases of the Two-Compartment First-Order Absorption Model

Two special cases are considered for the two-compartment first-order absorption model. First is the use of the one-compartment first-order absorption model to approximate plasma drug concentrations that follow two-compartment kinetics. The second case is when first-order drug delivery with rapid absorption can be modeled as an instantaneous absorption process.

10.12.5.1 *First-Order Drug Absorption with Rapid Absorption*

It was previously demonstrated in Section 10.9.5.3 that first-order drug absorption can be reasonably approximated by an instantaneous absorption model as long as the absorption process is completed in a short period of time relative to elimination. This holds true for both one- and two-compartment kinetics. Thus the two-compartment instantaneous absorption model provides a reasonable approximation when $k_a \geq 7 \cdot k$, which can be expressed equivalently as $7 \cdot t_{½,abs} \leq t_{½,elim}$. These criteria can be employed as a general rule of thumb, although the acceptable amount of difference between the models will depend on the required level of accuracy for a given application. When this approximation is used, the intravenous dose (D_{iv}) should be replaced by the total absorbed dose (FD) in the two-compartment bolus IV model equations.

10.12.5.2 *Approximation of Two-Compartment Drug by One-Compartment Model*

The two-compartment first-order absorption model is significantly harder to work with than the one-compartment first-order absorption model. Thus the one-compartment model often is used when it provides a reasonable approximation to the two-compartment values. In fact, the one-compartment model is often used even when a drug is known to significantly deviate from single compartment kinetics. Just as in the case of the two-compartment bolus IV injection model in Section 10.10.5.3, as a general rule of thumb the one-compartment model can be employed with reasonable accuracy for $B_1 \leq 2 \cdot B_2$. When this simplification is used, the one-compartment first-order absorption model equations can be used without modification.

10.13 GENERALIZED MULTICOMPARTMENT MODELS

One- and two-compartment PK models are adequate for the approximation of plasma concentrations for most drugs in most situations. There are some drugs or modeling situations, however, where more than two compartments are needed. It turns out that PK modeling equations follow particular patterns for a given type of drug delivery (instantaneous, zero-order, or first-order absorption). This allows the use of generalized modeling equations, which can be employed for any number of compartments. All generalized equations are written for a PK model containing n total compartments, where $n \geq 1$. When n is 1 or 2, the generalized equations give the same relationships as described previously for one- or two-compartment models, which does not provide any new information. The usefulness of the generalized equations is that they can be employed with three, five, or any other number of model compartments as needed for a particular drug modeling situation.

As with two-compartment models, the central compartment (compartment 1) always contains the systemic circulation. All other compartments (2, 3, . . . , n) are composed of different tissues and hence are all tissue compartments. Since distribution to and from any tissue always occurs by convective blood transport, all distribution processes are modeled as transport between the central compartment (containing the systemic circulation) and a tissue compartment. Standard multicompartment models do not include direct transport between tissue compartments.

10.13.1 Model Assumptions

As with previous PK models, deriving the multicompartment model equations requires several inherent assumptions. The multicompartment model equations described here require five inherent assumptions about the ADME processes during and after drug delivery. The specific nature and implications of each of these assumptions are described in this section.

10.13.1.1 Instantaneous, Zero-Order, or First-Order Absorption

Multicompartment model equations can be written for instantaneous absorption, zero-order absorption, or first-order absorption. For any of these particular absorption situations, the assumptions described previously for the corresponding absorption in one- and two-compartment models remains exactly the same for multicompartment models.

10.13.1.2 Instantaneous Distribution throughout the Central Compartment

This assumption is the same for all compartmental models with more than one compartment. See Section 10.10.1.2 for the details regarding this assumption.

10.13.1.3 Approach to Equilibrium is Similar throughout Each Tissue Compartment

The tissue compartments (compartment 2, 3, . . . , n) contain tissues that take a significant period of time to reach equilibrium with the systemic circulation. Although the tissues in these compartments do not reach equilibrium with the systemic circulation quickly, it is inherently assumed that all tissues within a given compartment approach equilibrium after a similar period of time. This doesn't mean that they all must approach equilibrium in an identical manner, merely that the approach to equilibrium is similar for all the tissues in a compartment.

10.13.1.4 First-Order Distribution Kinetics between Compartment 1 and Tissue Compartments

The rate of drug distribution transport between the central compartment (containing the systemic circulation) and any tissue compartment is taken to follow first-order or linear kinetics. This means that the rate of drug transport from compartment 1 to any other compartment is proportional to the amount of drug in compartment 1. Similarly, the rate of drug transport from any tissue compartment to compartment 1 is proportional to the amount of drug in that tissue compartment. This assumption is generally reasonable as long as active transport molecules are not involved in the distribution process. If active transport is involved, then the assumption is still reasonable as long as the drug concentration is lower than the transporter Michaelis-Menten K_t constant in the vicinity of the transporter molecules. Note that standard multicompartment models assume there is no distribution transport between any two tissue compartments.

10.13.1.5 First-Order (Linear) Elimination Kinetics

This assumption is essentially the same for all PK models described in this chapter. See Section 10.7.1.3 for the details regarding this assumption. Unlike the standard one- and two-compartment models, where the equations are written for elimination only from the central compartment (compartment 1), elimination can occur from any one or any combination of model compartments for the generalized multicompartment equations.

10.13.2 Mass Balance Equations

A separate mass balance equation is written in the form of Section 10.6.2 for each compartment in the model. Thus a total of n mass balance equations must be written and solved for an n compartment model. The details of these equations and their solution are not provided in this chapter. However, it will be noted that absorption, distribution, and elimination rates are written in the same form as in the previous one- and two-compartment models. The absorption rate for instantaneous, zero-order, or first-order absorption is identical to the previous forms for one- and two-compartment models. Distribution and elimination rates are written as first-order linear rate equations using micro rate constants. So the distribution rate from compartment 1 to compartment n is given by $k_{1n} \cdot A_1$, the distribution rate from compartment n back to compartment 1 equals $k_{n1} \cdot A_n$, and the elimination rate from any compartment is written $k_{n0} \cdot A_n$. A schematic diagram for the generalized n compartment model is illustrated in Figure 10.90.

10.13.3 Plasma Concentration versus Time Relationships

As with previous two-compartment models, the plasma concentration of drug (C_p) is given by dividing the amount of drug in compartment 1 (A_1) by distribution volume of compartment 1 (V_1). The generalized plasma concentration versus time equations are summarized in Table 10.2 for each type of drug absorption. Application of the generalized equations to one-, two-, and three-compartment models is provided to demonstrate the universality of these equations. For

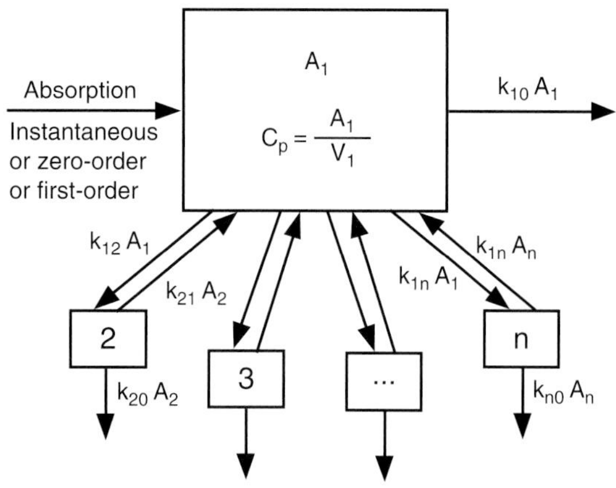

Figure 10.90 Generalized diagram for a PK model with n compartments.

a model with n compartments, the plasma concentration equation can be written as the sum of n exponential decay terms for instantaneous absorption or for the postexposure period following zero-order absorption, or alternatively as the sum of $n+1$ exponential decay terms for first-order absorption. The extra exponential decay term for first-order absorption represents the absorption phase. The coefficient (B_{n+1}) of this extra exponential decay term for first-order absorption is always negative, and all other coefficients are always positive.

10.13.3.1 Absorption, Distribution, and Elimination Phases

Each of the exponential decay terms in the generalized multicompartment models represent a distinct phase or change in shape of the plasma concentration versus time curve. The extra ($n+1$) exponential term for first-order absorption always has the absorption rate constant (k_a) in the exponent, and always represents an absorption phase. The exponential term with the smallest rate constant (λ_n) always represents the elimination phase, and this rate constant always represents the elimination rate constant and always equals the terminal line slope ($m = -\lambda_n$). All other exponential terms represent distinct distribution phases caused by the different rates of distribution to different tissue compartments.

10.13.3.2 Absorption, Distribution, and Elimination Half-Lives

As described in the previous section, each exponential term represents a distinct phase in the plasma concentration versus time curve. The term with the smallest rate constant (λ_n) represents the elimination phase, and hence

$$t_{1/2,elim} = \frac{\ln(2)}{\lambda_n} \approx \frac{0.693}{\lambda_n} \tag{10.325}$$

$$\lambda_n = \frac{\ln(2)}{t_{1/2,elim}} \approx \frac{0.693}{t_{1/2,elim}} \tag{10.326}$$

The extra exponential term in the first-order absorption equation represents the absorption phase, and hence the absorption half-life can be defined as

$$t_{1/2,abs} = \frac{\ln(2)}{k_a} \approx \frac{0.693}{k_a} \tag{10.327}$$

$$k_a = \frac{\ln(2)}{t_{1/2,abs}} \approx \frac{0.693}{t_{1/2,abs}} \tag{10.328}$$

All other exponential terms represent distribution phases, with the $n-1$ distribution half-lives given by

$$t_{1/2,dist,m} = \frac{\ln(2)}{\lambda_m} \approx \frac{0.693}{\lambda_m} \quad \text{where} \quad 1 \le m \le n-1 \tag{10.329}$$

$$\lambda_m = \frac{\ln(2)}{t_{1/2,dist,m}} \approx \frac{0.693}{t_{1/2,dist,m}} \quad \text{where} \quad 1 \le m \le n-1 \tag{10.330}$$

Given that $k_a > \lambda_1 > \lambda_2 > \ldots > \lambda_n$, it can readily be established that $t_{1/2,abs} < t_{1/2,dist,m} < t_{1/2,elim}$.

10.13.3.3 Estimating Plasma Drug Concentrations

It is not unusual for PK research articles to report model parameters for three-, four-, or five-compartment models for some drugs. If the multicompartment model parameters are known for a drug, then the plasma concentration at any time can be predicted by the equations in Table 10.2. Determining the time at which the plasma concentration reaches a particular value is generally a very laborious trial-and-error calculation, since the concentration equation contains multiple exponential decay terms. An exception occurs for plasma concentration (C_p) values at long enough times to be located on the terminal line. For this special case, the time at which a particular plasma concentration is reached is given by

$$t = \frac{-\ln\left(\frac{C_p}{B_2}\right)}{\lambda_n} \quad \text{for large } t \tag{10.331}$$

As a general rule of thumb, this equation can be used to estimate t as long as $t > 7 \cdot t_{1/2,dist,n-1}$.

10.13.4 Estimating Model Parameters from Measured Plasma Concentration Data

Estimation of multicompartment model parameters from measured plasma samples is typically performed utilizing specialized PK software. The general methods are very similar to that used for the previous models,

Table 10.2 Plasma Concentration (C_p) versus Time Relationships for Different Numbers of Model Compartments and Types of Absorption

Compartments	Instantaneous Absorption (e.g., Bolus IV Injection)	Zero-Order Absorption (e.g., IV Infusion)	First-Order Absorption (e.g., Oral Ingestion)
1	$C_p = B_1 e^{-\lambda_1 t}$ $B_1 = C_0 = \frac{FD}{V}$ $\lambda_1 = k$	$C_{p,0 \le t \le T} = B_1 \left(\frac{1 - e^{-\lambda_1 t}}{1 - e^{-\lambda_1 T}}\right)$ $C_{p,t > T} = B_1 e^{-\lambda_1 (t-T)}$ $B_1 = C_T = \frac{Fk_0}{V}(1 - e^{-\lambda_1 T})$ $\lambda_1 = k$	$C_p = B_1 e^{-\lambda_1 t} + B_2 e^{-k_a t}$ $B_2 = -(B_1) = -\frac{FD}{V}\left(\frac{k_a}{k_a - \lambda_1}\right)$ $B_2 = -(B_1)$ $k_a > \lambda_1$, $\lambda_1 = k$
2	$C_p = B_1 e^{-\lambda_1 t} + B_2 e^{-\lambda_2 t}$ $B_1 + B_2 = C_0$ $\lambda_1 > \lambda_2$	$C_{p,0 \le t \le T} = B_1 \left(\frac{1 - e^{-\lambda_1 t}}{1 - e^{-\lambda_1 T}}\right) + B_2 \left(\frac{1 - e^{-\lambda_2 t}}{1 - e^{-\lambda_2 T}}\right)$ $C_{p,t > T} = B_1 e^{-\lambda_1 (t-T)} + B_2 e^{-\lambda_2 (t-T)}$ $B_1 + B_2 = C_T$ $\lambda_1 > \lambda_2$	$C_p = B_1 e^{-\lambda_1 t} + B_2 e^{-\lambda_2 t} + B_3 e^{-k_a t}$ $B_3 = -(B_1 + B_2)$ $k_a > \lambda_1 > \lambda_2$
3	$C_p = B_1 e^{-\lambda_1 t} + B_2 e^{-\lambda_2 t} + B_3 e^{-\lambda_3 t}$ $B_1 + B_2 + B_3 = C_0$ $\lambda_1 > \lambda_2 > \lambda_3$	$C_{p,0 \le t \le T} = B_1 \left(\frac{1 - e^{-\lambda_1 t}}{1 - e^{-\lambda_1 T}}\right) + B_2 \left(\frac{1 - e^{-\lambda_2 t}}{1 - e^{-\lambda_2 T}}\right) + B_3 \left(\frac{1 - e^{-\lambda_3 t}}{1 - e^{-\lambda_3 T}}\right)$ $C_{p,t > T} = B_1 e^{-\lambda_1 (t-T)} + B_2 e^{-\lambda_2 (t-T)} + B_3 e^{-\lambda_3 (t-T)}$ $B_1 + B_2 + B_3 = C_T$ $\lambda_1 > \lambda_2 > \lambda_3$	$C_p = B_1 e^{-\lambda_1 t} + B_2 e^{-\lambda_2 t} + B_3 e^{-\lambda_3 t} + B_4 e^{-k_a t}$ $k_a > \lambda_1 > \lambda_2 > \lambda_3$ $B_4 = -(B_1 + B_2 + B_3)$
n	$C_p = B_1 e^{-\lambda_1 t} + B_2 e^{-\lambda_2 t} + \ldots + B_n e^{-\lambda_n t}$ $B_1 + B_2 + \ldots + B_n = C_0$ $\lambda_1 > \lambda_2 > \ldots > \lambda_n$	$C_{p,0 \le t \le T} = B_1 \left(\frac{1 - e^{-\lambda_1 t}}{1 - e^{-\lambda_1 T}}\right) + B_2 \left(\frac{1 - e^{-\lambda_2 t}}{1 - e^{-\lambda_2 T}}\right) + \ldots + B_n \left(\frac{1 - e^{-\lambda_n t}}{1 - e^{-\lambda_n T}}\right)$ $C_{p,t > T} = B_1 e^{-\lambda_1 (t-T)} + B_2 e^{-\lambda_2 (t-T)} + \ldots + B_n e^{-\lambda_n (t-T)}$ $B_1 + B_2 + \ldots + B_n = C_T$ $\lambda_1 > \lambda_2 > \ldots > \lambda_n$	$C_p = B_1 e^{-\lambda_1 t} + B_2 e^{-\lambda_2 t} + \ldots + B_n e^{-\lambda_n t} + B_{n+1} e^{-k_a t}$ $B_{n+1} = -(B_1 + B_2 + \ldots + B_n)$ $k_a > \lambda_1 > \lambda_2 > \ldots > \lambda_n$

however, and will be described for information purposes. If a multicompartment first-order absorption model is being used, then evaluation of the bioavailability requires comparison of AUC values to those for measured IV plasma concentrations just as with all previous first-order absorption models.

10.13.4.1 Linear Regression of Terminal Line Plasma Concentration Data

Estimation of multicompartment model parameters from measured plasma samples is very similar to the procedures described previously for the two-compartment first-order absorption model. The first step is to calculate $\ln(C_p)$ for each of the measured plasma sample concentrations. The values of $\ln(C_p)$ are then plotted versus time (t), and the points on the terminal line are identified. Linear regression analysis of the terminal line provides values for B_n ($B_n = e^b$) and λ_n ($\lambda_n = -m$). The first residual (R_1) values are then calculated as the difference between the measured plasma concentrations and the terminal line for points not used on the terminal line. A plot of $\ln(R_1)$ versus t is then employed to identify points on the next terminal line, with linear regression analysis of this line used to determine B_{n-1} and λ_{n-1}. Successive method of residuals analyses are then used to calculate the remaining B and λ values, with linear regression of the *n-1* residual (R_{n-1}) values providing the values of B_1 and λ_1. If a first-order absorption model is being used, then one more set of residuals (R_n) are calculated, and the linear regression analysis of these residuals then provides B_{n+1} and k_a. This type of analysis is typically performed by specialized PK software when the model contains more than two compartments.

10.13.4.2 Area under the Curve (AUC) and Bioavailability Calculations

First-order absorption processes require AUC values in order to evaluate the bioavailability (F). The AUC_{ev} for the multicompartment extravascular first-order absorption model can be calculated by the simple equation

$$AUC_{ev} = \frac{B_1}{\lambda_1} + \frac{B_2}{\lambda_2} + \ldots + \frac{B_n}{\lambda_n} + \frac{B_{n+1}}{k_a} \tag{10.332}$$

The AUC_{iv} for bolus IV injection can similarly be calculated by

$$AUC_{iv} = \frac{B_1}{\lambda_1} + \frac{B_2}{\lambda_2} + \ldots + \frac{B_n}{\lambda_n} \tag{10.333}$$

The bioavailability of the extravascular first-order absorption process is then given by

$$F_{ev} = \frac{AUC_{ev} \cdot D_{iv}}{AUC_{iv} \cdot D_{ev}} \tag{10.334}$$

Thus comparison to IV measurements provides the absolute bioavailability.

10.14 MULTIPLE DOSING MODELS

All the models in this chapter up to this point have been for plasma concentrations following a single drug dose. This section considers PK models for plasma concentrations after the administration of multiple doses of drug. These models are based on a principle called *superposition*, which states that the plasma concentration after multiple doses of a drug is equal to the sum of concentrations that would have resulted from each dose being given individually. Thus the single dose models described previously are still used to predict plasma concentrations for a particular drug dose, but the single dose models are applied multiple times or coupled with other single dose models to predict multiple dosing concentrations. Some multiple dosing situations involve drug delivery by two or more different delivery methods, such as an initial bolus IV injection (instantaneous absorption) followed by a prolonged IV infusion (zero-order absorption). However, most of the models considered are written for the repeated delivery of the same drug dose by the same administration route at regular time intervals (e.g., oral ingestion of a drug tablet every 24 hours). If the repeated doses are delivered at close enough intervals, then plasma drug concentrations can build up to levels substantially higher than those achieved with a single drug dose. The amount of drug accumulation that takes place during repeated dosing must be fully understood in order to design proper drug dosing regimens that achieve the desired therapeutic effect while minimizing unwanted side effects.

10.14.1 Model Assumptions

As with all previous PK models, multiple dosing models require a number of inherent assumptions. It turns out that the assumptions required for multiple dosing models are all derived from or identical to the assumptions already made in earlier single-dose models.

10.14.1.1 Single-Dose Model Assumptions

The multiple dosing models described here represent repeated application of previously described single-dose PK models. Thus the inherent assumptions for a multiple dosing model include all the assumptions made for each of the single-dose models that are being employed.

10.14.1.2 Superposition Principle Assumptions

The superposition principle, which forms the basis of all multiple-dose models in this section, is true only as long as all elimination processes follow first-order (linear) elimination kinetics. Since the assumption of first-order elimination kinetics has already been made for all the previous single-dose models that are being combined by superposition, the application of the superposition principle does not add any new model assumptions.

10.14.2 Superposition Principle

The superposition principle states that each drug dose behaves independently of all other drug doses that are administered. Thus for a given drug dose (D_1), the plasma concentrations (C_{D_1}) associated with this dose can be determined by the application of an appropriate single dose PK model to D_1, without consideration of other doses administered before, during, or after the administration of D_1. It also follows that the overall plasma concentration (C_p) after the administration of multiple drug doses (D_1, D_2, $D_3, \ldots$) is given simply by the sum of the plasma concentrations associated with each individual dose (C_{D1}, C_{D2}, $C_{D3}, \ldots$), which can be written

$$C_p = C_{D1} + C_{D2} + C_{D3} + \ldots \tag{10.335}$$

It should be kept in mind that the single dose model equations for a given dose are in terms of the time since that particular dose was administered, which is labeled t'. Thus if doses D_1, D_2, and D_3 are administered at times t_1, t_2, and t_3, respectively, then $t'_1 = t - t_1$, $t'_2 = t - t_2$, and $t'_3 = t - t_3$. This is illustrated in Figure 10.91 for three successive bolus IV injections (top graph) and three successive first-order absorption drug administrations (bottom graph). The drugs in each of these cases are taken to follow one-compartment models, with drug doses D_1, D_2, and D_3 administered at times t_1, t_2, and t_3, respectively. For the bolus IV injections (top graph in Figure 10.91), the plasma concentration versus time relationship is given by

$$C_p = C_{D1} + C_{D2} + C_{D3}$$
$$= \left(\frac{D_1}{V}\right) \cdot e^{-k(t-t_1)} + \left(\frac{D_2}{V}\right) \cdot e^{-k(t-t_2)} + \left(\frac{D_3}{V}\right) \cdot e^{-k(t-t_3)} \tag{10.336}$$

which can then be rewritten in terms of the t' values as

$$C_p = C_{D1} + C_{D2} + C_{D3}$$
$$= \left(\frac{D_1}{V}\right) \cdot e^{-kt'_1} + \left(\frac{D_2}{V}\right) \cdot e^{-kt'_2} + \left(\frac{D_3}{V}\right) \cdot e^{-kt'_3} \tag{10.337}$$

The plasma concentration for the first-order absorption drug deliveries (bottom graph in Figure 10.91) can then be written directly in terms of t' values as

$$C_p = C_{D1} + C_{D2} + C_{D3} = \left(\frac{FD_1}{V}\right) \cdot \left(\frac{k_a}{k_a - k}\right) \cdot [e^{-kt'_1} - e^{-k_a t'_1}]$$
$$+ \left(\frac{FD_2}{V}\right) \cdot \left(\frac{k_a}{k_a - k}\right) \cdot [e^{-kt'_2} - e^{-k_a t'_2}]$$
$$+ \left(\frac{FD_3}{V}\right) \cdot \left(\frac{k_a}{k_a - k}\right) \cdot [e^{-kt'_3} - e^{-k_a t'_3}] \tag{10.338}$$

The principles of superposition can be similarly applied for multiple drug doses administered by two or more different types of drug delivery. Figure 10.92 illustrates two different cases of combined drug delivery by a bolus IV injection and an IV infusion started at the same time as the injection. The top graph in Figure 10.92 represents a general case, where the plasma concentration during the infusion period ($0 \leq t' \leq T$) is given by

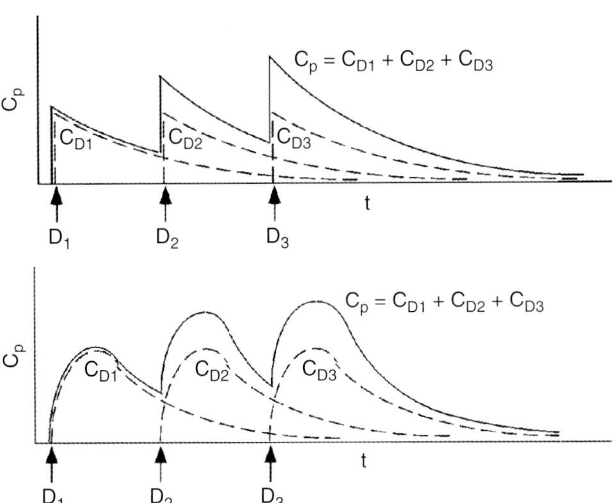

Figure 10.91 Plasma concentrations following three bolus IV injections (top graph) and three first-order absorption drug administrations (bottom graph) are given by the sum of the concentrations associated with each individual dose.

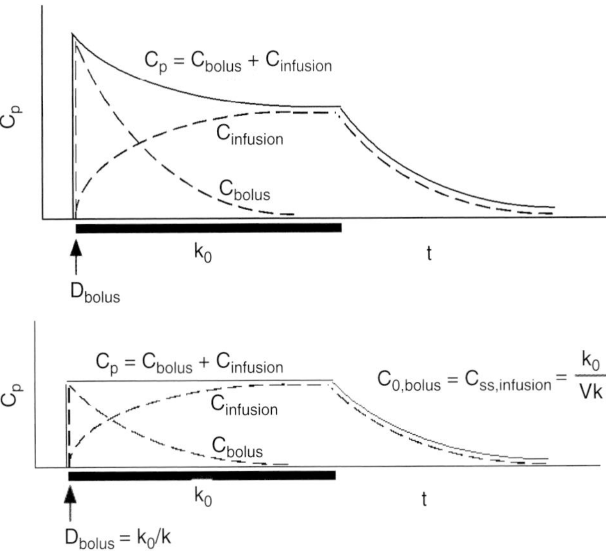

Figure 10.92 Plasma concentrations for drug delivery by both bolus IV injection and IV infusion for a general case (top graph) and for a special case where the bolus IV dose has been designed to be a loading dose for the infusion (bottom graph).

$$C_p = C_{bolus} + C_{infusion}$$
$$= \left(\frac{D_{bolus}}{V}\right) \cdot e^{-kt'} + \left(\frac{k_0}{Vk}\right) \cdot [1 - e^{-kt'}] \quad \text{for } 0 \leq t' \leq T \tag{10.339}$$

Note that t' is the same for both the bolus IV injection and the IV infusion since the reference starting time is the same for both. The bottom graph in Figure 10.92 illustrates the special case where the bolus IV injection dose has been designed specifically so that the initial bolus concentration ($C_{0,bolus}$) is exactly equal to the steady-state infusion concentration ($C_{ss,infusion}$). This is called a loading dose, which is sometimes used to bring plasma concentrations up to therapeutic levels more quickly. The correct loading dose for this situation is given by making D_{bolus} equal to k_0/k. The plasma concentration for this situation during the infusion period is then

$$C_p = C_{bolus} + C_{infusion} = \left(\frac{k_0}{Vk}\right) \cdot e^{-kt'} + \left(\frac{k_0}{Vk}\right) \cdot [1 - e^{-kt'}]$$
$$= \left(\frac{k_0}{Vk}\right) \quad \text{for } 0 \leq t' \leq T \tag{10.340}$$

Thus the plasma concentration for this special bolus loading dose situation is perfectly constant from the start to the finish of the infusion period.

10.14.3 Plasma Concentrations for Repeated Drug Dosing at Regular Time Intervals

A common therapeutic drug treatment approach involves the repeated delivery of a particular drug dose at regular time intervals. Most typical is the oral ingestion of a drug every 6, 8, 12, or 24 hours. Periodic IV infusions are also common for some antibiotic and chemotherapeutic drugs. The PK models described here for repeated drug dosing at regular time intervals assume that the individual doses are all identical, and the time between doses is always the same. The time between doses, or the dosing interval, is represented by the variable τ (pronounced "tau") in these equations. The time since the most recent drug administration (or the start of the most recent administration for first-order absorption) is represented by t'. Repeated drug dosing model equations are provided for instantaneous, zero-order, and first-order absorption for one-compartment models, as well as for instantaneous and first-order absorption with generalized multicompartment models.

10.14.3.1 One-Compartment Instantaneous Absorption

Repeated dosing for one-compartment instantaneous absorption is considered first. Although this model is most applicable to periodic bolus IV injections, it has been shown previously that the instantaneous absorption model provides a reasonable approximation to zero-order and first-order drug absorption processes as long as drug absorption is completed quickly compared to elimination ($T \leq t_{½,elim}$ for zero-order absorption, $7 \cdot t_{½,abs} \leq t_{½,elim}$ for first-order absorption). In order to accommodate these alternative drug delivery options, the instantaneous absorption equations are written here in terms of the absorbed dose (*FD*).

Plasma concentrations for a series of instantaneously absorbed drug doses (*FD*) administered at regular time intervals (τ) are illustrated in the top graph of Figure 10.93. As displayed in this graph, plasma concentrations rise immediately after each drug administration, then fall exponentially until the next dose is administered. During the first several dosing intervals, plasma concentrations rise steadily from one dosing interval to the next. After a longer period of time, however, the rise and fall of the plasma concentration during one dosing interval is essentially identical to the rise and fall during the next interval. This represents the approach to a steady-state condition after a sustained period of drug delivery, similar to the approach to steady-state after a prolonged IV infusion illustrated in the bottom graph of Figure 10.93. For the IV infusion case, steady-state is reached when the rate of drug absorption equals the rate of drug elimination. In an analogous manner, repeated drug dosing reaches steady-state conditions when the amount of drug absorbed during the dosing interval is equal to the amount of drug eliminated during the dosing interval. Repeated dosing approaches steady-state as a function of the elimination half-life ($t_{½,elim}$) in the exact same manner as an IV infusion does, so that in both cases the approach to steady-state is 50% complete at $t = t_{½,elim}$, 75% complete at $t = 2 \cdot t_{½,elim}$, about 99% complete at $t = 7 \cdot t_{½,elim}$, and about 99.9% complete at $t = 10 \cdot t_{½,elim}$. As a general rule of thumb, the plasma

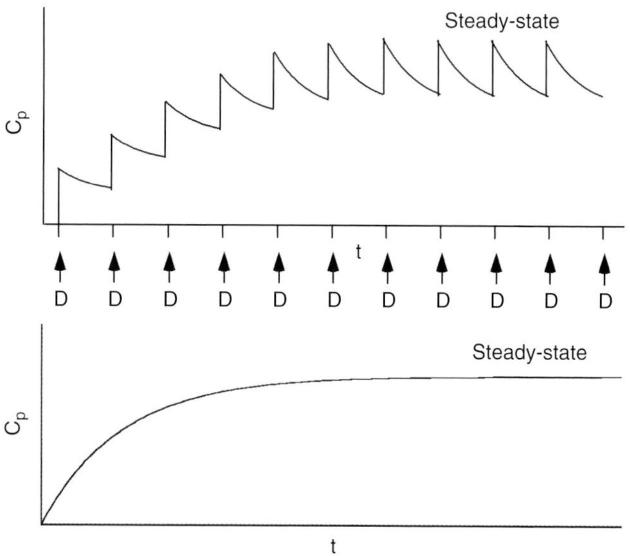

Figure 10.93 Approach to steady-state for repeated drug dosing at regular intervals (top graph) and for an IV infusion (bottom graph).

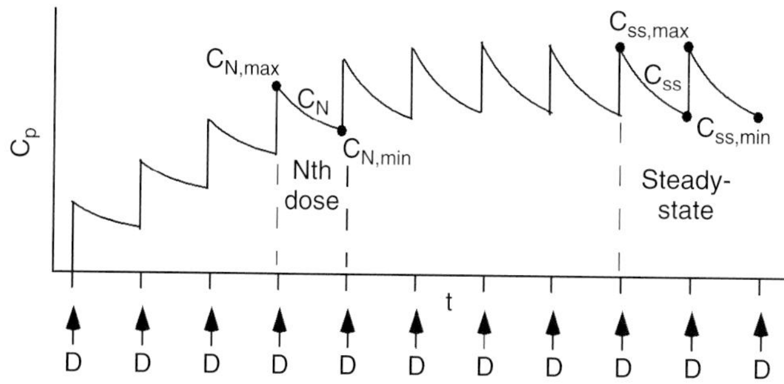

Figure 10.94 Plasma concentrations for repeated instantaneous absorption drug administration at regular time intervals.

concentrations can be taken to be essentially at steady-state for $t > 7 \cdot t_{½,elim}$.

The principle of superposition can be utilized to write equations for the plasma concentration (C_p) versus the time since the most recent dose administration (t') during any dosing interval. These equations can be written for the dosing interval after the Nth dose or alternatively for steady-state conditions, as illustrated in Figure 10.94. The plasma concentration versus t' over the entire interval for the Nth dose or at steady-state are given by

$$C_N = \frac{FD}{V}\left[\frac{1-e^{-Nk\tau}}{1-e^{-k\tau}}\right] \cdot e^{-kt'} \quad \text{for } 0 \le t' \le \tau \qquad (10.341)$$

$$C_{ss} = \frac{FD}{V}\left[\frac{1}{1-e^{-k\tau}}\right] \cdot e^{-kt'} \quad \text{for } 0 \le t' \le \tau \qquad (10.342)$$

The maximum concentration during any interval occurs when $t' = 0$, giving

$$C_{N,max} = \frac{FD}{V}\left[\frac{1-e^{-Nk\tau}}{1-e^{-k\tau}}\right] \qquad (10.343)$$

$$C_{ss,max} = \frac{FD}{V}\left[\frac{1}{1-e^{-k\tau}}\right] \qquad (10.344)$$

and the minimum concentration during any interval occurs at $t' = \tau$:

$$C_{N,min} = \frac{FD}{V}\left[\frac{1-e^{-Nk\tau}}{1-e^{-k\tau}}\right] \cdot e^{-k\tau} \qquad (10.345)$$

$$C_{ss,min} = \frac{FD}{V}\left[\frac{1}{1-e^{-k\tau}}\right] \cdot e^{-k\tau} \qquad (10.346)$$

The difference between the maximum and minimum steady-state concentrations is

$$C_{ss,max} - C_{ss,min} = \frac{FD}{V} \qquad (10.347)$$

The average plasma concentration at steady-state is given by

$$C_{ss,ave} = \frac{FD}{Vk\tau} = \frac{FD}{CL\tau} \qquad (10.348)$$

The equation for $C_{ss,ave}$ ends up being the same no matter what type of drug absorption or what type of single-dose model are being used. Finally, consider the cases illustrated in Figure 10.95, where dosing stops after the Nth dose (top graph) or after steady-state conditions have been reached (bottom graph). The plasma concentration after the final dose becomes

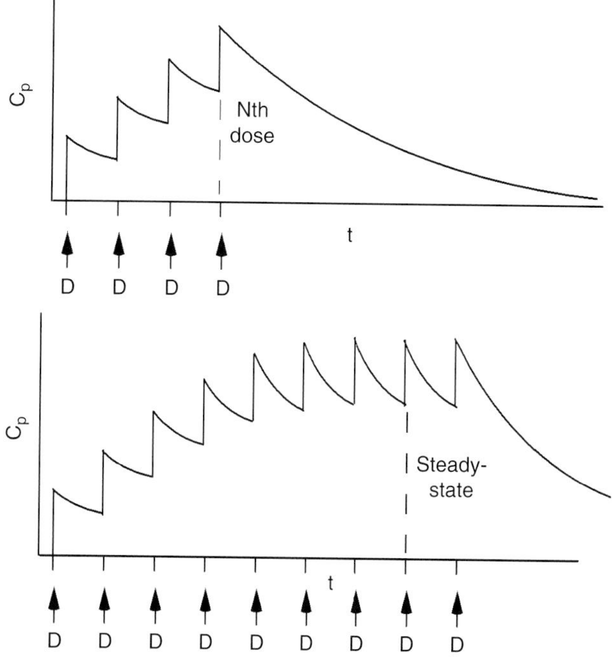

Figure 10.95 Plasma concentrations after dosing is stopped following the Nth dose (top) or after steady-state conditions have been reached (bottom).

$$C_{N,stop} = \frac{FD}{V}\left[\frac{1-e^{-Nk\tau}}{1-e^{-k\tau}}\right] \cdot e^{-kt'} \quad \text{for } t' \ge 0 \qquad (10.349)$$

$$C_{ss,stop} = \frac{FD}{V}\left[\frac{1}{1-e^{-k\tau}}\right] \cdot e^{-kt'} \quad \text{for } t' \ge 0 \qquad (10.350)$$

Note that the equations for plasma concentrations after dosing is stopped are identical to the equations for concentrations during the Nth interval or at steady-state conditions as given earlier in Equations (10.341) and (10.342). Thus as a general rule, plasma concentrations continue to follow the equations for the final dosing interval for all times ($t' \ge 0$) after last dose.

The term in square brackets in Equation (10.350) is called the accumulation factor. This factor accounts for the amount of drug remaining, or accumulated, from previous doses. The value of the accumulation factor depends on the relative size of the dosing interval (τ) and elimination half-life ($t_{½,elim}$). Values of the accumulation factor for different relative values of τ versus $t_{½,elim}$ are provided in Table 10.3. This table demonstrates that for $\tau < 2 \cdot t_{½,elim}$, there is a substantial amount of drug accumulation, resulting in concentrations climbing significantly higher than achieved for a single dose of the drug. Conversely, for $\tau > 4 \cdot t_{½,elim}$ there is little drug accumulation and hence drug concentrations are similar to those for a single drug dose. Additional accumulation factors appear in later

Table 10.3 Values of the Accumulation Factor for Different Relative Sizes of τ versus $t_{1/2,elim}$

Relative Size of τ versus $t_{1/2,elim}$	Accumulation Factor $\left[\frac{1}{1-e^{-k\tau}}\right]$
$\tau = t_{1/2,elim}/7$	10.6
$\tau = t_{1/2,elim}/4$	6.29
$\tau = t_{1/2,elim}/2$	3.41
$\tau = t_{1/2,elim}$	2.00
$\tau = 2 \cdot t_{1/2,elim}$	1.33
$\tau = 3 \cdot t_{1/2,elim}$	1.14
$\tau = 7 \cdot t_{1/2,elim}$	1.01

models, as there is generally an accumulation factor associated with each exponential decay term in the plasma concentration equations.

10.14.3.2 One-Compartment Zero-Order Absorption

Repeated zero-order absorption dosing is common for some antibiotic and chemotherapeutic drugs. Like the instantaneous absorption case, repeated zero-order absorption dosing also yields an approach to steady-state conditions after a sufficient duration of regular dosing intervals, as illustrated in Figure 10.96. Concentrations during each dosing interval rise during the infusion period, then drop back down each time infusion stops. Equations for the plasma concentrations versus t' (time since the start of the most recent infusion) during the infusion period ($0 \le t' \le T$) of the Nth interval or at steady-state become

$$C_N = \frac{k_0}{Vk}(1-e^{-kT}) \cdot \left[\frac{1-e^{-(N-1)k\tau}}{1-e^{-k\tau}}\right] \cdot e^{-k(\tau-T)}e^{-kt'} + \frac{k_0}{Vk}(1-e^{-kt'}) \quad \text{for } 0 \le t' \le T \qquad (10.351)$$

$$C_{ss} = \frac{k_0}{Vk}(1-e^{-kT}) \cdot \left[\frac{1}{1-e^{-k\tau}}\right] \cdot e^{-k(\tau-T)}e^{-kt'} + \frac{k_0}{Vk}(1-e^{-kt'}) \quad \text{for } 0 \le t' \le T \qquad (10.352)$$

Postinfusion ($T \le t' \le \tau$) plasma concentrations during the Nth interval or at steady-state become

$$C_N = \frac{k_0}{Vk}(1-e^{-kT}) \cdot \left[\frac{1-e^{-Nk\tau}}{1-e^{-k\tau}}\right] \cdot e^{-k(t'-T)} \quad \text{for } T \le t' \le \tau \qquad (10.353)$$

$$C_{ss} = \frac{k_0}{Vk}(1-e^{-kT}) \cdot \left[\frac{1}{1-e^{-k\tau}}\right] \cdot e^{-k(t'-T)} \quad \text{for } T \le t' \le \tau \qquad (10.354)$$

The maximum plasma concentration during each interval occurs when $t' = T$:

$$C_{N,max} = \frac{k_0}{Vk}\left(1-e^{-kT}\right) \cdot \left[\frac{1-e^{-Nk\tau}}{1-e^{-k\tau}}\right] \qquad (10.355)$$

$$C_{ss,max} = \frac{k_0}{Vk}\left(1-e^{-kT}\right) \cdot \left[\frac{1}{1-e^{-k\tau}}\right] \qquad (10.356)$$

The minimum plasma concentration during each interval occurs when $t' = 0$:

$$C_{N,min} = \frac{k_0}{Vk}\left(1-e^{-kT}\right) \cdot \left[\frac{1-e^{-(N-1)k\tau}}{1-e^{-k\tau}}\right] \cdot e^{-k(\tau-T)} \qquad (10.357)$$

$$C_{ss,min} = \frac{k_0}{Vk}\left(1-e^{-kT}\right) \cdot \left[\frac{1}{1-e^{-k\tau}}\right] \cdot e^{-k(\tau-T)} \qquad (10.358)$$

The average steady-state concentration is the same no matter what type of absorption occurs:

$$C_{ss,ave} = \frac{FD}{Vk\tau} = \frac{FD}{CL\tau} = \frac{k_0 T}{Vk\tau} = \frac{k_0 T}{CL\tau} \qquad (10.359)$$

If dosing stops after the Nth dose or after reaching steady-state, the plasma concentration equation for the postinfusion period of the final dosing interval applies for all later times ($t' \ge T$).

10.14.3.3 One-Compartment First-Order Absorption

Repeated first-order absorption dosing, particularly by oral ingestion, is the most common type of drug therapy dosing. As in previous repeated dosing models, plasma concentrations approach steady-state conditions after a sufficient duration of time, as illustrated

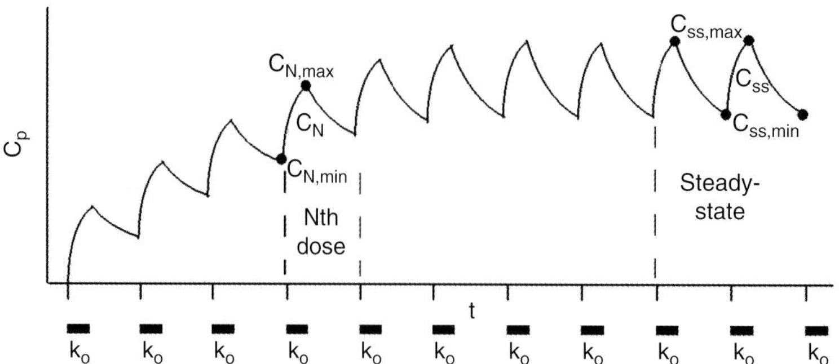

Figure 10.96 Approach to steady-state for repeated IV infusion drug dosing at regular intervals.

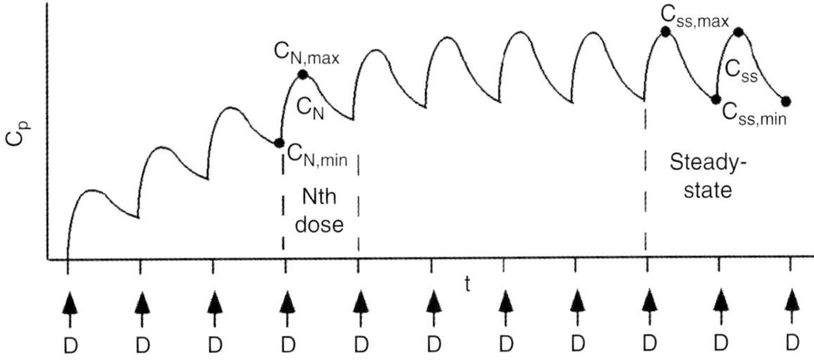

Figure 10.97 Approach to steady-state for repeated first-order absorption drug dosing at regular intervals.

in Figure 10.97. Concentrations during each dosing interval initially rise, then drop back down after the maximum concentration is reached. Equations for the plasma concentrations versus t' (time since the most recent dose administration) during the Nth interval or at steady-state become

$$C_N = \frac{FD}{V}\left(\frac{k_a}{k_a - k}\right)\left[\left(\frac{1-e^{-Nk\tau}}{1-e^{-k\tau}}\right)\cdot e^{-kt'} - \left(\frac{1-e^{-Nk_a\tau}}{1-e^{-k_a\tau}}\right)\cdot e^{-k_a t'}\right]$$

for $0 \leq t' \leq \tau$

(10.360)

$$C_{ss} = \frac{FD}{V}\left(\frac{k_a}{k_a - k}\right)\left[\left(\frac{1}{1-e^{-k\tau}}\right)\cdot e^{-kt'} - \left(\frac{1}{1-e^{-k_a\tau}}\right)\cdot e^{-k_a t'}\right]$$

for $0 \leq t' \leq \tau$

(10.361)

The maximum plasma concentration during each interval occurs when $t' = t'_{max}$:

$$t'_{max} = \frac{\ln\left[\frac{k_a}{k}\cdot\left(\frac{1-e^{-k\tau}}{1-e^{-k_a\tau}}\right)\right]}{k_a - k} \tag{10.362}$$

$$C_{N,max} = \frac{FD}{V}\left(\frac{k_a}{k_a - k}\right)\left[\left(\frac{1-e^{-Nk\tau}}{1-e^{-k\tau}}\right)\cdot e^{-kt'_{max}} - \left(\frac{1-e^{-Nk_a\tau}}{1-e^{-k_a\tau}}\right)\cdot e^{-k_a t'_{max}}\right] \tag{10.363}$$

$$C_{ss,max} = \frac{FD}{V}\left(\frac{k_a}{k_a - k}\right)\left[\left(\frac{1}{1-e^{-k\tau}}\right)\cdot e^{-kt'_{max}} - \left(\frac{1}{1-e^{-k_a\tau}}\right)\cdot e^{-k_a t'_{max}}\right] \tag{10.364}$$

The minimum plasma concentration during each interval occurs when $t' = 0$, giving

$$C_{N,min} = \frac{FD}{V}\left(\frac{k_a}{k_a - k}\right)\left[\left(\frac{1-e^{-Nk\tau}}{1-e^{-k\tau}}\right) - \left(\frac{1-e^{-Nk_a\tau}}{1-e^{-k_a\tau}}\right)\right] \tag{10.365}$$

$$C_{ss,min} = \frac{FD}{V}\left(\frac{k_a}{k_a - k}\right)\left[\left(\frac{1}{1-e^{-k\tau}}\right) - \left(\frac{1}{1-e^{-k_a\tau}}\right)\right] \tag{10.366}$$

The average concentration at steady-state is the same no matter what type of absorption occurs:

$$C_{ss,ave} = \frac{FD}{Vk\tau} = \frac{FD}{CL\tau} \tag{10.367}$$

If dosing stops after the Nth dose or after reaching steady-state, the plasma concentration equations for the final dosing interval can be used for all later times ($t' \geq 0$).

Note that the repeated dosing equations for one-compartment first-order absorption have two accumulation factors, one containing the elimination rate constant (k) and the other containing the absorption rate constant (k_a). As described previously, the accumulation factor containing k represents the amount of drug remaining from previous doses. The accumulation factor containing k_a then represents the amount of drug remaining to be absorbed from previous doses. The relationship between the absorption accumulation factor and the relative size of the absorption half-life ($t_{½,abs}$) versus the dosing interval (τ) is identical to that listed in Table 10.3 for the elimination half-life. Since the absorption half-life is generally substantially smaller than the elimination half-life, the amount of drug remaining to be absorbed from previous doses is generally much less than the amount of absorbed drug remaining from previous doses.

10.14.3.4 Generalized Multicompartment Model with Instantaneous or First-Order Absorption

As with all previous models, repeated instantaneous or first-order absorption dosing of a drug that follows multi-compartment kinetics gives plasma concentrations that

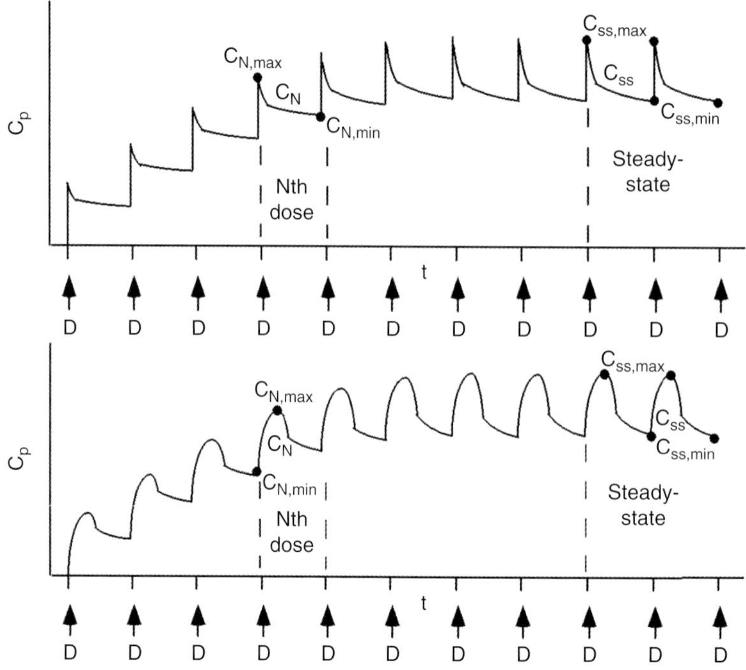

Figure 10.98 Approach to steady-state for repeated drug dosing at regular intervals (top) and for an IV infusion (bottom).

approach steady-state conditions after a sufficient duration of regular dosing intervals. This is illustrated in Figure 10.98 for instantaneous absorption (top graph) and first-order absorption (bottom graph). The shape of the concentration versus time during each dosing interval displays the characteristic distribution phase as expected for a drug following multicompartment kinetics. In order to simplify the multiple dosing equations in this section, the general single-dose multicompartment equations for instantaneous and first-order absorption are both expressed in the same form:

$$C_{singledose} = B_1 \cdot e^{-\lambda_1 t} + B_2 \cdot e^{-\lambda_2 t} + \ldots + B_z \cdot e^{-\lambda_z t} \quad (10.368)$$

where z is n for an instantaneous absorption model with n compartments, and z is $n+1$ for a first-order absorption model with n compartments. This notation allows the instantaneous and first-order absorption multiple dosing model equations to be written in the same form. Equations for the plasma concentrations versus t' (time since the most recent dose administration) during the Nth interval or at steady-state then become (for $0 \leq t' \leq \tau$)

$$C_N = B_1\left(\frac{1-e^{-N\lambda_1\tau}}{1-e^{-\lambda_1\tau}}\right)\cdot e^{-\lambda_1 t'} + B_2\left(\frac{1-e^{-N\lambda_2\tau}}{1-e^{-\lambda_2\tau}}\right)\cdot e^{-\lambda_2 t'} + \ldots + B_z\left(\frac{1-e^{-N\lambda_z\tau}}{1-e^{-\lambda_z\tau}}\right)\cdot e^{-\lambda_z t'} \quad (10.369)$$

$$C_{ss} = B_1\left(\frac{1}{1-e^{-\lambda_1\tau}}\right)\cdot e^{-\lambda_1 t'} + B_2\left(\frac{1}{1-e^{-\lambda_2\tau}}\right)\cdot e^{-\lambda_2 t'} + \ldots + B_z\left(\frac{1}{1-e^{-\lambda_z\tau}}\right)\cdot e^{-\lambda_z t'} \quad (10.370)$$

The maximum concentration during each dosing interval for instantaneous absorption can be readily calculated by setting $t' = 0$ in these equations. The time of the maximum concentration for first-order absorption cannot be solved directly and instead requires an extremely laborious trial-and-error determination (which means it is generally done with a computer). The minimum concentration for instantaneous absorption can be calculated by setting $t' = \tau$, and the minimum concentration for first-order absorption is given by setting $t' = 0$. The average concentration at steady-state, which has the same equation no matter what type of absorption or compartment model is used, becomes

$$C_{ss,ave} = \frac{FD}{CL\tau} \quad (10.371)$$

If dosing stops after the Nth dose or after reaching steady-state, the plasma concentration equations for the final dosing interval can be used for all later times ($t' \geq 0$).

10.14.4 Effect of Model Parameters on the Plasma Concentrations

As in single-dose models, the plasma concentrations can be substantially affected by changes in the values of the model parameters. The general effect of model parameter changes on multiple dosing plasma concentrations are summarized in Table 10.4.

10.14.5 Estimating Plasma Drug Concentrations

The model parameters utilized in multiple dosing models are identical to the model parameters used

Table 10.4 Effects of Model Parameters Value Changes on Multiple Dosing Plasma Concentrations

Parameter Change	Effect on Plasma Concentration	Explanation for Effect
Increase in FD (or k_0T)	Plasma concentrations increase	More drug is absorbed during each dosing interval
Increase in V (or V_1, V_{ss}, V_{AUC})	Plasma concentrations decrease	Drug is diluted into a larger volume in the body
Increase in k (or λ_z) or decrease in $t_{1/2,elim}$	Plasma concentrations decrease	More drug is eliminated during each dosing interval, less drug remains from previous dosing intervals
Increase in k_a or decrease in $t_{1/2,abs}$	Plasma concentrations rise more sharply during each interval, the maximum concentration is larger and occurs earlier	Absorption occurs faster and is completed more quickly during each dosing interval
Increase in τ with FD held constant	Plasma concentrations decrease	Less drug is delivered per unit of time
Increase in τ with FD/τ held constant	Average concentrations unchanged, bigger difference between maximum and minimum concentrations	Same amount of drug is delivered per unit of time, but drug is administered in larger doses (larger rise in concentration after dosing) with more time between doses (larger concentration drop over dosing interval)

with single-dose models. So as long as estimates of the single-dose parameters can be found in drug handbooks, text books, or literature articles, the plasma concentrations for multiple dosing situations can be estimated by the equations provided in this section.

10.15 ADVANCED PHARMACOKINETIC MODELING TOPICS

There are many other interesting and useful PK modeling topics that could not be included in this chapter due to their advanced nature or space limitations. This section is meant to provide a brief overview and general understanding of these topics. More detailed information on these topics can be found in the references listed at the end of this chapter.

10.15.1 Curve Fitting with Nonlinear Regression Analysis

All the methods for evaluating model parameters described previously in this chapter represent traditional PK analysis methods. These traditional methods rely on manipulating plasma concentration data so that some portion of the data falls on a terminal line that can be analyzed by simple linear regression. In most cases, the first stage of analysis is to identify the values of the natural logarithm of plasma concentrations that fall on a terminal line, and then evaluate a few initial parameters from the regression of these linear points. A method of residual analysis of the plasma concentration measurements not used in the first analysis stage then provides natural logarithm of residual values, some of which again fall on a terminal line. This yields a few more parameters after linear regression of the residual terminal line points. The method of residual analysis is then repeated as needed with the ever-dwindling number of measurements not used in previous stages of analysis. Thus this type of analysis utilizes the data in a piecewise fashion rather than considering all the data as a whole, and each stage of analysis involves fitting the data to an approximated linear form.

These traditional PK analysis methods do provide reasonable approximations for the model parameters, but more advanced nonlinear regression curve fitting approaches are available that offer a number of advantages. Nonlinear regression techniques allow the fitted equations to be written in any form, rather than only in the form of a straight line. Thus the complex equations for plasma concentration versus time for any of the models in this chapter can be utilized as the equation form to be fitted. The model parameters in these complex equations can also be fitted directly, rather than indirectly as some function of the linear slope or intercept. The fitting operations can also be performed using all the plasma concentration measurements simultaneously, rather than using different points for different parts of the analysis.

Nonlinear regression analysis does require purchasing and learning specialized software, rather than simply using a calculator and a piece of graph paper as can be done with traditional PK analysis methods. Many graphing and statistical analysis software packages can perform nonlinear regression analysis, however, and at least some of them are fairly easy to learn. KaleidaGraph® (Synergy Software, www.synergy.com) is a graphing program with a simple, straightforward nonlinear regression algorithm; Scientist® (Micromath Software, www.micromath.com) can perform powerful nonlinear regression fitting to any type of kinetic model. Specialized PK software packages are also available that perform nonlinear regression fitting for a variety of built-in PK models (including all the models discussed in this chapter). Commercial PK software packages include WinNonlin® (formerly PCNonlin®, Scientific Consulting Inc., Apex, NC), Kinetica® (Thermo Scientific, www.thermo.com), and PKAnalyst® (Micromath Software, www.micromath.com).

Nonlinear regression also requires fairly accurate preliminary estimates of the model parameter values.

If poor initial parameter estimates are used, it becomes likely that the nonlinear regression will not be able to find an acceptable fit, or it may stride off on a mathematical tangent and arrive at a nonsensical fit to the data. It turns out that the values determined by traditional methods of residual analyses typically offer excellent starting estimates for the model parameters. Hence the traditional data analysis methods described in this chapter remain highly useful, even when nonlinear regression curve fitting is employed as the final step of parameter evaluation.

A comparison of the two-compartment first-order absorption model fit to measured plasma concentration data from a traditional method of residuals analysis and a nonlinear regression analysis is provided in Figure 10.99. This figure illustrates the fact that both methods offer a very reasonable fit to the measured data. It also demonstrates that there is not a large difference between the fit provided by the two different techniques. Close examination does reveal, however, that the nonlinear regression analysis does provide a more universal fit to all the data points. This is likely due to the fact that nonlinear regression fits all the points simultaneously, whereas the method of residuals analysis fits the data in a piecewise manner with different data points used for different regions of the curve.

10.15.2 Noncompartmental Pharmacokinetic Analysis

The premise of noncompartmental PK analysis is to utilize a universal approach to analyze plasma concentration data without making assumptions about a specific number of model compartments or type of absorption process. This generally involves fitting the measured plasma concentration data to an equation in the form of a sum of multiple exponential terms:

$$C_p = B_1 \cdot e^{-\lambda_1 t} + B_2 \cdot e^{-\lambda_2 t} + \ldots + B_z \cdot e^{-\lambda_z t} \qquad (10.372)$$

where $\lambda_1 > \lambda_2 > \ldots > \lambda_z$. Note that this first step is not absolutely necessary, but is commonly used in this analysis. The next step is to calculate the area under the curve (AUC) from either the fitted exponential terms above, or by use of the trapezoidal rule. A related parameter called the area under the moment curve (AUMC) is also calculated. Whereas the AUC represents the integral of the plasma concentration with respect to time, the AUMC represents the integral of the product of the time multiplied by the plasma concentration. The value of the AUMC can be calculated from the fitted exponential terms, or by use of a modified version of the trapezoidal rule. If plasma concentration data is available from both IV and extravascular drug delivery, then the bioavailability (F), clearance (CL), and the AUC distribution volume (VAUC) can all be determined from the AUC values. The relative values of the AUC and AUMC can be used to evaluate the steady-state distribution volume (Vss), as well as the mean residence time (MRT) and mean absorption time (MAT) of the drug. The MRT represents how long the typical drug molecule remains in the body, and the MAT represents the average time it takes for a drug molecule to be absorbed. Thus noncompartmental PK analysis provides a straightforward means of evaluating general information about a drug's kinetics in the body. The commercial PK software packages WinNonlin® (formerly PCNonlin®, Scientific Consulting Inc., Apex, NC), Kinetica® (Thermo Scientific, www.thermo.com), and PKAnalyst® (Micromath Software, www.micromath.com) can all perform noncompartmental PK analysis in an automated manner.

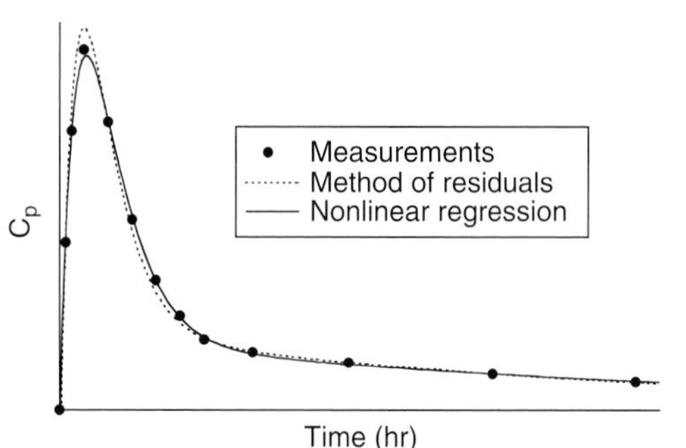

Figure 10.99 Comparison of the two-compartment first-order absorption model fit to measured plasma concentration data from a traditional method of residuals analysis and a nonlinear regression analysis.

10.15.3 Population Pharmacokinetic Analysis

Population PK analysis is an alternative method of evaluating PK model parameters that employs a very different approach from that of traditional PK analysis. In the traditional approach, a relatively large number of plasma concentration measurements (typically 5–15 samples) are made in a relatively small number of subjects (typically 5–20 volunteers). Data analysis is performed individually on each subject's plasma measurements to evaluate the model parameters for each subject. Variation in PK parameters between individuals is estimated by comparing the measured parameters for each subject.

Population PK analysis employs nearly the exact opposite approach. A small number of plasma concentration measurements (typically 1–2) are collected from a large number of subjects (typically 50–200). The concentration measurements often represent measurements made during routine monitoring of patients receiving drug therapy. The concentration measurements for all subjects are then analyzed simultaneously using a complex population-based PK model. The population-based PK model contains the same parameters and general form as a standard PK model, but also has extra terms that allow the parameter values to vary from one subject to another. Results from this analysis then provide values of not only the average values of each model parameter, but also indicate how much each parameter varies between subjects and whether parameter values are functions of other features such as subject age, body weight, and such. Thus population-based PK analysis provides a strong tool for understanding how drugs will behave in a general population of patients, but it also requires advanced statistical expertise as well as highly specialized statistical software. A specially designed statistical program called NONMEM® (GloboMax LLC, NONMEM Project Team, nminfo@globomaxnm.com) developed at the University of California, San Francisco is generally used for this type of analysis.

10.15.4 Excretion Pharmacokinetic Analysis

Although plasma (or blood) samples are most often employed in evaluating PK parameters, the amount of drug excreted in body wastes (most commonly urine samples) provide an alternative means of PK parameter evaluation. This can be accomplished by collecting urine and/or feces samples at varying time periods after drug administration, and then analyzing the amount of drug excreted in each sample. Dividing the amount of drug excreted in each sample by the length of time over which the sample was collected provides an estimate of the excretion rate for each sample collection period. Analysis of the excretion rate versus the time after drug delivery can then provide a reliable estimate of the elimination rate constant and the elimination half-life. Measured urinary excretion rates can also be used together with measured plasma concentrations to determine the renal clearance as described in Section 10.5.2.1. The total amount of drug excreted in the urine (or feces) can be determined by collecting excretion samples until drug can no longer be detected in the samples. The amount of drug excreted at different times after drug dosing can then be compared to the total amount of drug excreted to provide yet another means of determining the elimination rate constant and the elimination half-life. Thus though excretion analysis does not provide a means to estimate all PK model parameters, it can provide valuable information on the duration of drug in the body.

10.15.5 Estimation of Pharmacokinetic Parameters by Allometric Scaling

Allometric scaling is a method of interspecies extrapolation that is commonly used to estimate human PK parameters from PK parameters measured in animals. It makes use of the fact that many physiological parameters of different species can be empirically related to the relative size of the species (usually body weight, but other parameters such as the relative size of particular organs can also be useful for some parameters). The result is that PK parameter values (represented here by Y) for different species can often be correlated with species body weight (BW) by an equation of the form

$$Y = \alpha \cdot BW^{\beta} \tag{10.373}$$

where α and β are empirical constants for a given PK parameter. If the value of a PK parameter for a particular drug is measured in several animals of varying size (e.g., mouse, rat, rabbit, and sheep), then the empirical constants can be evaluated from the measured animal data. The human value for the PK parameter can then be predicted by substituting the human body weight into this equation. This approach is commonly employed with new experimental drugs, which typically are tested in several species prior to human testing. Allometric scaling is also valuable in estimating the PK parameters of toxic environmental or industrial chemicals, so that expected human plasma concentrations can be predicted for risk assessment.

10.15.6 Metabolite Kinetics

All the PK models in this chapter focus on the plasma concentration of the parent drug, with the formation of metabolites considered only in the sense that it represents the disappearance of parent drug molecules. This is a reasonable approach as long as the parent drug is the primary active form of the drug and metabolites are inactive as well as nontoxic. If the metabolite activity is similar to or greater than the parent drug, or if a metabolite causes unwanted or toxic side effects, then it becomes important to understand the metabolite kinetics. A prodrug, where drug is administered as an inactive parent form that is converted to an active metabolite after being absorbed, would be an obvious example where the plasma concentration and kinetics of the metabolite are more important than those of the parent drug. If a parent drug is delivered by bolus IV injection and both parent drug and metabolite follow one-compartment kinetics, then the shape of the plasma metabolite concentration (CM) versus time (t) is similar to a drug delivered by first-order absorption, as illustrated in Figure 10.100. The terminal slope of ln(CM) for this situation depends on the relative size of the elimination rate constants for the parent drug (kPD) and the metabolite (kM), as illustrated in Figure 10.101. If the parent drug is eliminated more slowly than the metabolite (kPD $<$ kM), then the parent drug and metabolite terminal lines are parallel with slopes of -kPD. If the metabolite is eliminated more slowly than the parent drug (kPD $>$ kM), then the metabolite terminal line

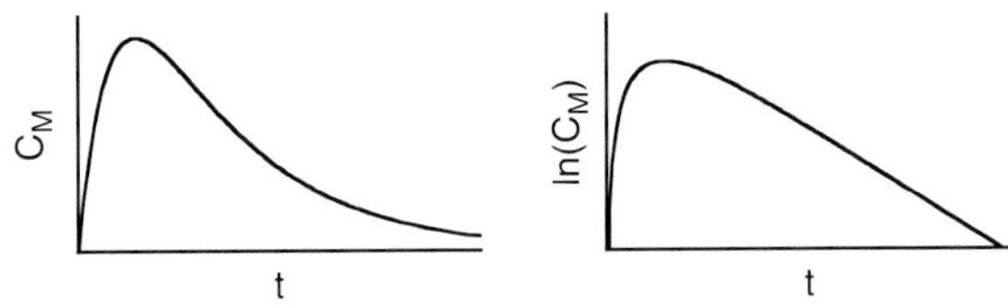

Figure 10.100 Graphical illustration of the general shape of plasma metabolite concentrations (CM) and ln(CM) versus time after a bolus IV injection of the parent drug.

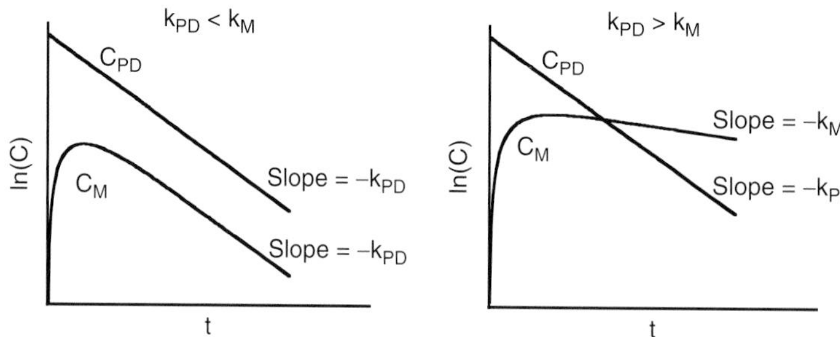

Figure 10.101 Graphical illustration of the relative shape of metabolite and parent drug concentrations (CM and CPD, respectively) following a bolus IV injection of the parent drug. The slope of the metabolite terminal line depends on the relative size of the metabolite elimination rate constant (kM) and the parent drug elimination rate constant (kPD).

has a slope of −kM and metabolite terminal line is not as steep as the parent drug terminal line. The latter case with slow metabolite elimination can lead to a buildup of the metabolite, particularly in multiple dosing situations, which can produce problems if the metabolite causes unwanted side effects or toxicity. PK metabolite models for other types of absorption or for multicompartment kinetics are more complicated and beyond the scope of this chapter.

10.15.7 Pharmacodynamic Models

Pharmacodynamic (PD) models describe the relationship between drug concentrations (in the plasma or target tissue) and the resultant pharmacological effect. Drug effects most commonly are caused by an interaction of drug molecules with a target protein or receptor. Drug molecules typically undergo reversible binding to the target receptor to form a drug-receptor complex. The intensity of the drug effect is then related to the amount of drug-receptor complex formed. When the drug concentration is low, there are many available open binding sites, and hence an increase in drug concentration under these conditions causes more drug-receptor complexes to form and yields an increase in effect. If drug concentrations are already high, most or all of the receptor binding sites are filled, and hence a further increase in drug concentration after receptors are saturated causes little or no increase in effect. The effect (E) versus plasma or target tissue drug concentration (C) can often be represented by an equation of the form

$$E = \frac{E_{max} \cdot C^{\gamma}}{EC_{50}^{\gamma} + C^{\gamma}} \tag{10.374}$$

where E_{max} is the maximum possible effect when all receptor binding sites are filled, EC50 is the drug concentration that produces 50% of the maximum effect, and γ (pronounced "gamma") is a fitted parameter that generally has a value of 0.5–3. Plotting the intensity of drug effect (E) versus ln(C) yields a sigmoid-shaped curve, as illustrated in Figure 10.102, where the curve flattens at high drug concentrations due to receptor saturation.

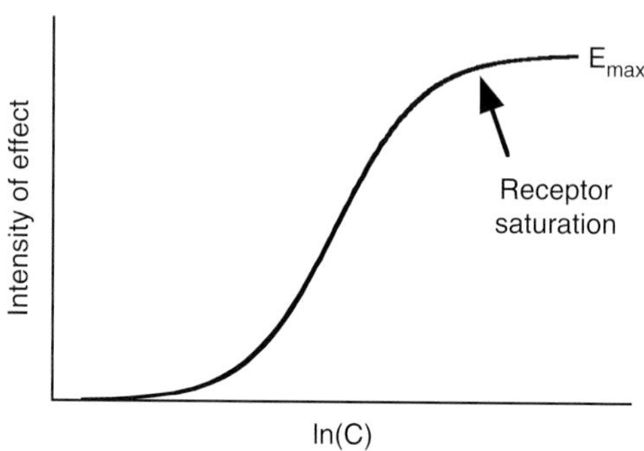

Figure 10.102 Graphical illustration of the typical relationship between drug concentration (in the plasma or the target tissue) and the intensity of the drug effect.

PK and PD models can be linked together to predict drug effect versus time. PK models are employed to predict plasma or target tissue drug concentrations, with PD models then used to estimate the effect at any time based on the current drug concentration.

10.15.8 Nonlinear Kinetics

Linear (or first-order) kinetics refers to the situation where the rate of some process is proportional to the amount or concentration of drug raised to the power of one (the first power, hence the name first-order kinetics). This is equivalent to stating that the rate is equal to the amount or concentration of drug multiplied by a constant (a linear function, hence linear kinetics). All the PK models described in this chapter have assumed linear elimination (metabolism and excretion) kinetics. All distribution processes have been taken to follow linear kinetics or to be instantaneous (completed quickly). Absorption processes have been taken to be instantaneous (completed quickly), follow linear first-order kinetics, or follow zero-order kinetics. Thus out of these processes, only zero-order absorption represents a nonlinear process that is not completed in too short of a time period to matter. This lone example of nonlinear kinetics in the standard PK models represents a special case since nonlinear absorption is relatively easy to handle mathematically. Inclusion of any other type of nonlinear kinetic process in a PK model makes it impossible to write the plasma concentration versus time in a simple, explicitly solved equation form.

The most common type of nonlinear kinetics arises when the rate of a process is determined by Michaelis-Menten kinetics. The concentration relationship for Michaelis-Menten kinetics can be written in the general form,

$$rate = \frac{V_{\max} \cdot f_u C}{K_m + f_u C} \qquad (10.375)$$

where V_{max} is the maximum possible rate, C is the local drug concentration, f_u is the unbound drug fraction (fraction of drug molecules not bound to macroproteins such as albumin) and K_m is the Michaelis-Menten metabolism constant representing the unbound drug concentration at which the rate is half of the maximal rate. The assumption that has been made for all PK models in this chapter is that the unbound drug concentration is much lower than the value of K_m, so that the rate equation can be simplified to

$$\text{for } f_u\, C << K_m,\ rate \approx \left(\frac{V_{\max}}{K_m}\right) \cdot f_u C \qquad (10.376)$$

Since V_{max}, K_m, and f_u can be considered constants in this equation, the rate becomes a first-order or linear function of the drug concentration. As stated previously, this assumption is generally very realistic for most drugs under most normal drug therapy situations. There are some drugs and some dosing situations for which this assumption is not valid, however, and this can then result in one or more of the PK processes becoming nonlinear in certain cases. One common and well-known example of nonlinear kinetics is the elimination of ethanol. Even modest levels of ethanol consumption can quickly saturate the primary metabolizing enzyme, resulting in nonlinear elimination kinetics. It is relatively easy to understand how the saturation of metabolizing enzymes results in nonlinear metabolism kinetics. It may not be quite as obvious, but any of the ADME processes can have nonlinear kinetics caused by the saturation of transporter proteins or other types of saturated protein binding.

There are a number of techniques available to check whether nonlinear kinetics occur for a given drug or dosing situation. One of the most common techniques is to measure plasma concentration levels after the administration of different doses of drug, and then calculate the AUC for each dose. A plot of AUC versus dose can then be used to check for nonlinear kinetics, as illustrated in Figure 10.103. If all kinetic processes remain linear for all doses tested, then the plot should yield points falling on or very near a straight line. If the points form a curve with an increasing slope at higher concentrations, then nonlinear kinetics are causing plasma concentrations to be higher than expected with linear kinetics. This type of relationship would be expected for saturated enzymes during metabolism or saturated secretion transporters during excretion. If the points form a curve with a decreasing slope at higher concentrations, then nonlinear kinetics are causing plasma concentrations to be lower than expected with linear kinetics. This type of relationship could be caused by saturated transporters involved in absorption or saturated reabsorption transporters involved in excretion. Other types of mechanisms can also cause one or the other type of curve through complex nonlinear interactions.

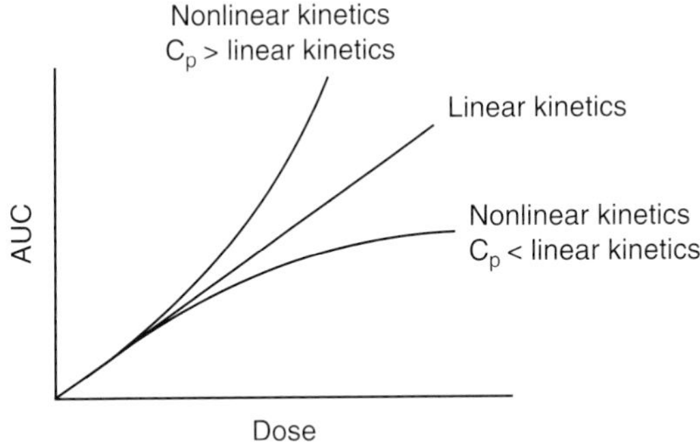

Figure 10.103 Illustration of how a plot of AUC versus drug dose can be employed to determine whether a drug follows linear or nonlinear kinetics.

As stated earlier, PK models for most nonlinear kinetic processes do not provide a simple relationship for plasma concentration versus time. Nonlinear kinetic modeling must often be performed using complex computer-based numerical method integrations that are beyond the scope of this text. More information about how to perform this type of modeling can be found in the references at the end of the chapter. Software packages that are useful for nonlinear kinetic modeling include Scientist® (Micromath Software, www.micromath.com) and WinNonlin® (formerly PCNonlin®, Scientific Consulting Inc., Apex, NC).

10.15.9 Physiologically-based Pharmacokinetic (PBPK) Models

Physiologically-based Pharmacokinetic (PBPK) models represent one of the most complex and powerful PK modeling approaches that are available. An example PBPK model is illustrated in Figure 10.104. PBPK models include a number of compartments, but unlike the previously described standard compartmental models, each compartment represents a specific tissue in the body. Thus the concentration of drug in a given tissue appears directly in the model. Transport of drug between compartments is also represented by realistic physiological processes. For example, perfusion-limited drug delivery to a tissue is written in terms of the blood flow to the tissue and the drug concentration in the blood. Permeation-limited drug delivery, such as across the blood–brain barrier, is then given directly in terms of the tissue and blood concentration on each side of the barrier along with the surface area and permeability of the barrier. Absorption from the intestines can be appropriately modeled as being carried by portal vein drainage directly to the liver. Metabolism or excretion occurring in a given tissue is represented

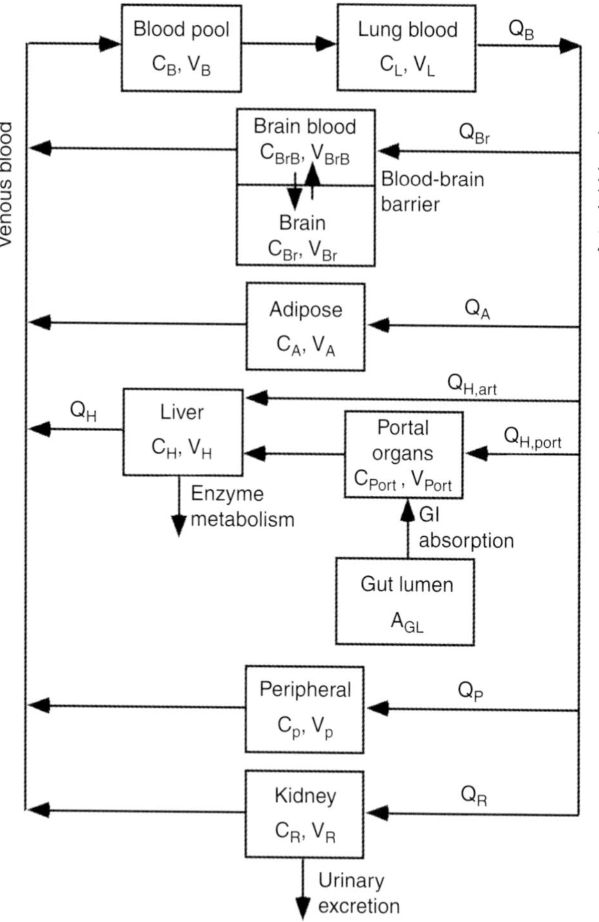

Figure 10.104 An example of a PBPK model diagram, where each tissue is represented by a separate compartment with a specific drug concentration, and transport between tissues is related to actual physiological parameters such as blood flow rates to each tissue.

by realistic kinetic models such as a Michaelis-Menten equation written in terms of the actual tissue concentration. Finally, the drug effect can be given as a direct pharmacodynamic function of the actual drug concentration within the target tissue.

These features demonstrate the realistic nature of PBPK models. These models can also be readily adjusted to reflect changes caused by a specific disease state. PBPK models also provide a much more accurate means of extrapolating animal measurements to predict human drug concentrations, as the actual organ sizes, enzyme levels, and blood flow rates can be adjusted specifically for different species. Inclusion of all these realistic features also makes PBPK models much more complex and laborious to use, with many more model parameters to evaluate, and computer-based numerical integration being absolutely necessary. Evaluation of the model parameters is simplified by the fact that many of these parameters represent real physiological features, such as the blood flow rates to different organs, which can be found in physiological tables and books. Software packages that are useful for PBPK modeling include Scientist® (Micromath Software, www.micromath.com) and PK-Sim® (Bayer Technology Services, www.bayertechnology.com). Thus PBPK models are very powerful tools for modeling and predicting drug disposition, but there is a very steep learning curve required for their use.

10.16 SUMMARY OF KEY POINTS

The key points that you should take away from this chapter can be summarized as follows:

- PK models are powerful tools that can be used to predict plasma concentrations when the model parameters are known for a drug, or can be utilized to evaluate model parameters from measured plasma drug concentrations.
- PK models can be valuable aids to the design of therapeutic drug dosing regimens, as the therapeutic effectiveness of drug treatment is generally closely related to drug concentrations.
- Plasma drug concentrations are determined by the relative rates of the ADME processes. ADME processes are represented in PK models by specific mathematical forms and parameters.
- All the standard PK models include a number of inherent assumptions about the ADME processes, including the universal assumption that elimination follows first-order or linear kinetics.
- Absorption in standard PK models is assumed to take place instantaneously, or by a zero-order or first-order absorption rate.
- Standard PK models represent the body as either a single compartment, which assumes instantaneous distribution to all tissues; or as two compartments, which assumes instantaneous distribution throughout the central compartment (containing the systemic circulation) and slower first-order distribution to the second compartment (representing tissues that equilibrate slowly).
- Generalized multicompartment models provide a means of representing highly complex PK situations with relatively simple plasma concentration equations.
- The model equations and shape of plasma concentration versus time is unique for each PK model. An appropriate PK model should then be selected based on the drug and the route of administration.
- Complex PK modeling cases can be represented by simplified model forms under certain specific circumstances.
- PK models for multiple dosing situations can be based on the principle of superposition as long as drug elimination follows linear kinetics. Superposition allows the concentration for each dose to be determined from single-dose PK models, and the overall resulting plasma concentrations for all combined doses to be taken as the sum of

the concentrations associated with each individual dose.

- Additional information is available for a number of very useful advanced PK topics in the references listed at the end of the chapter.

REVIEW QUESTIONS

1. What is the difference between using PK models to predict plasma concentrations and using PK models to evaluate model parameters?
2. What are the PK terms and model parameters associated with absorption processes? What are the different types of absorption in standard PK models? Provide examples of real world drug administration methods that can be represented by each of these types of absorption.
3. What are the PK terms and model parameters associated with distribution processes? What assumptions are made about distribution processes in standard one-compartment and two-compartment models?
4. What are the PK terms and model parameters associated with elimination processes? What assumptions are made about elimination processes in the PK models described in this chapter?
5. What shape would you expect for a plot of measured plasma concentrations versus time for each of the standard PK models? What shape would you expect for a plot of $\ln(C_p)$ versus time for each of the standard PK models?
6. What is a terminal line? Why do terminal lines form in the plot of $\ln(C_p)$ versus time? How are terminal lines used to evaluate model parameters from measured plasma drug concentrations?
7. What does a residual represent? How are residuals used to evaluate model parameters from measured plasma drug concentrations?
8. What are some advantages and disadvantages associated with the use of generalized multicompartment models?
9. What principle forms the basis of all multiple dosing PK models in this chapter? What model assumptions are required for this principle to be applicable?
10. What similar characteristics are found for a prolonged IV drug infusion and repeated dosing of a drug at regular time intervals?

ACKNOWLEDGEMENTS

My longtime colleague and close personal friend Dr. James P. Byers was writing this chapter when cardiovascular disease took him away at much too young an age. It has been my honor to finish this writing task in memory of my friend. I've done my best to complete the text using an organization and style consistent with the way Jim had started the chapter and the way he taught his courses. I'm sure Jim would wish to join me in dedicating this chapter to his wife Lisa and their children Sarah and John.

I would also be seriously remiss (and subject to numerous and humiliating practical jokes) if I failed to thank my diligent proofreaders, Dr. Jill Trendel, Crystal Bykowski, and Michael Reese, whose assistance has been invaluable in completing this chapter.

REFERENCES

The following references provide additional information on the topics discussed in this chapter.

Anderson, P. O., Knoben, J. E., & Troutman, W. G. (2001). *Handbook of Clinical Drug Data* (10th ed.). New York: McGraw-Hill.

Baselt, R. C., & Cravey, R. H. (1995). *Disposition of Toxic Drugs and Chemicals in Man* (4th ed.). Foster City, CA: Chemical Toxicology Institute.

Bonate, P. (2005). *Pharmacokinetic-Pharmacodynamic Modeling and Simulation.* New York: Springer.

Boroujerdi, M. (2001). *Pharmacokinetics: Principles and Applications.* New York: McGraw-Hill.

Burton, M. E., Shaw, L. M., Schentag, J. J., & Evans, W. E. (2005). *Applied Pharmacokinetics and Pharmacodynamics: Principles of Therapeutic Drug Monitoring* (4th ed.). Philadelphia, PA: Lippincott Williams & Wilkins.

Brunton, L. L., Lazo, J. S., & Parker, A. L. (Ed.). (2006). *Goodman and Gilman's The Pharmacological Basis of Therapeutics* (11th ed.). New York: McGraw-Hill.

Cooney, D. O. (1976). *Biomedical Engineering Principles.* New York: Dekker.

Fournier, R. L. (1998). *Basic Transport Phenomena in Biomedical Engineering.* Philadelphia, PA: Taylor & Francis.

Gabrielsson, J., & Weiner, D. (2007). *Pharmacokinetic and Pharmacodynamic Data Analysis: Concepts and Applications* (4th ed.). Stockholm, Sweden: Swedish Pharmaceutical Press.

Gibaldi, M., & Perrier, D. (1982). *Pharmacokinetics* (2nd ed.). New York: Dekker.

Ho, R. H., & Kim, R. B. (2003). Transporters and drug therapy: Implications for drug disposition and disease. *Clinical Pharmacology and Therapeutics, 78,* 260–277.

Kerb, R. (2006). Implications of genetic polymorphisms in drug transporters for pharmacotherapy. *Cancer Letters, 234,* 4–33.

Klaassen, C. (2007). *Casarett and Doull's Toxicology: The Basic Science of Poisons,* Columbus, Ohio: McGraw-Hill.

Macheras, P., & Iliadis, A. (2005). *Modeling in Biopharmaceutics and Pharmacodynamics: Homogeneous and Heterogeneous Approaches.* New York: Springer.

Notari, R. E. (1987). *Biopharmaceutics and Clinical Pharmacokinetics* (4th ed.). New York: Dekker.

Physician's Desk Reference (62nd ed.). (2008). Montvale, NJ: Thomson Healthcare.

Reddy, M., Yang, R. S., Andersen, M. E., & Clewell, H. J. (2005). *Physiologically Based Pharmacokinetic Modeling: Science and Applications.* Hoboken, NJ: Wiley-Interscience.

Rowland, M., & Tozer, T. N. (1995). *Clinical Pharmacokinetics: Concepts and Applications* (3rd ed.). Baltimore, MD: Williams & Wilkins.

Shargel, L., Wu-Pong, S., & Yu, A. B. C. (2004). *Applied Biopharmaceutics and Pharmacokinetics* (5th ed.). New York: McGraw-Hill.

Silverman, R. B. (1992). *The Organic Chemistry of Drug Design and Drug Action.* San Diego, CA: Academic Press.

Strauss, S., & Bourne, D. W. A. (1995). *Mathematical Modeling of Pharmacokinetic Data.* Boca Rotan, FL: CRC.

Tozer, T. N., & Rowland, M. (2006). *Introduction to Pharmacokinetics and Pharmacodynamics: The Quantitative Basis of Drug Therapy.* Philadelphia, PA: Lippincott Williams & Wilkins.

Wagner, J. G. (1993). *Pharmacokinetics for the Pharmaceutical Scientist.* Lancaster, PA: Technomic.

Winter, M. E. (2003). *Basic Clinical Pharmacokinetics* (4th ed.). Philadelphia, PA: Lippincott Williams & Wilkins.

Chapter

11

Bioanalytical Tools for Drug Analysis

Jim Bigelow

OUTLINE

11.1 INTRODUCTION

11.1.1 Overview

11.1.1.1 What Is a Drug?

The U.S. Food and Drug Administration (FDA) defines a drug as:

> *(A) articles recognized in the official United States Pharmacopeia, official Homeopathic Pharmacopeia of the United States, or official National Formulary, or any supplement to any of them; and (B) articles intended for use in the diagnosis, cure, mitigation, treatment, or prevention of disease in man or other animals; and (C) articles (other than food) intended to affect the structure or any function of the body of man or other animals; and (D) articles intended for use as a component of any articles specified in clause (A), (B), or (C). (http://www.fda.gov/opacom/laws/fdcact/fdcact1.htm, Chapter II – Definitions, (g)(1))*

Although this rather broad definition serves well for regulatory purposes, for this chapter, the term drug must be narrowed to that more appropriate to the disciplines of pharmacology, pharmacy, and medicine. In this context, we will define a drug as a specific chemical species able to cause specific changes in the functioning of living things. More specifically, we will further narrow the definition to relatively small (< 1500 Da) organic and occasionally inorganic compounds. This narrowed definition is not meant to indicate that the many macromolecular agents such as polyclonal or monoclonal antibodies or enzymes are of less value therapeutically, but merely recognizes the great difference between macromolecules and smaller discrete organic or inorganic molecules in terms of bioanalysis. Many herbicides, pesticides, and other poisons and pollutants would also qualify under this narrow definition because most are specific chemicals that do bring about specific biological responses, namely killing their target organism. There are rare instances, such as the drug warfarin, which is used as an anticoagulant and previously was used as a rat poison (employing the same mechanism of action in both cases), although these will not be explicitly considered in this chapter. Thus it is logical that the methods and techniques employed for drug analysis are often exactly the same as those employed in environmental analysis. In fact, drugs and their metabolites, excreted by both people and animals in their urine and feces, are increasingly being recognized as environmental pollutants. This should not be very surprising because drugs are discovered or designed for their very potent biological effects and many of their metabolites are also bioactive. If either parent drugs or metabolites are persistent in the environment, they would indeed be pollutants.

11.1.1.2 The Scope of Drug Bioanalysis

Drugs are used everywhere in our society and throughout the world. They have been used in one form or

Table 11.1 Industrial Uses of Drug Bioanalysis

Quality control	Research and development
Quality assurance	Manufacture
Instrument validation	Process development

another for all recorded history and certainly before man was even man. Their uses range from legitimate medical use (where the pharmaceutical industry prefers the term "medicine," believing it to have a less pejorative connotation) to illegal recreational use, as well as veterinary, animal husbandry, and sports-enhancement (both legal and illegal). Thus the scope of drug bioanalysis is very large. It includes clinical analysis for pharmacokinetics and therapeutic drug monitoring (see later) of patients receiving routine therapy. It also includes extensive use in drug discovery, development, and manufacture in the pharmaceutical and biotechnology industries (Table 11.1). Academic research in a wide range of fields also requires drug bioanalysis. Law enforcement requires highly accurate drug analysis for forensic investigation, for instance, in cases of poisoning, either accidental or deliberate. Finally, interdiction of illicit drug smuggling and use, including professional, national, and international athletics requires highly accurate and precise drug bioanalysis—to render a conviction or strip an athlete of a medal should be based only on the best evidence that drug bioanalysis can provide.

11.1.1.3 Pharmacokinetics and Therapeutic Drug Monitoring

Pharmacokinetics (PK) is the science of determining and quantitatively determining the time course of drugs throughout the body. When a drug is administered, it will follow a reasonably predictable course of *absorption* into the body, *distribution* throughout the body, possible enzymatic *metabolism* of the drug, and ultimate *excretion*. These processes, together with a drug's *toxicity*, constitute the common pharmaceutical acronym, *PK/ADMET*.

Although many drugs are very safe, some drugs can be quite toxic and even fatal at plasma concentration not far beyond their therapeutic levels. These include the mood stabilizer lithium (therapeutic range of 0.6 to 0.8 mEq/L, toxic above 1.2 mEq/L) and the anticonvulsant agent phenytoin (therapeutic range of 10 to 20 mg/L and often toxic above 20 mg/L). Drugs such as these are said to have a poor *therapeutic index* (*TI*), which is the ratio of the therapeutic level to the toxic level. Often in such cases and/or where there is much variability in the pharmacokinetics of a drug, either inter-patient or intra-patient, *therapeutic drug monitoring* (*TDM*) must be used. This involves taking a patient's blood sample and actually measuring the drug concentration in the sample. This allows for drug dosing adjustments to be made. In the most extreme case, that of inhaled anesthetics gas, the TI is so narrow and the consequences of failing to have a patient maintained in a therapeutic drug level window (death or insufficient anesthesia during surgery) that an entire medical specialty has arisen to administer this one class of drugs.

11.1.1.4 Polarity and Drug Properties

Pharmaceutical companies require certain properties of the drugs they discover, develop, and manufacture. Most importantly, drugs must be safe and effective. This is a trade-off. For some life-threatening diseases such as cancer or an acute serious infection, it is more important that a drug be effective than safe. Many anticancer drugs are very toxic as are some of the anti-infective agents. The very important drug amphotericin B, one of few drugs available for potentially fatal systemic fungal infections, is so toxic it has earned the moniker *amphoterrible*. On the other hand, drugs used very widely such as over-the-counter pain relievers or drugs taken regularly over years or decades for chronic conditions such as hypertension or osteoporosis are held to a much higher standard of safety.

Beyond safety and efficacy, drug manufacturers want drugs to be chemically stable, reasonably inexpensive, and easy to produce (this is often a fairly minor consideration since production costs often represent only a very small fraction of the consumer costs of a drug), have favorable pharmacokinetic and metabolic profiles, and importantly, that the drug be soluble to some extent in water or some aqueous formulation.

This aspect of drugs is dictated by the fact that they must function in living organisms, which are overwhelmingly composed of water. Although there are many means of drug administration, the two most important ones are intravenous injection and, most importantly, oral administration. For intravenous injection, a drug must either be soluble in a water-based formulation or must be able to be formulated as a stable suspension or colloid. For drugs taken orally, they ideally should have moderate solubility and be of moderate polarity. Highly polar molecules are generally very water soluble but pass very poorly through biological membranes via passive diffusion, whereas very nonpolar molecules pass readily through membranes but are essentially insoluble in the fluids of the stomach and intestines where drug absorption occurs.

11.2 SMALL MOLECULE CHEMICAL BIOANALYSIS

The general goal of small molecule chemical bioanalysis is to determine the concentration of a particular chemical species (or sometimes a closely related group of chemical species) in a mixture. This goal can be accomplished in one of two ways. Either the chemical species can be determined *in situ* via some high specific chemical interaction or the chemical species can be separated from one another and then be detected and measured separately. The former strategy very commonly employed high specific antigen-antibody interactions as embodied in such techniques as the Enzyme-Linked ImmunoSorbent Assay (ELISA), the Enzyme Multiplied Immunoassay (EMIT) RadioImmuno Assay (RIA), and the Fluorescence Polarization Immunoassay (FPIA). These assays are very important but are beyond the scope of this chapter. This chapter will instead focus on drug analysis utilizing *analytical* separations.

Analytical separations, including bioanalysis, seek only information—what is in the sample and how much. An important clarification must be made here. *Preparative* separations also exist and are very common but seek to recover a product from the separative process for later use and not necessarily any information about the components being separated. These form the basis of vast industries such as ore refining and preparative scale chromatographic purification of important chemicals and pharmaceuticals. Of course the two often are operated concomitantly, yielding both valuable information and material.

In general, the process of analytical separative drug bioanalysis requires some combination of *physical separation* of one analyte from another in a mixture and *detection* of the desired analyte(s). These are complementary processes. The better we can separate analytes, the less specific detection methods have to be. This represents a continuum in that if a detection method is so nonselective that it detects all analytes, then all analytes must be separated from one another. Alternatively, if a detector can detect only one analyte among all the others, then sometimes essentially no separation is required. In reality, bioanalysis methods usually lie somewhere in between; this can be well understood if we consider a drug analysis when the desired analyte is present at a high concentration and there are few other species present. This might be the case in the analysis of a production run of a pharmaceutical agent for the purposes of quality control. In this case a less specific detection method would likely suffice and the separation would likely be routine. Conversely, the drug analysis might be very challenging when the analyte is present at low concentration and the mixture is very chemically complex. This might be the case in determining the concentration of a trace level drug or metabolite in a biological fluid such as urine or plasma and would likely require both an excellent separation and a specific detection method.

11.2.1 Chromatography

One of the most important methods of bioanalysis is *chromatography*, literally color-writing. There are many chromatographic and chromatographic-like techniques that have been discovered—and sometimes rediscovered, developed, and refined—since 1900. A short list of those that have been most relevant to drug analysis at some point would include gas chromatography (GC), paper chromatography, thin layer chromatography (TLC), ion exchange chromatography (IEC), and capillary electrophoresis (CE), a chromatography-like technique. However one technique, high performance liquid chromatography (HPLC; also incorrectly though commonly called high pressure liquid chromatography or, somewhat factiously, high-priced liquid chromatography) has won out and is overwhelmingly the method of choice for drug analysis, particularly in the pharmaceutical industry.

Each technique has its advantages and disadvantages. Gas chromatography can analyze only compounds that are volatile, whereas CE and IEC generally are limited to ionic species. On the other hand, HPLC can analyze a very wide range of compounds provided they are liquid soluble. It is this property that makes HPLC the overwhelmingly preferred technique for drug analysis because the chemical nature of drugs and the analytical properties of HPLC are very closely matched.

Figure 11.1 shows a highly schematic view of a chromatographic system, which would be applicable to both HPLC and GC (and to related chromatographic techniques such as affinity chromatography and gel filtration chromatography). In chromatographic techniques, a discrete and very well controlled volume of the analyte sample is introduced, termed an *injection*, at the top or head of a *chromatographic column* in a very short period of time (milliseconds to no more than few seconds). The components in the sample are carried down the length of the column by forced fluid flow, where they are allowed to interact with fixed

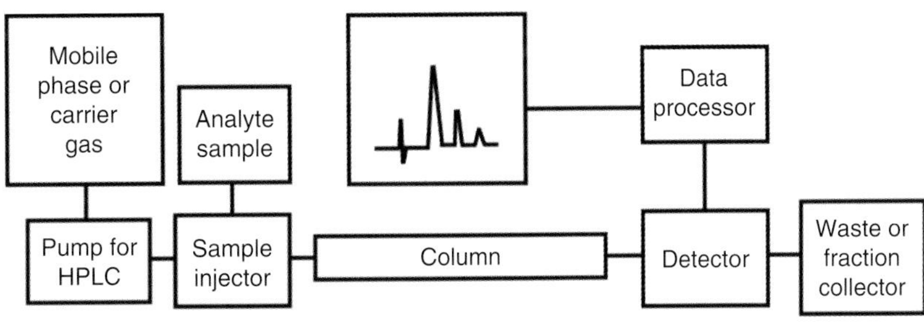

Figure 11.1 A highly schematic representation of a chromatographic system. In GC, the carrier gas is often in a gas cylinder, which has sufficient pressure to drive the gas through the column and no pump is required. In HPLC, a pump is required to force the mobile phase through the column. With exception of the data processor, the other components of GC and HPLC systems are often conceptually, although rarely instrumentally, similar.

surfaces present in the column, the *stationary phase.* Those sample components that interact more strongly with the stationary phase will be retained in the column for longer periods than components that interact less strongly with the stationary phase. The end result will be that the various sample components will become physically separated from one another.

Eventually, the sample components will *elute* or be carried out of the far end of the column and then be carried through one or more *detectors* (in tandem) that allow the concentration of the components to be determined. Detection of components, often by being passed through some form of *flow cell,* is done when the component is "interrogated" by the detection method that gives rise to a *signal* that is distinct from the carrier fluid. The signal is then passed to a computer and specialized software (the *data processor,* now present as part of all analytical instruments) for storage and analysis; the computer generally also allows for partial or complete control of the instrument. When all sample components have eluted (some may interact so strongly with the stationary phase they will never elute) or the desired information/material has been collected, the "chromatographic run" is terminated. The resultant temporal display of the signal information represents at what time, relative to the time of injection ($t = 0$), a given sample component eluted; this is termed a *chromatogram* (Figure 11.2).

The chromatogram contains a wealth of information. It will contain one or more peaks, usually of a slightly asymmetrical, normal (*Gaussian*) distribution (more on this later), indicating when each sample component eluted from the column and was detected. Each component has a *retention time* (t_R) that is specific for that component, and is reasonably consistent from one day to the next, run under a set of specific chromatographic conditions. The t_R is time of the maximum of the peak and is slightly longer than the true elution time because of the time delay between when a component actually elutes from the column and when it is detected. This delay is typically very short in well-designed instruments but it can be quite considerable in certain cases.

The height and area of the peak are proportional to the concentration or amount (mass) of the component contained in the peak. In most detectors, the proportionality is linear over a certain concentration range, which is to say that twice the concentration of an analyte injected will give rise to twice the detector response. This allows for the easy determination of the concentration of a drug in a complex mixture such as urine or plasma provided that a good separation is achieved. However, it is also very common for two or more sample components to elute at nearly the same time, known as *coelution,* which makes it impossible to determine the concentration of one from another using that detection method. Means do exist to determine when this has occurred but it remains a continuing problem in chromatographic analysis.

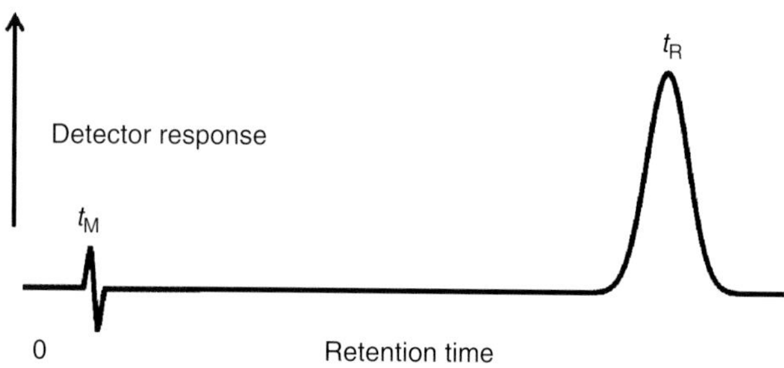

Figure 11.2 A highly schematic chromatogram of an analyte that has been injected and then eluted from the column and given rise to a detector signal. The analyte has a retention time of t_R whereas mobile phase or entirely unretained analytes will have retention times of t_M. The peak area and height are proportional to the concentration or amount present in the peak.

11.2.2 From LC to GC to HPLC—Comparisons and a History Lesson

Although conceptually and theoretically very similar, HPLC and GC differ in many important aspects, particularly in the nature of the column and the fluid that carries the analyte through the column, and to a lesser extent, the means by which this fluid is forced through the column. HPLC columns, particularly those used for analysis, nearly always start as empty tubes, typically of stainless steel, and are generally of considerable length in comparison to their internal diameter (ID); a length of 10 to 25 cm and an ID of 4.6 mm are typical. They are packed very carefully by their manufacturers with very fine (1 to 5 µm) particles. The particles themselves are usually not the stationary phase but serve instead merely as a solid support for a very thin (often a single molecular layer) chemical coating, which actually serves as the stationary phase. In contrast, the column in GC is usually a fused-silica hollow capillary and is much longer (up to 100 m) than an HPLC column. It is unpacked (although older types of packed GC column are still used) with an ID of 50 to 500 µm and the stationary phase is a very thin chemical coating on the column walls.

The fluid used to carry sample components through the column also differ greatly between HPLC and GC. In GC, the fluid is a very high-purity gas (the carrier gas) such as helium of hydrogen, which, although it can act as carrier for the analytes, rarely interacts with them chemically. In HPLC, the fluid is a liquid, referred to as the *mobile phase,* and is a very well-defined mixture of miscible solvent such as water and an organic solvent such as methanol or acetonitrile or organic solvents alone.

The means to drive the fluid through the column also differ substantially between HPLC and GC. In GC, the carrier gas usually is contained in a commercial gas cylinder, and the gas pressure in the cylinder, typically around 2500 pounds per square inch (PSI), is more than sufficient to force the carrier gas through the column (the gas pressure directly from the gas cylinder is generally far too high to feed directly into an GC instrument, and a gas pressure regulator attached to the cylinder is needed to reduce the pressure prior to the GC instrument).

In contrast, HPLC instruments require the liquid mobile phase be forced through the column and its dense packing of very fine particles. This can require pressure from 200 to 6000 pounds per square inch (PSI), depending on the column length and packing material; to generate these pressures is no trivial matter. To accomplish this many designs were developed at much effort and expense, and some of these will be discussed later. However, the first and simplest design was simply to raise the level of the liquid above that of the packing material and let gravity do the work of forcing a liquid, and the entrained analytes, through the packing material. This is a technique still used widely in research laboratories worldwide, but not for HPLC.

A sophisticated commercial HPLC or GC instrument now costs many thousands of dollars and requires a dedicated and skilled operator. It generally has very different applications with GC now generally rarely used in drug analysis but much more in environmental analysis (there are important exceptions). The analytical instruments are very different, employing very different carrier fluids (a carrier gas such as helium in GC versus a mobile phase such as a defined water/methanol mixture in HPLC), column types (packed columns in HPLC versus unpacked in GC), and different and distinct injection and detection methods.

Despite these many differences, chromatography, and in fact all separations, have a deep underlying unity that is reflected both theoretically and historically. Chromatography is now (arguably) the most widely used analytical technique. Highly sophisticated chromatographic instruments are available from many manufacturers, but of course this was not always so. In fact, the word chromatograph was first coined in 1906 by Mikhail Tswett (1872–1919).

> *The total chlorophyll can be extracted with petroleum ether containing alcohol.*
> *If a petroleum ether solution of chlorophyll filters through a column of an adsorption material (I use chiefly [finely ground] calcium carbonate which is firmly pressed into a narrow glass tube), the pigments will separate according to the adsorption series from above downward in differently colored zones.*
> *I call such a preparation a chromatogram and the corresponding method the chromatographic method. (Leicester, 1968, ref. 5.)*

With an appropriate mobile phase pump and colorimetric detector, Tswett's method would not be out of place in any separations laboratory today. However, the intervening calamities of the first half of the twentieth century, the First World War, the Great Depression, and the Second World War, resulted in Tswett's work largely being forgotten.

Instrumental development in separations and scientific progress in general began to recover as the Great Depression wore on. Much of this is attributable to gradually improving economic conditions in the late 1930s and various governmental efforts to prepare for what many saw was a coming war. In separation science however, much is attributable to the increasing importance of the petroleum industry in all facets of modern life. By the late 1930s, the petroleum industry in the United States was relatively mature in many respects. (The first truly commercially successful oil well in the United States was drilled by Edwin L. Drake in 1859, and the first real "gusher" in the United States occurred at an oil well on a small hill just outside of Beaumont Texas in January of 1901. This well, called Spindletop would, briefly, produce over 100,000 barrels per day and would, also briefly, drive oil prices until they were just three cents per barrel.)

By the late 1930s drilling techniques were relatively mature and drilling rigs capable of drilling below 15,000 feet (the bottom of the "oil window") were available for drilling on land. Finding the oil and understanding its source were still somewhat problematic and major advances in both fields would be made in the 1950s and 1960s. Artificial seismic techniques would go a long way toward solving the first problem and GC would go a long way toward solving the second; and the petroleum industry would provide both the need and means to do accomplish both. Gas chromatography gave a means of getting a chemical "fingerprint" of an oil sample from one oil-producing area versus another by separating and quantifying the volatile components in the sample. This, for instance, allowed petroleum geologists to determine that all oil in Wyoming comes from just two distinct geological formations (the Phosphoria Formation, about 280 million years old, and the Mowry Formation, about 90 million years old).

Gas chromatography was itself a conceptual derivative of the methods used to refine oil into gasoline, diesel fuel, and so on—a process that was (and is) essentially large-scale distillation. Gas chromatography would vastly reduce the scale and equally would vastly increase the separating power of distillation. The development of GC was intertwined with the development of an underling theoretical framework, which earned Martin and Synge the 1952 Noble Prize in Chemistry and gave rise to the concept of the *theoretical plate*, which will be discussed at length later in the chapter.

Chromatographic instruments began to be developed primarily after World War II, following the rapid success and popularity of GC in the early 1950s. The power of GC was not lost upon researchers in liquid-based separations, and much effort was expended to develop an LC equivalent of GC. Progress was incremental and eventuality was commercialized in the 1960s. Early companies such as Waters Inc. (1958) solved many of the problems of making (and selling) LC systems that could pressurize a mobile phase sufficiently to drive it through a packed column while allowing a small unpressurized sample plug to be introduced, very quickly, into the pressurized system, still giving reasonably reliable and reproducible results.

However, a solid theoretical framework was needed to allow the field to progress. Researchers such as J. Calvin Giddings (to be discussed later in the chapter) and Csaba Horváth in the mid-1960s provided profound insights into the separation process. In 1964, Giddings at the Department of Chemistry at the University of Utah (he would remain there until his untimely death from prostate cancer in 1996 at the age of 66) published a paper in *Analytical Chemistry* entitled *Comparison of the Theoretical Limit of Separating Ability in Gas and Liquid Chromatography.* Here he showed that there were benefits, potentially rivaling GC, an LC system might generate if the packing material consisted of small particles and increased flow pressures were used to drive the mobile phase; this paper would be a pivotal stimulus in the development of HPLC.

11.3 THEORETICAL FUNDAMENTALS OF CHROMATOGRAPHY

11.3.1 Equilibrium-Driven Separation

We will now consider how chromatography actually works. Separations are affected due to differences in analyte's relative affinities for the mobile phase and the stationary phase. To understand more fully the separation process we will now use a concept known as the *partition coefficient* (which has the symbol K). The partition coefficient is the equilibrium distribution of an analyte between the mobile phase and the stationary phase. It can be quantified as the simple ratio of the analyte molar concentration in the stationary phase ($C_{Stationary}$) versus the molar concentration in the mobile phase (C_{Mobile}) or

$$K = C_{Stationary}/C_{Mobile} \quad (11.1)$$

A large K value means the analyte spends more time in the stationary phase and thus spends more time on the column and has a longer retention time (Figure 11.3). The partition coefficient can be assumed to be constant for a compound under a given set of chromatographic conditions and represents the thermodynamic

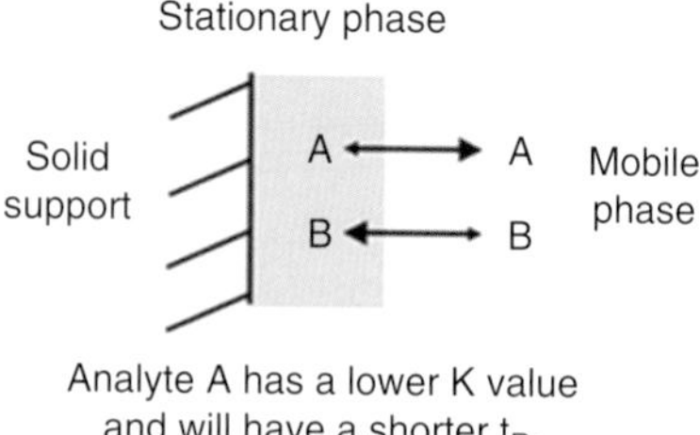

Figure 11.3 A depiction of partition effects in the context of chromatography. Analytes A and B have different partition coefficients, and this will influence how long they spend in the mobile phase relative to time spent in the thin band of stationary phase. Here analyte A has a lower K, and thus will spend more time in the mobile phase versus B and will have a shorter retention time.

contribution to a chromatographic separation (the kinetic contribution will be covered in the discussion of bandbroadening).

A more complete understanding of the explicit thermodynamic nature of K requires an understanding of the concept of *chemical potential.* The chemical potential for a given component i in an open system (in the thermodynamic sense) has the symbol μ_i and represents the intrinsic thermodynamic affinity of the component for a given phase as well as the dilution of the component in that phase. Chemical potential is analogous to gravitational potential energy when we consider, for instance, a rock at various heights above the ground. The larger the difference in chemical potential, the more strongly a component is attracted to a given phase. Just as the rock "seeks" to minimize its energy by falling to the ground, so will a chemical component, when forced to "choose" between the stationary or mobile phase, seek to lower its overall energy. At equilibrium the chemical potential of a given component is equal between the two phases or

$$\mu_i^A = \mu_i^B \quad (11.2)$$

Thus at equilibrium, component i has minimized its chemical potential by distributing between phases A and B. This does not mean, however, that the concentration of component i will be the same in phases A and B, and in fact that will rarely be the case, but only that the chemical potentials are the same. This is the fundamental basis of all chromatographic separations and the partition coefficient is related directly to the difference in the chemical potentials of a component between the stationary and mobile phase; thus all chromatographic separations are firmly rooted in equilibrium thermodynamics. A more thorough discussion of chemical potential would require a long detour into fundamental thermodynamics and is beyond the scope of this chapter. Interested readers are encouraged to consult the short and excellent book, *Unified Separation Science,* by J. Calvin Giddings, which is the best source on this matter (much material in this chapter is drawn directly from *Unified Separation Science*), or many books on physical chemistry (an older text, *Physical Chemistry with Applications to the Life Sciences* by David Eisenberg and Donald Crothers has an excellent discussion of chemical potential, the random walk model, and diffusion).

The interval between when an analyte has been injected on a column and when it exits the column is, as noted before, the retention time (t_R) and for a given set of chromatographic conditions, each analyte in a sample will have a characteristic t_R. The time it takes for the mobile phase, or an entirely unretained analyte, to pass through the column is called t_M or t_0 (*void time*) (Figure 11.2).

The retention time, however, is not a consistent measure of the relative affinity of the compound for the stationary versus the mobile phase and will vary with temperature, flow rate, column size and manufacturer, and so on. What is desired is a normalized measure of retention and thus we define a new term, *capacity factor* (k') (also referred to as the retention factor) where t'_R represents the adjusted retention time.

$$k' = (t_R - t_M)/t_M = t'_R/t_M \qquad (11.3)$$

The capacity factor is readily calculated from a chromatogram and is also related directly to the partition coefficient, where V_s and V_m are the volumes of the stationary phase and mobile phase, respectively.

$$k' = K(V_s/V_m) \qquad (11.4)$$

Provided V_s and V_m are known, this relationship can be used to measure K via chromatographic means very quickly and efficiently when that might otherwise be very difficult.

Here, an important point must be made with regard to Equation (11.4). The actual separative process is dependent on equilibrium thermodynamics, which assumes that sufficient time has elapsed to allow equilibrium to occur; thus there is no temporal component in the separative process. The means by which sample components are actually separated both physically and temporally from one another requires that equilibrium-driven separation be coupled with the physical flow of the mobile phase through the column that allows the differences in the stationary phase/mobile phase partition coefficients for two given analytes, perhaps a very small difference, to be amplified many times over as the two analytes move through the column as illustrated in Figure 11.4. Here, compound A has slightly greater affinity for the mobile phase than compound B, but this is magnified by the many interactions that are possible as the compounds move down the column. Given that many analytical HPLC columns are in the 15 to 25 cm range in length (or longer) and packed with 5 μm spheres, there are many such possible interactions indeed.

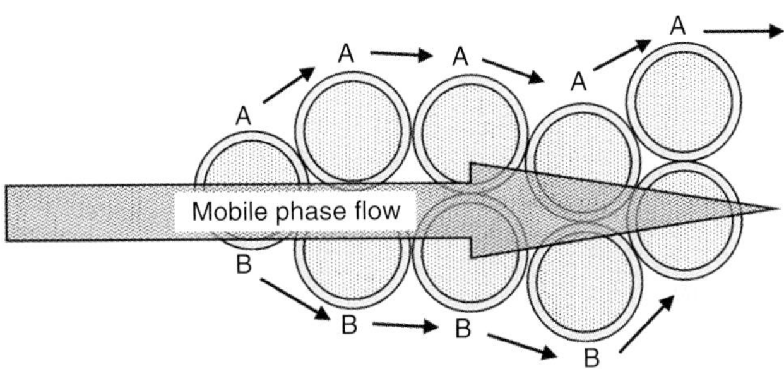

Figure 11.4 The chromatographic process at a microscopic scale. Analytes A and B each interact with the stationary phase (seen as the thin band on the spherical solid support spheres) and the mobile phase differently but not to a great extent. However these minor differences are amplified by the effects of flow. This allows analyte A, which has slightly greater affinity for the mobile phase versus the stationary phase in comparison to analyte B, to move ahead on average. Consider that if a series of 5 μm particles were stacked end-to-end down the length of a 25 cm column the stack would be 50,000 particles long, thus giving many chances for differential interactions.

11.3.2 Bandbroadening

If the fundamental basis of chromatographic separation is equilibrium thermodynamics, the fundamental *degrader* of a separation are *kinetic* processes. The art and science of all separation science, of which chromatography is just an important subset, is to maximize the separation and minimize the degradation. The degradation of the separation is also fundamentally thermodynamically based, but is also magnified by the effects of flow. The most important thermodynamic process for degradation of the separation is entropy, or the intrinsic tendency of all systems to increase their state of disorder.

This is best understood intially by considering the process of diffusion. Chromatographic peaks represent chemical species that have been concentrated in space and time and the process of diffusion will immediately disperse them in space as a function of time. The conceptual basis of diffusion lies in the concept of the *random walk model*, wherein particles/molecules in suspension or solution are being jostled continuously by collisions with other particles or molecules. This is also referred to as *Brownian* motion, and is readily apparent when observing small particles with a microscope, such as some pollen grains, that seem to be in constant and random motion as they gradually spread out from any center of concentration.

The degree of bandbroadening is statistical in nature in that a great many random events occur, some pushing the pollen grains (or analyte molecules) back toward the center of concentration and some away from the center of concentration. It can be shown that this statistical distribution, represented by the *variance*, σ^2, is equal to the product of the square of average step length, l, and the number of steps taken, n, or

$$\sigma^2 = l^2 n \qquad (11.5)$$

The time interval between when a particle has a new collision is Δt, which will give rise to a mean square displacement. The coupling between time and space in diffusion is seen in *Einstein's Diffusion Equation* (Eq. 12.6; not to be confused with a number of Einstein's other equations), where he showed that mean square displacement of a molecule is proportional to the time (Δt) where the proportionality constant is referred to as D, the diffusion coefficient with units of cm^2/sec.

$$\overline{x^2} = 2D \ \ \Delta t \qquad (11.6)$$

Equation (11.7) is a limiting form of Equation (11.6), in which Δt approaches t (a more complete explanation can be found in *Unified Separation Science*).

$$\overline{x^2} = 2Dt \qquad (11.7)$$

The relation between variance, diffusion, and time is shown in Equation (11.8) and follows a logical progression.

$$\sigma^2 = 2Dt \qquad (11.8)$$

However, the diffusion coefficient is not merely a proportionality constant joining bandbroadening and time, but is much more fundamental. This perhaps can be understood by considering the rather unchromatographic experiment of skydiving. If the skyjump starts from a sufficient altitude, the skydiver will soon reach a terminal velocity where the frictional force generated by moving through air exactly balances the gravitational force exerted by the Earth. When the parachute is deployed, the frictional force greatly and rapidly increases and a new, and much lower, terminal velocity is reached until the skydiver gently alights on the ground. Exactly the same phenomenon is seen anytime a particle (or molecule) is induced to accelerate in any viscous medium such as air, water, or a mobile phase. How much friction a particle (or skydiver) will generate depends on both the size and shape of the particle and gives rise to the coefficient of friction, f.

In the mid nineteenth century F.S.W. Stokes theoretically calculated the coefficient of friction for a sphere, f_0, given as Equation (11.9), and known as *Stoke's Law*:

$$f_0 = 6\eta\pi R \tag{11.9}$$

where R is the radius of the particle and η is the solvent *viscosity*. Viscosity is easily understood intuitively as a measure of how "thick" a solvent, solution, or suspension is; blood is thicker (more viscous) both physically (and metaphorically) than water and molasses flows slowly (especially in January) because it is very viscous. Viscosity is relatively easy to measure with a simple apparatus and this has been done for every solvent of interest in chemical separations.

Viscosity, however, is a deeper concept; it is the link between the macroscopic world of skydivers and the microscopic world of chemical separations as exemplified in Stoke's Law. There is clear connection between the motion of a particle (skydiver or analyte molecule) through its respective macroscopic medium (air or mobile phase) and the forces, submicroscopic in the case of the analyte, acting upon it. It represents all the forces that slow down, and eventually cease the acceleration of any body in any medium. Attention must turn now to the forces that impel that acceleration.

Brownian motion can readily be seen with a microscope as the erratic motion of small particles such as pollen grains in liquid suspension. However it has probably never been observed in any collection of bowling bowls in a similar setting—why? The answer lies in the relative forces involved. Observable Brownian motion arises when a pollen grain, for instance, encounters a random asymmetric force from a collection of nearby molecules in its suspension medium. These asymmetric forces must be sufficiently stronger than the many symmetric forces surrounding the grain it constantly encounters, to cause an observable movement of the grain. These symmetric forces, although no different from the asymmetric forces, will essentially cancel out each other and thus there will be no net observable motion. The random asymmetry gives rise to the observable erratic motion of pollen grains. But pollen grains are very small in comparison to bowling balls and the probability of a net asymmetric force arising that is sufficient to nudge a bowling ball is very much lower by many orders of magnitude than that for a pollen grain. Although it is possible (in the sense that any thermodynamically allowed event may be possible) that somewhere in the universe, sometime in the lifetime of the universe, Brownian motion of bowling balls (or something like them) might be observed owing only to a random asymmetric thermodynamic collection of, and then collision of, surrounding molecular species with said bowling balls, it is a highly unlikely event.

Brownian motion is an excellent bridge between the macroscopic world of skydivers and the submicroscopic world of analytic analysis. In this sense, we must consider the ultimate source of Brownian motion; the asymmetric random collisions of particles with the pollen grains. The ultimate source of the energy for these collisions is the heat in the medium in which the pollen grains are suspended. Thus diffusion represents a balance between accelerative forces and restrictive forces, which is seen in Equation (11.10), where T is absolute temperature in *Kelvins* and k_b is *Boltzmann's constant.*

$$D = \frac{k_b T}{f} \tag{11.10}$$

Boltzmann's constant is worth further consideration. In any collection of particles such as might occur in a chromatographic peak, there is a finite number (albeit a very large number) of possible arrangements of those molecules to achieve a given energy state. This number must be proportional to the total entropy, with greater possible numbers of arrangements leading to greater entropy. The proportionality constant between the number of possible arrangements and the entropy is Boltzmann's constant. Thus diffusion in Equation (11.10) reflects the balance between entropic forces ($k_b T$); forces that will disrupt any concentration of matter and the frictional forces that will oppose that disruption.

This returns us full circle to the link between diffusion and bandbroadening. Clearly diffusion will disperse chromatographic peaks. Chromatographic peaks represent chemical species that have been concentrated in space and time and are an inherently transient phenomenon. The shape of a chromatographic peak shows that it has the general form of a Gaussian distribution. Gaussian distributions arise naturally in any truly random process such as diffusion. (For more detail, consult any of variety of statistical texts.) A Gaussian peak is characterized by its *standard deviation* (the square root of variance), σ, which represents the peak width at the point of inflection where the slope of the curve of the peak reaches a maximum (on the upside) and then begins to decline to zero at the peak.

In the expanded form of Equation (11.11) many important elements relating temporally based formation of spatially apparent bandbroadening are evident including temperature (T), analyte size or molecular weight (R), mobile phase viscosity (η), time (t), and spatial distribution (σ).

$$\sigma^2 = 2\left(\frac{k_b T}{6\eta\pi R}\right)t \tag{11.11}$$

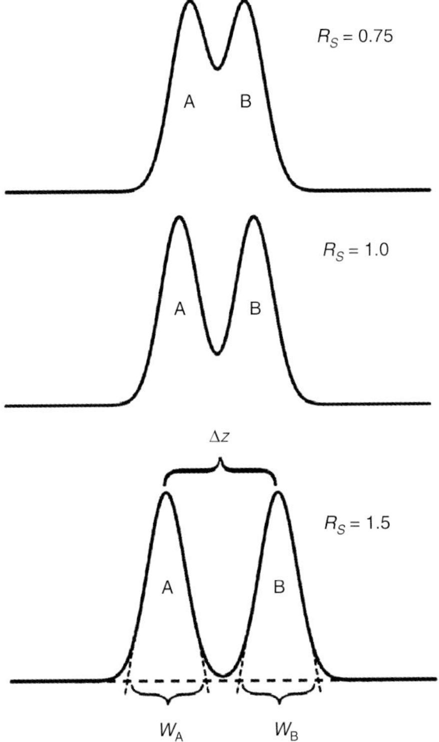

Figure 11.5 Chromatographic resolution in various states. A resolution of 0.75 is quite usable in terms of determining the presence of multiple analyte components but makes quantitation problematic. A resolution of 1.0 is suitable for quantitation. A resolution of 1.5 (approximately a 0.3% statistical peak overlap) is considered to be baseline resolved and allows for essentially complete quantitation in terms of both peak height and area.

Missing from Equation (11.11) is the very important amplifying effect of chromatographic flow. This requires that there be some quantitative means of determining how well, or how poorly, a separative process has achieved its goal. In Figure 11.5, the bottom trace is clearly the result of a better separation than the top two traces. The two bottom chromatographic peaks are said to be *baseline resolved,* in that they are clearly and completely separated from one another, whereas the two upper peaks overlap to a substantial degree, more so in the topmost trace. The degree of overlap is defined by a term referred to as *resolution* or R_s. Resolution can easily (although a little imprecisely) be calculated from a chromatogram based on the retention time and the peak width extrapolated from the relatively straight sides down to the baseline. Two forms of equations for resolution are:

$$R_s = 2((t_R)_B - (t_R)_A)/(W_A + W_B) \tag{11.12}$$

or

$$R_s = \Delta z/(^1/_2(W_A + W_B)) \tag{11.13}$$

Here W_A and W_B are the baseline extrapolated peak widths of peaks A and B, respectively. A resolution of 1.0 (resolution is unitless) is sufficient to give peaks that are separated from one another for reliable quantitation whereas a resolution of 0.75 can be problematic in that respect. A resolution of 1.5 indicates clear baseline resolution. Because peak separation is given a statistical definition, all peaks are assumed to extend to infinity in both directions, but a resolution of 1.5, or 0.3% peak overlap, is the accepted standard for complete resolution.

As with resolution, the ability of a given separative process to divide two analyte species from one another and limit their remixing should have a quantifiable metric; this is indeed so. A separative process that can perform that task well is said to be *efficient,* and this is quantified by a number, N. In a chromatographic separation wherein all the separation occurs on the column, an efficient column is given a high N value. The efficiency of a column is explicitly related to the peak width at the baseline with Equation (11.14); narrower peaks give rise to higher N values.

$$N = 16\left(\frac{t_r}{W}\right)^2 \tag{11.14}$$

The reciprocal of N is a quantity known as H, or very rarely now as *H.E.T.P.* These are all now referred to as *plate height* (H) or *theoretical plate height* or *height equivalent of (or to) a theoretical plate (H.E.T.P.).* The reasons for the older nomenclature can be found in the scientific literature dealing with distillation in general and petroleum distillation in particular, as discussed earlier, and now have much less relevance to a deeper understanding of separation science.

Plate height is very important both practically and theoretically; representing the most universal measure of bandbroadening. A peak moving down a column at a uniform velocity of v_p, will transverse, in time t, a distance of X, or

$$X = v_p t \tag{11.15a}$$

or

$$t = X/v_p \tag{11.15b}$$

Substituting into Equation (11.8) gives a modified expression for σ^2 in Equation (11.16).

$$\sigma^2 = \left(\frac{2D}{v_P}\right)X \tag{11.16}$$

This equation demonstrates that the distance traveled (X) down the column is directly proportional to the amount of zone broadening (σ^2) acquired along the journey. The ratioed proportionality constant, $2D/v_p$, reflects the role of diffusion and flow in contributing to bandbroadening. An efficient column will have a low H and thus a band will be able to travel a long distance (X) and generate little bandbroadening (σ^2). Plate height can now be defined by Equation (11.17).

$$H = \frac{\sigma^2}{X} \tag{11.17}$$

Plate height is often visualized as a chromatographic column consisting of a stack of physical plates, each of which contributes to the separation such that a column with "more or smaller plates" will give a better separation. This model, derived as previously noted from petroleum distillation columns, is not reflective of the continuous processes present in chromatography but is nonetheless conceptually useful and will yield useful Equations (11.18) that relate X to plate height (H) and column efficiency (N).

$$N = \frac{X}{H} \tag{11.18}$$

A simple substitution of Equation (11.17) into Equation (11.18) yields the important relationships

$$N = \frac{X^2}{\sigma^2} = \left(\frac{X}{\sigma}\right)^2 \quad \text{(11.19}a\text{ and 11.19}b\text{)}$$

and a further substitution of Equation (11.16) into Equation (11.17) yields Equation (11.20).

$$H = \left(\frac{2D}{v_P}\right) \tag{11.20}$$

This means that as an analyte band migrates down a column, the band acquires broadening for each conceptual down the column. Ideally we want a very small X value that will give a high N and the ultimate separation will be efficient. Both N and H are fundamental metrics of separation efficiency and readily related to their thermodynamic origins by their connection via the diffusion coefficient. In the limiting form when X is L we get the fundamental Equation (11.21).

$$N = \frac{L}{H} \tag{11.21}$$

The many relationships recently discussed can be collected in the following summary form (with the substitutions left as an exercise).

$$H = \frac{\sigma^2}{L} = \frac{l^2 n}{L} = \frac{L}{N} = \left(\frac{2D}{v}\right) \quad \text{(Summary Equation Series)}$$

This series shows the various relationships between the fundamental metrics of separation efficiency, N and H, diffusion, mobile phase flow rate, v, random walk step-length, l, step number, n, and column length, L.

11.3.2.1 *Components of Bandbroadening*

Bandbroadening is a very complex process but can be dissected into four essential components:

- Molecular or Longitudinal Diffusion (D)
- Eddy Diffusion (ED)
- Resistance to Mass Transfer (RMT)
- Extra-column Bandbroadening (ExC)

Each one contributes additively to the final Gaussian-like shape of a chromatographic peak because variances (σ^2) are additive (this is a fundamental principal of statistics and can be found more fully covered in standard statistical texts). Thus we can expect an overall equation describing total bandbroadening ($\sigma^2{}_T$) of a chromatographic peak to have the following form. (Note: the use of $\sigma^2{}_D$, $\sigma^2{}_{ED}$ etc. to represent the components of bandbroadening is not a general standard use in separation theory but is used herein for descriptive purposes only.)

$$\sigma_T^2 = \sigma_D^2 + \sigma_{ED}^2 + \sigma_{RMT}^2 + \sigma_{ExC}^2 \tag{11.22}$$

We will now sequentially replace these σ^2 values with values that reflect the physical values involved in a separation. Understanding these physical values allows them to be manipulated and thus the separation to be optimized.

Longitudinal Diffusion Longitudinal diffusion is simple diffusion as discussed previously. It occurs whenever chemical species are concentrated together, such as in a chromatographic peak, and are given time to diffuse away from one another. As $\sigma^2{}_T$ and diffusion are directly related to one another (see Eq. 11.8), the longer a peak stays on the column, the broader it will get (ignore for the moment the fact that the separation is developing as the peak moves down the column). Thus, the $\sigma^2{}_D$ will get larger, and bandbroadening worse, with analytes that have high diffusion coefficients and/or remain on the column for longer times showing increasing bandbroadening.

Although it is possible to reduce the analyte's diffusion coefficient by either increasing the mobile phase viscosity or reducing the mobile phase temperature (which also tends to increase the mobile phase viscosity), this has proven to be a generally ineffective and impractical means for a wide variety of reasons and is rarely done in either HPLC or GC. (In fact the mobile phase or carrier gas is often heated in HPLC and nearly always in GC.)

Manipulating the time an analyte spends on a column can be, and often is, as simple as adjusting the mobile phase or carrier gas flow rate by turning a dial or pressing a key. Because the mobile phase is usually much less viscous than the stationary phase, the amount of bandbroadening from longitudinal diffusion can be considered only in terms of diffusion in the mobile phase (correction terms exists for diffusion in the stationary phase). In this context, the longitudinal diffusion contribution to bandbroadening is shown in Equation (11.23), where D_m is the diffusion coefficient in the mobile phase, L is the column length, and v is the mobile phase flow rate.

$$\sigma^2 = \frac{2D_m L}{v} \tag{11.23}$$

The diffusion coefficient must be reduced in packed columns because there are obstructions that prevent simple linear diffusion. This is given a dimensionless measure as an *obstructive factor*, γ, with a value of approximately 0.6. Simple substitution into the Summary Equation Series gives the plate height contribution from longitudinal diffusion, H_D, which is conventionally represented as Equation (11.24), which shows the inverse proportionally between the contribution to bandbroadening and mobile phase flow rate where B is a conventional constant.

$$H_D = \frac{2\gamma D_m}{\upsilon} = \frac{B}{\upsilon} \tag{11.24}$$

Eddy Diffusion The second major term contributing to bandbroadening is *eddy diffusion*. This term arises because in a packed HPLC column, the mobile phase and any entrained analyte molecules may follow many different physical paths as they wind their way past the packing material. Although this may seem very difficult to model given the inherent complex nature of an analyte molecule's path, good generalization can be obtained and understood in terms of mobile phase flowrate, particle diameter, analyte diffusion coefficient, and particle diameter.

The first thing to recognize is that eddy diffusion is also fundamentally a statistical problem that can be best understood on the basis of the random walk. Particle diameter is of particular importance here, because, unlike the infinitesimal step lengths in the diffusional random walk, the particle diameter characterizes the step length in developing an expression for eddy diffusion.

At two conceptual extremes, we might envision that there are only two flow paths an analyte might take as it passes down the column, a slow path and fast path, and that at times the analyte may jump from one to another. There are also two conceptual extremes in traveling between the flow streams: (1) diffusion of the analyte molecule between flow streams and (2) a mobile phase flow-mediated transfer between flow streams. The former will be slow in comparison to the latter because diffusion mediated processes are much slower. In the case of eddy diffusion, flow-mediated transfer will overwhelmingly dominate the bandbroadening process.

To obtain a more quantitative understanding of eddy diffusion, consider that a molecule in a given path will proceed some average distance/time S, before it will transition into a new (slower or faster) path with each change from a slow to fast or fast to slow path representing a random walk step. In a column of length L, there will be n such steps (Eq. 11.25) with a length of l (Eq. 11.26):

$$n = \frac{L}{S} \tag{11.25}$$

$$l = \frac{\Delta\upsilon}{\upsilon_f} S \tag{11.26}$$

where v_f is the velocity of a fast (or slow) track analyte molecule and Δv is the difference between the average flow velocity and v_f. Because Δv and v_f are on the same scale in terms of particle size diameters, mobile phase flow rate, and such, they can be scaled together and treated as a constant.

The value of S is directly proportional to the column particle size, d_p. Noting that and substituting Equations (11.25) and (11.26) into $H = l^2 n/L$ from the Summary Equation Series we find that

$$H_{ED} = \lambda' dp = A \tag{11.27}$$

where λ' is grouped constant that reflects, in part, how well a column is packed. (This is a simplified version of λ'; a more detailed discussion can be found in *Unified Separation Science*.) Because a small plate height is desired, manufactures strive to pack columns in a very uniform fashion with very uniform and small particles, typically spheres in the 5 to 3 μm range.

Resistance to Mass Transfer The third element of bandbroadening is the mass transfer term. It results when an analyte molecule diffuses into the stationary phase. The diffusion coefficient of the analyte in the stationary phase will generally be considerably less than in the mobile phase and thus an analyte molecule will lag behind its fellow analyte molecules still entrained in the mobile phase. This process is also of course statistical in nature as the molecule will eventually leave the stationary phase, but some of the other analyte molecules are now delayed in the stationary phase. As such its magnitude should be directly proportional to the mobile phase flow rate, v, and inversely proportional to the diffusion coefficient of the analyte in the stationary phase, D_s. It should also be related to the thickness of the stationary phase, d. Because diffusing into and out the stationary phase is a random walk process, the time needed is exactly analogous to $\sigma^2 = 2DT$ and this time delay is magnified by effects of flow. Thus the plate height contribution from mass transfer will also be proportional to d^2. The squared dependence makes it particularly necessary to reduce the stationary phase thickness to minimize bandbroadening from mass transfer effects. The final form of the equation for H_{RMT} is in Equation (11.28) and a more common representation is in Equation (11.29), where C_s is the stationary phase plate height coefficient.

$$H_{RMT} = \mathrm{Const}\frac{d^2\upsilon}{D_S} \tag{11.28}$$

$$H_{RMT} = C_S\upsilon \tag{11.29}$$

Extracolumn Bandbroadening Extracolumn bandbroadening arises from processes independent of the separation process. It might arise, for instance, if there were a mixing volume between the end of column and the detector or if the sample was not introduced as a concentrated plug. Instrument manufacturers have greatly minimized extracolumn effects. This can be undone by end-users and thus actual hands-on training is *highly* recommended for any person intending to do HPLC analysis; it is possible for an untrained user to do considerable damage to a multithousand dollar instrument in a relatively short amount of time. For instance, although in general, only minimal lengths of very narrow-bore (0.005″ to 0.007″) tubing should be used to connect the column to the injector and to the detector(s) to minimize extracolumn bandbroadening, an example of that damage that could be done would be to connect a fluorescent detector "upstream" (before) and in tandem or series with a UV/Visible light absorbance detector using this narrow-bore tubing. Since many fluorescent detectors have optical cells that are delicate and do not tolerate high back-pressure, they might easily crack in such a circumstance requiring many hundred of dollars in repair costs (I personally know of at least three cases of something similar happening).

The van Deemter Curve and Equation The total plate height for a separation is equal to the sum of all its component plate heights. One such sum is known as the *van Deemter Equation*, originally published in 1956 by van Deemter and colleagues. In terms of the bandbroadening expression presented herein it takes the form where the first term represents bandbroadening contributions from eddy diffusion, the second term represents contributions from longitudinal diffusion, and the third term represents contributions from resistance to mass transfer.

$$H = A + \frac{B}{\upsilon} + C_S\upsilon \tag{11.30}$$

This is only one of a number of similar equations that relate summed plate heights to flow rates. It is generally most valid at high flow rates but is also the most well known, and when expressed schematically, the form of the van Deemter Curve (Figure 11.6) gives an excellent feeling for how variations in flow rate can effect separation efficiency.

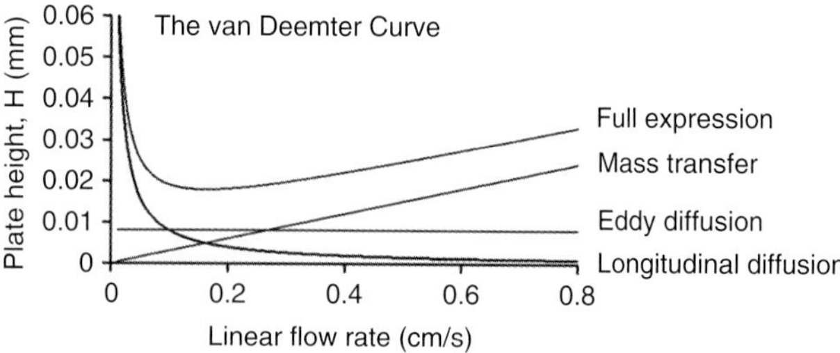

Figure 11.6 The van Deemter Equation plotted as a curve. The full expression is the sum of the three individual components. Eddy diffusion, the "A" term, a constant, does not change as the mobile linear flow rate changes. Bandbroadening from longitudinal diffusion steadily decreases the shorter the analyte remains on the column, in other words, the faster the flow rate is. Contributions from resistance to mass transfer of the analyte into and out of the stationary phase increase linearly with the mobile phase flow rate. The separation will be most efficient at the flow rate that minimizes plate height, in this case about 0.1 cm/s.

Contributions from longitudinal diffusion are greatest as the flow rate approaches zero at which point, of course, any separation would cease and the band would merely spread out gradually. Eddy diffusion (A) has no flow-related component but does contribute an absolute limit on the how small the overall plate height can be. Finally, the mass transfer term ($C_S\upsilon$) contributes increasing amounts of bandbroadening as the mobile phase flowrate increases.

Both mathematically and obviously graphically, it is possible to determine an optimal flow rate that minimizes bandbroadening. Mathematically this is easily obtained from taking the first derivative of the van Deemter Equation with respect to flow rate and setting it equal to zero or

$$\frac{dH}{d\upsilon} = -\frac{B}{\upsilon^2} + C = 0 \tag{11.31}$$

This gives an optimal flowrate of

$$\upsilon_{opt} = \left(\frac{B}{C}\right)^{1/2} \tag{11.32}$$

and a minimum plate height of

$$H_{min} = 2(BC)^{1/2} \tag{11.33}$$

11.4 ANALYTICAL SEPARATIONS IN PRACTICE

Manufacturers have taken this knowledge and designed columns to function under optimal conditions in a relatively limited range of flow rates. For instance most analytical HPLC columns work best around 1 mL/min and are rarely used outside the range of 0.5 to 2.0 mL/min. The column efficiency (for a given t_R) and often a "test" chromatogram are usually included with the column when it is purchased. The test is run by the manufacturer under a specified set of conditions with a small number (4 or 5) of readily obtained analytes to demonstrate to the purchaser that the column is performing as promised. It is a wise idea to periodically rerun those same conditions/analytes through the life of the column to monitor its performance and indicate when it should be retired. These indications include high backpressure (generally above 2500 to 3000 psi), substantial increases or decreases in retention time, peak doubling wherein a single known analyte appears to elute as two poorly resolved peaks or a "shoulder," loss of peak symmetry (i.e., fronting or tailing), very broad peaks or flat peaks.

Many major users of HPLC, particularly pharmaceutical companies working in an FDA regulated environment, will log every injection on a column through the column's lifetime and will have specific criteria (called Standard Operating Practices or SOPs) to indicate when a column should be retired. Many HPLC instruments also have bar code readers and the columns have corresponding bar codes to insure that documentation is correct. Major users will also maintain detailed and auditable records of the entire instrument life of any major instrument, including HPLC instruments, documenting all major (and minor) repairs and maintained procedures and will, usually annually, have instruments recertified to insure they are operating as originally specified.

For the actual user, the desire is to obtain well-resolved peaks in a short time period. How this might be done requires an understanding of how column properties, analyte equilibrium properties, t_R, and resolution are interrelated. To do this, first we will introduce a new term, α or the *selectivity factor*, which represents the equilibrium distribution between two analytes, A and B.

$$\alpha = (K_B/K_A) = (k'_B/k'_A) = (t'_B)_B/(t'_R)_A \qquad (11.34)$$

Assuming the peak widths are approximately the same, resolution can be expressed in terms of plate number, α and k' as

$$R_s = (N^{1/2}/4)((\alpha - 1)/\alpha)(k'_B/(1 + k'_B)) \qquad (11.35)$$

This equation can be used to direct the process of *methods development*, or how one goes about obtaining a suitable separation with a suitable resolution.

The first approach we might take is to increase the plate number. This could be done by optimizing mobile phase flowrate but, as noted, column manufacturers already have designed columns to operate at an optimal flowrate, thus little improvement could be expected by this means. We could also obtain a column with a lower overall plate number, perhaps a better packed column with a lower H_{ED}. However, for a given particle size, most commercial columns are fairly competitive in terms of efficiency and cost (a well-packed conventional HPLC column with a 4.6 mm internal diameter packed with 5 μm spheres can reach, and at times exceed, plate counts of 100,000 plates per meter, and a few HPLC columns much exceed 25 cm in length) and thus to substantially increase column efficiency the column will either need to be longer or have a smaller particle diameter. Increasing the column length (or linking two columns in series) will linearly increase N but with the disadvantages of increasing the total run time and the system backpressure.

It is also possible to use a column with a smaller particle size such as 3 μm (or even 1 μm) versus 5 μm. The reduction in particle size will typically yield a column that is twice as efficient without increasing (in principal) t_R although it will increase backpressure. This is a very common approach despite the higher costs (usually significantly higher) of the reduced-particle size columns. However, much of the increase in efficiency might be lost due to extracolumn bandbroadening in older instruments not designed for reduced-particle size columns (or in poorly designed or poorly operated newer instruments). However, perhaps the greatest disadvantage in attempting to improve resolution is the square-root dependence of resolution on N, which means doubling N will increase R_s by only a factor of 1.4.

An alternative strategy would be to increase k'. This might be done by altering the temperature, and though this is almost universally done in GC, it is, as noted previously, rarely done in HPLC. The alternative strategies are to alter either the mobile phase or the stationary phase, and these strategies are used widely in separations and drug bioanalysis.

11.4.1 HPLC Stationary Phases

To understand this strategy, we must understand the types of HPLC columns and their corresponding stationary phases available from the many commercial vendors. Early chromatographic columns were very similar to those employed by Tswett, packed with various inorganic materials such as silica and alumina. The surface chemistries of these materials are polar in that they attract, and polar compounds were typically used with nonpolar organic solvents as mobile phases. These types of column are referred as *normal phase* columns. Later in the development of HPLC a new type of stationary phase was - developed, *reversed-phase (RP)* columns, which both revolutionized the field and have come to dominate it. Reversed-phase columns are very simple in concept. The actual stationary phase itself is very commonly a single monolayer of an alkyl chain covalently linked, or *bonded phase*, to the surface of solid supporting beads.

Although there are many variations in terms of surface chemistry among the many manufacturers, the basic concept is illustrated in highly diagrammatic fashion in Figure 11.7. Depicted in this figure (obviously not to scale) is the most common alkyl bonded reversed-phase known as C_{18}, or octadecylsilane (ODS). The name derives from 18 carbon length of the alkyl chain. This is a very nonpolar phase and typically is used with mobile phases containing water and varying proportions of an organic modifier such as methanol or acetonitrile.

Manufacturers have developed a large variety of different stationary phases with different properties.

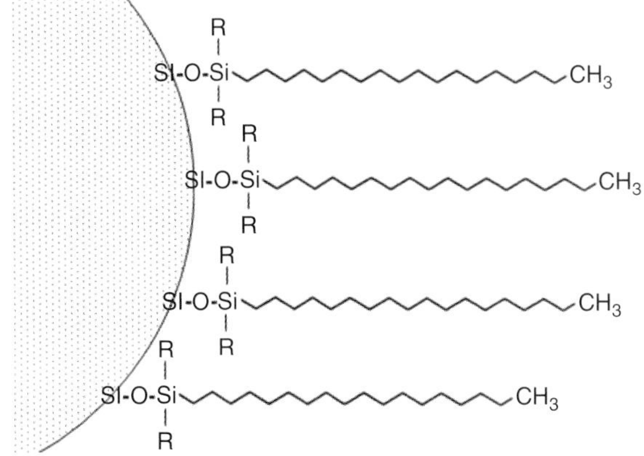

Figure 11.7 A highly diagrammatic representation of a C_{18} reversed-phase stationary phase. Carbon chains (18 long) are covalently bound to a silica support bead forming essentially a monolayer. The specific chemical details, particularly at the silica surface, vary from manufacturer to manufacturer. Although silica itself is very polar, the C_{18} mono-layer is the actual stationary phase, giving the column a very nonpolar characteristic.

Some of the more popular ones are phases with shorter alkyl chains such as C_8 (8 carbons) or C_4 (4 carbons). Specialized columns with chiral stationary phase are also available for the separation of enantiomers (mirror image isomers). Bonded stationary phases, which are polar, also exist; common ones are cyano, phenyl, and amino columns, which have respectively CN, phenyl, and NH_2 groups bonded to the silica support via short alkyl linker chains. These latter columns as well as HPLC columns packed with unbonded silica all have specialty uses but it is estimated approximately 80% of all HPLC separations are done using some form of reversed-phase, most commonly C_{18} because of its versatility and reproducibility.

With Figure 11.7 in mind, as well as previous discussions of the partition coefficient, it is easy to see how a separation might proceed. Analyte molecules can partition into the stationary phase; this is often referred to as *partition chromatography*. The relative affinities for the analyte molecule between the stationary phase and mobile phase will be strongly influenced by the nature of the mobile phase. As noted, in the case of reversed-phase, HPLC can have varying amount of an organic modifier such as methanol. Decreasing the amount of methanol, for instance, will cause all analytes to elute at longer times and thus have greater k' values. Similarly, using a column with a more nonpolar stationary phase, such a C_{18} instead of a C_8, would have much the same effect. However, it is nearly always easier to alter the mobile phase than to use a different column, and this is overwhelmingly the preferred choice.

This returns the discussion to how to optimize resolution by optimizing k'. A plot of resolution versus k' from Equation (11.35) (Figure 11.8) shows that very modest increases in k' can pay a great dividend in increased resolution, but a point of diminishing returns is rapidly reached and greater increases in k' lead to little improvement in resolution but result in a longer chromatographic run.

The alternative is to alter the selectivity factor between two analytes by either changing the mobile phase or the stationary phase. In an analogs fashion, a plot of resolution versus α from Equation (11.35) (Figure 11.9) shows that very modest increases in α can greatly increase resolution but a point of diminishing returns is also rapidly reached.

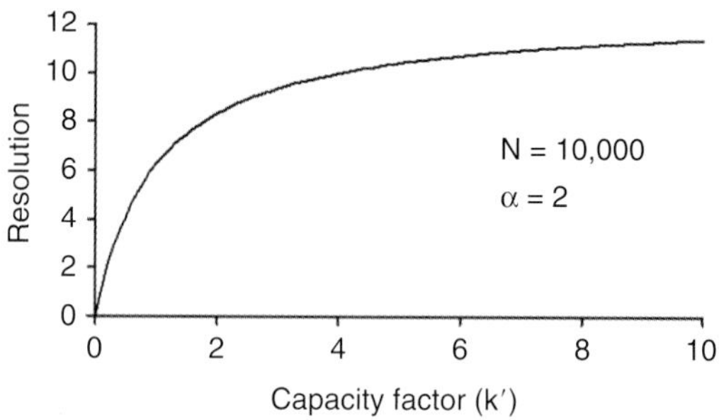

Figure 11.8 The relationship between capacity factor and resolution from a plot of Equation (11.35). A column efficiently of 10,000 theoretical plates and a selectivity factor of 2 was used. There is great increase in resolution for modest increases in capacity factor but this advantage is soon lost.

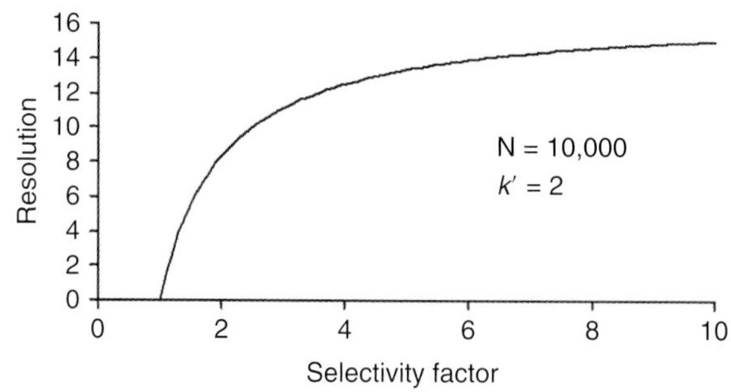

Figure 11.9 The relationship between the selectivity factor and resolution from a plot of Equation (11.35). A column efficiently of 10,000 theoretical plates and a capacity factor of 2 was used. There is great increase in resolution for modest increases in the selectivity factor but this advantage is soon lost.

11.4.2 Gradient versus Isocratic Elution

Isocratic elution refers to eluting analytes without changing the composition of the mobile phase during the course of the chromatographic run. Gradient elution refers to altering the composition of the mobile phase during the run. Isocratic elution is generally preferred; it gives more stable detector baselines and fewer artifactal peaks, can be performed with simpler and less expensive instrumentation and gives more reproducible results. Gradient elution has one great advantage, however; it allows the selectivity factor between two or more analytes to be altered during the run.

This can best be illustrated by an example. Figure 11.10 shows three chromatograms with three pairs of peaks, early eluting (1 and 2), middle eluting (3 and 4), and late eluting (5 and 6). These pairs for instance could be three pairs of chemically related compounds that are similar in polarity being separated via reversed-phase HPLC. In the top chromatogram (A) the mobile phase, for instance, might be composed of 75% water and 25% methanol. Here all are clearly resolved from one another but the chromatographic run time is too long and peaks 5 and 6 will be poorly quantitated because they are very broad. To solve this particular problem, the amount of organic modifier in the mobile phase could be increased to perhaps 75% methanol (CH_3OH) (and 25% water) for isocratic elution to sharply reduce the retention times of the peaks 5 and 6. However, this introduces another problem, the coelution (peak 1 and 2) and near coelution (peaks 3 and 4) seen in chromatogram (B). The attempted isocratic

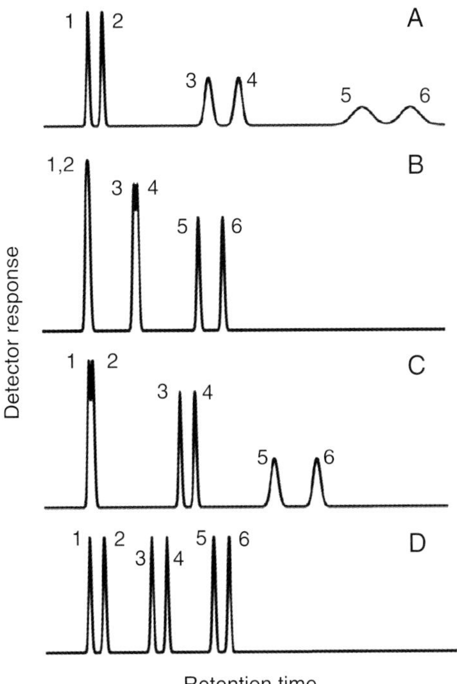

Figure 11.10 Diagrammatic illustration of the process of gradient elution in HPLC. In chromatogram (A) the mobile phase has a relatively low amount of organic modifier (25% methanol and 75% water) and isocratic elution is used. Although all peaks are well resolved, peaks 5 and 6 are too broad for good quantitation and the overall run time too long. Attempting to solve that problem isocratically by increasing the methanol concentration fails in both chromatograms (B) (25% water:75% methanol) and (C) 50% water:50% methanol) because of coelution. The use of gradient elution however, wherein the methanol content of the mobile phase is gradually increased from 25% to 75% over the course of the run, succeed in giving both good resolution and a reasonable run time as seen in chromatogram (D).

compromise of a mobile phase of 50% water and 50% methanol seen in chromatogram (C) still has peaks 1 and 2 nearly coeluting while peaks 5 and 6 still have long retention times.

The solution to this problem of having both adequate resolution and reasonable retention times lies in altering the composition of the mobile phase during the course of the run. By starting the run with a mobile phase that has a relatively small amount of organic modifier, perhaps 25% methanol and 75% water, peaks 1 and 2 will elute while still resolved. As the amount of the organic modifier is gradually increased, perhaps to 75% methanol (and 25% water), peaks 3 and 4 eluted followed by peaks 5 and 6, while retaining good resolution and reasonable retention time as seen in chromatogram (D).

11.4.3 Instrumental Aspects of HPLC

Many sophisticated HPLC instruments are currently manufactured and there are many variations in design and operation. All instruments do share some commonalities. First, all must have pumps (also know as solvent delivery systems) that can force the mobile phase through the column with its dense packing of very fine particles. This can require pressures from about 200 to 6000 pounds per square inch (psi; some other common pressure units are pascals (Pa) and atmospheres (atm); 1 atm = 14.7 psi and 1000 Pa = 0.145 psi) depending on the column. To accomplish this, a number of designs have been developed. Most instrument manufacturers now use a high precision piston design (Figure 11.11). In this design, unpressurized mobile phase enters a small piston chamber via the so-called *inlet check valve* from a solvent reservoir. Small pistons, often of synthetic sapphire, bring the mobile phase to high pressure in the piston chamber and force it out through the so-called *outlet check valve* and eventually through the column. Inlet check valves are designed to close off the flow of mobile phase from the solvent reservoir when the piston enters the piston chamber, thus preventing the mobile phase from returning to the solvent reservoir. Conversely, the outlet check valve will open as the piston enters the piston chamber and the mobile phase is pressurized and then forced through the column.

A common check valve design is to have a small synthetic ruby bead contained in a small cylinder that composes the check valve. On one end of the cylinder there is a centrally perforated funnel-like ceramic disk on which the bead can seat and block liquid flow. At the other end of the check valve, the ball can seat on a small ceramic highly porous disk (Figure 11.11). In the inlet check valve, as the piston enters the chamber and pressurizes the mobile phase, the bead will seat on the funnel-like disk and prevent any back-flow while the outlet check valve will open and allow the mobile phase to be forced through the column. As the piston is withdrawn from the chamber, backpressure will cause the outlet check valve to close and allow fluid to enter the piston chamber from the solvent reservoir via the inlet check valve. The cycle then repeats.

The sinusoidal nature of the piston movement causes pump pulsations. These both degrade the separation and can substantially decrease detector sensitivity by increasing undesirable detector signal (noise). To reduce this, several designs are employed. These include using two pistons that operate 180 degrees out of phase with one another (a double reciprocating design) so that the pump pulsations partially cancel each other out. A second common design is to have the intake stroke very short and fast (Fast Fill design) compared to the delivery stroke. In this design, the mobile thus is delivered mostly in a relatively steady fashion as the piston enters the piston chamber. The logical extension of this is a relatively uncommon design in which a single large piston or high pressure "syringe" that can hold hundreds of mLs of mobile phase is used. The mobile phase is delivered steadily from the syringe throughout the course of one or many chromatographic runs until empty. Because the contents of the syringe cannot be changed easily or rapidly (thus no gradient elution), this design is limited to specialized applications. A further design

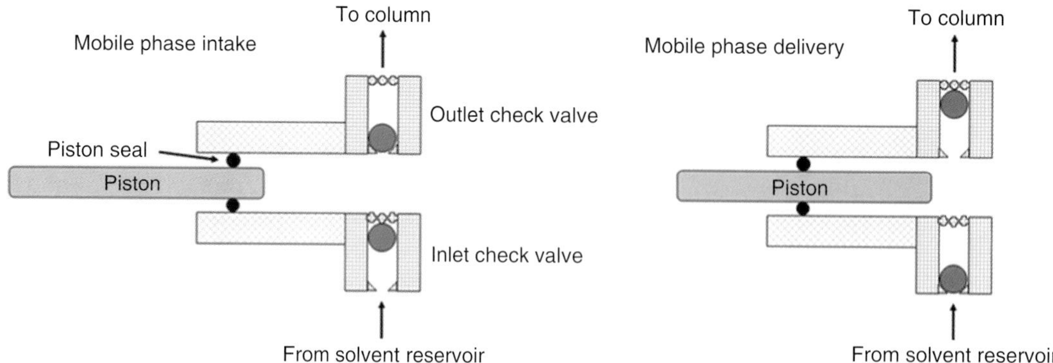

Figure 11.11 Schematic representation of a piston-driven HPLC pump. Check valves are designed to open and close in response to pressure. They do so by having fluid flow move a small ball, usually of synthetic ruby, from a place where it is firmly seated on a ceramic funnel-like cylindrical element that blocks fluid flow, to a position where it can rest against a highly porous screen-like ceramic element. During the intake phase of the pump stroke, as the piston withdraws from the piston chamber, back pressure (i.e., fluid pressure between the outlet check valve and the ultimate outlet of the detector(s)) forces the outlet check valve to close and allow mobile phase to enter the piston chamber. During the delivery phase, the piston enters the piston chamber and pressurizes it. This causes the inlet check valve to close and allows the outlet check valve to open once the back pressure in the system is exceeded by the fluid pressure in the piston chamber. This allows the mobile phase to be driven through the system. The piston seals prevent fluid from leaking past the piston into the piston drive motor mechanism.

employs a very fast pump cycle (seconds rather than the tens of seconds for other designs) combined with a small volume piston chamber. The high frequency pump pulsation noise is dealt with more easily by other means such as downstream pulse dampers. The latter devices employ some type of spring-like element such as a coil of thin-walled flexible tubing that can absorb some of the pulsation energy and release it as the pulse decreases. Pulse dampers can be employed on any HPLC instrument although they result in the introduction of a large fluid volume between the piston chamber(s) and the column. In isocratic elution this is of little consequence, but in gradient elution this may lead to poor reproducibly in gradient formation.

11.4.4 Gradient Formation

There are two basic strategies in forming a gradient: *high pressure mixing* and *low pressure mixing*. The first is accomplished by two or more independent high pressure pumps feeding different mobile phase components into a central mixing chamber at a point before the injector and the column. By varying the volumetric flow rates of the two high pressure pumps over time, the composition of the mobile phase can be changed in a reproducible fashion and gradient elution can be achieved. The second strategy has multiple mobile phase components entering a central mixing chamber before the high pressure pump. In this case the feed "pump" is usually gravity (although modest gas pressure sometimes is used to augment gravity). A simple valve is opened and closed for a specified period of time, thus allowing a certain percentage of a given mobile phase to enter the mixing chamber in a given time period (Figure 11.12).

In high pressure mixing, two (rarely more than two) independent high pressure pumps each deliver a mobile phase component to a central mixer. To control the final mobile phase compositions delivered to the column, the volumetric flow rate of each pump is controlled via computer or microprocessor. Thus, as earlier, an isocratic mobile phase of 75% water and 25% methanol delivered to the column at 1 mL/min would be obtained by having Pump A deliver water at 0.75 mL/min and Pump B deliver methanol at 0.25 mL/min. To effect the gradient as before, the flow rates of Pump A would be smoothly and continuously reduced from 0.75 mL/min to 0.25 mL/min over the course of the run whereas that of Pump B would increase from 0.25 mL/min to 0.75 mL/min over the same time period.

After the mobile phase exits the column, possibly carrying analytes, it will almost always go through one or more detectors (the only exception likely would be that the mobile phase might be collected in a fraction collector as might be done in preparative chromatography). Detection is the topic of the next section.

11.4.5 Detectors in HPLC

In this section, the most common (and some of the less common) HPLC detectors will be described, including their various advantages and disadvantages (for a summary see Table 11.2).

All chromatographic detectors, both for HPLC and GC (as well as for CE), seek to detect analytes based on some molecular property, which differs between the analyte and the carrier or mobile phase. An HPLC detector, for instance, might detect an analyte

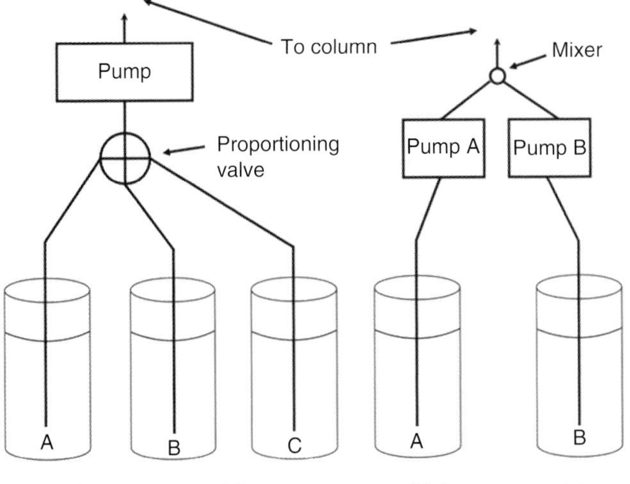

Figure 11.12 A schematic diagram illustrating the difference between low pressure mixing and high pressure mixing in mobile phase gradient formation. In low pressure mixing, mobile phase components drawn from solvent reservoirs A and B are brought, usually by gravity feed, to a proportioning valve. Reservoir A might perhaps hold water while reservoir B holds methanol. An isocratic mobile phase of 50% water and 50% methanol would be formed by having the valve open to A one-half the time and B one-half the time (with a valve switching time of a second or less). To form a gradient that changes the mobile phase composition from 75% water and 25% methanol to 25% water and 75% methanol (a common gradient in HPLC) the flow from reservoirs A or B would be altered for given amounts of time. Thus, the valve, under computer or microprocessor control, would initially be open on average for A for 75% of the time and for B for 25% of the time. The gradient would be formed by slowly altering the average amount of time input from A is open relative to input from B. Thus, at the end of the gradient, B would be open 75% of the time and A would be open 25% of the time with a smooth and continuous transition in between. The proportioning valve usually has the option for inputs from three (ternary; in this case it would be from reservoir C) or four (quaternary) solvents although in practice anything beyond a binary (two solvent) gradient is rarely used to effect a separation.

molecule because it absorbs ultraviolet (UV) or visible radiation at a given wavelength much more than mobile phase does (this is a very common HPLC detector and is discussed in more detail later) or it might detect analytes because they fluoresce, which is to say they emit light when exposed to light of a shorter (more energetic) wavelength; these are the processes of emission and excitation, respectively.

Detectors vary very widely in many important aspects including sensitivity and limit of detection (LOD) (see the following Glossary), lower limit of quantitation (LLOQ), dynamic range, selectivity, price, convenience, operating expense, principal of operation, and universality (their ability to detect any analyte). The ideal detector would be very sensitive, accurate, precise, stable, highly selective (or universal depending on the application); have a very wide linear dynamic range; be inexpensive, easy, and inexpensive to operate; and be robust and reliable. There is of course no such detector, and, as in everything, there are trade-offs.

11.4.5.1 A Glossary of Bioanalytical Terms (Source: Adapted from US Food and Drug Administration Guidance for Industry: Bioanalytical Method Validation)

Accuracy: The degree of closeness of the determined value to the nominal or known true value under prescribed conditions.

Precision: The closeness of agreement (degree of scatter) between a series of measurements obtained from multiple sampling of the same homogenous sample under the prescribed conditions.

Limit of detection (LOD): The lowest concentration of an analyte that the bioanalytical procedure can reliably differentiate from background noise.

Lower limit of quantification (LLOQ): The lowest amount of an analyte in a sample that can be quantitatively determined with suitable precision and accuracy.

Upper limit of quantification (ULOQ): The highest amount of an analyte in a sample that can be quantitatively determined with precision and accuracy. Its opposite is universality.

Quantification range: The range of concentration, including ULOQ and LLOQ, that can be reliably and reproducibly quantified with accuracy and precision through the use of a concentration-response relationship between the detector signal and the analyte concentration. If the relationship is linear, then the concentration range is the *linear dynamic range*.

Selectivity: The ability of the bioanalytical method to measure and differentiate the analytes in the presence of components that may be expected to be present.

Table 11.2 Comparison of HPLC Detectors (Adapted from Cunico et al., 1998)

Detector	Universality	Sensitivity	LOD (g)	Linear Dynamic Range	Cost
Fixed UV/Vis	Medium	High	10^{-10} to 10^{-11}	10^5	Low
PDA	Medium	High	3 ppb	>2 AU	Medium
Fluorescence	Low	High to very high	10^{-12}	10^3	Medium
MS	High	Medium	10^{-10}	Varies	High

11.4.5.2 The Ultraviolet-Visible Light Detector (the UV-Vis Detector)

The UV-Vis detector is one the most common and, historically, one of the earliest used in liquid chromatography, including HPLC. Its principal of operation is very simple. The analyte is carried by the mobile phase into a detector cell (Figure 11.13) through which light from a lamp is passing on its way to a photosensor. If the analyte absorbs more of the light than the mobile phase, there will be a diminution of light as measured by the photosensor. The associated electronics will record that diminution of light as a positive signal and pass it on to a computer for storage and analysis.

Many organic molecules, particularly if they have one or more double or triple bonds as is common in most drugs, will have reasonably strong absorption at some wavelength(s) and thus most can be detected by this means. There are important exceptions to this, particularly for mono- and small polysaccharides (small sugars) and most amino acids. These molecules generally absorb poorly in the UV or visible wavelengths although there are important exceptions to this such as the aromatic amino acids (phenylalanine, tyrosine, and tryptophan), which can be readily detected via UV absorption and are also naturally fluorescent. Specialized methods and detectors do exist to detect sugars and amino acids. For the carbohydrates in particular, these methods have great relevance in nutrition, agriculture, and food processing but less so for drug analysis.

These detectors are intrinsically linear because light absorption follows Beer's Law (Eq. 11.36):

$$A = \varepsilon LC \qquad (11.36)$$

where A is absorbance, ε is the molar extinction coefficient, L is the path length, in cm, of the flow cell (or cuvett in a spectrophotometer), and C is the analyte concentration in moles/L. Note this is a linear equation that follows the form of $A = mC + B$. These detectors deviate from linearity when the analyte concentration is so high that photosensor or associated electronics can no longer respond in a linear fashion (i.e., they exceed their linear dynamic range), in which case that detector is said to be *saturated*, something that can occur with any detector when the analyte concentration is sufficiently high. These detectors are also relatively inexpensive, sensitive, easy to operate and maintain, and robust and reliable. Their biggest drawback is their universal nature, which is to say their lack of selectivity in that they will detect all species that absorb at the designated wavelength. In complex biological fluids such as plasma and urine there can be hundreds of such interfering species, which usually necessitates prechromatographic sample preparation procedures (often extensive) to remove most of the potential interfering species (and often concentrate the analyte to facilitate further analysis). Nonetheless, UV-Vis detectors remain a mainstay of HPLC detection and a number of variants have been developed.

Fixed-Wavelength UV-Vis Detectors The UV-Vis detector can be an almost universal detector but to do so requires that the detection wavelength be one that the analyte will have markedly more absorbance than the mobile phase. Thus, there are a number of important variants of the UV-Vis detector that center on the wavelength of the light being passed through the detector. A very early, and still very common design, was to pass a single fixed-wavelength through the detector. This was (and is) most commonly done by having a single lamp, which produced one or a few intense emission wavelengths with optical filters being placed between the lamp and the flow-cell to allow the passage of the desired wavelength. The most common lamp was (and is) a small mercury lamp, where the mercury, as a vapor and upon electrical excitation, produces an intense emission wavelength at approximately 254 nanometers (nm). Most organic molecules, if they absorb UV light at all, will absorb at 254 nm whereas few mobile phase mixtures, especially for reversed-phase, absorb appreciably at that wavelength.

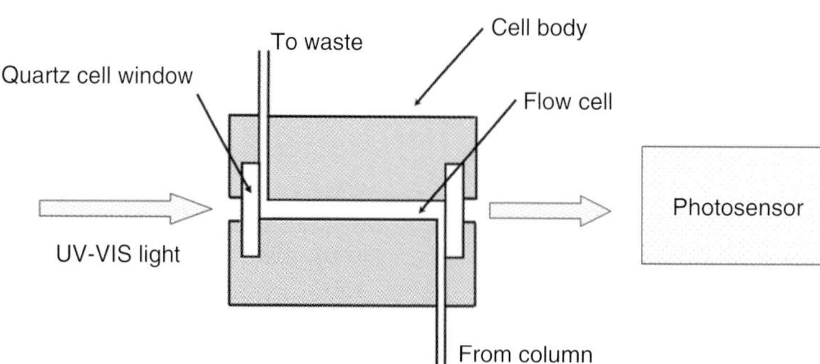

Figure 11.13 Schematic diagram of a UV-VIS detector. Mobile phase enters the flow cell through narrow-bore tubing. The flow cell volume is kept low to reduce the extra-column bandbroadening while the cell path length is designed to be as long as practical to increase sensitivity. Monochromatic light (UV or visible wavelengths) enters the flow cell through the quartz window (quartz does not appreciably absorb light in either the UV or visible wavelength ranges but conventional glass absorbs UV light). Any analyte passing through the cell that absorbs more light than the mobile phase will be measured as a decrease in radiation at the photosensor (which is often a photodiode).

This type of detector, although becoming increasingly uncommon in the product lines of major instrument manufacturers, is inexpensive (which may be why it is uncommon in those product lines), easy to operate, and robust and reliable.

Programmable Wavelength Detectors The fixed-wavelength UV-Vis detector suffers from the disadvantage that in order to change the detection wavelength you have to change the lamp and associated filters. This is not only inconvenient, it also requires that you own a wide variety of (often expensive) lamps, thus losing some of the initial price advantage of the detector. To avoid this problem, detectors were designed that used a lamp that generated fairly intense radiation over a broad spectrum (tungsten lamps for visible wavelengths and deuterium lamps for UV wavelengths). A monochromator was then used to select the appropriate detection wavelength that would be passed through the flow cell. Some very early designs used prisms as monochromators but now all designs use diffraction gratings. The desired wavelength could be selected with a manual control knob or button on the instrument, which physically moved the diffraction grating so that the correct wavelength would pass through the flow cell.

As electronic control of scientific instrumentation (and everything else) became more widespread (around the mid-1980s), detectors were designed where it was possible, either in the detector as a stand-alone unit, or integrated into a computer controlled instrument, to alter the detection wavelength during the course of the chromatographic run. They could also be programmed to subtract, either electronically or mathematically, any background absorbance from the mobile phase, a so-called *autozero*. This had a great advantage in that the optimal detection wavelength could be selected for each analyte, provided they were well resolved, during the course of the chromatographic run, thus improving the sensitivity of the detector.

Rapid-Scan Detectors There can be considerable information contained in the UV or UV-Vis spectrum of an analyte and it is desirable to obtain spectra "on the fly" during the course of the run. For instance, two analytes may have essentially the same retention time but may differ from one another because of differences in their respective spectra. Also, if they are coeluting, any spectrum obtained at the time of elution will be a composite of both (or all) spectra of coeluting species. By comparing that spectrum with those taken from pure analytes it is generally possible to determine if coelution is occurring, how many coelutants are present, and even their concentration and respective spectra. To determine if coelution is occurring from collected spectra, various (usually proprietary) computer algorithms are incorporated into the software packages of instrument manufacturers and will report *peak purity* (or something similar) and will give some measure of the statistical validity of the measurement. For these and other reasons, detectors were designed that could rapidly take a spectral scan during the course of the run by very rapidly moving or "scanning" the monochromator and collecting the resultant spectral data.

Photodiode Array (PDA) Detectors Rapid-scan detectors had a number of disadvantages. Because they required physical movement of the monochromator, they were both less reliable and robust in their operation and required greater maintenance and calibration than fixed-wavelength or programmable detectors operating at just a few wavelengths. They also generated considerably more, and more complex, data. Although stand-alone designs did, and do still exist, rapid-scan detectors are utilized best when their data can be sent to a computer for storage and analysis. But perhaps their biggest drawback in terms of scanning is the rate at which a spectrum can be taken because a rapid-scan detector actually has to scan by physically moving the monochromator. Thus, there is an upper limit on how fast a spectrum can be taken. If an analyte plug is moving through the detector while it is being scanned, the spectrum is distorted and desired goals such as peak purity analysis may not be obtained. Further, if a large spectral range must be scanned such as several hundred nanometers, then either the scan time must be long or the spectral resolution (data points per nm) must be low. Stop-flow valves, which divert the mobile phase flow away from the detector as soon as the analyte peak enters the detector and stops the flow of the analyte out of the flow cell, ameliorate this problem but come with their own problems including being usable on only very well-separated peaks. The ultimate solution to generating spectral data was the development of the *photodiode array (PDA) detector*.

The PDA detector does not scan at all, but instead continuously passes the entire spectral range of interest through the flow-cell. The light exiting the flow-cell is then spread out by a diffraction grating, which impinges on a linear array of photodiodes. This allows spectra to be taken continuously, with the only limitations being the speed of the electronics and computer storage and analysis, essentially negligible delays with current instruments. The PDA detector is a very powerful instrument and must be accompanied by a computer system to fully utilize that power. The output of a PDA detector is a three-dimensional chromatogram with retention time on one axis, absorbance signal intensity on a second axis, and wavelength on the third axis. The software allows for the spectrum of any given peak to be derived or a chromatogram at any give wavelength to be produced. Photodiode array detectors are heavily used in the pharmaceutical industry and, when coupled with mass spectral detectors (see later), represent one of the most powerful methods of drug analysis.

11.4.5.3 Fluorescence Detectors

Fluorescence detectors depend on the excitation of an analyte molecule with a specific excitation wavelength and the subsequent detection of the longer wavelength (less energetic) emitted light. Because fluorescence detectors are detecting a signal where previously there was none, they are very sensitive. This can be understood in the contrast with UV-Vis detectors, which may detect only a small decrease in light arriving at the photosensor. In selected applications they are the most sensitive of all HPLC detectors. Because relatively few molecules will naturally fluoresce (notable exceptions are the antimalarial agent quinine, its enantiomer quinidine, and the blood thinner, coumadine) they are not universal detectors.

Many important molecules, including drugs, have reactive functional groups to which a fluorescent agent can be covalently linked. If this linking process, referred to as *derivatization*, occurs before the analyte is chromatographically separated, the process is referred to as *precolumn* derivatization and if the linking process occurs after the analyte is separated, it is *postcolumn* derivatization. For fluorescence derivatization, the most important functional groups are reduced sulfhydryls (R-SH) and primary amines (R-NH_2), and to a lesser extent, secondary amine and derivatization of the former is an important means of analyzing amino acids. One such reaction is shown in Figure 11.14 where a derivatizing reagent, *ortho-phthalaldehyde* (*OPA*), is shown reacting with a primary amine (R_2NH_2) in the required presence of a reduced sulfhydryl (R_1SH) to generate and intensely fluorescent product. This particular reaction can be used to derivatize both primary amine analytes and sulfhydryl analytes, but not both in the same reaction mixture. However, the general strategy of chemically modifying the analyte to improve either detection sensitivity or chromatographic behavior is widely used with other types of HPLC detections. Derivatization is also widely used in GC to make analytes more volatile and thus amenable to GC analysis. As many derivatizing agents have been developed for various functional groups and for various reasons, students are highly advised to consult and carefully evaluate the primary literature in selecting appropriate derivatization procedures.

As with UV-Vis detection, there are a number of variants of fluorescence detectors that largely mirror those employed in UV-Vis. The simplest fluorescence detectors employ simple fixed wavelength lamps and optical filters to set both the excitation and emission wavelengths. Designs of intermediate complexity (and cost) use filters to set the excitation wave length and a monochromator to detect the emitted light, whereas the most complex designs have monochromators for both the excitation and emission. Because fluorescence sensitivity is enhanced by using more intense excitation radiation, xenon arc lamps or flash lamps are used, which produce very intense radiation. In very specialized instruments (not generally employed in drug analysis), lasers are used as the excitation source. For detection of the emitted radiation, *photomultiplier tubes* (*PMT*) are used. These tubes have a cascading series of metal plates held at very high voltages. When a photo strikes the first plate, it gives rise to a shower of electrons that strike other plates in the series, which in turn also give off many other electrons. This proceeds in a cascade, and the net effect is a very large (many orders of magnitude) amplification of the effect of the first photon. Because of the very close juxtaposition of an extremely intense excitation source and a extremely sensitive detector, the method can have very low LOQ values. Detection is performed at right angles to excitation. This is done so that the vast majority of excitation radiation will pass through the flow cell and only scattered light and background fluorescence from the mobile phase (usually very small) will become noise (unwanted signal not arising from the presence of the analyte) in the detector signal. A representation of a fluorescence detector is shown in Figure 11.15.

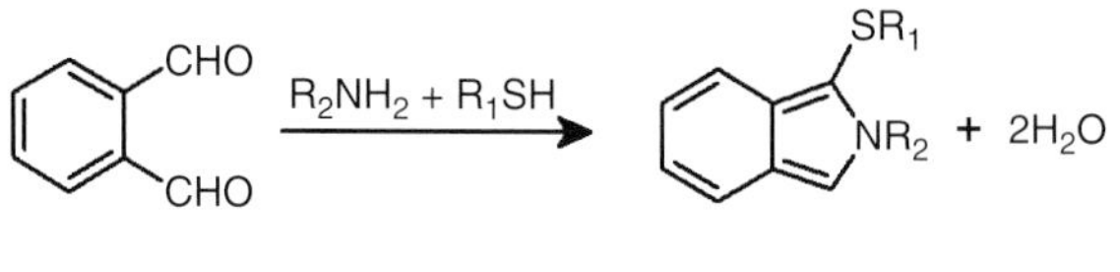

CHO, CHO $\xrightarrow{R_2NH_2 + R_1SH}$ SR$_1$, NR$_2$ + $2H_2O$

Figure 11.14 A derivatizing reaction (it could be either pre- or postcolumn) between the derivatization agent, ortho-phthalaldehyde (OPA), a primary amine (R_2NH_2), and a reduced sulfhydryl. The product is intensely fluorescent and is readily detected by using a fluorescence detector.

11.4.5.4 Mass Spectral Detectors

The final type of detector to be discussed is the mass spectral (MS) detector. This is a very common and very important type of detector, particularly in the pharmaceutical industry. It is used with both HPLC and GC but its most important application in drug analysis is when it is coupled to an HPLC, where it is refereed

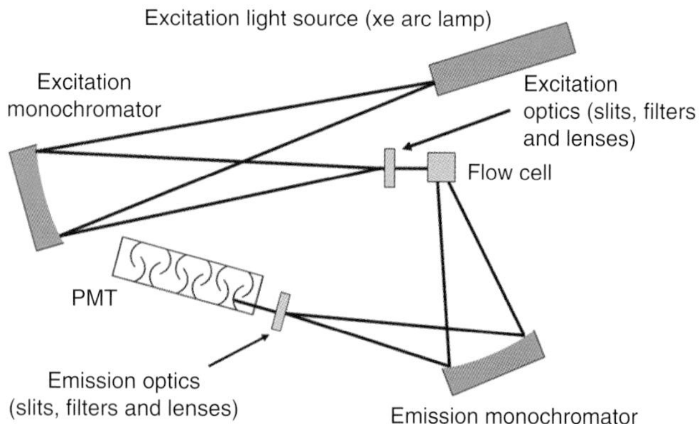

Figure 11.15 Schematic diagram of a fluorescence detector. Mobile phase enters a flow cell. Intense monochromatic light (UV or visible wavelengths) is used to excite analyte species in a flow cell. Emitted light at longer (less energetic) wavelengths are detected at right angles to the excitation light to reduce signal noise from scatter excitation light. The emitted light is greatly amplified by a photomultiplier (PMT) tube. Because one is detection signal (emission radiation) when normally none is present, fluorescence detection can be very sensitive. As relatively few molecules are naturally fluorescent, or can be chemically derivatized to become fluorescent, fluorescence detection can be very selective as well as very sensitive.

to as a *hyphenated technique*, HPLC-MS, or more commonly known as LC-MS (also commonly, LC/MS). The principal of MS is simple but both the theory and implementation are not.

In MS, analyte molecules must be in an ionized state under conditions of high vacuum. The *ion source* represents the interface between the sample *inlet*, which would be the end of a HPLC column in the case of LC-MS and the rest of the instrument. In the process of ionization both positive and negative ions can be formed in a given analyte molecule, which can adopt multiple charges in the process of ionization. Then under the influence of either electric or magnetic fields (neutral or uncharged molecules are not influenced by the fields present in a MS instrument) the ions are propelled through the instrument and then are separated from one another by one or more *mass analyzers.* This separation is based on their *mass-to-charge ratio*, known as the m/z of the analyte molecules, where m is the molecular weight of the analyte and z is the net charge. The high vacuum is necessary since analyte ions likely would collide with any residual gases before analysis could be completed (gases are introduced specifically to induce collision in a subtechnique of MS). They are then detected in a fashion entirely analogous to the PMT and the signal is appropriately processed by a computer. This instrument is illustrated in a highly schematic fashion in Figure 11.16.

Thus a very important point is that in both HPLC and GC, the analyte molecules are neither necessarily ionized nor are they in a high vacuum when they are being chromatographically separated. Thus they must be removed from the mobile phase or carrier gas, ionized, and then separated by the mass analyzer. Whereas the further discussion will concern only LC-MS as it is most relevant to drug analysis, many of the same principals apply to GC-MS.

Desolvation and Ion Generation In LC-MS, there are two very common means of removing the analyte species from the mobile phase, ionizing them, and introducing them into the high vacuum environment: *electrospray ionization* (*ESI*) and *atmospheric pressure chemical ionization* (*APCI*). (Another type of ionization, *matrix assisted laser desorption ionization* (*MALDI*) is used very commonly in the analysis of macromolecules, especially proteins, but has less relevance for small molecule drug analysis.)

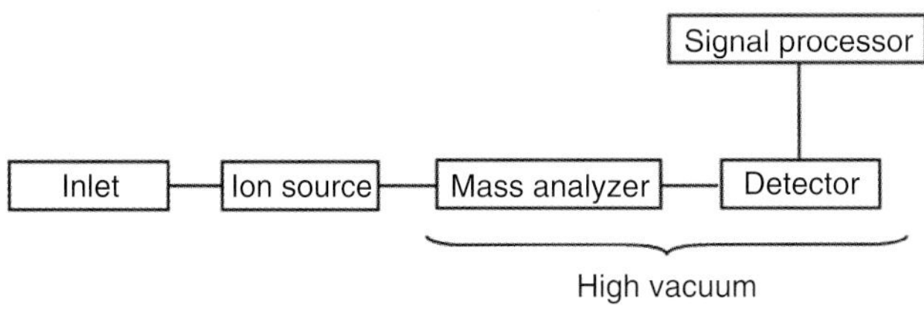

Figure 11.16 Highly schematic diagram of a mass spectral detector. The sample, perhaps entrained in the mobile phase of an HPLC system, enters an inlet region of the instrument where analyte molecules are ionized and mobile phase (in the case of HPLC) or carrier gas (in the case of GC) are removed. The ions enter the high vacuum region and are separated from one another on the basis of their mass-to-charge (m/z) ratio by one or more mass analyzers. The ions are detected and the signal passed to a computer system for storage and analysis (the signal processor).

Electrospray Ionization Electrospray ionization is illustrated in Figure 11.17. In this ionization technique, the mobile phase (or an infused solution) exiting from the HPLC is forced through a narrow capillary surrounded by a stream of nitrogen gas (not shown in the figure). The capillary is kept at high voltage. These result in the generation of a very fine mist of droplets carrying preformed ions in solution (only positive ions are shown in the figure). As the droplets move toward the entrance to the MS (which is only a centimeter away), solvent evaporates from the droplets, causing the net charge to become concentrated in a decreasing volume. The charge concentration results in the droplet "exploding" into even finer droplets, wherein the process repeats itself. At some point, essentially all solvent will have evaporated and what remains are isolated gas-phase ions and neutral molecules with only the ions being amenable to analysis by MS.

This ionization method is "soft" in that it does not cause the analyte molecule to fragment into multiple ions as older ionization methods often do. The use of the unfragmented, or *molecular ion*, greatly simplifies the resulting mass spectra, which greatly facilitates interpretation of the data. As ESI depends on preformed ions being solution, ion adducts are seen in the case of positive ion formation. In most cases these are proton (H^+) adducts, but sodium (Na^+) and potassium (K^+) are seen also. This form of ionization works with protic and polar analytes that readily form protonated species such as primary amines,

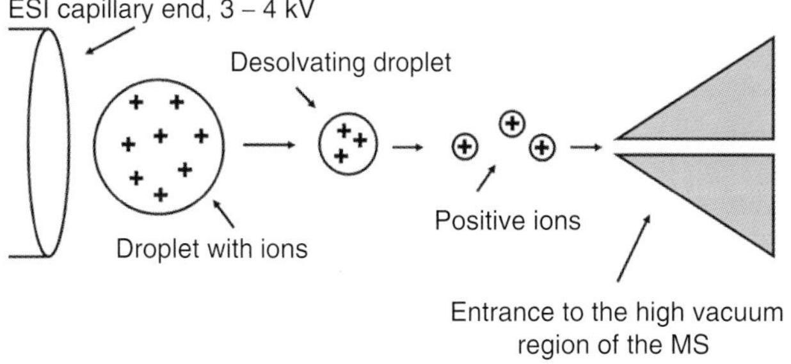

Figure 11.17 Schematic diagram of Electrospray Ionization (ESI) in LC-MS. Analytes in mobile phase exit the HPLC column and are directed through a narrow capillary entrained in flow of nitrogen gas (not shown). The capillary is maintained at a high voltage and the mobile phase exits the capillary as fine mist of very small droplets containing preformed analyte ions (only positive ions are shown but both positive and negative ions would be present). The droplets rapidly desolvate with a corresponding concentration of ions and charge. This results in disintegration of the droplets and the generation of even finer droplets. Eventually only essentially entirely desolvated gas-phase ions are left to enter the high vacuum region of the MS.

especially when the solution they are in has a pH below the pKa of the protonated functional group (pKa is the pH at which a functional group will be one-half ionized and one-half unionized). Multiproton adducts are nearly always seen in larger molecules such as peptides and proteins, as both type of molecules usually have many easily protonated groups such as amines. The resulting *m/z* value for such an analyte is readily determined as $(m + z)/z$. Thus a small polypeptide with a molecular weight of 1224 and two proton adducts would have a *m/z* value of $613 = (1224 + 2)/2$.

In Figure 11.17, the capillary is shown directly facing the very narrow orifice leading to the high vacuum region of the MS. This is done as a simplification. Many instrument designs now have the capillary oriented at right angles to the entrance to the MS. An appropriate voltage (positive for negative ions and negative for positive ions) is applied to the entrance zone of the MS to direct the ions into the MS while minimizing entrance of residual solvent and neutral species. This greatly reduces the burden on the pumps needed to maintain the high vacuum conditions necessary.

Atmospheric Pressure Chemical Ionization (APCI) In APCI, analyte molecules entrained in the mobile phase from an HPLC at the inlet are further entrained in an envelope of nitrogen gas in a heated quartz tube. Desolvation occurs in the heated quartz tube prior to ionization. Ionization occurs as a result of a gas-phase chemical reaction at the end of the tube. The corona needle depicted in Figure 11.18 produces a plasma or region of ionized gas by applying a high voltage to the needle in the vicinity of the analyte stream. The process of analyte ionization is both chemically and physically complex but ultimately positive ions are produced by a process of proton transfer to generate a $(A + H^+)$ ion adduct. Negative ions can be produced via transfer of a proton from the analyte to other molecules and can leave a $[M\text{-}H]^-$ ion. Addition of electrons to analyte molecules will also generate negative ions. Like ESI, APCI is a "soft" ionization source but works best with aprotic and more nonpolar species.

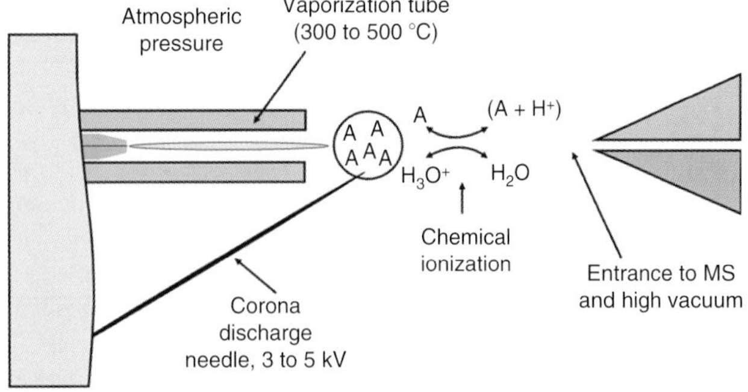

Figure 11.18 Schematic diagram of an APCI source. The analyte species are desolvated from the mobile phase in a stream of nitrogen gas in a heated quartz tube. The analyte species undergo a complex gas-phase chemical reaction produced by a gas-phase ionized environment (a plasma) generated by the high voltage of the corona discharge needle. The produced analyte ions can then enter the high vacuum region of the MS for further analysis.

Mass Analyzers There are a five predominate mass analyzers, each of which has both advantages and disadvantages but only two, the quadrupole and ion trap, are of significance in drug analysis. The action of neither mass analyzer is intuitively easy or obvious. The ion trap is essentially a small metal cylinder with metallic end-cap electrodes that utilizes oscillating electric fields to trap selected ions in an "electronic bottle." By adjusting the frequency of those fields, ions can be selectively held or ejected from the trap. The quadrupole mass analyzer is, as the name implies, a collection of four cylindrical or parabolicly shaped rods in a parallel configuration (Figure 11.19). A combination of positive and negative both fixed and oscillating electric fields applied to the rods can be adjusted such that only one ion of a given *m/z* can successfully pass down the axis between the rods and reach the detector. In both mass analyzers, electric field strengths and frequencies can be progressively adjusted (over a time span of mseconds) to allow a wide *m/z* range to be examined in a process known as *scanning*. This allows the mass spectrum to be taken. Alternatively, a single ion can be monitored in what is known as *single ion monitoring* (*SIM*), a procedure that improves sensitivity since the instrument is not spending time examining other ions.

Triple Quadrupole MS/MS The final topic to consider is the use of multiple mass analyzers in drug analysis. The most important is the *triple quadrupole* instrument. It is a very good method of drug measurement. It can be both very selective and sensitive. The principal is illustrated in Figures 11.20A and 11.20B. The instrument uses three quadrupole mass analyzers in tandem. The first mass analyzer is used to select a

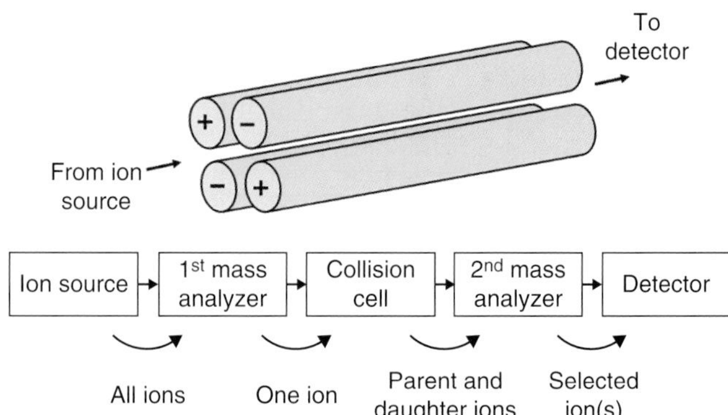

Figure 11.19 Schematic diagram of a quadrupole mass analyzer. Four cylindrical or parabolic metal rods are held in a parallel configuration with fixed or oscillating electric fields applied, as negative or positive, to opposing pairs of rods. The frequency and field strength can be so adjusted that only one ion of a given *m/z* can make the journey down the axis between the rods to the detector. The electric fields can be gradually adjusted or "scanned" (over a matter of mseconds) to allow a series of ions to reach the detector, thus giving the mass spectrum.

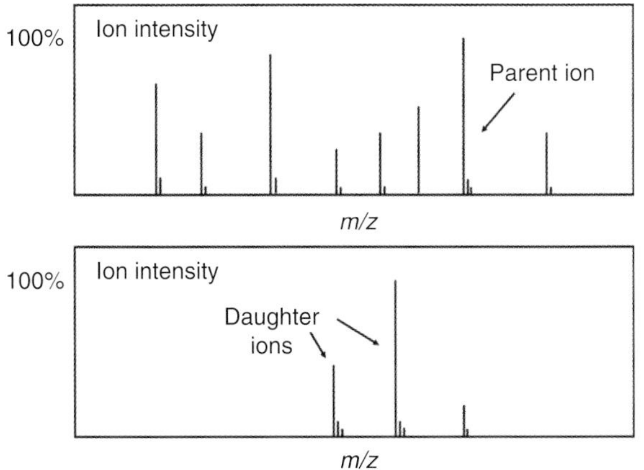

Figure 11.20 (A) A schematic diagram of a triple quadrupole during a selected reaction monitoring (SRM) or multiple reaction monitoring (MRM) experiment. (B) A multiple reaction monitoring (MRM) experiment. A single ion, the parent ion, is selected in the first mass analyzer and passed on the collision cell while all other ions are rejected. In the collision cell, the parent ion is fragmented into two daughter ions with a small amount of the parent ion remaining. The small lines adjacent to the large ion peaks represent stable isotopic variants of the large peaks (such as C_{13}) present in nearly all natural chemical species and are not drawn to scale.

given ion, the *parent ion* or *precursor ion*, for further analysis. The second mass analyzer is actually a collision cell, where the first ion is allowed to collide, a process known as *collision-induced dissociation* (*CID*), and fragment with a neutral *collision gas* such as argon, helium, or nitrogen. For any given analyte, under specific conditions, the resulting fragment ions, the *daughter ion(s)*, are going to be very characteristic. The third mass analyzer can be used to monitor one or more daughter ions. The former is known as *Selected Reaction Monitoring* (*SRM*) and the latter is *Multiple Reaction Monitoring* (*MRM*). This gives the technique a very high degree of selectivity. Even if an undesired ion having the same *m/z* of the desired analyte ion were admitted into the collision cell, it is highly unlikely (unless they were enantiomers) that the collision reactions would produce the same daughter ion(s). It also gives the technique a very high degree of sensitivity since, as in absence of analyte in the case of fluorescence detection, there is essentially no signal being generated in the absence of analyte.

11.5 KEY POINTS AND CONCLUSIONS

- The scope of drug bioanalysis is very large, ranging from medical drugs, illegal "recreational" drugs, law enforcement and forensics, academic and pharmaceutical research, and pharmaceutical manufacturing.
- Drugs in complex mixture can be analyzed *in situ*, usually via antigen-antibody interactions or by separating the drug from the other component of the mixture and detecting the drug via some means.
- The better analytes can be separated, the less specific detection methods need to be.
- Chromatographic separations are generally the best means of separating drugs.
- The basis of chromatographic separation is equilibrium thermodynamics.
- The basis of chromatographic bandbroadening is kinetics.
- Bandbroadening components can be treated as being additive and include contributions from longitudinal diffusion, eddy diffusion, and resistance to mass transfer.
- These contributions can be seen graphically in the van Deemter Curve.
- The most important stationary phase in HPLC is the reversed phase wherein a solid support (generally silica) is coated with a very thin layer of a nonpolar stationary phase.
- When k' values are low, increasing retention can substantially improve resolution but a point of diminishing returns is rapidly reached.
- Use of gradient elution is the best way to optimize both resolution and retention time.
- The two main ways to form gradients are high pressure mixing and low pressure mixing.
- Universality in a detector is a double-edged sword, valuable with less complex samples but prone to being overwhelmed with complex samples.
- Fluorescence detectors have the opposite problem. While they are very sensitive, their selectivity limits the range of compounds they can analyze.
- The two most important ionization for LC-MS are ESI and APCI.
- The two most important mass analyzers are the quadrupole and ion trap.
- Triple quadrupole LC-MS/MS is the method of choice from most drug analysis.

REVIEW QUESTIONS

1. How can a chemical be both a drug and a poison?
2. What does the acronym PK/ADMET stand for?
3. What is the difference between preparative and analytical chromatography?
4. How and why is the capacity factor of a peak calculated?
5. What is Brownian motion?
6. Sketch the van Deemter Curve and explain the contributions of each component of bandbroadening to it.
7. Explain how reversed-phase HPLC separations work.
8. Explain gradient elution.
9. How does a check-valve work?
10. Explain the difference between low pressure and high pressure mixing.
11. Discuss why fluorescent detection would be more sensitive than UV detection.
12. Explain the difference between ESI and APCI.
13. Explain SRM.

GLOSSARY OF MS TERMS

The following is adapted from a list compiled by Professor Anthony Mallet, University of Greenwich, London.

APCI (Atmospheric Pressure Chemical Ionization): Ionization by reaction with reagents formed with a plasma discharge in air.

Base Peak: The most intense ion detected in the spectrum.

CID (Collision Induced Dissociation): The fragmentation of an ion induced by collision with a neutral atom or molecule.

Collision Chamber: A region of relatively high pressure in a device where CID takes place.

Daughter Ion: Ion formed by decomposition of a parent ion.

ESI (Electrospray Ionization): Ionization produced by spraying a sample solution through a conducting capillary tube at a high voltage potential.

GC-MS (Gas Chromatography-Mass Spectrometry): The linking of mass spectrometry to a gas chromatographic system.

Ion-Trap: Ions are placed into a three "bottle" dimensional device where they are stored by a quadrupole field. They can then be ejected at defined *m/z* values by the application-appropriate secondary electric fields.

Isotopes: Most elements are composed of a mixture of isotopes. These will be separated in a mass spectrometer. Atoms or molecules containing such elements will display a cluster of ions reflecting the isotopic composition.

LC-MS (Liquid Chromatography-Mass Spectrometry): The linking of the effluent from a liquid chromatographic system to a mass spectrometer.

MS/MS: The use of two mass analyzers to detect parent ions and their product daughter ions.

m/z: The ratio of charge to mass of the ion detected.

Mass Spectrum: A plot of *m/z* or mass (x axis) versus the ion intensity, frequently normalized to 100% for the most intense ion detected (y axis). This is produced by scanning the analyzer to transmit ions (or release them from a trap) for a predefined range of *m/z* values over a fixed period of time.

Molecular Ion: The ion formed from the original molecule in the source.

Quadrupole: The application of a combination of DC and AC voltages to four parallel rods creates a filter through which only ions of any one defined *m/z* value can be transmitted.

SIM (Selected Ion Monitoring): In target analysis for defined analytes, the analyzer is operated so as to transmit only the calculated *m/z* values for the components present.

SRM (Selected Reaction Monitoring): In MS/MS, a specific dissociation of a parent to daughter ion is monitored.

IUPAC recommendations for terms for use in mass spectrometry can be found in (Todd 1991).

REFERENCES

Cunico, R. L., Gooding, K. M., & Wehr, T. (1998). *Basic HPLC and CE of Biomolecules.* Richmond, CA: Bay Bioanalytical Laboratory, Inc.

Eisenberg, D. S., & Crothers, D. (1979). *Physical Chemistry: With Applications to the Life Sciences.* Menlo Park, CA: Benjamin/Cummings Pub. Co.

Giddings, J. C. (1991). *Unified Separation Science.* New York, NY: John Wiley and Sons, Inc.

http://www.fda.gov

Leicester, H. M. (1968). *Source Book in Chemistry, 1900–1950.* Cambridge, MA: Harvard.

Todd, J. F. J. (1991). *Pure and Applied Chemistry* (Vol. 63). 1541–1566.

Tswett, M. (1906). Physical Chemical Studies on Chlorophyll Adsorptions. *Berichte der Deutschen botanischen Gesellschaft, 24,* 316–323.

Chapter

12

Drug–Drug Interactions with an Emphasis on Drug Metabolism and Transport

Kenneth Bachmann

OUTLINE

12.1 INTRODUCTION

12.1.1 Overview and History

Adverse drug reactions (ADRs) have been recognized as an important cause of morbidity and mortality and as a contributor to the spiraling costs of healthcare. The FDA's Center for Drug Evaluation and Research has reported that there are in excess of two million serious ADRs annually in the United States leading to over 100,000 deaths. They are responsible for about 20% of the injuries occurring annually to hospitalized patients, doubling the length of stay and cost of treatment of hospitalized patients. Nursing home ADRs occur at a rate of 350,000 per year. Costs of ADRs have been estimated at $136 billion per year. These estimates might underrepresent the outcomes and costs associated with ADRs likely to occur by the end of the first decade of the twenty-first century. That's because two out of three physician visits already result in a prescription. In 2000 there were 10 prescriptions written for every person in the United States. But the United States is in an exponential phase of growth of the very oldest segment of the population; a segment that tends to be composed of individuals requiring the greatest number of prescription drugs. Consider, too, that fewer than 20% of patients with either hypertension, diabetes, or hyperlipidemia are currently even treated at all. If access to healthcare improves and if diagnostic techniques improve it would follow that even more prescriptions will be issued in the years ahead, leading to more ADRs.

Although the purposeful coadministration of two drugs can be designed in such a way as to improve therapeutic outcomes or even to limit adverse effects, it is most often the case that unintended drug–drug interactions comprise a subset of ADRs. They represent between 3 and 5% of all preventable ADRs in hospitals. For decades the notion of drug–drug interactions (DDIs) was given short shrift in pharmacology, medicine, and pharmacy. Interactions were thought to be largely pharmacodynamic, and consequently largely preventable. The very first mention of drug interactions in *The Pharmacological Basis of Therapeutics* by Louis Goodman and Alfred Gilman didn't appear until the fourth edition was published in 1970. Drugs having opposite effects were said to exhibit functional antagonism. Drugs not sharing the same pharmacodynamic activity, but capable of altering one another's effects, were said to be heterergic. If two heterergic drugs combined to produce an effect greater than the effects of either one of them, then they were said to act synergistically. If two heterergic drugs elicited an effect less than that of either one of them, then the interaction was characterized as antagonistic. Heterergic drug interactions were then ascribed to the effect of one drug on the dispositional characteristics (absorption, distribution, metabolism, excretion) of the other.

The overall treatment of DDIs was given the space of one page in the fourth edition of the book. The eleventh edition of Goodman & Gilman's *The Pharmacological Basis of Therapeutics* was published more than 35 years later in 2006. The general treatment of DDIs expanded by that time to about two pages of text, however a section on drug interactions was written into many of the individual drug monographs. Today there are dozens of books available, each of which provides hundreds of monographs of DDIs. Searchable DDI databases are available online, permitting clinicians to generate DDI reports on virtually any combination of two drugs. These searchable databases allow the user to explore interactions between drugs and nutrients, and also interactions between drugs and herbal remedies.

There are circumstances that can increase the chance of ADRs developing from DDIs. One of those is the use of drugs with narrow therapeutic ranges. For these drugs it is possible that even relatively small changes in exposure to the drug will be met by either an ADR or therapeutic failure. Example of such drugs are:

- Aminoglycoside antibiotics (gentamicin, tobramycin)
- Anticoagulants (warfarin, heparins)
- Carbamazepine
- Estrogens
- Cyclosporine
- Digoxin
- Hypoglycemic agents
- Levothyroxine sodium
- Lithium
- Phenytoin
- Procainamide
- Quinidine
- Theophylline
- Valproic acid

Some disease states or conditions also predispose patients to experience ADRs, including those that result from DDIs. Examples are:

- Aplastic anemia
- Critical care/intensive care patients
- Patients with liver or renal dysfunction

12.1.1.1 Pharmacodynamic Interactions

DDIs that are rooted in the combined pharmacodynamic actions of the interacting drugs are referred to as pharmacodynamic interactions or pharmacodynamic DDIs. These interactions can be fairly obvious such as the interaction that might occur between caffeine and say, ramelteon or other sleep-inducing drugs. Ramelteon is a melatonin receptor agonist (both MT1 and MT2) that is used to treat insomnia, since it induces sleep. Caffeine is thought to produce CNS stimulation through adenosine receptor antagonism. Though ramelteon and caffeine interact with different receptors, they nevertheless produce opposite pharmacodynamic effects. Thus, it would not be difficult to understand how caffeine (in a cup of coffee, for example) might diminish the sleep-inducing effect of ramelteon. Though this interaction actually is not cited in DDI monographs, contemporary recommendations for good sleep hygiene, of course, do recommend against the use of CNS stimulants, including caffeine.

The foregoing interaction might be a subtle one that is dependent upon the amount of caffeine exposure (numbers of cups of coffee), and easily overlooked since caffeine is often not even regarded as a drug by anyone other than healthcare practitioners and pharmaceutical scientists. On the other hand, there are countless examples of very serious pharmacodynamic DDIs, some of which are actually quite well known even in popular culture. For example, the drugs for erectile dysfunction such as sildenafil (Viagra®) are vasodilators owing to their ability to inhibit phosphodiesterase 5 (PDE5). Nitroglycerin is a drug that is used to relieve the symptoms of angina by virtue of its vasodilatory effects. It is converted to nitric oxide (NO), which activates the enzyme guanylate cyclase, thereby promoting the synthesis of cyclic guanosine 3′,5′-monophosphate (cGMP) leading to increases in intracellular cGMP levels. The net downstream effect subsequent to kinase activation culminates in the dephosphorylation of the myosin light chain of smooth muscle fibers, the release of calcium from smooth muscle cells, smooth muscle relaxation, and vasodilation. The combined use of sildenafil or similar drugs for erectile dysfunction along with nitroglycerin or other nitrates or nitrites for angina ultimately was discovered to cause severe, even fatal, hypotension. Other fatal reactions have been reported for the combination of the opioid analgesic, meperidine, combined with monoamine oxidase inhibitors such as tranylcypromine. Accordingly the combination of meperidine and monamine oxidase inhibitors (MAOIs) is now contraindicated, and it is recommended that meperidine not even be administered within two weeks of an MAOI. MAOIs are used in depressive illness to increase CNS levels of neurotransmitters such as serotonin (5HT) by inhibiting the enzyme (MAO) that oxidatively deaminates 5HT. Though meperidine is used as a narcotic analgesic on account of its ability to stimulate kappa opiate receptors (OP2), it also interferes with the neuronal reuptake of serotonin. Thus, the combined use of meperidine with MAOIs can cause markedly elevated levels of 5HT leading to severe cardiovascular and/or neurologic adverse reactions, though there may be preexisting conditions such as hyperphenylalanemia that predispose patients to these outcomes.

Yet another example of a pharmacodynamic DDI would be the combined use of an adrenergic receptor agonist along with an adrenergic receptor antagonist. For example, men with benign prostatic hypertrophy (BPH) are likely to be treated with alpha 1 adrenergic receptor antagonists such as doxazosin (Cardura®). Doxazosin is a competitive inhibitor at postsynaptic alpha 1 adrenergic receptors in the sympathetic nervous system, and as a consequence it lowers blood pressure and also interferes with norepinephrine-induced stimulation of the prostatic stromal and bladder neck tissues. Thus the sympathetic tone-induced urethral stricture causing BPH symptoms is partially ameliorated by antagonists such as doxazosin. On the other hand, common over-the-counter (OTC) cough and cold remedies frequently contain the drug phenylephrine, which is used as a decongestant. Phenylephrine is an adrenergic agonist with some selectivity for the alpha 1 adrenergic receptor. Thus, patients with hypertension who take doxazosin may experience poorer blood pressure regulation when taking cold medications with phenylephrine, and patients with BPH who benefit from alpha 1 antagonists such as doxazosin, can experience relapses or worsening of symptoms if they should also use a cold product containing phenylephrine.

One final and more general example (of countless possible examples) of a pharmacodynamic DDI might be the combined use of aspirin and warfarin. Warfarin is an anticoagulant drug that can be taken orally for the treatment of thrombotic conditions such as deep vein thrombosis, or to prevent the risk of thrombus formation in patients who have recently had a myocardial infarction (MI) or who have atrial fibrillation (AF). Its anticoagulant activity derives from its ability to inhibit a hepatic enzyme, vitamin K epoxide reductase (VKOR), which plays a key role in the synthesis of four vitamin K-dependent clotting factors, factors II, VII, IX, and X. Aspirin shares indications in the management of post-MI patients to reduce the risk of a recurrent MI, and also for the reduction of the risk of stroke in patients with AF. Its value in these indications resides in its antiplatelet activity by virtue of its ability to inhibit cyclooxygenase enzymes and ultimately the production of thromboxane A2 by platelets, since thromboxane A2, an arachidonic acid metabolite, stimulates platelet aggregation. Thus, warfarin decreases the likelihood of thrombogenesis by slowing clot formation, and aspirin decreases the likelihood of thrombogenesis by limiting platelet aggregation. Another way of looking at it is that each drug independently also increases the risk of spontaneous bleeding, though the mechanisms are different. It follows, then, that the combined use of these two drugs, though sometimes warranted, nevertheless increases the risk of spontaneous bleeding more than the use of either drug alone. This risk is dose-dependent as well. Aspirin, in doses that might be used for treating the pain of arthritis, actually exhibits some anticoagulant activity that is mechanistically similar to that of warfarin. Thus the inadvertent use of high doses of aspirin by a patient who requires warfarin poses a serious risk of bleeding.

12.1.1.2 Pharmacokinetic Interactions

Pharmacokinetic (PK) interactions (PK DDIs) sometimes are also referred to as dispositional interactions. These interactions are characterized by the alteration of the PK or disposition (ADME) of one drug by another. Should these alterations be of sufficient magnitude, then significant changes in exposure to the affected drug can occur, ultimately leading to alterations in the effect of the drug. Exposure is quantified in PK terms by the area circumscribed by the plasma concentration versus time curve of a drug. That area is referred to as the area under the curve or AUC (see Chapter 10). If the exposure (i.e., AUC) is significantly increased, the pharmacological effects may become exaggerated and/or unwanted side effects may occur. If the exposure is significantly decreased, the therapeutic effects may fail to develop, and therapeutic failure may ensue. In some instances, changes in the peak plasma concentration (C_{max}) of one drug caused by another drug can be sufficient to elicit significant adverse consequences.

This is exemplified by drugs that are HERG channel blockers in cardiac cells. Spikes in the plasma concentrations of those drugs can cause cardiac arrhythmias marked by prolonged QT intervals on the EKG and Torsade de pointes, which is potentially fatal. Some of the earliest second-generation antihistamines (i.e., nonsedating antihistamines) such as astemizole and terfenadine were ultimately withdrawn from the market after it was discovered that inhibition of their metabolism by other drugs such as erythromycin could increase their plasma concentrations and increase their risks for causing fatal cardiac arrhythmias. Greenblatt and colleagues, a group of basic and clinical pharmacologists at Tufts University Medical Center who have characterized the mechanisms and magnitude of DDIs for decades, have often referred to the drug in a DDI whose disposition is altered as the "victim" drug, and the drug that causes the change in the victim's disposition as the "perpetrator."

By what mechanisms might a perpetrator alter the AUC of a victim drug? Simply put, a perpetrator might be expected to increase the AUC of a victim drug by:

- Slowing its metabolism in the liver or the intestine
- Blocking the efflux of the victim drug from hepatocytes into the bile
- Increasing its oral absorption; this could occur if the perpetrator slowed intestinal metabolism of the victim or blocked transporter-mediated efflux of the victim back from intestinal epithelial cells into the lumen of the intestine
- Slowing renal secretion of the victim drug into the urine
- Decreasing the protein or tissue binding of the victim drug

Contrariwise, a perpetrator could be expected to decrease the AUC of a victim drug by interfering with its absorption or bioavailability, accelerating its metabolism in the intestine or liver, or accelerating its efflux from intestinal cells into the lumen of the intestine or from hepatocytes into the bile. In theory, interference by a perpetrator drug with any facet of ADME of a victim drug could lead to an alteration in the AUC of the victim drug. For many years this broad mechanistic view of DDIs opened the door to predicting innumerable two-drug DDIs. Many of these potential DDIs were subsequently validated by case reports appearing in the medical and pharmaceutical literature that described adverse outcomes of small numbers of patients taking two drugs that had been predicted to exhibit dispositional interactions. Many times these case reports were not further validated (i.e., truly validated) with randomized control clinical trials, but they nevertheless became inscribed in the drug interaction literature, and ultimately included in DDI databases. The problem is that although many dispositional interactions can be predicted qualitatively on the basis of what is known about the ADME characteristics of interacting drugs, the quantitative changes in AUC are often too small to be clinically significant.

Dr. Benet of the University of California, San Francisco, has developed a compelling quantitative assessment of the clinical significance of DDIs arising from a perpetrator interfering with the plasma protein binding of a victim drug. That analysis makes it fairly clear that those types of DDIs will simply not likely be clinically significant. With regard to DDIs arising from the inhibition of hepatic metabolism of a victim drug, strategies that take into account the magnitude of AUC changes in predicting the clinical significance of DDIs weren't really codified in the DDI literature until the beginning of the twenty-first century. Quantitative treatment of perpetrator-induced AUC changes for victim drugs will be presented later in this chapter.

12.1.1.3 Sources of Drug Interaction Information

As the knowledge base pertaining to drug metabolism, especially hepatic drug metabolism, grew beginning in the middle of the twentieth century, so, too, did interest in DDIs. Numerous symposia have been organized around this topic. The clinical literature and clinical pharmacological literature became outlets for reviewing DDIs by therapeutic category and by mechanism. The collection of DDI monographs into hard-copy databases was undertaken to provide prescribers and pharmacists alike with handy reference guides to DDIs. A representative group of these DDI books is listed in the References. Some DDI databases have been cast in electronic versions for computer-based queries, or have been integrated into general pharmacy systems software that will flag DDIs for pharmacists prior to dispensing prescriptions that may interact. A problem, however, is that some DDIs enter these databases solely on the strength of small numbers of nonvalidated case reports so that it is possible that DDIs that will not lead to clinical consequences will inadvertently be flagged. DDI databases that are designed to allow user queries are somewhat more sophisticated in that they try to gauge the clinical severity of the interaction and may even characterize the reliability of the source data depending upon whether it arose from isolated case reports, randomly controlled clinical trials, or both. Examples of DDI database software that permits queries about virtually any two-drug combination include DrugIx, Epocrates Rx, iFacts, Lexi-Interact, mobileMICROMEDEX, Mosbylx, Clinical Pharmacology OnHand, and Tarascon Pocket Pharmacopoeia. The foregoing operate on handhelds as well as on PCs. Comparisons about the accuracy of these databases to predict true positive or true negative interactions (i.e., no DDI) have been published.

With regard to DDIs specifically associated with enzyme inhibition or enzyme induction (refer to Chapter 8) or with transporter inhibition or induction (refer to Chapters 7 and 9), searchable online databases can be accessed that permit the user to explore which enzymes or transporters process a given drug and additionally how a given drug is likely to affect the function of a particular enzyme or transporter. David Flockhart at Indiana University created a database table that lists drugs that are either substrates, inhibitors, or inducers of individual CYP isoforms. The table can be found at http://medicine.iupui.edu/flockhart/table.htm. Each drug listed is hyperlinked to literature references and abstracts thereof in the PubMed database. The table and associated links are available *gratis* to users. The Japanese pharmaceutical company Fujitsu maintains an online searchable database that permits users to explore which enzymes and/or transporters process a specific drug, and whether a given drug inhibits or induces enzyme or transporter activity. For drugs that are substrates of enzymes or transporters one can find links to literature citations. Many of those citations are further linked to tables that list enzyme kinetic parameters such as Vmax or Km (see Chapter 8) for a specific drug-enzyme or drug-transporter combination. Likewise, for drugs that are found to be inhibitors of individual enzymes or transporters, there are links that provide the user with the results of *in vitro* inhibition experiments that quantitatively characterize inhibition by either an IC50 value (see later) or a Ki value (see later). These parameters can be used to quantitatively predict AUC changes (see later). The Fujitsu ADME database is available online only with a paid subscription. Another searchable database providing Ki data is available from the University of Washington.

Much more sophisticated *in silico* predictors of DDIs are available to pharmaceutical scientists who are likely to have different objectives than healthcare practitioners. Here, the goal is to make a reasonable *a priori* prediction about the likelihood of clinically significant DDIs for NCEs even before the substance is placed into clinical trials. Even among these predictors there is a wide range of complexity and sophistication. One such program is Simcyp™, developed by experts in drug metabolism and PK in Great Britain. Simcyp™ combines quantitative *in vitro* data on drug processing, enzyme inhibition, and enzyme induction along with computer-based algorithms to predict quantitative AUC changes in humans for two-drug combinations. An example of the output is presented in Figure 12.1, which is modified from the Simcyp™ web site.

Predictions of drug interactions

Ritonavir and Viagra (n=14)

Ratio of AUC (after/before inhibition)

Trial number

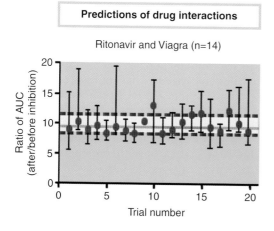

Figure 12.1 The results of twenty simulations resulting in predicted fold increases in the AUC of sildenafil (Viagra®) after the administration of ritonavir. Note the mean of all twenty trials approaches ten-fold. Redrawn from Simcyp website.

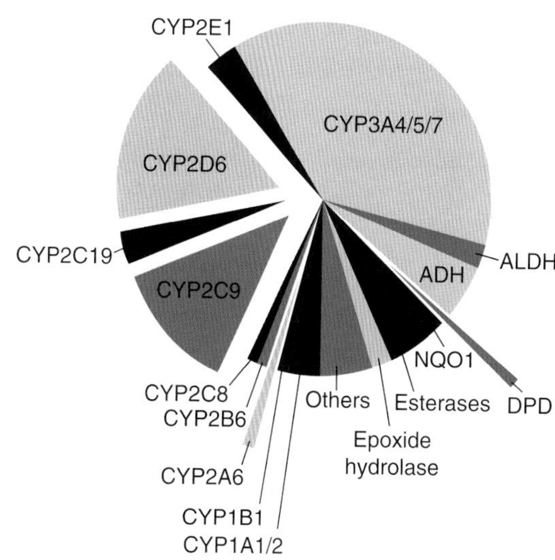

Figure 12.2 Relative importance of Phase I enzymes in drug metabolism.

Simcyp™ asserts that its quantitative predictions are accurate about 80% of the time. These quantitative predictions about the PK significance of DDIs enable developers of NCEs to make "go versus no-go" decisions about further drug development even before the DDI is actually studied in a clinical trial. A different approach is taken by Aureus Pharma, a knowledge base company that markets AurSCOPE® ADME/DDI. This is a structured knowledge database that is fully annotated. The knowledge base contains information on 10,360 parent compounds, 2700 metabolites, and 197,560 biological activities extracted from over 7000 published articles. That knowledge base is then used in comparison with novel drug structures to predict a novel drug's ADME and DDI characteristics. As with the Fujitsu database, both Simcyp and the AuroSCOPE™ ADME/DDI database can only be obtained through purchase or licensing agreements.

12.2 DDIs ASSOCIATED WITH ALTERED DRUG METABOLISM

Although, in theory, any inhibitor or any inducer of any drug metabolizing enzyme (see Chapter 8) could function as a perpetrator of DDIs, and any substrate of any drug metabolizing enzyme could become a victim, it is the inhibitors, inducers, and substrates of the cytochrome P450 enzymes (CYPs), for which the great majority of metabolic DDIs occur. To a large extent that is because CYPs are more prominent in the metabolism of drugs than any other type of enzyme, as shown in Figure 12.2.

12.2.1 DDIs Associated with Alteration of Cytochrome P450 Activity

As pointed out in Chapter 8, approximately three-fourths of all drugs are processed by CYPs, which are also the most abundant drug metabolizing enzymes in key clearing organs such as the intestines and the liver. Within the intestines the relative contributions of individual CYPs to total CYP content are: CYP3A, 82%; CYP2C9, 14%; CYP2C19, 2%; and CYP2D6, <1%. The relative contributions of individual CYPs to total CYP content in the liver are: CYP3A, 40%; CYP2C9 and 2C19 combined, 25%; CYP1A2, 10%; CYP2E1, 9%; CYP2A6, 6%; CYP2D6, 2%; and CYP2B6, <1%. The importance of CYP enzymes in metabolic DDIs is illustrated by the number of papers appearing in scientific and medical journals in which DDIs have been ascribed to the alteration of CYP activity. These papers numbered fewer than 10 per year since the time of the discovery of the CYPs until the mid-1980s. From the mid-1980s until 2000 the rate of publication of papers investigating the role of CYPs in DDIs increased exponentially with between 150 and 200 such papers published in 2000.

The strategy for *a priori* prediction of the clinical significance of DDIs evolved from a meeting of academic, regulatory, and pharmaceutical industry scientists who met under the auspices of the European Federation of Pharmaceutical Sciences (EUFEPS), and first published a consensus document in the European Journal of Pharmaceutical Sciences in 2001. Similar reports appeared shortly thereafter in the U.S. literature in key journals in clinical pharmacology and drug metabolism. The main focus of this strategy was to use *in vitro* drug metabolism data, particularly data pertaining to the inhibition of CYP enzymes by a potential perpetrator, in the prediction of the clinical significance of DDIs for this perpetrator. The *in vitro* enzyme inhibition data can be used alone or in combination with limited *in vivo* (clinical) data about the perpetrator as will be discussed shortly. The *in vitro* experiments are designed to quantitate the inhibition of a specific CYP enzyme by the potential perpetrator drug.

12.2.1.1 Predicting the Clinical Significance of DDIs Associated with CYP Inhibition from In Vitro *Data*

Ultimately, these *a priori* predictions rely on accurate *in vitro* estimates of the inhibition of specific CYP enzymes by perpetrators (inhibitors). The removal of a drug (substrate) from the blood by enzymatic metabolism (e.g., a specific CYP enzyme) occurring in a clearing organ such as the liver, is defined by the key quantitative characteristics of the (collective) enzymes that mediate that substrate's metabolism, namely Vmax and Km (see Chapter 8). If low enough substrate concentrations are used, then the ability of specific hepatic CYP enzymes to remove or clear drug from the blood can be quantitated as $\frac{V_{max}}{K_m}$, which would also be known as the *in vitro* CL_{int} or intrinsic clearance. Depending upon the nature of inhibition elicited by an inhibitor (perpetrator, in DDI terms), the addition of a perpetrator to an *in vitro* system might decrease V_{max}, increase K_m, or do both. Accordingly, it is possible to estimate a substrate's (victim, in DDI terms) intrinsic clearance in the absence (CL_{int}) and in the presence ($CL_{int,i}$) of a specified concentration of perpetrator (inhibitor) in *in vitro* experiments.

Alternatively we could measure the IC50 or the K_i (inhibitory constant) for the perpetrator. The K_i of a perpetrator that is capable of inhibiting an enzyme (or transporter) is the dissociation constant for the enzyme-inhibitor complex. Accurate estimation of the K_i requires, among other things, the appropriate definition or specification of the type of enzyme inhibition (e.g., competitive, noncompetitive, or uncompetitive). The appropriate *in vitro* experiments require that multiple concentrations of the inhibitor must be used as well as a range of substrate concentrations that embrace the substrate K_m, and from these experiments both the type of inhibition elicited by the perpetrator can be deduced and the K_i value for the perpetrator can be estimated. The K_i will have units of concentration. Alternatively, K_i values can be computed from IC_{50} values for an inhibitor. The IC_{50} is defined simply as the inhibitor concentration that decreases the biotransformation of a substrate at a single, specified concentration by 50%. This parameter obviously also has units of concentration (e.g., μM), and can be related to the K_i as follows.

For noncompetitive inhibition the IC_{50} and K_i values will be equal. For competitive inhibition $IC_{50} = K_i\left(1 + \frac{[S]}{K_m}\right)$, and if $[S]$ is much less than K_m, then $IC_{50} \sim K_i$. For competitive inhibition, if $[S]=K_m$, then $K_i \sim 0.5{*}IC_{50}$. This numerical approximation applies for uncompetitive inhibition as well, when $[S]$ approximates K_m. Armed with an experimental K_i for a perpetrator and an *in vitro* measure of CL_{int} for the substrate (victim) acquired in the absence of perpetrator, $CL_{int,i}$ can be calculated from:

$$CL_{int,i} = \frac{CL_{int}}{1 + \frac{[I]}{K_i}} \qquad (12.1)$$

where $[I]$ denotes the concentration of perpetrator (inhibitor) used.

The matrices for conducting these *in vitro* experiments have not been standardized. Some investigators prefer to use human hepatic microsomes, others prefer heterologous systems that express individual CYP enzymes, and others prefer fresh or cryopreserved human hepatocytes or even human liver slices. Quantitative outcomes can be affected by the choice of *in vitro* system and also by the substrate selected as the victim drug. Substrates that have been engineered to be highly selective for specific CYPs and highly fluorescent, making them suitable for use in HTP screens for enzyme inhibition, may not always yield, in the presence of perpetrator (inhibitor) drugs, K_i values that are comparable to those likely to occur when *bona fide* clinically used drugs are used as victim drugs in the assays. Indeed, The EUFEPS Conference Report recommended that the use of recombinant enzyme systems be limited to qualitative estimates of K_i owing to the variable expression of enzyme across systems as well as the variable stoichiometries of reductase and cytochrome b5 relative to enzyme levels across systems. These variabilities can at least be partially compensated by the application of relative activity factors (RAF). Alternatively, a normalized rate (NR) for a CYP reaction catalyzed by a recombinant enzyme can be computed by multiplying the reaction rate by the mean specific content of that CYP that is found in native human liver microsomes, and then summed for all CYPs to give a total normalized rate (TNR), and the percent TNR can be directly related to percent inhibition. Unfortunately, for some of the CYP enzymes the specific content within different human livers can vary by more than an order of magnitude.

Another approach that has been used to correct for differences in microsomes isolated from human livers versus individual enzymes expressed in heterologous expression systems involves the application of intersystem extrapolation factors, or ISEFs, that are empirically derived correction factors.

Regardless of the *in vitro* matrix used in the estimation of K_i and CL_{int}, another problem is the failure to account for nonspecific binding of the substrate and inhibitor (i.e., victim and perpetrator, respectively). Failure to account for nonspecific binding within cells, to microsomes, even to plates and other incubation vessels can lead to errant estimates of K_i.

Technical complications notwithstanding, how might the *in vitro* estimation of a victim drug's CL_{int} in the presence of a perpetrator ($CL_{int,i}$) be used to predict the clinical significance of a putative inhibitory DDI? If you'll recall, the underlying principle in predicting the clinical significance of a DDI is related to the prediction in the change in exposure (AUC) to the victim drug in the presence of the perpetrator drug (inhibitor). When there is no perpetrator involved, the AUC of the victim drug is inversely related to its intrinisic clearance (CL_{int}). In the presence of an inhibiting perpetrator drug the AUC of the victim drug (AUC_i) is inversely related to its intrinsic clearance ($CL_{int,i}$). Thus, the exposure or AUC to the victim in the presence of an inhibitor (AUC_i) relative to the exposure to the victim in the absence of an inhibitor (AUC) is given by:

$$\frac{AUC_i}{AUC} = \frac{CL_{int}}{CL_{int,i}} \tag{12.2}$$

Since $CL_{int,i}$ is determined by K_i and by the concentration of the inhibitor ([I]) as shown in Equation (12.1), if Equation (12.1) is substituted for $CL_{int,i}$ in Equation (12.2), then:

$$\frac{AUC_i}{AUC} = 1 + \frac{[I]}{K_i} \tag{12.3}$$

The ratio of $\frac{AUC_i}{AUC}$ is referred to as the AUC ratio. Once again, it denotes the increase in exposure to the victim in the presence of perpetrator relative to exposure in the absence of perpetrator. At this point there has *not* been a measurement of either AUC or AUC_i. These are *in vivo* measurements that could be measured only if the victim drug were administered to humans absent the perpetrator drug (AUC) and in the presence of the perpetrator drug (AUC_i). Nevertheless, the AUC ratio depends only on $[I]$ and K_i, and the K_i value, in fact, can be acquired from *in vitro* experiments. The strategy developed at the EUFEPS conference was to estimate the AUC ratio from K_i values obtained from *in vitro* experiments in accordance with Equation (12.3). The relationship between the AUC ratio and the K_i value for an inhibitory perpetrator is shown in Figure 12.3.

Actually, the predicted AUC ratio is plotted as a function of $[I]/K_i$, where $[I]$ denotes the concentration of the inhibitory perpetrator drug. But selecting an appropriate concentration or value for $[I]$ turns out to be a thorny issue. The AUC ratio is supposed to be predicted for the *in vivo* use of the victim drug in the presence of an *in vivo* concentration of the perpetrator. But, for predictive purposes, what *in vivo* concentration of perpetrator ($[I]$) ought to be selected? Should it be the average steady-state concentration? Should it be the peak steady-state concentration? Should it be measured in plasma? Should it represent the concentration in the liver? And, by the way, just how high should the predicted AUC ratio be predicted to be, before a DDI is thought to be clinically significant?

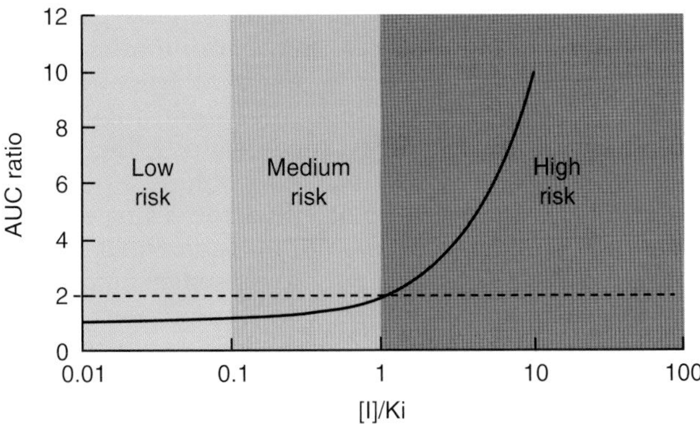

Figure 12.3 Relationship between AUC ratio and the ratio of $[I]/K_i$.

This last question has been addressed with a consensus opinion that a threshold AUC ratio of ≥2 is required before a DDI is considered a high risk DDI (Figure 12.3). Likewise an AUC ratio of ≤1.25 (for inhibitory DDIs) signifies low risk or no risk for a clinically significant DDI.

It would appear that by default AUC ratios that fall between 1.25 and 2 are viewed as posing moderate risk of a clinically significant DDI. Now, based on Equation (12.3) and Figure 12.3 it should also be apparent that the same risk (for a clinically significant DDI) analysis can be cast in terms of the $[I]/K_i$ ratio as well, only here the qualitative risk boundaries are as follows:

$[I]/K_i \leq 0.1$, small or no risk
$[I]/K_i$ between 0.1 and 1.0; moderate risk
$[I]/K_i \geq 1$; high risk of clinically significant DDI

Remember, the K_i is a parameter that can be derived strictly from *in vitro* experiments, and if the K_i is for a specific CYP enzyme, the experiments can be conducted using hepatic microsomes, cells, liver slices, or heterologous expression systems. The value for $[I]$, according to consensus, was supposed to be the steady-state peak plasma concentration (C_{max}) of the perpetrator in humans. However, in spite of the consensus opinion, some have found that C_{max} (i.e. $[I]_{max}$) does not always give the best prediction of the actual AUC ratio in humans. Various other fluid concentrations of the perpetrator have been proposed to be used in the computation of $[I]/K_i$, and some of them are listed in Table 12.1.

Indeed, Houston and colleagues at the University of Manchester in the U.K., who have been instrumental in establishing and refining the prediction of DDIs in humans from *in vitro* K_i data, have shown that not only will the predictive accuracy, which they refer to as qualitative zoning (e.g., low risk, moderate risk, and high risk), vary depending upon which value is selected for $[I]$, but the predictive accuracy will also vary depending on which value of $[I]$ is used even for a given CYP enzyme. In evaluating nearly 200 DDIs for which actual human AUC ratio data had been

Table 12.1 Representative Methods for the Selection or Computation of $[I]$

Choice of [*I*]	Computation of [*I*]
Average steady-state plasma concentration	$[I]_{av} = \frac{FD}{CL \times \tau}$
Peak steady-state plasma concentration	$[I]_{\max} = \frac{[I]_{av} k\tau}{(1 - \exp^{-k\tau})}$
Maximum hepatic input concentration	$[I]_{in} = [I]_{av} + \left(\frac{kaFaD}{Q}\right)$
Concentration in the hepatocytes	$[I]_{hep} = \frac{[I]_{in\ vitro}}{[I]_{medium}} \times [I]_{blood}$
Unbound concentration	$[I]_i \times f_u$

Table 12.2 The Percentage of True Positives, True Negatives, False Positives, and False Negatives as a Function of the Value for $[I]$[a]

	CYP3A4				CYP2D6				CYP2C9			
Result	$[I]av$	$[I]av_u^b$	$[I]max$	$[I]in$	$[I]av$	$[I]av_u^b$	$[I]max$	$[I]in$	$[I]av$	$[I]av_u^b$	$[I]max$	$[I]in$
True positives (%)	22	7	24	50	20	0	20	29	23	16	23	31
True negatives (%)	43	43	42	33	65	71	65	25	46	44	35	23
% correct[c]	65	50	66	83	85	71	85	54	69	60	58	54

[a]Values denote the percentage of data points in each category.
[b]This is $[I]_{av\ unbound}$ or $[I]_{av*fu}$.
[c]Denotes the sum of true positives plus true negatives.

determined in clinical trials and for which they had *in vitro* K_i data, they were able to actually pair true *AUC* ratios with $[I]/K_i$ data. One purpose for matching $[I]/K_i$ data with actual AUC ratios was to assess the accuracy of the entire predictive strategy discussed earlier. They tabulated the true positive predictions that were defined as all the data points for which the AUC ratio was ≥ 2 AND the $[I]/K_i$ ratio was ≥ 1 (Figure 12.3). They also tabulated the true negative predictions that were represented by AUC ratios ≤ 1.1 AND $[I]/K_i$ ratios ≤ 0.1. They did this for inhibitory DDIs involving three distinct CYPs, namely CYP3A4, CYP2D6, and CYP2C9. Their abridged findings are shown in Table 12.2.

The bottom line (literally) in Table 12.2 is merely the sum of the percentages of true positives and true negatives. Note, for example, for CYP3A4 the highest total percent correct AUC ratios that were predicted from $[I]/K_i$ ratios (83%) occurred when $[I]_{in}$ was used; that is, the computed concentration of perpetrator drug in the hepatic portal vein (Table 12.1). In contrast, for CYP2D6 the highest percent correct (sum of true positive plus true negative) predictions occurred when either $[I]_{max}$ or $[I]_{av}$ was used (85% for both). Interestingly, for inhibitory DDIs ascribed to CYP2C9 inhibition the predictive accuracy of an AUC ratio ≥ 2 or ≤ 1 was highest when $[I]_{av}$ was used in the $[I]/K_i$ ratio, however it only reached 69%.

What about the universality of the K_i value of a perpetrator for a particular CYP enzyme? Unfortunately the *in vitro* K_i value may vary depending on which victim drug is used as the substrate. There is evidence that some of the substrates engineered to be used (as victim drugs) with perpetrators (inhibitors) in HTP screens for assessing K_i values, yield K_i values for specific CYP enzymes that don't correlate very well with the K_i values computed when standard (clinically used) drugs are used as victim drugs. And, as mentioned earlier, K_i values can vary depending upon which *in vitro* matrix (isolated microsomes vs. heterologously expressed enzymes vs. hepatocytes) is used to study the DDI.

Yet another problem may arise from the increasingly apparent phenomenon of atypical enzyme kinetics of the substrate drug. One of the problems that has plagued the drug metabolism community until recently is the apparent lack of correlation between the clearance rates of multiple probes for the same CYPs. In part, at least, these poor correlations can now be ascribed to the allosteric kinetics of the CYP enzymes. For example, a single substrate for CYP3A4 may be capable of binding at either of two different locations in the broader binding site (see Chapter 8). Two molecules of substrate might bind simultaneously at two different locations within the broader binding site, which could lead to homotropic activation of the enzyme. Two different substrates might bind simultaneously at two different locations within the broader binding site leading to heterotropic activation of the enzyme. Allosteric kinetics occur among CYPs other than CYP3A, and they give rise to atypical enzyme kinetics that are not described by the simple Michaelis-Menten equation. Multiple binding arrangements for different CYP3A4 substrates may contribute to K_i values for a single inhibitor that vary by more than 10-fold, depending upon the substrate used. Carefully structured *in vitro* studies with more than one substrate and a range of substrate concentrations that enabled multisite kinetic analysis have demonstrated partial inhibition, cooperative inhibition, and concentration-dependent inhibition, but no mutual inhibition of CYP3A4 when combinations of nifedipine, midazolam, felodipine, and testosterone were used simultaneously. Clearly, the failure to account for atypical kinetics in *in vitro* experiments could give rise to errant values for K_m and K_i. The EUFEPS conference report recommended that the issue of enzyme cooperativity for CYP3A4 and CYP2C9 be addressed, at least partially, by the determination of IC_{50} values using at least two low (therapeutic) concentrations of at least two substrates, one of which is known to exhibit homotropic cooperativity, and by full characterization of activation kinetics when defining *in vitro* CL_{int} values.

It could be observed that in light of the vexing and variable issues such as the selection of *in vivo* perpetrator concentration ($[I]$), the experimental system for estimating K_i, the issue of nonspecific victim and perpetrator binding, and the sometimes atypical kinetics (see Chapter 8) of CYP enzymes associated with multiple substrate binding sites, heterotropic, and homotropic effects, that it is surprising that $[I]/K_i$ predictions of AUC ratios are as good as they are. After all, for DDIs involving inhibition of CYP2C9, CYP3A4, and CYP2D6 the accuracy of the clinical significance of DDIs from $[I]/K_i$ ratios computed from *in vitro* K_i values paired with *in vivo* perpetrator concentrations ($[I]$) was about 70%, 83%, and 85%, respectively (Table 12.2).

Refinements to the Prediction of the Significance of Inhibitory DDIs Based on *In Vivo* Values for [*I*] and *In Vitro* Values for K_i

Accounting for Mechanism-based Inhibition If a perpetrator elicits either competitive or noncompetitive inhibition of a CYP enzyme, then the *in vivo* AUC ratio can be predicted from an appropriately determined value for $[I]$ and for K_i in accordance with Equations (12.1), (12.2), and (12.3). On the other hand, if a perpetrator elicits mechanism-based inhibition (see Chapter 8) of a CYP, then the AUC ratio becomes:

$$AUC_{ratio} = \frac{k_{deg} + \dfrac{[I] \times k_{inact}}{[I] + K_{iapp}}}{k_{deg}} \tag{12.4}$$

where, as defined in Chapter 8, k_{inact} is the apparent inactivation rate constant for the enzyme; K_{iapp} is the concentration of inhibitor (perpetrator) that elicits a $k_{inact}/2$; and k_{deg} is the degradation rate constant for the enzyme.

There is some evidence that it may be possible to apply Equation (12.3) even in the case of mechanism-based inhibition so long as the inhibiting drug is preincubated for 30 minutes prior to the addition of the substrate.

Mechanism-based enzyme inhibition may be one of the more important types of DDIs, and examples of drugs that inhibit CYP enzymes in this fashion include paroxetine inhibition of CYP2D6, verapamil inhibition of CYP3A4, and the inhibition of CYP3A4 by protease inhibitors such as ritonavir. Some of the other drugs that cause mechanism-based inhibition of CYP enzymes include erythromycin, fluvoxamine, and ethinyl estradiol.

Accounting for the Fraction of Drug Metabolized by a Given CYP Enzyme How much of a victim drug must be metabolized by an enzyme, before enzyme inhibition by a perpetrator is likely to be clinically significant? Benchmarks have been set as low as 30%, but a good case can be made for 50%. For a drug that is cleared in part by metabolism via a CYP enzyme, its clearance in the presence of an inhibitor (perpetrator) of that enzyme can be defined as follows:

$$CL_{int,i} = CL_{int}(1 - fm_{cyp}) \tag{12.5}$$

where CL_{int} represents all clearance routes. Accordingly, the maximum impact on the AUC ratio that could occur if the metabolic contribution to drug clearance were completely stopped by a perpetrator (inhibitor) would be given by:

$$AUCratio = \frac{1}{1 - fm_{cyp}} \tag{12.6}$$

Thus, only if fm_{CYP} were 0.5 would the AUC ratio double by CYP inhibition. However, as described earlier, the extent of clearance inhibition associated with enzyme inhibition actually depends upon the K_i value for the perpetrator. If a victim drug is metabolized by a single CYP enzyme, and if metabolism accounts for $\geq$50% of the victim drug's total clearance, then the AUC ratio arising from inhibition of that enzyme by a perpetrator is given by the Rowland-Matin equation:

$$AUCratio = \frac{1}{\dfrac{fm_{cyp}}{1 + \dfrac{[I]}{Ki}} + (1 - fm_{cyp})} \tag{12.7}$$

If a victim drug (i.e., substrate) is subject to multiple metabolic pathways accounting for more than 50% of the total clearance of the victim drug, and if a perpetrator (inhibitor) affects those enzymes in quantitatively different ways, another layer of complexity is added to the estimation of the AUC ratio from $[I]/K_i$ data. If, say, two pathways are subject to inhibition by a particular inhibitor, the fraction of victim drug metabolized by each of the two pathways is known, and the K_i values for the perpetrator on each of the two pathways is known, then the AUC ratio can be described by:

$$AUCratio = \frac{1}{\left(\dfrac{fm_{cyp1}}{1 + \dfrac{[I]}{K_i, 1}}\right) + \left(\dfrac{1 - fm_{cyp2}}{1 + \dfrac{[I]}{K_i, 2}}\right)} \tag{12.8}$$

Accounting for Cooperativity In Chapter 8 it was noted that the kinetics of drug processing do not always occur in a manner that can be described by the Michaelis-Menten model, and that non-Michaelis-Menten kinetics can occur when an enzyme binding site accommodates more than one molecule at a time, opening the door to the phenomenon of cooperativity. Two identical molecules binding at the same time (homotropic) can be either positively or negatively cooperative. Two different molecules binding at the same time (heterotropic) can be positively or negatively cooperative. For an enzyme that can accommodate two molecules at the same time, the AUC ratio elicited by an inhibitor (perpetrator) can be described as follows:

$$AUCratio = \frac{\left(1 + \dfrac{[I]}{K_i}\right)^2}{1 + \dfrac{\gamma[I]}{\delta K_i}} \tag{12.9}$$

where γ is an interaction factor that denotes the change in catalytic efficacy in the presence of inhibitor, and δ is an interaction factor that denotes the change in binding affinity in the presence of inhibitor. When these two interaction factors are equivalent, Equation (12.9) simplifies to Equation (12.3).

Uncompetitive Inhibition As with mechanism-based inhibition, the failure to acknowledge the occurrence of uncompetitive inhibition could lead to errors in the prediction of the AUC ratio and risk of a DDI. Although there are, as yet, no prominent examples of uncompetitive inhibition of CYPs, the AUC ratio for the phenomenon would be given as:

$$AUCratio = 1 + \left(\frac{[I]}{K_i}\right)\left(\frac{[S]}{[S] + K_m}\right) \tag{12.10}$$

where $[S]$ and K_m are the concentration and Michaelis constant for the victim drug, and $[I]$ and K_i have their usual meanings for the perpetrator drug.

12.2.1.2 Interactions Resulting from Increased Enzyme Activity

In Chapter 8, the major role played by nuclear receptors as transcription factors in the increased expression of drug metabolizing enzymes was described. The key nuclear receptors in this regard are the AhR causing increased expression of CYP1A; PXR causing increased expression chiefly of CYP3A but also CYP2C9; and CAR causing increased expression of CYP2B6 and CYP2C. Actually, activation of PXR or CAR can lead to increased expression of some of the same enzymes due to their overlapping activities. Just as CYP3A plays a greater role in the oxidative metabolism of drugs compared to other CYP enzymes, PXR agonism is primarily responsible for the increased expression of enzymes, namely CYP3A4, and also for increased expression of P-glycoprotein (PgP), an efflux transporter. To be sure, CYP activities can be increased by mechanisms other than transactivation of CYP genes. For example, ethanol induces its own metabolism by CYP2E1 via stabilization of the protein thereby slowing its rate of degradation. And, as mentioned earlier and described in Chapter 8, some drugs can increase rates of drug metabolism by heterotropic or homotropic activation. However, it would appear that the majority of DDIs associated with perpetrator-elicited increases in the rate of metabolism of victim drugs is associated with perpetrator agonism of orphan receptors such as the PXR.

Long before the roles of AhR, PXR, or CAR in enzyme induction were known, it was recognized that numerous xenobiotics, including some drugs, were capable of increasing the activity of drug metabolizing enzymes; most notably the activity of CYPs. One of the earliest comprehensive compilations of information about the experimental induction of drug metabolizing enzymes by xenobiotics was compiled by Dr. A. H. Conney. Dozens of monographs and review papers about enzyme induction and DDIs have been published in both the clinical and scientific literature since Conney's review of enzyme induction and its pharmacological consequences in 1967. Some focus on therapeutic categories of drugs that are affected by enzyme induction. Others focus on the types of drugs that elicit enzyme induction such as the rifamycins. Still others focus on phytochemicals found within herbal remedies or nutraceuticals that can cause enzyme induction. Both the Flockhart database on DDIs and the Fujitsu database (vide supra) can both be searched for drugs that are CYP inducers.

If a perpetrator can, through transactivation of one or more CYP genes, increase the expression of CYP enzymes in, say, the liver, then might it be possible, as with inhibitory DDIs, to predict the clinical significance of that transactivation based on *in vitro* measures of transactivation? Possibly, but just how analogous to *in vitro* enzyme inhibition is the phenomenon of *in vitro* enzyme induction? For *in vitro* inhibitory experiments the key quantitative parameter denoting a perpetrator's ability to inhibit a specific enzyme is K_i. On the other hand, transactivation experiments typically measure the ability of, for example, a PXR agonist, to increase PXR activation in a reporter gene assay using luminescence intensity as the signal for PXR activation. The magnitude of transactivation is referenced to a positive control such as rifampin and also to a negative control such as DMSO. If transactivation is referenced only to a negative control such as DMSO, then induction could be quantitated as the luminescence response of the perpetrator relative to the luminescence response to DMSO, or $\frac{signal_{agonist}}{signal_{control}}$.

However, in the absence of a positive control, this data would be difficult to interpret. For example would a signal ratio of 1.4 indicate a low, medium, or high risk of a clinically significant *in vivo* interaction? If the signal were referenced to a positive control such as rifampin, the extrapolation of the *in vitro* findings to *in vivo* significance may also be difficult. For example, the positive control (e.g., rifampin) is typically used in a single concentration in the *in vitro* experiments (e.g., 10 μM). Suppose the positive control caused the luminescence signal to be 10 times higher than background (i.e., 10 × transactivation). The test perpetrator, however, causes the luminescence signal to be five times higher than background. This response is 50% of the response caused by rifampin. How should that be interpreted? Of course it's possible to combine both the negative and positive controls into the quantitation of the response of a perpetrator *in vitro*. One way of doing so is as follows:

$$\%\ \text{activation} = \frac{(signal_{agonist} - signal_{control})}{(signal_{rifampin} - signal_{control})} \times 100 \tag{12.11}$$

While taking account of the signal produced by a vehicle control such as DMSO, this method for quantitating transactivation is fundamentally still done in the context of the positive control (rifampin). Again, if the response were to be 50%, how should that be interpreted in a clinical sense? What if the response had been 20%? Such a response still might denote a twofold increase (compared to control) in PXR activation if, for example, the rifampin signal were 10 times higher than the control signal.

As in the *in vitro* inhibition experiments, the outcomes must be referenced to some *in vivo* concentration of the perpetrator. Michael Sinz and colleagues at Bristol-Myers Squibb Co. have evaluated the *in vitro* transactivation of the human PXR by 170 xenobiotics using Equation (12.11). They constructed dose-response curves for an entire range of concentrations for each perpetrator. Then they then asked the question, "What would be the expected *in vivo* percent transactivation for an *in vivo* concentration if perpetrator was the same as its expected peak plasma concentration, C_{max}? They delineated perpetrators with a high potential of inducing CYP3A4 *in vivo* as those that caused 40% transactivation *in vitro* at concentrations equal to the known *in vivo* C_{max}. Those that caused less than 15% transactivation *in vitro* at concentrations equal to the known *in vivo* C_{max} were said to have a low potential to cause enzyme induction *in vivo*. Compounds that caused between 15 and 40% transactivation *in vitro* at concentrations equal to the known *in vivo* C_{max} were deemed to have a moderate potential to cause enzyme induction *in vivo*. This is broadly similar to the qualitative zoning that evolved for the prediction of the clinical significance of inhibitor DDIs based on $[I]/K_i$ ratios. Using the qualitative zoning boundaries set forth by the group at Bristol-Myers Squibb, their analysis of 170 putative enzyme inducers revealed only nine that they predicted to have a high potential for clinically significant enzyme induction, and another four that they predicted to have a moderate potential. The rest had low or no potential.

Again, whether Equation (12.11) constitutes the best way to characterize *in vitro* transactivation, or whether activation referenced exclusively to a negative control would be more meaningful still remains to be determined. For example an alternative strategy might be to look at the ratio of $\frac{signal_{agonist}}{signal_{control}}$. Suppose this were 3.0 at an *in vitro* concentration equal to the known *in vivo* C_{max}? How could we rule out a significant *in vivo* enzyme induction effect? Moreover, any prediction that includes a value for an *in vivo* concentration of perpetrator raises the same issues that were discussed in Section 12.2.1.1. That is, should total concentration in plasma be used or should the unbound concentration be used? Should the concentration be a C_{max} as proposed by the group at Bristol-Myers Squibb, or should it be a concentration at the inlet of the liver or the concentration within hepatocytes? A group of Pfizer scientists suggest using the plasma C_{max} adjusted for binding (i.e., unbound C_{max}).

Just as these issues are still under investigation for the use of the $[I]/K_i$ paradigm in the prediction of the clinical significance of inhibitory DDIs, so, too, must they be evaluated in any predictive method aimed at inferring the clinical significance of enzyme induction-related DDIs that might be drawn from a mix of clinical drug concentrations and *in vitro* measures of enzyme induction. For inhibitory DDIs you may recall that a consensus opinion that perpetrator K_i values $\leq 1\mu M$ tend to be predictive of a high probability of a clinically significant DDI. There is insufficient analysis of induction-type experiments to permit a similar generalization about putative inducing agents.

Among the "high probability" inducers that produced *in vitro* transactivation greater than 40% of that produced by rifampin, all but one of the EC50 values for induction was less than 2 μM. However, only nine substances were high probability inducers, and even some low and medium probability inducers exhibited EC50 values less than 2 μM. On the other hand, the Pfizer group used both *in vitro* Emax and EC50 values to try and characterize the extent of induction. They first computed relative induction scores (RIS) for each of about two dozen inducers. The RIS was computed as $\frac{C_{max,unb} * E_{max}}{C_{max,unb} + \text{EC50}}$. Next they correlated the *in vitro* RIS with the percent reduction in AUC measured *in vivo*. This was done for two separate CYP3A4 substrates, namely midazolam and ethinyl estradiol. Though the curves were not identical for both substrates, the data points for both curves (one curve for midazolam and another for ethinyl estradiol) fit a three-parameter Hill function extremely well. Maximum *in vivo* induction plateaued once the RIS reached a value of about 0.5. From this analysis, we might infer that *in vitro* RIS values very much greater than 0.5 (e.g., 9 or 10) will produce no greater *in vivo* decreases in AUC than RIS values at approximately 0.5. Unfortunately, the slopes of the *in vivo* decrease in AUC versus RIS curves for midazolam and ethinyl estradiol were quite different from one another, making it hard to delineate the lowest RIS score that might define a clinically significant inductive DDI. If, for example, we were to assume that a 25% decrease in AUC would represent the least likely occurrence of a clinically significant DDI, then the RIS for inducers of midazolam metabolism would have to exhibit an RIS of approximately 0.02, whereas inducers of ethinyl estradiol metabolism would have to exhibit only an RIS of about 0.07.

It must also be recognized that there is not a linear correlation between the extent of *in vitro* induction or transactivation and in the magnitude of *in vivo* increases in clearance or decreases in AUC in humans. Though it represents a fairly crude attempt to match *in vivo* changes in drug metabolism (e.g., decreases in AUC, increases in clearance, or increases in metabolic ratios) to *in vitro* increases in transactivation or metabolic activity (expressed as fold increases), the nonlinearity between the two is exemplified in Figure 12.4. *In vitro* data was paired with *in vivo* data when both could be found for common perpetrator/victim pairs. For example, *in vivo* data for rifampin-induced changes in warfarin clearance was paired with *in vitro* data for induction of CYP2C9 by rifampin. The inducers for which both *in vivo* and *in vitro* data could be matched—typically *not* from the same study—were ritonavir, rifampin, sulfinpyrazone, phenobarbital, troglitazone, and either hyperforin or St John's wort. The victim drugs (or endobiotics) were warfarin, midazolam, erythromycin, alfentanil, and cortisol. As can be seen from the plot in Figure 12.4, even for perpetrators that could elicit more than 15-fold increases in *in vitro* metabolism or transactivation, those same perpetrators appeared to cause *in vivo* increases in clearance or metabolic ratios or decreases in AUC of not much more than two-fold.

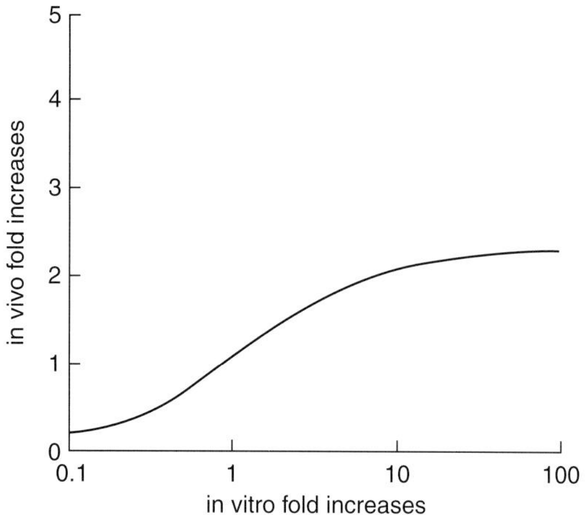

Figure 12.4 Increases in *in vivo* clearance or decreases in AUC correlated to *in vitro* fold increases in transactivation or enzyme activity.

As we get closer to being able to link EC50 and E_{max} values for PXR activation to the prediction of the significance of *in vivo* inductive DDIs, then even *in silico* approaches could also be used. Computer modeling methods are in place for computing EC50 values of transactivators on the basis of their fits to pharmacophore models of the human PXR (hPXR). As these models are refined and the computer-generated estimates of EC50 values begin to match more closely the actual *in vitro* EC50 values generated from reporter-gene transactivation assays, it may become possible to use these values along with, for example, *in vivo* C_{max} values in order to predict the clinical significance of enzyme induction interactions.

To get a sense of the xenobiotics that are known to cause clinically significant inductive DDIs in humans, check out the inducer table at http://medicine.iupui.edu/flockhart/table.htm.

12.2.2 Phase II Enzymes and DDIs

More is known about metabolic DDIs associated with CYP enzymes than any other drug-processing enzyme. This no doubt reflects the comparative extent to which these enzymes have been researched, the relative abundance of these enzymes, and their overall contribution to drug metabolism. Phase II enzymes have been less intensively studied, are collectively responsible for the metabolism of fewer drugs than the CYPs, and are often not responsible for the rate-limiting step in drug metabolism. It follows that less is known about their role in DDIs. Having said that, there are some very important Phase II reactions, and among the Phase II enzymes UDP-glucuronosyltransferases (UGTs) mediate more than one-third of the Phase II reactions of all drugs that are subject to Phase II metabolism. More information about UGTs and other Phase II enzymes can be found in Chapter 8.

As a quick reminder, though, the human UGTs comprise a superfamily of enzymes that play a role in the metabolism of numerous endobiotics and xenobiotics. They utilize UDP-glucuronic acid as a cofactor, and are bound to the internal membrane of endoplasmic reticulum. The human UGT superfamily consists of the UGT1 and UGT2 families and the UGT1A, UGT2A, and UGT2B subfamilies. As is the case with CYP enzymes, the UGTs tend to convert molecules to more hydrophilic metabolites, and—more often than not—less pharmacologically active molecules than their parent molecules. Although there is some evidence of substrate selectivity, in fact, most substrates are glucuronidated by multiple UGTs. The regulation of UGTs bears some similarity to the regulation of CYPs in that AhR, CAR, and PXR have been found to be involved in the increased expression of individual UGTs. Specifically, hPXR and CAR mediate UGT1A1 induction, whereas AhR regulates UGT1A6 and UGT1A9 induction.

UGTs are, like CYPs, inhibitible. However, unlike inhibitors of CYPs, there are very few known UGT inhibitors exhibiting *in vitro* K_i values ≤ 1 µM. Therefore, although ranitidine, propranolol, and cisapride have been shown to inhibit acetaminophen glucuronidation, it's not clear that this inhibition would be a clinically significant phenomenon. Likewise, although atovaquone, fluconazole, naproxen, and valproic acid have been shown to inhibit the glucuronidation of the antiretroviral drug, AZT, only the effects of fluconazole on the PK parameters of AZT (namely AUC and C_{max}) could be characterized as clinically meaningful. Tacrolimus, which elicits a K_i of 0.033 µM when mycophenolic acid is the UGT substrate in a kidney microsomal system, was shown to cause a 1.5-fold increase in the AUC for mycophenolate in 18 stable renal transplant patients. It's somewhat disconcerting that the two UGT inhibitors eliciting what might be considered clinically significant changes in victim drug PK (i.e., fluconazole inhibition of AZT glucuronidation and tacrolimus inhibition of mycophenolate glucuronidation) exhibit *in vitro* K_i values of 163 and 0.033 µM, respectively. Probenecid, better known for its inhibition of renal OATs, however, has been shown to inhibit UGT *in vitro*, and to significantly slow the clearance of lorazepam in humans.

Rifampin, carbamazepine, phenytoin, phenobarbital, and oral contraceptives have been studied for their ability to induce UGTs and alter PK characteristics of select victim drugs in humans. Rifampin caused a more than five-fold decrease in the AUC of codeine and a comparable increase in the oral clearance of codeine, though it didn't alter the AUC of morphine or either of the morphine glucuronides. Rifampin also doubled the clearance of lamotrigine and reduced its half-life comparably. It also caused a profound reduction in the oral bioavailability of propafenone. Estrogen-containing oral contraceptives caused a 65% increase in acetaminophen clearance, and shortened its half-life by about one-third. However, the effects of the anticonvulsant agents, phenytoin, carbamazepine, and phenobarbital, on acetaminophen PK were in the range of 25 to 33%, making it somewhat equivocal as to whether this represents a clinically significant effect.

12.2.3 Inhibition of Xanthine Oxidase

An interesting example of a DDI due to the inhibition of a non-CYP enzyme that can have serious clinical consequences is the inhibition of xanthine oxidase by allopurinol 6-mercaptopurine (6-MP) as an antimetabolite type of antineoplastic drug. One of its indications is in the treatment of inflammatory bowel disease. Actually, 6-MP is a prodrug whose active metabolite, 6-thioguanine (6-TG) is responsible for its therapeutic activity. Some nonresponders to 6-MP do not form sufficient amounts of 6-TG. A complementary pathway of 6-MP metabolism is oxidation to 6-thiouric acid (6TU), which is mediated by xanthine oxidase. Inhibition of this complementary pathway by allopurinol shunts the metabolism of 6-MP favoring increased formation of 6-TG.

12.2.4 Pharmacokinetic Considerations

For an inhibitory perpetrator, the magnitude of change in the plasma concentration versus time curve of the victim, or even in the AUC of the victim may not be well portrayed by Equations (12.3) through (12.9) even if the correct values of $[I]$ and K_i are used. Likewise, even if Equation (12.11) were ideally suited to estimate the extent of *in vitro* activation by an inducing perpetrator, and if the extent of *in vivo* induction or transactivation could be predicted from an *in vivo* C_{max} value of the perpetrator drug, the actual clinical impact of the perpetrator on the plasma concentration versus time curve of the victim drug might, nevertheless, be errantly predicted. Errant prediction of *in vivo* PK outcomes from *in vitro* data (K_i for inhibitory perpetrators and % maximum transactivation for inductive perpetrators) and *in vivo* data about the perpetrator (e.g., C_{max}) most likely would occur for victim drugs with high values for CL_{int}. These drugs (i.e., high clearance drugs) are subject to such rapid metabolic clearance that their total clearances are limited by organ blood flow rather than by metabolic clearance. The overriding contribution of organ blood flow to total clearance can be seen in the simple, well-stirred model of clearance:

$$CL = Q \times \frac{CL_{int}}{(CL_{int} + Q)} \tag{12.12}$$

where Q is organ blood flow rate and CL_{int} is intrinsic clearance mediated by the metabolic machinery of the organ (e.g., liver) and is the product of intrinsic unbound clearance, ($CL_{int,unb}$), and the unbound fraction of drug in the blood, f_u. Now, suppose CL_{int} of a victim drug was actually 10 times faster than hepatic blood flow, for example, $CL_{int} = 10\ Q$. The total organ clearance could be described as:

$$CL = Q \times \frac{10Q}{(10Q + Q)} \tag{12.13}$$

$$CL = .91Q \tag{12.14}$$

Next, suppose a perpetrator drug was added to the therapeutic regimen such that at its C_{max} value it was capable of doubling the rate of metabolism of the victim drug. In this case CL_{int} would double from $10Q$ to $20Q$. However total clearance would become:

$$CL = Q \times \frac{20Q}{(20Q + Q)} \tag{12.15}$$

or

$$CL = .95Q \tag{12.16}$$

Thus, the increase in CL would only be between 4 and 5%. If the victim drug were administered intravenously, it's not likely that there would be a detectable change in the plasma concentration versus time curve of the victim drug.

On the other hand, if the victim drug were given orally, there might be a significant change in the plasma concentration versus time curve. That's because the victim's hepatic extraction ratio is given by:

$$E = \frac{CL_{int}}{(CL_{int} + Q)} \tag{12.17}$$

If CL_{int} of the victim drug before treatment with a perpetrator were $10Q$, then the baseline extraction ratio, E, would be 0.91. For a victim drug processed only by the liver, the oral bioavailability, F, would simply be:

$$F = (1 - E) \tag{12.18}$$

or 9%. As shown earlier, if a perpetrator doubled the CL_{int} of the victim to $20Q$, then according to Equation (12.17), E would become 0.95, and F would become approximately 5%. Thus, for this high clearance victim drug a perpetrator capable of doubling the CL_{int} of the victim drug would decrease the AUC and the C_{max} of the victim drug by close to 50% if the victim drug were administered orally, but would fail to alter the AUC of the victim if the victim were given intravenously.

For the same high clearance victim drug, if a perpetrator were an inhibitor capable of decreasing the CL_{int} (initially $CL_{int} = 10Q$) of the victim by 50%, then the clearance of the victim drug would fall from $0.91Q$ to $0.83Q$ according to Equation (12.12). This would represent about an 8.8% decrease in the total clearance rate of the victim drug. However the extraction ratio, E, would go from an initial value (absent perpetrator) of 0.91 to a value of 0.83, and the oral bioavailability would just about double from the initial value of 9% to a value of 17%. Here, too, the impact of the perpetrator on the AUC and C_{max} of the victim would depend upon the route of administration of the victim. If the victim were administered intravenously, even reducing CL_{int} by 50% would not produce clinically significant changes in victim PK. However, if the victim were given orally, and if a perpetrator reduced the victim's CL_{int} by 50%, then the AUC of the victim and its C_{max} would nearly double. These examples are illustrated in the simulations depicted in Figure 12.5.

Dextromethorphan is a widely used cough suppressant. However, it is also known to possess neuroprotectant, anticonvulsant, and antinociceptive effects associated with NMDA receptor antagonism, calcium

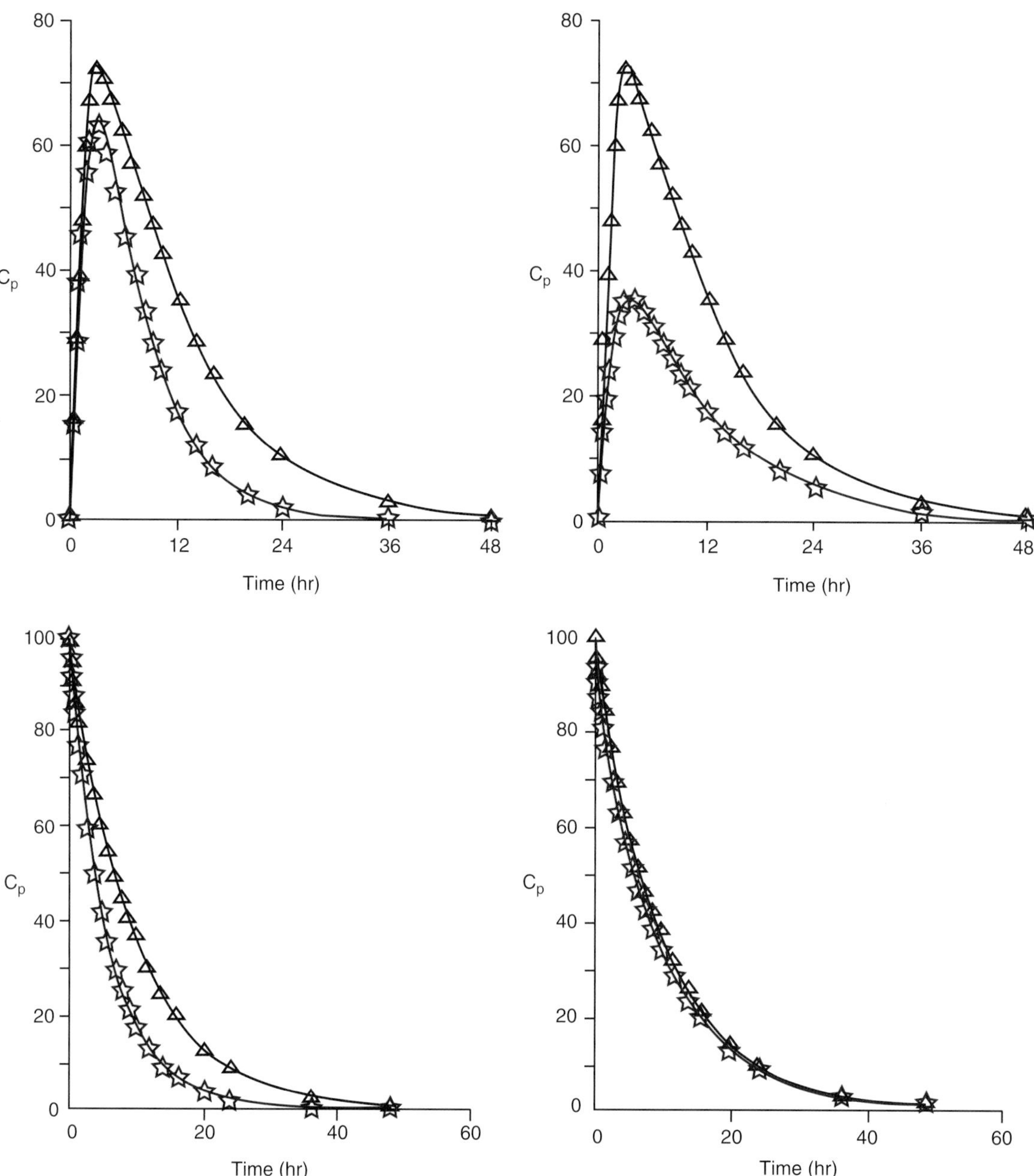

Figure 12.5 Plasma concentration time curves for DDIs if the victim drug is a low clearance drug (left panels) or a high clearance drug (right panels). The lower graphs depict likely outcomes if the victim drug is given intravenously. The upper panels depict likely outcomes if the victim drug is given orally. For a perpetrator acting as an enzyme inducer, the baseline conditions (before perpetrator) would be depicted by the upper curves, and the effect of the perpetrator would be depicted by the lower curves. For a perpetrator acting as an enzyme inhibitor, the baseline conditions (before the perpetrator) would be depicted by the lower curves, and the effect of the perpetrator would be depicted by the upper curves. Either way, note that in the lower right panel, significant changes in CL_{int} of the victim elicited by a perpetrator are not reflected in the shape of the plasma concentration versus time curve of the victim or the victim drug's AUC.

channel inhibition, and interactions with sigma-1 sites and voltage-gated sodium channels. However, the neuroprotectant effects that potentially could be useful in treating Parkinson's disease, amyotrophic lateral sclerosis, Huntington's disease, and neuropathic pain would require plasma concentrations considerably higher than those that develop after typical doses of dextromethorphan for cough. As it turns out, it's not easy to generate measurable plasma concentrations of dextromethorphan, even when doses many times higher than antitussive doses are given. The main reason is that dextromethorphan is cleared so rapidly by hepatic metabolism mediated largely by CYP2D6. Dextromethorphan clearance has been estimated at approximately 110.25 L/min. If hepatic blood flow is approximately 1.5 L/min, then dextromethorphan clearance is 73.5Q. Clearly, its metabolic clearance is flow-limited. Accordingly, its oral bioavailability would be expected to be very limited:

$$F = 1 - \left(\frac{73.5Q}{74.5Q}\right) \quad (12.19)$$

or 1−E. Thus, dextromethorphan would be expected to exhibit a bioavailability of about 1.5%. Quinidine is a highly selective and potent inhibitor of CYP2D6. It's use in a fixed dose combination with dextromethorphan is currently under investigation with a view that the combination might be used to generate high enough blood levels of dextromethorphan so that it could be used for its neuroprotectant effects. Since quinidine is such a potent CYP2D6 inhibitor, the dosages of quinidine could be kept low enough to be devoid of eliciting any effects of its own apart from inhibition of CYP2D6. In theory, if quinidine were used in doses that gave rise to plasma quinidine concentrations equal to its K_i (<0.1 μM or <0.03 mg/L) for CYP2D6 inhibition, then F would become

$$F = 1 - \left(\frac{36.75Q}{37.75Q}\right) \quad (12.20)$$

or 2.7%. It should be noted that the usual therapeutic concentration range of quinidine is approximately 2 to 5 mg/L. Thus the C_{max} of dextromethorphan would double. In fact, actual clinical trials in which capsules containing 30 mg each of dextromethorphan and quinidine have shown that 30 mg of quinidine for seven days can increase the dextromethorphan C_{max} from 15.9 ng/ml when dextromethorphan is given by itself, to 95.5 ng/ml when it is given with quinidine. This combination would be an example of a purposefully engineered drug–drug interaction.

Or consider the estrogen receptor blocking drug raloxifene, used in the treatment of breast cancer. Raloxifene exhibits an intrinsic clearance around 30Q. Thus its oral bioavailability is approximately 3%. It is metabolized by UGTs, which are inducible by drugs such as rifampin. If rifampin treatment were capable of doubling the intrinsic clearance of raloxifene to 60Q it only would increase raloxifene's oral clearance by about 1%. However it would decrease its bioavailability by 50%.

12.3 DRUG TRANSPORTERS AND DDIs

Just as the discovery of CYP enzymes in the mid twentieth century led to intensive research regarding their role in DDIs, the relatively recent discovery of the role of drug transporters in drug disposition (see Chapters 7 and 9) has led to increasingly intense investigation of transporters in DDIs. However, even before very much was known about the molecular features of drug transporters or the mechanisms by which they affected drug influx or efflux, it was widely recognized that an organic anionic drug transporter in renal proximal tubular epithelial cells played a significant role in the renal secretion of penicillin and most other ß–lactam antibiotics, and that the uricosuric agent, probenecid, was capable of inhibiting renal penicillin secretion by inhibiting the organic anion transporter. This observation led to the purposeful combined use of probenecid with certain ß–lactams for the express purpose of slowing their renal tubular secretion into the urine, increasing their blood levels, and extending their half-lives. This engineered DDI was used years before it was recognized that ß-lactams kill susceptible bacteria in a time-dependent manner rather than a concentration-dependent manner, and has been used clinically with good effect for many decades. The organic anion transporter that is responsible for renal penicillin secretion and that is inhibited by probenecid is OAT1 (see Chapter 9). Other transporters that are important in mediating the influx or efflux of drugs in ways that affect absorption and excretion are listed in Table 12.3.

12.3.1 Interactions Involving P-Glycoprotein (PgP)

PgP is expressed on the apical membrane of intestinal epithelial cells, the luminal membrane of proximal tubular epithelia, the apical (or bile canalicular) membrane of hepatocytes, and on the luminal membrane of brain capillary endothelial cells. Accordingly, it is situated to play a role in intestinal drug absorption, renal drug excretion, biliary drug excretion, as well

Table 12.3 Transporters Playing Key Roles in Drug Absorption and Excretion

Gene or Gene Family	Common Name
ATP Binding Cassette (ABC) Transporters	
ABCB1	PgP (P-glycoprotein)
ABCC1	MRP1
ABCC2	MRP2
ABCC3	MRP3
ABCC4	MRP4
ABCC5	MRP5
ABCC6	MRP6
ABCC11	MRP8, BSEP (bile salt exporter protein)
ABCG2	BCRP (breast cancer resistance protein), MXR
Solute Carrier Family Transporters (SLC)[†]	
SLC21	OATP (organic anion transporting polypetides)
SLC22	OAT (organic ion transporters)
	OCT (organic cation transporters)
SLC15A1	PEPT-1 (oligopeptide transporter)
SLC28& SLC29	NT (nucleoside transporters)

*There are 49 genes in the ABC superfamily.
[†]There are 43 families and ca. 300 genes in the SLC superfamily.

as drug extrusion across the blood–brain barrier. In a manner analogous to the CYPs in general and to CYP3A4 in particular, PgP exhibits a broad substrate specificity (i.e., nonspecificity), creating great opportunities for its involvement in DDIs. Digoxin is an inotropic cardiac steroid that is still used in the management of heart failure. It has a relatively narrow therapeutic margin of safety, and postdistribution serum or plasma concentrations above 2 ng/ml tend to be associated with serious ADRs including cardiac arrhythmias. Digoxin is essentially free from hepatic or intestinal metabolism by CYP enzymes. However, it is transported by PgP, therefore it has become a useful probe of PgP activity *in vivo*. Quinidine, as we have seen, is a very potent inhibitor of CYP2D6. It is also an inhibitor of PgP. The ability of quinidine to significantly increase blood levels of digoxin leading to serious ADRs has been known for many years, though the central role of PgP inhibition by quinidine is a more recent discovery. It is now recognized that quinidine can increase the absolute bioavailability of digoxin by at least 15% as a consequence of inhibiting intestinal PgP and bile canalicular PgP (which in the absence of quinidine would efflux digoxin into the intestinal lumen and the bile canaliculus, respectively). It also inhibits renal epithelial PgP, thus slowing digoxin's renal secretion. The net consequence can mean an increase in digoxin AUC by as much as 75%. Other drugs that have been reported to increase digoxin bioavailability and/or decrease its renal and biliary excretion are itraconazole and ritonavir.

Studies in *mdr1a*(-/-) mice who do not express PgP in brain capillary endothelial cells comprising the blood–brain barrier, exhibit much higher brain levels of numerous drugs compared to their wild type counterparts that do express PgP. In humans, brain endothelial PgP can be inhibited by quinidine, ketoconazole, or the immunosuppressant drug, cyclosporine A. Quinidine was shown to increase the respiratory depressant effects of loperamide in humans, and the effect was not due to the inhibition of loperamide metabolism by quinidine. Ketoconazole was shown to actually increase CSF levels of ritonavir and saquinavir by three- or four-fold in men and women with HIV. Elegant studies using positron emission tomography have shown that cyclosporine A can increase the penetration ratio of verapamil into the brain by 88%. Penetration ratio is defined as the AUC_{brain}/AUC_{blood}. However, the cyclosporine A levels required to limit the efflux of verapamil from the brain were supratherapeutic.

As occurs with the CYP enzymes, PgP expression is regulated by the PXR. Thus, PXR agonists such as rifampin and St. John's wort can be expected to increase PgP expression and the PgP-dependent efflux of its substrates. Accordingly, rifampin has been shown to decrease digoxin bioavailability approximately by half, and St. John's wort has been shown to decrease digoxin's AUC by almost 20%. Both of these effects could lead to therapeutic failure, since digoxin has a relatively narrow therapeutic range. Indeed, hyperforin in St. Johns wort was shown to decrease cyclosporine AUC and C_{max} values by more than 50%, and these changes have been associated with therapeutic failure of cyclosporine in renal transplant patients.

12.3.1.1 *Predicting Clinical DDI Outcomes from* In Vitro *DDI Data for PgP*

The general approach to these *in vitro/in vivo* predictions parallels the strategy used to predict the clinical significance of inhibitory metabolic DDIs from $[I]/K_i$ data. Here, too, it can be shown that if a transporter is responsible for $< 50\%$ of a victim drug's total clearance, then its inhibition will not increase the AUC ratio by two-fold. Endres and colleagues at the University of Washington, Seattle used the same model as shown in Equation (12.7), replacing fm_{cyp} with f_{tr} denoting fraction cleared by transport, and representing both passive diffusion as well as transporter-mediated transport. Thus Equation (12.7) becomes:

$$AUCratio = \frac{1}{\dfrac{f_{tr}}{1+\dfrac{[I]}{K_i}} + (1 - f_{tr})} \tag{12.21}$$

And if the victim drug's clearance were mediated entirely by transport (e.g., biliary or renal excretion), then Equation (12.21) would simplify to its Equation (12.3) counterpart as follows:

$$AUCratio = 1 + \frac{[I]}{K_i} \tag{12.22}$$

Only now the K_i would be the inhibition constant for perpetrator inhibition of transporter function *in vitro*, and $[I]$ would still denote some appropriate *in vivo* concentration of the perpetrator, for example, C_{max}. Log transformations of the AUC ratios based on their data are plotted in Figure 12.5 with calculations referenced to both total $[I]$ and unbound $[I]$ (i.e., $fu * [I]$). The standard two-fold prediction ranges are shown parallel

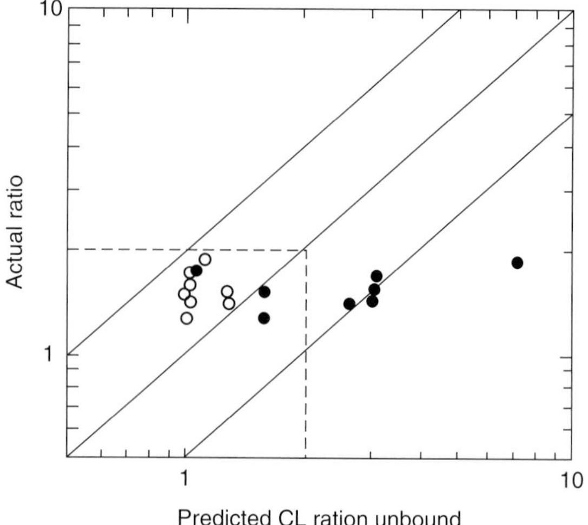

Figure 12.6 Actual versus predicted AUC ratios for transporter inhibition. Open symbols denote predictions based on unbound [*I*]. Closed symbols denote predictions based on total [*I*].

Table 12.4 Examples of Clinically Significant DDIs Associated with Inhibition of Transporters Other Than PgP

Transporter	Perpetrator	Victim	Outcome	Mechanism
BCRP (ABGC2)	GF120918	Topotecan	> 2-fold increase in bioavailability and AUC	Inhibition of intestinal BCRP and PgP
OATP1B1 (SLCO)	Gemfibrozil	Rosuvastatin Pravastatin Simvastatin Lovastatin	~ 2-fold increase in AUC	Inhibition of hepatic sinusoidal OATP1B1 and also inhibition of MRP2?, BCRP?
OATP1B1 (SLCO)	Gemfibrozil	Cerivastatin	> 5-fold increase in AUC	Inhibition of hepatic sinusoidal OATP1B1 & also inhibition of MRP2? & BCRP? & CYP2C8
OATP1B1 (SLCO)	Cyclosporine A	Rosuvastatin	7-fold increase in AUC	Inhibition of hepatic sinusoidal OATP1B1 & and also inhibition of CYP2C? & BCRP?
OAT1 (SLC22A6)	Probenecid	Penicillins Cephalosporins	~ 2-fold increase in AUC	Inhibition of renal proximal tubular basolateral OAT1
OAT1 (SLC22A6)	Probenecid	Cidofovir	Decrease renal CL by 27%, which is sufficient to reduce cidovovir nephrotoxicity	Inhibition of renal proximal tubular basolateral OAT1
OCT1 (SLC22A1) and OCT2 (SLC22A3)	Cimetidine	Procainamide Metformin	34–43% increase in AUC	Inhibition of renal proximal tubular basolateral OCTs

to the identity line for the AUC ratios. The bounded region denotes a true negative region in which both predicted and actual AUC ratios are <2. Notice that when unbound [*I*] was used in the predictions, none of the predicted AUC ratios reached or exceeded a value of 2. However when total [*I*] was used two-thirds of the predicted AUC ratios were greater than 2 even though none of the actual AUC ratios exceeded 2.

12.3.2 DDIs Due to Inhibition of Other Transporters

The study of the influence of transporters on drug disposition is still pretty much in its infancy; however, it is becoming increasingly clear that the inhibition or induction of transporters other than PgP can significantly influence the absorption and/or excretion of many (victim) drugs. Table 12.4 provides some examples of clinically significant DDIs associated with the alteration of transporter function by some perpetrator drugs.

12.3.3 Predicting DDIs When Victim Drugs Are Processed Both by CYPs and PgP, and When Perpetrators Inhibit Both

We have learned that it is possible to predict with about 80% accuracy (i.e., true positive and true negative predictions) clinically significant inhibitory metabolic DDIs arising from *in vitro* determination of the perpetrator's K_i for a specific CYP and a reasonable estimate of the perpetrator's *in vivo* concentration, [*I*]. Furthermore, it is likely that the accuracy rate can be increased by refining the selection of [*I*] (e.g., bound vs. unbound), accounting for parallel metabolic pathways and the fraction of metabolic clearance for each CYP involved, and also accounting for (if possible) molecular cooperativity within the broader enzyme binding site (see Eq. 12.9). The same general strategy can be applied to the prediction of clinically significant outcomes associated with the inhibition of transporters as shown for PgP. It should be noted that all throughout this chapter (and generally throughout the literature as well) the term "clinically significant" implies a two-fold change in the victim drug's AUC in the presence of a perpetrator (i.e., a two-fold increase in the AUC in the presence of an inhibitor or a 50% decrease in the presence of an enzyme inducer). However, even changes of this magnitude may not truly be clinically significant for drugs that have very large therapeutic ranges and/or wide margins of safety. That is to say, doubling the AUC for a relatively nontoxic drug will not likely increase the likelihood of ADRs.

In any case, to what extent can these *in vitro*-to-*in vivo* predictions be relied upon if a drug is both metabolized by CYP enzymes and effluxed by PgP, and if a perpetrator inhibits both of these pathways? We might envision that the combined inhibitory effects could be estimated from:

$$AUCratio = \frac{1}{\left[\dfrac{fm_{cyp}}{1+\dfrac{[I]}{Ki_{cyp}}}+[1-fm_{cyp}]\right]}\cdot\frac{1}{\left[\dfrac{f_{TR}}{1+\dfrac{[I]}{Ki_{TR}}}+[1-f_{TR}]\right]} \quad (12.23)$$

where fm_{cyp} denotes the fraction of victim drug clearance due to CYP metabolism, K_{icyp} is the corresponding metabolic K_i elicited by the perpetrator, fm_{TR} denotes the fraction of victim drug clearance due to transport (e.g., biliary excretion), and Ki_{TR} is the corresponding K_i for the perpetrator inhibition of the transporter. However, these two processes may not be entirely independent with inhibition of efflux transporter function giving rise to greater enzyme activity (liver) or less enzyme activity (intestine) in the presence of perpetrator than would be expected if the perpetrator inhibited only the enzyme and not the efflux transporter. The issue becomes more complex and it becomes accordingly more difficult to predict outcomes if a perpetrator inhibits enzymes and transporters in both the intestines and the liver, or if a perpetrator inhibits enzymes, efflux transporters, and influx transporters and does so in more than one clearing organ.

12.3.4 Using the Biopharmaceutics Classification System (BCS) to Assist in the Prediction of the Clinical Significance of CYP-based and Transporter-based DDIs

In the past few years a substantial effort has been invested in understanding the combined complex roles of transporters and drug metabolizing enzymes in *in vitro*-to-*in vivo* (*iv/iv*) predictions of drug clearance and DDIs. Some of these efforts have been described in the work of Leslie Benet and colleagues at the University of California, San Francisco; K. Sandy Pang and colleagues at the University of Toronto; and Yuichi Sugiyama and colleagues at the University of Tokyo; some of which is cited in the bibliography at the end of this chapter. Adapting the BCS to create a Biopharmaceutics Drug Disposition Classification System that segregates drugs by their permeability and solubility characteristics, Wu and Benet at UCSF defined the relative roles of transporters and metabolism on a drug's disposition (Table 12.5). One of the values in segregating drugs by this classification system is that it becomes easy to discern, *a priori*, the types of drugs for which *iv/iv* predictions about the clinical significance of DDIs should be the easiest. Class 1 substances (high permeability and high solubility compounds) tend to be extensively metabolized, but not particularly subject to processing by transporters. Therefore, *iv/iv* DDI predictions should be relatively uncomplicated for Class 1 substances. Likewise *iv/iv* DDI predictions for Class 3 substances (low permeability and high solubility) that are likely to be processed chiefly by influx transporters (e.g., penicillin influx via OATs in the kidney) should be relatively uncomplicated. On the other hand, *iv/iv* DDI predictions may not be quite so easy for Class 2 substances (high permeability and low solubility) that are both extensively metabolized (e.g., CYP3A4) and subject to significant cellular efflux (e.g., PgP). Likewise, since Class 4 substances (low permeability and low solubility) are subject to both influx and efflux transport, *iv/iv* prediction of DDIs may be somewhat complicated.

12.4 DDIs ASSOCIATED WITH PROTEIN BINDING

The drug interaction literature is replete with warnings about the potential increase in pharmacological activity or ADRs associated with the displacement of a victim from its plasma protein binding sites by a perpetrator that also has affinity for the same binding sites. The major plasma proteins to which most drugs bind are albumin and α1-acid glycoprotein; the former typically binds acidic, anionic drugs whereas the latter typically favors basic drugs (see Chapter 7). Dr. James Gillette working at the NIH was one of the first people to explore the clinical significance of so-called binding-displacement interactions; interactions in which a perpetrator was postulated to interfere with the binding of a victim drug, thereby increasing the circulating unbound concentration of the victim. Since the pharmacodynamic effects of drugs correlate with their unbound concentrations, it follows that increases in unbound concentrations will be associated with increases in desired therapeutic effects or with ADRs. Dr. Gillette formulated a very simple analysis that

Table 12.5 Transporter and Metabolic Contribution to Drug Disposition Depending upon the Drug's Solubility and Permeability

Characteristic	Class 1 Substances	Class 2 Substances	Class 3 Substances	Class 4 Substances
Permeability	High	High	Low	Low
Solubility	High	Low	High	Low
Metabolism	Extensive*	Extensive*	Poor	Poor
Renal or biliary excretion	Minor	Minor	Major	Major
Significant efflux transporter effects	No	Yes	No	Yes
Significant influx transporter effects	No	No	Yes	Yes

*at least 70% metabolized

stipulated how extensively a victim drug had to be bound to plasma proteins in order for there to be a significant change in its pharmacodynamic effects on account of the phenomenon of protein binding displacement by some perpetrator (binding displacer). The very simplest case of his explanation follows.

Suppose that a victim drug bound only to the protein, albumin, in the blood. Its volume of distribution throughout the body would be described by its distribution in the albumin space, ~ 5.5 liters, plus its distribution throughout total body water, ~ 50 liters.

The total body burden of the drug could then be described by the following:

$$A_T = C_b \times 5.5 + C_u \times 50 \qquad (12.24)$$

where A_T is the total amount of drug in the body, C_b is the concentration of drug bound to albumin in the blood (assuming virtually all albumin binding occurs in the blood), and C_u is the unbound concentration of the drug in all body water. Now, if the fraction of the victim drug circulating in the blood as unbound drug (f_u) is 50%, then the fraction bound (f_b) will also be 50%. The unbound concentration will be $C \times f_u$, and bound concentration will be $C \times f_b$. Substituting $C \times f_u$ for C_u and $C \times f_b$ for C_b in Equation (12.24), and using 0.5 for both f_u and f_b (the drug exhibits a free fraction of 50%), then:

$$A_T = (C \times 0.5 \times 5.5) + (C \times 0.5 \times 50) \qquad (12.25)$$

Now, the percent of the total amount of bound drug in the body (not the plasma) would be:

$$\frac{(C \times 0.5 \times 5.5)}{(C \times 0.5 \times 5.5) + (C \times 0.5 \times 50)}$$

or approximately 10%. Therefore the total amount of unbound drug in the body (not the plasma) would be about 90%. Assuming the perpetrator were capable of displacing every molecule of victim drug from its albumin binding sites in the plasma, then the very most that the pharmacodynamic effect could be expected to increase would be 10% as virtually all the drug in the body became unbound. Furthermore, it is likely that in order to effectively displace all the victim from its albumin binding sites, the perpetrator drug would have to achieve a concentration in the plasma of about 0.6 μM, which is approximately the molar concentration of albumin. According to this line of reasoning it would seem that for a victim drug that exhibits a bound fraction (in blood or plasma) of 50%, and for a perpetrator that could elicit the complete binding displacement of the victim drug, there would not be much expected change in the pharmacodynamic effect of the victim drug. This same approach can be used to predict outcomes for other extents of victim binding to plasma proteins. Table 12.6 is also based on Equation (12.24).

According to this simple analysis, a victim drug would have to approach exhibiting a bound fraction of 90% (f_u ~ 10%) before a perpetrator likely would cause a large enough change in the unbound amount of drug in the body to cause a significant alteration in the victim drug's pharmacodynamic effect.

Table 12.6 Possible Increase That Plasma Protein Binding Displacement Could Make in a Victim Drug's Pharmacodynamic Effect as a Function of the Extent of Plasma Protein Binding of the Victim Drug

Maximum Fraction Bound in Plasma ($ß_{max}$)	Fraction of Total Drug Bound in the Body	Maximum Possible Increase in Pharmacodynamic Effect Due to Complete Binding Displacement
50%	10%	10%
90%	49.6%	~ two-fold
99%	91.5%	~ 12-fold

There's also a pharmacokinetic way to analyze the likely outcome of binding displacement interactions on pharmacodynamic outcomes. Steady-state unbound plasma concentrations can be defined in terms of a drug's clearance (*CL*), the fraction of drug absorbed (*F*), the dose (*D*), and the dosing interval, τ,

$$\overline{C}_{ss} = \frac{FD}{CL \times \tau} \qquad (12.26)$$

The total organ clearance (e.g., liver) will depend upon the intrinsic clearance (e.g., metabolic clearance) and the unbound fraction of the drug, f_u.

$$CL = CL_{int} \times f_u \qquad (12.27)$$

Substituting into Equation (12.26),

$$\overline{C}_{ss} = \frac{FD}{CL_{int} \times f_u \times \tau} \qquad (12.28)$$

now, the average steady-state unbound concentration, $\overline{C}_{SSunb}$, is related to the total average steady-state concentration as follows:

$$\overline{C}_{SSunb} = \overline{C}_{ss} \times f_u \qquad (12.29)$$

Notice in Equation (12.28), that if you multiply both sides by f_u the following expression develops:

$$\overline{C}_{ss} \times f_u = \frac{FD}{CL_{int} \times \tau} \qquad (12.30)$$

or

$$\overline{C}_{SSunb} = \frac{\mathrm{FD}}{CL_{int} \times \tau} \qquad (12.31)$$

This means that $\overline{C}_{SSunb}$ is strictly a function of metabolic intrinsic clearance, the dose, the fraction of dose absorbed, and the dosing interval. Furthermore,

$$\overline{C}_{SSunb} = \frac{AUC_{unb}}{\tau} \quad (12.32)$$

Therefore the unbound AUC will only be a function of metabolic intrinsic clearance, dose, and fraction of dose absorbed as follows:

$$AUC_{unb} = \frac{F \times D}{CL_{int}} \quad (12.33)$$

It will not at all depend upon the fraction of drug that is unbound in the blood.

This means that overall exposure to unbound drug can't be affected by plasma binding or plasma protein binding displacement interactions. Furthermore, if the drug is a high hepatic extraction-ratio drug, such that $CL_{int} >>> Q$, then Q, hepatic blood flow rate, becomes limiting, and Equation (12.31) becomes:

$$\overline{C}_{SSunb} = \frac{FD}{Q \times \tau} \quad (12.34)$$

Thus, for a high (hepatic) extraction ratio victim drug the AUC_{unb} will be solely a function of hepatic blood flow rate, fraction of dose absorbed, and dose. Again, plasma protein binding, and therefore changes in plasma protein binding associated with binding displacement, will not affect total exposure to unbound drug.

The total exposure to unbound drug (AUC_{unb}) is not a function of the fraction of drug unbound, f_u, but rather the fraction of dose absorbed, the dose, and CL_{int} for low clearance drugs or hepatic blood flow rate, Q, for high clearance drugs, therefore changes in f_u caused by protein-binding displacement interactions would not be expected to have significant outcomes. Even though AUC_{unb} would not be affected by f_u, there could be times within each dosing cycle when exposure to unbound drug would, in fact, be determined by the unbound fraction of drug. Dr. Gerhard Levy at SUNY, Buffalo illustrated this many years ago. Suppose a highly bound low clearance drug exhibited very rapid distribution throughout the body. Its unbound plasma concentrations at steady-state might be depicted by Figure 12.6. Suppose, too, that if this victim drug were coadministered with another drug (i.e., perpetrator) that in fact was capable of displacing the victim drug from plasma protein binding sites, f_u for the victim drug increased. This is shown for the dashed curve in Figure 12.6. The increase in f_u for the victim drug subsequent to protein-binding displacement by the perpetrator drug gives rise to (1) an increase in the clearance of the victim as evidenced by a steeper disappearance curve; (2) an increase in the peak plasma concentration of unbound drug; and (3) a decrease in the trough plasma concentration of unbound drug. So, the AUC_{unb} (i.e., total exposure to unbound victim drug) would not be altered fundamentally (as shown in Equations 12.26–12.34). But it is nevertheless possible that the peak plasma concentrations of unbound drug at steady-state would be higher than prior to the addition of the perpetrator (dashed lines vs. solid lines), and also that the trough concentrations would

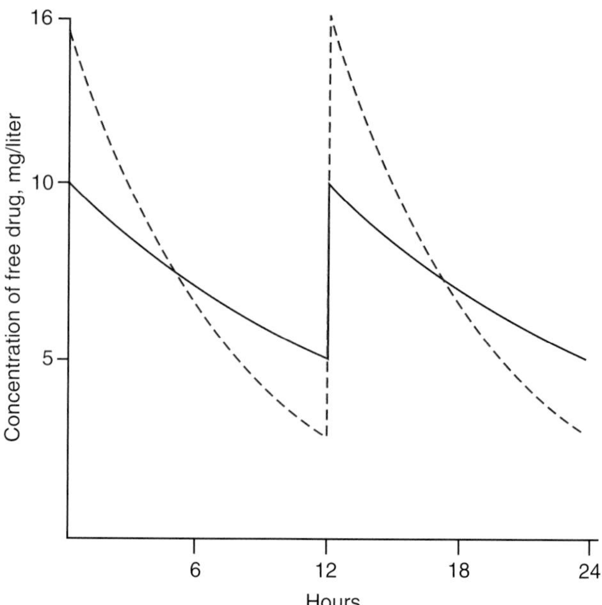

Figure 12.7 Steady-state unbound plasma concentrations of an extensively bound low-clearance victim drug before (solid line) and after (dotted line) its displacement (decrease in plasma protein binding) caused by a perpetrator.

be lower. Even though the total exposure to unbound drug would not have changed, it is possible that ADRs could develop soon after the dose of the victim drug (peak), and it is simultaneously possible that therapeutic failure could occur immediately before each next dose of the victim drug (trough). It's actually possible that a binding displacement interaction involving a low clearance, extensively bound victim drug could result in both an increased chance of ADRs and also therapeutic failure.

12.5 CONCLUSIONS AND KEY POINTS

Drug–drug interactions constitute a significant fraction of avoidable ADRs. The frequency with which they occur depends, in part, on the number of different drugs that are used simultaneously. Since the population is aging, and therefore it is expected that the number of drugs used per person in an aging population will increase, it may well be that the risk of DDIs leading to ADRs will increase sharply. On the other hand, some DDIs can be engineered purposefully to improve dosing schedules or therapeutic outcomes. For the purpose of drug management in general and in an aged population in particular, it is important to be able to identify DDIs that are likely to lead to clinically significant adverse outcomes marked either by ADRs or therapeutic failure. To assist clinicians in identifying risks associated with the combined use of two drugs, drug-interaction books and searchable drug-interaction databases are available. These resources exhibit varying degrees of sophistication and accuracy, and both include some interactions that have never been validated by controlled clinical trials.

Pharmaceutical scientists engaged in drug development require predictive tools to enable them to ascertain whether a drug under development is likely to cause clinically significant drug interactions with marketed drugs. Recognizing the likelihood of clinically significant drug interactions is an important determinant in decisions about continuing further with drug development. Though predictions might be made from analogies to what is known about drug interactions of currently marketed drugs, these analogous predictions can be completely wrong. For example, the anti-infective drug, ciprofloxacin, is a fluoroquinolone and a known inhibitor of CYP1A2. It can sufficiently slow the clearance of theophylline, a drug with a relatively narrow margin of safety, to cause ADRs including seizures. On the other hand, apart from enoxacin, most of the fluoroquinolones that have been marketed since ciprofloxacin do not inhibit CYP1A2, and would not be expected to interact with theophylline. Placing all fluoroquinolones into a probable risk category for an adverse reaction with theophylline based on the findings with ciprofloxacin would lead to bad predictions. Along these lines the macrolide antibiotic, triacetyloleandomycin (TAO), is a reasonably good inhibitor of CYP3A4. Erythromycin and clarithromycin are less effective inhibitors, but have been shown to be capable of causing serious clinical adverse effects associated with CYP3A4 inhibition. On the other hand, neither dirithromycin nor azithromycin, both of which are also macrolide antibiotics, inhibit CYP3A4. They do not share the same risks of DDI-related ADRs as erythromycin, clarithromycin, or TAO.

Beginning at the start of this century an attempt was made to bring together regulatory scientists, those in the pharmaceutical industry, and those in academia to agree upon predictive strategies for characterizing the clinical significance of DDIs. These efforts focused primarily on predicting the clinical significance of inhibitory metabolic and inhibitory transporter-based DDIs, and established the paradigm of using $[I]/K_i$ ratios for this purpose. In this paradigm, DDIs with a high probability of being clinically significant would be those in which the AUC ratio (AUCi/AUC) ≥ 2, and an $[I]/K_i$ ratio ≥ 1 would predict an AUC ratio ≥ 2. Likewise, an AUC ratio ≤ 1 would suggest that there would be little or no likelihood of a clinically significant DDI, and an $[I]/K_i$ ratio ≤ 0.1 would predict an AUC ratio ≤ 1.1. There are many subtleties that must be taken into consideration, however, including the matrix or system in which K_i is estimated, the type of *in vitro* victim or substrate that is used, nonspecific binding of the victim, the most representative value for the *in vivo* concentration of $[I]$ for the perpetrator, metabolism of the victim drug by parallel pathways, the issue of cooperativity, and others. Remarkably, even when these subtleties are simply ignored, the predictive accuracy of the $[I]/K_i$ paradigm is between 70 and 85%. The same strategy can be applied to predicting the clinical significance of DDIs associated with transporter inhibition. In view of the relatively high level of predictive accuracy of the $[I]/K_i$ paradigm, flaws notwithstanding, it may not be too soon to begin applying it to the evaluation of DDIs when the only data at hand is case report data. For example, authors of case reports of putative inhibitory DDIs should include $[I]/K_i$ data when it is available, to support any contention of an inhibitory DDI.

Other factors currently limit the predictive accuracy of inhibitory DDIs. For example, although there is some consensus about the drugs that should be used as representative victim drugs of each of the CYP enzymes, such a consensus about representative victim drugs for transporters or for non-CYP enzymes doesn't exist. The exception to this might be for the transporter, P-glycoprotein, for which digoxin may be the victim of choice. By comparison, the study of the function of OATs, OCTs, MRPs, OATPs, and other transporters, their substrates, and their inhibition, is still in its early stages. In addition, some drugs can be substrates for both influx and efflux transporters as well as for CYP or other enzymes. Some drugs can inhibit both CYP enzymes and transporters, for example, PgP, whereas other drugs can induce the activity of CYP enzymes and transporters. The multiplicity of dispositional processes to which a given victim drug might be subject and the multiplicity of processes that a perpetrator drug might affect promise to make our ability to improve on the predictive accuracy of inhibitory DDIs a significant challenge.

Strategies for predicting the clinical significance of enzyme-inducing or transporter-inducing DDIs are not quite as far advanced as for the inhibitory DDIs. To be sure, many of the same issues that limit the predictive accuracy of inhibitory DDIs suffuse predictions for inductive DDIs. However, early work in this field suggests that relatively few perpetrators capable of stimulating, for example, the PXR, will cause clinically meaningful (victim) exposure (AUC) decreases in humans. Moreover, there are currently very few examples of clinical increases in victim clearance that are much greater than two-fold, regardless of the extent of PXR agonism or CYP induction *in vitro*. Unless a victim has a very narrow therapeutic range, it could be that these types of interactions are simply overrated.

One of the issues that has not been explored extensively in connection with *iv/iv* predictions of the clinical significance of DDIs is the impact of the victim drug's clearance (before the interaction) on the clinical significance of an interaction in humans. Whether the interaction is one of inhibition of the victim drug's metabolism or whether it is induction of the victim drug's metabolism, even a predicted outcome based, for example, on $[I]/K_i$ ratios might errantly predict real-life clinical consequences if the victim's baseline clearance isn't considered. Remember, it is possible that the pharmacokinetics of a high clearance drug given intravenously will not be substantially affected even in the face of an $[I]/K_i$ ratio of ~ 1, although the pharmacokinetics of the same drug given orally might be substantially affected.

Finally, it would appear that most putative protein-binding displacement interactions should not have meaningful clinical consequences, since the AUC_{unb}

will not be affected by changes in protein binding. However, there could still be instances in which the displacement of an extensively bound drug could result in both higher peak plasma concentrations of unbound drug and also lower trough plasma concentrations of unbound drug. Detecting the clinical consequences would take very careful clinical observations, since under these circumstances it is possible for such a DDI to cause both an increase in intermittent ADRs and some evidence of intermittent therapeutic failure.

REVIEW QUESTIONS

1. What are the essential features about two drugs that you would have to know in order to determine whether there was a chance that they could (1) interact pharmacodynamically and (2) interact pharmacokinetically?
2. How can the *in vitro* determination of a perpetrator drug's K_i value along with knowledge about its C_{max} in humans permit a prediction as to the clinical significance of its interaction with a victim drug?
3. Use of $[I]/K_i$ ratios to predict the clinical significance of inhibitory metabolic DDIs in humans (qualitative zoning) has been shown to be over 80% accurate for interactions involving CYP3A4 inhibition and approximately 70% accurate for interactions involving CYP2C9 inhibition. What are some of the reasons why the accuracy rates aren't, say, 95%?
4. How can *in vitro* transactivation assays be used to predict the clinical significance of inductive DDIs? What are some of the drawbacks or limits to this strategy?
5. How could the $[I]/K_i$ strategy for predicting the clinical significance of DDIs be used to strengthen or refute case reports about the significance and/or mechanism of inhibitory DDIs in humans?
6. How would you use the bipharmaceutics classification system (BCS) to enable you to predict the clinical significance of a pharmacokinetic DDI from *in vitro* data?
7. A new chemical entity has the following properties: (1) it has been shown to inhibit CYP enzymes in heterologous expression systems expressing human CYP enzymes; (2) it has been shown to be selective for CYP2C9; and (3) though three different substrates were used, the mean (range) for its K_i for CYP2C9 inhibition was 0.5 (0.2–0.8) μM. The C_{max} in early clinical trials was 4 μM. Would a clinically significant interaction with the anticonvulsant drug, phenytoin (Dilantin®) be anticipated based on the foregoing data? Why or why not?
8. Valproic acid is an anticonvulsant drug that binds principally to plasma albumin, and at therapeutic plasma concentrations the extent of its binding is 93%. Gemfibrozil is a drug used to lower LDL cholesterol and triglycerides. Its peak plasma concentration at usual doses is about 100 μM, and it also binds principally to plasma albumin. Would you expect that gemfibrozil would promote a binding-displacement interaction with valproic acid? Why or why not? What would the consequences be of such an interaction?

REFERENCES

Books

Bachmann, K., Lewis, J., Fuller, M., & Bongiglio, M. (2004). *Lexi-Comp's Drug Interactions Handbook* (2nd ed.). Hudson, OH: Lexi-Comp, Inc.

Brunton, L., Lazo, J., & Parker, K. (2006). *Goodman & Gilman's The Pharmacological of Therapeutics* (11th ed.). New York: McGraw Hill.

Cozza, K., Armstrong, S., & Oesterheld, J. (2003). *Concise Guide to Drug Interaction Principles for Medical Practice. Cytochrome P450s, UGTs, P-Glycoproteins* (2nd ed.). Arlington: American Psychiatric Publishing.

Goodman, L., & Gilman, A. (Eds.). (1970). *The Pharmacological Basis of Therapeutics* (4th ed.). New York: Macmillan Co.

Hansten, P., & Horn, J. (2006). *The Top 100 Drug Interactions: A Guide to Patient Management.* Freeland: H&H Publications.

Hansten, P., & Horn, J. (2006). *Drug Interactions Analysis and Management. Facts and Comparisons.* St. Louis, Mo: Wolters Kluwer Health.

Levy, R. H., Thummel, K. E., Trager, W. F., Hansten, P. D., & Eichelbaum, M. (Eds.). (2000). *Metabolic Drug Interactions.* Philadelphia: Lipincott Williams & Wilkins.

Rodrigues, A. D. (Ed.). (2002). *Drug-Drug Interactions.* New York: Marcel Dekker.

Sandson, N. (2003). *Drug Interactions Casebook. The Cytochrome P450 System and Beyond.* Arlington: American Psychiatric Publishing.

Stockley's Drug Interactions (7th ed.). (2005). Chicago: Pharmaceutical Press.

Tatro, D. (2007). *Drug Interaction Facts. Facts and Comparisons.* St. Louis: Wolters Kluwer Health.

Monographs, Reviews, and Original Articles

Abernathy, D., Greenblatt, D. J., Ameer, B., & Shader, R. (1985). Probenecid impairment of acetaminophen and lorazepam clearance: Direct inhibition of ether glucuronide formation. *The Journal of Pharmacology and Experimental Therapeutics, 234,* 345–349.

Anon. (2006). *Preventing Medication Errors.* Institute of Medicine.

Anon. (2006). www.fda.gov/cder/drug/drugReactions. Accessed November, 2006.

Anon. (2006). *Guidance for industry: Drug Interaction Studies—Study design, data analysis, and implications for dosing and labeling.* U.S. Dept. Health and Human Services, Food and Drug Administration, CDER, 1–55.

Aronson, J. K. (2006). Classifying drug interactions. *British Journal of Clinical Pharmacology, 58,* 343–344.

Bachmann, K. (2006). Inhibition constants, inhibitor concentrations and the prediction of inhibitory drug-drug interactions: Piftalls, progress, and promise. *Current Drug Metabolism, 7,* 1–14.

Balayssac, D., Authier, N., Cayre, A., & Coudore, F. (2005). Does inhibition of P-glycoprotein lead to drug-drug interactions? *Toxicology Letters, 156,* 319–329.

Bertelsen, K., Venkatakrishnan, K., von Moltke, L., Obach, R. S., & Greenblatt, J. (2003). Apparent mechanism-based inhibition of human CYP2D6 in vitro by paroxetine: Comparison with fluoxetine and quinidine. *Drug Metabolism and Disposition: The Biological Fate of Chemicals, 31,* 289–293.

Brown, C. H. (2005). *Overview of Drug Interactions. US Pharmacist.* www.uspharmacist.com/index.asp (accessed November, 2006).

Brown, H., Ito, K., Galetin, A., & Houston, J. (2005). Prediction of *in vivo* drug-drug interactions from *in vitro* data: Impact of incorporating parallel pathways of drug elimination and inhibitor absorption rate constant. *British Journal of Clinical Pharmacology, 60,* 508–518.

Budnitz, D., Pollock, D., Weidenbach, K., Mendelsohn, A., Schroeder, T., & Annest, J. (2006). National surveillance of emergency department visits for outpatient adverse drug events. *JAMA: The Journal of the American Medical Association, 296*, 1858–1866.

Egnell, A., Houston, J., & Boyer, C. (2005). Predictive models of CYP3A4 heteroactivation: In vitro-in vivo scaling and pharmacophore modeling. *The Journal of Pharmacology and Experimental Therapeutics, 312*, 926–937.

Endres, C., Hsiao, P., Chung, F., & Unadkat, J. (2006). The role of transporters in drug interactions. *European Journal of Pharmaceutical Sciences: Official Journal of the European Federation for Pharmaceutical Sciences, 27*, 501–517.

Gillette, J. R. (1971). Factors affecting drug metabolism. *Annals of the New York Academy of Sciences, 179*, 43–66.

Gurwitz, J., Field, T., Harrold, L., Rothschild, J., Debellis, K. L., Seger, A. et al. (2003). Incidence and preventability of adverse drug events among older persons in the ambulatory setting. *JAMA: The Journal of the American Medical Association, 289*, 1107–1116.

Halkin, H., Katzir, I., Kurman, I., Jan, J., & Malkin, B. (2001). Preventing drug interactions by online prescription screening in community pharmacies and medical practices. *Clinical Pharmacology and Therapeutics, 69*, 260–265.

Ito, K., Hallifax, D., Obach, R. S., & Houston, J. (2005). Impact of parallel pathways of drug elimination and multiple cytochrome P450 involvement on drug-drug interactions: CYP2D6 paradigm. *Drug Metabolism and Disposition: The Biological Fate of Chemicals, 33*, 837–844.

Kanjanarat, P., Winterstein, A., Johns, T., Hatton, R., Gonzalez-Rothi, R., & Segal, R. (2003). Nature of preventable adverse drug events in hospitals: a literature review. *American Journal of Health-System Pharmacy: AJHP: Official Journal of the American Society of Health-System Pharmacists, 60*, 1750–1759.

Khaliq, Y., Gallicano, K., Venance, S., Kravick, S., & Cameron, W. (2000). Effect of ketoconazole on ritonavir and saquinavir concentrations in plasma and cerebrospinal fluid from patients infected with human immunodeficiency virus. *Clinical Pharmacology and Therapeutics, 68*, 637–646.

Kiang, T., Ensom, M., & Chang, T. (2005). UDP-glucuronosyltransferases and clinical drug-drug interactions. *Pharmacology & Therapeutics, 106*, 97–132.

Lundkvist, J., & Jönsson, B. (2004). Pharmacoeconomics of adverse drug reactions. *Fundamental & Clinical Pharmacology, 18*, 275–280.

Mai, I., Bauer, S., Perloff, E., Johne, A., Uehleke, B., Frank, B., et al. (2004). Hyperforin content determines the magnitude of the St John's wort-cyclosporine drug interaction. *Clinical Pharmacology and Therapeutics, 76*, 330–340.

McGinnity, D., Tucker, J., Trigg, S., & Riley, R. (2005). Prediction of CYP2C9-mediated drug-drug interactions: A comparison of data from recombinant enzymes and human hepatocytes. *Drug Metabolism Disposition, 33*, 1700–1707.

Metabolism and transport drug interaction database. http://depts.washington.edu/didbase (accessed 2003 Mar 24).

Obach, W., Walsky, R., Venkatakrishnan, K., Gaman, E., Houston, J., & Tremaine, L. (2006). The utility of in vitro cytochrome P450 inhibition data in the prediction of drug-drug interactions. *The Journal of Pharmacology and Experimental Therapeutics, 316*, 336–348.

Obach, R., Walsky, R., Venkatakrishnan, K., Houston, J. (2005). In vitro cytochrome P450 inhibition data and the prediction of drug-drug interactions: Qualitative relationships, quantitative predictions, and the rank-order approach. *Clinical Pharmacology and Therapeutics, 78*, 582–592.

Paine, M., Hart, H., Ludington, S., Haining, R., Rettie, A., & Zeldin, D. (2006). The human intestinal cytochrome P450 "pie". *Drug Metabolism Disposition, 34*, 880–886.

Rostami-Hodjegan, A., & Tucker, G. (2004). In silico simulations to assess the in vivo consequences of in vitro metabolic drug-drug interactions. *Drug Discovery Today, 1*, 441–448.

Ripp, S., Mills, J., Fahmi, O., Trevena, K., Liras, J., Maurer, T., et al. (2006). Use of immortalized human hepatocytes to predict the magnitude of clinical drug-drug interactions caused by CYP3A4 induction. *Drug Metabolism Disposition, 34*, 1742–1748.

Sadeque, A., Wandel, C., He, H., Shah, S., & Wood, A. J. J. (2000). Increased drug delivery to the brain by P-glycoprotein inhibition. *Clinical Pharmacology and Therapeutics, 68*, 231–237.

Sinz, M., Kilm, S., Zhu, Z., Chen, T., Anthony, M., Dickinson, K., et al. (2006). Evaluation of 170 xenobiotics as transactivators of human pregnane X receptor (hPXR) and correlation to known CYP3A4 drug interactions. *Current Drug Metabolism, 7*, 375–388.

Sparrow, M., Hande, S., Friedman, S., Lim, W., Reddy, S., Cao, D., et al. (2005). Allopurinol safely and effectively optimizes tioguanine metabolites in inflammatory bowel disease patients not responding to azathiopurine and mercaptopurine. *Alimentary Pharmacology & Therapeutics, 22*, 441–446.

Tirona, R., & Bailey, D. (2006). Herbal product-drug interactions mediated by induction. *British Journal of Clinical Pharmacology, 61*, 677–681.

Ucar, M., Neuvonene, M., Luurila, H., Dahlqvist, R., Neuvonen, P., & Mjörndal, T. (2004). Carbamazepine markedly reduces serum concentrations of simvastatin and simvastatin acid. *European Journal of Clinical Pharmacology, 59*, 879–882.

Venkatakrishnan, K., von Moltke, L., Obach, R., & Greenblatt, D. (2003). Drug metabolism and drug interactions: Application and clinical value of in vitro models. *Current Drug Metabolism, 4*, 423–459.

Walsky, R., Gaman, E., & Obach, R. (2005). Examination of 209 drugs for inhibition of cytochrome P4502C8. *Journal of Clinical Pharmacology, 45*, 68–78.

Wang, Y. H., Jones, D. R., & Hall, S. D. (2005). Differential mechanism-based inhibition of CYP3A4 and CYP3A5 by verapamil. *Drug Metabolism Disposition, 33*, 664–671.

Wienkers, L., & Heath, T. (2005). Predicting in vivo drug interactions from in vitro drug discovery data. *Drug Discovery, 4*, 825–833.

Williams, J., Hyland, R., Jones, B., Smith, D., Hurst, S., Goosen, T., et al. (2004). Drug-drug interactions for UDP-glucuronosyltransferase substrates: pharmacokinetic explanation for typically observed low exposure (AUCi/AUC) ratios. *Drug Metabolism Disposition, 32*, 1201–1208.

Wrighton, S. A., Schuetz, E. G., Thummel, K. E., Shen, D. D., Korzekwa, K. R., & Watkins, P. B. (2000). *Drug Metabolism Reviews, 32*, 339–361.

Wu, C., & Benet, L. (2005). Predicting drug disposition via application of BCS: Transport/absorption/elimination interplay and development of a biopharmaceutics drug disposition classification system. *Pharmaceutical Research, 22*, 11–23.

Yuan, R., Madani, S., Wei, X., Reynolds, K., & Huang, S. (2002). Evaluation of cytochrome P450 probe substrates commonly used by the pharmaceutical industry to study in vitro drug interactions. *Drug Metabolism Disposition, 30*, 1311–1319.

Zhou, S., Chan, S., Goh, B., Chan, E., Duan, W., Huang, M., et al. (2005). Mechanism-based inhibition of cytochrome P450 3A4 by therapeutic drugs. *Clinical Pharmacokinetics, 44*, 279–304.

Chapter

13 Adverse Drug Reactions

Miles Hacker

OUTLINE

13.1 INTRODUCTION

Adverse drug reactions (ADR) are far more commonplace than one would think. It is estimated that ADRs represent the fourth leading cause of death in the United States and Canada behind heart disease, cancer, and stroke. Further, it is estimated that ADRs are the sixth leading cause of death worldwide. Recent meta-analysis of prospective ADR studies estimates that over 180,000 Americans will die from ADRs and over one million will be injured from ADRs in 2008. Although these data are controversial and the actual incidence of ADRs is impossible to assess, there is no doubt that ADRs have a significant impact on both the healthcare delivery and the drug development industries.

The monetary costs to society due to these ADRs are equally hard to assess accurately, but recent studies have estimated the costs to range from $75 to $180 billion each year for adults alone. When compared to the costs of treating diseases such as diabetes ($45 billion), cardiovascular disease ($120–150 billion), or cancer ($130–195 billion) we begin to truly realize the impact of this aspect of pharmacology on healthcare delivery. Yet another way to demonstrate the impact of ADRs is to realize that approximately 5% of all hospital admissions are a direct result of ADRs, and unfortunately incidence has not changed over the past 30 years.

If ADRs are such a drain on our healthcare delivery system, what are ADRs? The World Health Organization has put forth the definition of ADR as "any response to a drug which is noxious and unintended, and which occurs at doses used in man for prophylaxis, diagnosis or treatment." In other words, an ADR could be an unexpected or unwanted effect that is a direct extension of the mechanism of drug action; in an organ system that is not the target of drug therapy; an allergic response; a hypersensitive response; an idiosyncratic response (one totally unpredictable); or a drug interaction with unexpected results. In each case the ADR represents an unwanted toxic effect as a result of taking a given drug or set of drugs. The purpose of this chapter is discuss in detail the various types of ADRs using specific examples to demonstrate the types of ADRs that can be encountered when drugs are administered as well as factors that may affect the incidence or severity of a given ADR.

13.2 TYPE A ADRs

13.2.1 How Are Type A Reactions Caused?

Type A reactions represent approximately 70 to 80% of all ADRs and are both dependent on the dose of drug administered and related to the desired pharmacological effect of the drug administered. Since these types of ADRs are in fact a direct extension of the desired drug action, such ADRs are often preventable and predictable. A classic and predictable form of toxicity is one that results from a direct extension of the therapeutic mechanism of action of the drug. If a patient is taking an immunosuppressant following organ transplantation and the patient suffers an increased incidence of infection, this is a predicted adverse effect or toxicity since the drug is designed to lower the immune system of the patient. Similarly, a patient taking a drug to treat hypertension suddenly suffers from orthostatic hypotension; this too is a direct extension of the therapeutic use of the drug and the dizziness may well have resulted from drug-induced hypotension.

The major step forward that moved organ transplantation from a potentially important therapeutic modality to a routinely used surgical technique was the development drugs that could suppress the immune system of the patient. With the advent of this class of drugs it is now possible to control the recipient's immune system such that the donated organ is far less likely to be rejected by the recipient. Unfortunately, the suppression of the immune system hampers the ability of the organ recipient to fend off infectious diseases and increases the risk of infection for this individual. Thus, increased number of infections following organ transplantation would be expected.

In a related vein, most anticancer drugs kill cells in mitosis. Although these drugs have had a dramatic effect in certain tumors, they do have very serious ADRs and are considered the most dangerous of drugs given to humans with respect to toxicities. One such toxicity is immunosuppression due to the killing of actively dividing immune cells by the drugs and the increased risk of serious infections. In this case however the immunosuppression is an unwanted side effect, not desired pharmacological effect as described for the immunosuppressants.

Hypertension is often referred to as the silent killer since a person can be totally unaware of dangerously high blood pressure. If life style changes do not control hypertension, then pharmacological approaches are required. Since blood pressure is a product of the amount of blood pumped by the heart (cardiac output) and the force required to push the blood through the vasculature (peripheral resistance), drugs have been developed to modify both components of blood pressure. Drugs can decrease cardiac output or lower peripheral resistance to lower blood pressure and in either case there is the potential of lowering either parameter excessively and inducing hypotension. In fact, with the case of certain vasodilators (decreasing peripheral resistance) there is a risk of orthostatic hypotension in which patients standing too quickly can actually suffer dizziness or even loss of consciousness. Here again, the ADR is a direct extension of the desired effect of the drug.

Patients with congestive heart failure must have increased cardiac output while decreasing the workload on the damaged heart. The cardiac glycosides are most frequently used to enhance cardiac output. This class of drugs appears to work by increasing the calcium concentration of the myocardiocyte and thus increase the force of contraction by the cardiac muscle. Thiazide diuretics enhance urine output and thereby decrease peripheral resistance and workload placed on the heart. The thiazides function by increasing potassium and water excretion from the body and can induce hypokalemia, which can result in serious ADRs in patients treated with the cardiac glycosides. The reason for this rests on the fact that as extracellular potassium concentrations decrease (hypokalemia), the effect of the cardiac glycosides on calcium levels in the heart increases. With hypercalcemia in the cardiac muscle comes the risk of cardiac arrhythmias and even cardiac fibrillations. These ADRs can occur if a patient ingests excessive amounts of the cardiac glycoside (here a direct extension of the desired pharmacological effect the cardiac glycosides); however, the combination of cardiac glycosides and the thiazide diuretics can also increase the risk of such ADRs through the mechanism just described.

We recently reported on yet another type of ADR resulting from drug interactions. Second-generation antihistamines are less sedative than first-generation antihistamines because the levels of the former drug in the CNS are less than that of the latter type of antihistamine. It has been reported that the second-generation antihistamines do not cross the blood–brain barrier (see Chapter 12 for a discussion of this anatomical feature). However, when we administered desloratidine (a second-generation antihistamine) to mice in combination with verapamil (drug that inhibits a membrane protein found in the blood–brain barrier that effluxes drug from the CNS back into the blood), it resulted in a sedation of mice that was equivalent to that seen in mice treated with a classic first-generation, sedating antihistamine. Here the effects of one drug resulted in an ADR not thought to occur in the other drug.

Although this is a relatively mild ADR, such interactions have the potential to cause catastrophic ADRs. For example, an important anticancer drug is the plant product vincristine, which stops cells from dividing by interrupting microtubule polymerization. This prevents chromosomal segregation and cell division in the M phase of the cell cycle. A significant ADR with vincristine is a potentially irreversible neurotoxicity, thought to be related to the microtubular effects of the drug (thus an extension of the desired drug activity). Approximately two to three times per year vincristine is administered accidentally intrathecally in cancer patients and is a uniformly fatal ADR. Vincristine is an excellent substrate for the membrane-bound efflux pump discussed. This protein is also expressed on the plasma membrane of certain drug resistant cancer cells and is thought to be a mechanism of multidrug resistance (MDR) by preventing intracellular drug accumulation (see Chapter 15 for a discussion of drug resistance). Our results suggest that the use of inhibitors of the membrane pump such as that discussed earlier has the very possibility of increasing CNS levels of vincristine and could result in serious neurotoxicities (thus a toxic risk enhanced through drug interactions).

13.2.2 How Are the Risks of Type A ADRs Reduced?

During the preclinical and premarketing testing of the drug under study, a great deal of information has been accumulated regarding the doses to be used, the schedule and duration of drug administration, the route of administration, drug absorption, pharmacokinetics, and pharmacodynamics. From these data, the dose, the route of administration, and treatment schedule are designed to provide the greatest therapeutic benefit with the least risk of toxicity to the individual taking the drug. Further, during the development of a given drug, the therapeutic index (discussed elsewhere in the text) can be calculated for that drug. A drug with a small therapeutic index is one in which the serum concentration required to attain a therapeutic benefit is close to the serum level expected to cause some toxicity. A drug with a large therapeutic index has a much larger difference between serum levels needed for therapeutic benefit and the toxic serum levels. Thus, a drug with a small therapeutic index is much more likely to cause adverse effects during therapeutic use (the best examples here are the anticancer drugs) whereas the drug with a large therapeutic index (drugs such as penicillin) are much safer to use.

Keep in mind, however, that there can be a wide variance in response to a given drug among a given population. These variances can be related to a number of factors including gender, age, race, genetics, diet, underlying diseases, and so on. Associated with these variances in response within a given population is the variance in dose needed to provide therapeutic benefit in a given member of that population and a dose that can cause an ADR in that individual.

13.2.3 The Concept of Dose Response in Type A ADRs

A characteristic described in detail elsewhere in this text is the concept of dose response. Briefly, as the dose of a given administered drug increases, the pharmacological effect likewise increases (Figure 13.1). Note that once a specific dose has been exceeded no further increase in the desired pharmacological effects is expected. This plateau is dependent upon a number of factors and is critical to remember because once the plateau dose is reached the only possible outcome of increasing the dose administered is an increased likelihood of ADR incidence and severity. There is another equally important dose response curve to take into consideration when evaluating the use of a given drug and that is the toxicity dose response curve. Note that in this figure the shape of the efficacy dose response curve is identical to that of the toxicity dose response curve, but the curve is shifted to the left with respect to the toxicity dose response curve. This situation usually indicates that the efficacy and the toxicity arise from the same mechanism. Therefore this ADR is a direct extension of the desired efficacy of the drug.

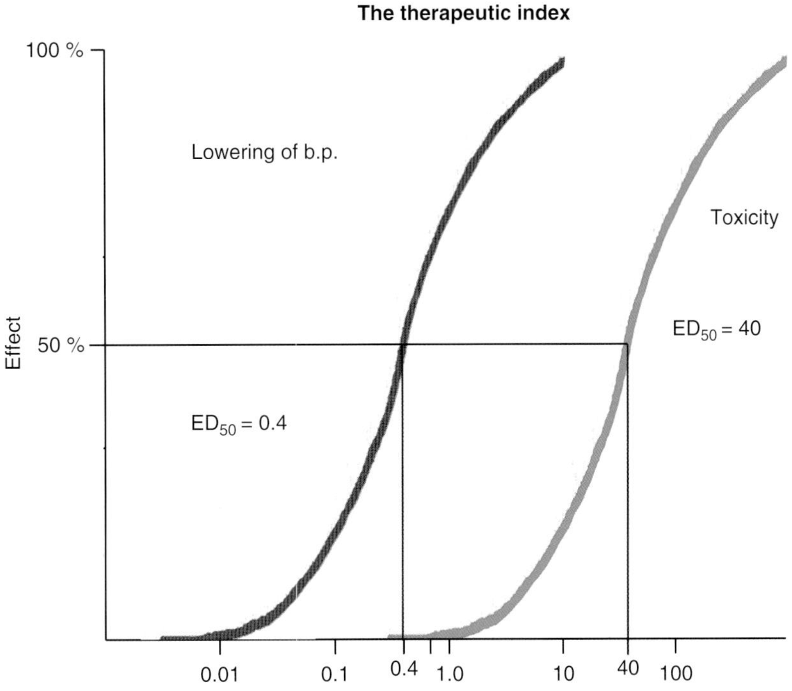

Figure 13.1 Dose response curve for both efficacy and toxicity.

13.2.4 The Importance of the Therapeutic Index in Type A ADRs

The therapeutic index for a given drug can be calculated using a variety of ratios of efficacy and toxicity. As shown in this example the Therapeutic Index (TI) would be:

TI = TD50/ED50 in this case ED50 = 0.4 mg/kg and TD50 = 40 mg/kg thus 40/0.4 = 100
TI = TD10/ED 90 in this case TD10 = 10mg/kg and ED90 = 4 mg/kg and TI = 2.5

As is shown here, the more conservative approach results in a much smaller TI, which indicates that the drug is much less safe than the previous calculation, but may be a more realistic assessment of the risk of a given drug to cause an ADR in a given population.

13.2.5 Population Distribution and Drug Sensitivity

The therapeutic index is calculated for the average person taking the drug, and for approximately 95% of the patients treated with the drug, we can anticipate the type and extent of drug toxicity that might be encountered. For the remaining 5% of the patients, half will be resistant to the therapeutic benefit of the drug, thus requiring increased drug dosage to attain the desired response, if possible. These individuals are referred to as hyporesponsive. For these individuals there may an equal resistance to the toxic effects of the drug, and thus no increased risk of toxicity exists. In other patients hyporesponsiveness to the therapeutic benefit is *not* accompanied by a hyporesponsiveness to the toxic effects of the drug; in these patients increased dosage is risky or even inappropriate. The remaining 2.5% of the population is referred to as hyperresponsive and require significantly less drug to elicit a given response. These individuals are at risk of ADRs at doses recommended for the general population.

During the clinical development of a drug through Phase 1, 2, and 3 studies the range of sensitivity to the drug from hypo- to hypersensitivity is identified and dose range is well defined prior to marketing the drug. Unfortunately, this is not always the case and unexpected ADRs are encountered. With the advent of pharmacogenomics, it is possible that within the foreseeable future these problems will be overcome as we design individualized therapies based on the genomic information for a given patient.

The reasons for hypo- and hypersensitivity are discussed elsewhere in the textbook; however, the terms are based on population distribution as shown in Figure 13.2.

Within any given population there exists variation in the sensitivity of the individual to a given drug. Figure 13.2 describes the typical bell-shaped curve and indicates a Gaussian distribution of the population with respect to the response of that population to a given dose of drug administered to that population. This figure could also describe the dose of drug required to attain a given response to that drug (this is the basis of the dose response curve shown earlier) within any population there are individuals who respond to low doses of the drug whereas others require a much higher dose of drug to attain the same response, but approximately two-thirds of the population respond similarly to a relatively narrow dose range. The reasons for this variation were described previously.

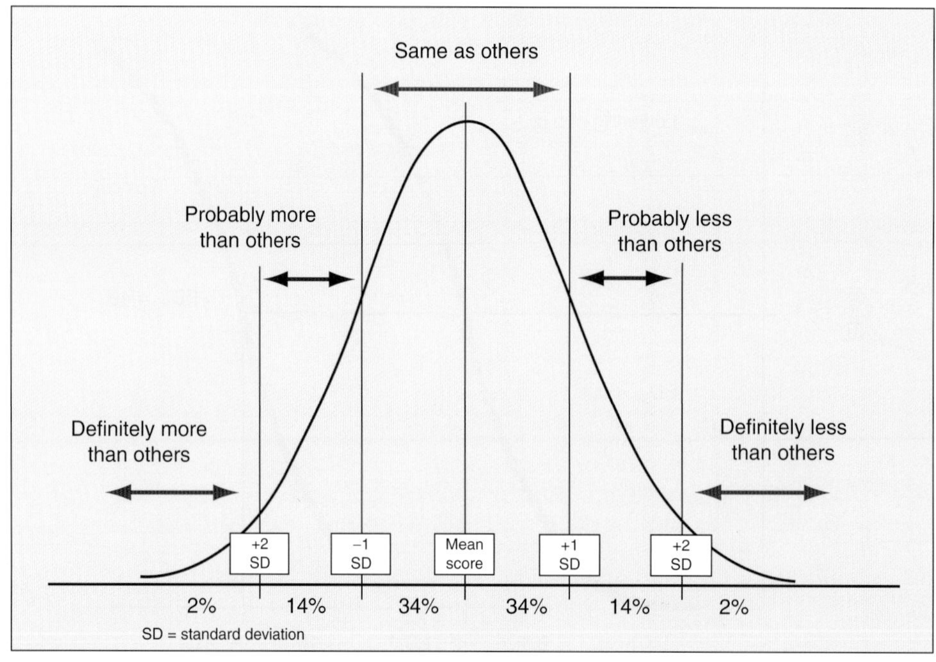

Figure 13.2 Population distribution with respect to drug sensitivity.

13.3 EXAMPLES OF TYPE A ADRs

As stated earlier, Type A ADRs are often extensions of the desired pharmacological effects and can often be predicted. The actual dose or duration of exposure to the drug required to induce an ADR cannot be accurately predicted given the Gaussian distribution of a human population. A perfect example of Type A ADRs, sometimes with life-threatening consequences, is myelosuppression following cytotoxic chemotherapy. Most anticancer drugs are designed to kill dividing cells, and since the bone marrow has a large population of dividing cells, it is not surprising that patients treated with such drugs are at risk of myelosuppression. Noncytotoxic drugs may also cause myelosuppression, but these toxicities most often are categorized as Type B ADRs.

The bone marrow must maintain proper levels of circulating peripheral blood cells. The average sized adult human has about 3.5 kg of marrow tissue distributed throughout the axial skeleton, which produces some 2.5×10^9 red cells, 2.5×10^9 platelets, and 1×10^7 white blood cells daily. There can be considerable daily fluctuations according to demand and these fluctuations are regulated by a variety of growth and maturation factors. The therapeutic efficacy of most anticancer drugs relies on interference with cellular mitotic activity. Nonmalignant cells usually recover from these toxic effects if drug is removed and subsequent rounds of therapy can be initiated following recovery.

During the interval of myelosuppression the patient is at risk of anemia, bleeding problems, and loss of immune protection, depending on the drug(s) being administered to the patient. Although these toxicities are dangerous, they are reversible and as stated previously, once the patient has recovered subsequent drug regimens can be administered. The therapeutic advantage of these drugs may rest in the fact that most malignant cells recover from the toxic effects of anticancer drugs more slowly than do nonmalignant cells, hence the concept of aggressive therapy followed by a rest period. During the aggressive stage cell kill both malignant and nonmalignant cells are killed, whereas during the rest period nonmalignant cell levels return to normal and the malignant cells remained suppressed.

As will be discussed under Type B ADRs there are other toxicities associated with selected cytotoxic drugs that damage tissues without a high mitotic index. These types of toxicities are unexpected, occur in specific organs depending on the drug in question, most often are irreversible, and most often are referred to as organ directed dose limiting toxicities. Since these toxicities were not expected as they occur in organs with a low mitotic index, these organ directed toxicities were not appreciated until a large number of patients had been treated with the drug. Once these toxicities were recognized, ways to prevent or at least minimize the risk or extent of toxicity were developed, but the overall efficacy of anticancer drugs causing organ directed toxicities remains compromised.

This raises an interesting problem regarding the classification of such toxicities. Some apparently Type B toxicities may become more appropriately classified as predictable Type A ADRs for individuals having certain constitutional risk factors, once the mechanism of toxicities are elucidated and risk factors become better understood. An in-depth discussion of such is beyond the scope of this textbook, but the role of genetic make-up and drug toxicity, especially those exceedingly rare types of toxicity, are becoming increasingly better understood as our appreciation and understanding of the human genome increases. Again, this is another excellent example of how pharmacogenomics will play an increasingly important role in the treatment of disease.

Aspirin, or acetylsalicylic acid, has been used for more than 100 years for its analgesic, antipyretic and anti-inflammatory activities. More recently an array of NSAIDs have been developed and introduced into the clinic. For the most part these drugs are well tolerated, but a variety of Type A ADRs, some of which can be life threatening, have been reported for these drugs. An important mechanism of action of the NSAIDs efficacy is the inhibition of the enzyme cyclo-oxygenase 2 (COX-2), which prevents the overproduction of prostaglandins and decreases the pain, fever, and inflammation associated with COX-2 activity.

Until recently all NSAIDs inhibited both COX-1 and COX-2 enzymes. The problem with this effect is the that COX-1 produces low levels of prostaglandins associated with homeostasis whereas COX-2 produces high levels of prostaglandins associated with the inflammatory process. As a result conventional NSAIDs have the capacity to cause such side effects as peptic ulcers and gastritis due to the inhibition of COX-1 and thus are an extension of the drug action. Less frequent ADRs but still Type A ADRs include respiratory distress, NSAID-induced asthma and rhinitis, and urticaria in individuals with no underlying risk factors. These remain type A ADRs since these toxicities appear to be related to the decreased prostaglandin levels resulting from COX-1 inhibition.

Given that the overwhelming evidence indicates that the most frequent toxicities observed with traditional NSAIDs are a consequence of COX-1 inhibition, the industry has struggled to develop a COX-2 selective inhibitor. To date four such drugs have been approved: These drugs entered the market with a great deal of fanfare but as clinical use increased a troubling increase in cardiovascular-related disorders, including strokes, clots, and heart attacks was noted. Vioxx subsequently has been removed from the market but the remaining two are still marketed. These relatively rare toxicities are considered to be Type B ADRs and are discussed later in this chapter. Other Type B ADRs associated with NSAID use are cutaneous and pulmonary in nature. These ADRs appear to mediated through IgE production and are also discussed later in the chapter.

An important consideration when discussing ADRs is the role of drug metabolism in drug toxicity. Often, the parent drug is vastly different from its metabolites with respect to efficacy and toxicity. Due to large number of such events we will not discuss all metabolically induced ADRs. Rather we will provide a limited number to provide some insight into interaction between drug metabolism and Type A ADRs (a similar discussion will be presented later in the chapter regarding Type B ADRS).

Cholesterol-lowering drugs have been a major mainstay for controlling the cholesterol levels in patients presenting with hypercholesterolemia. The tolerability of these drugs during long-term administration is an important issue since hypercholestolremia is a chronic disease. Adverse reactions involving skeletal muscle are not uncommon, and sometimes serious adverse reactions involving skeletal muscle such as myopathy and rhabdomyolysis may occur, requiring discontinuation of the drug. Occasionally, arthralgia, alone or in association with myalgia, has been reported. We will focus on HMG-CoA reductase inhibitor-related musculoskeletal system toxicities. Cytochrome P450 (CYP) 3A4 is the main isoenzyme involved in the metabolic transformation of HMG-CoA reductase inhibitors. Individuals with both low hepatic and low gastrointestinal tract levels of CYP3A4 expression may be at an increased risk of myotoxicity due to potentially higher HMG-CoA reductase plasma concentrations.

The next example addresses two issues regarding metabolic-induced drug toxicity—the role of drug metabolism in ADRs and the effect of age on metabolism. ADRs can vary depending on the age of the individual. For example children often respond differently to a drug than do adults. Some of these differences are related to differences in liver metabolism. Altered drug disposition in the developing child occurs as a result of both biochemical and physiological changes. The clearance of many drugs is dependent on their biotransformation in the liver and small bowel and consequently is developmentally determined by a number of factors including both the activity and abundance of enzymes involved in Phase 1 and 2 drug metabolism. Altered drug metabolism can lead to the development of adverse effects in neonates and small infants that are not generally seen in the adult population. For instance, the altered metabolism of sodium valproate in children under 3 years of age is thought to be responsible for a higher incidence of hepatotoxicity; the impaired metabolism of chloramphenicol in neonates has resulted in the grey baby syndrome (cyanosis and respiratory failure); and metabolic acidosis following the use of propranolol in the critically ill child may be due to altered drug metabolism.

On the other extreme the elderly represent a challenge regarding the prediction of ADRs. Older people are major consumers of drugs and because of this, as well as comorbidity and age-related changes in pharmacokinetics and pharmacodynamics, they are at risk of associated adverse drug reactions. Although age does not alter drug absorption in a clinically significant way, and age-related changes in volume of drug distribution and protein binding are not of concern in chronic therapy, reduction in hepatic drug clearance is clinically important. Liver blood flow falls by about 35% between young adulthood and old age, and liver size decreases by about 24 to 35% over the same period. First-pass metabolism of oral drugs avidly cleared by the liver and clearance of capacity-limited hepatically metabolized drugs fall in parallel with the fall in liver size, and clearance of drugs with a high hepatic extraction ratio falls in parallel with the fall in hepatic blood flow. In normal aging, in general, activity of the cytochrome P450 enzymes is preserved, although a decline in frail older people has been noted, as well as in association with liver disease, cancer, trauma, sepsis, critical illness, and renal failure. Because the contribution of age, comorbidity, and concurrent drug therapy to altered drug clearance is impossible to predict in an individual older patient, it is wise to start any drug at a low dose and increase this slowly, monitoring carefully for beneficial and adverse effects.

13.4 AVOIDING TYPE A ADRs

Here the adage "an ounce of prevention is worth a pound of cure" rings so true. That means careful defining of dose, treatment schedule, and likely toxicities during the development of a drug is vitally important. These values are defined during drug development using data obtained from a number of clinical trials usually performed throughout the world. Careful and accurate reporting of all data obtained from such studies is essential to minimize ADRs once the drug has been approved for marketing. Further, continued surveillance for ADRs following drug marketing approval (Phase 4 of drug development) is equally essential to minimize the risk of ADRs that may have been overlooked or never occurred due to the rarity during premarketing. For physicians in the hospital or office practice using an approved drug the filing of ADRs is purely voluntary, which can lead to underreporting of ADRs. In contrast the pharmaceutical industry is required to report all ADRs.

Recently, Hazell and Shakir reviewed the incidence of ADR underreporting in 37 spontaneous reporting system studies from 12 countries that used a variety of surveillance methods and found an underreporting rate of 94% (interquartile range 82–98%) with drugs that were in the postmarketing phase. There was no difference in underreporting when private practice studies were compared to hospital-based studies. Although underreporting was less for ADRs considered to be serious to severe, the underreporting rate was still greater than 80%. The implications of these results are obvious—the incidence and types of ADRs encountered are not adequately quantified in postmarketing studies. Why would such a problem exist given the importance of ADR reporting? Physicians state that it is lack of time, lack of ability to ascribe the ADR to the drug, poor understanding of the report forms, and lack of understanding of the role of the spontaneous reporting system (SRS).

Even more troubling would be underreporting of ADRs observed during premarketing clinical trials. During these studies it is vital to report all likely ADRs as they provide an important profile of potential ADRs that may be encountered later. During the tightly controlled and carefully regulated premarketing clinical trials, ADRs are negative events and often result in the cessation of further clinical development of a drug. Given the amount of time and money invested in a given drug, especially those drugs that have reached Phase 3 clinical trials, reporting ADRs to the FDA is a necessary but difficult endeavor for any pharmaceutical company sponsoring the clinical development of a drug. Reporting ADRs during preclinical trials is much more controlled than in postmarketing clinical studies described previously, but even in these preclinical trials underreporting ADRs is possible.

A number of strategies have been proposed to encourage and facilitate the reporting of ADRs such as greater accessibility to the SRS database through electronic and online reporting, including the pharmacist and nurse in the reporting cadre, increased understanding for the purpose and importance of pharmacovigilance by the physician, and continued training of the medical profession to maintain the quality and quantity of ADR reporting.

How do we assess the likelihood that the adverse event noted in a given study in fact is related to the drug under study? This question is a major contributor to underreporting of ADRs in drug studies. The most logical approach is to develop an algorithm that enables the observer to determine with a higher degree of certainty that the adverse effect is drug-related. Such an algorithm has been proposed by Koh and Li (Table 13.1).

The degree of likely causal relationship between drug administration and ADR is based on the total number of points accrued by the given ADR. Scores greater than 12 = definite; 8 to 11 = probable; 0 to 7 = possible; less than 0 = unlikely. This algorithm is actually a modified form of the 56-question Kramer algorithm, and is considered the gold standard for these types of assessment when compared to the Kramer algorithm in a total of 450 different ADR reports. The algorithm was found to have a greater than 98% congruency with the far more time-consuming and bulky Kramer algorithm.

Another approach to proper reporting of ADRs is systematic reviews of clinical trials. Although it would seem logical to have experts review the clinical data to quantify ADRs, there are some significant obstacles facing the experts conducting such reviews. First, the methodology for performing such reviews mostly results from poor indexing of ADRs in medical databases. Second, interpretation of ADR reporting in randomized clinical trials is hampered by the poor quality of the reports. Although database searching of the literature has improved dramatically during the last few years, searching for relevant articles remains a challenge.

A more recent approach to controlling the quality and quantity of ADR reporting is at the publication stage. Several medical journals are requiring that the clinical trial data conform to CONSORT (consolidated standard of reporting clinical trials), a newly developed way to systematize ADR reporting in clinical data, in order to be published in the journal. Given that these journals include the British Medical Journal, JAMA, Lancet, and New England Journal of Medicine there is a good chance that CONSORT will have a positive impact on the ADR activities.

13.5 PHARMACOVIGILANCE AND ADR

While premarketing clinical trials are important it must be remembered that upon completion of all premarketing studies, only a limited number of individuals, usually less than 3000, have been treated with the test drug. This small subset of the entire population can often miss important but infrequent ADRs. Once a drug has been awarded an NDA, marketing is now possible. The drug can now be prescribed for use in all appropriate patients and vast numbers of humans can be treated with the drug. Now an accurate profile of toxicities can be developed if rigorous good postmarketing surveillance process (GPMSP) is properly carried out. GPMSP is essential if good pharmacovigilance practices are to be effective.

During this time of GPMSP, data accrual is dependent on accurate and complete spontaneous adverse reaction report submission. As described earlier, this is at best a questionable state of affairs as underreporting is widespread. However, there is an increasing awareness among all involved in drug discovery, development, and use that the only way to lower the ADR

Table 13.1 Determining Cause of ADR

Questions	Yes	No	Unknown	NA[a]
Is the time between dosing and ADR reasonable?[b]	2	−4	0	—
Has the ADR been associated with this drug before?	2	−2	0	—
Could the ADR be related to an existing clinical condition?	0	4	0	—
Is there an overdose of the drug?	2	0	0	—
If the drug is withdrawn does the ADR disappear?	1	−2	0	0
Did the ADR resolve with continued treatment?	−2	0	0	0
Did the ADR occur if a specific antagonist was administered?	4	0	1	0
Did the ADR recur if the drug was re-administered?	4	−2	0	0

a = not applicable; *b* = depending on the drug and the ADR rate is to maintain careful pharmacovigilance processes. Successful pharmacovigilance requires both careful planning and strict adherence to the described standard operating procedures (SOP).

Spontaneous reports have been the cornerstone of pharmacovigilance; the central goal of these efforts is to develop scientifically strong indicators of ADR and accurately identify rare, serious, unusual, or unexpected ADRs as soon as possible after marketing launch. The basic principles of this activity include:

- Effectiveness, including rigorous alerting of suspected ADRs, signal detection, and handling of reports
- Efficiency focusing on the important reactions
- Consistency providing a unified corporate opinion on type and severity of the ADR
- Validity insuring that the tools utilized yield correct results

How do we reduce these principles into practice? Pharmacovigilance should be a stepwise approach:

- Data triage
- Information acquisition
- Single case assessment
- Technical checks
- Case series
- Interpretation
- Communication

The goal of data triage is to sort reports that are likely of clinical importance from those that are less likely to be important. Given the volumes of reports submitted, especially on drugs with a large market, it is vital to have an efficient and accurate means to triage data. What makes a set of data important includes the potential severity of the ADR, the medical significance of the ADR, and whether the ADR is "usually related to drug ADRs." Only those reports labeled as important require a clinical review at the individual case level. Those reports considered less important can be handled in aggregate and carefully data mined. Only those less important reports that meet an alerting threshold as described next need individual case review.

As stated previously, underreporting is a significant problem in any effort to identify ADRs quickly and accurately. Thus enhanced acquisition of important data is essential. All reports deemed important need an active query with the reporter to increase the likelihood of making a causality determination. For a subset of these important reports, which are related to organ systems that are historically linked to drug toxicity, there exist a set of data collection instruments that provide an efficient, effective, and structured query. Given that such reports can result in the removal of a drug from the market it is critical that all such reports and the reporter are accurate. Further, it is recommended in such situations, the company selling the drug has a team in place that can be mobilized to travel to the site of the report to obtain the relevant laboratory or biopsy samples.

The third step in the process of pharmacovigilance has two parts—single case assessment and signal-based evaluation. The initial step is to add a quality score using algorithms such as that discussed earlier, which enables the reviewers to sort the reports into three levels of quality reports. This evaluation is done prior to regulatory submission. After the report is submitted to the regulators, the main pharmacovigilance assessment and evaluation occurs. The risk assessor compares these new data to similar cases and assigns a level of importance to the report. All reports deemed important at this point warrant an issuance of an alert, which is simply an initial warning to look at the data carefully. If the data have sufficient substance to require further investigation then a signal is issued.

Yet another series of checks are now required in technical checks. The primary purpose of the technical checks is to send alerts to the reviewers for assessment and judgment as to whether the alert warrants a signal status. There must be in place methodologies, such as the FDA Baysian ratio technique discussed elsewhere in the text, to evaluate the reports since most reports are not evaluated on an individual basis.

The next step in data analysis is the case series, which remains the clinical mainstay. There is more to be learned from a carefully assembled series of like cases than can be extracted from the isolated review of an individual case. This is the first time that the risk assessors view the data both clinically and epidemiologically. Here the quality of reports probably exceeds the quantity of reports, and underreporting of spontaneous reports becomes less important. It is at this point that the signal determination can be assessed, which results in informing the proper level of corporate management, and a full signal work-up and report is required. Once a signal determination has been issued the work-up begins. Factors to consider include epidemiological context, exposure data, age and gender demographics, natural history of the disease and the observed outcome, alternative risk factors, plausibility of results, and whether they employed good pharmacoepidemiological practices.

Finally, if the risk assessors evaluation results in the assessment of a true signal indicator, it requires notification of the corporation, the medical field, and business stakeholders. At this point the ADR may be placed on the label as a risk of drug ADR. A sufficiently severe ADR may result in the "black box" label on the drug. The name refers to the black box placed around that specific ADR and is considered the most serious of possible ADRs.

13.6 TYPE B ADRs

This class of ADRs includes drug allergies (hypersensitivity reactions), idiosyncratic responses, or intolerance. These types of ADRs are difficult if not impossible to predict and are therefore unavoidable until sufficient knowledge of the drug and the patients taking this drug allows the development of characteristics that increase the risk of Type B ADRs. Obviously, although we discussed the importance of pharmacovigilance in the preceding portion of this chapter, diligent reporting of Type B ADRs is even more critical as these ADRs are difficult to predict and most often encountered in the postmarketing clinic. In this section of the chapter we will discuss examples of Type B ADRs based on different organ systems of the body.

13.6.1 Drug Allergies

The importance of this drug toxicity is probably best exemplified by penicillin, a drug that revolutionized the treatment of bacterial infections, converting what had been potentially lethal diseases into manageable diseases with excellent clinical outcomes. This class of drugs is the closest thing we have to the silver bullet described by Ehrlich in the 1800s as there is virtually no Type A ADR associated with penicillin. However, it soon became apparent that penicillin does cause a drug allergy that can range from a mild itching of the skin to life threatening anaphylactic shock. Other drugs that cause drug allergies include the nonsteriodal anti-inflammatories, the thiazides, sulfa drugs, anticonvulsants, barbiturates, and iodine as well as the protein-based formulations such as vaccines, insulin, and TSH. In fact, drug allergies account for approximately 20% of all reported ADRs. In this portion of the chapter we will discuss the types of drug allergies, mechanism of drug allergies, and specific examples of important drug allergies.

A controversial aspect of drug allergies is one commonly referred to as multiple drug allergy syndrome, in which patients have experienced allergic reactions to two or more noncross-reacting medications. It has been hypothesized that such a reaction results from an individual's underlying heightened propensity to develop allergic responses (both IgE- and non IgE- mediated).

13.6.1.1 Classification of Drug Allergies

The term hypersensitivity is often associated with drug allergy. However, as was discussed earlier, the term hypersensitivity has a different connotation in pharmacology that it does in immunology. Drug hypersensitivity is considered to be a dose-related response to a drug such that the hypersensitive individual responds to a much lower dose of the drug than does the general population. The immune system plays no role in drug hypersensitivity. Drug allergies on the other hand are not dose related and do involve the immune system centrally in this type of ADR, but are often called hypersensitivity reactions. A hypersensitive individual is quite different from an individual suffering a hypersensitive reaction.

Allergies are mediated by a variety of immune responses and because of this, allergies are most commonly classified based on immune response mechanisms responsible for the allergic response. In 1963, Gell and Coombs divided allergic responses into four subtypes; this classification remains virtually intact today (Table 13.2).

13.6.1.2 Activation of the Immune System

The immune system is designed to eliminate foreign proteins, invading organisms, and damaged or malignant cells and is composed of macrophages or antigen presenting cells and lymphocytes. In the case of an allergic response the mast cell, basophil, and/or eosinophil provide the histamine to help drive the allergic response. The general scheme for activation of the humoral immune response, the branch of the immune system response for allergic responses, is shown in Figure 13.3.

Antigen presenting cells (APC) ingest a foreign protein and present a portion of the protein (the antigen) on the surface of the APC through a surface receptor known as the HLA II (human leukocyte antigen II). T-Helper cell (Th) binds to the antigen through the T Cell Receptor (TCR), and this initiates the response. A second costimulatory signal is then activated by two proteins on the surface of the APC (CD80 and CD86) binding to a Th cell surface molecule (CD28). These cosignals then activate the Th cell to release the protein cytokine IL-4, which then activates a subset of the helper T cells, Th 2 cells, to produce more IL-4. In the presence of antigen and the released IL-4, B cells then mature to plasma cells that recognize the antigen and produce antibodies on subsequent exposure to the antigens. There exist a number of different classes of antibodies including IgA, IgG, IgM, IgD, and IgE. With immediate allergic responses the critical antibody class is IgE. The IgE then binds to high

Table 13.2 Allergic Response Subtypes

Allergic Response	Involves	Characteristics
Type 1	IgE and T-helper 2 cells orchestrate response Maximal response within 30 minutes	Immediate hypersensitivity Hay fever, urticaria, atopic asthma
Type II	Cytotoxic autoantibodies	Antibody-dependent cytotoxic hypersensitivity
Type III	Tissue damage secondary to immune complex formed Maximal response 3–8 hrs post exposure	Immune complex mediated hypersensitivity (Arthus reaction)
Type IV	Erythema and induration T-helper 1 cells mediated Seen 24–48 hrs post exposure	Delayed hypersensitivity. Contact hypersensitivity, TB dermal test, poison ivy

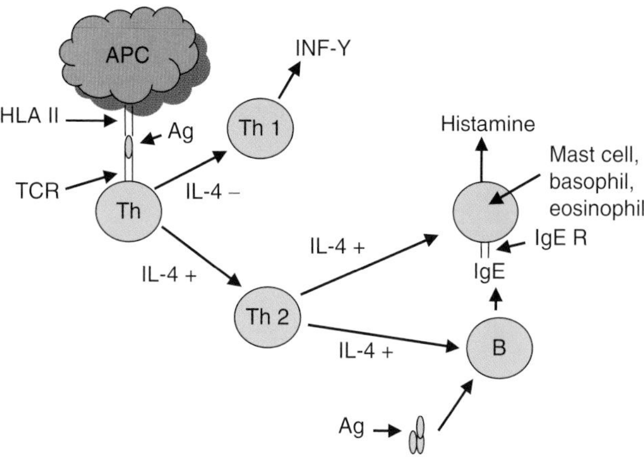

Figure 13.3 Allergic response to drug (Ag).

affinity IgE receptors on the surface of histamine releasing cells including mast cells, basophils, and eosinophils.

The IgE molecule cross links two IgE receptors on the histamine releasing cell, which signals the cell to release histamine into the extracellular fluid. Histamine is rapidly deactivated by the enzymes histamine N-methyl transferase or diamine oxidases, which normally limits the effect of histamine to the cells near the histamine releasing cell. The released histamine diffuses into the ECF and binds to histamine receptors, of which the two most studied are H1 and H2. Binding of histamine to its receptor initiates the physiological effect of histamine, which is dependent on the cell type activated by the histamine. Typical effects of histamine binding to H1 receptors include bronchoconstriction, vasodilation, allergic rhinitis, itching, pain, and edema formation. In contrast, binding of histamine to H2 receptors initiates increased acidity of the stomach. Thus as will be demonstrated, drug allergies have a large variability in pathophysiological pathways, clinical signs and symptoms, severity, and in the drugs that can elicit these responses.

13.6.1.3 Latency Period in Drug Allergies

Drug allergies are classified by the latency period between drug exposure and the onset of allergic reactions and include immediate, late, and delayed. The symptoms of an immediate type reaction are urticaria, angioedema, rhinitis, asthma, and anaphylaxis. Thus, the immediate onset type of drug allergy can range from mild itching of the skin to the life-threatening anaphylaxis. What dictates the degree of allergic reaction is, as discussed earlier, directly related to extent and sites of histamine release. In urticaria, histamine release is limited to the skin whereas in anaphylaxis histamine release is generalized resulting in alterations in pulmonary and cardiovascular function.

Late reactions can present as allergic vasculitis (characterized by damage to the blood vessels and skin), pupura pigmentosa (a discoloration of the skin), erythema multiforme (lesions of the skin leading to open sores that may or may not have systemic symptomatology), and serum sickness (characterized by hives, rash, itching of the skin, joint pain, fever, and malaise). Unlike the immediate reaction, which is solely driven by rapid onset histamine release, the pathogenesis of the late reaction is the complexation of an antibody, most frequently IgG, with antigen. These complexes can then lead to the activation of complement or binding of the complex to cells with cytotoxic effects. Keep in mind that the late reaction may also have an IgE-histamine component leading to rhinitis or skin reactions, but these occur much later than would be expected of an immediate reaction and appear to be a result of histamine release by the basophil rather than mast cells. Drugs known to cause this type of reaction are the oral contraceptives, pyrazolones, and sulfonamides.

The delayed type reaction presents as allergic contact dermatitis (as seen after exposure to poison ivy in 85% of the population) and morbilliform exanthemas (lesions that burst forth on the skin or mucous membranes). The delayed type reaction can result in far more serious consequences such as TEN (Toxic Epidermal Necrosis), a skin erosion that can affect large patches of skin including mucous membranes of the eyes, oropharynx, and genitalial and has a 30% mortality rate or SJS (Stevens-Johnson Syndrome, which includes fever, malaise, myalgia, arthralgia, and extensive erythema multiforme of the trunk and face). A surprisingly large number of drugs are capable of causing this type of drug allergy:

Antituberculous drugs, Barbiturates, Carbamazepine, Cephalosporins, Erythromycin, Frusemide, Gold, Gentamicin, Isoniazid, Nitrofurantoin, Penicillins, Phenothiazines, Phenylbutazone, Phenytoin, Sulphonamides, Thiazides.

Fortunately, the incidence is low. The cause of this reaction appears to be an activation of the CD8+ T-cell, the immune cell responsible for cellular immunity, which then attacks and destroys autologous epidermal keratinocytes.

How do small molecular weight chemicals such as the vast majority of drugs cause an immune-mediated drug allergy?

13.6.1.4 Development of Drug Allergies

There are two models put forth for the development of drug allergies—the hapten model and the direct recognition model. The hapten model, which states that a drug must attach to a protein to become an allergen, is the more established explanation. The direct recognition model states that the T cell recognizes the drug itself together with the MHC/peptide complex to initiate the drug allergy. The direct recognition model does not require metabolism and may provide a more straightforward explanation as to why the skin plays such a prominent role in drug allergies.

Hapten Model Antigens are commonly thought of as portions of proteins metabolized by the APC and are recognized by the T cell only after being attached to the MHC on the surface of the APC. Given that drugs are often considered too small to act as antigens in this manner an alternative pathway for Th cell activation must be considered. A drug (direct hapten) or drug metabolite (indirect hapten) binds covalently to an extracellular or intracellular protein (haptenization). If the haptenization occurs extracellularly then the APC can endocytose the haptenized protein, digest the complex in the lysosome, and then couple the antigens to MHC II prior to the complex migrating to the surface of the APC. This MHC II bound complex can then interact with the Th cell as described earlier. The Th cell can then interact with T cells to activate either the Th 1 or Th 2 pathways or can activate B cells to initiate the humoral response to the antigen.

As shown earlier, the Th 1 pathway results in the release of the pro-inflammatory molecule INF-γ and is involved primarily in the Type IV delayed hypersensitivity responses, which includes allergic contact dermatitis, exanthemas, TEN, or SJS. Activation of the drug specific Th 2 cells can result in the activation and attraction of eosinophils, which reflects the prevalence of eosinophils present in allergic skin eruptions seen in late drug allergies. Finally, activated Th cells can stimulate mature plasma cells in the presence of the drug antigen to release antibodies that result in antibody-antigen complexes and the resulting late drug hypersensitivity, or in the release of histamine seen in either rapid onset hypersensitivity or late drug reactions.

The Direct Recognition Model This model was developed in an attempt to explain how APC that have been fixed and metabolically inactive could activate an immune response to a drug. In this situation the APC presents an intact drug molecule or a metabolite of the drug *without* being covalently linked to a protein and activation of the T cells can still occur. This is a fairly recent observation and more work is required to better understand the mechanism of this reaction and the significance of the reaction in drug-induced allergies.

13.6.2 Hypersensitivity Reactions to β-lactam Antibiotics

Allergies to this class of drugs are the most commonly reported of all drug-related allergies, with a reported incidence of penicillin allergy of around 10% of all patients. A complicating feature of penicillin allergies is the fact that more than 90% of patients who claimed to have penicillin allergy lack the penicillin-specific IgE antibodies seen in patients with true immediate onset penicillin allergy. Further, most allergic patients do not respond to classic skin tests for allergic sensitivity. What is the basis of the discrepancy between "claimed" and "true" penicillin allergy is not completely understood. Drug-induced ADRs observed when hypersensitivity to β-lactams is encountered are summarized in Table 13.3.

Table 13.3 Drug Allergy Induced ADRs with β-lactams

Multisystem	Skin
Anaphylaxis	Maculopapular/morbilliform eruptions
Serum sickness-like reaction	Urticaria/angioedema
Drug fever	SJS
Vasculitis	TEN
Generalized lymphadenopathy	Contact dermatitis
Bone Marrow	**Lung**
Hemolytic anemia	Eosinophilic pulmonary infiltrates
Thrombocytopenia	
Neutropenia	
Aplastic anemia	
Eosinophilia	
Heart	**Liver**
Myocarditis	Hepatitis
Kidney	
Interstitial nephritis	
Nephrotic syndrome	

As can be seen from Table 13.3, the β-lactams have been implicated in a wide variety of allergic ADRs, but in many cases these reactions do not fit into the traditional Gell and Coombs classification. As was discussed earlier these ADRs are more than likely a result of both IgE- and T-cell mediated reactions and constitute potential immediate, late, and delayed hypersensitivity responses. For the remainder of this chapter we will focus on the IgE-related reactions since we have the greatest understanding of the pathogenesis of such ADRs in β-lactam antibiotics.

13.6.2.1 Epidemiology of Beta Lactam Drug Allergies

As stated earlier, the β-lactams are reported in 10% of all patients treated with penicillin, yet 90% of patients claiming to be allergic to penicillin do not have the penicillin-specific IgE. What could account for the glaring discrepancy? Several factors, including the previous reaction attributed to the administration of the drug may actually have been related to the disease and not the drug, the reaction may have been a predictable reaction and not an allergic response at all, or patients tend to lose IgE antibody titers with time following drug exposure. Unfortunately, there has been no prospective study to evaluate the sensitization rate of patients during a course of therapy. Retrospective studies have supported the claim that β-lactams cause the greatest number of cutaneous ADRs (between 1 and 5% of patients treated, depending on the β-lactam administered) but it is unknown how many of these reactions were accompanied by a rise in IgE titer. Further, with surprising consistency, retrospective studies also have demonstrated that penicillin-induced anaphylactic responses are rare (1–4/10,000 patients treated) and are seen most frequently in patients receiving multiple parental treatments. Finally, though not well studied, the data accumulated with the cephalosporins suggest that the incidence of immune-mediated ADRs are approximately one order of magnitude lower for the cephalosporins than that observed with the penicillins.

13.6.2.2 Risk Factors for the Development of β-lactam Allergies

Patients between 20 and 49 appear to be at greatest risk of developing acute allergic reactions to penicillin. It is interesting that children, who receive significant antibiotic therapy, have a lower incidence of allergic reactions. It is possible that the discrepancy in age may be related to immune response differences in different age populations. Children with allergies to bee stings lose venom IgE far more rapidly than do adults. It is possible that a similar mechanism exists for penicillin allergy.

Patients suffering from atopy (the genetic susceptibility to develop allergies) were at one time thought to be at a significantly higher risk to develop penicillin allergies. Meta-analysis of large scale studies have proven this to be inaccurate although asthmatics may be more likely to develop anaphylactic reactions to penicillin.

An interesting phenomenon is the fact that patients treated with penicillin while infected with Epstein Barr virus are more likely to develop mobilliform eruption, but at the same time lack penicillin-specific IgE antibodies. Further, these patients appear to tolerate future course of penicillin therapy quite well. The actual mechanism of this infection-associated phenomenon is unknown but viral infection is associated with increased release of interferons. Interferons have been reported to increase MHC expression on the surface membranes of APC in the skin and thus increase activity of dermal immune activity.

Given that the route of antigen exposure is known to be important in determining the type of immune response initiated, it is perhaps not surprising that parentally administered penicillin (either IM or IV) is far more likely to develop Type 1 allergic response than those receiving oral penicillin. The frequency of treatment may also play a role as patients with cystic fibrosis who undergo frequent IV antibiotic treatments are particularly prone to developing IgE mediated penicillin allergies.

13.6.3 Multiple Drug Allergy Syndrome

This term refers to patients who have experienced allergic reactions to two or more noncross-reacting medications, and is controversial. One theory concerning this syndrome states that a patient who develops an allergy to one drug is more likely to develop an allergy to a second unrelated drug due to the patient's propensity to develop allergic reactions (both IgE and non-IgE related). Limited studies are available to state conclusively that such a syndrome exists and if so, the mechanism of the multidrug allergies. In fact, several investigators have published studies contradicting the multidrug allergy syndrome. Khoury et al., using age and sex matched groups of patients that were either positive or negative to penicillin skin tests, reported that penicillin reactive patients were least likely to react to other antibiotics.

13.6.4 Mechanisms of Allergic Responses

As discussed earlier in this chapter, the most widely accepted concept for the development of drug-induced allergies is that the drug (hapten), too small to initiate an immune response on its own, must first covalently bind to a carrier protein (haptenation). This newly formed multivalent complex can then elicit an immune response, which in the case of penicillins is most frequently the immediate type and correlates with the presence of IgE antibodies. An interesting feature of β-lactam allergies is that the route of administration seems to play a role in the type of allergic response seen. Although not conclusively demonstrated in prospective studies there is a significant body of literature to suggest that the parental route of administration is more likely to induce Type 1 allergies and more likely to cause anaphylaxis than the oral route of administration.

There is at best limited data to support or refute the role of heredity in the susceptibility to antibiotic allergies. Few reports have been published regarding this phenomenon and unfortunately those that have been reported lack confirmatory testing or provocative testing but rely almost exclusively on patient histories. Even more confounding is the fact that these reports do not separate IgE mediated from non-IgE mediated allergic responses. Further these studies focused on drug allergies and not purely on antibiotic drug allergies and reported a familial predilection for drug allergies across drug classes. One explanation for an apparent but not yet proven familial predilection for drug allergies across drug classes is that these individuals are likely to mount a humoral immunological response to drug protein complexes formed during therapy. Since we lack the necessary data to clarify whether heredity plays a distinct role of beta-lactam antibiotic allergies, further research is needed.

Although it well accepted that drug allergies are the most common with beta-lactam antibiotics, other drug classes have the potential of inducing such an immunological response. Sulfonamide-induced allergic reactions occur in as many 20 to 30% of AIDS patients. Often AIDS patient allergies present as skin rashes. Yet another nonurticarial rash hypersensitivity (Stevens-Johnson syndrome discussed elsewhere in the chapter) are thought to be a response reactive to metabolites such as the hydroxylamines, N-acetylated sulfonamides, or the nitroso-metabolites. Given the interesting history of the sulfa-based compounds and the variety of nonantibiotic uses of these compounds there is a very real concern about cross-allergic responses to nonantibiotic sulfa compounds in sulfonamide allergic patients. To date no such increased incidence has been noted in sulfonamide allergic patients.

13.6.4.1 NSAIDs Allergic Responses

Even nonantibiotic drugs can induce allergic responses. Aspirin and nonselective NSAIDs can cause an idiopathic urticaria and upon rechallenge 20 to 30% will develop urticaria or angioedema. For this reason, such drugs are contra-indicated in patients developing such skin reactions following drug therapy. In contrast, if a patient is rechallenged with a COX-2 selective drug no skin reactions are noted in the vast majority of patients. There are interesting reports that a patient may develop skin reactions to one nonselective NSAID but have no reaction to a different NSAID. The mechanism of this selective reactivity is very poorly understood at the present time but may be related to the pharmacological effects of these drugs.

In addition to skin eruptions aspirin can cause a syndrome referred to as aspirin exacerbated respiratory disease (AERD) in which the classic triad of asthma, rhinitis, and aspirin sensitivity was first described by Samter. It is important to note that AERD has as its precursor an underlying respiratory disease such as asthma that is exacerbated by aspirin but not caused by aspirin. Briefly, the natural history of this disease indicates that the patient first develops an upper respiratory tract inflammation that persists rather than subsides. Sinusitis develops, which progresses to pansinusitis with nasal polyps and asthma noted. At some point the patient takes aspirin or some other COX-1 inhibitor and an AERD reaction occurs. Although this is truly an idiopathic reaction to NSAIDs, adult patients with chronic sinusitis and nasal polyps should be observed carefully for the potential development of AERD.

At present there is very little that can be used to identify individuals with NSAID sensitivity using *in vitro* tests. Consequently challenges to the patient must be used and in this case only oral challenges are approved in the United States. Such tests are risky and should be performed only by well-trained physicians who are ready to rapidly and aggressively treat a variety of responses including severe bronchospasm, cutaneous, GI, and vascular effects.

The pathogenesis of AERD is confusing because the symptoms of AERD mimic those of a true immediate hypersensitivity reaction; no antibody-antigen mechanism has ever been established. Rather, it appears as though the initiation may be related to the inhibition of intracellular COX enzymes causing a rapid decrease in prostaglandin production and the leukotriene pathway becoming dominant. Given that prostaglandins induce bronchodilation and leukotrienes induce bronchoconstriction, the subsequent bronchoconstriction is not surprising. However, if this were the only cause then all individuals taking an NSAID would be at risk of AERD. Recent data suggest that AERD susceptible individuals have upregulated leukotriene receptors in the bronchiolar tree. Another potential explanation for this AERD response in a select number of individuals is the observation that following NSAID exposure urine levels of leukotriene metabolites increase two- to 10-fold. In summary, NSAID-induced AERD is of interest because it represents a class A ADR (since inhibition of COX, the pharmacologic target of NSAIDs appears to induce the response) but since it is so rare it is classified as an idiosyncratic response or class B ADR.

13.6.4.2 Allergies to Cancer Chemotherapeutic Drugs

Discussion of all hypersensitivity reactions is beyond the scope of this chapter, however one more example will be discussed—that being the case of hypersensitivity to anticancer drugs. At present there are more than 85 drugs used to treat cancer, yet few drugs are actually associated with hypersensitivity responses. These drugs include bleomycin, platinum complexes, epipodophyllotoxins, taxanes, anthracyclines, and asparginase. It is of interest that each of these examples, with the notable exception of the platinum complexes, are drugs derived from a microbial or plant source (natural products). As with previous examples of drug-induced hypersensitivity, we must be careful in defining hypersensitivity. Here we define hypersensitivity as signs and symptoms not normally associated with those given that occur within hours of drug administration, almost always following a parenteral drug administration. Symptoms most commonly observed include skin flushing, bronchospasm, altered cardiac activity, dyspnea, fever, back pain, nausea and vomiting, and skin rashes of all types. Although these responses are most frequently associated with specific drugs, there also exist responses to drug formulations such as the excipient Cremaphor EL or pegylation of the drug.

L-Asparaginase L-asparaginase is an enzyme used to treat acute lymphocytic leukemia (ALL) and is associated with a high frequency of hypersensitivity responses. Route of administration plays a significant role in the incidence of hypersensitivity as IV administration causes a significant number of hypersensitive responses (6–43%) whereas IM or subcutaneous routes cause far lower incidences (6–14%). Because of the high incidence of hypersensitivity it is prudent to test a patient for hypersensitivity before the first dose or any dose that an interval of one week or more has elapsed between doses. The actual mechanism responsible for the immediate hypersensitivity response remains unclear. Studies have shown that a pegylated form of L-asparaginase is tolerated by many who have had hypersensitivity responses to native L-asparaginase, suggesting that it may not be a simple reaction to the enzyme protein. Further, production of L-asparaginase in a different bacteria (*Erwinia*) rather than *E.* coli results in a protein that can be administered to patients previously shown to be hypersensitive to the *E.* coli product. These results suggest that the hypersensitivity may be related to the bacterial source of the enzyme.

The mechanism of this drug-induced hypersensitivity remains unknown but IgE antibodies have been identified in some but not all patients. In others, complement activation has been reported but no clear-cut mechanism can be identified. A study in children reported that 35% had IgG specific for L-asparaginase and 50% of these children had hypersensitivity responses to the drug but only 18% of the children not expressing IgG had similar hypersensitivity response. Patients suffering hypersensitivity to *E.* coli derived L-asaparaginase could be treated safely with pegylated drug or L-asparaginase from *Erwinia.* It is highly encouraged that any patient should be skin tested prior to receiving L-asparaginase.

Platinum-based Drugs The platinum complexes have been a mainstay of cancer chemotherapy for more than 25 years. The complexes consist of a central platinum-two stable ammines and leaving groups as shown in Figure 13.4.

The proposed mechanism of action for the platinum complexes is that the leaving groups hydrolyze from the central platinum in a process known as aquation, enabling the drug to form intrastrand crosslinks with DNA, thereby inhibiting DNA synthesis. Cisplatin was the first platinum complex to be used clinically but is being replaced by carboplatin. Cisplatin can cause typical type A ADRs such as marrow depression and GI problems but is associated with significant type B toxicities including hypersensitivity (discussed now) and neurological and renal toxicities (discussed later in this chapter). Unfortunately, the incidence of hypersensitivity responses for carboplatin are approximately equivalent to that of cisplatin.

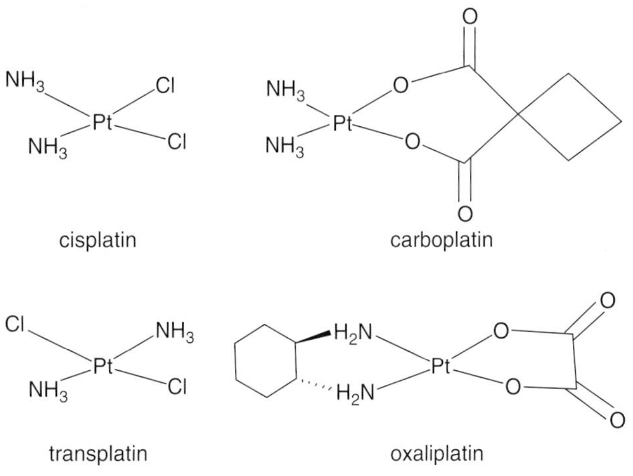

Figure 13.4 Chemical structures of platinum complexes.

Oxaliplatin was developed in an attempt to circumvent the problem of cisplatin resistance noted in patients treated with cisplatin who subsequently relapse and are retreated with cisplatin. This drug and the resistance to cisplatin are described in Chapter 15. Transplatin was included to demonstrate one of the primary structural requirements of the platinum complexes, that being that the stable ammines must be in the cis configuration. Ammines in the trans configuration, as in the case of transplatin, result in platinum complexes that lack antitumor activity.

Anaphylactic responses have been reported in 10 to 30% of patients treated with the platinum complexes. Symptoms, including facial edema, bronchoconstriction, hypotension, and tachycardia, occur within minutes of drug administration in patients previously exposed to the platinum complexes. The incidence of hypersensitivity increases with increasing courses of platinum therapy. There appears to be cross-reactivity among the platinum complexes in that patients reactive to cisplatin have a much higher incidence of hypersensitivity to carboplatin than do previously non-treated patients.

The severity of reactions ranges from mild pruritis and erythema to immediate life-threatening generalized anaphylaxis. Those patients with mild reactions most often are able to complete a given treatment schedule. Interestingly, patients treated intraperitoneally with the drug, most often used to treat metastatic ovarian cancer, seemed to develop platinum complex hypersensitivity far less frequently and with far less severity than patients treated intravenously with the same platinum complex. Once again showing that drug hypersensitivity can be depend on the route of drug administration. The explanation for this dependence on route of administration remains an enigma for most drugs but may be related to hypersensitivity to drug metabolites for some drugs as discussed previously in this chapter.

Epipodophyllotoxins The epipodophyllotoxins, VM-26 and VP-16, used in selected tumor types, are semisynthetic derivatives of the podophyllotoxin isolated from the Mayapple plant. Both drugs inhibit the enzyme topoisomerase II and block DNA replication in dividing tumor cells. Again, these drugs cause both type A ADRs such as marrow depression and type B ADRs such as hypersensitivity and possible hepatotoxicity.

Hypersensitivity responses occur shortly after rapid IV drug perfusion and include hypotension, fever, chills, urticaria, and bronchospasm. The fact that about a third of all reactions occur following the first exposure to the drug and that the severity of the responses is dose related suggest that this is not a true immune response to the drug but may be related to a drug-induced histamine release.

Given that the incidence and severity of these responses can by diminished dramatically by administering the drug via slow infusion over a period of 30 to 60 minutes rather than a one- or two-minute bolus injection has led to the hypothesis that the vehicle, cremophor, rather than the drug itself may be causing these responses. Factors arguing against this are that both drugs cause hypersensitive response yet only teniposide utilizes cremophor and second, teniposide formulated in a vehicle other than cremophor also induces the hypersensitivity.

Taxanes Taxanes are a class of anticancer drugs first isolated from the bark of the Yew tree. Subsequently semi-synthetic derivatives have been introduced and proved to be very important anticancer drugs. These drugs languished for quite some time until they were shown to be mechanistically distinct from the established anticancer drugs vincristine and vinblastine. The vincas prevent the polymerization of microtubules and thus prevent mitosis by inhibiting the segregation if chromosomes during the M-phase of the cell cycle. The taxanes, paclitaxel and docetaxel, prevent the depolymerization of microtubules and thus prevent the progression of cells through the M-phase of the cell cycle, albeit through a completely different effect on microtubular function.

Severe anaphylactic reactions occur in 2 to 4% of patients treated with these drugs. The symptoms are similar to those previously discussed and can range from minor discomfort to life-threatening crises. Patients with atopy have a higher incidence of hypersensitivity than the normal population of patients but the reaction to the taxanes does not appear to be IgE related. Experimental evidence supports the idea that these reactions are caused by drug-induced histamine release from basophils. Because of the potential severity of these reactions, all patients are pretreated with a steroid, an H1 blocker, and an H2 blocker within 60 minutes of drug administration. If a patient has had a hypersensitive response to paclitaxel yet needs further paclitaxel, the patient can either be desensitized to the drug or be treated with docetaxel. Desensitization appears quite effective but there are a limited number of clinical trials supporting this. Patients are usually not cross-reactive to these two taxane drugs.

13.6.5 Nonallergic Type B ADRs

A comprehensive discussion of all nonhypersensitive type B ADRs is beyond the scope of this chapter. Rather, we will discuss a limited number of toxicities as examples of the types of type B ADRs that can be encountered.

13.6.5.1 Myelosuppression

A type B ADR encountered with a number of drugs from varying classes of therapeutic agents is drug-induced myelosuppression. Although myelosuppression is an accepted type A ADR of cytotoxic chemotherapy, type B ADR class of myelosuppression is usually far more insidious and may occur up to several months following the last course of drug therapy.

Examples of type B ADR myelosuppression are shown in Table 13.4.

Table 13.4 Type B ADR Myelosuppression

Antimicrobials	Chloramphenical, sulfonamides, nitrofurantoin, Ziodvudine, quinacrine, amodiaquine, mepacrine, pyrimethamine, chloroquine, mebendazole
Antirheumatics	Gold, penicillamine, indomethacin, oxyphenbutazone, phenbutazone, piroxicam, sulfsalazine, diclofenac, suldinac, allopurinol
Antithyroid drugs	Carbimazole, thiamazole, thiouracils
Anticonvulsants	Phenytoin, carbamazepine, felbamate
Psychotropic drugs	Phenothiazines, dothiepin, clozapine, mianserin
Cardiovascular drugs	Methyldopa, captopril, lisinopril, ticlopidine
Other drugs	Tolbutamide, acetazolamide, interferon-alpha

13.6.5.2 Aplastic Anemia

Quinacrine is an antimalarial drug that has proven correlation between drug administration and aplastic anemia. Used widely as a prophylactic against malaria infection during WWII, enough patients were studied to provide statistical significance to clinical observations. Although the incidence of aplastic anemia was approximately one to two cases per 100,000 in soldiers stationed in the European theater, the incidence increased to two to 28 cases per 100,000 troops treated with quinacrine. The actual mechanism of aplastic anemia appears to be immunologically related as quinacrine appears to serve as a hapten that induces antibody production. Surprisingly this antibody is directed toward bone marrow stem cells and prevents normal bone function.

Chloramphenicol is a broad spectrum antibiotic that has direct effects on the bone marrow, probably related to the drug's inhibitory effects on the mitochondria. This reversible depression of marrow function is considered to be a type A ADR and is not the same toxicity as chloramphenicol-induced aplastic anemia. Chloramphenicol-induced aplastic anemia occurs weeks to months following drug treatment and does not appear to be related to dose or length of treatment. The oral route of administration most commonly is associated with the development of aplastic anemia, leading some investigators to speculate that a nitrosylated derivative formed by intestinal bacterial metabolism is the causative agent for aplastic anemia. This hypothesis has been supported recently by clinical studies with topically administered drug, particularly ocular use of the drug to treat conjunctivitis in which no increase in the incidence of aplastic anemia above control populations were observed. Although chloramphenicol does cause aplastic anemia the actual mechanism remains unknown.

13.6.5.3 Agranulocytosis

In addition to aplastic anemia, more bone marrow selective drug-induced hypoplasias have been reported. For example, clozapine-induced agranulocytosis occurs in approximately 1% of the patients receiving this drug. Clozapine is an important psychotropic drug used to treat schizophrenia. The major advantage of this drug is its low propensity to cause the extrapyramidal effects commonly associated with long-term use of earlier antipsychotics.

The mechanism of clozapine-induced agranulocytosis has been under intensive investigation but has yet to be conclusively identified. It appears likely that activation of clozapine, to norclozapine and/or a further metabolite, clozapine N-oxide, to electrophilic nitrenium ions is the initial step in the events leading to neutropenia/agranulocytosis. Oxidation of clozapine by neutrophil-generated hypochlorous acid (HOCl) via the NADPH oxidase/myeloperoxidase system has been demonstrated, which could then lead to granulocyte death.

Antineutrophil antibodies, possibly generated by reaction of nitrenium ions with neutrophil proteins resulting in hapten formation, may also be involved in the etiology of clozapine-induced neutropenia. There is likely to be an immune component since the reaction occurs more quickly and is more severe on rechallenge of patients who have developed clozapine-induced neutropenia.

It should be noted that other chemically related antipsychotic drugs such as olanzepine and quetiapine have the potential to undergo similar metabolic pathways and cause agranulocytosis, but the incidence of these ADRs is less than that of clozapine. Given the importance of clozapine in long-term management of patients it is possible that a patient could be rechallenged with the drug. In such cases, only about 60% of the patients will be able to continue clozapine following rechallenge. Switching to one of the less toxic drugs such as olanzepine may provide benefit, but once a patient has developed clozapine-induced neutropenia or agranaulocytosis, the risk of a repeat toxic event using a drug such as olanzapine appears to be significantly increased.

13.6.5.4 Sideroblastic Anemia

Sideroblastic anemia is characterized by a pattern of morphological marrow abnormalities in which there is an accumulation of perinuclear granules in nucleated red blood cell precursors. These granules, referred to as siderotic granules, are a result of disordered hemoglobin synthesis. The antitubercular drugs such as isoniazid and cycloserine can cause such dysplasias. The extent of damage is exacerbated in patients with underlying vitamin B6 deficiency.

Why isoniazid causes this type of anemia is not well understood but it is well established that the toxic effects of long-term isoniazid therapy of tuberculosis can be significantly diminished by coadministration of Vitamin B6. This is somewhat surprising since the primary anti-TB mechanism of action for isoniazid appears to be the inhibition of mycolic acid, an important substituent in Mycobacteria cell walls, which is not Vitamin B6 dependent. However, Vitamin B6 does play an important role in heme synthesis. Since the administration of Vitamin B6 with isoniazid can reverse the formation of sideroblastic anemia it seems likely that isoniazid affects Vitamin B6 in a number of important metabolic pathways.

13.6.6 Idiosyncratic Hepatotoxicity

This form of type B ADR is again difficult to study as it is a rare event and it is human specific. This type of toxicity results from a series of multiple discrete events that eventually is expressed as hepatoxicity. The key determinant events are the chemical in question, type and length of exposure, and environmental and genetic factors. The chemical properties critical to idiosyncratic drug toxicity are identified via a review of the common properties of drugs that cause idiosyncratic liver toxicity. These properties include:

- Formation of reactive metabolites
- Metabolism by P450 isoforms
- Preponderance of P450 inducers
- Occurrence of clinically significant pharmacokinetic interactions with coadministered drugs

Although idiosyncratic hepatotoxicity is a relatively rare event, a number of drugs have the potential of inducing such a toxicity (Table 13.5).

As can be seen from Table 13.5, a number of drugs used to treat a wide variety of diseases are included. Recognize that other drugs can also affect liver function in an idiosyncratic manner; the drugs listed in Table 13.5 are but examples of drugs with the greatest potential of inducing idiosyncratic hepatotoxicity. Again, discussion of each of these drugs is beyond the scope of this chapter. Rather, we will discus diclofenac as a representative of drugs capable of inducing idiosyncratic hepatotoxicity.

Of the drugs listed, 25 are capable of undergoing hepatic metabolism, generating reactive metabolites that can form protein adducts. The enzymes responsible for these metabolic processes are primarily cytochrome P450 isoforms and the UDP glucuronosyltransferase isoforms. It is possible that the adducted proteins could serve as neoantigens leading to autoimmune diseases of the liver. Of the drugs listed in Table 13.5, 15 can induce the cytochrome P450 enzymes. Although there is no evidence as yet that enzyme induction can lead to hepatotoxicity, enzyme induction does cause altered gene expression. As toxicogenomics, the study of gene expression and toxicity, increases as a research tool, the role of enzyme induction in drug toxicity may become better understood. In its most simplistic terms it is not unreasonable to hypothesize that the induction of these metabolic enzymes leads to more reactive metabolites and hence increased neoantigen formation.

An interesting correlation between drug and dose is noted from Table 13.5. Most of the drugs listed in that table could be thought of as high-dose drugs administered according to prolonged regimens. This continued exposure to high levels of drug and metabolites could enhance the likelihood of hepatotoxicity. Perhaps the development of low-dose drug equivalents may lower the risk of idiosyncratic hepatotoxicities.

13.6.6.1 Diclofenac as a Model of Idiosyncratic Hepatotoxicity

Diclofenac is an NSAID widely used in the treatment of rheumatoid diseases such as osteoarthritis, rheumatoid

Table 13.5 Drugs Known To Be Associated with Idiosyncratic Hepatotoxicity

Drug	Purpose
Acetaminophen	Antipyretic analgesic
Alpidem	Antianxiety
Amineptine	Antidepressant
Amodiaquine	Antimalarial
Bromfenac	Analgesic
Carbamazepine	Anticonvulsant
Combination	Anti-HIV therapy
Cyproterone acetate	Androgen antagonist
Diclofenac	NSAID
Dideoxyinosine	Anti-HIV
Dihydralazine	Antihypertensive
Ebrotidine	H2-receptor antagonist
Enalapril	Antihypertension
Felbamate	Antiepileptic
Flutamide	Nonsteroidal antiandrogen
Halothane	Anesthetic
Isoniazid	Anticonvulsant 300
Ketoconazole	Antifungal
Methotrexate	Anticancer/antipsoriatic
Methoxyflurane	Anesthetic
Minocycline	Antibiotic
Nefazodone	Antidepressant
Phenobarbital	Anticonvulsant
Phenprocoumon	Anticoagulant
Phenytoin	Antiepileptic
Procainamide	Antiarrhythmic
Pyrazinamide	Antibacterial
Rifampicin	Antimicrobial
Salicylate	Analgesic
Sulfasalazine	Crohn's disease
Tacrine	Alzheimer's disease
Tienilic acid	Diuretic
Troglitazone	Diabetes
Valproate	Anticonvulsant

arthritis, and alkylosing spondylitis. Although the incidence of idiosyncratic hepatotoxicity is rare on a per patient basis, given the large numbers of patients being treated with the drug the absolute number of patients developing this toxicity is quite impressive. Obtaining exact numbers of patients developing this toxicity is very difficult as there is significant underreporting, a problem addressed earlier in the chapter.

The symptomatology of this toxicity is similar to other idiosyncratic drug toxicities in that the onset is delayed, usually after four to six weeks of treatment and may be accompanied by rashes, fever, and/or eosinophilia. Further, blood tests reveal that alterations in serum enzymes such as aminotranserase rise slightly and remain elevated in about 25% of the patients developing this toxicity. Taken together diclofenac-induced idiosyncratic hepatotoxicity is not an acute toxicity but appears to be a result of multiple insults that once a threshold level of damage is reached liver toxicity occurs rapidly primarily to the hepatobiliary region of the liver.

Diclofenac is extensively metabolized by the cytochrome P450 3A4 and 2C8 isoforms to generate reactive metabolites capable of interacting with protein and nonprotein –SH groups.

Diclofenac can also undergo glucuronidation to form diclofenac 1-acyl-glucuronide, which then attacks nucleophilic sites on proteins to form yet another class of protein adducts. These adducts could result in the formation of neoantigens, thus inducing an autoimmunity as described earlier, or in fact could inhibit the CYP enzymes and enhance significantly the risk of drug–drug interactions. Yet another potential role for diclofenac metabolism in idiosyncratic hepatotoxicity is the generation of free radicals during drug metabolism and the subsequent effect of these free radicals on

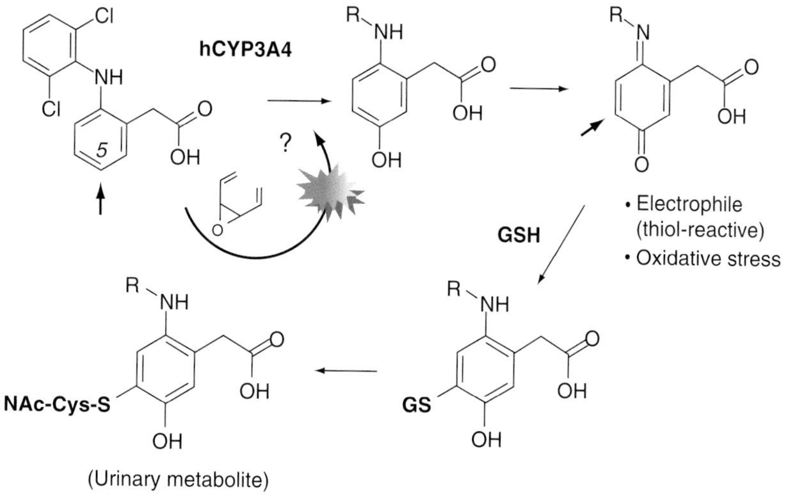

Figure 13.5 Liver metabolism of diclofenac.

mitochondrial function. This latter hypothesis is supported by experimental data demonstrating that diclofenac can decrease ATP production by 20 to 40%. Further, drug-induced ROS have been reported to alter mitochondrial membrane function in other ways such as elimination of the inner transmembrane potential.

Although much has been learned regarding this toxicity much still remains unknown. We do not understand the role of the genetic makeup of the patient, the role of the environment regarding sensitivity of this toxicity, nor the actual mechanism of the toxicity. Until the mechanism of toxicity and relevant factors affecting susceptibility to the toxicity are known, prevention of the toxicity will remain on an individual basis. Again, the role of genotoxicity and pharmacogenomics could very well play a pivotal role in unraveling this and many other idiosyncratic toxicities.

13.6.7 Idiosyncratic Cardiotoxicity

The list of drugs known to cause idiosyncratic cardiotoxicity is significantly smaller than that of drugs known to cause idiosyncratic hepatotoxicity. The reason for this may rest in the fact that many drug metabolites are responsible for the unexpected toxicities, and the liver is the primary site of drug metabolism. Thus the concentration of these reactive metabolites is highest in the liver. Be that as it may, the list in Table 13.6 clearly demonstrates that a number of noncardiac drugs are capable of inducing or worsening cardiomyopathies. Note that there are at least four major ways in which drugs cause this type of type B ADR.

Table 13.6 Noncardiac Drugs Known to Induce or Worsen Heart Damage

Cardiomyopathy	
Cytotoxic drugs	Doxorubicin, epirubicin, and other anthracyclines, mitoxantrone, cyclophosphamide, 5-fluorouracil, capecitabine, gleevec, sunitinib
Immunomodulating drugs/antibodies	Trastuzumab, interferon-α-2, interleukin-2, infliximab, etanercept
Antifungal drugs	Itraconazole, amphotericin B
Antipsychotic drugs	Clozapine
Pulmonary Hypertension	
Antimigraine drugs	Methysergide, ergotamine
Appetite suppressants	Fenfluramine, dexfenfluramine, phentermine
Heart-valve Abnormalities	
Antimigraine drugs	Methysergide, ergotamine
Appetite suppressants	Fenfluramine, dexfenfluramine, phentermine
Antiparkinsonian drugs	Pergolide
Fluid Overload	
NSAIDs	All
Antidiabetic drugs	Rosiglitazone, pioglitazone, troglitazone
Glucocorticoids	All

13.6.7.1 Anthracycline Cardiotoxicity

The anthracyclines have been by far the most studied of all cardiotoxic drugs and doxorubicin is by far the most studied of the anthracyclines. Doxorubicin is a microbial derived natural product that has proven clinical activity in a wide array of tumors. The mechanism of action ascribed to this drug is the inhibition of topoisomerase II following DNA intercalation, thus interfering with cell division. Not surprisingly this drug causes reversible marrow suppression and GI disturbances. However, once entered into the clinic a disturbing pattern of cardiotoxicity was observed in cancer patients.

These toxicities are not related to the mechanism of antitumor activity and in point of fact are not completely understood. What is known is that patients treated with doxorubicin can display an acute type of cardiac alteration and/or a chronic type of cardiac toxicity. The acute toxicities are most often expressed as myocardial arrhythmias and decreased left ventricular ejection fraction. Both effects are reversible once drug administration stops and are not considered to be a reason to discontinue the use of doxorubicin. Whether there is a correlation between these acute events and subsequent chronic cardiac toxicity is not known since individuals who never displayed acute toxicities ultimately developed chronic toxicities including fatal congestive heart failure. A reversible and nontreatment-limiting pericarditis is also observed within weeks of doxorubicin administration.

The most severe cardiotoxic effect of doxorubicin is chronic and dose-related cardiomyopathy. Because of the progressive nature of this toxicity is it recommended that no patient receive a cumulative dose of drug exceeding 450 to 550 mg/m^2. Once this total dose is reached the risk of drug-induced digitalis nonresponsive congestive heart failure (with a fatality rate approaching 50%) becomes too great and further treatment with doxorubicin is ceased. Morphological changes include loss of mitochondrial structure integrity, loss of myofibrils, and altered cellular shapes all detected by electron microscopy. At present a great deal of effort is being placed on developing noninvasive clinical methods such as echocardiograms and radionuclide cineographic techniques to predict the development of these cardiomyopathies.

Given the importance of this drug, if the toxicity could be prevented the patient could receive the benefit of this drug for longer periods of time. A number of chemical analogs have been tested either preclinically or clinically but unfortunately no approved drug has proven to be a significant step forward in diminishing this dangerous ADR. Liposome encapsulation of doxorubicin appears to decrease the cardiac toxicity of doxorubicin but it is still early to state confidently that this approach has obviated the concern of doxorubicin-induced cardiac toxicity.

The exact mechanism of doxorubicin-induced cardiomyopathy remains unknown but there is a considerable body of evidence supporting the hypothesis that doxorubicin-induced free radicals may play an important role. The current working hypothesis is that the drug is distributed to tissues throughout the body. The drug can generate reactive oxygen species (ROS) through redox recycling of the drug. Further, doxorubicin can bind iron and deliver the iron to DNA through intercalation, and this iron can undergo its own redox recycling further generating ROS. Both pathways are shown in Figure 13.6.

Why is the heart selectively damaged if the drug is distributed widely in the body? Studies have clearly demonstrated that the heart is far less capable of protecting itself from ROS than are other tissues in the body and is therefore far more sensitive to drug-induced ROS. This sensitivity of heart tissue to drug-induced ROS is substantiated through a number of experimental studies. First, at least in nonclinical studies, antioxidants such as cytochrome Q10, vitamin E, and the flavinoids have protected the heart for some of doxorubicin-induced cardiotoxicity. One free-radical scavenger, dexrazoxane, has been shown clinically to reduce the cardiotoxic risk of doxorubicin and is currently undergoing broad clinical testing to establish its efficacy.

In summary, doxorubicin, an important anticancer drug, causes a dose-limiting toxicity to an organ that we would not predict to be a target for toxicity with this drug. The mechanism of toxicity is different from the mechanism of antitumor activity, and this toxicity was totally unexpected. Although the toxicity is fairly common in cancer patients, it does not truly fit into the type A ADR and is therefore included in the type B ADR.

13.6.7.2 NSAIDs and Cardiotoxicity

Another unexpected cardiotoxicity following drug administration is the increased risk of myocardial infarction in patients taking one of the COX-2 (cyclooxygenase-2) selective NSAIDs for rheumatoid arthritis. NSAIDs have been a long-standing class of drugs to help treat inflammation, pain, and fevers. Until recently, all NSAIDs inhibited both COX-1 and COX-2. A problem with these drugs is the potential for GI complications, including gastric mucosal ulceration, hemorrhage, or perforation. The mechanism of this toxicity is most commonly ascribed to the inhibition of COX-1, which has an important role in the production of prostaglandins needed to provide GI protection. Thus the search for a COX-2 selective NSAID was a major undertaking for the pharmaceutical industry.

Several years ago a new family of NSAIDs, the coxibs, were developed and were the desired COX-2 selective drugs. This class of drugs has been discussed previously but in this section we focus on the perplexing problem of NSAID-induced myocardial damage. Clinical trials have demonstrated that these new drugs provide equivalent analgesic and anti-inflammatory effect but with fewer GI complications. However, recent studies have reported an association been coxib use and increased cardiovascular disease. This association is strongest between rofecoxib and cardiovascular disease. When administered 50 mg/day for nine months and comparing the results to patients receiving 500 mg naproxen (a nonselective COX inhibitor) for nine months, a higher incidence of myocardial infarction was noted in the rofecoxib group.

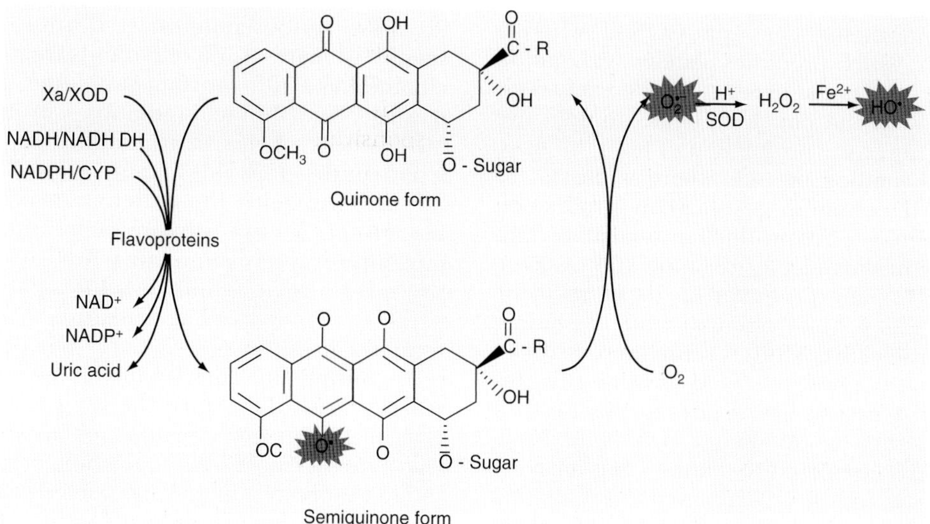

Figure 13.6 Redox cycling of doxorubicin.

Initially this increased risk of myocardial infarction was attributed to the myocardial protective properties of the nonselective COX inhibitors. COX-2 selective inhibitors may lack this protective capability. Later meta analysis suggested that the degree of myoprotection associated with naproxen could not account for the difference in the incidence of myocardial infarction. Merck, the maker of rofecoxib, withdrew the drug from the market because of this association. The other two coxibs, celecoxib and lumiracoxib, remain on the market as no similar increase in myocardial infarction has been associated with these drugs. It must be stated here that there is controversy regarding this issue and only time will provide the ultimate answer regarding the cardiotoxic potential of these two coxibs.

Another potential use for these drugs was to prevent the formation of adenomatous polyps in patients with a history of colorectal adenomas. Rofecoxib and celecoxib were both tested in this disease. It was the results of this test that prompted Merck to withdraw their drug from the market since this study clearly established the increased risk of cardiovascular events when rofecoxib is used. The results were sufficiently strong to have the safety monitoring board reevaluate the data for a similar trial with celecoxib. On the basis of these data the study with celecoxib was also terminated. Interestingly, another study in which celecoxib was used to prevent polyp formation resulted in no increase in cardiovascular events. The only difference between the two studies was that in the latter case celecoxib was given once a day whereas in the prior study celecoxib was administered at the same dose but twice a day. How this difference in treatment schedules affected the toxic outcomes is unknown at the present time.

Why these drugs apparently increase the risk of cardiovascular problems in patients remains unknown. One interesting hypothesis rests on the fact that COX-1 and COX-2 both metabolize arachadonic acid to protanoinds, protacyclins, and thromboxane A2. Prostacyclins help prevent platelet aggregation and induce vasodilation and are produced primarily in the vascular endothelial cells via COX-2, whereas thromboxane A2, which promotes platelet aggregation and vasoconstriction, is the product almost exclusively of COX-1 activity in the platelets. Thus, nonselective COX inhibitors lower the production of both the prostacyclins and thromboxane A2, whereas the COX-2 selective NSAID diminish prostacyclin production but leave thromboxane A2 production unabated. This imbalance promotes platelet aggregation and vasoconstriction. There remain a number of questions to be answered regarding this phenomenon including whether the nonselective NSAIDs cause increased cardiovascular problems, how the NSAIDs cause this toxicity, what the risk factors are regarding this toxicity, and whether there is a therapeutic benefit in using one type of NSAID compared to another. It is amazing given the extensive use of NSAIDs over the years that such toxicities are now being considered and so many questions remain. But of course that is the nature of the beast when evaluating type B ADRs.

13.6.8 Idiosyncratic Pulmonary Damage

The number of drugs with a demonstrated propensity to cause an idiosyncratic lung disease are far fewer than either hepatotoxicity or cardiotoxicity. One such drug is yet another anticancer drug called bleomycin. This drug is a natural product of microbial origin that intercalates DNA and causes DNA damage through free-radical generation. There are two important regions to this molecule, shown in Figure 13.7.

A metal binding site is on left-hand side of the molecule and a spermidine tail on the right-hand side of the molecule. The metal binding site traps the metal (iron or cobalt have been the two commonly cited metals) and provides the ROS generation site for the molecule. The spermidine tail enables the drug to interact with DNA through intercalation and delivers the metal to the DNA to maximize ROS-induced DNA damage. Loss of either portion of the molecule results in complete loss of antitumor activity.

As with doxorubicin we might ask why the lung is particularly affected when the drug is distributed throughout the body. Further, if bleomycin kills cells through ROS production then why isn't a significant amount of cardiotoxicity seen in patients treated with bleomycin since we just established that doxorubicin-induced cardiotoxicity results from insufficient ROS protection in the heart? The reason rests in the fact that most tissues are endowed with an enzyme bleomycin hydrolase, which forms a metabolite lacking the metal binding site and the loss of ROS production. In contrast, the lung lacks sufficient quantities of the enzyme to protect it from ROS damage. Thus, the duration of exposure to the ROS producing bleomycin is significantly longer than it is in almost any other tissue in the body. Interestingly, another organ with limiting amounts of the enzyme is the skin, which is also susceptible to bleomycin-induced ROS damage.

Bleomycin-induced lung damage begins as a pneumonitis that can either be resolved or progress to a far more serious pulmonary fibrosis. This toxicity is seen in as many as 5% of patients treated with bleomycin and has a 10% mortality rate. Age, underlying lung damage, and thoracic radiation can increase the risk and severity of this treatment-limiting toxicity. Once a patient develops this toxicity, regardless of the severity of the toxicity, the patient can no longer receive bleomycin. Unlike doxorubicin-induced cardiotoxicity, there is no cumulative toxicity and therefore there is no total cumulative dose that can be used to predict an increasing likelihood of pulmonary toxicity.

Including this toxicity in the area of idiosyncratic toxicity is justified since the lung is not thought of a typical target for cytotoxic chemotherapy. Rather, the toxicity results from an unexpected organ differential that results in an unexpected but not rare toxicity. Further, there are few indicators that will provide insight into if and when this toxicity will be encountered.

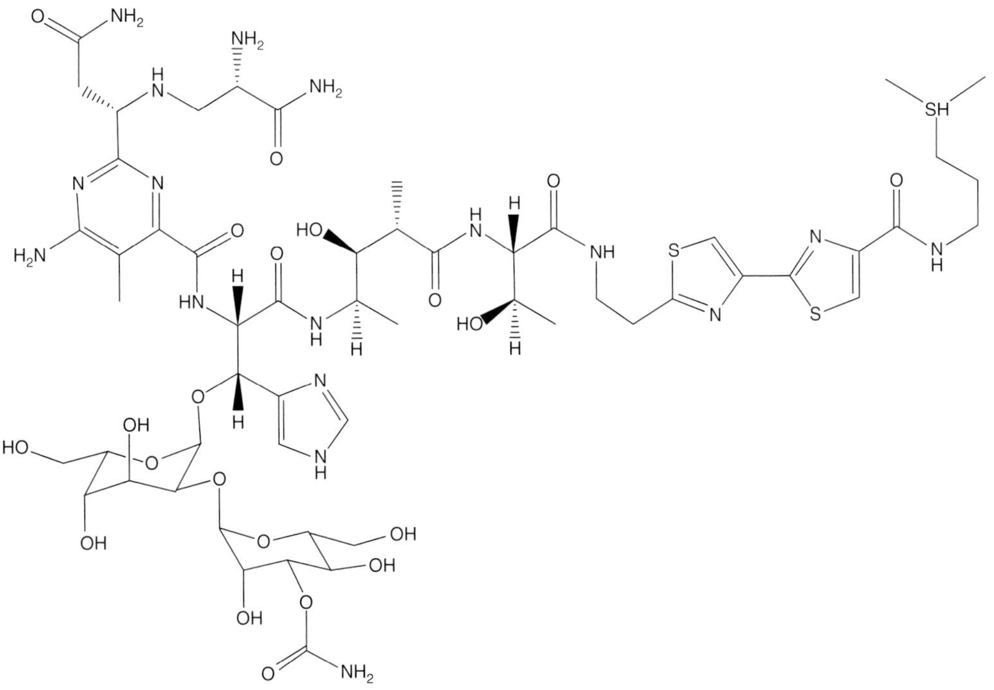

Bleomycin

Figure 13.7 Chemical structure of bleomycin.

13.6.9 Idiosyncratic Renal Toxicity

To address this organ-directed idiosyncratic toxicity we will highlight two drugs, cisplatin and streptomycin, which are chemically distinct (see structure in Figure 13.8) yet have an intriguing similarity of spectrum of activities.

13.6.9.1 Cisplatin-induced Renal Toxicity

Cisplatin, as described earlier, is a heavy metal-based anticancer drug with absolutely no chemical features, mechanism of action, or spectrum of activity in common with streptomycin, yet both drugs cause loss of hearing, peripheral neuropathies, and renal toxicities.

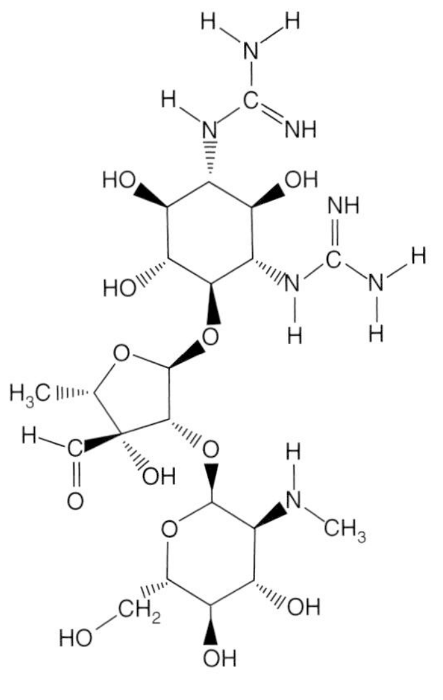

Figure 13.8 Chemical structure of streptomycin.

Approximately 25% of patients treated with cisplatin would develop a renal toxicity primarily of the proximal convoluted tubules when cisplatin was first used clinically. As with doxorubicin and bleomycin, once a patient developed tubular nephritis, no further cisplatin could be administered, regardless of the responsiveness of the tumor to cisplatin. The toxicity is associated with hypomagnesemia, loss of urinary concentration, loss of electrolyte control, and proteinuria. Cisplatin administration is associated with increases in creatinine and BUN levels, two indicators of renal toxicity. In addition, histopathology revealed that the damage was primarily to the epithelial cells lining the tubules and included mitochondrial damage, nuclear damage, and major alterations of epithelial morphology. Although many of these drug-induced changes in renal morphology and function are apparently reversible, a patient remains much more susceptible to platinum toxicity.

The toxicity is thought to be related to other heavy metal renal toxicity. In spite of the clinical importance and the relative frequency of this toxicity the mechanism of the toxicity remains unknown. A number of hypotheses have been put forward including altered mitochondrial function, activation of cisplatin, and inappropriate cellular binding, concentration of the heavy metal in the kidney, induction of apoptosis in tubular epithelial cells, but as yet no clear-cut mechanism has been identified.

In spite of the lack of understanding of the mechanism of toxicity, treatment regimens have been developed that have diminished renal toxicity associated with cisplatin. Briefly, patients are infused with hypertonic saline solutions prior to administration and hydration and elevated urine output maintained during cisplatin administration. The mechanism of protection is not completely understood but it is believed that the hypertonic saline slows the activation of cispatin in the renal tubules, which lowers inappropriate cellular binding. The increased urine output is thought to lower cisplatin accumulation in the kidneys. Whatever the mechanism, cisplatin-induced nephrotoxicity has decreased significantly following the introduction of this protective clinical protocol.

More recently, the clinical introduction of the cisplatin analog, carboplatin, appears to be far less renal damaging that its precursor yet maintains equivalent antitumor activity. Why this is so is under investigation. Encouraging data further demonstrate that this newer platinum anticancer drug is far less nauseating and far less neurotoxic than cisplatin. This is very important since cisplatin is considered to be the most nauseating drug ever given to humans. Further, continued therapy with cisplatin results in an ever-increasing likelihood of a potentially significant and even paralyzing neurotoxicity.

This story of the development of carboplatin in an attempt to develop a less toxic platinum-based drug demonstrates clearly the importance of continued drug development. Remember that one of the most important considerations in the use of a drug is its therapeutic index and risk versus benefit. The smaller the TI the greater the risk of using a given drug. When treating a headache or common cold, we would not accept a high risk since the benefit is low. In contrast when treating cancer, we accept a much higher risk since the potential benefit is much greater. In spite of this, the development of a drug with an increased TI is the goal of even anticancer drug discovery. We can increase the TI of a drug by increasing efficacy, decreasing toxicity, or both. Carboplatin is an improved drug because it has a lowered toxicity potential and can be used much more safely than cisplatin. We must keep this concept in mind when involved in drug discovery; improvements come not only from developing a more active analog but also by developing a less toxic analog.

13.6.9.2 Streptomycin-induced Renal Toxicity

The class of antibiotics called the aminoglycosides, of which streptomycin is a member, was an important addition to our arsenal of drugs to treat infectious diseases. First used to treat TB, the drugs soon expanded in importance and spectrum of activity. The use of these drugs has decreased dramatically in the Western nations as they have been replaced by safer and more effective drugs. Worldwide, however, the use of aminoglycosides remains important because these drugs are relatively inexpensive when compared to many of the newer less toxic antibiotics.

This continued use of the aminoglycosides warrants a discussion of the toxicities associated with their use. Surprisingly, many of the toxicities of the aminoglycosides are similar to those ascribed to cisplatin, that being nephrotoxicity, neurotoxicity, and hearing loss. Why these two disparate classes of drugs cause similar toxicities is unknown.

After only a few days of administration, streptomycin induces characteristic changes in lysosomes of proximal tubular cells consistent with the accumulation of polar lipids (myeloid bodies). These changes are preceded and accompanied by signs of tubular dysfunctions or alterations (release of brush-border and lysosomal enzymes; decreased reabsorption of filtered proteins; wasting of K^+, Mg^{2+}, Ca^{2+}, and glucose; phospholipiduria; and cast excretion). In humans, the occurrence of these signs may be followed by the development of overt renal failure characterized mainly by a nonoliguric and even often polyuric hypoosmotic fall in creatinine clearance. Progression to oliguric or anuric renal failure is infrequent, and recovery upon drug discontinuation is most often observed. Occasionally, a Fanconi's syndrome or a Bartter's-like syndrome has been observed. A correlation between the development of these clinical signs and the severity or rate of progression of the subclinical alterations remains difficult to establish, mainly because of large interpatient variations. Consequently, the usefulness of monitoring the subclinical changes to detect individuals at risk has remained questionable. In animals, tubular alterations have clearly been associated with the development of focal necroses and apoptoses in the tubular epithelium, together with an extensive tubular and peritubular cell proliferation, without an apparent change in kidney function.

As with platinum complexes a great deal of effort has gone into preventing this toxicity. Streptomycin is concentrated in lysosomes and Golgi bodies. Decreasing or preventing streptomycin accumulation by the kidneys would represent one of the most simple approaches to reduce streptomycin-induced nephrotoxicity. Streptomycin accumulation could be reduced either by impairing drug uptake or by enhancing its excretion. Two strategies have been used to reduce drug uptake: (1) to complex the drug extracellularly, and (2) to compete with or decrease drug binding to the brush-border membrane. Unfortunately, these approaches could not be translated into clinical applications because of a lack of efficacy and/or because of intrinsic toxicity. Another approach has been to develop ways to minimize lysosomal concentration of the drug either by the use of lysosomotropic drugs or by structural modification of the aminoglycoside to lower lysosomic trapping. Again, neither approach has met with significant clinical success.

Significant effort has been expended in an attempt to develop less toxic analogs of the initial aminoglycosides with the focus on two properties of the aminoglycosides. The first was described earlier—lowered potential to accumulation on the lysosomes. At present it must be concluded that this approach has met with some success but not significant success. A lowered nephrotoxic potential of such drugs has been reported but the impact has been relatively small in clinical trials. The other approach has been to develop drugs with less ability to bind renal phospholipids, a proposed mechanism of streptomycin nephrotoxicity. Several compounds have undergone clinical trials but unfortunately none has shown to be a breakthrough drug. Thus, the search goes on to prevent or at least decrease the nephrotoxic potential of the aminoglycosides. Unfortunately, this search has not met with the same success as the platinum story. Given the importance of these drugs this search will continue and hopefully someday the efforts will bear fruit for this important class of drugs.

13.7 SUMMARY

In summary, ADRs remain a very significant problem in pharmacology. It seems as though every day a new problem is identified that has raised concerns about the safety of drugs that we take. As discussed in this chapter there are a number reasons why this is so. With type A ADRs the concern is that during the development of the drug, both preclinical and clinical, we must maintain a rigorous pharmacovigilance to insure these toxicities are identified early to limit the risk of untoward effects in large numbers of individuals taking the drug. Careful reporting, recording, and analyses of all type A ADRs must occur. These toxicities are far more predictable than type B ADRs, and it is incumbent upon our health delivery system to prevent or at least minimize the incidence of these effects. Type B ADRs are far more difficult to predict and prevent because they are rare and/or idiosyncratic in nature. The identification of these types of toxicities rely even more heavily on careful observations and record keeping. As can be seen from the examples presented in this chapter, ADRs represent a significant problem in pharmacology but also provide a vast array of research opportunities for the experimentalist.

REVIEW QUESTIONS

1. Discuss the differences between type A and type B ADRs.
2. What is pharmacovigilance?
3. Discuss potential difficulties in identifying ADRs and assuring that these ADRs in fact are related to the drug under testing.
4. A drug that is being developed to lower blood pressure is in Phase 1 clinical trials. While the subject is taking the drug, a calcium channel blocker, you note the following symptoms: decreased cardiac output, significant vasodilation, and a weakening of skeletal muscle strength. In addition as the study is continued a worrisome elevation of SGPT and SGOT are noted. Which of these would you ascribe to type A and which to type B ADRs? Defend your decisions.
5. Why is it that a drug may progress to postmarketing clinical trials before certain toxicities are identified?
6. What is the difference between a hypersensitivity response and a hypersensitive individual?
7. What is the therapeutic index and how does it come into play in the drug discovery process? Weave the concept of risk versus benefit in your answer.
8. How might drug metabolism play a role in both type A and type B ADRs? How might pharmacogenomics come to play a role in this process?
9. What is the concept of a rechallenge in a hypersensitive patient? What are potential risks involved in such a process?
10. Discuss how a small molecular weight molecule such as a typical drug induce an immunological response.
11. How might a drug induce a hypersensitive response without induced IgE antibody production? What role could IgE play in a hypersensitive response?

REFERENCES

Aagaard, L., Soendergaard, B., Stenver, D. I., & Hansen, E. H. (2008 Mar). Knowledge creation about ADRs—Turning the perspective from the rear mirror to the projector? *British Journal of Clinical Pharmacology, 65*(3), 364–376.

Agbabiaka, T. B., Savović, J., & Ernst, E. (2008). Methods for causality assessment of adverse drug reactions: A systematic review. *Drug Safety: An International Journal of Medical Toxicology and Drug Experience, 31*(1), 21–37.

Aithal, G. P., & Day, C. P. (2007 Aug). Nonsteroidal anti-inflammatory drug-induced hepatotoxicity. *Clinics in Liver Disease, 11*(3), 563–575.

Almenoff, J. S. (2007). Innovations for the future of pharmacovigilance. *Drug Safety: An International Journal of Medical Toxicology and Drug Experience, 30*(7), 631–633

Almenoff, J. S., Pattishall, E. N., Gibbs, T. G., DuMouchel, W., Evans, S. J., & Yuen, N. (2007 Aug). Novel statistical tools for monitoring the safety of marketed drugs. *Clinical Pharmacology and Therapeutics, 82*(2), 157–166.

Alugupalli, K. R. (2008). A distinct role for B1b lymphocytes in T cell-independent immunity. *Current Topics in Microbiology and Immunology, 319*, 105–130.

Andrade, R. J., Robles, M., Fernández-Castañer, A., López-Ortega, S., López-Vega, M. C., & Lucena, M. I. (2007 Jan 21). Assessment of drug-induced hepatotoxicity in clinical practice: A challenge for gastroenterologists. *World Journal of Gastroenterology: WJG, 13*(3), 329–340.

Arany, I., & Safirstein, R. L. (2003 Sep). Cisplatin nephrotoxicity. *Seminars in Nephrology, 23*(5), 460–464.

Arber, N., Eagle, C. J., Spicak, J., Rácz, I., Dite, P., Hajer, J., Zavoral, M., Lechuga, M. J., Gerletti, P., Tang, J., et al. (2006 Aug 31). Celecoxib for the prevention of colorectal adenomatous polyps. *The New England Journal of Medicine, 355*(9), 885–895.

Aronson, J. K., Derry, S., & Loke, Y. K. (2002 Feb). Adverse drug reactions: Keeping up to date. *Fundamental & Clinical Pharmacology, 16*(1), 49–56.

Aronson, J. K., & Ferner, R. E. (2005). Clarification of terminology in drug safety. *Drug Safety: An International Journal of Medical Toxicology and Drug Experience, 28*(10), 851–870.

Atuah, K. N., Hughes, D., & Pirmohamed, M. (2004). Clinical pharmacology: Special safety considerations in drug development and pharmacovigilance. *Drug Safety: An International Journal of Medical Toxicology and Drug Experience, 27*(8), 535–554.

Averbeck, M., Gebhardt, C., Emmrich, F., Treudler, R., & Simon, J. C. (2007 Nov). Immunologic principles of allergic disease. *Journal der Deutschen Dermatologischen Gesellschaft = Journal of the German Society of Dermatology: JDDG, 5*(11), 1015–1028.

Azambuja, E., Fleck, J. F., Batista, R. G., & Menna Barreto, S. S. (2005). Bleomycin lung toxicity: Who are the patients with increased risk? *Pulmonary Pharmacology & Therapeutics, 18*(5), 363–366.

Baliga, R., Ueda, N., Walker, P. D., & Shah, S. V. (1999 Nov). Oxidant mechanisms in toxic acute renal failure. *Drug Metabolism Reviews, 31*(4), 971–997.

Bennett, C. L., Nebeker, J. R., Lyons, E. A., Samore, M. H., Feldman, M. D., McKoy, J. M., et al. (2005 May 4). The Research on Adverse Drug Events and Reports (RADAR) project. *JAMA: The Journal of the American Medical Association, 293*(17), 2131–2140.

Berthiaume, J. M., & Wallace, K. B. (2007 Jan). Adriamycin-induced oxidative mitochondrial cardiotoxicity. *Cell Biology and Toxicology, 23*(1), 15–25.

Biro, L., & Leone, N. (1965 Nov). Aplastic anemia induced by quinacrine. *Archives of Dermatology, 92*(5), 574.

Brockow, K., & Romano, A. (2008). Skin tests in the diagnosis of drug hypersensitivity reactions. *Current Pharmaceutical Design, 14* (27), 2778–2791.

Brown, E. G. (2003). Methods and pitfalls in searching drug safety databases utilizing the Medical Dictionary for Regulatory Activities (MedDRA). *Drug Safety: An International Journal of Medical Toxicology and Drug Experience, 26*(3), 145–158.

Brown, J. S., Kulldorff, M., Chan, K. A., Davis, R. L., Graham, D., Pettus, P. T., et al. (2007 Dec). Early detection of adverse drug events within population-based health networks: application of sequential testing methods. *Pharmacoepidemiology and Drug Safety, 16*(12), 1275–1284.

Bryson, E. O., Frost, E. A., & Rosenblatt, M. A. (2007 Oct). Management of the patient reporting an allergy to penicillin. *Middle East Journal of Anesthesiology, 19*(3), 495–512.

Buchanan, F. G., Holla, V., Katkuri, S., Matta, P., & DuBois, R. N. (2007 Oct 1). Targeting cyclooxygenase-2 and the epidermal growth factor receptor for the prevention and treatment of intestinal cancer. *Cancer Research, 67*(19), 9380–9388.

Buchmiller, B. L., & Khan, D. A. (2007 Nov). Evaluation and management of pediatric drug allergic reactions. *Current Allergy and Asthma Reports, 7*(6), 402–409.

Cavani, A., & De Pità, O. (2006 Feb). The role of T cells in drug reaction. *Current Allergy and Asthma Reports, 6*(1), 20–24.

Clark, R. C., Maxwell, S. R., Kerr, S., Cuthbert, M., Buchanan, D., Steinke, D., et al. (2007). The influence of primary care prescribing rates for new drugs on spontaneous reporting of adverse drug reactions. *Drug Safety: An International Journal of Medical Toxicology and Drug Experience, 30*(4), 357–366.

Cresswell, K. M., Fernando, B., McKinstry, B., & Sheikh, A. (2007). Adverse drug events in the elderly. *British Medical Bulletin, 83*, 259–274.

Demiroglu, H., & Dündar, S. (1997 Jan-Feb). Vitamin B6 responsive sideroblastic anaemia in a patient with tuberculosis. *The British Journal of Clinical Practice, 51*(1), 51–52.

Demoly, P., Pichler, W., Pirmohamed, M., & Romano, A. (2008 May). Important questions in Allergy: 1—Drug allergy/hypersensitivity. *Allergy, 63*(5), 616–619.

Etminan, M., Carleton, B., & Rochon, P. A. (2004). Quantifying adverse drug events: Are systematic reviews the answer? *Drug Safety: An International Journal of Medical Toxicology and Drug Experience, 27*(11), 757–761.

Fanikos, J., Cina, J. L., Baroletti, S., Fiumara, K., Matta, L., & Goldhaber, S. Z. (2007 Nov 1). Adverse drug events in hospitalized cardiac patients. *The American Journal of Cardiology , 100*(9), 1465–1469.

Fietta, P. (2007 May-Aug). Life-or-death fate in the adaptive immune system. *Rivista di Biologia, 100*(2), 267–283.

Gell, P. G. H., & Coombs, R. R. A. (Eds.). (1963). *Clinical Aspects of Immunology* (1st ed.). Oxford, England: Blackwell.

Greenberger, P. A. (2006 Feb). Drug allergy. *The Journal of Allergy and Clinical Immunology, 117*(2 Suppl. Mini-Primer), S464–S470.

Gruchalla, R. S. (2003 Feb). Drug allergy. *The Journal of Allergy and Clinical Immunology, 111*(2 Suppl.), S548–S559.

Gunzer, M. (2007). Migration, cell-cell interaction and adhesion in the immune system. *Ernst Schering Found Symp Proc,* (3), 97–137.

Hammond, I. W., Gibbs, T. G., Seifert, H. A., & Rich, D. S. (2007 Nov). Database size and power to detect safety signals in pharmacovigilance. *Expert Opinion on Drug Safety, 6*(6), 713–721.

Handler, S. M., Altman, R. L., Perera, S., Hanlon, J. T., Studenski, S. A., Bost, J. E., et al. (2007 Jul-Aug). A systematic review of the performance characteristics of clinical event monitor signals used to detect adverse drug events in the hospital setting. *Journal of the American Medical Informatics Association: JAMIA, 14*(4), 451–458.

Hanigan, M. H., & Devarajan, P. (2003). Cisplatin nephrotoxicity: Molecular mechanisms. *Cancer Ther, 1*, 47–61.

Hartford, C. G., Petchel, K. S., Mickail, H., Perez-Gutthann, S., McHale, M., Grana, J. M., et al. (2006). Pharmacovigilance during the pre-approval phases: An evolving pharmaceutical industry model in response to ICH E2E, CIOMS VI, FDA and EMEA/CHMP risk-management guidelines. *Drug Safety: An International Journal of Medical Toxicology and Drug Experience, 29*(8), 657–673.

Hauben, M., Horn, S., & Reich, L. (2007). Potential use of data-mining algorithms for the detection of 'surprise' adverse drug reactions. *Drug Safety: An International Journal of Medical Toxicology and Drug Experience, 30*(2), 143–155.

Hazell, L., & Shakir, S. A. (2006). Under-reporting of adverse drug reactions: A systematic review. *Drug Safety: An International Journal of Medical Toxicology and Drug Experience, 29*(5), 385–396.

Hilário, M. O., Terreri, M. T., & Len, C. A. (2006 Nov). Nonsteroidal anti-inflammatory drugs: Cyclooxygenase 2 inhibitors. *Jornal de Pediatria, 82*(5 Suppl.), S206–S212.

Hopstadius, J., Norén, G. N., Bate, A., & Edwards, I. R. (2008). Impact of stratification on adverse drug reaction surveillance. *Drug Safety: An International Journal of Medical Toxicology and Drug Experience, 31*(11), 1035–1048.

Ingelman-Sundberg, M. (2004 Jan). Human drug metabolising cytochrome P450 enzymes: Properties and polymorphisms. *Naunyn-Schmiedeberg's Archives of Pharmacology, 369*(1), 89–104.

Jain, V. V., Perkins, D. L., & Finn, P. W. (2008 Mar). Costimulation and allergic responses: Immune and bioinformatic analyses. *Pharmacology & Therapeutics, 117*(3), 385–392.

Jensen, B. V. (2006 Jun). Cardiotoxic consequences of anthracycline-containing therapy in patients with breast cancer. *Seminars in Oncology, 33*(3 Suppl. 8), S15–S21.

Jordan, S., Knight, J., & Pointon, D. (2004 Dec). Monitoring adverse drug reactions: Scales, profiles, and checklists. *International Nursing Review, 51*(4), 208–221.

Karch, S. B. (2007 Feb). Peer review and the process of publishing of adverse drug event reports. *J. Forensic Leg. Med., 14*(2), 79–84.

Kellogg, V. A., & Havens, D. S. (2003 Oct). Adverse events in acute care: An integrative literature review. *Research in Nursing & Health, 26*(5), 398–408.

Keystone, E. C. (2005 Mar). Safety of biologic therapies—An update. *The Journal of Rheumatology. Supplement, 74*, 8–12.

Khan, A., Hill, J. M., Grater, W., Loeb, E., MacLellan, A., & Hill, N. (1975 Oct). Atopic hypersensitivity to cis-dichlorodiammineplatinum(II) and other platinum complexes. *Cancer Research, 35*(10), 2766–2770.

Koh, Y., & Li, S. C. (2005). A new algorithm to identify the causality of adverse drug reactions. *Drug Safety: An International Journal of Medical Toxicology and Drug Experience, 28*(12), 1159–1161.

Lassere, M. N., Johnson, K. R., Woodworth, T. G., Furst, D. E., Fries, J. F., Kirwan, J. R., et al. (2005 Oct). Challenges and progress in adverse event ascertainment and reporting in clinical trials. *The Journal of Rheumatology, 32*(10), 2030–2032.

Leviton, I. (2003). Separating fact from fiction: The data behind allergies and side effects caused by penicillins, cephalosporins, and carbapenem antibiotics. *Current Pharmaceutical Design, 9* (12), 983–988.

Lièvre, M. (2006 Dec). Evaluation of adverse treatment effects in controlled trials. *Joint, Bone, Spine: Revue du Rhumatisme, 73*(6), 624–626.

Malkin, D., Koren, G., & Saunders, E. F. (1990 Winter). Drug-induced aplastic anemia: Pathogenesis and clinical aspects. *The American Journal of Pediatric Hematology/Oncology, 12*(4), 402–410.

Martin, E., Mayorga, C., Rodriguez, R., Torres, M. J., & Blanca, M. (2005 Jun). Drug hypersensitivity: Insights into pathomechanisms. *Eur Ann Allergy Clin Immunol, 37*(6), 207–212.

Martínez-Salgado, C., López-Hernández, F. J., & López-Novoa, J. M. (2007 Aug 15). Glomerular nephrotoxicity of aminoglycosides. *Toxicology and Applied Pharmacology, 223*(1), 86–98.

McGettigan, P., Han, P., Jones, L., Whitaker, D., & Henry, D. (2008 Jun). Selective COX-2 inhibitors, NSAIDs and congestive heart failure: Differences between new and recurrent cases. *British Journal of Clinical Pharmacology, 65*(6), 927–934.

Meisel, C., Gerloff, T., Kirchheiner, J., Mrozikiewicz, P. M., Niewinski, P., Brockmöller, J., et al. (2003 Mar). Implications of pharmacogenetics for individualizing drug treatment and for study design. *Journal of Molecular Medicine (Berlin, Germany), 81*(3), 154–167.

Mercier, C., Ciccolini, J., Pourroy, B., Fanciullino, R., Duffaud, F., Digue, L., Tranchand, B., Monjanel-Mouterde, S., Guillet, P., et al. (2006 Apr). Dose individualization of carboplatin after a 120-hour infusion schedule: Higher dose intensity but fewer toxicities. *Therapeutic Drug Monitoring, 28*(2), 212–218.

Millington, O. R., Zinselmeyer, B. H., Brewer, J. M., Garside, P., & Rush, C. M. (2007 Oct). Lymphocyte tracking and interactions in secondary lymphoid organs. *Inflammation Research: Official Journal of the European Histamine Research Society... [et al.], 56*(10), 391–401.

Min, B., & Paul, W. E. (2008 Jan). Basophils and type 2 immunity. *Current Opinion in Hematology, 15*(1), 59–63.

Minotti, G., Recalcati, S., Menna, P., Salvatorelli, E., Corna, G., & Cairo, G. (2004). Doxorubicin cardiotoxicity and the control of iron metabolism: Quinone-dependent and independent mechanisms. *Methods in Enzymology, 378*, 340–361.

Miraglia del Giudice, M., Decimo, F., Leonardi, S., Maioello, N., Amelio, R., Capasso, A., et al. (2006 Nov-Dec). Immune dysregulation in atopic dermatitis. *Allergy and Asthma Proceedings: The Official Journal of Regional and State Allergy Societies, 27*(6), 451–455.

Montastruc, J. L., Sommet, A., Lacroix, I., Olivier, P., Durrieu, G., Damase-Michel, C., et al. (2006 Dec). Pharmacovigilance for evaluating adverse drug reactions: Value, organization, and methods. *Joint, Bone, Spine: Revue du Rhumatisme, 73*(6), 629–632.

Moodley, I. (2008 Mar-Apr). Review of the cardiovascular safety of COXIBs compared to NSAIDS. *Cardiovasc J Afr, 19*(2), 102–107.

Moreno, E., Macías, E., Dávila, I., Laffond, E., Ruiz, A., & Lorente, F. (2008 May). Hypersensitivity reactions to cephalosporins. *Expert Opinion on Drug Safety, 7*(3), 295–304.

Nebeker, J. R., Yarnold, P. R., Soltysik, R. C., Sauer, B. C., Sims, S. A., Samore, M. H., et al. (2007 Oct). Developing indicators of inpatient adverse drug events through nonlinear analysis using administrative data. *Medical Care, 45*(10 Suppl. 2), S81–S88.

Nelson, R. C., Palsulich, B., & Gogolak, V. (2002). Good pharmacovigilance practices: Technology enabled. *Drug Safety: An International Journal of Medical Toxicology and Drug Experience, 25*(6), 407–414.

Opgen-Rhein, C., & Dettling, M. (2008 Aug). Clozapine-induced agranulocytosis and its genetic determinants. *Pharmacogenomics, 9*(8), 1101–1111.

Page, R. L. 2nd, & Ruscin, J. M. (2006 Dec). The risk of adverse drug events and hospital-related morbidity and mortality among older adults with potentially inappropriate medication use. *The American Journal of Geriatric Pharmacotherapy, 4*(4), 297–305.

Pålsson-McDermott, E. M., & O'Neill, L. A. (2007 Dec). Building an immune system from nine domains. *Biochemical Society Transactions, 35*(Pt 6), 1437–1444.

Panjrath, G. S., & Jain, D. (2006 May-Jun). Monitoring chemotherapy-induced cardiotoxicity: Role of cardiac nuclear imaging. *Journal of Nuclear Cardiology: Official Publication of the American Society of Nuclear Cardiology, 13*(3), 415–426.

Park, M. A., & Li, J. T. (2005 Mar). Diagnosis and management of penicillin allergy. *Mayo Clinic Proceedings. Mayo Clinic, 80*(3), 405–410.

Park, M. A., Matesic, D., Markus, P. J., & Li, J. T. (2007 Jul). Female sex as a risk factor for penicillin allergy. *Annals of Allergy, Asthma & Immunology: Official Publication of the American College of Allergy, Asthma, & Immunology, 99*(1), 54–58.

Patrignani, P., Capone, M. L., & Tacconelli, S. (2008 Apr). NSAIDs and cardiovascular disease. *Heart (British Cardiac Society), 94*(4), 395–397.

Phillips, K. A., Veenstra, D. L., Oren, E., Lee, J. K., & Sadee, W. (2001 Nov 14). Potential role of pharmacogenomics in reducing adverse drug reactions: A systematic review. *JAMA: The Journal of the American Medical Association, 286*(18), 2270–2279.

Posadas, S. J., & Pichler, W. J. (2007 Jul). Delayed drug hypersensitivity reactions—New concepts. *Clinical and Experimental Allergy: Journal of the British Society for Allergy and Clinical Immunology, 37*(7), 989–999.

Rahman, S. Z., Khan, R. A., Gupta, V., & Uddin, M. (2007 Jul 24). Pharmacoenvironmentology—A component of pharmacovigilance. *Environmental Health: A Global Access Science Source, 6*, 20.

Redegeld, F. A., & Wortel, C. H. (2008 Nov). IgE and immunoglobulin free light chains in allergic disease: New therapeutic opportunities. *Current Opinion in Investigational Drugs London, England: 2000), 9*(11), 1185–1191.

Reidenberg, M. M. (2006 Jul). Improving how we evaluate the toxicity of approved drugs. *Clinical Pharmacology and Therapeutics, 80*(1), 1–6.

Romano, A., & Demoly, P. (2007 Aug). Recent advances in the diagnosis of drug allergy. *Current Opinion in Allergy and Clinical Immunology, 7*(4), 299–303.

Rosário, N. A., & Grumach, A. S. (2006 Nov). Allergy to beta-lactams in pediatrics: A practical approach. *Jornal de Pediatria, 82*(5 Suppl.), S181–S188.

Roujeau, J. C. (2006 Mar). Immune mechanisms in drug allergy. *Allergology International: Official Journal of the Japanese Society of Allergology, 55*(1), 27–33.

Roychowdhury, S., & Svensson, C. K. (2005 Dec 9). Mechanisms of drug-induced delayed-type hypersensitivity reactions in the skin. *The AAPS Journal, 7*(4), E834–E846.

Sandhiya, S., & Adithan, C. (2008 Jul). Drug therapy in elderly. *The Journal of the Association of Physicians of India, 56*, 525–531.

Scharf, O., & Colevas, A. D. (2006 Aug 20). Adverse event reporting in publications compared with sponsor database for cancer clinical trials. *Journal of Clinical Oncology: Official Journal of the American Society of Clinical Oncology, 24*(24), 3933–3938.

Schwab, S. R., & Cyster, J. G. (2007 Dec). Finding a way out: lymphocyte egress from lymphoid organs. *Nature Immunology, 8*(12), 1295–1301.

Sebti, S. M., Mignano, J. E., Jani, J. P., Srimatkandada, S., & Lazo, J. S. (1989 Aug 8). Bleomycin hydrolase: Molecular cloning, sequencing, and biochemical studies reveal membership in the cysteine proteinase family. *Biochemistry, 28*(16), 6544–6548.

Seoane-Vazquez, E. (2008). Drug selection and adverse drug reactions: Balancing outcomes and costs. *Electron J Biomed, 2*, 3–5.

Sitkauskiene, B., & Sakalauskas, R. (2005 Apr). The role of beta(2)-adrenergic receptors in inflammation and allergy. *Current Drug Targets. Inflammation and Allergy, 4*(2), 157–162.

Smith, R. G. (2008 Nov-Dec). Penicillin and cephalosporin drug allergies: A paradigm shift. *Journal of the American Podiatric Medical Association, 98*(6), 479–488.

Solensky, R. (2003 Jun). Hypersensitivity reactions to beta-lactam antibiotics. *Clinical Reviews in Allergy & Immunology, 24*(3), 201–220.

Takemura, G., & Fujiwara, H. (2007 Mar-Apr). Doxorubicin-induced cardiomyopathy from the cardiotoxic mechanisms to management. *Progress in Cardiovascular Diseases , 49*(5), 330–352.

Thien, F. C. (2006 Sep 18). Drug hypersensitivity. *The Medical Journal of Australia, 185*(6), 333–338.

Trotti, A., Colevas, A. D., Setser, A., & Basch, E. (2007 Nov 10). Patient-reported outcomes and the evolution of adverse event reporting in oncology. *Journal of Clinical Oncology: Official Journal of the American Society of Clinical Oncology, 25*(32), 5121–5127.

Uetrecht, J. (2006). Evaluation of which reactive metabolite, if any, is responsible for a specific idiosyncratic reaction. *Drug Metabolism Reviews, 38*(4), 745–753.

Uetrecht, J. (2007). Idiosyncratic drug reactions: current understanding. *Annual Review of Pharmacology and Toxicology, 47*, 513–539.

Uzel, I., Ozguroglu, M., Uzel, B., Kaynak, K., Demirhan, O., Akman, C., et al. (2005 Jul). Delayed onset bleomycin-induced pneumonitis. *Urology, 66*(1), 195.

van Adelsberg, J., Gann, P., Ko, A. T., Damber, J. E., Logothetis, C., Marberger, M., et al. (2007). The VIOXX in Prostate Cancer Prevention study: cardiovascular events observed in the rofecoxib 25 mg and placebo treatment groups. *Current Medical Research and Opinion.*

Walgren, J. L., Mitchell, M. D., & Thompson, D. C. (2005 Apr-May). Role of metabolism in drug-induced idiosyncratic hepatotoxicity. *Critical Reviews in Toxicology, 35*(4), 325–361.

Waller, P. C. (2006 Mar). Making the most of spontaneous adverse drug reaction reporting. *Basic & Clinical Pharmacology & Toxicology, 98*(3), 320–323.

White, W. B. (2007 Apr). Cardiovascular risk, hypertension, and NSAIDs. *Current Rheumatology Reports, 9*(1), 36–43.

Wilczynski, J. R., Radwan, M., & Kalinka, J. (2008 Jan 1). The characterization and role of regulatory T cells in immune reactions. *Frontiers in Bioscience: A Journal and Virtual Library, 13*, 2266–2274.

Wong, B. B., Keith, P. K., & Waserman, S. (2006 Aug). Clinical history as a predictor of penicillin skin test outcome. *Annals of Allergy, Asthma & Immunology: Official Publication of the American College of Allergy, Asthma, & Immunology, 97*(2), 169–174.

Zandieh, S. O., Goldmann, D. A., Keohane, C. A., Yoon, C., Bates, D. W., & Kaushal, R. (2008 Feb). Risk factors in preventable adverse drug events in pediatric outpatients. *The Journal of Pediatrics, 152* (2), 225–231.

Zarraga, I. G., (2007 Jan 2). Schwarz, E.R., (2007 Jan 2). Coxibs and heart disease: What we have learned and what else we need to know. *Journal of the American College of Cardiology, 49* (1), 1–14.

Zopf, Y., Rabe, C., Neubert, A., Gassmann, K. G., Rascher, W., Hahn, E. G., et al. (2008 Oct). Women encounter ADRs more often than do men. *European Journal of Clinical Pharmacology, 64*(10), 999–1004.

Chapter

14 Risk Assessment

Bill Bress

OUTLINE

14.1 HISTORY

Risk assessments have been performed for a variety of topics, from accidents in the workplace, to lifestyle choices and natural catastrophes. This chapter will focus on evaluating human risk primarily from chemical and radiological exposure. Risk assessment as defined by the National Academy of Science is "the use of the factual base to define the health effects of exposure of individuals or populations to hazardous materials and situations." Risk assessment determines if a chemical has a toxic effect, estimates the exposure to this chemical and identifies the adverse effects of the chemical. The combination of the toxicity influenced by the level of exposure estimates what the likelihood of the adverse effect would be in a given population.

Recognition of the toxicity of chemicals can be traced back thousands of years. Natives in South America recognized the toxicity of curare and used it on their arrow tips for hunting. The ancient Greeks described the toxic effects of mercury and lead. Paracelsus wrote in 1567, "All substances are poisons: There is none which is not a poison. The right dose differentiates a poison from a remedy." Paracelsus learned this firsthand, because he believed a poison in the body can be treated with a similar poison. Dosing for him was trial and error. He believed animal testing of chemicals would be valuable in estimating their toxicity.

In the 1930s, the Food and Drug Administration approved tolerances for food additives. These tolerances had to meet a standard of reasonable certainty of no harm when used as intended.

In 1910, the National Bureau of Mines was established; it was charged with, among other things, enhancing the safety, health, and environmental impact of mining. They performed measurements of exposures to chemicals by workers, and noted effects at certain concentrations. Using these studies they recommended when safety equipment was needed.

In 1954, the Food and Drug Administration published a paper that defined the basis for the acceptable daily intake (ADI). The ADI was a threshold for intake of a chemical for a large population, below which there should be no significant toxic risks. The paper not only defined a procedure for the ADI, but also described the use of safety factors and how animal data could be used to estimate risk to humans. A no effect level was determined from animal studies and a safety factor of 100 was used to establish a safe level. Tolerances for chemical additives and pesticides were calculated, comparing the safe level to the residue concentration of these chemicals in crops (e.g., wheat) and that crop's contribution to the individual's daily diet.

The Food Additive Amendment of 1958, the Color Additives Amendment of 1960, and the Animal Drugs

Amendment of 1968 all contained a "Delaney Clause," which states that any additive shall not be deemed safe if it is found, after appropriate tests, to induce cancer in man or animal. Since testing technology was becoming very sophisticated, the FDA decided that not detecting a carcinogen in food was not a practical way to regulate. They developed a cancer risk assessment method, which they used to describe a risk of cancer from that chemical so infinitesimal, that any incremental cancer risk that might occur due to the residue would be essentially zero. FDA eventually defined as "essentially zero" to a one in one million risk of getting cancer in a lifetime of exposure.

The Environmental Protection Agency in the 1980s expanded the techniques for risk assessment. EPA established guidelines for evaluation of risk at Superfund sites, which are contaminated sites that EPA has set as priorities for investigation and remediation.

EPA's Risk Assessment Guidelines were developed to help guide EPA scientists in assessing risks to human health from chemicals or other agents in the environment. They also inform EPA decision makers and the general public about these procedures. EPA published an initial set of five risk assessment guidelines (relating to cancer, mutagenic effects, developmental effects, exposure assessment, and chemical mixtures) in 1986 as recommended by the National Academy of Sciences. EPA continues to revise its risk assessment guidelines and to develop new guidelines as experience and scientific understanding evolve. The Guidelines include Mutagenicity Assessment (1986), Developmental Toxicity Risk Assessment (1991), Exposure Assessment (1992), Reproductive Toxicity Risk Assessment (1996), Neurotoxicity Assessment 1998, and Carcinogen Risk Assessment (2005).

EPA in the mid 1990s decided there was a need for short-term air contaminant guidelines. The impetus for this was the Bowpal, India, chemical plant tragedy, where over a thousand people died from exposure to methyl isocyanate. There were no evacuation level standards for the chemical produced at the factory. EPA established a national advisory committee for Acute Exposure Guideline Levels (AEGL), which has since produced 10-minute to 8-hour exposure limits for over a hundred chemicals, with a goal of 400 different chemicals. These guidelines are used by factories and fire departments as evacuation standards for communities adjacent to chemical facilities. The national advisory committee for AEGLs develops the guidelines, which are then presented to a subcommittee of the National Research Council (NRC). When concurrence by the NRC/AEGL Subcommittee is achieved, the AEGL values are considered final and are published by the NRC. Final AEGL values may be used on a permanent basis by all federal, state, and local agencies, and private organizations. When new data becomes available that challenges the scientific credibility of final AEGLs, the chemical can be resubmitted to the NAC/AEGL Committee and recycled through the review process.

14.2 HAZARD IDENTIFICATION

Hazard identification is the process of determining whether exposure to an agent can be linked to an increase in the incidence of an adverse health effect and characterizes the nature and strength of the evidence of causation. The basis of hazard identification is founded on epidemiology, animal studies, and/or *in vitro* studies, and structure-activity relationships. A risk assessment might not progress further than hazard identification. If the agent does not possess an adverse effect, or if there is legislation or regulatory policy that requires no further action, then the risk assessment would stop there.

14.2.1 Epidemiology

Well-conducted human studies that can show an association between exposure to a chemical and health outcomes are few. However, for those that exist, they are invaluable for assessing risk. An important limitation of epidemiological studies is that they provide evidence of adverse effects, only after exposure and onset of disease. There is also often a latency period for many environmentally caused diseases. A large number of occupational studies exist, but many are accidental exposure and in most cases accurate measurements are lacking. Often, the number of people exposed to an agent is low and the incidence of disease is small. It is not unusual to have published studies from the early 1900s, where a college professor and a few of his graduate students exposed themselves to various gases and aerosols in a room. They would measure how long they could stay in the environment and describe their symptoms. Use of such human studies is limited.

In larger epidemiological studies, populations may include infants, the elderly, and healthy young adults. As a result, the effect on sensitive populations is difficult to estimate. Benzene is a chemical, for which there is a considerable body of epidemiological studies in workers. The dose and disease ratio from these studies has been used to calculate the risk of developing leukemia. There have also been studies conducted on children who develop leukemia and the distance their homes are from power lines. These project directors were looking to see if there was a correlation between power line electromagnetic fields and cancer. Some of the studies indicate a possible connection, and others do not. One problem with epidemiology studies of this type is the question of actual exposure. Most of the conclusions are based on distance from a power line and not actual measurements inside the homes. Appliances in homes generate electromagnetic fields also. Therefore the true dose that the children received remains unknown.

One of the most thoroughly researched epidemiology studies has been conducted at Fallon, Colorado. There was a belief that the number of childhood cancers (acute lymphocytic leukemia) in that town was above expected values. CDC sampled soil, air, water, and many other mediums looking for a cause. They even used biomonitoring (blood and urine sampling) looking for contaminates in the body. CDC conducted genetic testing on the children, to see if there was a common trait. To date, no cause has been found, but genetic studies saw an association between a *SUOX* gene locus and disease status in the presence of high tungsten and arsenic levels. CDC feels this warrants further investigation. Although epidemiology studies are valuable when looking at risk, we must realize their limitations. Humans are not a homogenous strain, unlike the rats and mice used in toxicity studies, and they are exposed to many different chemicals in the air and in food, whereas in animal bioassays, rodents are given one substance during a study. Finally, people do not always live in the same location, they move constantly, so trying to analyze a population for exposure can be daunting.

There has been speculation that chlorinated disinfection byproducts lead to an increase in bladder cancer in the communities that use chlorine as a disinfectant. After examining these studies, the Environmental Protection Agency has singled out trihalomethanes (THMs) as the byproduct causing this increase. They also believe other disinfection byproducts of chlorination, specifically haloacetic acids, could lead to some birth defects. Based on these studies the EPA has rewritten their drinking water regulations to lower the allowable concentrations of these chemicals in public drinking water supplies. When it comes to risk versus benefit, EPA believes the benefit of disinfection of public water supplies, which prevents diseases such as giardia, cryptosporidium, and Norwalk's virus, outweighs the risk of bladder cancer and birth defects.

A well-conducted and controlled epidemiological study of a population is the first choice for a risk assessment. An epidemiological study with good exposure response data is used and animal data for the same compound are used as supporting data. Sometimes human data is useful in showing a qualitative relationship between environmental exposure and heath outcomes. In this case the human data is used as support for animal studies.

Epidemiology generally looks at populations, however new developments in genomic research can target individuals and should have a large impact on risk assessments in the future. Experiments have been designed to evaluate responses to toxicants to determine if known mechanisms of toxicity could be associated with characteristic gene expression profiles and evaluate the utility of this technology for risk assessment applications. The genetic testing techniques will allow identification of sensitive subpopulations and ultimately could allow personalized risk profiling for an individual. There are ethical concerns about using this data. If there is not a clear understanding of gene-environment interactions, differences in individual responses, and the qualitative and quantitative association between toxicity and disease, there is real potential for misinterpretation of data where risk assessment is concerned.

14.2.2 Animal Bioassay Studies

The database for toxicity for most chemicals is sparse for toxic effects on humans. In such cases, we may infer the potential for a substance to cause adverse effects in humans from information drawn from studies conducted on animals. Animal studies have been shown to be reliable indicators of adverse health effects including development of cancer and birth defects. Consistent positive results in both sexes and in several different species and also the presence of a dose effect is an effective indicator of the possibility of also causing cancer in humans. Some of these animals include the rat, mouse, guinea pig, hamster, dog, and monkey. There is an inference that humans and mammals are similar in susceptibility to toxic chemicals, and data from these animals can be used as a surrogate to data from humans. This is the basic premise for toxicology of the present and is important in regulation of toxic chemicals. There are times, however, when effects in animals are not relevant to humans, due to physiological differences. EPA considers that if an agent has an adverse effect in animals the effects will, in general, be the same in humans across strains, sexes, species, and routes of exposure.

Some examples of toxicological animal studies include:

- LD50—Establishing the lethal dose in 50% of animals tested
- Acute—Two-week exposure rodent study
- Subchronic—Four- to 15-week exposure rodent study
- Chronic toxicity—Six-month rodent study
- Lifetime carcinogenicity—Two-year rodent study

Animal studies can include the following routes of administration: inhalation, dermal, oral gavage, feeding, and intraperitoneal, intravenous, and subcutaneous. Studies can include looking at developmental and reproductive toxicity, neurotoxicity, histopathology, and carcinogenic end points.

14.3 DOSE RESPONSE ASSESSMENT

Dose response assessment explores the relationship between the dose of an agent administered or received and the incidence of an adverse health effect on humans or animals. It is a quantitative relationship derived between the dose and the probability of induction of a carcinogenic effect. The incidence of the adverse dose is estimated as a function of the exposure to the chemical. Factors involved with dose assessment are age, exposure, pattern of exposure, gender, genetics, and socioeconomic conditions. Dose response assessment is usually performed on animals. Typically they are given the highest dose that they can tolerate and two doses at lower concentrations. Control animals are not exposed to the agent. If the agent's adverse effects intensify with a larger dose, there is an indication that the agent has a positive dose response.

14.3.1 Uncertainty in Dose Response Assessment

There are a number of reasons to use this data cautiously. Due to differences in metabolism between humans and rodents, the total dose consumed does not necessarily correlate with the total dose delivered to the target organ. Humans are usually exposed to much lower doses of a chemical, compared to the rodents in these studies; the dose response curve is an extrapolation from a high animal dose to a low human dose. Some factors that affect uncertainty are:

- Experimental design and conduct
- Variability in commercial mixture composition
- Variability across strains
- Variability between sexes
- Variability across experiments
- Experimental uncertainty (sample size)
- Potential for other carcinogenic effects
- Animal-to-human extrapolation
- High-to-low-dose extrapolation
- Route-to-route extrapolation
- Difference between commercial and environmental mixtures
- Persistence and exposure duration
- Human variability in sensitivity
- Human variability in exposure
- Few relevant studies

14.3.2 Supporting Data

There are other types of studies that can be used to support the likelihood of occurrence of adverse health effects on people. There are metabolic and pharmacokinetic studies, which can describe the mechanism of action of a compound. If we look at the metabolism of an animal versus a human, evidence for toxic effects in humans may be deduced. Considerable species variation exists with respect to benzene metabolism. Metabolism studies of benzene showed that mice metabolize benzene faster than rats and convert more of the benzene to toxic metabolites than do rats, primarily at exposure levels up to about 200 ppm. This is partly due to increased inhalation per unit body weight but also due to a higher activity of hepatic metabolism. From *in vitro* experiments with hepatocytes or liver microsomes it was shown that the range of metabolite production from human tissue more or less spans the range between mice and rats.

14.3.3 *In Vitro* Studies

Evidence of the association between carcinogens and mutagens leads to the presumption that mutagenic substances will also be carcinogenic. Studies with microorganisms or cell cultures may be used to provide access to a compound's potential for biological activity. There are tests for point mutations, DNA damage/repair, chromosome aberrations, both numerical and structural cell transformation. These techniques may give information on mechanisms of carcinogenicity. Lack of positive results in short-term tests for genotoxicity should not be considered as a basis for eliminating a compound for long-term carcinogenicity testing. Although these quick and relatively inexpensive tests are valuable for screening potential carcinogens, they do not supply sufficient evidence to conclude that the agent in question is a carcinogen.

14.3.4 Structure-Activity Studies

Structure related activity (SAR) is based on a chemical's structure as another potential source of supporting data. The chemical structure of a substance can, in some cases is used to predict its toxicity. An example of this is the family of dioxin compounds. Toxicity of tetra-substituted dioxins and furans are predicted based on what chemical groups are present at the active sites of the molecule. The tetra-substituted 2,3,7,8 TCDD is more toxic and persistent than an octa-substituted dioxins structure. Unfortunately, overall, this method has so far proved to be of little help in identifying and predicting carcinogenic potential of many chemicals.

14.4 EXPOSURE ASSESSMENT

Exposure assessment determines the type and magnitude of exposure to a chemical or chemicals exposure. Exposure assessments identify the exposed population, describe its composition and size, and present the magnitude, frequency, type, and duration of exposure. It is used to predict effects of exposure and recommend strategies for reducing that exposure. Once the exposure assessment has been determined, the results are combined with toxicity information to characterize potential risks.

Exposure is defined as the contact of an organism with a chemical or physical agent. The exposure is determined by estimating the amount of a chemical available to the lungs, skin, or stomach during a determined time period.

Exposure assessment is equal to the magnitude, duration, frequency, and route of exposure. Exposure assessments may be used to consider past, present, and future exposures. In many cases it is impossible to know what the exact past exposures were; in those cases we may use current exposure as a surrogate, or conduct a purely qualitative exposure scenario. We can also use tissue chemical concentrations of people exposed. An example of this would be tooth analysis for radioisotopes for children living near nuclear power plants.

Exposure estimates of the present can be based on actual laboratory measurements or exposure models of the chemicals. Future exposures can be based on modeling future conditions.

Ambient concentrations of chemicals to which people may be exposed can be estimated by emission rates, transport, and persistence. Exposure assessment is also complicated by the presence of many different chemicals in a community and many different sources of pollutants.

As analytical technology progresses, chemicals are now being detected at much lower concentrations than in the past. New chemicals, especially degradation by-products and reagent contaminants are being detected in soil, air, and groundwater. Many of these chemicals have no toxicity testing history and create a challenge to risk managers.

Preliminary identification of potential human exposure provides much needed information for a site assessment plan. This activity involves the identification of the media of concern, the area of concern, the types of chemicals expected at the site, and the potential routes of contaminant transport through the environment. In order to perform a preliminary assessment, sample collection and analysis must occur.

14.4.1 Pattern of Sampling

Pattern of sampling involves not only the contaminate site but also background location sampling. Most naturally occurring agents are present in measurable quantities in air, water, and soils. Some areas of the country contain naturally occurring high concentrations of potentially toxic substances (arsenic, uranium). Without a background test, the risk assessor might be misled into believing a particular agent is a contaminant rather than a natural part of the site's geology. Statistics may be used to evaluate background sampling data. Because the number of background samples collected is important for statistical hypothesis testing, a statistician should be consulted when planning background sampling. Many decisions must be made by the risk assessor related to the appropriate sample size for an investigation. A statistician cannot estimate an appropriate sample size without the supporting information provided by a risk assessor. These considerations include the following factors: logistics and cost, number of areas of concern that will be sampled, statistical interpretation to be used, and the statistical interpretation of the data that will be collected.

14.4.2 Soil Sampling

A large problem in soil sampling is that soil is usually heterogeneous in nature. Therefore larger numbers of samples must be taken compared to a medium (e.g., water), which can be homogeneous. Taking composite samples may reduce the number of samples needed to calculate an exposure concentration, but using composites will mask hot spots in the soil. A *hot spot* is an area of very high concentrations and could present a risk to the public from direct exposure. Sample depth is important when determining risk. If a contaminant is capable of leaching from the surface into ground water, then subsurface sampling is valuable. Assessment of surface exposures may be conducted at zero to 6″. Results from this depth can be used for risk scenarios involving sites like baseball fields and playgrounds.

Subsurface soil samples are important, however, if soil disturbance is likely or if leaching of chemicals to ground water is of concern, or if the site has current or potential agricultural uses. For subsurface testing, depths of one to two feet can be used. Another item of concern is the determination of the types of samples to be collected. Basically, two types of samples may be collected at a site: grab and composite. Grab samples represent a single part of a medium collected at a specific location and time. Composite samples (sometimes referred to as continuous samples for air) combine subsamples from different locations and/or times. Composite samples may misrepresent or dilute concentrations at specific points and, therefore, should be avoided as the only inputs to a risk assessment.

14.5 RISK CHARACTERIZATION

Risk characterization is defined as the estimate of the magnitude of the public health problem. It is determined by combining the information gathered from hazard identification and exposure assessments. These produce a quantitative risk estimate in which the major assumptions, strengths, weaknesses, judgments, and estimates of uncertainty are examined. Determining the characteristics of the site is an important part of exposure assessment. Vegetation, soil, climate, surface, and ground water are identified in this step. Outdoor playgrounds in a tropical climate would have a more frequent use than one in an artic climate. Next, the populations that occupy this area are identified and examined for their potential for use of the media in this area and the frequency with which they use the site. Sensitive subpopulations are also identified at this time.

A risk assessment requires a characterization of exposure setting. In this step, the assessor characterizes the exposure setting with respect to the general physical characteristics of the site and the characteristics of the populations on and near the site. Basic site characteristics such as climate, vegetation, groundwater hydrology, and the presence and location of surface water are identified in this step. Populations are also identified and are described with respect to those characteristics that influence exposure, such as location relative to the site, activity patterns, and the presence of sensitive subpopulations. The characteristics of the current population, as well as those of any potential future populations are considered.

Those pathways by which the previously identified populations may be exposed are examined by the identification of exposure pathways. Exposure pathways are identified based on the release, source, and locations of chemicals at the site. Some sites have chemicals that were deposited decades ago, therefore, present surface contamination may be low today, but may have been significant in the past. The environmental fate of a chemical depends on a number of factors: transport, persistence, partitioning, and media transfer. Some chemicals degrade with time, and present exposure may be limited to these degradation products and not to the parent chemical. Some examples are tetrachloroethylene converted to dichloroethylene, DDT to DDE and thorium to radon gas. Points of potential contact with the chemical and possible routes of exposure such as ingestion, inhalation, and dermal, are identified for each exposure pathway.

Quantification of exposure is measured by examining the quantity, magnitude, frequency, and duration of exposure for each pathway identified and are followed by estimation of exposure and calculation of intakes. In the estimation of exposure, chemical concentrations, monitoring data, chemical transport and environmental fate models can be utilized. Modeling is useful if there is no current data and future use is uncertain. A risk assessor is interested in the calculation of intakes. Exposure estimates are expressed in terms of the mass of substance in contact with the body per unit body weight per unit time (e.g., milligram (mg) chemical per kilogram (kg) body weight per day is expressed as mg/kg-day). This is a daily intake. Chemical intakes are calculated using equations that include variables for exposure concentration, exposure duration, contact rate, exposure frequency, body weight, and exposure averaging time. The values of these variables will change with different populations (age group, dietary habits, etc.). After all the intakes have been calculated, the sources of uncertainty are considered. These include, but are not limited to quality of analytical data, behavioral assumptions, and modeling results.

The exposure assessment concludes with a summary of the estimated intakes for each pathway evaluated. The reasonable maximum exposure (RME) is defined as the highest exposure that is reasonably expected to occur at a site. RMEs are estimated for individual pathways or a combination of exposures across pathways. In the past, all routes of exposures were generally estimated for an average and an upper-bound exposure case, instead of a single exposure case. The disadvantage of this approach is that the upper-bound estimate of exposure may be above the range of possible exposures, whereas the average estimate is lower than exposures potentially experienced by much of the population. The intent of the RME is to estimate a conservative exposure that is still within the range of possibility.

14.5.1 Exposure Setting

In evaluating exposure at a hazardous site, the assessor tries to characterize the site with respect to its physical characteristics as well as those of the human populations on and near the site. This results in a qualitative evaluation of the site and the potentially exposed populations with respect to the characteristics that influence exposure. Information gathered during this step will support the identification of exposure pathways. In addition, the information on the potentially exposed populations will be used to determine the values of some intake variables. An exposure pathway generally consists of four elements, a source and mechanism of chemical release, a retention or transport medium, a point of potential human contact with the contaminated medium, and an exposure route (e.g., ingestion) at the contact point. A medium contaminated as a result of a past release can be a contaminant source for other media (e.g., soil contaminated from a previous spill could be a contaminant source for ground water or surface water).

14.5.1.1 Characterizing the Physical Setting

This step characterizes the exposure setting with respect to the general physical characteristics of the site. Important site characteristics include the following: climate, meteorology, geologic setting, vegetation, soil type, ground-water hydrology, and location and description of surface water.

Information gathered can come from county soil surveys, wetlands maps, aerial photographs, and reports by the National Oceanographic and Atmospheric Association (NOAA) and the U.S. Geological Survey (USGS).

14.5.1.2 Exposed Populations

First, we need to determine the location of current populations relative to the site with regard to distance and direction Then, we can attempt to identify those populations that are closest to the site and that have the greatest potential for exposure. Included are populations that could be exposed in the future to chemicals that have migrated from the site. Potential sources of this information include site visits, population surveys, topographic maps, and commercial and recreational fishing data.

14.5.1.3 Current Land Use

Land use can be residential, commercial/industrial, and recreational. The best way to determine the current land use or uses of a site and surrounding area is with a site visit. Determine if there are playgrounds, parks, businesses, industries, or other land uses on or in the vicinity of the site.

14.5.1.4 Activity Patterns

Determine the percent of time that the potentially exposed population(s) spends in the contaminated area. For people in a commercial or industrial area, a reasonable maximum daily exposure period is likely to be eight hours. If the population is residential, a maximum daily exposure period of 24 hours is possible. We should determine if activities occur primarily indoors, outdoors, or both. Determine how activities change with the seasons.

14.5.2 Cancer and Noncancer Endpoints

14.5.2.1 Choosing Toxicity Information

Calculation of risk from carcinogens and noncarcinogens are conducted differently. EPA uses a three-tiered approach for using data for risk assessments. They are:

Tier 1: EPA's IRIS Integrated Risk Information System—www.epa.gov/iris/

Tier 2: EPA's Provisional Peer Reviewed Toxicity Values (PPRTVs)—The Office of Research and Development/National Center for Environmental Assessment/Superfund Health Risk Technical Support Center (STSC) develops PPRTVs on a chemical-specific basis when requested by EPA's Superfund program.

Tier 3: Other Toxicity Values—Tier 3 includes additional EPA and non-EPA sources of toxicity information. Priority should be given to those sources of information that are the most current, the basis for which is transparent and publicly available, and which have been peer reviewed. The California Environmental Protection Agency (Cal EPA) toxicity values are peer reviewed and address both cancer and noncancer effects. Cal EPA toxicity values are available on the Cal EPA Internet web site at www.oehha.ca.gov/risk/chemicalDB//index.asp.

The Agency for Toxic Substances and Disease Registry (ATSDR) Minimal Risk Levels (MRLs) are estimates of the daily human exposure to a hazardous substance that is likely to be without appreciable risk of adverse noncancer health effects over a specific duration of exposure. The ATSDR MRLs are peer reviewed and are available at http://www.atsdr.cdc.gov/mrls/index.html on the ATSDR web site.

14.5.2.2 Noncarcinogens

There are a number of methods available for evaluating noncancer toxicity of chemicals. One is using a no-observed effect level with uncertainty factors and the other is the benchmark dose. Both methods can be used to calculate a chronic reference dose.

Chronic Reference Dose (RfD) RfD is an estimate (with uncertainty spanning perhaps an order of magnitude) of a daily oral exposure for a chronic duration (up to a lifetime) to the human population (including sensitive subgroups) that is likely to be without an appreciable risk of deleterious effects during a lifetime. It can be derived from a NOAEL, LOAEL, or benchmark dose, with uncertainty factors generally applied to reflect limitations of the data used. The RfD is generally used in EPA's noncancer health assessments.

An RfD is derived from the no-observed adverse effect level (NOAEL) by consistent application of uncertainty factors (UFs) that reflect various types of data sets used to estimate RfDs. For example, a valid chronic animal NOAEL is normally divided by a UF of 100. This represents an uncertainy factor of 10 for interspecies variability and 10 for intraspecies variabiltiy. In addition, a modifying factor (MF), may be used based on a professional judgment of the entire database of the chemical. These modifying factors generally vary from 3 to 10.

Chronic Reference Concentration (RfC) RfC is an estimate (with uncertainty spanning perhaps an order of magnitude) of a continuous inhalation exposure for a chronic duration (up to a lifetime) to the human population (including sensitive subgroups) that is likely to be without an appreciable risk of deleterious effects during a lifetime. It can be derived from a NOAEL, lowest observed adverse effect level (LOAEL), or benchmark concentration, with uncertainty factors generally applied to reflect limitations of the data used.

The RfD is determined by use of the following equation:

$$\mathrm{RfD} = \mathrm{NOAEL}/(\mathrm{UF} \times \mathrm{MF})$$

The no-observed adverse effect level is determined from a critical study of the agent in question.

For some volatile chemicals, EPA has calculated RfC, reference concentrations of the chemical in air. RfCs are represented in mg/m^3.

Benchmark Dose EPA and California EPA may use an alternative method to calculate the reference dose. One is called the benchmark dose. The benchmark dose (BMD) or concentration (BMC) is a dose or concentration that produces a predetermined change in response rate of an adverse effect (called the benchmark response or BMR) compared to background.

Benchmark dose level (BMDL)or benchmark concentration level(BMCL) is a statistical lower confidence limit on the dose or concentration at the BMD or BMC, respectively. Benchmark response (BMR) is an adverse effect, used to define a benchmark dose from which an RfD (or RfC) can be developed. The change in response rate over background of the BMR is usually in the range of 5 to 10%, which is the limit of responses typically observed in well-conducted animal experiments.

The use of the benchmark dose requires using data from multiple studies. EPA has benchmark dose software available for free on its Internet site.

Example of USEPA Benchmark Dose Model for Continuous Data

$$\text{Linear model } u(dose) = b + c_1 d$$

Used for body weight gain where:

U(dose) = the expected value of the response
b = background
c = polynomial coefficient
d = dose

14.5.2.3 Carcinogens

EPA uses two methods to calculate cancer potency. One is the nonlinear dose response, which is a pattern of frequency or severity of biological response that does not vary directly with the amount of dose of an agent. The second is the linear dose response, which is a pattern of frequency or severity of biological response that varies directly with the amount of dose of an agent. Linear extrapolation is approriate when an agent has a mutagenic mode of action or acts through another mode of action expected to be linear at lower dose. Nonlinear extrapolation is appropriate when there is no evidence of linearity and there is sufficient information to support a mode of action that is nonlinear at low doses.

A cancer slope factor is an upper bound, approximating a 95% confidence limit, on the increased cancer risk from a lifetime exposure to an agent. This estimate, usually expressed in units of proportion (of a population) affected per mg/kg-day, is generally reserved for use in the low-dose region of the dose-response relationship; that is, for exposures corresponding to risks less than 1 in 100. EPA uses a number of different types of mathmatical models to calculate cancer slope factors. These include the Weibull model, Probit model, and Logistic model, a dose-response model used for low-dose extrapolation. The Multistage model is a mathematical function used to extrapolate the probability of cancer from animal bioassay data; the Multistage Weibull model is a dose-response model for low-dose extrapolation that includes a term for decreased survival time associated with tumor incidence; and the One Hit model is a dose-response model based on a mechanistic argument that there is a response after a target site has been hit by a single biologically effective unit of dose within a given time period. EPA publishes its calculated reference doses and cancer slopes on its Integrated Risk Information System and will show the calculations and models used to determine the RfDs and slope factors.

EPA has been redefining its classification system for carcinogens. The traditional system was:

Group A: Human Carcinogen

This group is used only when there is sufficient evidence from epidemiologic studies to support a causal association between exposure to the agents and cancer.

Group B: Probable Human Carcinogen

This group includes agents for which the weight of evidence of human carcinogenicity based on epidemiologic studies is "limited" and also includes agents for which the weight of evidence of carcinogenicity based on animal studies is "sufficient". The group is divided into two subgroups. Usually, Group B1 is reserved for agents for which there is limited evidence of carcinogenicity from epidemiological studies. It is reasonable, for practical purposes, to regard an agent for which there is "sufficient evidence of carcinogenicity" in animals as if it presented a carcinogenic risk to humans. Therefore, agents for which there is "sufficient" evidence from animal studies and for which there is "inadequate evidence" or "no data" from epidemiologic studies would usually be categorized under Group B2.

Group C: Possible Human Carcinogen

This group is used for agents with limited evidence of carcinogenicity in animals in the absence of human data. It includes a wide variety of evidence, e.g., (a) a malignant tumor response in a single well-conducted experiment that does not meet conditions for sufficient evidence, (b) tumor responses of marginal statistical significance in studies having inadequate design or reporting, (c) benign but not malignant tumors with an agent showing no response in a variety of short-term tests for mutagenicity, and (d) responses of marginal statistical significance in a tissue known to have a high or variable background rate.

Group D: Not Classifiable as to Human Carcinogenicity

This group is generally used for agents with inadequate human and animal evidence of carcinogenicity or for which no data are available.

Group E: Evidence of Non-Carcinogenicity for Humans

This group is used for agents that show no evidence for carcinogenicity in at least two adequate animal tests in different species or in both adequate epidemiologic and animal studies.

The designation of an agent as being in Group E is based on the available evidence and should not be interpreted as a definitive conclusion that the agent will not be a carcinogen under any circumstances.

Source: ***U.S. EPA (1986) Guidelines for Carcinogen Risk Assessment.***

A new set of definitions has been suggested by EPA. Using a weight of evidence descriptor these are:

1. Carcinogenic to humans
2. Likely to be carcinogenic to humans
3. Suggestive evidence of carcinogenic potential
4. Inadequate information to assess caecinogenic potential
5. Not likely to be carcinogenic to humans

These descriptions should contain key evidence supporting these conclusions, a summary of key default options used, and a summary of potential modes of action.

There is also a guidance for assessing early life exposure to carcinogens. This recommends a quantitative adjustment of cancer slope factors only for chemicals having a mutagenic mode of action (MOA). The conclusion is there can be a greater susceptability in early life for the development of cancer as a result of exposures to chemicals with a mutagenic MOA compared to later in life.

14.5.3 Hazard Index

The hazard index is used for mixtures of chemicals. The concentration of a chemical is divided by a health-based standard or guideline and its ratio is added to the ratios of the other chemicals in the mixture.

$$HI = C_1/HS1 + C_2/HS_2 + \ldots\ldots + Cn/HSn$$

where:

HI = Hazard index
C_1 = the first contaminant concentration
HS_1 = the first health based standard

U.S. EPA Risk Assessment Guidelines recommend generating a separate hazard index for each group of chemicals defined by a common toxicity endpoint. All carcinogens fall under one endpoint: cancer. The endpoints for noncarcinogenic, or systemic, toxicants are the affected organ or organ system. U.S. EPA uses the same studies to calculate the reference doses that were used to identify the toxicological endpoints for the systemic toxicants.

Some examples of these toxicological endpoints for systemic toxicants include liver, stomach, kidney; developmental effects; and male reproductive, cardiovascular, endocrine, and nervous systems.

We would not use the additive model for contaminants to substances or chemicals in a mixture that do not share a common toxic endpoint. A hazard index equal to 1.0 for a mixture is analogous to the HS for an individual contaminant. Therefore, a hazard index greater than 1.0 indicates that the mixture exceeds the health risk limit. Contaminants that have more than one toxicological endpoint listed should be included in all the appropriate toxicological endpoint groups. Group the contaminants in the mixture according to the health effects they cause.

Example

Well water contains 1,2-dibromoethane at .002 mg/L at and carbon tetrachloride at .003 mg/L. Both are liver toxins, therefore they will be added together using the Hazard Index formula. The EPA RfDs can be used as the health-based standard. For 1,2-dibromoethane it is 9×10^{-3} mg/kg/day and for carbon tetrachloride it is 7×10^{-4}-mg/kg/day.

For a 70 kg man the HS for 1,2 dibromomethane would be $9 \times 10^{-3} \times 70$ kg, or 0.63mg. The HS for carbon tetrachloride would be $7 \times 10^{-4} \times 70$ kg or 0.05 mg.

Drinking two liters of water a day, the total daily concentration of 1,2-dibromomethane would be .004 mg and carbon tetrachloride would be .006 mg. Therefore:

HI = .004 mg/.63 mg + .006 mg/.05 mg
HI = .0063 mg + .12 mg
HI = .126 mg

The mixture total is less than 1, therefore it has not exceeded liver endpoint for toxicity. Note that using the hazard index does not take into account synergistic or antagonist effect of multiple chemicals. A hazard index is not used for carcinogenic risk for chemical mixtures. If the chemicals are carcinogenic, their cancer slopes can be added together when calculating risk.

14.5.4 Calculating Exposure Doses

The EPA, on their Mid Atlantic Risk Assessment website, publishes a list of preliminary remediation goals (PRGs). These are risk-based tools for evaluating contaminated sites. These goals incorporate exposure through inhalation, ingestion, and dermal exposure from ground water, surface water, and soil. Table 14.1 is a list of the default factors used by EPA Region 9.

Instead of using the generic approach in assessing sites, many risk assessors prefer to generate their own site specific data. In such cases, calculations are carried out to develop independent assessments.

14.5.4.1 Generic Exposure Dose

The generic exposure dose equation is

$$D = C \times IR \times AF \times EF/BW$$

where:

D = exposure dose (total dose of agent to person)
C = contaminant concentration (measured amount of agent in medium)
IR = intake rate of contaminated medium (how much of medium is exposed to body)
AF = bioavailablity factor (percent of total agent ingested, inhaled, or enters body)
EF = exposure factor (EF = (F × ED)/ AT)
F = frequency of exposure in days/year
ED = exposure duration (years)
AT = averaging time (ED × 365 days/year)
BW = bodyweight (exposed person's weight in kilograms. Standard defaults are listed in Table 14.1)

In most cases the bioavailabilty factor is assumed to be 1 (100%) unless there are well-conducted studies that have determined what percent of a substance has actually entered the blood stream after exposure through inhalation, ingestion, or skin contact.

Many risk assessors calculate their own default values for parameters particular to the population and location of the affected site. For example some use a woman's bodyweight instead of a man's as a default. Some standard default values for various parameters are noted here:

Bodyweight (BW) adult = 70 kg, child 1–6 years 16 kg, infant 10 kg
Exposure duration (ED) 70 years = lifetime, 30 years; upper bound time (90th percentile) spent at one residence, 9 years; median time spent at one residence, 6 years; child 1–6 years old.
Water intake rates = 2 liters/day for an adult and 1 liter/day for a child.

An example of calculating an exposure factor follows:
A child plays on contaminated soil in a playground five days a week, for three months each summer over a two-year period.

EF = (F × ED)/AT
EF = ([5 days/week × 12 weeks/year] × 2 years)/ (2 years × 365 days/year)
EF = 0.027

Site-specific exposure conditions should be used to determine the exposure factor.

When calculating drinking water exposure, the total dose comes from not only drinking the water, but if the substance is a volatile organic compound, also from inhalation and skin contact. The magnitude of these exposures depends on how much water is consumed,

Table 14.1 Standard Default Factors (Source: EPA Region 9)

Symbol	Definition (units) Default	Reference
CSFo	Cancer slope factor oral (mg/kg-d)-1	IRIS, PPRTV, HEAST, NCEA, or California
CSFi	Cancer slope factor inhaled (mg/kg-d)-1	IRIS, PPRTV, HEAST, NCEA, or California
RfDo	Reference dose oral (mg/kg-d)	IRIS, PPRTV, HEAST, NCEA, or California
RfDi	Reference dose inhaled (mg/kg-d)	IRIS, PPRTV, HEAST, NCEA, or California
TR	Target cancer risk 10^{-6}	
THQ	Target hazard quotient 1	
BWa	Body weight, adult (kg) 70	RAGS (Part A), EPA 1989 (EPA/540/1–89/002)
BWc	Body weight, child (kg) 15	Exposure Factors, EPA 1991 (OSWER No. 9285.6-03)
ATc	Averaging time – carcinogens (days) 25550	RAGS(Part A), EPA 1989 (EPA/540/1–89/002)
ATn	Averaging time – noncarcinogens (days) ED*365	
SAa	Exposed surface area for soil/dust (cm_2/day) – adult resident 5700 – adult worker 3300	Dermal Assessment, EPA 2004 (EPA/540/R-99/005)
SAc	Exposed surface area, child in soil (cm_2/day) 2800	Dermal Assessment, EPA 2004 (EPA/540/R-99/005)
AFa	Adherence factor, soils (mg/cm_2) – adult resident 0.07 – adult worker 0.2	Dermal Assessment, EPA 2004 (EPA/540/R-99/005)
AFc	Adherence factor, child (mg/cm_2) 0.2	Dermal Assessment, EPA 2004 (EPA/540/R-99/005)
ABS	Skin absorption defaults (unitless):	
	– semi-volatile organics 0.1	Dermal Assessment, EPA 2004 (EPA/540/R-99/005)
	– volatile organics	Dermal Assessment, EPA 2004 (EPA/540/R-99/005)
	– inorganics	Dermal Assessment, EPA 2004 (EPA/540/R-99/005)
IRAa	Inhalation rate – adult (m_3/day) 20	Exposure Factors, EPA 1991 (OSWER No. 9285.6-03)
IRAc	Inhalation rate – child (m_3/day) 10	Exposure Factors, EPA 1997 (EPA/600/P-95/002Fa)
IRWa	Drinking water ingestion – adult (L/day) 2	RAGS(Part A), EPA 1989 (EPA/540/1–89/002)
IRWc	Drinking water ingestion – child (L/day) 1	PEA, Cal-EPA (DTSC, 1994)
IRSa	Soil ingestion – adult (mg/day) 100	Exposure Factors, EPA 1991 (OSWER No. 9285.6-03)
IRSc	Soil ingestion – child (mg/day), 200	Exposure Factors, EPA 1991 (OSWER No. 9285.6-03)
IRSo	Soil ingestion – occupational (mg/day) 100	Soil Screening Guidance (EPA 2001a)
EFr	Exposure frequency – residential (d/y) 350	Exposure Factors, EPA 1991 (OSWER No. 9285.6-03)
EFo	Exposure frequency – occupational (d/y) 250	Exposure Factors, EPA 1991 (OSWER No. 9285.6-03)
EDr	Exposure duration – residential (years) 30[a]	Exposure Factors, EPA 1991 (OSWER No. 9285.6-03)
EDc	Exposure duration – child (years) 6	Exposure Factors, EPA 1991 (OSWER No. 9285.6-03)
EDo	Exposure duration – occupational (years) 25	Exposure Factors, EPA 1991 (OSWER No. 9285.6-03)
Age-Adjusted Factors for Carcinogens:		
IFSadj	Ingestion factor, soils ([mg-yr]/[kg-d]) 114	RAGS (Part B), EPA 1991 (OSWER No. 9285.7-01B)
SFSadj	Dermal factor, soils ([mg-yr]/[kg-d]) 361	By analogy to RAGS (Part B)
InhFadj	Inhalation factor, air ([m_3-yr]/[kg-d]) 11	By analogy to RAGS (Part B)
IFWadj	Ingestion factor, water ([L-yr]/[kg-d]) 1.1	By analogy to RAGS (Part B)
VFw PEF	Volatilization factor for water (L/m_3) 0.5	RAGS(Part B), EPA 1991 (OSWER No. 9285.7-01B)
VFs	Particulate emission factor (m_3/kg). See below.	Soil Screening Guidance (EPA 1996a,b)
	Volatilization factor for soil (m_3/kg). See below.	Soil Screening Guidance (EPA 1996a,b)
sat	Soil saturation concentration (mg/kg). See below.	Soil Screening Guidance (EPA 1996a,b)

[a]Exposure duration for lifetime residents is assumed to be 30 years total. For carcinogens, exposures are combined for children (6 years) and adults (24 years).

how often someone bathes or showers, and air exchange rates inside the home. Although in many cases the inhalation and dermal exposures may not be known, it is safe to assume they can contribute as much total absorbtion as the ingestion of drinking water alone.

Drinking water ingestion is:

$$D = (C \times IR \times EF)/BW$$

where:

D = exposure dose
C = contaminant concerntration (mg/L)
IR = intake rate of contaminated water (L/day)
EF = exposure factor (unitless)
BW = bodyweight (kg)

Use default drinking water value.

For example, a man has a well contaminated with tetrachloroethylene at a concentration of 100 micrograms/L:

D = (C X IR X EF)/BW
D = (0.1 mg/L x 2/L day x 1)/70 kg
D = 2.8 micrograms of tetrachloroethylene per kilogram bodyweight per day

For a child with the same concentration in the water, the result would be

D = (0.1 mg/L x 1L x 1)/10
D = 10 micrograms of tetrachloroethylen per kilogram bodyweight per day.

You can see that a child will consume more chemical per bodyweight than an adult using the same water supply.

14.5.4.2 Dermal Contact

As mention previously, dermal absorption of contaminants in water can be significant. The permeability of the skin to a chemical is influenced by an agent's molecular weight, electrostatic charge, hydrophobicity, and solubility in aqueous and lipid media. Chemicals that can penetrate the skin easily, are generally nonionized, lipid soluble, low molecular weight substances. Chemical-specific permeability coefficients should be used to estimate dermal absorption of a chemical from water.

Water Dermal Contact Dose Equation

$$D = (C \times P \times SA \times ET \times CF)/BW$$

D = dose (mg/kg/day)
C = contamination concentration (mg/L)
P = permeability coefficient (cm/hr)
SA = exposed body surface area (cm^2)
ET = exposure time (hours/day)
CF = conversion factor (1 Liter = 1000 cm^3)
BW = bodyweight (kg)

Dermal absorption of contaminants from soil is dependent on the area of contact, the duration of contact, the chemical adherence to the soil, and the degree to which the contaminant can penetrate the skin. Lipophilic properties, polarity, molecular weight, volatility, and solubility also affect dermal absorption from soil. A typical scenario for residential risk is a young child playing in the back yard on contaminated soil.

Soil Dermal Contact Calculation

$$D = (C \times A \times AF \times EF \times CF)/BW$$

where:

D = dose (mg/kg/day)
C = contaminant concentration (mg/kg)
A = total soil adhered (mg)
AF = bioavailability factor (unitless)
EF = exposure factor (unitless)
CF = conversion factor (10^6kg/mg)
BW = body weight (kg)

14.5.4.3 Inhalation

Experimental studies have demonstrated that volatile organic chemicals (VOCs) can be transferred from water to air, especially in showers and dishwashers where the water is heated. VOCs released to the air eventually pervade the rest of the house. Modeling has been used to calculate the concentration of VOCs in air in various parts of the house as a result of VOC release during indoor water use. Be aware the models that exist can over- or underestimate exposure. Another type of exposure in the home can come from a house sitting above an aquifer contaminated with a volatile compound. This compound can migrate through the soil into the home. This is an important route of exposure for radon gas.

Exposure Doses from Inhalation of Contaminated Air

$$D = (C \times IR \times EF)/BW$$

where:

D = exposure dose (mg/kg/day)
C = contaminant concentration (mg/m^3)
IR = intake rate (m^3)/day)
EF = exposure factor (unitless)
BW = body weight (kg)

Some generic default air intake rate examples:

10m^3/day for a child 6–8 years old
15.2m^3/day male, 19–65+ years old

14.5.5 Plant Models

For a complete analysis of food chain exposures for humans, it is necessary to estimate concentrations of contaminants in plants directly consumed by humans and in plants consumed by animals that are then eaten by humans. Plants may be exposed to contaminants as a result of direct deposition onto plant surfaces (wet and dry deposition, including resuspension), root uptake from soil, and irrigation with contaminated water.

Resuspension accounts for contaminants deposited on soil that are resuspended in air by wind, rainsplash, or physical disturbance and subsequently deposited on plant surfaces. When possible, samples of plants or plant products should be used to estimate exposure concentrations (EPA 1989c).

14.5.5.1 General Model

As noted previously, the general model for estimating contaminant concentrations in and on plants includes root uptake and foliar deposition from air and resuspended soil. Where irrigation is a significant management practice, components accounting for root uptake and resuspension of contaminants originating in irrigation water and direct deposition of irrigation water on plant surfaces can be added. Therefore, the comprehensive plant model for a site where irrigation is a consideration is:

$$\text{Cplant} = \text{Cplant-us} + \text{Cplant-da} + \text{Cplant-rs} + \text{Cplant-ui} + \text{Cplant-di} + \text{Cplant-ri}$$

where:

Cplant = concentration in and on plant estimated based on root uptake and foliar deposition (mg/kg or pCi/kg)
Cplant-us = concentration in plant tissue resulting from root uptake from soil (mg/kg or pCi/kg)
Cplant-da = concentration in edible parts of plant as a result of direct deposition of airborne contaminants (mg/kg or pCi/kg)
Cplant-rs = concentration in edible parts of plant as a result of resuspension of contaminants associated with soil (mg/kg or pCi/kg)
Cplant-ui = concentration in plant tissue associated with root uptake of contaminants resulting from irrigation F-6 (mg/kg or pCi/kg)

Table 14.2 Distribution Factors for Total Skin Surface Area/Body Weight Ratio by Age

Age	Arithmetic mean (cm^2/kg)	Standard deviation (cm^2/kg)
0–2	641	114
2–18	423	76
>18	248	28

Cplant-di = concentration in edible parts of plant as a result of direct deposition of contaminants in irrigation water (mg/kg or pCi/kg)

Cplant-ri = concentration in edible parts of plant as a result of resuspension of contaminants associated with irrigation water (mg/kg or pCi/kg)

The last three terms of this model are set to zero if irrigation is not a consideration.

14.5.5.2 Surface Area

EPA's recommended value for an average surface area of a male adult body is 1.94 m^2. Since surface area is a function of the body weight, Finley developed a relationship between skin surface area, body, weight, and age based on lognormal distributed factors. These factors are presented in Table 14.2.

Sometimes the solution for reducing the risk at a site actually introduces new risks to the population. Some things to keep in mind when coming up with a site clean-up plan are as follows.

Comparison of the baseline human health risk assessment and the risk evaluation of alternatives. Baseline Human Health Risk Assessment (quantitative):

- Contaminant sources
- Uncontrolled site remedial activity and residual contamination
- May include chemicals not present under baseline conditions (e.g., those created during remediation)
- Timing of releases
- Releases due to natural processes (e.g., leaching, weathering)
- Releases due to implementation of remedy
- Exposed populations
- Current and potential future current, remediation workers, and potential future (if residual risks are present)
- Duration: includes lifetime exposure; long-term includes lifetime exposure, short-term includes only less-than-lifetime exposure

14.6 RADIOLOGICAL RISK ASSESSMENTS

Radiological risk assessments differ from conventional chemical assessments. Radiation toxicology is well researched and EPA has set preventative action guidelines (PAGS) to be used in a radiological emergency. Health effects from radiation range from severe (death, cancer, immune system destruction) to less severe (hematological deficiencies, nausea, vomiting, hair loss, and chromosomal changes) Thyroid, skin, and fetal cancers are the most common cancers associated with radiation poisoning.

Radiation exposure is called a Roentgen. This exposure is a measure of the ability of photons to produce ionization in air. Most commonly available instruments give the exposure rate in Roentgen per hour (R/hr). Absorbed dose (rad) is a measure of energy imparted per unit mass. One rad is the dose delivered to any material that receives 100 ergs of energy per gram.

Dose equivalent (rem) is a measure of biological damage that is calculated by multiplying absorbed dose by quality factor for the type of radiation involved. The unit of dose is the *rem*. The TEDE (total dose equivalent) is a term that combines the effects of both the internal and external exposures.

There are three phases of a radiological accident: early, intermediate, and late. The *early* phase of an incident is characterized by a need to make immediate decisions about protective actions. These actions are based on a nuclear power plants status and dose projections. Recommendations may be shelter in place or evacuation if the dose is greater than 1 rem.

The *intermediate* phase is used to determine the need to relocate from an area where contamination levels exceed 2 rem TEDE in the first year following cessation of a release. Long-term goals include relocation of individuals if the second year or any subsequent year TEDE dose would exceed 0.5 rem and the 50-year projected dose would exceed 5 rem TEDE.

Nuclear reactor accident assessments consider the five R's:

Restricted zone is an area with controlled access from which the population has been evacuated. People may be permitted back temporarily into a restricted zone (farmers to milk their cows).

Relocation is the removal or continued evacuation of people from contaminated areas, to prevent chronic radiation exposure.

Return is the reoccupation of areas that have been remediated and cleared for unrestricted use.

Reentry is the temporary entry into a restricted zone under controlled conditions.

Recovery is the process of reducing radiation exposure rates and concentrations to acceptable levels.

Emergency workers during nuclear emergencies, have their own set of dose thresholds, in order to perform their jobs. These are found in Table 14.3. Risk assessment of a radioactive event must take into account exposure from *cloudshine*, which is direct exposure through the air of gamma radiation; *inhalation of particles* contaminated with radioactive iodine; and *groundshine*, which is the radiation given off from deposition and which is the reflection of radiation from contaminated soils and consumption of contaminated food and water.

The Food and Drug Administration has developed derived intervention levels (DIL) for food. A DIL is

Table 14.3 EPA/Department of Energy Dose Limits for Workers Performing Emergency Services (EPA Manual of Protective Actions, 1992)

TEDE Dose Limit (rem)	Eye Dose Limit (rem)	Organ, Thyroid, Skin Dose Limit (rem)	Activity	EPA/DOE Dose Limits for Workers Performing Emergency Services
5	15	50	All	
10	30	100	Protecting major/valuable property	Where lower dose limit is not practicable
25	75	250	Lifesaving or protection of large populations	Where lower dose limit is not practicable
>25	>75	250	Lifesaving or protection of large populations	Only on a voluntary basis by persons fully aware of the risks involved

Table 14.4 Cancer Risk to Average Individuals from 25 rem Effective Dose Equivalent Delivered Promptly

Age at Exposure (years)	Approximate Risk of Premature Death (deaths per 1000 persons exposed)
20 to 30	9.1
30 to 40	7.2
40 to 50	5.3
50 to 60	3.5

Source: EPA92, Table 2–4 FRMAC (2005)

the concentration in food that equals the PAG if ingested over the relevant period of time.

$$\text{DIL} = \text{PAG (f) (food intake) (DC)}$$

where:

DIL = derived intervention level Bq/kg
PAG = protective action guideline, mSv
F = fraction of food assumed contaminated
Food intake = quantity of food consumed kg
DC = dose received per unit of activity mSv/Bq
Sv = Seivert = 100 rem
Bq = Becquerel = quantity of radioactive material in which one atom is transformed per second or undergoes one disintegration per second

The risk from consuming radioactively contaminated food can be calculated by actually analyzing the food or using field soil and air measurements in conjunction with computer modeling.

14.7 RISK MANAGEMENT

Risk management is the process of weighing policy alternatives and selecting the appropriate regulatory action. Figure 14.1 shows that all previous calculations lead eventually to risk management (Figure 14.2) and risk

Risk assessment process and use

Hazard identification
Exposure assessment
Dose-response assessment
Risk characterization
Risk management and risk communication

Figure 14.1 Risk Assessment Process and Use.

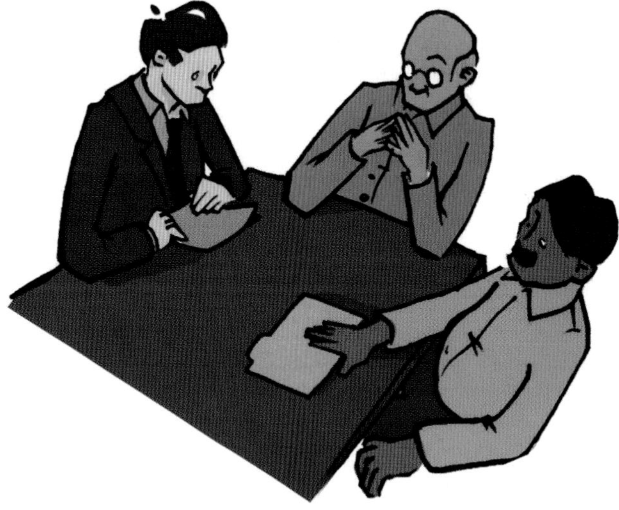

Figure 14.2 Risk Management Planning. With permission of Ira Marcks.

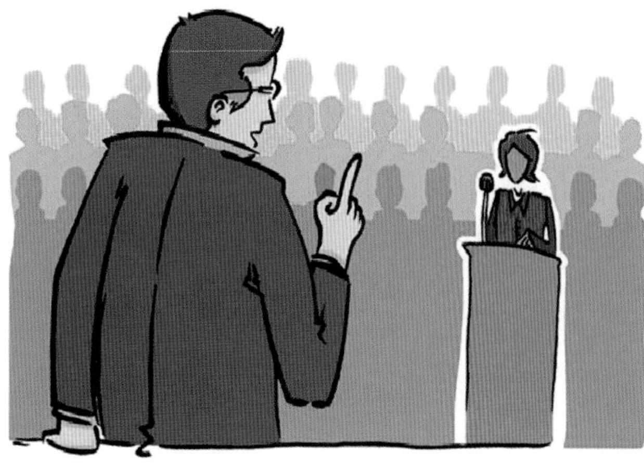

Figure 14.3 Risk Communication at public meeting. With permission of Ira Marcks.

communication (Figure 14.3). A risk manager will take the information provided by the risk assessor, and also consider social, economic, political, and engineering factors. Sometimes risk management is constrained by regulatory legislation. The role of the risk manager is to find a practical solution for cleaning up a contaminated site, while protecting human health to the greatest degree and keeping the project economically feasible. Table 14.5 shows sources of contamination and types of remediation available to counteract the hazards.

As a risk manager you have a small town of 24,000 people with a public water system that is contaminated with trichloroethylene. It has been determined that the concentration of chemicals will cause an increase in cancer over a lifetime, to the average user, of five in 10,000. This is determined to be an unacceptable risk. The engineering cost of finding and developing a new water source is \$3 million. This should remove all risk from exposure to this chemical. Engineering the existing system using certain equipment will reduce the cancer risk to one in 1,000,000 at a cost of \$25,000 annually, adding hundreds of dollars to everyone in town's yearly water bills. Another, simpler engineering solution, at a cost of \$6,000 a year will reduce the risk to one in 100,000. The town knows they don't have \$3 million, so option one is not considered. The town may decide that a small reduction in risk, at a huge cost is not worth it; therefore, the town opts for the third solution.

Table 14.5 Remedial Technologies and Associated Source Type Categories

Source Type Category	Associated Remedial Technologies
VOC point sources	Air strippers, soil vapor extraction units, thermal desorption units Thermal destruction units (incinerators)
Particulate point sources	Thermal destruction units (incinerators), thermal desorption units
VOC area sources	Excavation, dredging, solidification/ stabilization,
Particulate area sources	Excavation, materials handling, solidification/stabilization

Another solution for reducing risk at a contaminated site is to restrict access. A town may have a contaminated property, for example, the site of an old machine factory. The cost of digging up the contaminated soils and transporting them to a hazardous waste landfill is prohibitive. One option is to put a fence around the site, to keep the public off the land. Another is to cap the site with a layer of clay and clean soil. As long as the fence is maintained and the cap is not disturbed, the hazard of the site still remains, but the exposure to the hazard has been removed. Therefore the risk from the site has been eliminated as long as the institutional controls are maintained.

Sometimes, the risk to the public does not come from the area where the public resides. An example is the migration of mercury from coal-fired plants in the Midwest being carried into the atmosphere and deposited into lakes the Northeast. The mercury converts to methyl mercury and then bioaccumulates and eventually concentrates in fish in those lakes. This results in the issuance of fish consumption advisories in the affected areas. In developing the Clean Air Mercury Rule, the U.S. EPA modeled the location of mercury deposition using a spatially explicit air quality model to assess the magnitude of fish contamination and a behavioral model to assess population consumption patterns of these fish. EPA reported monetized benefits from implementing the Clean Air Mercury Rule, measured as decreases in IQ.

14.7.1 Risk Management Factors in Cost and Feasibility

There are a number of drinking water standards for chemicals that are based on best available technology for removing the chemical. This does not always coincide with a health-based standard. The Environmental Protection Agency developed a health-based drinking-water standard for uranium at 20 ug/L. Due to costs associated with public water systems achieving this number, EPA settled on a standard of 30 ug/L.

Another approach of risk management is cost–benefit. Cost calculations can be based on number of lives saved or additional years of life. Burnett and Hahn examined the proposed EPA rule to lower the arsenic drinking water standard from 50 ug/ to 10 ug/L. They stated that EPA used the value of a human life at \$6.1 million dollars. EPA determined that people are willing to pay up to \$6.1 million dollars per life saved to implement a policy to reduce safety and health risks. EPA's model showed 28 lives saved, which translated into a benefit of \$170 million dollars, but the costs of saving those 28 lives was \$210 million dollars. Therefore, the cost effectiveness of the reduction was \$7.5 million dollars a life.

14.8 RISK COMMUNICATION

Risk assessment is of no use if it can't be explained to the public in an understandable manner. The attack on the World Trade Center buildings brought questions from the public about the air quality in the surrounding area. After the WTC terrorist attack, people received information from many different sources, and many factors could have influenced their actions and the actions of responders and clean-up crew. *Risk communication* is a critical component in aiding the public to minimize their exposure to potential health hazards. Risk communication is an interactive process of exchange of information among individuals and groups that involves multiple messages about the nature of risk. On September 18, 2001, seven days after the towers fell, the Environmental Protection Agency pronounced that the air was "safe" to breathe. Airborne dust from the collapse of the towers dispersed outdoors and indoors around Lower Manhattan. The mixture of building debris and combustion by-products contained such ingredients as asbestos, glass fibers, lead, and concrete dust. Some residences had rooms covered in dust for months after the incident. EPA monitored the air for some contaminants before they made their assessment that the air was safe to breathe, but they believed there were qualifications to this statement that the air was acceptable. These were the caveats for the "air was safe" statement:

1. For long-term health effects, not short-term or acute health effects
2. For the general public, not Ground Zero workers
3. For outdoor air, not indoor air
4. For healthy adults, not sensitive subpopulations such as children and the elderly
5. For asbestos, not other air pollutants

With the exception of caveat 2, most press releases did not contain these caveats.

The risk assessment process was incomplete because there was a lack of test results for many pollutants, and many test results were not completed for a number of days after sampling. There was also an absence of short-term health benchmarks for asbestos and other pollutants, and problems with asbestos monitoring. EPA did not have monitoring data to support reassurances made in their early press releases, because they lacked monitoring data for several contaminants, such as PCBs, particulates, dioxin, and polyaromatic hydrocarbons.

Obviously, an important component of risk communication is if you do not know an answer or are uncertain, acknowledge it and do not hesitate to admit mistakes or disclose risk information. The Centers for Disease Control, to their credit, did admit they made mistakes about the information they supplied initially about anthrax, during the anthrax exposures to postal workers during October 2001. They stated that only workers who opened the letters contaminated with anthrax were at risk. It turned out that the spores could migrate out of the unopened letters, which ended up exposing other postal workers.

The public gets their risk information from the media, governmental agencies, or industry. Based on this information they can react with dread (fear, voluntary vs. no choice, threat to future) and knowledge (how well a risk is understood). Several authors have examined risk judgment as a two-part phenomenon, heuristic and systematic. A heuristic approach is a superficial reaction to risk information, whereas in a systematic mode, a person takes more time processing information before forming an opinion on the level of risk.

Risk communication, if done properly, will not necessarily alarm the public. Given information and education, the public can then express concerns, ask questions, and get accurate answers. Education is achieved through effective communication. Risk communicators shouldn't feel that the issues are too technical for the public. Covello and Allen established five rules for building trust and credibility:

1. Accept and involve the public as a partner. Work with and for the public to inform, dispel misinformation, and, to every degree possible, allay fears and concerns.
2. Appreciate the public's specific concerns. Statistics and probabilities don't necessarily answer all questions. Be sensitive to people's fears and worries on a human level. Your position does not preclude your acknowledging the sadness of an illness, injury, or death. Do not overstate or dwell on tragedy but do empathize with the public and provide answers that respect their humanity.
3. Be honest and open. Once lost, trust and credibility are almost impossible to regain. Never mislead the public by lying or failing to provide information that is important to their understanding of issues.
4. Work with other credible sources. Conflicts and disagreements among organizations and credible spokespersons create confusion and breed distrust. Coordinate your information and communications efforts with those of other legitimate parties.
5. Meet the needs of the media. Never refuse to work with the media. The media's role is to inform the public, which will be done with or without your assistance. Work with the media to ensure that the information they are providing the public is as accurate and enlightening as possible.

The two goals of risk communication are to ease the public's concern and to give guidance on how to respond to the risk.

REVIEW QUESTIONS

1. What are the six components of carrying a risk assessment from start to finish?
2. What are the some of the benefits and pitfalls of epidemiology studies?

3. What are some of the uncertainties with dose response assessments?
4. Why is exposure assessment vital to a risk assessment?
5. When conducting risk characterization, what are some important considerations for collecting soil samples?
6. Name some site-specific characteristics a risk assessor looks at and what tools can be used to identify those characteristics.
7. Name two methods for calculating RfDs.
8. How is a Hazard Index calculated?
9. Name three types of routes of entry into the body for volatile chemicals in a water supply.
10. What are the three phases of a radiological accident?
11. What is risk management?
12. What are some important features of successful risk communication?

REFERENCES

Bruckner, J. V., Keys, D. A., & Fisher, J. W. (2004). The Acute Exposure Guideline Level (AEGL) program: Applications of physiologically based pharmacokinetic modeling. *Journal of Toxicology and Environmental Health, 67*(8), 621–634.

Burnett, J. K., & Hahn, R., A Costly Benefit, Regulation pp. 44–49 Fall 2001.

Calabrese, E. J., Pastides, H., Barnes, R., et al. (1989). How much soil do young children ingest: An epidemiologic study. In E. J.Calabrese & P. T.Kostecki (Eds.), *Petroleum Contaminated Soils* (Vol. 2, pp. 363–417). Chelsea, MI: Lewis Publishers.

California EPA. (1994). *Preliminary Endangerment Assessment Guidance Manual (PEA)*. Sacramento, CA: Department of Toxic Substances Control.

California EPA. (1996). *Guidance for Ecological Risk Assessment at Hazardous Waste Sites and Permitted Facilities, Part A: Overview*. Sacramento, CA: Department of Toxic Substances Control.

Covello, V., & Allen, F., Seven Cardinal Rules of Risk Communication USEPA Office of Policy Analysis (1988).

Cowherd, C., Muleski, G., Engelhart, P., & Gillette, D. (1985). *Rapid Assessment of Exposure to Particulate Emission from Surface Contamination*. EPA/600/8–85/002. Prepared for Office of Health and Environmental Assessment, Washington, DC: U.S. Environmental Protection Agency, NTIS PB85-1922197AS.

Davis, S., Waller, P., Buschom, R., Ballou, J., & White, P. (1990). Quantitative estimates of soil ingestion in normal children between the ages of 2 and 7 years: Population-based estimates using Al, Si, and Ti as soil tracer elements. *Archives of Environmental Health, 45*, 112–122.

Emergency Management Institute, National Emergency Training Center. (October 2000). *Radiological Accident Assessment Concepts (E341) Precourse Workbook*.

EPA Final Evaluation Report: EPA's Response to the World Trade Center Collapse Report No. 2003-P-00012 (2003).

EPA Risk Assessment Guidelines A1 1989 5401/1-89/002.

EPA Supplemental Guidance for Assessing Susceptibility from Early-Life Exposure to Carcinogens. (2005). EPA/630/R-03/003F.

EPA Guidelines for Carcinogen Risk Assessment (Final). (2005). Washington, DC: U.S. Environmental Protection Agency, EPA/630/P-03/001F.

EPA Manual of Protective Action Guidelines and Protective Actions for Nuclear Incidents 1992 400R92001.

EPA Regulatory Impact Analysis of the Clean Air Mercury Rule. (2005). EPA-452/R-05-003. Washington, DC: Office of Air Quality Planning and Standards Environmental Air Quality Strategies and Standards Division, U.S. Environmental Protection Agency.

EPA Superfund Exposure Assessment Manual. (1988). EPA/540/1–88/001. Washington, DC: Office of Emergency and Remedial Response.

EPA Subsurface Contamination Reference Guide. (1990a). EPA/540/2–90/011. Washington, DC: Office of Emergency and Remedial Response.

EPA Exposure Factors Handbook. (1990b). EPA/600/8089/043. Washington, DC: Office of Health and Environmental Assessment.

EPA Risk Assessment Guidance for Superfund Volume 1: Human Health Evaluation Manual (Part B, Development of Risk-Based Preliminary Remediation Goals. (1991a). Publication 9285.7-01B. Washington, DC: Office of Emergency and Remedial Response, NTIS PB92-963333.

EPA Human Health Evaluation Manual, Supplemental Guidance: Standard Default Exposure Factors. (1991b). Publication 9285.6-03. Washington, DC: Office of Emergency and Remedial Response, NTIS PB91-921314.

EPA Technical Support Document for Land Application of Sewage Sludge. (1992a). Vols. I and II. Washington, DC: Office of Water. 822/R-93-001a,b.

EPA Dermal Exposure Assessment: Principles and Applications. (1992b). EPA/600/8–91/011B. Washington, DC: Office of Health and Environmental Assessment.

EPA Soil Screening Guidance: Technical Background Document. (1996a). EPA/540/R-95/128. Washington, DC: Office of Emergency and Remedial Response, PB96-963502.

EPA Soil Screening Guidance: User's Guide. (1996b). EPA/540/R-96/018. Washington, DC: Office of Emergency and Remedial Response, PB96-963505.

EPA Superfund Chemical Data Matrix. (1996c). EPA/540/R-96/028. Washington, DC: Office of Solid Waste and Emergency Response, PB94-963506.

EPA Ecological Risk Assessment Guidance for Superfund: Process for Designing and Conducting Ecological Risk Assessments, Interim Final. (1997b). EPA/540/R-97/006. Washington, DC: Office of Solid Waste and Emergency Response, PB97-963211.

EPA Supplemental Guidance for Developing Soil Screening Levels for Superfund Sites, Interim Guidance. (2001a). OSWER 9355.4–24.

EPA Guidance for Characterizing Background Chemicals in Soil at Superfund Sites (Draft) June 2001. (2001b). EPA/540/R-01/003. Washington, DC: Office of Solid Waste and Emergency Response.

EPA Evaluating the Vapor Intrusion to Indoor Air Pathway from Goundwater and Soils. Draft EPA/530/F/02/052.

EPA Risk Assessment Guidance for Superfund Volume I: Human Health Evaluation Manual (Part E, Supplemental Guidance for Dermal Risk Assessment), Final. EPA/540/R/99/005. Washington, DC: Office of Solid Waste and Emergency Response, PB99-963312, 2004.

EPA Health Effects Assessment Summary Tables (HEAST): Annual Update, FY. (1997). Washington, DC: National Center For Environmental Assessment (NCEA), Office of Research and Development and Office of Emergency and Remedial Response.

FRMAC Assessment Manual, Pre-Assessed Default Scenarios, The Federal Manual for Assesssing Environmental Data During a Radiological Emergency. (April 2003). (Vol. 3). SAND2003-1073P.

FRMAC Operations Manual. (2005). December DOE/NV/11718-080-Rev.2.

Henderson, R. F., Sabourin, P. J., Bechtold, W. E., Griffith, W. C., Medinsky, M. A., Birnbaum, L. S., et al. (1989). The effect of dose, dose rate, route of adminsitration, and species on tissue and blood levels of benzene metabolites. *Environmental Health Perspectives, 82*, 9–17.

Howard, P. H. (1990). *Handbook of Environmental Fate and Exposure Data for Organic Chemicals*. Chelsea, MI: Lewis Publishers.

Kahlor, L., et al. Studying Heuristic- Systematic Processing of Risk Communication, Risk Analysis, Vol. 23, No. 2, pp. 355–368, 2003.

Medinsky, M. A., Kenyon, E. M., Seaton, M. J., & Schlosser, P. M. (1996). Mechanistic considerations in benzene physiological model development. *Environmental Health Perspectives, 104*(Suppl. 6), 1399–1404.

Rinsky, R. A., Young, R. J., & Smith, A. B. (1981). Leukemia in benzene workers. *American Journal of Industrial Medicine, 2*, 217–245.

Rinsky, R. A., Smith, A. B., Horning, R., et al. (1987). Benzene and leukemia: An epidemiologic risk assessment. *The New England Journal of Medicine, 316*, 1044–1050.

Steinberg, K. K., Relling, M. V., Gallagher, M. L., Greene, C. N., Rubin, C. S., French, D., et al. (2007). Genetic Studies of a Cluster of Acute Lymphoblastic Leukemia Cases in Churchill County. *Nevada Environmental Health Perspectives, 115*(1), 158–164.

Tumbo, C. W., & McComas, K. A. The Function of Credibility in Information Processing for Risk Perception, Risk Analysis Vol. 23, No. 2, pp. 343–353, 2003.

Van Wijnen, J. H., Clausing, P., & Brunekreef, B. (1990). Estimated soil ingestion by children. *Environmental Research, 51*, 147–162.

Chapter

15

Drug Resistance

Lori Hazlehurst ▪ Miles Hacker

OUTLINE

15.1 INTRODUCTION

The need to increase drug dosage to maintain the desired pharmacological effects can result from the phenomenon known as drug tolerance (discussed elsewhere in the textbook) or as a result of drug resistance. The former is considered to result from changes in the host whereas the latter arises from changes in the target organism—most frequently cancer or infectious diseases. The purpose of this chapter is to define and describe mechanisms of drug resistance encountered in the treatment of infectious diseases or cancers. Drug resistance can lead to a complete loss of drug efficacy because the target organism no longer responds to pharmacologically relevant doses of the drugs. When drug resistance develops in cancer cells, the drug is often rendered useless because increasing the dose of the drug even slightly can lead to unacceptable host toxicity.

15.2 CANCER CELL DRUG RESISTANCE

Most cancers will initially respond to standard chemotherapy. However, failure to eliminate the entire tumor population (often referred to as minimal residual disease) and the subsequent emergence of drug resistance currently limits the cure rate of many malignancies. It is thought that genetic instability characteristic of tumors as well as the tumor microenvironment can contribute to the emergence of clinical drug resistance. Investigators have developed drug resistant tumor cell lines to aid in the identification of drug resistant mechanism and targets. These resistant cell lines have revealed that cancer cells can employ multiple mechanisms of drug resistance including (Figure 15.1):

- Altered drug transport
- Altered drug metabolism
- Altered drug target
- Enhanced repair of drug induced damage
- Altered apoptotic pathway

In this chapter we will discuss each of these mechanisms, and possible ways to overcome these forms of resistance, where available.

15.2.1 Drug Transporters and Drug Resistance

15.2.1.1 Drug Efflux Proteins

Exposing a parental tumor cell line to increasing amounts of a chemotherapeutic agent, until a drug resistant population emerges is a classic way to induce drug resistance. Once a resistant cell line has been created, investigators can use biochemical, pharmacological, and molecular techniques within an isogenic system to identify drug resistant mechanisms (Figure 15.2).

One of the most frequent phenotypic changes observed in drug resistant cell line models is a decrease in the intracellular concentration of the drug. Most anticancer drugs are designed to diffuse passively through the cell membrane. However, it must be noted that some anticancer agents use existing transport systems to enter the cell. For example, melphalan, an agent that covalently cross-links DNA, contains a phenylalanine group and is reported to use the large neutral amino acid transporter, which is

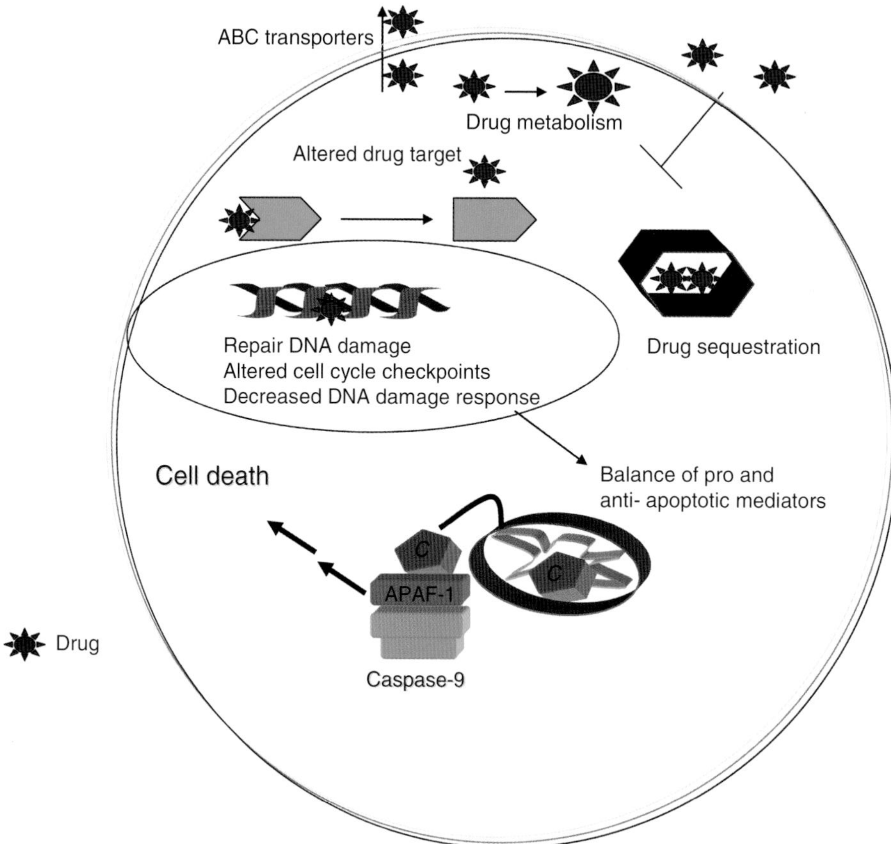

Figure 15.1 A cancer cell can evade drug-induced cell death by several mechanisms, making therapeutic intervention inherently challenging.

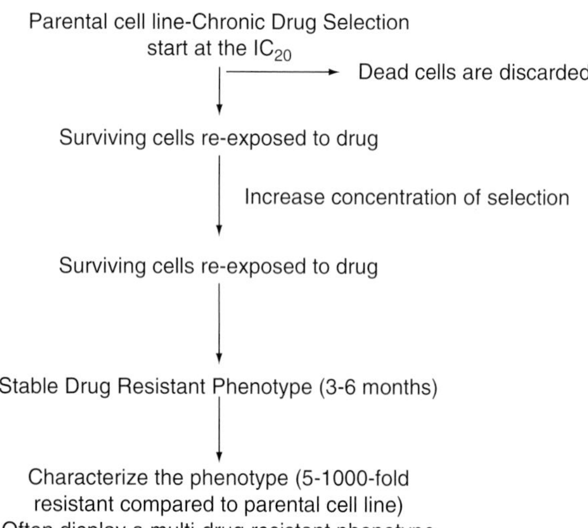

Figure 15.2 Typical method for developing acquired drug-resistant cells lines.

critical for proper nutrition and cell growth. Other examples of membrane transporters include methotrexate, which uses the folate transport system, and nucleoside analogs, which enter the cell via nucleoside transport proteins. Passive membrane diffusion is usually a slower process than is the carrier-mediated transporter system. Remember, however, that passive diffusion is an unsaturable concentration-driven process whereas carrier-mediated transport is saturable and dependent on the number of transporter proteins present in the cell membrane. Further, the carrier-mediated process can exist in at least two forms—facilitated transport, which can shuttle chemicals across the membrane but can not shuttle against a concentration gradient, or active transport, which is an ATP-dependent transporter capable of moving chemicals against a concentration gradient.

Decreased intracellular concentration of a carrier-mediated drug accumulation can result from mutated carrier protein such that drug recognition is decreased, and there is loss of membrane bound carrier or decreased rate of drug transport across the membrane. Another mechanism of drug resistance resulting from lowered intracellular drug accumulation also relies on a membrane protein, but in this case the pump serves as an efflux mechanism. In this case the drug most often enters the cell by simple passive diffusion, but as the drug diffuses across the cell membrane the efflux protein shuttles the drug out of the cell at sufficient rate to prevent drug accumulation to the cytotoxic level.

The first phenotypic demonstration of efflux transporters was reported in 1973 when Dano noted that daunorubicin was actively pumped out of daunorubicin-resistant Erhlich ascites tumor cells. Three years later it was reported that a 170 kd protein localized to the cellular membrane of drug resistant cells but not the parental cells; this newly identified protein was called P-glycoprotein or Pgp. Subsequently, laboratories reported that tumor cells that had elevated levels of the Pgp were cross-resistant to a number of chemically divergent anticancer drugs. Overexpression of membrane-bound Pgp has since been named multidrug resistance (MDR).

With the advent of powerful molecular tools it has been possible to identify the mRNA sequence of Pgp and show a striking similarity to drug transporters seen in many infectious diseases to be discussed later in this chapter. Pgp is an ATP-binding cassette (ABC) transporter protein composed of two homologous halves, each containing a transmembrane domain (TMD), a total of 12 transmembrane regions, and a nucleotide binding domain (NBD), separated by a flexible linker region.

Transport of one drug molecule requires the hydrolysis of two ATP events (H and R). The binding of substrate to the transmembrane regions results in the hydrolysis of one ATP causing a conformational change in the protein and the release of substrate to the outer leaflet of the membrane. Hydrolysis at the second ATP site is required for the transporter to bind another substrate. Thus it appears that ATP hydrolysis occurs sequentially rather than simultaneously to export one molecule of substrate.

Upon binding of ATP to the NBDs, Pgp undergoes conformational changes and the TMDs reorganize into three compact domains. This reorganization opens the central pore and allows transport of hydrophobic drugs (transport substrates) directly from the lipid bilayer into the central pore of the transporter.

The ability of this protein to efflux drug out of the tumor cell provides the tumor cell a significant means of protection. Further, the lack of chemical specificity of the protein provides the tumor cell protection from a variety of drugs once the membrane protein is expressed. An obvious question to be asked at this point is, If the protein pumps drugs out of the cell could we not inhibit the pump and thereby obviate the resistance factor the protein provides? Yet another approach would be to develop anticancer drugs not affected by the Pgp. In fact there exist a variety of drugs that are not substrates of the membrane pump but unfortunately some of our most important anticancer drugs such as doxorubicin, vincristine, and taxol are affected by this pump.

Investigators have attempted to identify drugs capable of just such a pharmacological activity. To date a number of Pgp inhibitors have been identified and are currently classified as first-, second-, or third-generation MDR inhibitors. The first-generation inhibitors had other unwanted pharmacological features and were not developed as they were not specific MDR inhibitors. Clinical trials revealed that such drugs were limited in activity and had rather significant toxicological potential.

Second-generation MDR inhibitors were more effective than their precursors but problems remained. Many of these drugs were substrates for the cytochrome P450 3A4 xenobiotic metabolizing enzyme and as a result caused unpredictable rises in plasma levels of the actual anticancer drug. Given the extraordinarily small therapeutic index for these drugs, any unanticipated elevation of drug plasma levels could have significant effects on host toxicity. Further, these drugs seemed to inhibit all the ABC transporter proteins. Given that this family of proteins has important roles in removal of xenobiotics from the host and limiting chemical access to the CNS, testes, and placenta inhibition of this family of proteins could lead to undesirable consequences as anticancer drugs would now have access to these previously protected tissue compartments.

Third-generation MDR inhibitors have been developed. These drugs do not affect cytochrome P450 3A4 nor do they appear to inhibit the normal ABC transporters. To date several such drugs have been tested but none have received FDA approval. Thus, the search for a chemical means to overcome MDR continues.

Reports of multidrug resistance in tumor cells that did not express the class Pgp form of MDR led investigators to search for alternate mechanisms of MDR. In 1992, Cole and Deeley identified MRP1 as being overexpressed and sharing homology to MDR1 in a human small cell lung carcinoma cell line selected for resistance to doxorubicin. This protein has three membrane spanning domains, two nucleotide binding domains, and an extracellular N-terminal. Both the structure and drug resistance spectra of MRP1 and Pgp are similar with the exception of the taxanes, which are poor substrates for MRP1. Following this initial observation an additional five MRP-related proteins have been described, and each has its own substrate and protein characteristics. As with the Pgp protein, each of these MRP proteins seems to have important physiological roles other than serving as anticancer drug efflux pumps.

Doyle et al. first identified BCRP (breast cancer resistance protein) following exposure of breast cancer cells to an anticancer drug called mitoxantrone, a chemical relative of daunomycin and doxorubicin. This dimeric protein requires either homo- or Homo-dimerization for the protein to function as a membrane-bound pump. Once dimerized the protein can shuttle drug extracellularly from the membrane in a manner similar to that of the other ABC cassette proteins such as Pgp.

Finally, a protein has been identified that is unique from the previously discussed ABC proteins. This protein, called lung resistance protein or major vault protein, has a molecular weight of 110 kD and is found not in the cell membrane but rather the nuclear membrane or the cytoplasm. The role of this protein is to prevent the drug from accessing the nucleus by trapping the drug in vesicles called vaults. The vaults then shuttle the drug to the cell membrane where the drug is then removed from the cell. An alternative pathway for the drug is that the LRP shuttles the drug to the lysosome where the drug is removed by exocytosis.

With these discoveries it became apparent that multiple drug transporters were likely to exist and function *in vivo.* Indeed the subsequent sequencing of the human genome revealed that the ABC transport family consists of 49 members, which are now organized into seven subfamilies (A-G).

Most of the 49 transporters recognize and transport a variety of xenobiotics as well as physiological substrates that include bile acids, peptides, steroid ions, and phospholipids. However, of these 49 transporters MRP1, Pgp and BCRP are the best documented for their role in conferring anticancer drug resistance and for this reason will be the focus of our discussion in this portion of the chapter.

Pgp, MRP1, and BCRP belong to the ABCB, ABCC, and ABCG family, respectively. Pgp (gene symbol ABCB1) has two nucleotide binding regions (NBD) that are separated by two membrane spanning domains (MSD). Each MSD is comprised of six transmembrane regions (Figure 15.3). MRP1 (gene symbol ABCC1) contains three MSD domains and the NH2 terminus is located on the extracellular surface; in

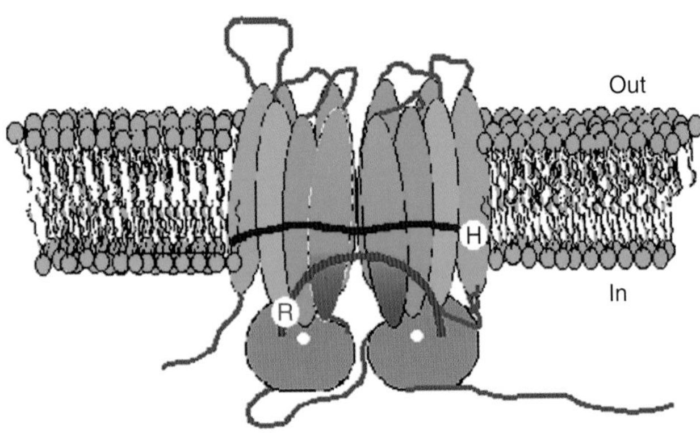

Figure 15.3 Pgp protein in cell membrane.

contrast, BCRP (ABCG2) has only one MSD region and one NBD and is thought to require homodimerization or possibly even a homotetramer to function as a drug efflux pump. As shown in Table 15.1, some overlap with respect to substrate recognition exists between the identified transporters. Despite the overlap in substrate recognition (Table 15.1), differences between individual transporters include tissue distribution and substrate preference. Thus, these ABC transporters are not functionally redundant molecules. Pgp is considered to prefer large hydrophobic, either uncharged or slightly charged compounds. MRP1 also can extrude large uncharged compounds but it also exports hydrophobic anionic conjugates. MRP1, although ATP-dependent, transports via a cotransport mechanism in which drug molecules are transported with reduced glutathione (GSH), whereas both Pgp and BCRP transport one molecule at a time. Moreover, MRP1 has been shown to export glutathione-conjugated endogenous metabolites including cysteinyl leukotriene and prostaglandin, which might provide an important role in regulating arachodonic acid metabolites. In addition, MRP1 has been shown to export glutathione conjugated anticancer agents such as melphalan, doxorubicin, and cyclophosphamide (see Chapter 9 for an in-depth discussion of drug excretion).

Finally, MRP1 plays in important role in transporting glutathione conjugated toxins such as alflatoxin B_1, which could provide a protective mechanism against xenobiotic toxins and carcinogens. The substrate preference of BCRP is still under investigation, and literature reports are complicated by the observation that polymorphic variants of BCRP alter the substrate recognition of this transporter. However, recent evidence suggests that, similar to MRP1, BCRP can recognize and export metabolites including sulfated estrogens and methotrexate and folate polyglutamates.

As discussed earlier, Pgp, MRP1, and BCRP are expressed in normal tissues and are thought to be important for protecting normal cells from the accumulation of xenobiotics. The tissue distribution of MRP1 is the most ubiquitous and is expressed in most tissues with high

Table 15.1 Substrate Recognition

Common Name	Systematic Name	Anticancer Agents	Other Substrates
Pgp	ABCB1	Vincristine Vinblastine Doxorubicin Etoposide Imanitib	Neutral and cationic organic compounds, many commonly used drugs
MRP1	ABCC1	Vincristine Doxorubicin Etoposide methotrexate	Organic anions Glutathione conjugated-doxorubicin, melphalan, aflatoxin B1 Gluthathione
BCRP	ABCG2	Mitoxantrone Topotecan Doxorubicin Imanitib Gefinitib	Sulphated oesterogens Methotrexate-polyglutamates Prazosin

levels found in the lung, testis, kidneys, skeletal muscle, and peripheral blood mononuclear cells but at relatively low levels in the liver. The tissue distribution of Pgp and BCRP expression is more limited compared to MRP1. High expression of Pgp in normal tissue is found in the intestine, liver, kidney, placenta, and the blood–brain barrier. BCRP is found most frequently in the placenta, intestine, breast, and liver. All three transporters are thought to form an intestinal barrier for the absorption of drugs. Pgp plays an integral role in preventing xenobiotics from entering past the blood–brain barrier, whereas MRP1 is localized to the basolateral membrane of the chorid plexus and serves to pump xenobiotics from the blood-cerebrospinal-fluid into the blood. In summary, in addition to conferring drug resistance to tumor cells, ABC transporters are a major determinant of absorption, distribution, and toxicology of drugs.

As can be seen from this overview of transport-related drug resistance, there are myriad ways in which the tumor cell can overcome effects of anticancer drugs via drug efflux. The problem with this is the fact that these transport proteins not only provide resistance for the tumor cell, they also serve important physiological roles for the host. Simple inhibition of such proteins will not likely provide a significant therapeutic advantage for a drug. These and similar problems will be discussed in the section on drug resistance in infectious diseases. Ways to modulate such resistance will be an important focus of pharmacological research for the foreseeable future.

15.2.1.2 Drug Uptake Proteins in Drug Resistance

The classic antifolate methotrexate MTX continues to be an important component of the chemotherapeutic armamentarium for a variety of cancers including pediatric ALL, osteogenic sarcoma, lymphoma, and breast cancer. Raltitrexed, another anti-folate, is used throughout much of the world outside of the United States for advanced colorectal cancer. Finally, Pemetrexed was approved in 2004 for the treatment of pleural mesothelioma and shortly thereafter as a second line treatment for nonsmall cell lung cancer. These drugs mimic the natural folate molecule and in so doing utilize the membrane-bound reduced folate carrier (RFC) protein system to gain entry into the cell.

The RFC must actively transport sufficient levels of unbound drug to provide intracellular drug concentrations adequate to sustain inhibition of the target enzyme dihydrofolate reductase (DHFR) and for the synthesis of polyglutamated antifolates, the storage form of these drugs. Indeed, antifolate resistance due to decreased RFC expression has been cited in the literature since 1962 and has since emerged as an important mechanism of resistance to classical antifolates.

Loss of RFC function can occur by decreased expression of the protein and thus decreased levels of membrane-bound RFC. Once the RFC was cloned it became evident that profound losses of RFC transport and antifolate resistance were associated with mutations in the RFC. These mutations resulted in decreased transport of the drug or no loss of drug transport and tremendous increase in folate transport. Since the antifolates compete for the binding of DHFR with normal reduced folates, the increased transport of folates provided the cells as much benefit as did the decreased antifolate transport.

15.2.2 Glutathione and Drug Resistance

Increased intracellular glutathione levels can contribute to drug resistance by either direct conjugation of the drug and/or by preventing oxidative stress induced by redox cycling drugs such as doxorubicin (refer to Chapters 8 and 9 for an excellent review of glutathione and drugs). Glutathione conjugation to electrophillic anticancer agents are catalyzed by glutathione s-transferases (GSTs) (Figure 15.4). Glutathione conjugation can render compounds biologically inactive as the reactive group is now neutralized and may lead to the inability of the drug to bind the target. For cross-linking agents, such as melphalan glutathione, conjugation inhibits DNA cross-linking, which is considered to be the initiating cytotoxic event of melphalan induced cell death. In addition, glutathione conjugated melphalan is now a good substrate for MRP1 mediated drug efflux. Increased glutathione levels have also implicated resistance platinum analogs as the conjugation of the platinum analog prevents activation of the drug thus preventing drug-DNA interactions.

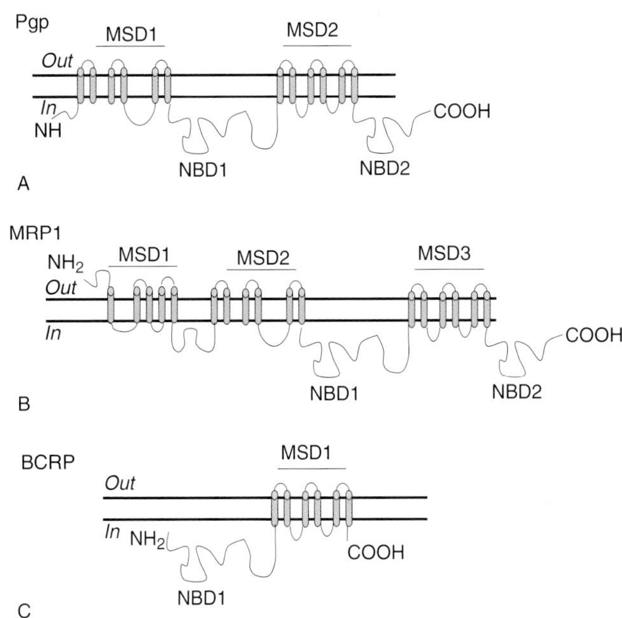

Figure 15.4 Predicted secondary structure of Pgp, MRP 1, and BCRP. Pgp contains two membrane spanning domains (MSD) and two nucleotide binding domains (NBD). In contrast, MRP 1 contains MSD and two NBD. Finally BCRP is considered a half-transporter and contains one MSD and one NBD, and requires dimerization to function as transporter.

In support of the importance of glutathione levels as a mechanism of drug resistance, several investigators have shown that acquired drug resistant cell lines contain elevated levels of glutathione. The rate-limiting step of *de novo* glutathione synthesis is glutamylcysteine synthase. Depletion of glutathione levels with the pharmacological inhibitor of glutamylcysteine synthase L-buthionine-[S,R]-sulfoximine (BSO) is reported to increase the sensitivity of cells to melphalan in several cell line models. Previous work has demonstrated that the catalytic subunit of glutamylcysteine synthase is increased in acquired melphalan resistant cell lines. The gene expression profiling correlated with our earlier finding showing that melphalan resistant cell lines demonstrated increased glutathione levels. Thus current experimental data suggest that increased glutathione levels and regulation of *de novo* synthesis of glutathione may be important for mediating resistance to melphalan and other alkylating agents.

15.2.3 Alterations in Drug Target

15.2.3.1 Structural Modifications

Assuming the access of the drug to the target is unaltered, the next temporal point along the cell death pathway which can influence cell survival following drug treatment, is the drug target itself. Documented alterations in the target include point mutations, amplifications, alterations in the localization, and activity of the target. Since discussing all anticancer drug targets is beyond the scope of this chapter, for purposes of illustration we will discuss documented alterations in Bcr-Abl. The discovery that Bcr-Abl was the transforming event associated with chronic myelogenous leukemia (CML) provided an ideal target for drug discovery. Indeed Bcr-Abl inhibitors first discovered in 1996, remain the best success story of target-directed drug development in the field of cancer chemotherapy. Typically 90% of CML patients will express Bcr-Abl, which is created by a reciprocal translocation between chromosome 9 and 22, creating a fusion protein consisting of Bcr (breakpoint cluster region) and the proto-oncogene c-abl. The end result of this is the expression of a chimeric fusion protein referred to as Bcr-Abl. This hybrid protein contains functional domains from both Bcr and Abl.

Within the Bcr region there exist two regions, which are causally linked to the oncogenic properties of Bcr-Abl. Phosphorylation of tyrosine 177 is critical because this event appears necessary for binding of Grb2 and the subsequent activation of the Ras pathway. The second region of Bcr is the coiled-coil domain located in the n-terminus (amino acids 1-63). This region is required for dimerization of Bcr-Abl and is crucial for Abl kinase activity. Abl is classified as a nonreceptor tyrosine kinase and normally the kinase activity of Abl is tightly regulated. In normal cells Abl is expressed largely in the nucleus, but can be found in the cytoplasm as well. Cellular functions associated with Abl are complex and include regulation of cell cycle progression and DNA repair. Similar to other tyrosine kinases, Abl contains an SH3 and SH2 domain at the N-terminal region of the protein. SH3 and SH2 domains allow for docking of proteins containing proline rich domains (SH3 domain) and tyrosine domains that interact with the SH2 domain. Abl also contains nuclear localization signals (NLS) that allow for nuclear import as well as a nuclear export signal, and this is consistent with the observed nuclear and cytoplasmic localization of Abl.

The fusion protein Bcr-Abl demonstrates increased constitutive kinase activity compared to Abl and is located predominately in the cytosol. The uncontrolled kinase activity of Bcr-Abl interacts with effector proteins resulting in disregulated cellular proliferation and reduced sensitivity to apoptotic stimuli. Bcr-Abl is known to activate multiple survival pathways including the PI3 kinase/AKT survival pathway and Stat5. Stat5 is a transcriptional regulator of the anti-apoptotic Bcl-2 family members MCL-1 and Bcl-xl. Current data suggest that the transforming capabilities of Bcr-Abl are the culmination of the activation of multiple survival and growth pathways. In summary, Bcr-Abl is a constitutively active tyrosine kinase and is generally accepted as the initiating step in CML. CML typically begins with an indolent chronic phase, which is associated with the gradual expansion of myeloid cells with normal differentiation, and over time will proceed to a

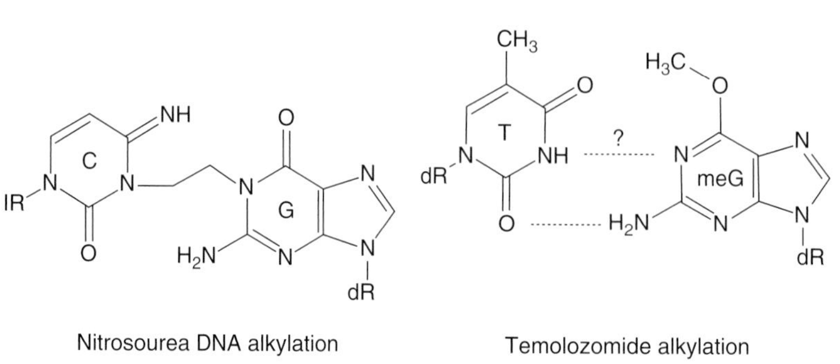

Figure 15.5 Alkylation of DNA.

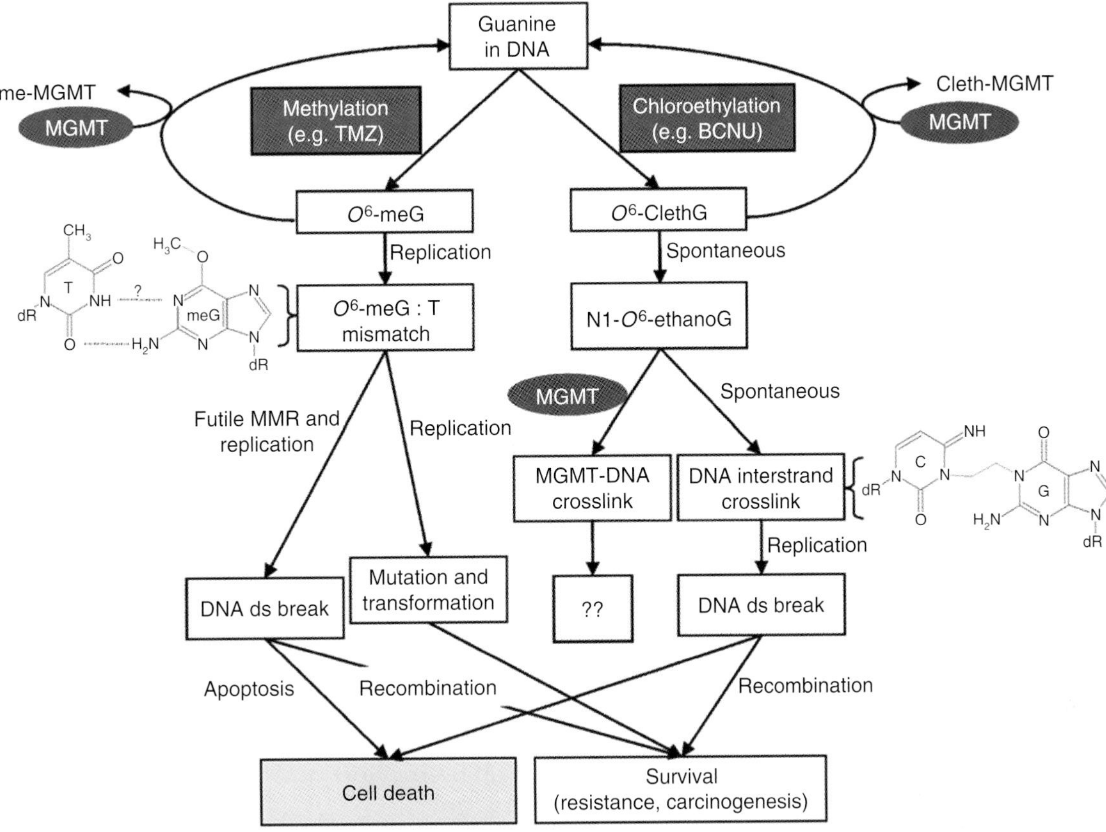

Figure 15.6 MGMT role in cell death and cell survival.

terminal blastic stage. Disease progression is usually associated with additional genetic abnormalities as well as impaired differentiation.

Although most patients will respond to Imatinib it is not curative as minimal residual disease can be detected at the molecular level in the bone marrow. Mutations within the kinase domain of Bcr-Abl which can inhibit drug binding is known to contribute to clinical resistance. Additional mechanisms of resistance include the activation of Bcr-Abl independent survival pathways and overexpression of drug transporters. Finally an active area of research is to determine the contribution of the microenvironment of the bone marrow were minimal residual disease is typically found. Determining whether specific soluble factors or extracellular matrixes produced by the bone marrow microenvironment contributes to imanitib resistance may lead to combination therapies targeting minimal residual disease within the bone marrow compartment.

Despite the lack of complete molecular understanding of how Bcr-Abl transforms cells into a malignant phenotype, Bcr-Abl provided an ideal target for drug development. In 1996, STI571 or Imanitib was discovered as an inhibitor of Bcr-Abl kinase activity. Imanitib is a competitive inhibitor of the ATP binding domain located in the tyrosine kinase domain of Bcr-Abl. The result of Imanitib binding to Bcr-Abl is the inhibition of the kinase activity and eventual cell death in Bcr-Abl positive cells. Clinically Imanitib rapidly became the first-line treatment for CML.

15.2.3.2 Altered Levels of Drug Target

Methotrexate binds to DHFR and inhibits the cell's ability to maintain the stores of tetrahydrofolates (THF) necessary for cell survival and division. More than 30 years ago studies were performed that clearly demonstrated that acquired methotrexate resistance resulted from DHFR gene amplification and DHFR enzyme overexpression. Gene amplification can result from a stable expanded chromosome region known as a homogeneous staining region (HSR). This type of gene amplification is stable and replicated with cell division. The other type of gene amplification is an unstable formation of double minutes (DM) in which the DMs are acentromeric and cannot participate in equal chromosome segregation at mitosis. The end result is the potential loss of the gene amplification in daughter cells and the loss of methotrexate resistance.

Whether the stable mutation HSR or the unstable DM, cells that overexpress DHFR have a consistent level of resistance depending upon the amount of DHFR present. As the level of DHFR increases, the fraction of active DHFR needed to maintain cellular stores of THF decreases. For example, if 5% of the catalytically active DHFR is needed to maintain THF and DHFR, amplification results in a 100-fold increase in DHFR, then only 0.05% of the total enzyme is necessary to maintain THF. In this case methotrexate must now inhibit greater than 99.95% of the available DHFR to negatively impact THF pools.

Given that the antifolates enter cells by a nonconcentrating RFC transport system, attaining 99.95% inhibition of DHFR would be virtually impossible without also attaining highly toxic or even lethal blood levels of the antifolate.

Newer antifolates have been developed that are THF antagonists, which potently inhibit the enzyme thymidylate synthase (TS). Again, cells exposed to increasing levels of the antifolates resulted in an increased resistance to these antifolates. In this circumstance the increased resistance was related to increased expression of TS and not DHFR. Similarly cells made resistant to classical TS inhibitors such as 5-fluorouracil were cross-resistant with the TS inhibitor antifolates.

15.2.4 DNA Repair and Drug Resistance

Many anticancer drugs kill tumor cells by forming covalent bonds with DNA. This class of compounds is known as the alkylating agents and can form interstrand crosslinks, intrastrand crosslinks, or can modify the basic structure of nucleotides making up DNA. Such drug DNA interactions stop DNA synthesis, and tumor cells die when the number of DNA lesions exceeds the capacity of the cell to correct these lesions. Hence an obvious mechanism of drug resistance would be to increase DNA repair processes in the target cell. Previously we discussed the role of glutathione in drug resistance. In that case the glutathione prevented formation of DNA lesions. The present mechanism of resistance relies on the ability of the cell to correct the actual DNA damage caused by the alkylating agents.

Alkylation of guanines at the O^6 position is common for nitrosoureas and temozolomide. However, the actual product formed is quite different depending on the drug in question. Whereas temozolomide forms a methylated O^6 product, the nitrosoureas form a chloroethylated O^6 product, which then undergoes a spontaneous rearrangement for an interstrand crosslink.

An enzyme, O methyl guanine DNA-methyltransferase (MGMT), was first identified in bacteria, but subsequently a human equivalent was shown to provide cancer cells protection from the lethal effects of the drugs. MGMT can remove the alkylation product before DNA damage can occur. For the drugs such as temolozomide, lethality occurs when the mismatch repair system (MMR) causes a futile replication and double-stranded DNA breaks occur. For the nitrosourea alkylation products, MGMT removes the chloroethyl group prior to the spontaneous formation of the interstrand crosslinks. Interestingly, it appears as though the drug itself induces tumor cell drug resistance as these drugs induce the production of MGMT (thus increasing DNA repair) and at the same time suppress the production of MMR (thus decreasing the formation of lethal ds DNA breaks).

One way to overcome this form of resistance is to decrease the effectiveness of MGMT. Pseudosubstrates

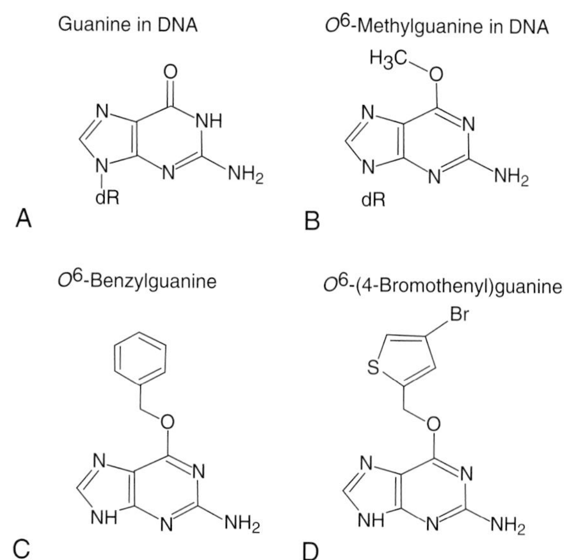

Figure 15.7 Alkylation of guanine at the O6 position.

(as shown in Figure 15.7) that have been synthesized inhibit the enzyme and thereby prevent the repair process. The problem with this approach is that the MGMT inhibitors provide an unacceptable collateral toxicity.

The alkylating agent Cisplatin forms intrastrand crosslink DNA adducts that trigger a series of intracellular events that ultimately results in cell death. If the cell can process and repair these lesions before the apoptotic pathway is initiated, the cell can survive the effects of cisplatin. One of the repair processes thought to have a major impact on resistance to alkylating cytotoxicty is nucleotide excision repair (NER).

NER is a highly conserved DNA repair pathway that can deal with a wide variety of DNA damaging agents; most commonly studied are UV T-T dimmers and agents such as the nitrogen mustards, cisplatin, and aryl mutagens. The basic mechanism is shown in Figure 15.8, using the UV dimerization as the model.

This process, although simple in description, is a complex process using a number of proteins to complete the process. Initially, proteins must recognize the damaged DNA and bind to the lesion, which then complexes with the damaged DNA binding factor. The damaged area is then demarcated and verified by a complex of proteins referred to as TFIIH. Yet another complex of proteins then binds to the site, readying the lesion for incision. The lesion is then cut, forming a 24-32 nucleotide oligomer, which is then released and the gap filled by DNA polymerases. Finally the DNA ligase enzyme reanneals the repaired sequence with the undamaged DNA sequence.

By increasing the amount and/or activity of the DNA repair process the cell can withstand increasing amounts of DNA damage and repair these lesions before the cell process is begun. Given the number of proteins involved in this process it would appear

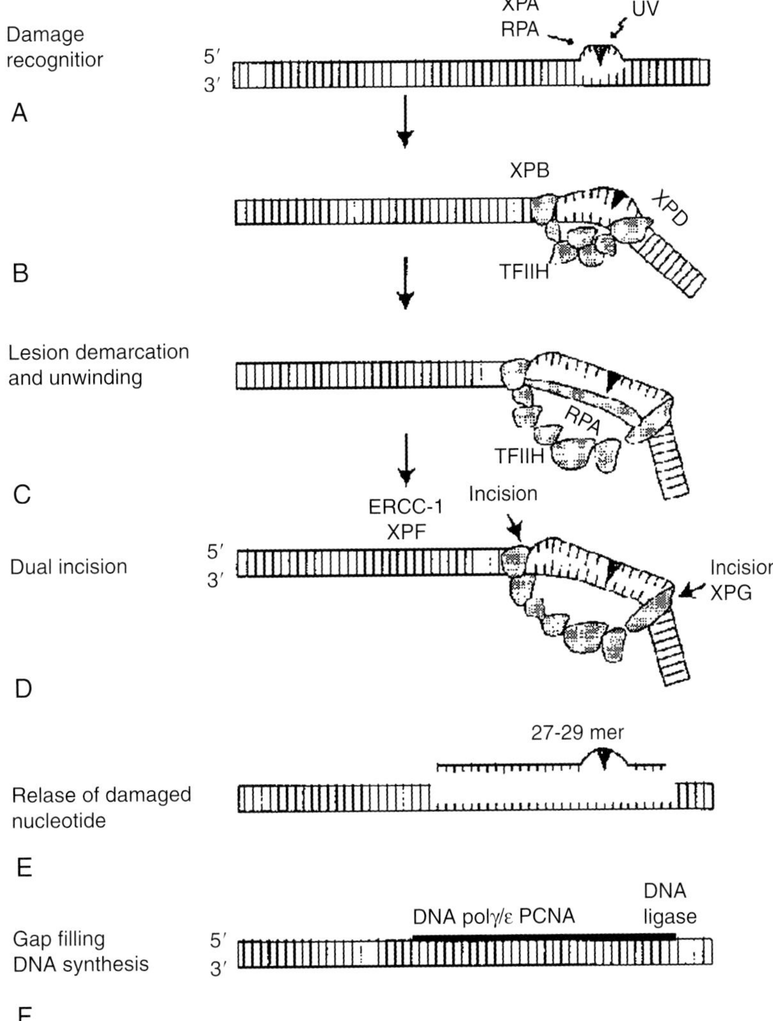

Figure 15.8 Nucleotide excision repair (NER).

likely that there exists a number of potential targets for drug discovery and overcoming this form of drug resistance.

15.3 DRUG RESISTANCE IN INFECTIOUS DISEASES

With the advent of drugs that could effectively treat previously lethal or severe infectious diseases, the era of infectious diseases was naively declared over in the 1970s. Unfortunately, the inaccuracy of this statement was demonstrated shortly thereafter as more and more drug resistance was noted in an ever-increasing number of infectious diseases. The halcyon days of living in an infectious disease-free world never developed, and now we are faced with counter-attack by the drug resistant infectious agents. In the remainder of this chapter we will discuss ways in which these organisms have been able to avoid the toxic effects of drugs used today.

15.3.1 Resistance to Penicillin: A Story of Two Mechanisms

Almost immediately after the introduction of penicillin to the clinic the value of the drug was evident. Different penicillins were developed with differing pharmacological properties, routes of administration, and spectrum of activities, but all penicillins worked in the same manner and required one particular chemical moiety, that being an intact beta-lactam ring (Figure 15.9).

Opening of the beta-lactam ring results in the complete loss of pharmacological activity of the drugs. Basically, the bacterial cell wall has layers of peptidogylcans that are then linked together by crosslinking the peptide chains (transpeptidation) of the peptidogylcan building blocks. The crosslinking of these building blocks strengthens and stabilizes the bacterial cell wall. The penicillins inhibit the peptide crosslinking process and thus do not allow the building blocks to polymerize, thus destabilizing and weakening the cell wall. The bacterial membrane being highly permeable now

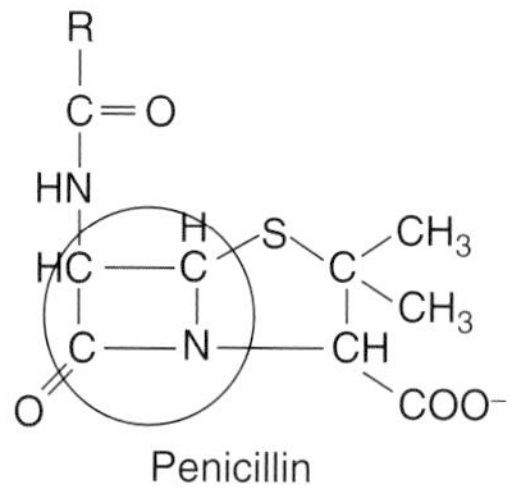

Figure 15.9 Beta lactam ring of penicillin.

expands rapidly, without the support of cell wall lyse. The pharmacologic target for the penicillins is a family of proteins called the penicillin binding proteins (PBP), which play a critical role in transpeptidation. Penicillins bind to these proteins, block transpeptidation, and prevent cell wall synthesis.

From this brief description of penicillin mechanism of action and structural requirements, two likely sites of drug resistance stand out. First, if the bacteria were able to break open the beta-lactam ring then the drug would lose its pharmacological activity. Second, if mutations of PBP were to occur, preventing penicillins from binding to the PBP, the penicillins would lose their pharmacological activity. Both have been described in clinical isolates and will be discussed next.

15.3.1.1 Drug Inactivation by Beta-Lactamases

The first described mechanism of a bacterial resistance was the production of a beta-lactamase enzyme capable of opening the beta-lactam ring and rendering the penicillins inactive. There exist hundreds of beta-lactamases, but there are only two primary ways in which these enzymes attack the drug. One class of beta-lactamases, the serine-beta-lactamases, is divided further into four categories: group 1 is poorly inhibited by clavulanic acid (a drug designed to prevent or lessen penicillin inactivation by the beta-lactamases); group 2 beta-lactamases are clavulanic acid sensitive and include a family of enzymes called the extended spectrum beta-lactamases; group 3 beta-lactamases are thought to be metallo beta-lactamases that work through activation of water via a Zn center; and group 4 includes clavulanic resistant beta-lactamases, which do not fit into the other categories.

The serine beta-lactamases work in a mechanism similar to serine proteases and esterases, where the Ser center performs a ring opening electrophilic attack on the beta-lactam ring. Water then enters the site and enables the hydrolysis of the enzyme drug intermediate. The inactive penicillin is released and the enzyme is ready to attack another ring. This group of beta-lactamases is by far the more clinically important form of drug inactivation.

Most gram-positive bacteria are capable of producing and secreting beta-lactamase into the medium surrounding the organism. Thus, if the antibiotic is sensitive to the enzyme, drug inactivation will occur primarily extracellularly. On the other hand, gram-negative bacteria secrete less enzyme into the medium and as a result less extracellular drug inactivation is observed with these organisms. However, many gram-positive bacteria do produce the enzyme but retain the enzyme in the periplasmic space. In this way the drug is inactivated after it has diffused across the cell wall but before it binds to its target PBP.

It should be noted that another class of beta-lactam antibiotics that also inhibit PBPs has been developed. These drugs, the cephalosporins (Figure 15.10) also require an intact beta-lactam ring to be active and are therefore susceptible to beta-lactamase inactivation. However, given the structural differences from penicillin, the sensitivity of the cephalosporins to the beta-lactamases differs from that of the penicillins.

Note that the cephalosporins six-member dihydrothiazine ring is attached to the beta-lactam ring. Note also that whereas the penicillin backbone has but one site for chemical modification, there are two sites for the cephalosporins. As with the penicillins there is a wide array of clinically available cephalosporins with varying sensitivities to the beta-lactamases. There are a number of excellent reviews for in-depth discussions regarding antibiotic sensitivity to the beta-lactamases.

A number of approaches have been taken to overcome beta-lactamase-driven drug resistance, but the two that have been most successful have been developing drugs less sensitive to enzymatic degradation and the coadministration of an enzyme inhibitor such as clavulanic acid with the beta-lactam drug. Given the fact the more than 200 different beta-lactamases have been reported it is not surprising that neither approach has been totally successful. Further, as new beta-lactam drugs are developed the bacteria respond by producing enzymes capable of overcoming the advantages of the new drugs. Remember that the developing resistance is a result of a selection process placed on the bacteria in which the drug selects for bacteria that have the ability to survive the chemical effects of the drug. There is no true adaptive response by the bacteria; rather it is simply a mutational process that enables the organism to live in an environment otherwise toxic to the organism.

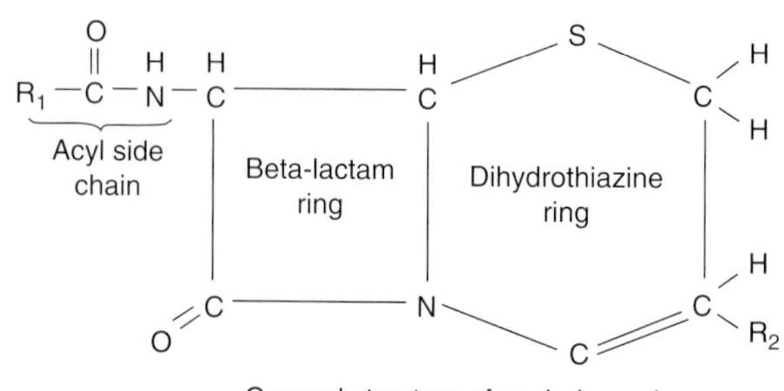

Figure 15.10 General structure of cephalosporins.

15.3.1.2 Altered Drug Target

As stated earlier, the target for the beta-lactams is the transpeptidase family of enzymes, commonly referred to as the PBP. It should be noted, however, that PBP is at times loosely employed in the literature. Some PBP in fact do bind to the beta-lactams but have yet to be shown to play a role in cell wall synthesis. Further, a bacteria more than likely will contain several types of PBP and only recently has their physiological roles in cell division begun to be understood.

PBPs are serine acyltransferases. Once the beta-lactam has bound to the PBP it interacts with the active site serine. The resulting acyltransferase-drug complex can only be hydrolyzed at a very slow rate, thus effectively lowering the enzyme available for cell wall synthesis. Interestingly, the PBP also inactivates the drug by cleaving the beta-lactam ring, but the turnover is so slow that the drug effectively inhibits transpeptidation in a suicide-like mechanism. In contrast, the beta-lactamases also bind the beta-lactams through a serine in the active site of the enzyme but in this case there is an extremely high turnover rate and the enzyme inactivates the drug rather than the drug inactivating the enzyme.

There have been approximately 800 PBPs identified thus far. These proteins have been divided into class A and class B proteins, depending primarily on the number of reactions the protein is capable of catalyzing. Class A PBPs are bifunctional and catalyze both the polymerization of the glycan subunits (GT) and the transpepditation (TP) of the peptide chains, whereas the Class B PBPs are monofunctional and serve as transpeptidase enzymes only. Both classes of PBPs are susceptible to beta-lactam attack and inhibition. Once the PBP is acylated by the beta-lactam it is incapable of further hydrolysis of the covalent acyl-enzyme intermediate and transpeptidation is inhibited.

Resistance to the beta-lactams can occur through mutation of the PBPs. Although this mechanism is far less studied than the beta-lactamase mechanism, interesting observations have been made. Thus far, there have been reported mutations in PBPs that cause pneumococcal resistance to the beta-lactams. One mechanism has been the mutation in which the serine binding site for the beta-lactams is distant from the active site of the enzyme. Thus, the drug binds to the Ser site, but this site is no longer associated with the active site of the enzyme. The other mechanism has been reported to be a charge modification of the active site, thus preventing the drug access to the active site.

Yet another mechanism has been the increased expression of one or more PBP in *Enterococcus faecium*. This overproduction of the PBP enables the overly produced PBP to take over the functions of the beta-lactam inhibited PBPs. A similar mechanism has been reported for methicillin-resistant *Staphylococcus aureus*. However where the *E. faecium* is a naturally occurring type of PBP related resistance, the MRSA results from a horizontal transfer of genetic material. Once transferred, the PBP production can be induced to overproduction following exposure to a beta-lactam. Again, this overly produced PBP can take over the function of the inhibited PBPs.

The future of PBP-targeted antibiotics remains active. A new approach is to develop transpeptidase inhibitors that lack the beta-lactam ring, such as the carbapenems, which are resistant to Ser-based transpeptidases but can be inactivated by the metallo-transpeptidases. Still others are searching for transpepditase inhibitors that do not resemble the beta-lactams. At present a limited number of nonbeta-lactam inhibitors have been identified, but the arylalkylidene-related molecules appear to be excellent precursors for active drug discovery. Another approach has been to not target the transpepditase function of the PBPs, but rather to develop inhibitors of the GT function of the PBPs. GT is essential for bacterial survival and recent molecular studies have clearly demonstrated that GT domains are distinct from the TP domains.

15.3.2 Malaria and Drug Resistance

Probably no disease has killed more humans throughout history than malaria. Malaria is transmitted by the bite of an *Anopheles* mosquito. There are four different parasites that can infect humans, but *Plasmodium falciparum* is the most virulent. The parasite first migrates to the liver where after several replications the parasites are released into the bloodstream. The parasite then invades the red blood cells and feeds off the hemoglobin. Survival of the parasite relies on the ability of the parasite to package the toxic heme metabolites formed during hemoglobin metabolism in nontoxic hemazoin particles. The parasite causes anemia, fevers, chills, veno-occlusive disorders, liver damage, and death.

With the discovery of effective antimalarial drugs and DDT, an amazingly effective mosquitocide, it was felt that malaria could be a disease of the past. Unfortunately, due to environmental concerns, the use of DDT was dramatically curtailed and at about the same time the development of new antimalarial drugs was basically stopped. As a result the mosquito vector of this disease came back strong and as we relied on the same drugs for a prolonged period of time, drug resistance developed in the parasites. In fact, chloroquine, the gold standard for malaria treatment, is rapidly becoming useless as resistance is flourishing worldwide. Similarly, resistance to other drugs such as the antifolates and even the newly introduced arteminisins is becoming problematic.

15.3.2.1 Resistance to Chloroquine: Another Membrane-bound Transporter Protein

Chloroquine is a semisynthetic derivative of quinine, the first drug used effectively to treat malaria. Chloroquine was used for decades as the drug of choice to treat malaria because it was a safe, highly effective, and relatively inexpensive drug. The effectiveness of chloroquine was first clearly demonstrated during World War II when in the Pacific Theater more GIs were hospitalized by malaria than by the Axis forces. By 1957, the first reports of chloroquine resistance were coming from Thailand, followed shortly thereafter in South America. By 1988, chloroquine resistance was encountered worldwide, and today the drug is essentially useless in all but a few areas of the world.

Chloroquine kills by concentrating in the food vacuole of the parasite and preventing the formation of the nontoxic heme metabolite hemazoin by the parasite. The parasite then dies from the toxic by-products of its own metabolism of hemoglobin. In the resistant parasite far less chloroquine is maintained in the acidic food vacuole and the parasite is able to detoxify the heme moieties. The exact mechanism of chloroquine action in the food vacuole is not understood, but there are experimental data supporting the idea that chloroquine binds to a heme moiety that both enables high concentrations of chloroquine to develop within the food vacuole and interferes with normal hemoglobin metabolism. The once-touted hypothesis of proton trapping of chloroquine in the acidic food vacuole, which then alters the pH of the organelle, appears inaccurate.

How the parasite removes chloroquine from the food vacuole appears to be related to mutations of a specific gene, named *pfcrt* for "plasmodium falciparum chloroquine resistance transporter." The protein product of this gene (CRT) is a 49 kD transmembrane protein that has a predicted 10 transmembrane domains. The key mutation seems to be K76T since no chloroquine resistant isolate carries the wild type lysine at position 76. It should be noted that usually a number of other mutations are noted in chloroquine resistant malaria, but only the K76T amino acid switch is seen consistently in the chloroquine resistant malaria.

What is the function of the CRT and how does the K76T affect the protein? Bioinformatics place this CRT in a super-family of drug and metabolite membrane transports. Currently it is thought that in the wild type parasite the chloroquine enters the food vacuole as nonprotonated, but is converted to the diprotonated form within the acidic environment and thus prevents the efflux of the drug by the normally positively charged CRT at the K76 site. However, the K76T mutation results in a CRT that can now transport the chloroquine out of the food vacuole. Recent results further suggest that the CRT protein is *not* an active transporter but rather a gated channel or pore that allows the chloroquine to escape from the vacuole in an energy-independent process.

The membrane of the food vacuole has other transporter proteins associated with it. One such protein, encoded by the *pfmdr1* gene, shows structural similarity to the human PGP that was discussed earlier in this chapter. This malaria protein has a molecular weight of 162 kD, and is an ABC transporter with 12 transmembrane domains and two ATP binding folds. The mammalian PGP pumps drug out of the cell but the malarial MDR1 actually pumps drugs into the food vacuole. Although this protein can add to the resistance associated with K76T mutation of the CRT protein, by itself it does not provide a chloroquine resistant phenotype. However, numerous reports find a reciprocal relationship between chloroquine resistance and resistance to other drugs that act on the food vacuole such as mefloquine and halofantrine. Exactly how the MDR1 protein affects parasite sensitivity to food vacuole poisons remains a mystery.

15.3.2.2 Antifolate Resistance

Assessment of resistance to the antifolates has been much more straightforward than it has for chloroquine, since the molecular targets for this class of drugs have been known since the 1930s. The malaria parasite relies on the intracellular synthesis of the folate molecule since the parasite cannot effectively scavenge folates from the surrounding environment. These organisms have an enzyme dihydropteroate synthase (DHPS). They also contain dihydrofolate reductase (DHFR) to insure sufficient levels of tetrahydrofolates needed for many cellular processes. The DHPS is an enzyme unique to the malaria parasite but both the host and the parasite have DHFR. Fortunately drugs that target the parasitic DHFR do so at affinities 100 times greater than that of the mammalian DHFR.

Antifolates with clinically important activity include the sulfa drugs, which target DHPS, as well as pyrimethamine and proguanil, which target DHFR. The most commonly used clinical formulation of the antifolates is to use a combination of a sulfa drug such as sulfadoxine and pyrimethamine to inhibit both enzymes involved in folate metabolism. The primary goal of this combination is to inhibit DNA synthesis when the parasite begins DNA synthesis for cell replication.

The genetic basis for antifolate resistance relies almost exclusively on mutations found in the protein targets such that the drug no longer binds with sufficient affinity to allow inhibition of the enzyme. There need be but a few point mutations in these enzymes to result in loss of drug affinity. The most common DHFR mutations are S108N, N51I, and C59R. Similarly, point mutation patterns appear common for the DHPS. Further these mutations seem geographically related in that sulfadoxine resistance in Africa is commonly associated with A437G/K540E mutations, whereas sulfadoxine resistance in Southeast Asia is associated with A437G/A581G or A437G/A581G/K540E mutations. In Southeast Asia and South America a fourth mutation, I164L, in DHFR in combination with the three mutations just cited results in an organism completely resistant to antifolate resistance.

Surprisingly, a method of antifolate resistance commonly cited in tumor cells is gene amplification resulting in increased target protein and decreased anti-folate efficacy, which has yet to be identified in any clinically relevant isolate. A further difference in antifolate resistance between mammalian cells and the parasitic cell is altered polyglutamation of the antifolate drugs. In mammalian cells, folates are taken up by a folate transport system and once inside the cell are polyglutamated to trap the folates intracellularly. A reported mechanism of resistance in the cancer cell is the loss of polyglutamation of the antifolate, and cells can no longer concentrate and store the antifolate. Cytotoxic levels of the drug cannot be attained and the cell becomes resistant to drug. There does not appear to be such a process in the parasite and thus antifolate trapping is not an important process in the parasite.

15.3.2.3 Recent Drugs, Drug Resistance, and Overcoming Resistance

Unfortunately, as new drugs are finally entering the clinic for the treatment of malaria, resistance is developing rapidly against these drugs. Two such drugs are atovaquone and artemisinins. One approach that is gaining traction is to end monodrug therapy and incorporate multidrug therapy to treat malaria. The concept behind drug combination is that a simple point mutation may not provide the protective cover that the parasite needs when two drugs are used simultaneously. This approach is being considered in the therapy of all infectious diseases. Whether this approach does in fact slow the development of drug resistance is at present unknown. Obviously the other approach to overcoming drug resistance is to identify new parasitic targets and develop drugs to affect these targets. Here again, unless something such as multidrug therapy is used when these drug are introduced, clinical drug resistance will develop and will develop rapidly.

15.3.3 Tuberculosis Drug Resistance through Decreased Drug Activation

Tuberculosis (TB) is an infectious disease that remains a leading killer (>2 million/year) primarily in individuals in poor living conditions. Further, one to two billion people are latently infected worldwide. Fortunately, less than 15% of latenyl infected people will go on to develop clinical TB; this represents a vast storehouse of potential cases of TB. The most important causative agent of this disease is *Mycobacterium tuberculosis*, a slim, aerobic, acid-resistant bacterium. Since 1945 a number of drugs have been developed and proved effective in TB. Unfortunately, due to inappropriate therapy and poor knowledge of the disease we have not been able to control TB. Of the many drugs used to treat TB, isoniazid (INH: isonicotinic acid hydrazide) has been the most widely used and is most effective. The structure for INH is shown in Figure 15.11.

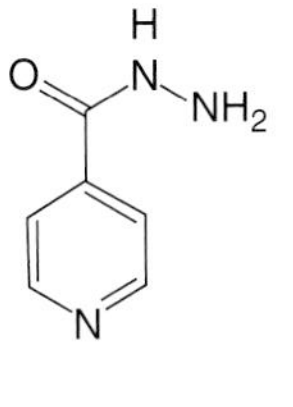

Figure 15.11 Structure of isoniazide.

The exact mechanism(s) of action has not been identified for INH, but it has been well established that INH serves as a prodrug. The drug gains access inside the bacterium through small water-filled pores by passive diffusion. Once inside the cell the nontoxic INH is thought to undergo metabolic activation. A multifunctional catalase/peroxidase, KatG, is responsible for the activation of INH. The physiological role for KatG is thought to be protection against host phagocytic NADPH oxidase-derived peroxides and nitroxides. Interaction between INH and KatG could have two deleterious consequences for the bacterium. First, the enzyme converts the inactive prodrug to a variety of metabolites with tuberculocide activities; and second, the binding of INH to the KatG decreases the efficacy of this protective enzyme against peroxides and nitroxides. It is currently believed that in addition to the generation of a number of INH-derived radicals, the activated INH inhibits the enzyme enoyl-ACP reductase, an enzyme critical for the formation of mycolic acid, a precursor essential for mycobacterial cell wall synthesis. The activated INH is capable of acylation or oxidation of a number of amino acids in a variety of proteins. What impact these reactions have on protein function is still being determined. Interesting, INH has little activity in bacteria other than Mycobacterium.

Given that INH is a prodrug that requires intracellular activation for anti-TB activity, a logical site for drug resistance would be a mutation of the KatG protein. A correlation between INH activation and peroxidase enzyme dates back to the 1960s, when it was reported that INH resistant M tuberculae also lacked peroxidase/catalase activity.

Subsequently molecular techniques have confirmed this observation and have identified mutations in the KatG gene that render the bacterium resistant to INH. Most frequently point mutations have been described such as S315T, but a range of other mutations have been identified. Crystal structure analysis of the wild type KatG and the S315T mutated KatG have provided a possible explanation for the INH resistance. In the wild type protein the heme access pore is 7 angstroms; in the mutated form the pore is 4.7 angstroms, suggesting decreased INH access to the oxidizing site of the mutated protein. This mutation prevents that activation of INH but does not affect the ability of KatG to serve as a peroxidase catalase. It must be noted here that more than 40 additional point mutations in the KatG gene have been correlated with INH resistance, but the S315T is the most commonly identified mutation in clinical isolates.

Other sites of mutation associated with INH resistance include the inhA gene, which codes for the enoyl-ACP reductase, the putative target for activated INH. Since this type of resistance is to the activated drug and the activation of a prodrug, this mechanism of resistance will not be discussed in detail here. The combination of KatG and inhA mutations account for approximately 80% of all INH-resistant clinical isolates. The remaining resistance phenotypes have yet to be identified.

15.3.4 Drug Resistance through Drug Transport

As was discussed with cancer cell drug resistance, infectious diseases also express drug resistance through decreased drug uptake or increased drug efflux. In the late 1970s, tetracycline resistance was first attributed to an efflux mechanism. Since then efflux-based mechanisms of antibiotic resistance has been described for a wide range of antibacterial agents. Based on what we discussed earlier in the chapter it is not surprising that some of these efflux mechanisms are relatively drug specific, but many accommodate an array of drugs. One point to keep in mind is the fact that there are gram-negative and gram-positive bacteria. The former have a complex cell envelope surrounding the organism. This cell envelope limits the access of many drugs and as a consequence drug resistance in gram-negative bacteria in many cases is attributable to a synergy between the membrane-bound drug efflux pumps and the cell envelope mediated poor drug uptake.

Bacterial drug efflux transporters are classified into five families:

- The major facilitator family (MFS)
- The ATP binding cassette superfamily described previously for cancer cells and the malaria parasite
- The small multidrug resistance family (SMR)
- Resistance nodulation cell division superfamily (RND)
- The multidrug and toxic compound extrusion family (MATE)

Of these families the ABC and MFS families are by far the largest. Gram-positive bacteria usually require only a single component efflux mechanism to pump the drug out of the cytoplasmic membrane whereas gram-negative bacteria have a multicomponent efflux mechanism including the membrane efflux pump (MFP) and an outer membrane protein component (OMP) to efflux out of the cytoplasmic membrane and across the cell envelope.

15.3.4.1 Major Facilitator Superfamily

The MFS is an ancient and diverse set of proteins numbering more than 1000 sequenced membranes that are involved in transporting sugars, metabolites, anions, and drugs. Most MFSs are single-component systems, but a few multicomponent systems have been described for gram-negative bacteria. The MFP proteins have 12 to 14 TMD and catalyze drug efflux using at least different subfamilies of drug/H+ antiporters (DHA). DHA 1 and 2 are found in both prokaryotes and eukaryotes whereas DHA 3 is prokaryote specific. Members of the DHA 1 family export a variety of chemicals including sugars, polyamines, monamines, acetylcholine, paraquat, and methylglyoxal. DHA 2 has a more limited spectrum of substrates, which includes dyes and bile salts. DHA 3 is known to efflux a number of antibiotics including the macrolides and tetracyclines. The tetracycline efflux pumps are the best studied of the MFS family and are present in both gram-negative and gram-positive bacteria.

15.3.4.2 ABC Transporter Superfamily

This superfamily of transporters contains both uptake and efflux transporter systems and requires the hydrolysis of ATP to provide the energy to shuttle drug across membranes. The pumps are multiprotein complexes with six TMD, and associate on the cytoplasmic faceoff the inner membrane with two ATPase subunits. Although there are significant similarities between the proteins and the mammalian ABC efflux proteins involved in MDR, drug efflux pumps belonging to the ABC transporter superfamily are rare in prokayotes.

15.3.4.3 Small Drug Resistance Family (SMR)

This family of transported proteins consists of proteins having approximately 110 amino acids, four TMD, and are powered by a proton motive force similar to mitochondria. These proteins must form tetramers to function as transporters. These pumps are capable of effluxing drugs, dyes, and cations.

15.3.4.4 Resistance Nodulation Cell Division Superfamily (RND)

These proteins are encoded in chromosomal genes, but an RND protein recently was found encoded in a plasmid. These transporters serve as antiporters and have been shown to be important in acquired and intrinsic resistance in gram-negative bacteria. All RND described thus far serve as multidrug efflux transporters.

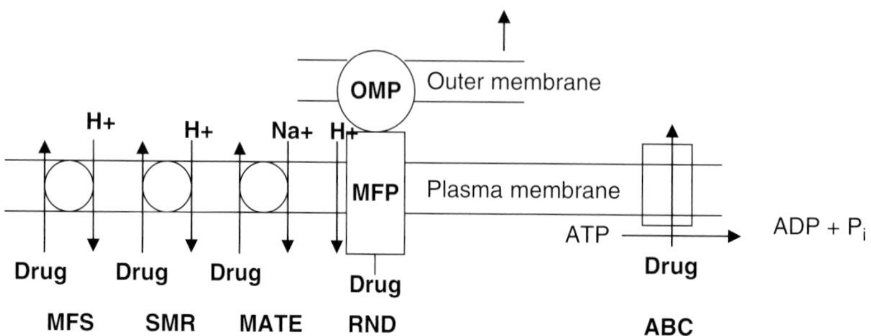

Figure 15.12 Membrane bound drug transporters.

In gram-negative bacteria, a unique arrangement must be established between the cytoplasmic RND consisting of RND transmembrane protein with 12 TMD, an MFP, and an OMP. A characteristic feature of the RND topology is the presence of two large periplasmic loops between TMD 1 and 2 and TMD 7 and 8. The N-terminus halves of the RND family of proteins are identical to the C-terminus halves. It is thought that these proteins arose from an intragenic duplication process that occurred before the divergence of the RFD family.

15.3.4.5 Multidrug and Toxic Compound Extrusion (MATE)

This family of proteins was at one time thought to be a member of the MFS superfamily due to similar membrane topology. However, they show no sequence homology and are now described as a separate family of transporter proteins. Proteins in this family use a sodium gradient as the energy source for effluxing drugs such as the fluoroquinolines and other dyes.

The combination of these families of drug transporters has resulted in a variety of resistant phenotypes in both gram-negative and gram-positive bacteria. However, this type of drug resistance is far less common in bacteria than it is in cancer cell drug resistance.

15.4 SUMMARY

We have discussed examples of drug resistance reported for both cancer cells and infectious diseases. There are myriad ways in which both populations of cells develop drug resistance depending upon the drug type and the cell type. Although this phenomenon of drug resistance is, on the surface, a roadblock to effective chemotherapy, it provides the pharmacologist newer targets for drug development as well as a better understanding of drug action and cell response to the drugs. Hopefully, this chapter has provided more insight into drug resistance and encourages you to learn more about this fascinating phenomenon.

REVIEW QUESTIONS

1. What is the difference between inherent (natural) and acquired drug resistance?
2. Compare and contrast the MDR and MRP1 with respect to structure, function, and drug selectivity.
3. Discuss some of the unwanted potential consequences when we try to inhibit MDR to overcome drug resistance.
4. Describe the role of RFC in drug resistance.
5. How are BER and NER used as means to drug resistance? How do they differ and how are they similar? How might these pathways be important in normal cell function?
6. What are PBPs? How are they important in drug action and drug resistance?
7. Membrane-bound drug transporter proteins are important in drug resistance. What types of transporters are used in chloroquine resistance and what do they do?
8. Antifolates are important in the treatment of cancer and infectious diseases. Discuss mechanisms of antifolate drug resistance in cancer and malaria.
9. Discuss the rationale of using multidrug therapy rather than monotherapy if monotherapy is effective at present.
10. How does isoniazide kill *M. tuberculae* organisms? What is a common mechanism of drug resistance to INH?
11. Cytosine arabinoside (Ara-C) is an anticancer drug, and an example of host effects causing the need for large doses of drug to have a clinical effect far greater than would have been predicted from *in vitro* studies. What is the reason for this? How is it overcome?

Chapter

16 Ion Channels

Georgi V. Petkov

OUTLINE

16.1 INTRODUCTION

The cell membrane facilitates the diffusion of nonpolar hydrophobic molecules between intracellular and extracellular compartments; it also serves as a major barrier to ion migration. Mechanisms that utilize specialized integral membrane proteins or protein complexes have evolved to enable regulated transport of ions across this barrier. There are two basic classes of cell membrane transporters:

1. Carriers bind to specific cargo molecules, including organic compounds (e.g., sugars and amino acids) and inorganic ions, and transfer them across the membrane. Carrier-mediated transport may be further subdivided into passive transport, which does not require energy and provides for the selective passage of specific ions or ion classes down their *electrochemical gradient* (Section 16.2); and active transport, which uses energy, typically in the form of ATP hydrolysis, to transport ions against their electrochemical gradient. The most important active transport-based carriers are the *ion pumps* (also known as *ion ATPases*), including the sodium-potassium and calcium pumps.
2. Ion channels form pores in the plasma membrane and, like passive transporters, facilitate the flow of ions, typically inorganic ions such as sodium (Na^+), potassium (K^+), calcium (Ca^{2+}), and chloride (Cl^-), down their electrochemical gradients. Unlike carriers, which have limited flux capacity, a single ion channel can permit 1 to 100 million ions per second across the cell membrane. Ion channels are not simply pores in the membrane that indiscriminately provide free passage to charged molecules; they exhibit varying degrees of ion selectivity—some allow broad classes of ions (e.g., cations) to pass whereas others effectively restrict transmembrane movement to a single ionic species (Section 16.2.2.1). Ion channel-mediated transport is subject to complex modulation by membrane potential (voltage), protein interactions, posttranslational modification (e.g., phosphorylation by protein kinases), and binding of extracellular or intracellular ligands. Different cell types express unique assemblages of various ion channels, each of which allows for ions to pass down their electrochemical gradient until they reach their ionic equilibrium, defined

by the Nernst equation (Section 16.2). This electrochemical equilibration process, in conjunction with the action of ion pumps and other carriers, defines the standing voltage difference across the cell membrane, known as the *membrane potential*. The membrane potential is relatively stable when the cells are at rest, thus it often is referred to as a *resting* membrane potential. Although the value of the resting membrane potential is a distinct property of each given cell type, all cells maintain a negative resting membrane potential (i.e., the interior of the cell membrane is negative compared to the extracellular surface) in the millivolt range (from −80 mV to about −30 mV). Many cell types referred to as *excitable cells*, such as nerve and muscle cells, can exhibit (spontaneously or in a response to stimuli) rapid and transient changes in their resting membrane potential, which are called *action potentials*.

Ion channels are fundamental to cell existence and control a broad range of essential physiological processes, including nerve and muscle excitation, action-potential generation and shaping, muscle contraction, sensory transduction, blood pressure regulation, cell proliferation, hormone secretion, learning and memory, cell volume regulation, fertilization, maintenance of salt and water balance, and cell death. Approximately 340 human genes are thought to encode individual ion channel proteins. Defects or alterations in ion channel structure or function can lead to serious consequences, including life-threatening diseases (Section 16.6). The fact that more than 60 drugs that modulate ion channels are currently marketed for multiple therapeutic uses is a testament to the importance of ion channels as therapeutic targets.

16.1.1 Overview and History

The electrical excitability of nerve and muscle tissue has attracted scientific attention since the eighteenth century. As early as 1791, Galvani suggested that animals used electrical signals in their nervous system, a hypothesis that was corroborated in the mid-1800s by du Bois-Reymond. The word *ion*, which in Greek means "wanderer," was first introduced by Michael Faraday in 1834. Faraday also proposed the terms *cation* and *anion* for the positively and negatively charged ions, respectively. During the nineteenth century, studies by scientific luminaries including Luigi Galvani, Hermann von Helmholtz, Ernst von Brücke, Emil du Bois-Reymond, Jöns Jakob Berzelius, Leopoldo Nobili, and Carlo Matteucci explored the physicochemical processes underlying nerve and muscle excitability. In the 1880s, Sidney Ringer showed that an isolated frog heart would continue beating for an extended period of time only in a solution that contained Na^+, K^+, and Ca^{2+} in specific proportions. Thus, they were identified as the three most important cations for proper physiological function of the organism. In the early twentieth century, Walter Nernst and Max Planck formulated the concept of electro-diffusion, combining diffusion and conductance into a single kinetic and equilibrium theory. The understanding of electro-diffusion led scientists to the idea that ion mobility differences and diffusion potentials could account for the cell membrane excitability.

Another central concept regarding the cell membrane structure was developed during this time period. This idea of living cells being surrounded by a lipid bilayer was presented formally in 1935 and is referred to as the Danielli-Davson model. In the beginning of the twentieth century, Julius Bernstein proposed his famous "membrane hypothesis" for resting potential and action potential (Figure 16.1). By applying the Nernst equation (Section 16.2) to the study of the resting potential, he concluded that the cell membrane of a neuron at rest was selectively permeable only to K^+. Starting with the knowledge that the interior of nerve cells was negative compared to the outside of the cell under resting conditions, Bernstein measured changes in the membrane potential during an action potential, which normally lasts only a few milliseconds. Bernstein found that over the course of the action potential, the membrane potential became transiently positive, changing briefly from about −60 mV to 0 mV. His explanation for this was that a resting membrane was selectively permeable to K^+, but when the cell was stimulated it somehow became "disorganized" and then would allow any ion to pass through it in either direction. Though this tentative step was in the right direction, the "disorganized membrane" concept did not clarify the actual mechanism by which ions crossed the cell membrane.

In 1939, British physiologists Alan Hodgkin and Andrew Huxley (Figure 16.1) showed that during an action potential, the transient membrane potential depolarization, although qualitatively similar to that described by Bernstein, actually reversed such that the interior of the cell became much more positive (up to +40 mV), an event that is termed *overshoot* (Figure 16.2). Subsequent groundbreaking studies on neuronal membrane conductivity, using giant squid axons, by Hodgkin and Huxley published in 1952 in *The Journal of Physiology*, laid the groundwork to suggest the existence of ion channels. They showed that the action potential could be described by two separate, voltage- and time-dependent membrane permeability changes for Na^+ and K^+ ions. This research revolutionized the understanding of the ionic mechanisms involved in membrane electrophysiology, and would earn Hodgkin and Huxley the Nobel Prize in Physiology or Medicine in 1963.

A series of pharmacological and biophysical experiments conducted in the 1960s and 1970s provided additional evidence that the Na^+- and K^+-conducting elements were separate entities. By the early 1960s, it was becoming clear that ion channels were composed of proteins. The first actual ion channel to be identified at the molecular level was the nicotinic acetylcholine receptor (nAChR) in 1983. The cloning of nAChR subunits within the laboratories of Patrick, Heinemann, and Numa established the primary structure of the channel and for the first

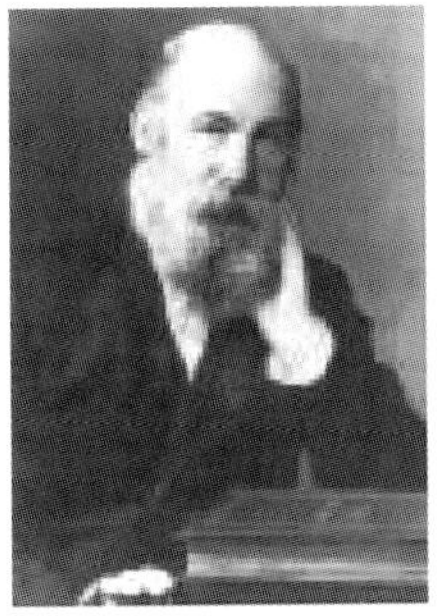

Julius Bernstein

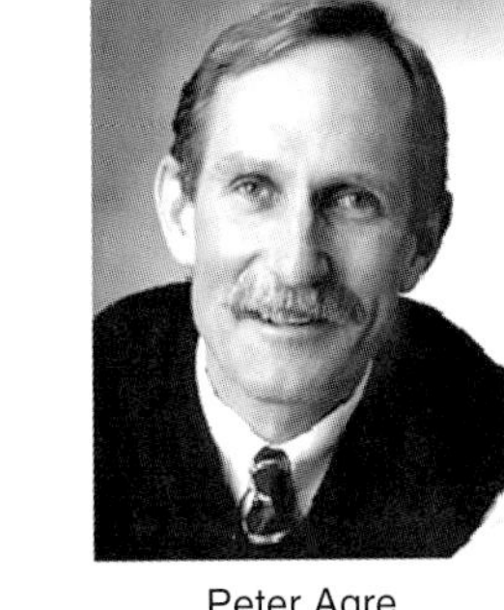

Peter Agre

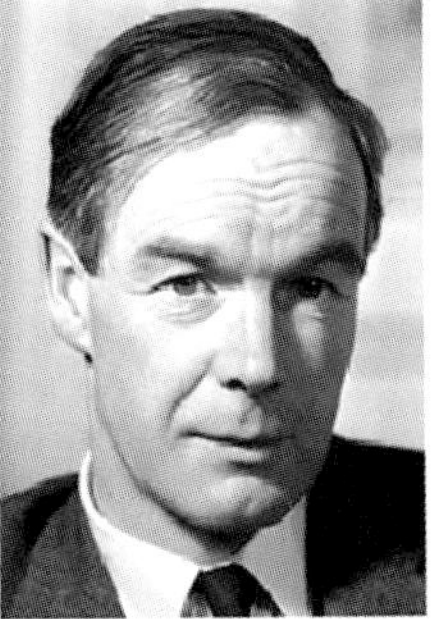

Alan Hodgkin

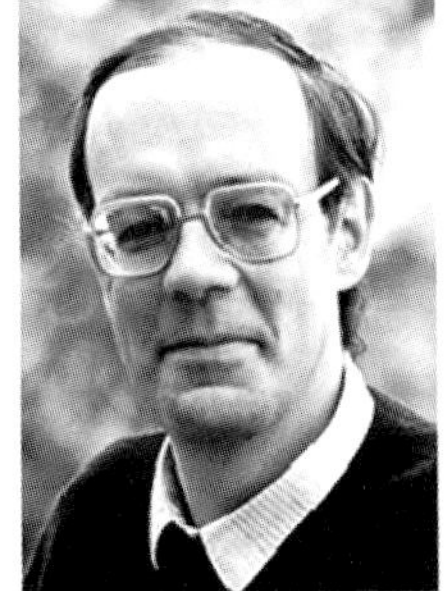

Bert Sakmann

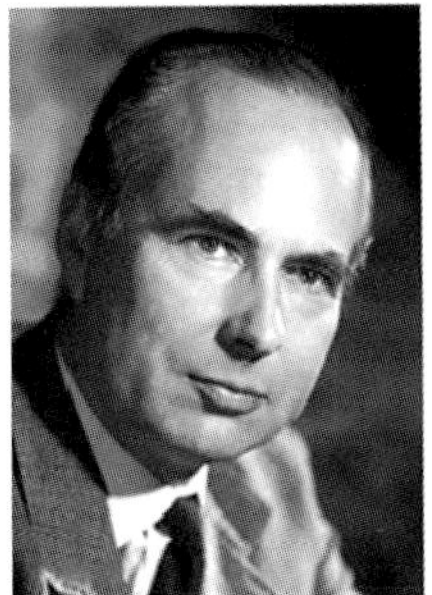

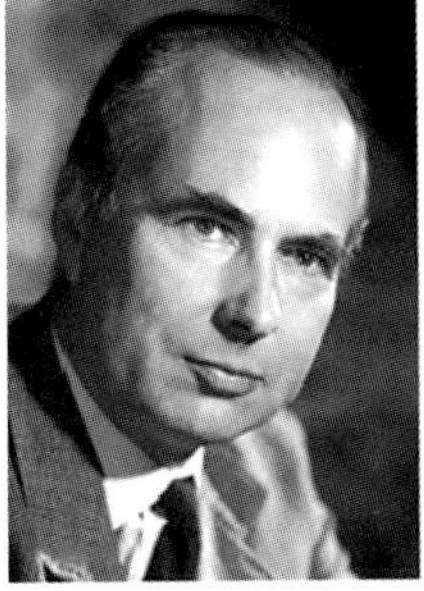

Andrew Huxley

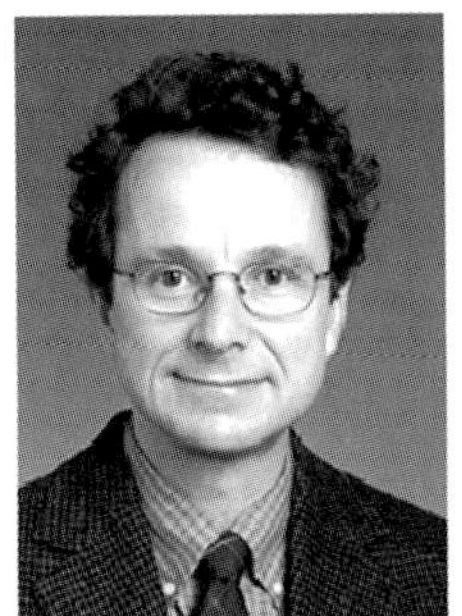

Roderick MacKinnon

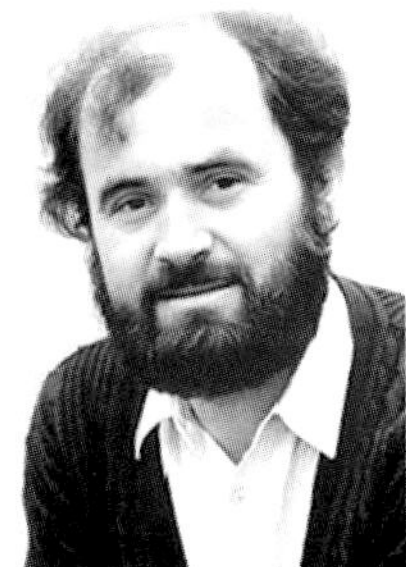

Erwin Neher

Figure 16.1 Scientists who made significant contributions to ion channel science.

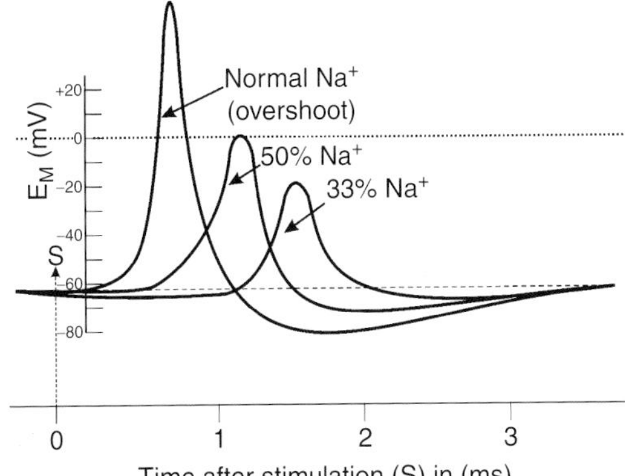

Figure 16.2 Illustration of the squid giant axon action potential and its dependence on external Na^+. The resting membrane potential (E_M) is about −60 mV. Following stimulation (S), the initial Na^+-dependent depolarization phase of the action potential that rises above 0 mV (overshoot) is gradually reduced in amplitude and delayed in time with reduction in extracellular Na^+. Similar experiments were originally conducted by Hodgkin, Huxley, and Katz in the 1930s/1950s using the voltage clamp technique (Section 16.5.1.1).

time provided an opportunity to characterize the ion channel functional properties.

Also, during the late 1970s and early 1980s, the **patch-clamp** technique (Section 16.5.1.3) was developed by two German scientists from the Max Planck Institute—Neher and Sakmann (Figure 16.1). This sophisticated technique provided the means for recording the tiny electrical currents flowing through an ion channel, allowing scientists to explore the function of ion channels in native cells down to the single channel level. First described in detail in *Pflügers Archiv* in 1981, the patch-clamp technique would become the quintessential method, incorporating the use of modern technology, for the study of electrophysiology. In 1991, Sakmann and Neher received the Nobel Prize in Physiology or Medicine for this technical milestone in ion channel discovery.

The concept of ion channels had evolved from the vague "disorganized membrane" of Bernstein's hypothesis, through the identification of discrete Na^+ and K^+ conducting elements of Hodgkin and Huxley, and finally to the elucidation of membrane proteins, whose molecular identity and functional properties could be probed with molecular and electrophysiological techniques. In the late 1990s, the biophysicist Roderick MacKinnon (Figure 16.1), provided high-resolution images of an individual ion channel. Working at Cornell and the Brookhaven National Laboratory, MacKinnon and colleagues used X-ray analysis to reveal the architecture of a bacterial K^+ channel (KcsA) from *Streptomyces lividans* (Figure 16.3). For this work, originally published in *Science* in 1998, and related independent investigations on water channel structure by Peter Agre of Johns Hopkins University School of Medicine (Figure 16.1), these investigators would share the 2003 Nobel Prize in Chemistry.

16.1.2 Ion Channel Classification and Nomenclature

Ion channels initially were classified on the basis of their most important **permeant** ion. In Hodgkin and Huxley's classic analysis of membrane ion conductivity,

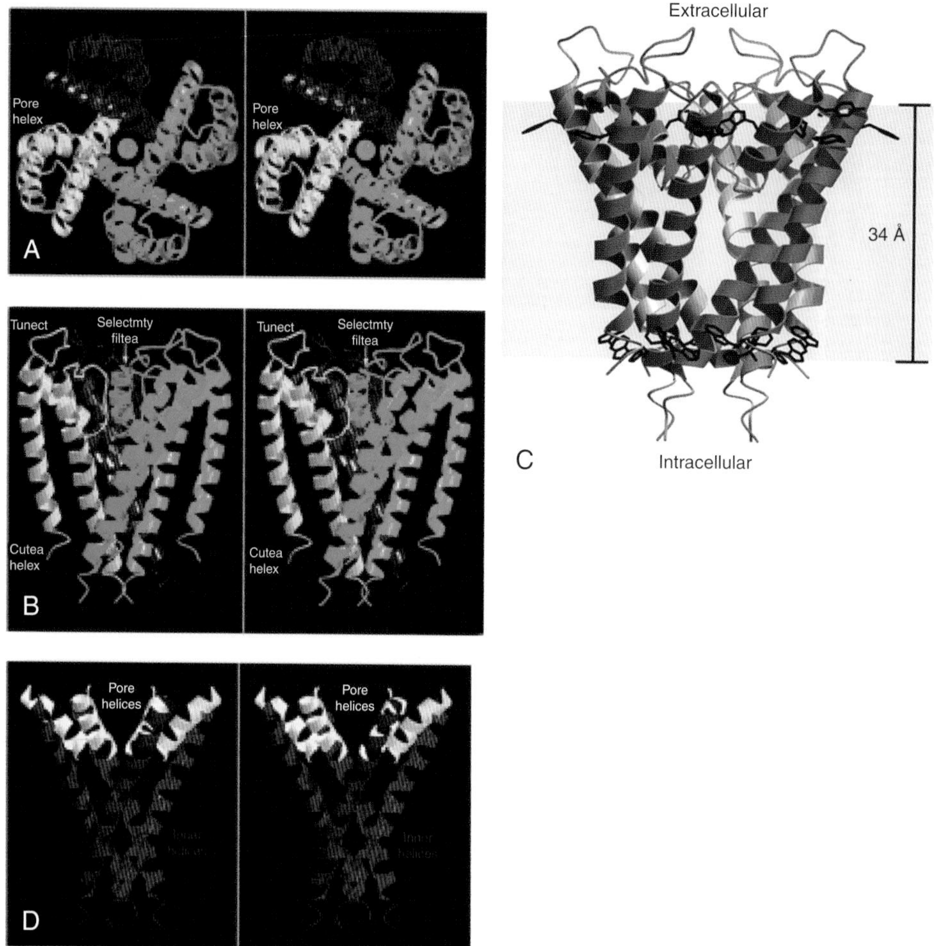

Figure 16.3 Images illustrating the architecture of a bacterial K^+ channel (KcsA). (A) Stereoview of a ribbon representation of the three-dimensional fold of the KcsA tetramer viewed from the extracellular side. The four subunits are distinguished by color. (B) Stereoview from another perspective, perpendicular to that in (A). (C) Ribbon representation of the tetramer as an integral-membrane protein. Aromatic amino acids on the membrane-facing surface are displayed in black. (D) Inverted cone-like architecture of the tetramer. With permission from American Association for the Advancement of Science.

two specific components of the current were recognized—Na^+ and K^+; a third component, termed *leak current*, completed the mathematical analysis. Thus, for the corresponding classes of ion channels, the names **Na^+ channel** and **K^+ channel** were given, and are still in use today. After that initial finding, it was further established that four main ions, Na^+, K^+, Ca^{2+}, and Cl^-, are responsible for controlling the electrical excitability of the cell membrane. The classification of ion channels into one of four main types on the basis of their ion selectivity—Na^+ channels, K^+ channels, Ca^{2+} channels, and Cl^- channels—was initially sufficient, but this simple scheme proved inadequate when it became clear that molecularly diverse channels were selective for the same ion. Furthermore, some channels lack clearly defined ion selectivity, acting instead as nonselective cation channels (Section 16.4.6).

For a time, as in the case of the moluscan ganglion cells, different channels with the same permeant ion were assigned to subgroups designated by letters A, B, C, and so on. In other cases, a descriptive approach was used to name channels. Channels were named for their responsiveness to specific neurotransmitters, such as the nAChR and glycine receptors, which bind to acetylcholine (ACh) and glycine, respectively. Channels also were named for the phenotype caused by their deletion, like the "Shaker" K^+ channel, which, when absent, produced a distinctive ataxic behavior. With the detection of the association of channel defects and disease, another nomenclature specific to the channels responsible for the disease arose—for example, the cystic fibrosis transmembrane conductance regulator (CFTR). Another naming policy originated from the use of inhibitors of channel function; the channels took their names from the particular inhibitors used to block their activity—for example, the amiloride-sensitive Na^+ channel. Some channels, like the Gardos channel, a Ca^{2+}-activated K^+ channel of intermediate conductance involved in red blood cell volume regulation, have taken on the name of the investigator that first described them.

It has become clear that there are hundreds of distinct, genetically encoded channels belonging to dozens of molecular families and superfamilies. The explosive increase in the number of individual channels identified, made possible by the widespread use of molecular cloning techniques, has resulted in the proliferation of channel names and naming systems. Many channels retain multiple common names, reflecting the near simultaneous identification—and naming—by researchers working independently of one another. To avoid confusion due to duplicated names, the International Union of Pharmacology (IUPHAR) has recently introduced standardized nomenclature for the voltage-gated Na^+, K^+, and Ca^{2+} channels (Section 16.4). This nomenclature is comparable to the enzymes nomenclature adopted by the Enzyme Commission, and uses a numerical system to define families, subfamilies, and individual members based on evolutionary and structural relationships of the ion channel genes. According to the IUPHAR system, the name of an individual voltage-gated channel consists of the chemical symbol of the main permeant ion (Na, K, or Ca) followed by the primary ion channel regulator (voltage) indicated in a subscript (Na_V, K_V, Ca_V). The number following the subscript indicates the gene subfamilies: Na_V1; K_V1, $K_V2 \ldots K_V12$; Ca_V1, Ca_V2, Ca_V3; and the number following the dot indicates the individual channel member, for example, $K_V3.1$, $Ca_V2.2$. Splice variant isoforms can be indicated by lowercase letters at the end—$K_V1.1a$, $K_V1.1b$, and so on. The Ca^{2+}-activated ($K_{Ca}1$–$K_{Ca}5$) and inwardly rectifying K^+ channels ($K_{ir}1$–$K_{ir}7$) use the same system for classification. Although IUPHAR has developed this unified nomenclature for some ion channels and is formalizing a new system for channel clones, as it had done previously for membrane receptors, the coexistence of multiple nomenclature systems is a challenge for researchers, and will likely remain a source of confusion for students of ion channel pharmacology.

16.2 ION CHANNEL STRUCTURE AND FUNCTION: BASIC PRINCIPLES AND MECHANISMS

The directional movement of ions through an ion channel is an electrical phenomenon because any net flow of charge, by definition, is electrical current, measured in amperes (A). One ampere is the steady flow of one coulomb (C) per second, where coulomb is a quantity of charge. For reference, the charge of one proton is 1.6×10^{-19} C. Ionic current through a single channel is determined by the electrochemical gradient, which consists of two factors: (1) the concentration of ions in the intracellular and the extracellular space; and (2) the potential difference across the cell membrane. Na^+ and K^+ ions are the two most abundant cations in most organisms. Na^+ is in high concentration outside the cell membrane, whereas K^+ is in high concentration inside the cell. Therefore, under physiological conditions, the currents flowing through the Na^+ channels are inward currents and those flowing through the K^+ channels are outward currents.

Although the extracellular Ca^{2+} concentration is relatively low (about 1.5 μM), there is still a high chemical gradient for Ca^{2+}, as its intracellular concentration is only about 100 nM at rest. Because of this, the currents flowing through a Ca^{2+} channel are also inward currents, like the Na^+ currents. In general, the ionic current that flows through a single ion channel is typically in the picoampere (pA) range; ionic current measured across an entire cell's membrane representing the ensemble current of many individual channels may be in the nanoampere range. These are small currents that require specific electronic equipment for detection (Section 16.5.1). Potential difference is measured in volts (V) and is defined as the work needed to move a unit test charge in a frictionless manner from one point to another. The potential difference across the cell membrane of a living cell is in the millivolt (mV) range. The ease of flow of current between two points is called conductance, and it is measured in Siemens (S). The conductivity (which is a channel property reflecting conductance) of a single ion channel is in the picoSiemens (pS) range.

Ohm's law, one of the most important laws in physics, is also a central law in the ion channel function. Ohm's law relates the potential (voltage) difference (E), conductance (g), and current (I), and is usually expressed as $I = g_x E$, which means that the current (I) equals the product of conductance (g) and potential difference. Ohm's law can also be expressed in the terms of Resistance (R), which is the reciprocal of conductance (see earlier), and is measured in ohms (Ω). In this case, Ohm's law is written as $E = I_x R$. Ohm's law plays a central role in ion channel research because each ion channel is an elementary conductor, with its own conductivity, passing through an electrically insulating cell membrane. The total electrical conductivity of a membrane is the sum of all ion channel single conductivities in parallel. It is a measure of how many ion channels are open, how many ions are available to go through them, and how easily the ions pass.

The second most important equation in ion channel research, which tells us about the equilibrium potential (E_s), is the Nernst equation:

$$E_s = \frac{RT}{z_s F} \ln \frac{[S]_o}{[S]_i}$$

R is the universal gas constant
T is the temperature in Kelvin
F is the Faraday constant
S is the particular ion type with charge z_s
$[S]_o$ is the ion concentration outside the cell membrane
$[S]_i$ is the intracellular ion concentration

The *equilibrium potential*, also known as *reversal potential*, is the cell membrane potential at which there is no net flow of ions (for a particular ion type) through the membrane. Equilibrium reflects the fact that the net ion flow, for the particular ion, at the given voltage, is zero. Reversal reflects the fact that further change of the membrane potential can reverse the direction of ion flux for the particular ion type. In other words, at very positive values of the membrane potential (over $\sim$+60 mV), the Na^+ and Ca^{2+} currents can become outward currents and at very negative values (less than $\sim$−100 mV) the K^+ current can become an inward current. Under physiological conditions, the cells maintain a negative resting membrane potential because, overall, they have more K^+ channels open than Na^+ or Ca^{2+} channels.

16.2.1 Ion Channel Structural Properties

A functionally defined channel is rarely a single polypeptide chain. Instead, ion channels are usually composed of one or more pore-forming subunits that are often associated with accessory subunits that regulate channel-gating behavior (activation/inactivation kinetics) and/or ligand binding. In general the pore-forming subunits are referred to as α subunits, whereas the accessory subunits are designated by subsequent letters in the Greek alphabet (β, γ, δ, ϵ, etc.).

16.2.1.1 Ion Channel Pore Structure

All ion channels form a pore that allows selective flow of ions through the membrane. Most channels have two transmembrane segments (TMs), called M1 and M2, linked by a *pore loop*, a region of the protein pore structure that loops back into the cell membrane to form the **selectivity filter** (Section 16.2.2.1). Interestingly, from an evolutionary perspective, all pore-loop channels resemble the KcsA channel, whose crystal protein structure was recently revealed through the work of the MacKinnon's group (Figure 16.3). The inwardly rectifying K^+ (K_{ir}) channel is the simplest of all channels, representing this basic structure (Figure 16.4). Among K_V and Ca^{2+}-activated K^+ (K_{Ca}) channel families, the most common arrangement is that of four such subunits assembling (tetramer) to form the channel pore (Figure 16.4). This tetrameric structure of the pore-loop channels contributes to channel diversity, as closely related subunits can associate to form heteromeric structures with novel functional properties, as in the case of the K_V channels (Section 16.4.4). An alternative to this basic channel structure is the two-pore domain K^+ channels (for example, the K_{2P} channel), which most likely have developed from a duplication of the original individual subunit. Two such subunits (a dimer) create a pore tetrameric structure.

Another basic pore structure is represented by the S4 channel superfamily, which involves the voltage-gated Na_V, Ca_V, and K_V channels (Figure 16.4). Members of this family possess an additional four (five in the case of the $K_{Ca}1.1$ [BK] channel) TM segments at the amino-terminal of the protein. The fourth TM segment (S4) is positively charged and serves as a voltage sensor. In some channels of the S4 family, such as the voltage-gated Ca^{2+} (Ca_V) and Na^+ (Na_V) channels, the entire pore is composed of a single polypeptide chain of about 250–500 kDa that forms the tetrameric pore structure alone (Figure 16.4).

There are also many other channel structures referred to as nonpore-loop channels, which are a diverse and dissimilar group. The essential transmembrane topology and subunit stoichiometry of the basic ligand-gated channel families are illustrated in Figure 16.9.

16.2.1.2 Ion Channel Accessory Proteins

In addition to the pore-forming structure, most channels possess tightly associated accessory subunits, which tremendously increase ion channel diversity. In general, these accessory subunits determine ion channel tissue specificity. They can also modulate channel functional properties, including channel-gating mechanisms, channel sensitivity to endogenous ligands and pharmacological agents (Figures 16.5 and 16.6). Accessory ion channel subunits may facilitate the trafficking of pore-forming subunits to the cell membrane. Accessory proteins may also be crucial to ion channel function, and in their absence, the channels could completely cease functional activity. For example, the sulphonylurea receptor (SUR) subunit of the K_{ir} (K_{ATP}) channel, which belongs to the "ATP-binding cassette" (ABC) family of ATP-driven pumps that transport nutrients, drugs, and solutes across the membrane using the energy of ATP hydrolysis, plays a key role in the metabolic regulation of the channel by stimulating ATP-dependent channel opening and determining the sensitivity to therapeutic drugs known as K^+ channel openers (Section 16.4.4). The inactivation properties of many voltage-gated channels are controlled by their accessory subunits. Accessory subunits may even serve as kinases that phosphorylate the pore-forming subunit or other proteins.

In addition to these ion channel structural considerations, it should be noted that channels can be expressed in different isoforms encoded by distinct genes or as different splice variants that may be selectively expressed in certain cell types or during certain developmental stages of an organism. These structural variations dramatically increase the level of channel functional diversity.

16.2.2 Ion Channel Functional Properties

The two most essential ion channel properties are ion selectivity and gating. **Selectivity** is the property of the channels to discriminate among different ions, allowing some to pass through the pore while arresting the flow of others. **Gating** is the process by which the ion channel is physically opened or closed to permit the transit of ions.

16.2.2.1 Ion Selectivity

With the exception of some channel groups, such as the nonselective cation channels (Section 16.4.6), most ion channels are very selective for their particular

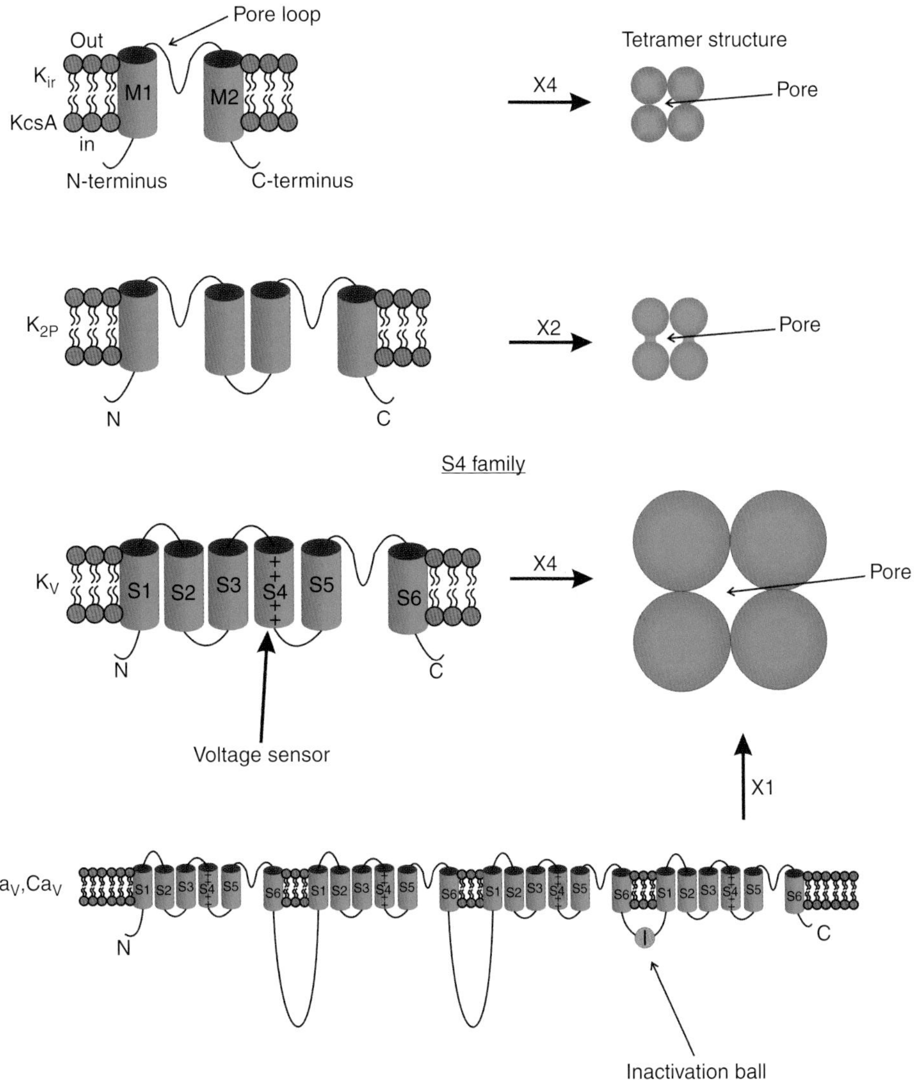

Figure 16.4 Cartoon illustrating the hypothetical transmembrane topology (left side) and subunit stoichiometry (right side) of the basic pore-loop ion channel types. K_{ir}, inwardly rectifying K^+ channel, is the simplest ion channel structure with two transmembrane segments connected by a pore loop. Four such subunits form a functional channel pore (tetramer). The two-pore domain K^+ (K_{2P}) channels make a tetrameric pore structure from two subunits-dimers. The S4 channel family is presented by the K_V, voltage-gated K^+ channel; Na_V, voltage-gated Na^+ channel; and Ca_V, voltage-gated Ca^{2+} channel. The S4 transmembrane domain is the voltage-sensor. The numbers above the arrows refer to the number of subunits that make up the tetramer channel pore.

permeant ion. This is especially valid for the four major channel families—Na^+, K^+, Ca^{2+}, and Cl^- channels. The distinction between separate ions takes place at a specialized structure of the ion channel pore, known as the selectivity filter.

The best studied **selectivity filter** is that of the K^+ channels. These channels are about 10,000 times more permeable to K^+ than Na^+. Differences in the ion's size and its crystallographic (Pauling) radius—Na^+ (0.96 Å radius), K^+ (1.33 Å radius), Ca^{2+} (0.99 Å radius), Cl^- (1.81 Å radius)—is apparently one possible explanation for the mechanism of the selectivity filter (Table 16.1). Interestingly, K^+ ion selectivity is

Table 16.1 Differences in the Atomic Radii and Hydration Shield Diameters of Cation Species

Cation Species	Na^+	K^+	Ca^{2+}
Cation radius (Pauling radius)	0.96 Å	1.33 Å	0.99 Å
Number of water molecules	6–8	4–6	8–10
Diameter of the first hydration shield	~8 Å	~6 Å	~12 Å

achieved despite the fact that the Na^+ ion is smaller than K^+. In a solution, however, ions are surrounded by water molecules, and therefore are hydrated. This changes their total diameter, as the first hydration shell of a K^+ and Na^+ ion contains 4–6 and 6–8 water molecules, respectively, and those of Ca^{2+} have 8–10. Taking into account the diameter of the water molecule (about 2 Å), the hydrated Na^+, K^+, and Ca^{2+} have diameters of approximately 8 Å, 6 Å, and 12 Å, respectively (Table 16.1). Therefore, the ion selectivity is not simply based on the ion size.

In the past decade, X-ray crystallography studies on the bacterial K^+ channel by MacKinnon's group have provided insight into the molecular basis of the K^+ channel selectivity filter, demonstrating that it is the narrowest part of the channel, which has an inverted, cone-like shape made by four identical K^+ channel subunits (Figures 16.3 and 16.5). In order for the K^+ ions to pass through the selectivity filter, which is only 12 Å long and about 2.70–3.08 Å in diameter, the hydrated K^+ ions must be completely dehydrated. This process takes place in another unique structure, known as the central cavity, which is about 10 Å in diameter and is located on the intracellular side, just before the selectivity filter. The K^+ ion needs to be dehydrated prior to entering the selectivity filter. Dehydration is an energy-consuming process that depends on the ion size. As the ionic radius decreases, the interaction with water molecules becomes stronger because its positively charged nucleus can approach more closely to the negatively charged oxygen atoms of the water molecules. Na^+ (0.96 Å radius) and Ca^{2+} (0.99 Å radius) are both excluded from the K^+ selectivity filter because their dehydration energies are much higher than those of the K^+ (1.33 Å radius).

The K^+ selectivity filter has two conformational states, controlled by the K^+ concentration. High K^+ concentration maintains a conductive state, whereas low K^+ concentration locks the filter and the whole channel in a nonconductive state. This has an important physiological relevance as the intracellular K^+ concentration is high and may relate to the channel-gating mechanism (Section 16.2.2.2). MacKinnon's X-ray crystallographic studies also revealed that a chain of carbonyl oxygen atoms span along the selectivity filter forming four K^+-binding sites (Figure 16.5). Eight oxygen atoms form each K^+-binding site. These carbonyl residues replace the water molecules of hydration and the binding sites they form are a perfect match for the K^+ ion. This structure facilitates a mechanism allowing the K^+ ions to pass through the filter by jumping from one binding site to the next. The oxygen atoms of the carbonyls are far enough and cannot interact directly with the smaller Na^+ ions, which do not appear to be a good match for these K^+ binding sites. Thus, Na^+ is effectively excluded from the K^+ selectivity filter. While in the filter the dehydrated K^+ ions are so close together that they repel each

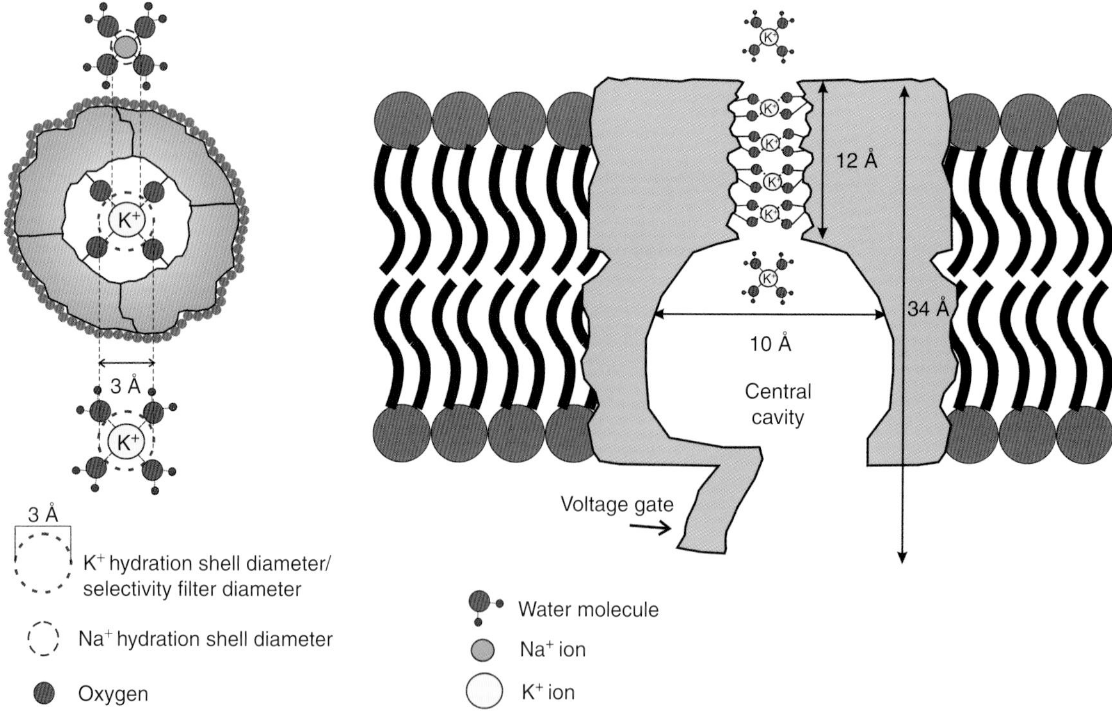

Figure 16.5 Illustration of the structure and mechanism of the K^+ channel selectivity filter with views from above (left side) and as transmembrane protein structure with a gate, central cavity, and a selectivity filter (right side). To pass through the filter, the K^+ needs to be dehydrated. The K^+ selectivity filter holds and stabilizes four dehydrated K^+ ions by using carbonyl oxygen atoms (red) that resemble the K^+ hydration shell. The smaller Na^+ ion cannot stabilize in this structure that fits uniquely to the size of the K^+ ions only. Based on MacKinnon's X-ray crystallographic studies and proposed mechanism.

other. They push each other through the filter quickly by overcoming the attractive forces between K^+ ions and the carbonyl oxygen atoms of the selectivity filter. This unique mechanism and distinctive structure of the selectivity filter provide for the high K^+ conductivity and selectivity (Figure 16.5).

Na^+ and Ca^{2+} channels most likely use different mechanisms to achieve their selectivity. Although their crystal structure is still unknown, it is believed that Na^+ and Ca^{2+} channels also use negatively charged oxygen residues to coordinate the cation flow. A highly conserved amino acid sequence—aspartate, glutamate, lysine, and alanine (DEKA) in the pore loops of each domain (I, II, III, and IV) is believed to form the selectivity filter of the Na channel (Figures 16.4 and 16.10). Studies indicate that Na^+ channels have wider selectivity filters (4–6 Å) than that of K^+ channels (about 3 Å). Theoretically, the selectivity filter of the Na^+ channel is large enough to allow an Na^+ ion in partially dehydrated form through, but stops the larger hydrated K^+ ion.

It is believed that the Ca^{2+} channel also contains negatively charged binding sites to provide for cation selective transport. Ca^{2+} ion selectivity is not simply based on ion hydration size, because Ca^{2+} is better hydrated than Na^+ and the unhydrated diameters of Ca^{2+} and Na^+ are about the same. Although the permeability of monovalent cations in the Ca^{2+} channel is quite low at physiological ionic concentrations, increased monovalent cationic permeability occurs in the absence of Ca^{2+} and other divalent cations (e.g., Mg^{2+}). This suggests that in its essence the Ca^{2+} channel is permeable to both divalent and monovalent cations, but the selectivity arises from competition between ions. Under physiological ionic concentrations, the monovalent cations simply cannot compete with Ca^{2+}. It is important to note that through all the speculation and theories surrounding their functions, the precise ion selectivity mechanisms that work in the Na^+ and Ca^{2+} channels remain undiscovered.

The nAChR, P2X receptors (Section 16.4.1), and the nonselective cation channels (Section 16.4.6), as their names indicate, permit flux of different cations, mainly Na^+ and Ca^{2+}. These channels have a relatively large water-occupied pore through which cations move fully hydrated or in a partially dehydrated state. Negatively charged residues in the pore exclude all anions, allowing cation flux only.

As a simple alternative to the mechanisms described earlier, anion selective channels such as the Cl^- channels (CLC) have rings of positively charged residues in their pore, which helps to exclude all cations.

16.2.2.2 Gating

Opening and closing of ion channels are essentially random processes often referred to as ion channel open probability. **Open probability** usually is indicated by a number reflecting the time the channel is open divided by the entire time of single channel recording (Section 16.5.1.3). Theoretically, the open probability value can be anything between zero (the channel is closed 100% of the time) and one (the channel is open 100% of the time). An open probability value of 1 is never achieved under physiological conditions. The transition rate between open and closed states is in the range of several microseconds and the flux rate through the transiently open pore ranges from several hundreds of thousands to 100 million ions per second. Structural and functional studies have revealed that most channels are closed by a gate that acts as a physical barrier to ion movement (Figure 16.6). Although in some channels the selectivity filter itself may act as an additional gating mechanism, the protein structures that make up ion channel gates are physically distinct from those that form the selectivity filter (Figures 16.5 and 16.6).

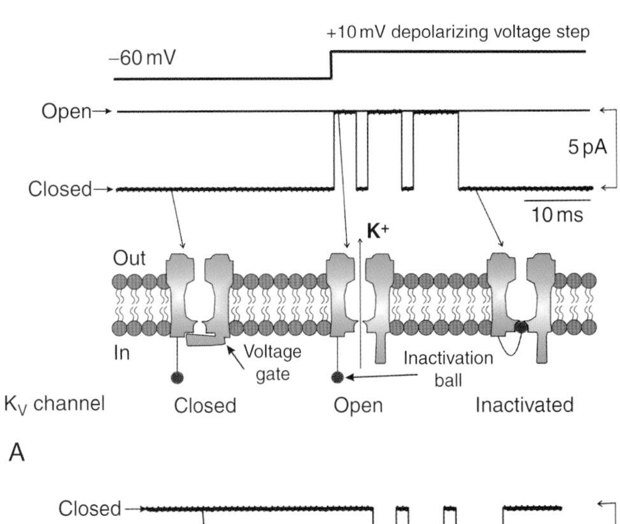

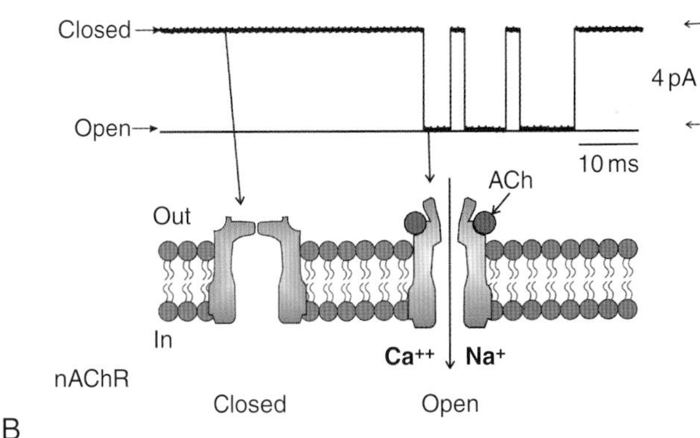

Figure 16.6 Illustration of the voltage-gated (A) and ligand-gated (B) ion channel mechanism. A. A voltage-gated channel such as the K_v channel, opens under depolarization. Illustrated are the associated single-channel recordings during a depolarizing stimulation from −60 mV to +10 mV (Section 16.5.1.3). After opening, the K_v channel (and some other voltage-gated channels) enters an inactivated nonconducting conformational state, which involves a separate gating mechanism. B. The nAChR, a ligand-gated channel, opens upon acetylcholine (ACh) allosteric binding to the channel proteins. nAChR has two ACh binding sites and after opening conducts both Ca^{2+} and Na^+ ions. Associated single-channel recordings are also illustrated.

The predominant influences on the frequency of ion channel opening and closing are transmembrane voltage (cell membrane potential) and ligand binding. The ion channel opening and closing can also be modulated by a number of other processes including protein–protein interactions, posttranslational modifications, mechanical stress, and changes in temperature. Accordingly, ion channels typically are classified as voltage-gated or ligand-gated. Some channels, such as the large conductance voltage-gated and Ca^{2+}-activated K^+ (BK, MaxiK, or $K_{Ca}1.1$) channel, have dual mechanisms of regulation and are both voltage- and ligand-gated.

Voltage Gating As the name implies, the activity of voltage-gated channels is regulated by changes in the transmembrane voltage. Voltage sensing requires a specialized structure that is capable of detecting the transfer of an electrical charge through the cell membrane in response to changes in transmembrane voltage. Based on similar structural elements, the voltage-gated Na_V, Ca_V, and K_V channels are classified as the S4 channel superfamily. In this S4 family, the voltage sensor consists of several positively charged residues in the fourth TM segment (S4). Transmembrane voltage changes produce conformational modifications in the pore region through movement of these conserved S4 segment residues (Figures 16.4 and 16.6A). This increases the ion channel's open probability. In the case of CLC, the voltage-gated mechanism is driven by charged ligand activators bound to sites deep within the protein.

Following activation and opening, some voltage-gated channels, mainly K_V, Na_V, and Ca_V, are subject to inactivation and can adopt a separate inactivated state. This ion channel state is distinct from the closed state of the channel and is characterized as a nonconducting state refractory to subsequent cell membrane depolarization. Inactivation of some K_V channels is produced by an N-terminus intracellular region of the channel and for that reason is termed *N-type inactivation* (also known as fast inactivation). This tethered protein structure, acting much like a ball-and-chain, swings into the pore and physically plugs it (Figure 16.6A). Some K_V channels have an additional mechanism for inactivation, located at the C-terminus, called *C-type inactivation* (also known as slow inactivation). Inactivation of voltage-gated CLC is based on very subtle conformational changes where even the rotation of a single amino acid can be responsible for the inactivation process leading to inhibition of ion permeation.

Ligand Gating In the context of ion channels, a ligand is any molecule that interacts with an ion channel or with a receptor linked to an ion channel, and regulates channel opening and closing by producing conformational changes (Figure 16.6B). Channel ligands are commonly extracellular small organic molecules including neurotransmitters such as ACh, glutamate, glycine, γ-aminobutyric acid (GABA), or nucleotides. The ligand-binding sites typically are located at the boundary between two adjacent channel subunits and may lie at some considerable distance from the channel gate. Such examples are the ACh-binding site of nAChR, glutamate-binding site of the glutamate receptor (GluR) channel, the cyclic-nucleotide-binding site of cyclic-nucleotide-gated (CNG) channels, and the ATP-binding site of Kir6.2 (K_{ATP}) channels (Section 16.4.4).

Another interesting feature of some ligand-gated channels is that they may have more than one ligand-binding site; two for example in the case of nAChR (Figure 16.6). The CNG channels have four cyclic nucleotide binding sites. This is important from a functional perspective as it provides multiple degrees and levels of regulation. In some cases, however, the conformational and functional changes could be initiated by ligand binding to only one site of two or more available. For example, the four inhibitory ATP-binding sites of the K_{ATP} channel act independently and the binding of only one ATP molecule to any of the four available sites is sufficient to close the channel. Sometimes ligands bind at the intracellular side of the channel. Inorganic ions (e.g., H^+, Ca^{2+}) may also act as intracellular ligands. Examples include proton (H^+)-gated channels and $K_{Ca}1.1$ (BK) channels, which respond with an increase in activity upon binding the intracellular inorganic ligand, H^+ or Ca^{2+}, respectively.

A fundamental principle of ligand gating is that ligands bind differently to open and closed channel conformations. Ligand binding to the open state usually contributes to channel activation, whereas binding to the closed configuration most often leads to channel inhibition. Ion channels may also be regulated by endogenous peptides—ligands—but by far the most important role that peptide ligands play in ion channel pharmacology is as highly selective inhibitors of channel function (Section 16.3).

And finally, it is important to consider that ion channels are surrounded and directly associated with membrane phospholipids that influence the channel gating. However, the exact mechanisms of channel-gating modulation by membrane lipids remain to be discovered.

16.3 ION CHANNEL PHARMACOLOGY: PRINCIPLES AND MECHANISMS

Ion channel pharmacology is concerned with the mechanisms of ion channel inhibition, activation, and modulation by different compounds. These compounds include a wide variety of chemicals, inorganic and organic ions, drugs, plant alkaloids, and other polyamines, peptides, toxins, venoms, and neurotransmitters. Highly specific ion channel inhibitors have enabled researchers to selectively isolate individual ion channels and determine their contribution to complex physiological processes. In fact, the Na^+ and K^+ channels were identified first as two distinct molecular entities based on their sensitivities to two separate selective inhibitors—tetrodotoxin (TTX) and tetraethylammonium (TEA) (Figure 16.7). TTX is a paralytic

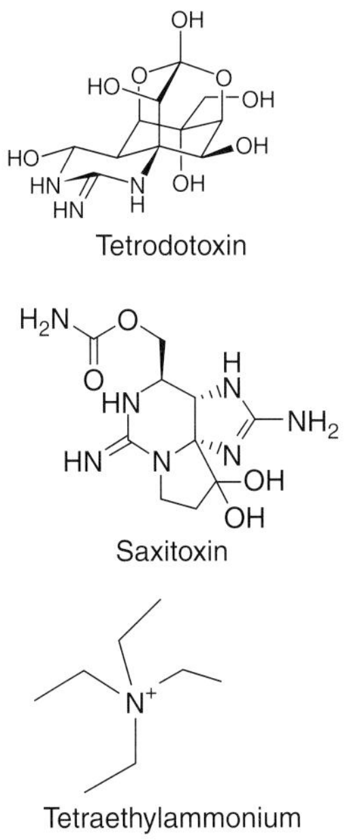

Tetrodotoxin

Saxitoxin

Tetraethylammonium

Figure 16.7 Chemical structure of tetrodotoxin (TTX), saxitoxin (STX), and tetraethylammonium (TEA).

toxin extracted from *Tetraodontiformes* fish (pufferfish, porcupinefish, ocean sunfish, and triggerfish). These fish are culinary delicacies in some countries, but if prepared improperly, they have been known to kill consumers. In the mid-1960s, voltage-clamp experiments (Section 16.5.1.1) on lobster giant axons by Narahashi and colleagues showed, for the first time, that TTX is a highly specific and potent Na_V channel inhibitor. Also in the 1960s, another toxin, saxitoxin (STX), isolated from *Dinoflagellate* plankton, was demonstrated to inhibit the Na_V channel in the same manner (Figure 16.7). In the late 1950s/early 1960s, TEA was shown to block the voltage-dependent K^+ current component, and therefore the K_V channel. Thus, these three highly specific ion-channel inhibitors would become the fundamental element enabling the emerging field of ion-channel pharmacology.

16.3.1 Mechanism of Ion Channel Inhibition

Ion channel inhibitors make use of different mechanisms to inhibit ion channels, but their modes of action can roughly be classified into two major categories: (1) pore plugging; and (2) allosteric binding. The precise mechanisms of ion channel inhibition remain controversial and it is often difficult to determine which mechanism is used by a particular inhibitor.

The pore plugging inhibitors enter the channel pore, bind somewhere in the pore region, and physically obstruct the ion transport through the pore. In general, channel pore plugging inhibition is a reversible process, and washing out the inhibitor restores the normal function of the channel. This mechanism does not involve allosteric binding, by comparing it to a cork stopping the flow of wine from a bottle. TTX and STX bind (nonallosterically) and plug the Na_V channel from the extracellular side of the pore. Most often, however, the plugging takes place from the intracellular part of the channel, which requires the inhibitor first to pass through the cell membrane. TEA and other K^+ channel inhibiting quaternary ammonium ions (QA) use this mechanism acting from the intracellular side of the channel.

The original evidence for this mechanism came in the late 1960s from experiments showing that TEA and QA are more effective in inhibiting the outward K^+ current versus the inward K^+ current. It should be mentioned that TEA has a second binding site at the extracellular mouth of the channel providing an additional inhibition for the K channels. Sometimes the channel inhibition can occur only when the channel is open and not in a closed state. This is referred to as open channel inhibition. TEA and QA use this approach to inhibit the K_V channels from the intracellular side. When the cell membrane is depolarized, the voltage gate opens, TEA enters the enlarged section of the channel known as the central cavity (Section 16.2.2.1), and becomes lodged, thereby plugging the channel (Figure 16.8). Local anesthetics, which inhibit the neuronal Na_V channels, use the same mechanism and require the Na_V channel to be open. Moreover, under repeated depolarizations of the membrane, local anesthetics exert cumulative inhibition of the Na_V channel, a mechanism termed *use-dependent* (state-dependent or phasic) inhibition. The inhibitory mechanism of phenalkylamines on the L-type Ca^{2+} channels (Ca_V1) is also use-dependent.

Allosteric binding requires a specific binding site, often found, but not limited to, the extracellular side of the pore where the allosteric inhibitor binds to the channel and causes conformational changes that prevent the normal function of the channel. This mechanism is analogous to the way agonists and antagonists bind to other membrane receptors, and is similar to that of ligand-binding in the case of nAChR (Figure 16.6A). Usually, the allosteric inhibitors bind to and lock the channel in a nonconducting conformational state. Dihydropyridines (DHPs), L-type Ca^{2+} channel (Ca_V1) inhibitors, and most natural toxins (Section 16.3.2) use the allosteric mechanism of channel inhibition.

In the case of voltage-gated channels, a "favorite" binding site for inhibitors and channel modulators is often located somewhere on the voltage-sensor domain (S4) or the inactivation ball. The voltage-sensor domain is partially exposed to the extracellular space, which makes the binding easier. Such modulators interfere with the voltage-sensor, and thus modulate the ion channel gating. For this reason they are often referred to as voltage-sensor modulators or gating modifiers. Gating modifiers can have different effects, including but not limited to sustained channel activation or inhibition, or increased or delayed inactivation. They can also inhibit the inactivation process completely.

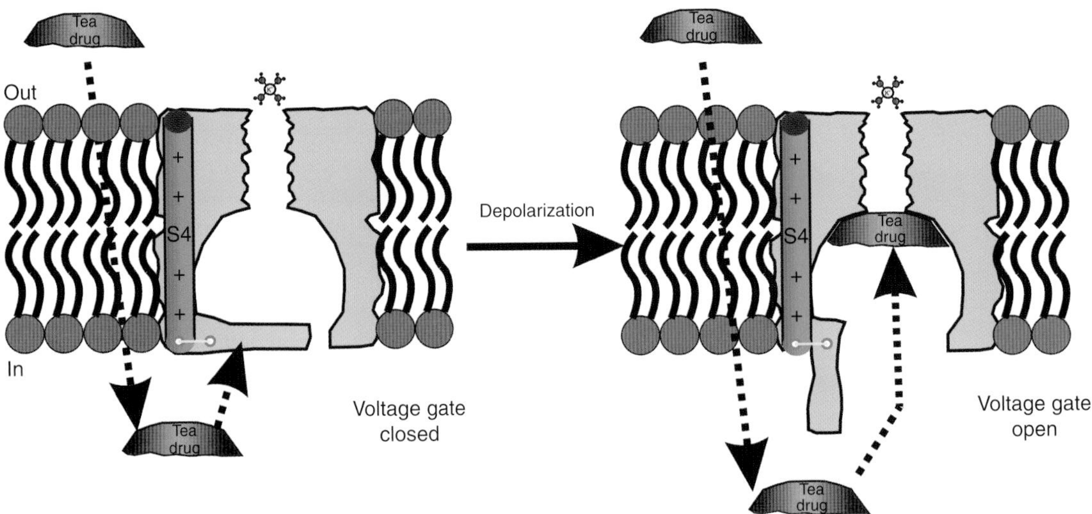

Figure 16.8 Illustration of open channel inhibition. Tetraethylammonium (TEA) penetrates the cell membrane and acts from the intracellular side of the K_V channels. Channel inhibition occurs only under membrane depolarization when the voltage gate opens. TEA or a structurally related drug enters the central cavity and occludes the channel. The voltage sensor (S4 domain) that opens and closes the voltage gate is also illustrated.

16.3.2 Natural Toxins as Ion Channel Research Tools

Since the discovery of TTX and STX inhibitory effects on Na_V channels, a number of natural toxins have been shown to be highly specific ion channel inhibitors. Due to their relatively small molecular size, compact and rigid structure, high potency and selectivity, ion channel inhibitors isolated from poisonous species have emerged as highly valuable pharmacological tools for ion channel research. To capture prey, poisonous creatures use a vast arsenal of biologically active venom compounds. Although venom components may target different cellular mechanisms, their high effectiveness is directly related to the fact that they specifically target ion channels that are key regulators of cell membrane excitability. The degree of pharmacological diversity accumulated during their evolution has resulted in extremely complex mixtures of thousands of active ion channel compounds that have been isolated from snakes (α-bungarotoxin), snails (ω-conotoxin), newts, spiders (ω-agatoxin), scorpions (iberiotoxin, charybdotoxin), bees (apamin), molluscs, fish (TTX), sea anemones, and plants (D-tubocurarin, ryanodine). For example, a single type of spider venom might contain up to several hundred peptides, some of which are very specific ion channel modulators.

Toxins isolated from venomous animals are usually small peptides, ranging from several amino acids to around 70 amino acids. Their various pharmacological advantages include high ion channel specificity, high activity, and relative insensitivity to proteases. The names of these peptides usually begin with a Greek letter, such as ω for Ca channels or for Na channels, followed by the name of the venomous species, and finishing with numbers and letters related to the position of the peak in the eluate from a separation column; for example, "ω-conotoxin GVIA" and "μ-conotoxin GIIIA." In general, venom toxins use allosteric binding mechanism and are effective in nanomolar or even picomolar concentrations. Most of these toxins are rich in disulfide bonds and target primarily cation-selective channels. Toxin channel selectivity is achieved by additional protein–protein interactions. Therefore, information on the three-dimensional structure of both the channel and toxin helps to better understand how the toxins discriminate between close structurally related channels. In the next sections we will review some of the more common venom toxins that are used as inhibitors or modulators for each specific ion channel family.

16.4 ION CHANNEL GROUPS: FUNCTIONAL IMPLICATIONS AND PHARMACOLOGICAL MODULATORS

In this section we will review the major groups and families of ion channels, their basic characteristics and physiological roles, inhibitors and activators, and their pharmacological significance. The subsections about the Na channels, Ca channels, and K channels are focused primarily on the voltage-gated Na_V, Ca_V, and K_V channels, which are structurally similar and belong to one big superfamily of voltage-gated channels.

16.4.1 Ligand-Gated Channels

The ligand-gated channels, also known as agonist-gated, are a group of ion channels that open or close in response to binding of a chemical messenger (ligand), as opposed to voltage-gated ion channels (see earlier). Although structurally and functionally diverse, the ligand-gated channels have a great degree of homology at the genetic level. Based on their structural properties they are classified into three major superfamilies: (1) cys-loop channels, (2) glutamate receptor (GluR) channels, and (3) ATP-gated/purinergic receptor channels (Figure 16.9, Table 16.2).

The cys-loop superfamily, also know as pentameric fast ligand-gated receptors, consists of two subgroups: (1) cationic channels—serotonin/5-hydroxytryptamine (5-HT_3) receptors and nAChRs, and (2) anionic (Cl^-) channels—$GABA_A$ and glycine receptors. The receptors of the cys-loop superfamily are made of five homologous subunits arranged in a ring that forms a pore (pentramer). Each subunit contains an extracellular domain, followed by four transmembrane segments (Figure 16.9). All cys-loop channels are allosterically inhibited by Zn^{2+}, believed to be due to a block of the channel-gating mechanism.

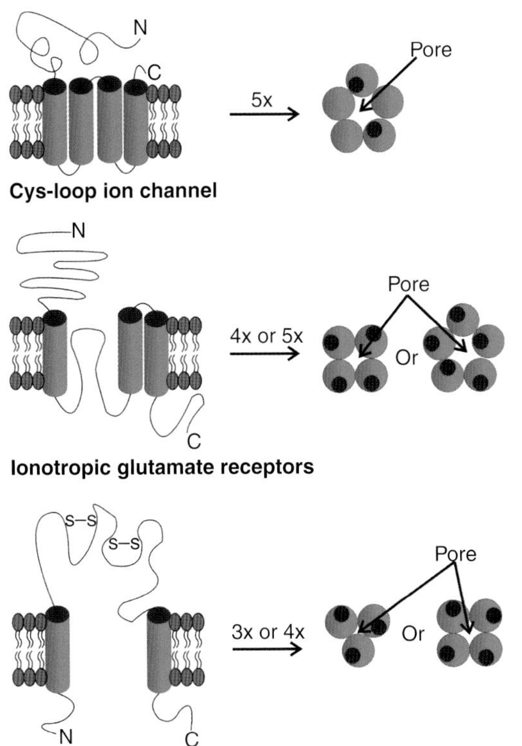

Figure 16.9 Cartoon illustrating the hypothetical transmembrane topology (left side) and subunit stoichiometry (right side) of the three basic ligand-gated channel superfamilies: (1) cys-loop channels; (2) glutamate receptor channels; and (3) ATP-gated/P2X purinergic receptor channels. The numbers above the arrows refer to the number of subunits that make up the channel pore. The hypothetical ligand-binding sides are indicated in red.

A classic example of a ligand-gated ion channel from the cys-loop superfamily is the nAChR. The *nicotinic* AChRs are named so because they can be activated by the tobacco alkaloid *nicotine* in the same way they are activated by ACh. It should be mentioned that the *muscarinic* AChRs, which respond to the alkaloid *muscarine*, are not ion channels, and therefore not discussed in this chapter. The nAChR is made up of five subunits ($\alpha1$, $\beta1$, γ, δ, and ϵ) with two binding sites for ACh (Figures 16.6B and 16.9). The nAChRs are expressed in nerves and skeletal muscle (but not smooth muscle) and play an important role in the fast synaptic transmission in synaptic neuronal-neuronal and neuromuscular junctions. nAChR is a nonselective cation channel that allows the flow of many cations, but not anions. After ACh binds to the nAChR it allows Na^+ and also Ca^{2+}, to flow down their electrochemical gradient into the cell, which depolarizes the cell membrane and generates an action potential (Figure 16.6B).

Two powerful nAChR inhibitors, the plant alkaloid *D-tubocurarine* (also known as *curare*) and the snake venom peptide *α-bungarotoxin*, have helped to reveal the function of nAChR. Interestingly, as early as the 1940s, D-tubocurarine was used as a muscle relaxant in surgeries. And finally, an important characteristic of the nAChR is its ability to desensitize. **Desensitization** is a process whereby after initial stimulation with ACh, or with a related agonist like nicotine, the channel loses its agonist sensitivity and shuts down after a short period of stimulation. This process is analogous to the inactivation process of the voltage-gated channels (see earlier, and Figure 16.6A).

The $GABA_A$ receptor is a Cl^--selective, ligand-gated ion channel that mediates the fast synaptic inhibition

Table 16.2 Basic Classification of Ligand-Gated Ion Channels, Their Inhibitors and Activators

Superfamilies	Major Family Members	Inhibitors (Antagonists)	Activators (Agonists)
Cys-loop receptors	nAChRs	α-bungarotoxin, D-tubocurarin (curare)	ACh, nicotine
	5-hydroxytryptamine (5-HT3)/ serotonin receptors	—	Serotonin
	$GABA_A$	Picrotoxin, bicuculline	Alcohol, barbiturates, steroids (estrogens, progesterone), benzodiazepines (diazepam)
	Glycine receptors	Strychnine	Glycine, taurine, β-alanine
Glutamate receptors	NMDA	APV (AP5), MK- 801, phencyclidine, external Mg2+,	Glutamate, NMDA
	Kainate	CNQX	Glutamate, kainate
	AMPA	CNQX	Glutamate, AMPA, quisqualate
ATP-gated channels/ purinergic receptors	P2X receptors	α,β-methyleneATP (>10 μM)	Extracellular ATP, α,β-methyleneATP (<10 μM)

in the central nervous system (CNS). For comparison, the $GABA_B$ receptor is not an ion channel. The $GABA_A$ receptor has a very complex pharmacology and many different binding sites for pharmacological modulators. Its two major inhibitors are the plant alkaloids *picrotoxin* and *bicuculline*. Picrotoxin is a pore-plugging, noncompetitive inhibitor. In contrast, bicuculline is a competitive channel inhibitor using a separate binding site. Alcohol, barbiturates, some steroids such as estrogens and progesterone, and benzodiazepines (diazepam) exert their effects via activation of the $GABA_A$ receptor. All these agents modulate $GABA_A$ receptors indirectly by increasing the channel open probability but not the single channel conductance.

L-Glutamate is a major excitatory neurotransmitter in the mammalian CNS, acting mainly via cationic ligand-gated ion channels, also referred to as ionotropic GluR (iGluR). For comparison, the metabotropic GluR receptors are not ion channels. The iGluR are multimeric assemblies of four or five subunits, and are divided into three subgroups based on their pharmacological and structural similarities (Table 16.2):

- N-methyl-D-aspartate (NMDA)
- α–amino-3-hydroxyl-5-methyl-4-isoxaspartate (AMPA)
- Kainate receptors

Ionotropic GluRs are involved in excitatory synaptic transmission and synaptic plasticity, and thus implicated in learning and memory. The iGluR are also potential targets for therapies for CNS disorders such as Alzheimer's disease and epilepsy.

The ATP-gated purinergic receptor channel superfamily is represented mainly by the P2X receptors, which are nonselective cation-permeable channels that open in response to extracellular ATP. They are part of a larger family of receptors known as purinergic receptors. However, not all purinergic receptors are ion channels. At least three ATP molecules are required to activate a P2X receptor, suggesting that ATP needs to bind to each of the three subunits in order to open the channel pore (Figure 16.9). The precise mechanism by which the binding of ATP leads to the opening of the P2X receptor channel pore is not well understood. Seven separate genes ($P2X_1$–$P2X_7$) encode the functional P2X receptors that are formed by three or four separate subunits (Figure 16.9). The P2X receptors are involved in a variety of physiological processes, such as mediation of nociception and synaptic transmission. They also contribute to contraction of cardiac, skeletal, and various smooth muscle tissues, including the vasculature, vas deferens, and urinary bladder.

16.4.2 Sodium Channels

The essential physiological processes, which enable us to see, hear, move, sense, think, and experience emotion are completely dependent on the voltage-gated Na^+ (Na_V) channels. Na_V channels are the major and most important group of Na channels. The Na_V channels are involved in the generation of the rapid upstroke of the action potential in neurons (Figure 16.2), cardiac and skeletal muscle, and neuroendocrine cells. The classic studies of Hodgkin and Huxley led to identifying the three key features of the Na_V channels: voltage-dependent activation, rapid inactivation, and high Na^+ selectivity. The Na_V channels have a single channel conductance of about 20 to 25 pS and their open probability is very low at the levels of the resting membrane potential. However, only several millivolts of membrane depolarization is needed to quickly (1–2 milliseconds) activate and then inactivate the Na_V channels. At a membrane potential of 0 mV or higher, these channels are almost completely inactivated.

Molecular cloning experiments have revealed a family of nine different α-subunits of the Na_V channels, and a tenth member has been suggested to be a related protein. The pore-forming α-subunit is a single polypeptide chain (~260 kDa) that folds into four homologous domains (D I–D IV), each consisting of six TM segments (Figure 16.10). The short intracellular loop connecting D III and D IV forms the inactivation ball-and-chain, which is capable of inactivating the Na_V channel within 1 to 2 milliseconds after the channel is activated. During this short time period, the inactivation ball-and-chain folds over and blocks the intracellular mouth of the pore (Figure 16.4, but see also Figure 16.6A).

In 2001, using cryo-electron microscopy and single particle analysis, Sato and colleagues provided the first three-dimensional view of the Na_V channel isolated from the eel *Electrophorus electricus*. The channel was found to have a bell-shaped extracellular surface structure with square-shaped intracellular base and a spherical top (Figure 16.10). In addition to the pore-forming α-subunits, the Na_V channels have four additional accessory subunits ($Na_V\beta_1$–$Na_V\beta_4$), each measuring

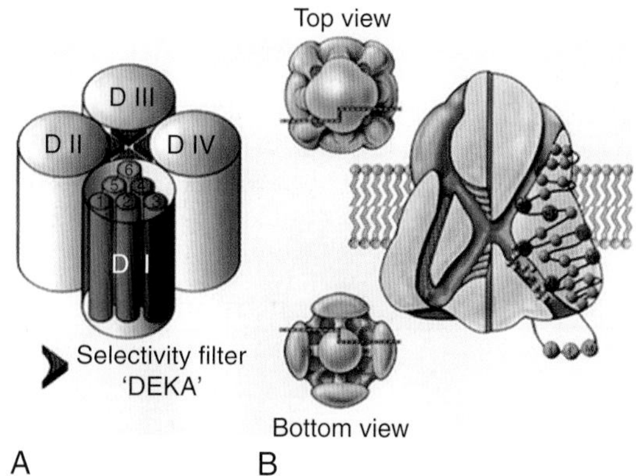

Figure 16.10 Cartoon illustrating the hypothetical structure of the Na_V channel α-subunit. A. Illustration of the four domains D I–D IV, each consisting of six TM segments (see also Figure 16.4). The four amino acids—aspartate, glutamate, lysine, and alanine (DEKA) from the pore loop links between S5 and S6 TM segments that form the selectivity filter are illustrated as red triangles. B. Three-dimensional illustrations of the Na_V channel with views from the top, bottom, and cross-section through the S4 segment. Residues that are colored in red are essential for the local anesthetics binding. Used with permission from Catterall, *Nature* **409**, 988–991 – Nature Publishing Group.

about 33 to 36 kDa. They influence the activation and inactivation properties of the pore-forming α-subunits and are involved in channel localization as well as interaction with cell adhesion molecules.

Table 16.3 summarizes the major genetic, molecular, physiological, and pharmacological characteristics of the Na_V channels. As key elements in membrane excitability, Na_V channels are targeted by a broad range of venom toxins that modulate their function upon binding to specific sites. The most important are TTX and STX, which bind reversibly and with high affinity to specific sites at the extracellular mouth of the Na_V channels. As an indication of the specificity of the interaction between TTX and the channel, the first isolation of the Na_V channel was based on its ability to bind TTX. Interestingly, TTX inhibits the neuronal Na_V channels but has almost no effect on the skeletal and cardiac muscle Na_V channels.

Studies coming mainly from Catterall's group have established that all the pharmacological modulators acting on the Na_V channels bind to defined sites on the α-subunit only. Na_V channels have important pharmacological significance because they appear to have six separate binding sites for neurotoxins and one additional binding site for local anesthetics, antiarrhythmic, and antiepileptic drugs (Table 16.4). $Na_V1.6$, $Na_V1.8$, and $Na_V1.9$ family members are also targets for analgesic drugs. The pharmacological knowledge about the different Na_V channel toxin/drug-binding sites provides important information for development of Na_V channel subtype-specific drugs to control different disorders, such as epilepsy, periodic paralysis, neuropathic pain, inflammation, and cardiac long QT (LQT) syndrome (Section 16.6).

A special class of epithelial Na channels (ENaC), located in the apical epithelial membranes, mediate the active Na^+ reabsorption in kidney, colon, lung, and sweat glands; they are essential for the maintenance of the body's salt and water balance. The ENaC are completely different from the Na_V channels and are not sensitive to TTX. Instead, they are inhibited with high affinity by amiloride, which is an established diuretic drug. ENaC form four channel subfamilies: α, β, γ, and δ. Structurally they are 510 to 920 amino acid proteins with two TM segments separated by a large extracellular loop and have a single channel conductance of 4 to 5 pA.

16.4.3 Calcium Channels

The voltage-gated Ca^{2+} channels (Ca_V) are ubiquitous and have two fundamental physiological functions: electrogenic and regulatory. Ca_V channels trigger the action potential in smooth muscle and in cardiac pacemaker cells, analogous to the Na_V channels in neurons. The Ca^{2+} ion plays a role as a second messenger and is implicated in key signal transduction pathways relevant to neurotransmission, secretion, and even gene expression. The Ca^{2+} ion also activates muscle contraction. Thus, the Ca_V channels translate the changes of the cell membrane excitability into local intracellular Ca^{2+} transients that control different physiological processes. The Ca_V channel family has 10 members, encoded by 10 distinct genes (Table 16.5). Analogous to the Na_V channels, the Ca_V channel consists of a pore-forming α_1-subunit (190–250 kDa) that folds into homologous domains (I–IV), each with six TM segments (Figure 16.4). The α_1-subunit incorporates not only the gating mechanism and the voltage sensor, but also the binding sites for venom toxins and drugs. Although accessory subunits, including a disulfide-linked $\alpha_2\delta$ subunit complex (Table 16.5), can modulate the properties of the Ca_V channels to some extent, the channel's pharmacological diversity is determined mainly by the pore-forming α_1-subunit.

Ca_V channels are closed at the level of the resting membrane potential and open upon membrane depolarization like the Na_V channels. Some Ca_V channels, however, require much more positive voltages (–30–+20 mV) for activation compared to the Na_V channels. In the 1970s and 1980s they were initially called high-voltage activated channels, to distinguish them from another group of low-voltage activated Ca channels. Richard Tsien's group further subdivided the high-voltage activated channels into L-type (from long-lasting current), N-type (from neuronal), P/Q-type (sensitive to ω-agatoxin IVA), and R-type (resistant to toxins); and called the low-voltage activated channels T-type (from tiny conductance and transient current). Although the contemporary IUPHAR nomenclature (Section 16.1.2) is based on the three distinct gene subfamilies—Ca_V1 (L-type), Ca_V2 (N-type, P/Q-type, and R-type), and Ca_V3 (T-type) (Table 16.5)—Tsien's classic classification is still widely used.

The Ca_V1 (L-type) channels are expressed in skeletal, cardiac, and smooth muscle, in which they initiate contraction, and in endocrine cells, in which they initiate secretion. These channels are also implicated in the Ca^{2+} regulation of gene expression. Two unique features of the Ca_V1 (L-type) channels are their dual voltage and Ca^{2+} inactivation. The Ca^{2+} inactivation component provides self-regulation because the same Ca^{2+} that enters the channel also inactivates it. The neuronal Ca_V2 group (N-type, P/Q-type, and R-type) channels, similar to the L-type channels, also require higher levels of membrane depolarization for activation. They are responsible for the initiation of neurotransmission in most fast neuronal synapses. The Ca_V3 (T-type) are transient, low-voltage-activated channels that control Ca^{2+} entry in a variety of excitable cells during small degrees of depolarization around the level of the resting membrane potential. Thus, they play an important role in shaping the action potential, and are involved in many pacemaker mechanisms.

The pharmacology of the three Ca_V channel subfamilies is quite distinct and exceptionally complex (Table 16.5). The Ca_V1 (L-type) channels can be inhibited by three separate groups of organic, lipid-soluble, compounds: 1,4-dihydropyridines (DHPs) (e.g., nifedipine), phenylalkylamines (e.g., verapamil, D-600), and benzothiazepines (e.g., diltiazem) (Figure 16.11). These inhibitors traditionally are known in the pharmacological literature as Ca-antagonists, and the Ca_V1 (L-type) channel activators are often called Ca-agonists. The interaction of DHPs with the L-type (Ca_V1) channels

Table 16.3 Major Characteristics and Pharmacological Modulators of the Na_V Channel Family Members

Name	Human Gene	Human Chromosome	Accessory Subunits	Tissue Distribution	Inhibitors (Antagonists)	Activators (Agonists)	Gating Modifiers
$Na_v1.1$	SCN1A	2q24.3	$Na_V\beta_1$, $Na_V\beta_2$, $Na_V\beta_3$, $Na_V\beta_4$	CNS, spinal cord, cardiac myocytes	TTX (10 nM), STX (2 nM), local anesthetics, antiepileptics, antiarrhythmic drugs	Veratridine, batrachotoxin, aconitine, grayanotoxin, β-scorpion toxins	α-Scorpion toxins, sea anemone toxins, δ-conotoxins
$Na_v1.2$	SCN2A	2q22-23	$Na_V\beta_1$, $Na_V\beta_2$, $Na_V\beta_3$, $Na_V\beta_4$	CNS, spinal cord	TTX (10 nM), STX (2 nM), local anesthetics, antiepileptics, antiarrhythmic drugs	Veratridine, batrachotoxin, aconitine, grayanotoxin, β-scorpion toxins, kurtoxin	α-Scorpion toxins, sea anemone toxins, δ-conotoxins
$Na_v1.3$	SCN3A	2q23-24	$Na_V\beta_1$, $Na_V\beta_3$	CNS, spinal cord	TTX (10 nM), STX (2 nM), local anesthetics, antiepileptics, antiarrhythmic drugs	Veratridine, batrachotoxin, aconitine, grayanotoxin, β-scorpion toxins	α-Scorpion toxins, sea anemone toxins, δ-conotoxins
$Na_v1.4$	SCN4A	17q23-25	$Na_V\beta_1$	Skeletal muscle	TTX (10 nM), STX (2 nM), μ-conotoxin GIIIA, μ-conotoxin PIIIA, local anesthetic, antiepileptic, antiarrhythymic drugs	Veratridine, batrachotoxin, grayanotoxin, β-scorpion toxins	α-Scorpion toxins, sea anemone toxins
$Na_v1.5$	SCN5A	2q24	$Na_V\beta_1$, $Na_V\beta_2$, $Na_V\beta_3$, $Na_V\beta_4$	Cardiac muscle, embryonic neurons	TTX-resistant (>1 μM), STX, local anesthetics, antiepileptics, antiarrhythmic drugs	Veratridine, batrachotoxin, aconitine	β-Scorpion toxins, sea anemone toxins, δ-conotoxins
$Na_v1.6$	SCN8A	12q13	$Na_V\beta_1$, $Na_V\beta_2$	CNS neurons, cardiac muscle, Purkinje cells	TTX (10 nM), STX, local anesthetics, antiepileptics, antiarrhythmic drugs	Veratridine, batrachotoxin	α-Scorpion toxins, sea anemone toxins
$Na_v1.7$	SCN9A	2q24	$Na_V\beta_1$, $Na_V\beta_2$	Glia, peripheral sympathetic neurons, dorsal root ganglion	TTX (10 nM), STX, local anesthetics, antiepileptics, antiarrhythmic drugs	Veratridine, batrachotoxin	α-Scorpion toxins, sea anemone toxins
$Na_v1.8$	SCN10A	3p21-24	Unknown	CNS, spinal cord, dorsal root ganglion	TTX-resistant (>50 μM), lidocaine	Unknown	Unknown
$Na_v1.9$	SCN11A	3p21-24	Unknown	C-type dorsal root ganglion neurons	TTX-resistant (>50 μM)	Unknown	Unknown

Table 16.4 Na_V Channel Binding Sites for Venom Neurotoxins and Drugs

Binding Site	Domain/TM Segment	Neurotoxin or Drug	Channel Effect
Binding site #1	I S2–S6, II S2–S6 III S2–S6, IV S2–S6	Tetrodotoxin Saxitoxin μ-Conotoxin	Pore plugging
Binding site #2	I S6, IV S6	Veratridine Batrachotoxin Grayanotoxin, aconitine	Sustained increase in activation and inhibition of activation
Binding site #3	I S5–IS6, IV S3–S4 IV S5–S6 II S1–S2, II S3–S4	α-scorpion toxins Sea anemone toxins β-scorpion toxins	Delayed inactivation
Binding site #4	II S1–S2, II S3–S4	β-scorpion toxins	Increased activation
Binding site #5	I S6, IV S5	Brevetoxins Ciguatoxins, versutoxin	Increased activation and inhibition of inactivation
Binding site #6	IV S3–S4	δ-Conotoxins, pyrethoid insecticides	Delayed inactivation and increased activation
Local Anesthetics Binding site	I S6, III S6, IV S6	Local anesthetic drugs Antiarrhythmic drugs (class I) Antiepileptic drugs	Open channel inhibition

Based on data from Catterall's group—*Pharmacol. Rev.*, 2005, **57**(4): 397–409 and *Toxicon*, 2007, **49**(2): 124–141.

is quite complex as they may act either as channel inhibitors or activators, as in the case of nitrendipine and Bay K8644. This was an enigma until it was realized that these compounds were a racemic mixture of two optical enantiomers, with agonist properties of one isomer, (*S*)-(−)-Bay K8644, and antagonist activity of the other, (*R*)-(+)-Bay K8644. Furthermore, it was established that DHP antagonists bind much better to the inactivated state of the Ca_V1 (L-type) channels than to the resting state, and therefore the properties of the DHP-binding site depend on the gating state of the channel. For these reasons, DHPs were thought to act allosterically, moving the channel toward an open or closed state rather than plugging the pore. Now it is known that the DHP binding site includes amino acid residues in the S6 TM segments of D III and D IV and in the S5 TM segment of D III. Phenylalkylamines act by plugging the pore from the intracellular side and have a binding site in the S6 TM segments of D III and D IV, analogous to the local anesthetic site of Na_V channels. Benzothiazepines, such as diltiazem, bind allosterically to a third site that also partially overlaps the phenylalkylamine binding site.

Ca_V2 (N-type, P/Q-type, and R-type) channels are relatively insensitive to Ca_V1 (L-type) channel antagonists and are blocked by specific polypeptide toxins isolated from snail and spider venoms. The Ca_V3 (T-type) channels can be inhibited by some nonspecific inhibitors (Ni^{2+}, mibefradil) and are resistant to both Ca-antagonists (e.g., nifedipine) and to snake and spider toxins. Figures 16.12 and 16.13 illustrate simultaneous recordings of Ca^{2+} currents through Ca_V1 (L-type) and Ca_V3 (T-type) channels and their pharmacological dissection by nifedipine and Ni^{2+}, which reveals their high- and low-voltage-activated biophysical properties, respectively.

16.4.4 Potassium Channels

K^+ channels are the largest and most diverse group of ion channels, encoded by about 70 to 80 different genes. It is believed that all cell types possess K^+ channels. As the K^+ ion has a negative equilibrium potential close to the level of the resting membrane potential, the K^+ channels play a critical role in establishing the cell's membrane potential. In general, the opening of these channels decreases membrane excitability. K^+ channels also shape the cell's action potential by securing repolarization after an episode of depolarization. They control the rhythmic activity of excitable cells, and have complex mechanisms of regulation. Some of the most important physiological functions controlled by the K^+ channels are neurotransmitter release, insulin secretion, differentiation, proliferation, apoptosis (programmed cell death), and many others. All known K^+ channels are inhibited by TEA from inside, outside, or both, as well as by Cs^+ ions. In fact, Cs^+ is a large ion that can barely pass through the K^+ channel, getting stuck in the selectivity filter, thus inhibiting the channel. This phenomenon was illuminating regarding the mechanism of the K^+ channel's selectivity filter (Section 16.2.2.1; Figure 16.5), as the filter diameter (~3 Å) was approximately the same as the Cs^+ ion diameter (~3.3 Å).

Structurally, all K^+ channels form a pore-loop and can have a 2TM, 6TM, 7TM, or 8TM segment architecture (Figure 16.4). Functionally, the K^+ channels form four major families:

- Voltage-gated K^+ channels (K_V) with 6TM architecture
- Ca^{2+}-activated K^+ channels (K_{Ca}) with 6TM or 7TM architecture
- Inward-rectifying K^+ channels (K_{ir})—with 2TM architecture
- K_{2P} family—with 2TM architecture

Among all K^+ channels, the K_V family is the most diverse, with pronounced mechanisms of activation and inactivation (see earlier, and Figure 16.6A). This family is represented by 40 different genes (Table 16.6), each K_V gene encoding a 6TM subunit, four of which form a functional channel tetramer (Figure 16.4).

Table 16.5 Major Characteristics and Pharmacological Modulators of the Ca_V Channel Family Members

Name	Human Gene	Human Chromosome	Accessory Subunits	Inhibitors (Antagonists)	Activators (Agonists)	Gating Modifiers
$Ca_v1.1$ (α_{1S}; L-type)	CACNA1S	0.1q32	$Ca_v\alpha_2\delta$, $Ca_v\beta$, $Ca_v\gamma$	Cd^{2+}, verapamil, devapamil, (+)-cis-diltiazem, calcicludine, calciseptine, kurtoxin, TaiCatoxin	DHP-agonists, (*S*)-(−)-Bay K8644, FPL64176	DHP-antagonists, (*R*)-(+)-Bay K8644, kurtoxin
$Ca_v1.2$ (α_{1C}; L-type)	CACNA1C	12p13.3	$Ca_v\alpha_2\delta$, $Ca_v\beta$, $Ca_v\gamma$	Cd^{2+}, devapamil, diltiazem, calcicludine, calciseptine, kurtoxin, TaiCatoxin	DHP-agonists, (*S*)-(−)-Bay K8644, FPL64176	DHP-antagonists, (*R*)-(+)-Bay K8644, kurtoxin
$Ca_v1.3$ (α_{1D}; L-type)	CACNA1D	3p14.3	$Ca_v\alpha_2$, $Ca_v\beta$, $Ca_v\delta$	Cd^{2+}, calcicludine, calciseptine, kurotoxin, TaiCatoxin	DHP-agonists, (*S*)-(−)-Bay K8644,	DHP-antagonists, (*R*)-(+)-Bay K8644
$Ca_v1.4$ (α_{1F}; L-type)	CACNA1F	Xp11.23	Unknown	Cd^{2+}, calcicludine, calciseptine, kurtoxin, TaiCatoxin	DHP-agonists, (*S*)-(−)-Bay K8644,	DHP-antagonists, (*R*)-(+)-Bay K8644, D-*cis*-diltiazem, verapamil, kurtoxin
$Ca_v2.1$ (α_{1A}; P/Q-type)	CACNA1A	19p13	$Ca_v\alpha_2\delta$, $Ca_v\beta$	Piperidines, piperazines, substituted diphenylbutylpiperidines, volatile anesthetics, gabapentin, mibefradil, DW13.3, ω-conotoxins: MVIIC and SVIB, ω-agatoxins: IVA and TK, kurtoxin	None	ω-agatoxin IVA, ω-agatoxin IVB, kurtoxin
$Ca_v2.2$ (α_{1B}; N-type)	CACNA1B	9q34	$Ca_v\alpha_2\delta$, $Ca_v\beta_1$-β_3	ω-conotoxins: GVIA, MVIIA, MVIIC, SVIA, SVIB, and CVID, piperidines, substituted diphenylbutylpiperidines, long alkyl chain molecules, aliphatic monoamines, tetrandine, gabapentin, peptidylamines, volatile anesthetics, SNX-325 and DW13.3	None	None
$Ca_v2.3$ (α_{1E}; R-type)	CACNA1E	0.1q25–31	$Ca_v\alpha_2\delta$, $Ca_v\beta$	SNX-482, ω-grammotoxin SIA, Ni^{2+}, mibefradil, volatile anesthetics	None	None
$Ca_v3.1$ (α_{1G}; T-type)	CACNA1G	17q22	Unknown	Mibefradil, penfluridol, pimozide, Ni^{2+}, amiloride, kurtoxin	None	Kurtoxin
$Ca_v3.2$ (α_{1H}; T-type)	CACNA1H	0.16p13.3	Unknown	Ni^{2+}, mibefradil, U92032, penfluridol, pimozide, amiloride, nimodipine, kurtoxin	None	Kurtoxin
$Ca_v3.3$ (α_{1I}; T-type)	CACNA1I	22q13.1	Unknown	Mibefradil, U92032, penfluridol, pimozide, Ni^{2+}	None	None

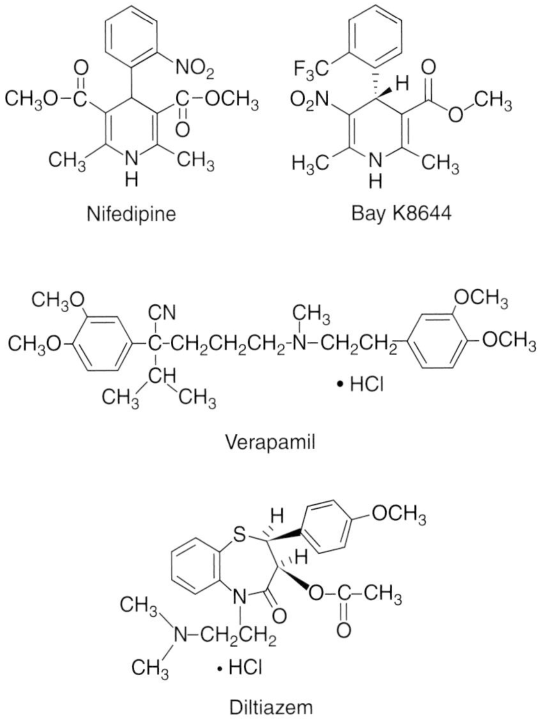

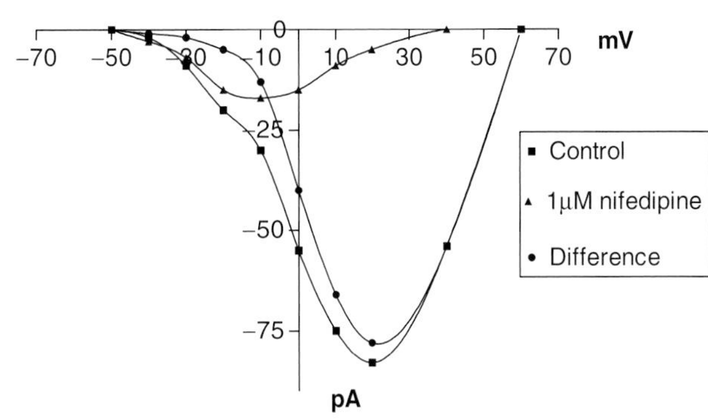

Figure 16.13 Current-voltage relationship for the Ca_V1 (L-type) and Ca_V3 (T-type) currents pharmacologically dissected by nifedipine, as related to the original recordings in Figure 16.12. The maximum peak of the nifedipine-insensitive Ca_V3 (T-type) current is at low negative voltages, whereas the maximum peak of the nifedipine-sensitive Ca_V1 (L-type) current is at high positive voltages (+10, +20 mV). Used with permission from Petkov et al., 2001b, *Acta Physiologica Scandinavica*, **173**(3), 257–265 – Bleckwell Publishing (new journal name is *Acta Physiologica*).

Figure 16.11 Chemical structure of the three most important representatives of the Ca_V1 (L-type) channel organic antagonists: DHPs (nifedipine), phenylalkylamines (verapamil), and benzothiazepines (diltiazem). The DHP derivative, Bay K8644, can be either agonist or antagonist depending on the optical enantiomer.

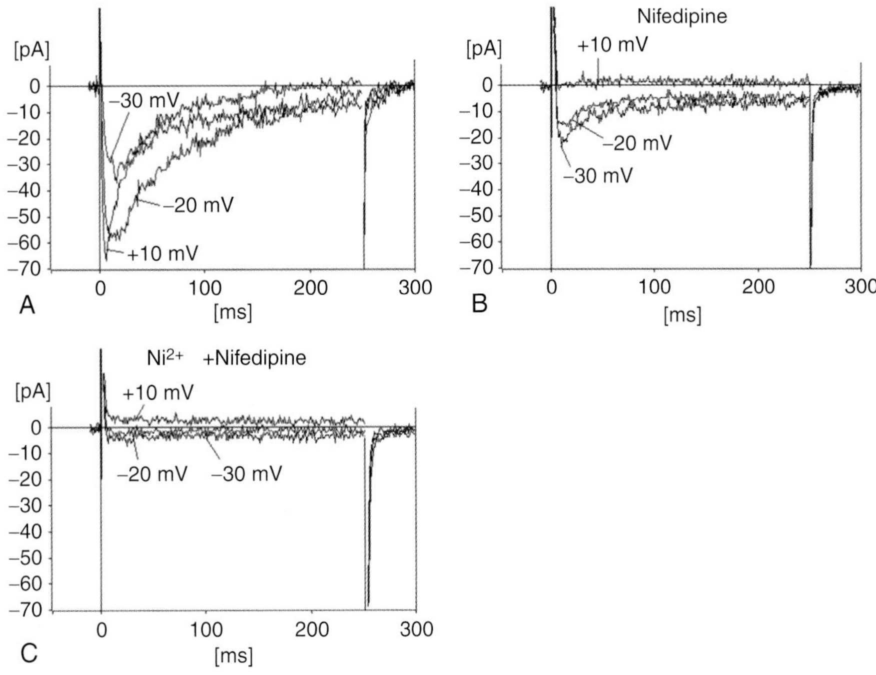

Figure 16.12 Ca_V1 (L-type) and Ca_V3 (T-type) currents from an arterial smooth muscle cell expressing both Ca_V1 (L-type) and Ca_V3 (T-type) channels. A. Original current recordings in whole cell patch-clamp configuration during different depolarizing potentials (−30, −20, and +10 mV) with 200 ms duration (Section 16.5.1.3). Inward T-type Ca^{2+} currents are activated at low voltages (−30, −20 mV), whereas Ca_V1 (L-type) currents are activated at higher voltages (−20, +10 mV). B. Nifedipine inhibits the Ca_V1 (L-type) current recorded at −20 and +10 mV, but not the Ca_V3 (T-type) currents recorded at −30 and −20 mV. C. Subsequent addition of Ni^{2+}, a non-specific Ca_V3 (T-type) channel inhibitor, causes inhibition of the remaining Ca_V3 (T-type) current. Used with permission from Petkov et al., 2001b, *Acta Physiologica Scandinavica*, **173**(3), 257–265 – Bleckwell Publishing (new journal name is *Acta Physiologica*).

Table 16.6 Major Characteristics and Pharmacological Modulators of the K_V Channel Family Members

Name	Human Gene	Human Chromosome	Accessory Subunits	Tissue Distribution	Inhibitors (Antagonists)	Activators (Agonists)
$K_v1.1$	KCNA1	12p13.3	$K_v\beta_1$, $K_v\beta_2$, PSD95, SAP97, SNAP25	Brain, heart, eye, skeletal muscle, pancreas	TEA, DTX, DTX-K, ShK, 10-*N*-methylcarbamoyl-3,7-bis(dimethylamino)phenothiazine, 4-AP, capsaicin, resiniferatoxin, flecainide, nifedipine, diltiazem, kaliotoxin, margatoxin, hongotoxin-1	None
$K_v1.2$	KCNA2	1p13	$K_v\beta_1$, $K_v\beta_2$, PSD95, SAP97, SNAP25, Caspr2, RhoA	Brain, spinal cord, heart, pancreas, eye, smooth muscle, Schwann cells	4-AP, capsaicin, resiniferatoxin, flecainide, nifedipine, diltiazem, 10-*N*-methylcarbamoyl-3,7-bis(dimethylamino)phenothiazine, DTX, charybdotoxin, margatoxin, natrexone, TEA, H37, picrotoxin-Kα, OsK2, BgK, HgTx, anandamide	None
$K_v1.3$	KCNA3	1p13.3	$K_v\beta$, hDlg, β_1 integrin, KChaP	Brain, lung, pancreas, spleen, testis, thymus	4-AP, TEA, charybdotoxin, naltrexone, MgTX, kaliotoxin, AgTX2, Pi1, Pi2, Pi3, HsTx1, ShK, BgK, ShK-Dap22, quinine, diltiazem, verapamil, CP339818, UK78282, correolide, sulfamidbenzamidoindane, capsaicin, resiniferatoxin, nifedipine, H37	None
$K_v1.4$	KCNA4	11p14.3-15.2	$K_v\beta$, PSD95, SAP97, SAP90, α-actinin-2, KChaP, σ receptor	Brain, skeletal muscle, heart, pancreas	4-AP, TEA, UK78282, riluzole, quinidine, nicardipine	None, but phosphorylation/dephosphorylation of CaMKII/calcineurin causes inactivation to become Ca^{2+} dependent
$K_v1.5$	KCNA5	12p13.3	$K_v\beta_1$, $K_v\beta_2$, KCNA3B, Src tyrosine kinase, fyn, KChaP, α-actinin-2, caveolin, SAP97	Heart, colon, kidney, stomach, smooth muscle, Schwann cells	S9947, 4-AP, capsaicin, resiniferatoxin, flecainide, nifedipine, diltiazem, TEA, clofilium inside, bupivacaine, propafenone, quinidine	None
$K_v1.6$	KCNA6	12p13.3	$K_v\beta_1$, $K_v\beta_2$, Caspr2	Brain, colon, heart, lung, ovary, testis, smooth muscle	α-Dendrotoxin, 10-*N*-methylcarbamoyl-3,7-bis (dimethylamino)phenothiazine, 4-AP, TEA, ShK, HgTX, BgK	None
$K_v1.7$	KCNA7	19q13.3	None	Placenta, pancreas, skeletal muscle, heart, pulmonary arteries	Flecainide, quinidine, verapamil, amiodarone, 4-AP, TEA	None
$K_v1.8$	KCNA10	1p13.1	KCNA4B	Kidney, brain, heart, skeletal muscle, adrenal gland	Ba^{2+}, TEA, 4-AP, charybdotoxin, ketoconazole, pimozide, verapamil	CGMP
$K_v2.1$	KCNB1	20q13.2	$K_v5.1$, $K_v6.1$-6.3, $K_v8.1$, $K_v9.1$-9.3, KChaP, Fyn SH2 domain	Brain, heart, skeletal muscle, eye, lung, Schwann cells	TEA, tertrapentylammonium, Ba^{2+}, Mg^{2+}, 4-AP, halothane, hanatoxin, stromatoxin-1	Linoleic acid
$K_v2.2$	KCNB2	8q13.2	$K_v8.1$, K_v9, KChaP	Brain, tongue, smooth muscle, heart	Quinine, TEA, 4-AP, phencyclidine, stromatoxin-1	None

$K_v3.1$	KCNC1	11p15	Unknown	Brain, skeletal muscle, lung, testis	4-AP, capsaicin, resiniferatoxin, flecainide, nifedipine, diltiazem, cromakalin, TEA	None
$K_v3.2$	KCNC2	12q14.1	None	Brain, pancreas, heart, Schwann cells	TEA, 4-AP, 8-bromo-cGMP, 3-isobutyl-1-methylxanthine, D-NONOate, verapamil, ShK	None
$K_v3.3$	KCNC3	19q13.3-4	None	Brain, eye	TEA, 4-AP, hypoxia	None
$K_v3.4$	KCNC4	1p21	MiRP2	Brain, prostrate, parathyroid, skeletal muscle	BDS-I, TEA	None
$K_v4.1$	KCND1	Xp11.23	KChIP1	Brain, heart, lung, colon, stomach, testis, liver, kidney, pancreas	4-AP, TEA	None
$K_v4.2$	KCND2	7q31	KChIP1, PSD95, filamin, frequenin, DPPX, DPP10	Brain, heart	4-AP, heteropodatoxins, PaTX, arachidonic acid	None
$K_v4.3$	KCND3	1p13.3	KChIP1, KChIP4a, KChAP, DPP10, $K_{v\beta}2$	Heart, brain, smooth muscle	4-AP, bupivacaine, PaTX1,2, nicotine	None
$K_v5.1$	KCNF1	2p25	$K_v2.1$, $K_v2.2$	Brain, heart, skeletal muscle, liver, kidney, pancreas	Not a functional channel	
$K_v6.1$	KCNG1	20q13	K_v2 family	Brain, skeletal muscle, uterus, ovary, kidney, pancreas, prostate, testis	Not a functional channel	
$K_v6.2$	KCNG2	18q22-23	K_v2 via N termini	Fetal brain, heart	Not a functional channel	
$K_v6.3$	KCNG3	2p21	$K_v2.1$	Brain, spinal cord, testis, small intestine	Not a functional channel	
$K_v6.4$	KCNG4	16q24.1	$K_v2.1$	Brain, liver, small intestine, colon	Not a functional channel	
$K_v7.1$	KCNQ1	11p15.5	KCNE1, KCNE3	Heart, kidney, ear, pancreas, lung	Chromanol 293B, L735821, mefloquine, azimilide, HMR-1556, XE991, linopiridine	R-L3, mefenamic acid, niflumic acid, 4,4′-diisothiocyanostilbene-2,2′-disulfonic acid
$K_v7.2$	KCNQ2	20q13.3	KCNQ3, KCNE2	Brain, lung, testis, heart, breast, small intestine	TEA, XE991, linopiridine, L735821	Retigabine, BMS204352
$K_v7.3$	KCNQ3	8q24	KCNQ2, KCNQ5	Brain, testis, eye, colon	TEA, linopiridine	Retigabine, BMS204352
$K_v7.4$	KCNQ4	1p34	KCNQ3	Brain, placenta	TEA, linopiridine, bepridil	Retigabine, BMS204352
$K_v7.5$	KCNQ5	6q14	KCNQ3	Brain, skeletal muscle	TEA, linopiridine, linopiridine KCNQ5/KCNQ3, XE991	Retigabine, BMS204352
$K_v8.1$	KCNV1	8q22.3-24.1	K_v2 family	Brain, kidney	Not a functional channel	
$K_v8.2$	KCNV2	9q24.2	K_v2 family	Lung, liver, kidney, pancreas, soleen, prostate, testis, ovary, colon	Not a functional channel	

Continued

Table 16.6 Major Characteristics and Pharmacological Modulators of the K_V Channel Family Members—cont'd

Name	Human Gene	Human Chromosome	Accessory Subunits	Tissue Distribution	Inhibitors (Antagonists)	Activators (Agonists)
K_v9.1	KCNS1	20q12	K_v2 family	Brain	Not a functional channel	
K_v9.2	KCNS2	8q22	K_v2 family	Brain, retina, spinal cord	Not a functional channel	
K_v9.3	KCNS3	2p24	K_v2 family	Brain, breast, colon, eye, heart, kidney, lung, testis, uterus	Not a functional channel	
K_v10.1 (eag1)	KCNH1	1q32-41	Hk, CaM, Slob, epsin, KCR1	Brain, skeletal muscle	Quinidine, calcium/calmodulin	None, but speed of activation affected by polarization
K_v10.2 (eag2)	KCNH5	14q23.1	Hk, CaM, Slob, KCR1	Brain	Quinidine, calcium	None
K_v11.1 (erg1)	KCNH2	7q35-36	minK, MiRP1	Brain, heart, kidney, liver, lung, ovary, pancreas, testis, prostate, uterus, small intestine	Astemizole, BeKM-1, ergtoxin, sertindole, dofetilide, cisapride, pimozide, terfenadine, halofantrine, BRL32872, E-4031, CT haloperidol, imipramine, cocaine, ketoconazole	None
K_v11.2 (erg2)	KCNH6	17q23.3	K_v11.1, K_v11.2, K_v11.3	Brain, uterus	Sipatrigine	None
K_v11.3 (erg3)	KCNH7	2q24.2	K_v11.1, K_v11.2, K_v11.3	Brain	Sertindole, pimozide	None
K_v12.1 (elk1, elk3)	KCNH8	3p24.3	Unknown	Brain, testis, colon, lung, uterus	Ba^{2+}	None
K_v12.2 (elk2)	KCNH3	12q13	Unknown	Brain, lung, eye	None	None
K_v12.3 (elk1)	KCNH4	17q21.2	None	Brain, lung, esophagus	Ba^{2+}	None

Normally, the K_V channels form homotetramers. A unique feature of the K_V subunits is their ability to form heterotetramers—channels composed from different 6TM subunits within the same family (e.g., within K_V1, K_V7, K_V10), which are also functional K_V channels but with totally new properties. Another difference comes from the fact that K_V5, K_V6, K_V8, and K_V9 channels do not make their own homotetramers but rather form heterotetramers with the K_V2 subunits. Splice variance, posttranslational modification (e.g., modified by phosphorylation), and a large variety of accessory K_V subunits make the K_V family the most diverse one in the ion channel world (Table 16.6).

The *ether-a-go-go* (*eag*) K_V channel subfamily is the most recently discovered, with three structurally similar representatives: the *eag* (K_V10) with two members, and the *eag* related channels (*erg* or K_V11) and the *eag*-like K^+ channels (*elk* or K_V12) with three members each (Table 16.6). The *erg* or Kv11 includes Kv11.1 (also known as *erg1*, hERG, or KCNH2), $K_V11.2$ (also known as *erg2* or KCNH6), and $K_V11.3$ (also known as *erg3* or KCNH7) channels. The best studied is $K_V11.1$, which regulates the duration of the cardiac action potential, gastrointestinal smooth muscle membrane excitability, and is involved in cell and cancer proliferation.

The Ca^{2+} activated K^+ ($K_{Ca}1$–$K_{Ca}5$) channels are regulated by intracellular Ca^{2+}. They are represented by three major groups (Table 16.7):

- Large conductance ($K_{Ca}1.1$ or BK or MaxiK)
- Small conductance ($K_{Ca}2$ or SK)
- Intermediate conductance ($K_{Ca}3$ or IK or SK4) channels

The large conductance Ca^{2+}-activated and voltage-gated K^+ channel ($K_{Ca}1.1$, BK, or MaxiK, slo) is the only member of the K^+ channel family that is activated by both voltage and Ca^{2+}, and thus is uniquely suited to serve as a Ca^{2+}/voltage signal integrator in the modulation of membrane excitability. With the exception of the cardiac muscle, the $K_{Ca}1.1$ channels are distributed in all different cell types and have fundamental physiological roles in shaping action potential repolarization. These channels have a single-channel conductance of 100 to 250 pS, hence the name "big K^+ channel" (BK), and are blocked with high affinity by the scorpion venom iberiotoxin (Figure 16.14). The $K_{Ca}1.1$ channel's α-subunit has the structure of the K_V channel's α-subunit with the addition of an S0 TM segment (providing a 7TM architecture) and a

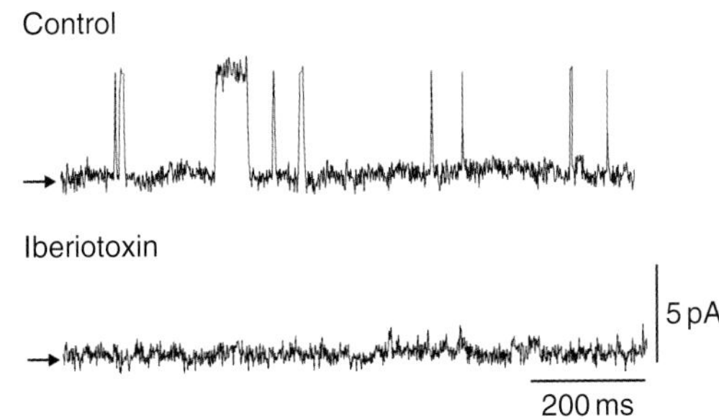

Figure 16.14 Original $K_{Ca}1.1$ (BK) single channel recordings and the inhibitory effect of iberiotoxin. Currents were recorded from a guinea pig urinary bladder smooth muscle cell using the whole cell (cell-attached), perforated patch-clamp technique at 0 mV holding potential (Section 16.5.1.3.). Shown is a series of $K_{Ca}1.1$ (BK) channel openings recorded before (upper trace) and after application of 200 nM iberiotoxin (lower trace). Iberiotoxin completely inhibits the single channel activity. Arrows indicate the closed channel level. Used with permission from Georgi V. Petkov and Mark T. Nelson. Differential regulation of Ca^{2+}-activated K^+ channels by -adrenoceptors in guinea pig urinary bladder smooth muscle, *Am J Physiol Cell Physiol* **288**: C1255–C1263, 2005.

Table 16.7 Major Characteristics and Pharmacological Modulators of the K_{Ca} Channel Family Members

Name	Human Gene	Human Chromosome	Accessory Subunits	Inhibitors (Antagonists)	Activators (Agonists)
$K_{Ca}1.1$ (BK, MaxiK, slo)	KCNMA1	10q22	$K_{Ca}1.1\beta_1$, $K_{Ca}1.1\beta_2$, $K_{Ca}1.1\beta_3$, $K_{Ca}1.1\beta_4$	Iberiotoxin, paxilline, charibdotoxin, α-KTx, TEA (1 <mM)	NS1619, NS1608
$K_{Ca}2.1$(SK1)	KCNN	19p13	Calmodulin	Apamin, scyllatoxin, curare, TEA	1-EBIO, NS309, riluzole, chlorzoxazone
$K_{Ca}2.2$(SK2)	KCNN2	5q23	Calmodulin	Apamin, scyllatoxin, curare, TEA	1-EBIO, NS309, riluzole, chlorzoxazone
$K_{Ca}2.3$(SK3)	KCNN	1q21	Calmodulin	Apamin, scyllatoxin, curare, TEA	1-EBIO, NS309, riluzole, chlorzoxazone
$K_{Ca}3.1$(IK, SK4)	KCNN4	19q13	Calmodulin	Charbybdotoxin, TRAM-34, clotrimazol, TEA	1-EBIO, NS309, riluzole, chlorzoxazone
$K_{Ca}4.1$(Slack)	KCNMB2	9q34	Unknown	Unknown	Unknown
$K_{Ca}4.2$	Unknown	1q31	Unknown	Unknown	Unknown
$K_{Ca}5.1$(slo-3)	KCNMC1	8p11	Unknown	Unknown	Unknown

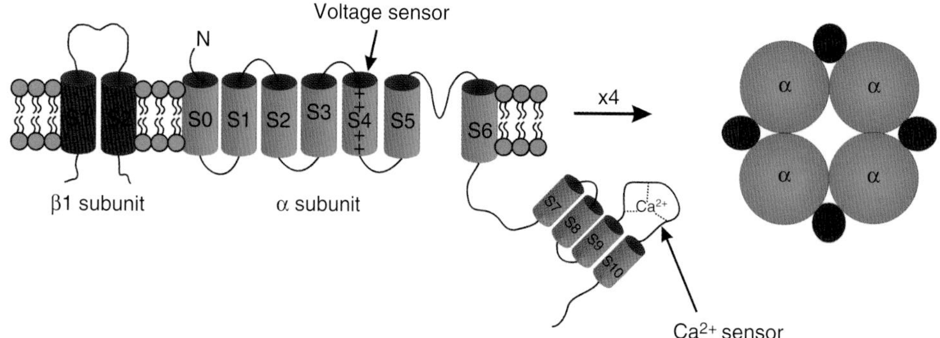

Figure 16.15 Illustration of the $K_{Ca}1.1$ (BK) channel molecular structure.

long intracellular domain (S7–S10) at the C-terminus that contains the Ca^{2+} sensor (Figure 16.15).

In addition to the pore-forming α-subunits, the $K_{Ca}1.1$ channels have four tissue-specific accessory subunits ($K_{Ca}1.1\beta_1$–$K_{Ca}1.1\beta_4$) with $K_{Ca}1.1\beta_1$ being smooth muscle-specific and $K_{Ca}1.1\beta_4$ neuronal-specific. Data from $K_{Ca}1.1\beta1$-subunit knockout (KO) mice indicate that the β1-subunit increases the apparent Ca^{2+} and voltage sensitivity of the $K_{Ca}1.1$ channels and is particularly enriched in urinary bladder smooth muscle (Figure 16.16). $K_{Ca}1.1$ channels are under the local control of so-called "Ca^{2+} sparks" caused by Ca^{2+} release from the sarcoplasmic reticulum, adjacent to the plasma membrane. The concept of **Ca^{2+} sparks** having a role in smooth muscle relaxation through the local activation of $K_{Ca}1.1$ (BK) channels, and thus spontaneous transient outward currents (STOCs), was first proposed by Nelson's group in 1995 (Section 16.4.8; Figure 16.17).

The small conductance Ca^{2+}-activated K^+ ($K_{Ca}2$; SK) channels (single channel conductance 5–20 pS) play an important role in the after-hyperpolarization phase of the action potential. They are specifically inhibited by the bee venom apamin. The intermediate conductance Ca^{2+}-activated K^+ ($K_{Ca}3$; IK) channels (single-channel conductance 20–80 pS) are largely expressed in nonexcitable (erythrocytes, endothelial) cells and smooth muscle. These channels, first identified in erythrocytes in the 1950s, are also known as Gardos channels, named for the investigator who first described them.

The inward-rectifying K^+ (K_{ir}) channels are another large family ($K_{ir}1$–$K_{ir}7$) of K^+ channels that have inward rectification properties and are voltage-independent. Inward rectification refers to the fact that the inward K^+ current, under hyperpolarizing conditions (below the K^+ equilibrium potential) has a much higher amplitude compared to the outward K^+ current elicited under equivalent depolarizing conditions. The K_{ir} channels play a critical role in maintaining the cell's resting membrane potential in neuronal and all muscle cell types. The most important representative of the K_{ir} channel family is the ATP-sensitive K^+ channel (K_{ATP}, $K_{ir}6$), which is composed of four inwardly rectifying K^+ channel subunits ($K_{ir}6$) and four regulatory sulphonylurea receptor (SUR) subunits. The K_{ATP} channels are inhibited by intracellular ATP and by sulphonylurea agents. They are activated when the intracellular ATP concentration is low and ADP concentration high, thus linking the cell's metabolic state with the cell's membrane excitability. Activation of K_{ATP} channels and the associated membrane hyperpolarization closes the Ca_V channels, which leads to a

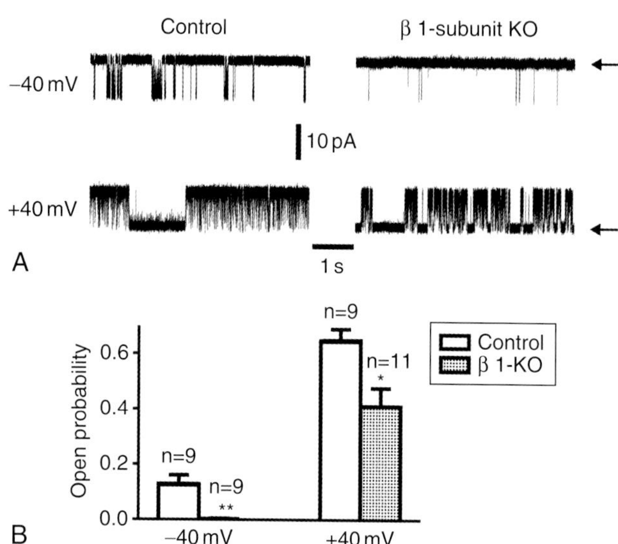

Figure 16.16 Data from $K_{Ca}1.1\beta1$-subunit knockout (KO) mouse urinary bladder smooth muscle cells indicate that the $K_{Ca}1.1$ (BK) channels from β1-subunit KO mice have a reduced open probability compared to control (normal wild type) mouse. (A) illustrates single channel recordings from excised inside-out membrane patches (Section 16.5.1.3.) held at −40 and +40 mV in 10 μM free Ca^{2+} and symmetrical 60 μM K^+ concentration. Arrows indicate the closed state of the channels. (B) illustrates BK channel open probability in control and β1-subunit KO animals at two different voltages (−40 and +40 mV). Data were obtained from n=9–11 cells of each animal group. Asterisks indicate statistically significant difference. Used with permission from Petkov et al., 2001a, *J. Physiol.* **537**: 443–452 – © Copyright 2001 The Physiological Society.

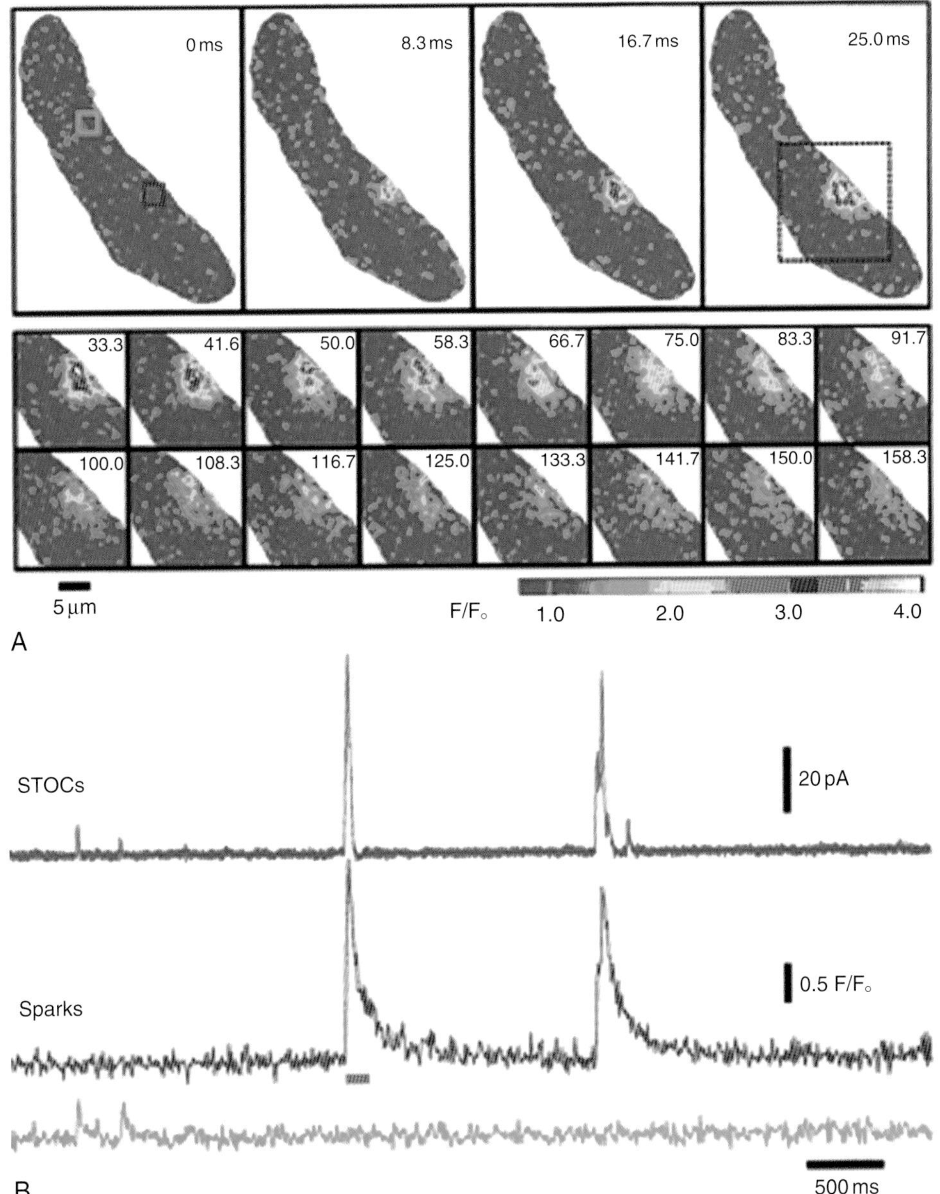

Figure 16.17 Simultaneous recordings of Ca^{2+} sparks and spontaneous transient outward $K_{Ca}1.1$ (BK) channel currents (STOCs). Each spark generates a single STOC. A. Original sequence of two-dimensional confocal images obtained every 8.33 ms of an entire smooth muscle cell isolated from rat basilar cerebral artery (top), followed by subsequent images of the region of interest (dotted box) illustrating the time course of the fractional increase in fluorescence (F/F_o) and decay of a typical Ca^{2+} spark. The images are color-coded as indicated by the bar. B. Simultaneous STOC (pA) and spark (F/F_o) measurements, at −40 mV, illustrating temporal association. (Blue) current, (red and green) the F/F_o average of the red and green boxes (2.2 μm/side) indicated in A, respectively. The pink bar indicates the segment of the trace illustrated in A. Used with permission from Perez et al., *J Gen Physiol.* **113**(2): 229–238, 1999 – The Rockefeller University Press (http://www.jgp.org/misc/terms.shtml)

reduction in Ca^{2+} entry into the cells. This fundamental mechanism controls the insulin secretion and muscle contractility. A large group of chemically unrelated compounds, known as K_{ATP} channel openers (cromakalim, pinacidil, diazoxide, ZD6169) bind directly to the channel proteins and activate K_{ATP} channels.

The K_{2P} channel members ($K_{2P}1$–$K_{2P}15$), also known as "leak K^+ channels," consist of two 2TM subunits linked in tandem, forming a functional channel-dimer (Figure 16.4). These channels play an important role in stabilizing the cell's membrane potential and are involved in many physiological processes. They are regulated by lipids, volatile anesthetics, heat, oxygen, protons, and membrane tension, and may become important therapeutic targets in the future.

16.4.5 Chloride Channels

From all anion selective channels, the Cl^- channel (CLC) family is of key importance, as the Cl^- ion is the most abundant physiological anion. In general, similar to the K^+ channels, the CLCs oppose excitability and help stabilize the resting membrane potential. There are three major groups of the CLC family with diverse structures and functions:

- The voltage-gated CLC
- The voltage-independent group of cystic fibrosis transmembrane conductance regulator (CFTR) channel
- The ligand-gated CLC, reviewed in Section 16.4.1

Interestingly, the voltage-gated CLC has classic channel characteristics, whereas CFTR has characteristics of an ion channel and a carrier. Apparently, in the case of CLC, the classical definition for channels and carriers is mixed, suggesting that the two types of ion transport mechanisms share common features.

The voltage-gated CLC family in mammals contains at least nine different genes, encoding CLC-1–CLC-7, CLC-0, CLC-Ka (CLC-K1), and CLC-Kb (CLC-K2). All voltage-gated CLCs have a common structure, with intracellular N- and C-termini and 10 to 12 TM domains. Mutations in the skeletal muscle-specific CLC-1 lead to increased excitability, suggesting that CLCs control the resting membrane potential in excitable cells. The ubiquitously expressed CLC-3 participates in cell volume regulation. In epithelial cells, CLC-Ka (CLC-K1) mediates Cl^- transport and is essential for the concentration of urine, while CLC-Kb (CLC-K2) is a basolateral Cl^- channel found in distal nephron segments that is necessary for Cl^- reabsorption. The kidney-specific CLC-5 is located in the endosomal membrane and provides Cl^- for intravesicular acidification, which is necessary for endocytosis. Voltage-gated CLCs are inhibited by both external Zn^{2+} and low pH. Many of the known CLC inhibitors are aromatic acids, including anthracene-9-carboxylic acid (9-AC), niflumic acid, 4,4′-diisothiocyanostilbene-2,2′-disulfonic acid (DIDS), 5-nitro-2-(3-phenylpropylamino) benzoic acid (NPPB), and tamoxifen. It is important to note that these inhibitors are not very specific.

A unique representative of the CLC family is the epithelial CLC, CFTR, which is similar to the SUR subunit that regulates $K_{ir}6$ of the K_{ATP} channel complexes. The CFTR is a unique CLC that transports Cl^- across epithelial cells membranes and has ATPase activity that is used to drive the protein between open and closed conformations (Figure 16.18). To function, the CFTR requires phosporylation by cAMP-protein kinase (PKA). CFTR mutations lead to cystic fibrosis (Section 16.6).

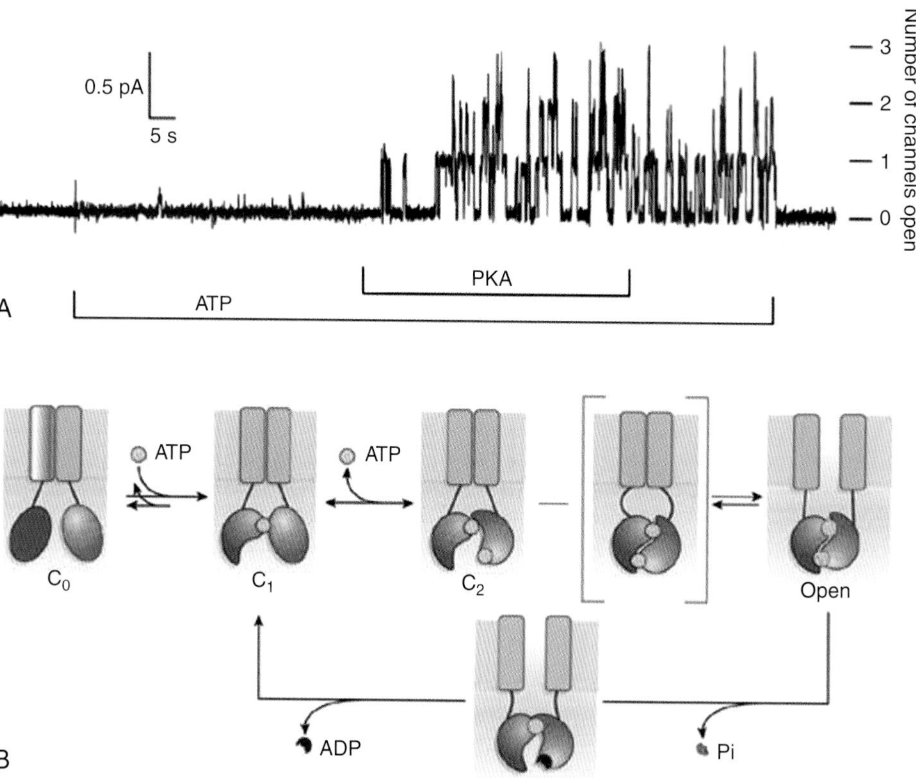

Figure 16.18 Illustration of the CFTR channel mechanism, which requires both ATP energy and PKA phosphorylation for channel opening. (A) illustrates single channel recordings activated by ATP and PKA. (B) illustrates the hypothetical channel structure and the different conformational stages. Used with permission from Gadsby et al., *Nature* **440**, 477–483, 2006 – Nature Publishing Group.

16.4.6 Nonselective Cation Channels and TRP Channels

In the late 1960s, Cosens and Manning identified a *Drosophila* mutant with a transient rather than sustained response to prolonged illumination, which in 1975 was named by Minke as transient receptor potential (*trp*) because of its unique phenotype and its physiological implications to the photoreceptor cells. It was established that the TRP protein is a new type of Ca^{2+}-permeable, nonselective cation channel; the discovery of mammalian homologues of the *Drosophila* TRP channels soon followed. Transient receptor potential (TRP) channels are a superfamily of functionally versatile, nonselective, cation-permeant ion channels that are present in most cell types of the human body. These channels mediate the transmembrane influx of cations down their electrochemical gradients, thereby raising intracellular Ca^{2+} and Na^{+} concentrations and depolarizing the cell membranes. Although TRP channels originally were proposed to be responsible for "store-operated Ca^{2+} entry," recent studies indicate a broad spectrum of roles for TRP channels.

In the past 10 years, independent studies from different laboratories revealed the TRP superfamily. The commonly accepted nomenclature for TRP channels subdivides the 28 known channel genes into seven subfamilies termed TRPA (ankyrin), TRPC (canonical), TRPM (melastatin), TRPML (mucolipin), TRPN (NOMPC), TRPP (polycystin), and TRPV (vanilloid). Mammals express representatives from all subfamilies except TRPN, which is found in *Drosophila, C. elegans* (worm) and zebra fish. All the channels are permeable to monovalent cations (mainly Na^{+}) and most are also permeable to Ca^{2+}.

Although TRP channel-gating mechanisms remain ill defined, certain physiological functions and signaling mechanisms are known. TRP channels are involved in mechanotransduction (TRPV), transduction of taste (TRPM) and odor (TRPV), osmoregulation (TRPV), thermosensation (TRPV, TRPA, TRPM), nociception, and auditory processes (TRPA). Members of the TRPC subfamily are activated by G protein-coupled receptor/phospholipase C signaling (e.g., by diacylglycerol) and may act as store-operated Ca^{2+} channels. The prototypical member of the TRPV subfamily, TRPV1, is the receptor for capsaicin, the active ingredient in hot chili peppers. TRPM channels are activated by intracellular Ca^{2+}, and several TRP channels, including members of the TRPV and TRPM families, are regulated by membrane potential and inositol phosphates.

The study of TRP channels is a newly emerging field. Many of the fundamental features of channel structure, function, and pharmacology that are well defined in other ion channel families remain unexplored. The development of selective pharmacological activators and inhibitors, currently unavailable for most TRP channels, would substantially improve our ability to study this newly discovered ion channel family.

16.4.7 Water Channels

Almost all cell membranes exhibit some water permeability. Our understanding of the movement of water through cell membranes has been greatly advanced by the discovery of a family of water-specific, membrane-channel proteins—the *aquaporins.* At least 12 different aquaporins (0 to 11) have been identified. These proteins are present in organisms at all levels of life, and their unique permeability characteristics and distribution in numerous tissues indicate diverse roles in the regulation of water homeostasis. Agre (Figure 16.1) of Johns Hopkins University School of Medicine received the 2003 Nobel Prize in Chemistry for the discovery of the water channels.

16.4.8 Intracellular and Gap-Junction Ion Channels

Ion channels are found not only in the cell membrane but also in the membranes of the intracellular organelles such as mitochondria, lysozymes, nucleus, and secretory, endocytotic, and synaptic vesicles, as well as in the endoplasmic/sacroplasmic reticulum (ER/SR). Two major intracellular Ca^{2+} channels, the inositol 1,4,5-trisphosphate (IP_3) receptor and the ryanodine receptor (RyR), are located in the ER/SR membranes and contribute to changes in intracellular Ca^{2+} concentration. Based on their mechanism of activation, these two channels are classified as ligand-gated channels (Section 16.4.1).

IP_3 receptors are important downstream targets of G-protein coupled receptors (GPCR). Activation of this class of GPCR leads to stimulation of phospholipase C, which hydrolyzes phosphatidylinositol 4,5-biphosphate (PIP2) to 1,2-diacylglicerol (DAG) and IP_3. IP_3 activates ligand-gated IP_3 Ca^{2+} receptor channels, release of Ca^{2+} from ER/SR stores, and an increase in Ca^{2+} concentration throughout the cell. Ca^{2+} is an important second messenger in all cell types that regulates many intracellular events, including neurotransmission, cell growth and proliferation, secretion, and gene transcription. In muscle cells, Ca^{2+} is required for contraction.

The RyR has allosteric binding site for the plant alkaloid ryanodine (hence the name RyR), which locks the RyR channel in an open state and inhibits the channel. In muscle cells, the coordinated opening of a cluster of RyR in the SR membrane leads to local transient Ca^{2+} release events termed Ca^{2+} sparks. Ca^{2+} release from ryanodine receptors in the SR membrane is more difficult to detect compared to the IP_3-receptor mediated Ca^{2+} release, displaying important cell type-specific differences. In cardiac myocytes, in which Ca^{2+} sparks were first described by Lederer's group in 1993, RyR are activated by a triggering pulse of Ca^{2+} entering through Ca_V1 (L-type) channels. This process, known as Ca^{2+}-induced Ca^{2+}-release, leads to the rapid and progressive opening of a large number of RyR clusters and a cell-wide increase in Ca^{2+}. This global increase in Ca^{2+} is required for myocyte contraction, and when summed across coordinately regulated ventricular myocytes, underlies a single heartbeat. Unlike cardiac myocytes, in which RyR are in close juxtaposition to cell membrane Ca_V1 (L-type) channels, in smooth muscle, RyR are positioned near Ca^{2+}-activated $K_{Ca}1.1$ (BK) channels, which are not expressed in cardiac myocytes. Because of these differences in protein expression and cellular architecture, RyRs play a completely different role in smooth muscle than in cardiac muscle. In smooth muscle, RyR activity is closely related to SR Ca^{2+} load, with increased SR Ca^{2+} resulting in increased RyR activity. RyR-mediated Ca^{2+} release in smooth muscle produces a highly localized increase in Ca^{2+} that does not activate other RyRs and therefore does not spread to the rest of the cell. Instead, the smooth muscle Ca^{2+} spark, as shown by Nelson's group, acts directly on the nearby $K_{Ca}1.1$ channel to stimulate transient outward $K_{Ca}1.1$ (BK) currents (STOCs) (Figure 16.17). The resulting membrane hyperpolarization decreases the activity of Ca_V1 (L-type) channels, resulting in a decrease in Ca^{2+} influx, a decrease in global intracellular Ca^{2+} levels, and a reduction in Ca^{2+}-dependent contraction. Thus, in smooth muscle, RyR-mediated Ca^{2+} release acts as a negative feedback mechanism to oppose contraction—a result that is diametrically opposed to the function of these channels in the heart.

Gap-junction channels are a unique type of intercellular junction that connects the cytoplasm of adjacent cells within a tissue, and whose presence is essential for the normal function of many organs. They are the largest known channels, permitting not only ions but also larger molecules to pass through. The main gap-junction channel proteins, **connexins**, are a family of highly homologous proteins named for their approximate molecular weight (e.g., connexin30, connexin37, connexin43, etc.). Human genome studies suggest that all existing members of the connexin family have now been identified. Structurally, gap-junction channels are comprised of two hemichannels, each formed by the assembly of six connexins. Since each connexin member has unique gating as well as permeability and selectivity properties, some combinations of connexins produce intermediate or new properties, analogous to the K_V channel heterotetrameric structure, which provide a huge diversity to the interconnecting properties between cells. In some gap-junction channels, the gating mechanism acts like the iris diaphragm of a camera, and discriminates solely on the basis of size. Furthermore, gap-junction channels follow other various gating mechanisms, including voltage-gating and ligand-gating, where channel phosphorylation could act as an additional modulator.

An important consequence of the connectivity provided by gap junctions in excitable cells is that individual cells are electrically coupled such that a signal generated in one cell is rapidly communicated to connected cells. In both excitable and nonexcitable cells, gap junctions provide a means for communicating Ca^{2+} signals between cells. These ubiquitous channels play critical roles in many signaling processes by allowing rapid intercellular communication and synchronization of coupled cell activities, including coordinated cardiac and smooth muscle contractions, neuronal excitability, neurotransmitter release, insulin secretion, and epithelial electrolyte transport. In contrast to most other channels, no natural toxin or synthetic specific inhibitor of gap-junction channels has been identified yet.

16.5 METHODS FOR THE STUDY OF ION CHANNELS

This section summarizes the main techniques and methods used to study ion channels. These techniques range from the measurement of ionic current flow through a single-ion channel to investigating ion-channel function in whole-animal experiments, including the use of genetically engineered mouse models with altered ion-channel structure, or that either lack or overexpress a particular channel type. Although some of these techniques are very well established, various methods for examining the structure and function of ion channels are still being developed.

16.5.1 Electrophysiological Techniques

All electrophysiological techniques that are used to study ion channel activity are based on the fact that ion channels conduct electrical current carried by ions (Section 16.2) that can be detected with highly sensitive electronic equipment.

16.5.1.1 Voltage Clamp Techniques

The voltage clamp is a classic electrophysiological technique to measure ion currents across the cell membrane. Under voltage clamp conditions, voltage-gated ion channels open and close as normal, but the voltage clamp apparatus compensates for the changes in the ion current to maintain a constant membrane potential. The investigator sets a desired holding membrane potential, also referred to as holding voltage or command potential, and the voltage clamp uses negative feedback to maintain the cell at this desired holding potential (Figure 16.19).

The voltage clamp was first applied by Cole in the 1930s to 1940s, and then further developed by Hodgkin and Huxley (Figure 16.1). The original two electrodes that Cole, Hodgkin, and Huxley used were fine wires that could be inserted only into extremely large cells such as the squid giant axon, which are as large as 1 mm in diameter. Hodgkin and Huxley used the squid giant axon to determine the ionic basis of the action potential (Figure 16.2), as described in a landmark set of papers in 1952.

16.5.1.2 Conventional ("Sharp") Microelectrodes

This technique is the same as the voltage clamp, but the electrodes are made of glass with very sharp tips (<1 μM in diameter) filled with a KCl solution (2–3 μM). For

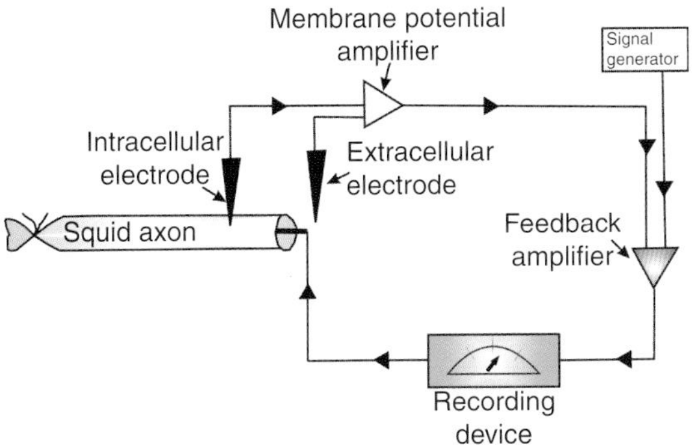

Figure 16.19 Diagram illustrating the voltage-clamp technique applied to the giant squid axon. The voltage clamp operates by negative feedback. The membrane potential amplifier measures membrane potential and outputs to the feedback amplifier. It subtracts the membrane potential from the holding potential, which it receives from the signal generator. This signal is amplified and output is sent into the axon via the current electrode. Whenever the cell diverges from the holding potential, an error signal is generated, which is the difference between the holding potential and the actual cell membrane potential. The feedback circuit passes current into the cell to reduce the error signal to zero. Thus, the voltage-clamp circuit produces a current equal and opposite to the ionic current.

this reason, the conventional microelectrodes are also known as "sharp" microelectrodes. Unlike Cole's original voltage-clamp approach, the microelectrodes can be applied to cells much smaller than the squid giant axon (Figure 16.20). There are two variations of this technique: (1) two-electrode voltage clamp and (2) single-electrode voltage clamp. The latter variation uses one impaling electrode only, which serves as both a current-passing and voltage-recording electrode. The single-electrode can be applied to very small cells that would be impossible to impale with two electrodes. The disadvantage of the sharp microelectrode is that it does not conduct as well as the wire, and sometimes cannot pass current rapidly enough to compensate for the cell membrane current. Another disadvantage involves space clamp issues. Cole, Hodgkin, and Huxley's voltage clamp employed a long wire inserted throughout the squid giant axon that allowed for uniform voltage clamping of the axon along its entire length (Figure 16.19). The current passed through a sharp microelectrode, however, decreases gradually from the impaling point to the more distant parts of the cell membrane. In other words, the current supplied by a microelectrode may not uniformly affect different parts of a larger or irregularly shaped cell (e.g., neurons with complex dendritic structure).

16.5.1.3 Patch-Clamp Technique

This technique allows the study of single-ion channels as well as whole-cell ion channel currents. Essentially, the patch-clamp technique is an improved and refined version of the voltage-clamp technique. It requires a low electrical noise borosilicate glass electrode, also known as a patch electrode or patch pipette, with a relatively large tip (>1 μm) that has a smooth surface rather than a sharp tip as with the conventional microelectrodes. This is a major difference between the patch electrode and the sharp electrode used to impale cells directly through the cell membrane (Figure 16.20).

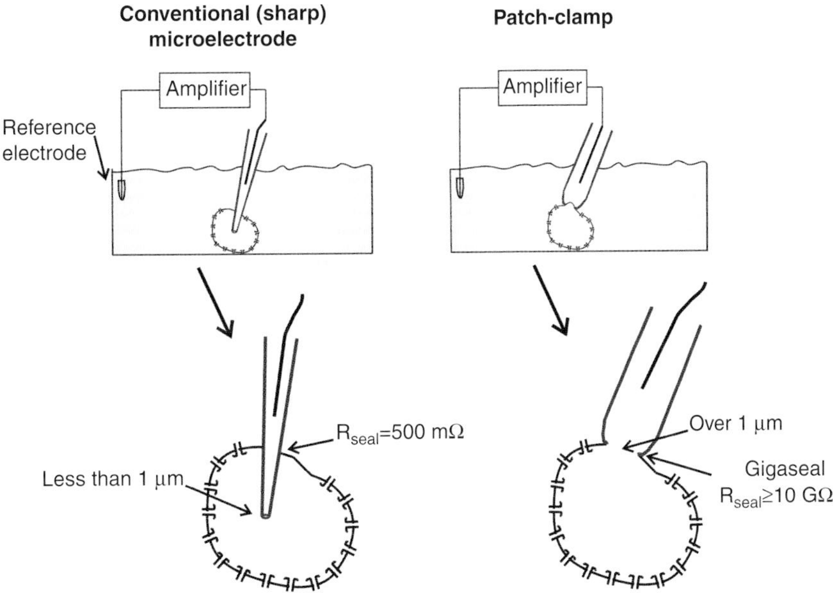

Figure 16.20 Comparison between the conventional (sharp) microelectrode and patch-clamp technique. The sharp microelectrode is less than 1μm at the tip and impales the cell, whereas the patch-clamp electrode is over 1μm at the tip and forms a gigaseal (>10 GΩ) with the cell membrane.

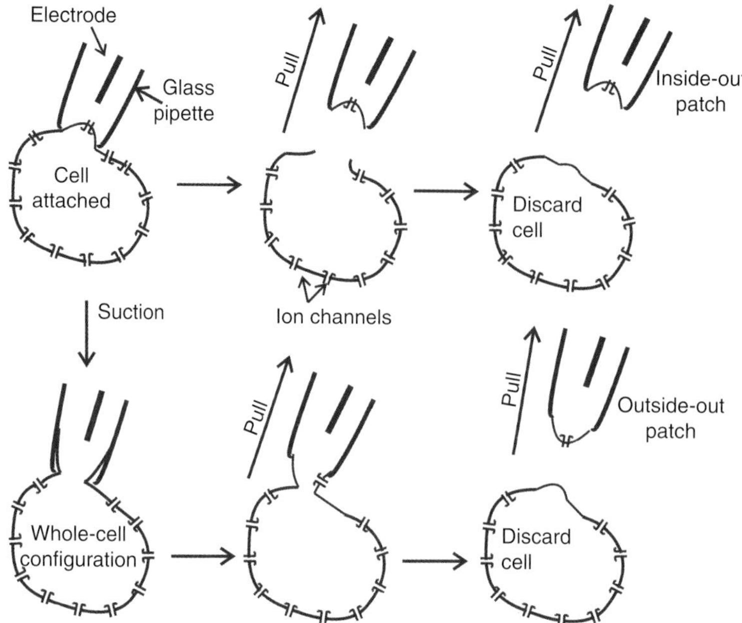

Figure 16.21 Illustration of the different modes and configurations of the patch-clamp technique.

The patch-clamp electrode is pressed against a cell membrane and suction is applied to pull the cell membrane inside the electrode tip. The suction causes the cell to form a tight, high-resistance seal with the rim of the electrode, usually greater than 10 giga Ohms, which is called a *gigaseal* (Figures 16.20 and 16.21).

There are several variations of the patch-clamp technique (Figure 16.21). Ion channel currents can be recorded from a whole cell or from small membrane pieces called excised patches, which are sections that are physically excised and removed from the cell membrane. The excised patch can be either in inside-out or outside-out configuration. The different patch-clamp configurations are described later.

Cell-attached mode. With this mode, the patch electrode remains sealed to the cell membrane, permitting the recording of currents through single-ion channels from the patch of membrane surrounded by the tip of the electrode. Some original single-channel recordings in cell-attached mode are shown in Figure 16.14.

Whole-cell mode—conventional. From the initial cell-attached configuration, additional suction is applied to rupture the cell membrane, thus providing access to the intracellular space of the cell. The larger opening at the tip of the patch electrode, compared with the sharp microelectrode, provides lower resistance and thus better electrical access to the cell. Because the volume of the patch electrode is much bigger than the cell, the soluble contents of the cell will slowly be replaced by the contents of the electrode, referred to as "dialyzing" the cell contents. Whole-cell mode records currents through all channels from the entire cell membrane at once (Figure 16.12). Therefore, the recorded currents are significantly larger compared to the single-channel recordings from excised membrane patches (Figure 16.16).

Whole-cell mode—perforated. This mode is similar to the conventional whole-cell mode but the cell membrane is not ruptured. Instead, small amounts of an ionophore, such as amphotericin B, nystatin, or gramicidin, are added into the electrode solution, which produce very small perforations in the membrane patch surrounded by the electrode. Only small ions (K^+, Na^+) and not larger ones (Ca^{2+}) or any other molecules can move freely through the formed membrane holes. This mode allows ion current recordings while the internal content of the cell is kept intact.

Inside-out mode. From the cell-attached configuration, the electrode is quickly pulled out from the cell, thus ripping the patch of membrane from the cell. This leaves the patch of membrane attached to the electrode exposing the intracellular surface of the membrane to the external environment, allowing pharmacological manipulations to the intracellular side of the ion channels (Figure 16.21). Some original inside-out recordings are shown in Figure 16.16.

Outside-out mode. After achieving cell-attached configuration, the electrode is slowly withdrawn from the cell, allowing a membrane patch to be excised, which will then reorganize on the edge of the electrode with the original interior of the cell membrane facing inside the electrode solution (Figure 16.21). Outside-out mode allows researchers to examine ion channel properties while the channel is exposed to the outside environment, but not in contact with its native cellular environment. This mode allows studying effects of membrane nonpermeable molecules (when included in the patch electrode solution) on the intracellular part of the channel.

Current clamp mode. In this mode the current is kept constant by the patch-clamp amplifier while voltage is measured, allowing recordings of the membrane potential.

The patch-clamp technique requires very sophisticated equipment (Figure 16.22). Sakmann and Neher (Figure 16.1) received the Nobel Prize in Physiology or Medicine in 1991 for the development of this method. A detailed description of the electrophysiological techniques can be found in the following books and monographs:

- *Single Channel Recording*, edited by Sakmann and Neher
- *Patch Clamping: An Introductory Guide to Patch Clamp Electrophysiology*, by Molleman
- *Patch-Clamp Analysis*, edited by Waltz, Boulton, and Baker
- *Axon Guide*, published by Axon Instruments

16.5.2 Pharmacological Techniques

The electrophysiological techniques, as well as functional studies on whole animals or isolated tissues

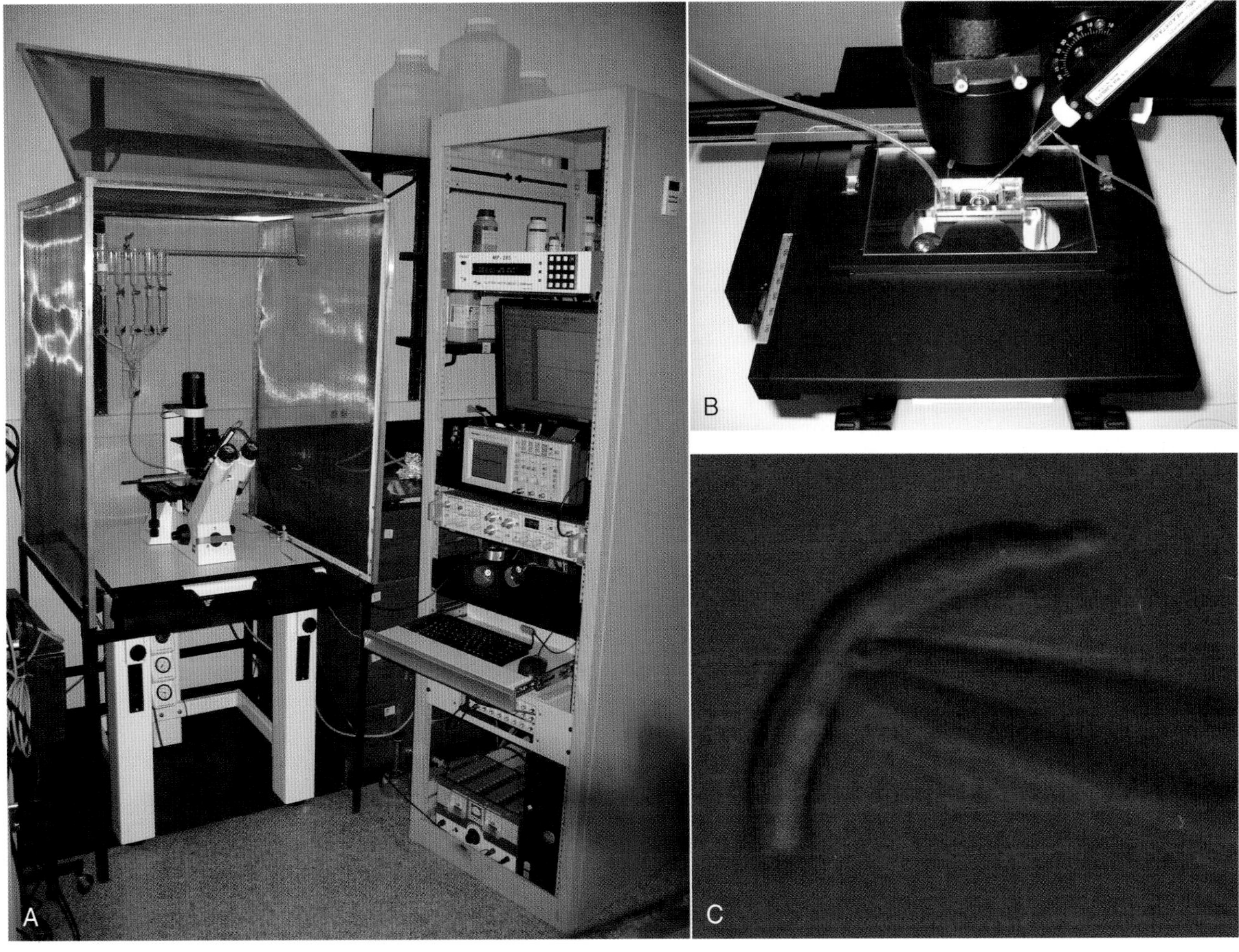

Figure 16.22 Patch-clamp setup. A. A typical patch-clamp setup consists of a high resolution inverted microscope positioned on a vibration isolation table and surrounded by a Faraday cage, which serves to isolate the contaminating electrical noise. On the right-hand side of the picture is an electrophysiological rack, which holds the patch-clamp amplifier, a PC with interface and specialized software, micromanipulator controller box, an oscilloscope, and an external power supply for the microscope used to reduce the contaminating electrical noise. B. Illustration of the amplifier headstage with the borosilicate glass patch pipette (electrode) positioned on a micromanipulator. The microchamber, which is positioned in the middle of the inverted microscope stage, is connected to a perfusion system that helps to control the external media. C. The patch pipette is approaching a single urinary bladder smooth muscle cell located at the bottom of a microchamber.

and organs, can be combined with pharmacological approaches when the channel is tested by various ion channel inhibitors or activators (Section 16.3). The smooth muscle tissue builds up the walls of all internal organs of the human body, including blood vessels, and is enriched in various ion channels that control excitability and contractility. One classic pharmacological technique is the isometric muscle-force recording (contractility) from isolated smooth muscle strips (or blood vessel rings) from different organs (Figure 16.23). Numerous ion channel modulators can be tested on the smooth muscle contractility, thus examining the role of individual ion channels. This technique is used largely by the pharmaceutical industry.

16.5.3 Crystallographic and Spectroscopic Techniques

These methods are based on the use of light waves to probe the macromolecular nature of ion channels and are useful for obtaining structural information about ion channel proteins. Without enough valid structural information, all data gleaned from traditional protein chemistry techniques are simply

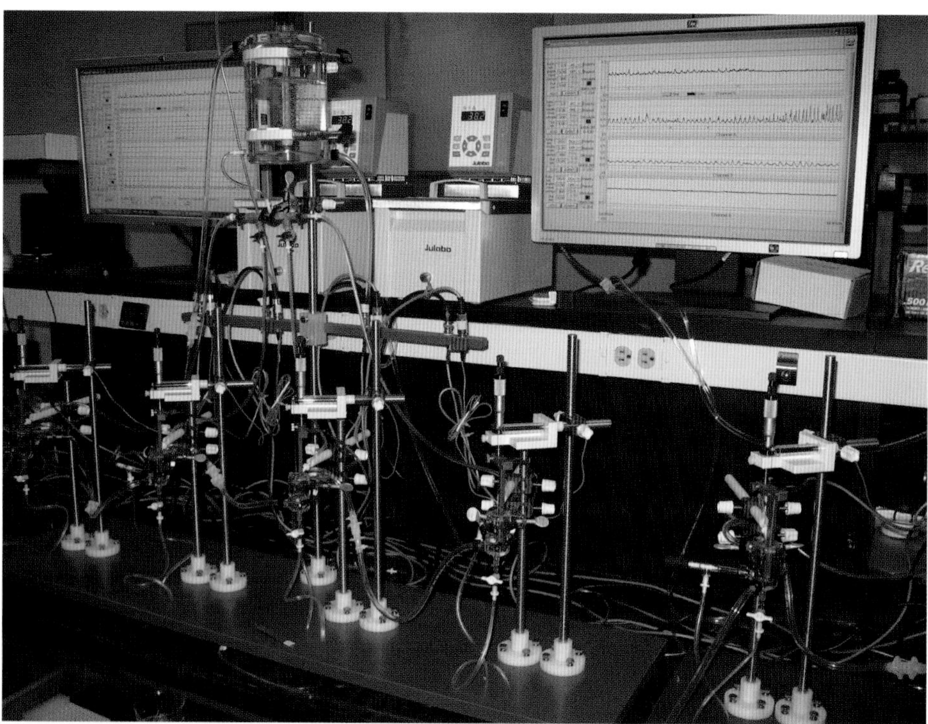

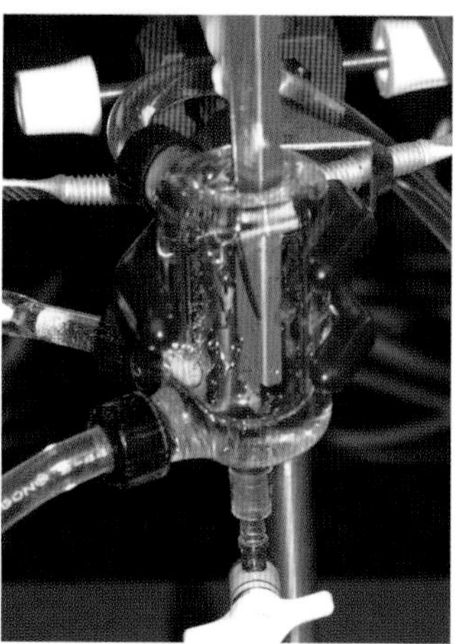

Figure 16.23 Pharmacological setup for isometric tension (contractility) recordings of isolated smooth muscle preparations under the influence of ion channel modulators (inhibitors and activators). Smooth muscle strips (as visible on the second enlarged picture) or rings are placed in thermostatically controlled tissue baths and are connected to a force displacement transducer for isometric recording. The force signal (contractions) is recorded electronically via specialized software and displayed on a monitor.

conjecture. In the late 1960s, one of the first methods applied to ion channel research, which showed that ion channels are proteins, was called *limited proteolysis*. Unfortunately, many established protein chemistry methods are not applicable, simply because ion channels require a natural lipid environment to function normally. X-ray crystallography studies solved the molecular structure of the K^+ channel (Figure 16.3) and earned MacKinnon (Figure 16.1) a Nobel Prize in Chemistry in 2003.

16.5.4 Molecular and Cell Biology Techniques

In general, all molecular and cell biology techniques used in protein research can be applied to ion channels. The major obstacle is that the ion channels' membrane proteins are of limited quantities. Thus, prior to the advent of modern molecular biology techniques, ion channel studies were restricted to the availability of ion channel proteins. The molecular biological techniques are used not only as a way to discover new ion channels, but also to provide ion channel material in larger quantities, increasing their convenience. Isolation of ion channel membrane proteins requires solubilization with detergents and purification on the basis of their ability to bind specific markers with high affinity. For example, the Na_V channels can be isolated based on their ability to bind TTX with high affinity, and the Ca_V channels likewise are isolated based on their affinity to dihydropyridines. The first ion channel to be studied in purified form was nAChR, which could be easily isolated in relatively large amounts from readily available tissue sources.

Currently, it is standard procedure to develop ion channel-specific antibodies for immunocytochemistry, to perform Western and Northern blot analyses, ion channel *in situ* hybridization, or reverse transcription polymerase chain reaction (RT-PCR). The introduction of the single-cell RT-PCR in combination with the patch-clamp method in the 1990s made it possible to identify gene transcripts and to correlate them with functional data for the same individual cell. Finally, one of the most powerful cell biological techniques in the study of ion channels is based on artificial expression systems such as microinjection of mRNA encoding channel subunits into *Xenopus* oocytes and selective expression of native ion channels or with different subunit composition (e.g., K_V channel subunits). Because the *Xenopus* oocytes are large, they are a perfect model to study artificially expressed channels. Another good model for artificial ion channel expression is the Chinese hamster ovary (CHO) cell line.

16.5.5 Genetically Engineered Animal Models

The ability to genetically manipulate the mouse genome by deleting or overexpressing specific genes allows researchers to evaluate the significance of certain ion channel gene products and to study their functional effects from the cellular level to the whole-animal level. The mouse is the predominant model of choice for genetic engineering, due to its short gestation cycle, low maintenance costs, the relative ease of introducing foreign genetic material into their genomes, and the extensive mouse genetics literature. There are two basic approaches to mouse genomic manipulation. In the first approach, the exogenous DNA transgene is introduced into a fertilized oocyte by microinjection, resulting in random chromosomal integration. This technique commonly is used to generate "gain-of-function" transgenic animals in which the expression—usually overexpression—of the exogenous gene is under the control of a specific promoter. Variations on this theme allow for spatial and/or temporal control of gene expression, through the use of tissue-specific promoters and inducible regulatory cassettes. In the second approach, which involves introduction of exogenous DNA into pluripotent mouse embryonic stem cells (ES), homologous recombination of foreign DNA with its genomic target leads to selective disruption of the endogenous gene, producing a so-called knockout animal. In most cases, this approach targets only a portion of the target gene that is critical for function, although techniques are available that allow the gene to be replaced in its entirety.

One limitation to the genetic ablation approach is the problem of developmental compensation, in which protein products of other, usually closely related, genes functionally substitute for a deleted gene, resulting in the absence of obvious phenotypic abnormalities. A classic example of this phenomenon is the knockout for SUR1—the regulatory subunit of the pancreatic beta cell $K_{ir}6$ (K_{ATP}) channel, which is responsible for insulin secretion and is essential to life. Contrary to expectation, the mice carrying the deletion were capable of regulated insulin secretion and managed to maintain glucose at near-normal levels. Although the precise compensatory mechanism is not clear, the developing embryo had managed a "fix" for what should have been a lethal defect. The trend in genetic engineering is toward strategies that allow for both spatial and temporal control of transgene expression and target gene knockout/knockdown, as a way of bypassing the potentially confounding effects of developmental compensation.

The number of genetically engineered mouse lines for ion channel research has grown rapidly. Some examples for knockouts lacking K^+ channels include the $K_{Ca}1.1$ (BK), $K_{Ca}2.2$ (SK2), and $K_{Ca}3.2$ (SK3) channels; knockouts lacking TRP channels include TRPC2, TRPC4, TRPC6, TRPV1, TRPV4, TRPV5, TRPM5 channels, and so on. Knockouts for accessory ion channel subunits such as $K_{Ca}1.1\beta$-1-subunit, $Ca_v\beta$-2, and so on have also been studied extensively. Examples of single $K_{Ca}1.1$ (BK) channel current recordings from control and $K_{Ca}1.1\beta$-1-subunit knockout mice are illustrated in Figure 16.16. An interesting transgenic animal model is one that possesses tetracycline-based genetic switches and can either overexpress or suppress a particular ion channel expression, depending on orally administered tetracyclines such as doxycycline.

Genetically engineered animal models offer an important method to evaluate the significance of certain ion channel proteins *in vivo* and evaluate their role at the organism level. For cases in which selective pharmacological agents are not available for a given channel, TRP for example, knockout animals are often the only effective tool for determining a channel's physiological role. A comprehensive discussion of genetic models relevant to ion channel function would constitute a chapter in itself, but many of the disease associations described in the next section have been studied or established using various genetic models.

16.6 ION CHANNELS AND DISEASE

Diseases resulting from alterations or mutations in ion channel structure and function are known as *channelopathies*. Identified mutations in more than 60 different ion channel genes have been revealed to cause human disease, indicating the importance of ion channels in human physiology. Channelopathies may be due to mutations either in the α-pore-forming subunit or in the ion-channel accessory subunits. Mutations may affect the gating mechanism, selectivity filter, channel conductance, or single-channel open probability. Sometimes these mutations may be very subtle when only one single amino acid is affected. Alternatively, some channelopathies are due to mutations in multiple genes simultaneously. Mutations that prevent ion channel protein synthesis, called loss-of-function mutations, can lead to some disorders. Increase of ion channel function (gain-of-function) may also cause diseases. The degree to which a mutation is revealed functionally also depends on the channel's tissue distribution as well as the relative importance and contribution of the particular channel to membrane excitability. The same mutation may have different effects on different genetic backgrounds. Ion channel disease could occur due to abnormalities in regulatory mechanisms such as protein kinase-mediated channel phosphorylation. Channelopathies may be caused not only by ion channel mutations but also by autoimmune disorders in which antibodies target critical ion channels.

Ligand-gated channels. Decreased expression of the nAChR in the postsynaptic membrane of the neuromuscular junction leads to myasthenia gravis syndrome (skeletal muscle weakness). Most often, the decreased number of the skeletal muscle nAChRs is caused by T-lymphocyte-dependent autoimmune reaction against nAChR. Sometimes, however, myasthenia gravis may also occur due to hereditary mutations in the ε-subunit of the nAChR.

Na^+ channels. Mutations in the α-subunit of the neuronal Na_V ($Na_V1.1$, $Na_V1.2$, or $Na_V1.3$) channels lead to epilepsy, whereas mutations in $Na_V1.3$, $Na_V1.6$, $Na_V1.7$, $Na_V1.8$, or $Na_V1.9$ channels cause chronic pain. Genetic malfunctions of the skeletal muscle $Na_V1.4$ channels disabling the channel to inactivate normally are the origin for periodic paralysis, a disorder that leads to periodic muscle weakness. Mutations in the heart $Na_V1.5$ channels are the root for an abnormal cardiac action potential with prolonged repolarization phase, known as LQT syndrome, because of its unusual long QT interval that appears on the electrocardiogram. Increase of function mutations in the amiloride-sensitive ENaC (Section 16.4.2) lead to enhanced Na^+ uptake in the kidney tubules. Because plasma Na^+ concentration regulates blood pressure, this can cause inherited *hyper*tension (Liddle's syndrome). Alternatively, ENaC loss-of-function mutations can cause hereditary *hypo*tension (pseudohypoaldosteronism type-1).

Ca^{2+} channels. Mutations in the α-subunit of the skeletal muscle Ca_v1 channel lead to hypokalaemic periodic paralysis, a disorder associated with episodic attacks of muscle weakness that are related to low serum K^+ concentrations. Mutations in the α-subunit of the neuronal Ca_v2 channels are the cause for familial hemiplegic migraine, episodic ataxia type-2, and spinocerebellar ataxia type-6.

K^+ channels. The Kir6 (K_{ATP}) channel is distributed in pancreatic beta cells, nerve, and muscle cells. This channel, however, is the most predominant regulator of the resting membrane potential in the pancreatic beta cells, and therefore the most severe effect of K_{ATP} channel mutations is seen in the pancreas. Mutations in the Kir6 (K_{ATP}) channel lead to neonatal diabetes and congenital hyperinsulinemia. Loss-of-function mutations in the SUR regulatory subunit of the Kir6 (K_{ATP}) channel cause congenital hyperinsulinemia as well. Mutations in some K_V channels in the cochlea may lead to deafness. K_V channels also have a role in cancer. For example, $K_V1.3$ triggers lymphocyte activation and is overexpressed in various tumors. Mutations in the Kv11.1 channel, which participates in the last repolarization phase of the cardiac action potential, causes one form of inherited LQT syndrome, which can lead to cardiac arrhythmias and sudden death. LQT syndrome, however, may also be due to mutations in the K_V accessory subunits or the Na_V channel. Overall, mutations in up to eight different genes, either alone or in concert, may cause LQT syndrome.

CLC. A classic example of an inherited channelopathy is a mutation in CFTR leading to cystic fibrosis, a disease that causes the human body to produce unusually thick and sticky mucus, which clogs the lungs and leads to life-threatening lung infections. Cystic fibrosis affects about 30,000 people in the United States and about 70,000 worldwide.

TRP channels. Some human diseases and important pathological conditions are now being associated with TRP channel dysfunction. At this point, four channelopathies have been identified in which a defect in a TRP channel encoding gene is the direct cause of disease. TRPs also are involved in some systemic diseases because they can be modulated by xenobiotic toxins, irritants, and inflammation products. Other indications of the involvement of TRPs in several diseases come from both the correlation between the level of channel expression to disease symptoms and from the mapping of encoding genes for TRP channel.

Intracellular channels. Mutations of the genes encoding intracellular ion channels may also cause disease. Mutations in the RyR (Section 16.4.8) lead to malignant hyperthermia, a disorder in which common inhalation anesthetics produce unrestrained muscle contractions and a lethal increase in body temperature. Connexin mutations may lead to different pathologies, such as peripheral neuropathies, cardiovascular diseases, deafness, dermatological diseases, and cataracts.

Some of the major channelopathies with relevant diseases or conditions are summarized in Table 16.8. Collective studies on the channelopathies have led to new insights into ion channel mechanisms and their potential roles as therapeutic targets. Further advances in ion channel research will help to illuminate how ion channel mutations predispose individuals to common genetic diseases such as type 2 diabetes, obesity, hypertension, and cardiac disease. This will advance the development of new therapeutic strategies, and even new drugs targeting one's individual genetic profile could be discovered.

Table 16.8 Major Channelopathies with Relevant Diseases or Conditions and the Particular Ion Channel Involved

Ion Channel	Disease/Condition
nAChR	Myasthenia gravis
$GABA_A$	Juvenile epilepsy
$Na_V1.1$, $Na_V1.2$, or $Na_V1.3$	Epilepsy
$Na_V1.3$, $Na_V1.6$, $Na_V1.7$, $Na_V1.8$, or $Na_V1.9$	Chronic pain
$Na_V1.4$	Periodic paralysis
$Na_V1.5$	LQT syndrome and other arrhythmias
ENaC	Hypertension (Liddle's syndrome) or Hypotension (pseudohypoaldosteronism type-1)
Neuronal Ca_V2	Ataxia, migraine, epilepsy
$Ca_V1.2$	Timothy Syndrome
$K_{ir}1.1$	Bartter's syndrome
$K_{ir}6.2$, K_{ATP}	Diabetes
SUR1 of the Kir6.2, K_{ATP}	Diabetes
hERG	LQT syndrome
MinK	LQT syndrome
$K_{Ca}1.1$ (BK)	Epilepsy, seizures; maybe urinary incontinence
CFTR	Cystic fibrosis
CLC2	Epilepsy
CLC5	Dent's disease and other kidney stone diseases
CLC7	Osteopetrosis
CLC-Ka	Bartter's syndrome
TRPP2	Kidney disease
TRPC6	Glomerulosclerosis, defective Mg reabsorption
TRPML1	Mucolipidosis IV
Skeletal muscle RyR channel	Malignant hyperthermia, central core
Cardiac RyR channel	Cardiac arrhythmia

16.7 ION CHANNELS AS DRUG TARGETS

Due to their structural heterogeneity, membrane localization, tissue specificity, and fundamental functional roles, ion channels are attractive targets for drug therapy. Many currently existing drugs, such as blood pressure regulators, local anesthetics, sedatives, antianxiety agents, antidiabetic drugs, and even antiviral therapies, exert their effects by interacting with ion channels. The ion channel drugs that are currently on the market, with their particular channel target and mechanism of action, are summarized in Table 16.9.

A large variety of drugs had been in use for many years before we knew that their effects were caused specifically by targeting ion channels. For example, benzodiazepines have been available since the early 1960s, before the discovery of the $GABA_A$ receptor channels. Cocaine was used as a local ophthalmic anesthetic as early as the 1880s, and lidocaine, currently an extensively used local anesthetic, was synthesized in the 1940s. We now know that local anesthetics target the neuronal Na_V channels in a voltage-dependent or use-dependent manner (Section 16.3.1). The L-type (Ca_V1) channels are targets of the organic **Ca-antagonists**, which are commonly used in the therapy of hypertension and cardiovascular diseases.

Looking at the booming pharmaceutical industry that exists today, it is important to note that in addition to the big pharmaceutical companies such as Merck, Pfizer, GlaxoSmithKline, and Bristol-Myers Squibb, which have had established ion channel research groups for many years, emerging small biopharmaceutical companies such as Icagen, Hydra, Scion Pharmaceuticals, and many others have focused their entire effort on the discovery, development, and commercialization of novel small molecule drugs that exclusively modulate ion channel targets. By integrating a number of scientific and drug development disciplines, these small companies are able to efficiently discover and develop small molecular compounds that are more specific for the relevant disease ion channels, and therefore have

Table 16.9 Currently Available Ion Channel Drugs Used for Multiple Indications

Generic Drug Name*	Disease/Condition	Ion Channel Targeted	Mechanism
Amiloride (13)	Hypertension and congestive heart failure	ENaC	Blocks ENaC
Bepridil (2)	Angina	Ca_V1 (L-type) and Ca_V3 (T-type) channels	Has antiarrhythmic and antihypertensive properties; it is not related to any other Ca^{2+} channel blocker
Cinnarizine (41)		Ca_V1 (L-type) and Ca_V3 (T-type) channels	Inhibits L-type and T-type Ca^{2+} channels in vascular smooth muscle
Ibutilide fumarate	Atrial fibrillation	hERG potassium channels, delayed inward rectifier potassium (Kir) channels and L-type (Ca_V1) Ca^{2+} channels	Class III antiarrhythmic drug
Dihydropyridines: 1) amlodipine (13) 2) felodipine (30) 3) isradipine (19) 4) lercanidipine (2) 5) nicardipine (5) 6) nifedipine (108) 7) nimodipine (5) 8) nitrendipine (11) 9) nisoldipine (9)	Hypertension; angina	Ca_V1 (L-type) channels	Inhibits L-type Ca^{2+} channels in cardiac and vascular smooth muscle cells by modulating ion channel gating mechanisms; decreases systemic blood pressure and heart contractility
Phenylalkylamines: verapamil (33)	Angina; hypertension; some forms of cardiac arrhythmias	Ca_V1 (L-type) channels	Inhibits L-type Ca^{2+} channels in cardiac and vascular smooth muscle cells; more selective for the myocardium with minimal vasodilatory effects compared with dihydropyridines; class IV antiarrhythmic agents
Benzothiapines: diltiazem (39)	Hypertension; angina; some forms of cardiac arrhythmias	Ca_V1 (L-type) channels	Inhibits L-type Ca^{2+} channels in cardiac and vascular smooth muscle cells by modulating ion channel gating mechanisms; decreases systemic blood pressure and heart contractility
Pregabalin (2)	Seizure; neuropathic pain	Ca^{2+} channels	Binds with high affinity to the alpha2-delta subunit of voltage-gated Ca^{2+} channels in CNS; anticonvulsant drug
Local anesthetics: 1) benzocaine (32) 2) bupivacaine (22) 3) chloroprocaine (50) 4) cocaine (89) 5) levobupivacaine (1) 6) lidocaine (39) 7) mepivacaine (17) 8) mexiletine (5) 9) oxybuprocaine (27) 10) prilocaine (7) 11) procainamide (15) 12) procaine (25) 13) propafenone (7) 14) ropivacaine (6)	Local and spinal anesthetic; also used for treatment of status epilepticus; migraine and cluster headaches; ventricular arrhythmias, ventricular fibrillation; cardiac arrest; neuropathic pain, postherpetic neuralgia	Na_V channels	Inhibits neuronal fast Na_V channels, and thus blocks the action potential; inhibits also cardiac Na_V channels
Sulfonylurea derivatives: 1) acetohexamide (14) 2) chlorpropamide (31) 3) gliclazide (11) 4) glimepiride (8) 5) glipizide (31) 6) gliquidone (2) 7) glyburide (108) 8) tolazamide (3) 9) tolbutamide (38)	Diabetes Mellitus type 2 (noninsulin-dependent)	$K_{ir}6$ (K_{ATP})channel	Binds to the regulatory SUR subunit of the K_{ATP} channel in pancreatic ß-cells and inhibits the channel

Continued

Table 16.9 Currently Available Ion Channel Drugs Used for Multiple Indications—cont'd

Generic Drug Name*	Disease/Condition	Ion Channel Targeted	Mechanism
Nateglinide (5)	Diabetes Mellitus type 2 (noninsulin-dependent)	$K_{ir}6$ (K_{ATP})channel	Inhibits K_{ATP} channels in the pancreatic ß-cells; the mechanism is highly tissue selective with low affinity for heart and skeletal muscle; enhances insulin secretion; works differently than sulfonylureas
Repaglinide (6)	Diabetes Mellitus type 2 (noninsulin-dependent)	$K_{ir}6$ (K_{ATP})channel	Inhibits K_{ATP} channels in the pancreatic ß-cells; works differently than sulfonylureas
Barbiturates: over 12 drugs currently in use	Seizure disorders; insomnia; anesthetics	1) $GABA_A$ receptor neuronal ligand gated Cl^- channels in the CNS; 2) Na_V channels	Activates $GABA_A$ Cl^- channels, which causes hyperpolarization of the postsynaptic membrane and decrease in neuronal activity; may inhibit Na_V channels
Benzodiazepines: 1) alprazolam (21) 2) chlordiazepoxide (50) 3) clonazepam (11) 4) diazepam (123) 5) flurazepam (11) 6) lorazepam (29) 7) nitrazepam (9) 8) oxazepam (54) 9) temazepam (22) 10) triazolam (13)	Anxiety, insomnia, seizures, muscle spasms	$GABA_A$ receptor neuronal ligand gated Cl^- channels in the CNS	Activates $GABA_A$ Cl^- channels, which causes hyperpolarization of the postsynaptic membrane and decrease in neuronal activity
Imidazopyridines (unrelated to benzodiazepines): zolpidem (8)	Insomnia	$GABA_A$ receptor neuronal ligand gated Cl^- channels (CNS)	Activates $GABA_A$ Cl^- channels; selective for the alpha-1 receptor

*The number in parenthesis after a drug name indicates the total number of different brand names and drug synonyms. Some drugs have multiple pharmacological targets. Only ion channel effects and related diseases are indicated here.

a reduced likelihood of clinical failure and adverse side effects. Key elements of the ion channel drug discovery technology include cloning of the known 340+ human ion channel genes, which are believed to represent the majority of the human ion channel genome, expertise in developing high throughput screens for ion channel targets, ion channel focused chemistry libraries of hundreds of thousands of different compounds, computational chemistry methods, and an extensive ion channel database that integrates biological and chemical information about the ion channel targets and the compounds. In this strategic approach, all ion channels are considered in order to identify applications to the treatment of various diseases by searching small molecule modulators for a particular ion channel target. Automated patch-clamp devices such as *PatchXpress* and *OpusXpress*, originally developed by Axon Instruments (now Molecular Devices), are used for high throughput ion channel screening using these small molecules. Animal models of disease are then used to further confirm the particular target. If a small molecule demonstrates activity in the animal model, it both confirms the target and provides a starting point for further chemical modification to increase ion channel specificity.

A number of ion channel-specific compounds have recently been approved by the Food and Drug Administration (FDA) as therapeutics, and others are currently in various stages of clinical trials as potential drugs for a number of indications, including pain, cardiovascular, and neurological pathologies. For example, the current development of specific and high-affinity drugs targeting the Ca_V2 channel subfamily may help control synaptic transmission. Compounds that are thought to inhibit gap-junction channels show cardio- and neuroprotective effects, suggesting that modulation of intercellular communication is a potential pharmacological target. Future discovery of gap-junction channel modulators might be a promising avenue for drug development.

The ion-channel accessory subunits are also the targets of various compounds, indicating their importance to the pharmaceutical industry. The smooth muscle-specific β-1 subunit of the $K_{Ca}1.1$ (BK) channel has profound effects in regulating vascular smooth muscle tone, and thus blood pressure, as well as urinary bladder (where it is most heavily expressed) contractility. Targeting the $K_{Ca}1.1$ channel β-1 subunit may lead to novel therapeutics to control blood pressure and urinary incontinence. The $K_{Ca}1.1$ channel has a fundamental role in regulating penile erection and urinary bladder function, and has been identified as a potential target for the development of therapies for erectile dysfunction and urinary incontinence. Currently, there is a need to develop better therapies for erectile dysfunction because sildenafil is effective in only about 50% of patients, and has serious side effects. The current antimuscarinic drugs used to treat overactive bladder are largely ineffective and have many adverse side effects. Ion channel targeting could be the new therapeutic approach for erectile and bladder dysfunction in the near future.

Recent discoveries indicate that a number of the adverse effects of different drugs are due to their effects on ion channels in various tissues. For example, drugs that cause ventricular arrhythmia as a side effect do so by blocking the cardiac Kv11.1 channel. This phenomenon has been named Acquired LQT Syndrome, as opposed to the inherited syndrome (see previous section). For these reasons, the FDA now requires testing of all new drugs for their potential Kv11.1 inhibitory effects.

16.8 KEY POINTS AND CONCLUSIONS

Ion channels are integral membrane proteins that span through the cell membranes to form a pore that can be penetrated by selected ions at a rate of up to 100 million per second. They are found in virtually all organisms from viruses and bacteria to plants and animals, and in all cell types of the human body. The ion channels consist of pore-forming and, sometimes, accessory subunits. Most ion channels have specialized gate mechanisms, capable of making transitions between conducting and nonconducting states. Channel function can be modulated by changes in membrane potential, ligand binding, intracellular second messengers and metabolites, protein–protein interactions, phosphorylation, and many other factors.

The possible existence of specialized mechanisms for selective ion conductance was first hypothesized by Hodgkin and Huxley in the early 1950s within their Nobel-Prize winning action potential theory. The existence of ion channels then was confirmed in the 1970s to 1980s with a tiny electrical current recording technique known as the patch-clamp. Our understanding of ion channel function has been illuminated by recent breakthroughs in high-resolution ion channel structure determination. In the past decade, a series of *Science* and *Nature* papers by MacKinnon's group has provided solutions for the three-dimensional ion channel structure and the mechanisms of ion selectivity. Many other researchers worldwide continue to pursue a more detailed understanding of how ion channel proteins can be used as targets for drugs.

In order to develop new ion channel targeted drugs, we must clearly understand ion channel structure-to-function relationships. We now know the crystal protein structure of the bacterial KcsA channel, but soon we will have additional crystal ion-channel structures. In the past several decades, ion channel research has been one of the most rapidly developing biomedical fields of importance for drug discovery. Due to their high potency and ion-channel selectivity, different natural toxins and venom peptides have recently emerged as invaluable tools for drug discovery and drug development. In the coming years, key structural elements that distinguish ion channels from other pharmacological targets most likely will be discovered. We will better understand how accessory subunits regulate channel structure, how gating mechanisms work, and how phospholipids interact with channel proteins and modulate their function. In the past two to three decades, advances in molecular genetics made it possible to clone individual channels. Presently, with the sequencing of the entire human genome, we can finally recognize all human ion channel genes and are approaching the time when we will have a full list of all channels from all cell types of the human body.

Finally, this chapter outlines only some basic ion channel principles and mechanisms. Those students who would like to expand their knowledge in this exciting field should start with two valuable ion channel books—*Ionic Channels of Excitable Membranes*, by Bertil Hille, and *Single-Channel Recording*, edited by the Nobel Prize winners Bert Sakmann and Erwin Neher.

ACKNOWLEDGMENTS

I am indebted to my mentor Mark Nelson who provided many insights to this chapter. I am thankful to my students from the lab, Sean Brown and Whitney Kellett, for their invaluable help. I am also grateful to Whitney for drawing most of the original figures and diagrams. Special thanks are extended to Dr. Jennifer Schnellmann, who helped with reviewing the final version of the chapter.

REVIEW QUESTIONS

1. What is the difference between an ion channel and ion carrier?
2. What are the most essential characteristics of ion channels?
3. What is ion channel selectivity? Describe the mechanism of the ion channel selectivity filter.
4. How does the ion channel-gating mechanism work?
5. What is the role of the ion channel accessory proteins and how do they modulate ion channel function?
6. Describe the major ion channel families.
7. Why are the K^+ channels the most diverse ion channel family?
8. How do local anesthetics act?
9. What are Ca-antagonists and how do they exert their effects?
10. What are the major techniques used to study ion channels?
11. What is a voltage clamp? What is a patch-clamp?
12. What are channelopathies?
13. Why are ion channels important targets for therapeutic drugs?

GLOSSARY

Action potential—Rapid and transient change of the cell resting membrane potential.

Aquaporins—Proteins assembling the water channels.

Ca-antagonists—Group of organic Ca_V1 (L-type) channel inhibitors.

Ca^{2+} spark—Local transient intracellular Ca^{2+} release event due to coordinated opening of RyR Ca^{2+} release channel in the SR membrane.

Channelopathies—Diseases caused by mutations in the genes encoding ion channel subunits or regulatory proteins.

Connexins—Proteins that make gap-junction channels.

Desensitization—A process whereby an ion channel loses its agonist sensitivity after initial agonist stimulation.

Electrochemical gradient—Gradient that combines the two forces of the ion concentration and the potential (voltage) difference across the cell membrane.

Equilibrium potential—The value of the cell membrane potential at which there is no net flow of a particular ion type across the membrane.

Excitable cells—Cells that are capable of generating action potential. By definition these are cells expressing Na_V or Ca_V channels; generally neuronal and muscle cells.

Gating—The intrinsic mechanism responsible for ion channel opening or closing.

Inactivation—Process of ion channel transition from a conductive activated state to an inactivated nonconducting state, which is a separate conformational state of the channel.

Ligand—Any molecule that interacts with an ion channel and regulates channel opening and closing by producing conformational changes.

Open probability—The fraction of time an ion channel stays in an open (conductive) state.

Patch-clamp—Technique for recording tiny electrical currents flowing through a single or multiple ion channels.

Permeable—Ion channel capability of being permeated (by an ion).

Permeant—Ion capability of permeating (an ion channel). This term is often mistaken for **permeable**. An ion is *permeant*, an ion channel is *permeable.*

Resting membrane potential—Potential (voltage) difference across the cell membrane, while the cell is at rest and not active; it is always negative in the millivolt range.

Reversal potential—see **Equilibrium potential**.

Selectivity filter—The narrowest region of an ion channel pore that determines which type of ion can pass through the channel.

Voltage clamp—Electrophysiological technique for measuring ion currents across the cell membrane, while a constant membrane potential (voltage) is maintained by the apparatus.

ABBREVIATIONS

ABC—ATP-binding cassette

ACh—acetylcholine

AChR—acetylcholine receptor

nAChR—nicotinic acetylcholine receptor (ion channel)

4-AP—4-aminopyridine

APV (AP5)—D-2-amino-5-phosphonovalerate

BK—large conductance voltage-gated/dependent and Ca^{2+}-activated K^+ channel

Ca_V—voltage-gated (dependent) Ca^{2+} channel

CLC—Cl^- channel

CFTR—cystic fibrosis transmembrane conductance regulator

CNG—cyclic-nucleotide-gated channel

CNQX—6-cyano-7-nitroquinoxaline-2,3-dione

CNS—central nervous system

DHP—1,4-dihydropyridines

DAG—1,2-diacylglicerol

DEKA—amino acid sequence of aspartate, glutamate, lysine, and alanine

D—domain

ENaC—epithelial Na channels

ER—endoplasmic reticulum

FDA—Food and Drug Administration

GABA—γ-aminobutyric acid

GluR—glutamate receptor channel

GPCRs—G-protein coupled receptors

5-HT_3—5-hydroxytryptamine/serotonin

IP_3—inositol 1,4,5-trisphosphate

IP_3R—inositol 1,4,5-trisphosphate receptor

K_{ir}—inwardly rectifying K^+ channel

KcsA—bacterial K^+ channel from *Streptomyces lividans*

K_V—voltage-gated/dependent K^+ channel

LQT syndrome—Long QT syndrome, which could be congenital or acquired

Na_V—voltage-gated/dependent Na^+ channel

PIP2—phosphatidylinositol 4, 5-biphosphate

PKA—cAMP-protein kinase

PLC—phospholipase C

QA—quaternary ammonium ions

RyR—ryanodine receptor

RT-PCR—reverse transcription polymerase chain reaction

SK—small conductance Ca^{2+}-activated K^+ channel

SR—sacroplasmic reticulum

STOCs—spontaneous transient outward currents mediated via BK channels

STX—saxitoxin

SUR—sulphonylurea

TEA—tetraethylammonium

TM—transmembrane
TRP—transient receptor potential channel
TRPA—TRP ankyrin receptor subfamily
TRPC—TRP canonical receptor subfamily
TRPM—TRP melastatin receptor subfamily
TRPML—TRP mucolipin receptor subfamily
TRPN—TRP NOMPC receptor family
TRPP—TRP polycystin receptor subfamily
TRPV—TRP vanilloid receptor subfamily
TTX—tetrodotoxin
IUPHAR—International Union of Pharmacology

REFERENCES

Books

Aidley, D. J., & Stanfield, P. R. (1996). *Ion Channels: Molecules in Action.* Cambridge University Press.

Ashcroft, F. M. (2000). *Ion Channels and Disease: Channelopathies.* New York: Academic Press.

Chung, S. H., Andersen, O. S., & Krishnamurthy, V. (2006). *Biological Membrane Ion Channels: Dynamics, Structure, and Applications (Biological and Medical Physics, Biomedical Engineering).* Springer.

Hille, B. (2001). *Ionic Channels of Excitable Membranes* (3rd ed.). Massachusetts: Sinauer.

Molleman, A. (2002). *Patch Clamping: An Introductory Guide to Patch Clamp Electrophysiology.* John Wiley & Sons.

Sakmann, B., & Neher, E. (Eds.). (1995). *Single-Channel Recording* (2nd ed.). Springer.

Stockand, J. D., & Shapiro, M. S. (2006). *Ion Channels: Methods and Protocols (Methods in Molecular Biology* (1st ed.). Humana Press.

Soria, B., & Cena, V. (Eds.). (1998). *Ion Channel Pharmacology* (1st ed.). USA: Oxford University Press.

Triggle, D. J., Gopalakrishnan, M., Rampe, D., Zheng, W., Mannhold, R., Kubinyi, H., et al. (Eds.). (2006). *Voltage-Gated Ion Channels as Drug Targets.* Weinheim: Wiley-VCH.

Waltz, W., Boulton, A. A., & Baker, G. B. (Eds.). (2002). *Patch-Clamp Analysis: Advanced Techniques.* Totowa, NJ: Humana Press.

Watling, K. J. (Ed.). (2006). *The Sigma-RBI Handbook of Receptor Classification and Signal Transduction* (5th ed.). St. Louis, MO: Sigma-Aldrich Group.

Monographs, Review Articles, and Original Papers

Agre, P. (2004). Nobel Lecture. Aquaporin water channels. *Bioscience Reports, 24*(3), 127–163.

Agre, P. (2006). The aquaporin water channels. *Proceedings of the American Thoracic Society, 3*(1), 5–13.

Ashcroft, F. M. (2006). From molecule to malady. *Nature, 440,* 440–447.

Benarroch, E. E. (2007). Sodium channels and pain. *Neurology, 68*(3), 233–236.

Bernstein, J. (1902). Untersuchungen zur Thermodynamik der bioelektrischen ströme I. *Pflügers Archiv fur die Gesamte Physiologie des Menschen und der Tiere, 92,* 521–563.

Brayden, J. E., & Nelson, M. T. (1992). Regulation of arterial tone by activation of calcium-dependent potassium channels. *Science, 256*(5056), 532–535.

Brenner, R., Pérez, G. J., Bonev, A. D., Eckman, D. M., Kosek, J. C., Wiler, S. W., et al. (2000). Vasoregulation by the β1 subunit of the calcium-activated potassium (BK) channel. *Nature, 407,* 870–877.

Brown, S. M., Bentcheva-Petkova, L. M., Lei, L., Kellett, W. F., Meredith, A., Aldrich, R. W., Nelson, M. T., & Petkov, G. V. (2008). Large conductance Ca^{2+}-activated K^+ channel mediates smooth muscle relaxation in response to beta-adrenergic receptor stimulation in mouse urinary bladder. *American Journal of Physiology. Renal Physiology, 295*(4), F1149–F1157.

Cannell, M. B., Cheng, H., & Lederer, W. J. (1995). The control of calcium release in heart muscle. *Science, 19, 268*(5213), 1045–1049.

Catterall, W. A. (2001). Structural biology: A 3D view of sodium channels. *Nature, 409,* 988–991.

Catterall, W. A., Cestele, S., Yarov-Yarovoy, V., Yu, F. H., Konoki, K., & Scheuer, T. (2007). Voltage-gated ion channels and gating modifier toxins. *Toxicon: Official Journal of the International Society on Toxinology, 49*(2), 124–141.

Catterall, W. A., Goldin, A. L., & Waxman, S. G. (2005). International Union of Pharmacology. XLVII. Nomenclature and structure-function relationships of voltage-gated sodium channels. *Pharmacological Reviews, 57*(4), 397–409.

Catterall, W. A., Perez-Reyes, E., Snutch, T. P., & Striessnig, J. (2005). International Union of Pharmacology. XLVIII. Nomenclature and structure-function relationships of voltage-gated calcium channels. *Pharmacological Reviews, 57*(4), 411–425.

Chen, M. Y., & Petkov, G. V. (2009). Identification of large conductance Ca^{2+}-activated K^+ channel accessory β4 subunit in rat and mouse urinary bladder smooth muscle. *Journal of Urology,* 182.

Desai, B. N., & Clapham, D. E. (2005). TRP channels and mice deficient in TRP channels. *Pflügers Archiv: European Journal of Physiology, 451*(1), 11–18.

Doyle, D. A., Cabral, J. M., Pfuetzner, R. A., Kuo, A., Gulbis, J. M., Cohen, S. L., et al. (1998). The structure of the potassium channel: molecular basis K+ conduction and selectivity. *Science, 280* (5360), 69–77.

Filosa, J. A., Bonev, A. D., Straub, S. V., Meredith, A. L., Wilkerson, M. K., Aldrich, R. W., et al. (2006). Local potassium signaling couples neuronal activity to vasodilation in the brain. *Nature Neuroscience, 9*(11), 1397–1403.

Gadsby, D. C., Vergani, P., & Csanády, L. (2006). The ABC protein turned chloride channel whose failure causes cystic fibrosis. *Nature, 440,* 477–483.

Gutman, G. A., Chandy, K. G., Grissmer, S., Lazdunski, M., McKinnon, D., Pardo, L. A. et al. (2005). International Union of Pharmacology. LIII. Nomenclature and molecular relationships of voltage-gated potassium channels. *Pharmacological Reviews, 57*(4), 473–508.

Hamill, O. P., Marty, A., Neher, E., Sakmann, B., & Sigworth, F. J. (1981). Improved patch-clamp techniques for high-resolution current recording from cells and cell-free membrane patches. *Pflügers Archiv: European Journal of Physiology, 391*(2), 85–100.

Hardie, R. C. (2007). TRP channels and lipids: from Drosophila to mammalian physiology. *The Journal of Physiology, 578*(Pt 1), 9–24.

Herrera, G. M., Pozo, M. J., Zvara, P., Petkov, G. V., Bond, C. T., Adelman, J. P., et al. (2003). Urinary bladder instability induced by selective suppression of the murine small conductance calcium-activated potassium (SK3) channel. *The Journal of Physiology, 551,* 893–903.

Hristov, K. L., Cui, X. L., Brown, S. M., Lei, L., Kellett, W. F., & Petkov, G. V. (2008). Stimulation of β3-adrenoceptors relaxes rat urinary bladder smooth muscle via activation of the large conductance Ca^{2+}-activated K^+ (BK) channels. *American Journal of Physiology. Cell Physiology, 295*(5), C1344–C1353.

Huxley, A. (2002). From overshoot to voltage clamp. *Trends in Neurosciences, 25,* 553–558.

Huxley, A. L., & Huxley, A. F. (1952). A quantitative description of membrane current and its application to conduction and excitation in nerve. *The Journal of Physiology, 117*(4), 500–544.

Huxley, A. L., & Huxley, A. F. (1939). Action potentials recorded from inside a nerve fibre. *Nature, 144,* 710–711.

Jaggar, J. H., Porter, V. A., Lederer, W. J., & Nelson, M. T. (2000). Calcium sparks in smooth muscle. *The American Journal of Physiology, 278,* C235–C256.

Ledoux, J., Werner, M. E., Brayden, J. E., & Nelson, M. T. (2006). Calcium-activated potassium channels and the regulation of vascular tone. *Physiology (Bethesda), 21,* 69–78.

Meredith, A. L., Thorneloe, K. S., Werner, M. E., Nelson, M. T., & Aldrich, R. W. (2004). Overactive bladder and incontinence in the absence of the BK large conductance Ca^{2+}-activated K^+ channel. *The Journal of Biological Chemistry, 279,* 36746–36752.

Minke, B. (2006). TRP channels and Ca^{2+} signaling. *Cell Calcium, 40*(3), 261–275.

Narahashi, T., Moore, J. W., & Scott, W. R. (1964). Tetrodotoxin blockage of sodium conductance increase in lobster giant axons. *The Journal of General Physiology, 47*, 965–974.

Nelson, M. T., Cheng, H., Rubart, M., Santana, L. F., Bonev, A. D., Knot, H. J., et al. (1995). Relaxation of arterial smooth muscle by calcium sparks. *Science, 270*, 633–637.

Nilius, B., Voets, T., & Peters, J. (2007). TRP channels in disease. *Science STKE, 295*, re8.

O'Rourke, B. (2007). Mitochondrial Ion Channels. *Annual Review of Physiology, 69*, 19–49.

Pedersen, S. F., Owsianik, G., & Nilius, B. (2005). TRP channels: an overview. *Cell Calcium, 38*(3-4), 233–252.

Perez, G. J., Bonev, A. D., Patlak, J. B., & Nelson, M. T. (1999). Functional coupling of ryanodine receptors to KCa channels in smooth muscle cells from rat cerebral arteries. *The Journal of General Physiology, 113*(2), 229–238.

Petkov, G. V., Balemba, O. B., Nelson, M. T., & Mawe, G. M. (2005). Identification of a spontaneously active, Na+-permeable channel in guinea pig gallbladder smooth muscle. *American Journal of Physiology. Gastrointestinal and Liver Physiology, 289*(3), G501–G507.

Petkov, G. V., Bonev, A. D., Heppner, T. J., Brenner, R., Aldrich, R. W., & Nelson, M. T. (2001a). β1-subunit of the Ca2+-activated K+ channel regulates contractile activity of mouse urinary bladder smooth muscle. *The Journal of Physiology, 537*, 443–452.

Petkov, G. V., Fusi, F., Saponara, S., Gagov, H. S., Sgaragli, G., & Boev, K. K. (2001b). Characterization of plasma membrane calcium currents in freshly isolated smooth muscle cells from rat tail main artery. *Acta Physiologica Scandinavia, 173*(3), 257–265.

Petkov, G. V., Heppner, T. J., Bonev, A. D., Herrera, G. M., & Nelson, M. T. (2001c). Low levels of KATP channel activation decrease excitability and contractility of urinary bladder. *American Journal of Physiology. Regulatory, Integrative and Comparative Physiology, 280*, R1427–R1433.

Petkov, G. V., & Nelson, M. T. (2005). Differential regulation of Ca2+-activated K+ (BK) channels by β-adrenoceptors in guinea pig urinary bladder smooth muscle. *American Journal of Physiology. Cell Physiology, 288*(6), C1255–C1263.

Quayle, J. M., Nelson, M. T., & Standen, N. B. (1997). ATP-sensitive and inwardly rectifying potassium channels in smooth muscle. *Physiological Reviews, 77*(4), 1165–232.

Ramsey, S., Delling, M., & Clapham, D. E. (2006). An introduction to TRP channels. *Annual Review of Physiology, 68*, 619–647.

Sato, C., Ueno, Y., Asai, K., Takahashi, K., Sato, M., Engel, A., et al. (2001). The voltage-sensitive sodium channel is a bell-shaped molecule with several cavities. *Nature, 409*, 1047–1051.

Scholz. (2002). Mechanisms of (local) anaesthetics on voltage-gated sodium and other ion channels. *British Journal of Anaesthesia, 89*, 52–61.

Taylor, M. S., Bonev, A. D., Gross, T. P., Eckman, D. M., Brayden, J. E., & Bond, C. T., et al. (2003). Altered expression of small-conductance Ca2+-activated K+ (SK3) channels modulates arterial tone and blood pressure. *Circulation Research, 93*(2), 124–131.

Thorneloe, K. S., & Nelson, M. T. (2005). Ion channels in smooth muscle: Regulators of intracellular calcium and contractility. *Canadian Journal of Physiology and Pharmacology, 83* (3), 215–242.

Szewczyk, A., Skalska, J., Glab, M., Kulawiak, B., Malinska, D., Koszela-Piotrowska, I., et al. (2006). Mitochondrial potassium channels: from pharmacology to function. *Biochimica et Biophysica Acta, 1757*(5-6), 715–720.

Valiyaveetil, F. I., Leonetti, M., Muir, T. W., & Mackinnon, R. (2006). Ion Selectivity in a Semisynthetic K+ Channel Locked in the Conductive Conformation. *Science, 314*(5801), 1004–1007.

Useful Ion Channel Related Web Sites

www.alomone.com
www.ionchannels.org
www.iuphar-db.org/iuphar-ic/index.html
www.moleculardevices.com/pdfs/Axon_Guide.pdf
http://nerve.bsd.uchicago.edu/
www.rockefeller.edu/labheads/mackinnon/mackinn-lab.php
http://depts.washington.edu/pbiopage/people_fac_page.php?fac_ID=17

Chapter

17

Targeting the Cell Cycle to Kill Cancer Cells

William R. Taylor ▪ Aaron Grabovich

OUTLINE

17.1 INTRODUCTION

Cancer cells are characterized by the ability to progress through the cell cycle under conditions where normal cells stop dividing. Also, cancer cells exhibit less fidelity in the duplication and equal segregation of cellular contents to daughter cells. This can lead to losses and gains of chromosomes or chromosomal regions resulting in deregulation of gene expression. Mammalian cells have multiple pathways that respond to DNA damage caused by environmental factors and by-products of normal metabolism. It is common for cancer cells to have defects in the pathways that respond to DNA damage, which can further disrupt the genes that encode proteins that drive cells to divide. Many standard cancer treatments impact the cell cycle by damaging DNA. Normal cells delay cell cycle progression to provide time to fix the damage. Defects in cell cycle arrest pathways that develop in cancer cells can make them more susceptible to die when DNA is damaged, although this is not universally true.

Tumors are actively dividing tissues, which renders them susceptible to drugs and treatments that cause DNA damage in specific phases of the cell cycle. Although this provides a level of tumor specificity, many host tissues contain actively proliferating cell populations and as such are damaged during cancer treatment. Additional cancer therapies target the mitotic spindle, a structure needed for chromosomes to be segregated before cells divide. These drugs do not directly cause DNA damage and are effective against a number of cancers. Spindle-targeting drugs invoke a cellular response, whose normal function is to ensure that each daughter cell receives a copy of each chromosome at division. This response normally delays the cell cycle, however the anti-spindle drugs cause a prolonged cell cycle block that ultimately leads to cell death. Knowledge of the proteins that drive cells through the cell cycle has opened up a new avenue for developing cancer treatments. These drugs target protein kinases needed for cell cycle progression and do not directly cause DNA damage. Ongoing clinical trials should uncover the potential of this new class of inhibitors to treat cancer.

One way or another, the majority of current cancer treatments involve targeting what cancer cells do best—divide. This includes traditional radiation and chemotherapies and newer agents that attack proteins involved in signaling cell division. To gauge the impact of classical therapies on cell division, one only needs to look at some of the common side effects of these drugs. Suppression of the immune system, damage to the gastrointestinal epithelium, and hair loss are the results of indeterminate damage to host tissues with rapidly growing cells. Clearly, other critical toxicities involve nonproliferative tissues such as cardiac muscle and peripheral nerves. Still many of the treatments in use today kill cancer cells not for some unique activity; normal cells must also proliferate. Instead, current treatments target a process that occurs universally in cancer cells since tumors in general are formed and maintained by new cell division.

Uncontrolled cell division, the hallmark of cancer, is relatively inefficient at inflicting morbidity. Single tumors are very often amenable to complete surgical removal. It is the metastatic spread of tumors that renders surgical removal ineffective. Successful metastatic spread of a cell to a new site requires activities that have little to do with uncontrolled proliferation. However, once at a new site, the tumor cell must divide, in order to create a secondary tumor with adverse consequences for the host. Thus, cell division is at the foundation of tumor formation at the initial site and at new secondary sites. It is for this reason that cell division provides an important target for the treatment of cancer.

17.2 THE CELL CYCLE

The cell cycle traditionally is separated into the G1, S, G2, and M phases. During G1, cells synthesize and modify proteins in preparation for DNA synthesis during S phase. With chromosomes and centrosomes duplicated during S phase, the cell arrives in G2 where additional modifications occur in preparation for mitosis. G1 is a major control point in the cell cycle. For example, when growth factors are limiting, cells exit the cycle from G1 and do not continue to divide. Cells exiting the cell cycle from G1 enter a state named G_0, where they are metabolically active, but unable to proliferate. Many of the cells in fully developed tissues reside in G_0 permanently. G_0 can be reversible with cells reentering G1 when the need arises. One of the major defects in cancer cells is that they are unable to enter G_0 under conditions where normal cells do, such as when growth factors are withdrawn. In both normal and cancer cells, G1 and G2 are major stopping points when DNA is damaged. This can allow repair before further progression through the cell cycle.

17.2.1 CDKs, Cyclins, CDKIs

Movement of cells from one phase of the cell cycle to the next is controlled by the Cyclin-dependent kinases (CDKs). There are currently 12 known CDKs although many of these enzymes are not involved in cell cycle regulation. The hallmark of a CDK is that it can be active only when bound to its cognate Cyclin subunit. The Cyclin family consists of 16 members (Cyclins A through M, Cyclin S, Cyclin T, and Cyclin Y) and there is overlap in CDK binding. For example, Cyclins D1, D2, and D3 can bind either CDK4 or CDK6; however, an active complex contains only a single CDK and a single Cyclin. The core Cyclin-CDK complexes for cell cycle progression include CDK4/6 bound to the D-type Cyclins, which controls progression through G1 and into S phase. CDK2 in complex with Cyclin E coordinates late and early S phase events, and when bound to Cyclin A is a key regulator of late S and early G2 events. CDK1 (also called CDC2) binds Cyclin A early during the G2/M transition and then to a B-type Cyclin to bring cells into and through mitosis (Figure 17.1).

In general, the levels of CDKs do not vary through the cell cycle, however the Cyclins may oscillate, and this provides a major level of regulation. Periodic expression of a specific Cyclin at a specific point in the cell cycle contributes to cell cycle regulated activation of various CDKs. For example, Cyclin B is rapidly degraded during G1 and S phase. When cells enter G2, the level of Cyclin B rises, providing the needed subunit for CDK1 to be active. This oscillation is intrinsic to the cell cycle and drives cells into mitosis once per cycle. On the other hand, the levels of D-type Cyclins are controlled in large part by signals received from outside of the cell. Extracellular growth factors induce the transcription of D Cyclins, and also accelerate the translation of the mRNA. These effects provide a link between growth factors and movement from G1 into S phase, since high levels of D-Cyclins are needed for CDK4/6 to be active. An extensive literature describes the alterations in growth factor signaling pathways in cancer. These alterations render many tumor cells independent of extracellular growth factors for cell cycle progression. In the case of the EGF receptor, ERB2, this has spawned the development of the drug Herceptin/Trastuzumab, which binds to the overexpressed ERB2 receptor in breast cancer cells and targets them for death. Similarly, the drug Imatinib/Gleevec was selected for its ability to inhibit the activity of the BCR-ABL kinase whose hyperactivation is a driving force in chronic myelogenous leukemia. Clinical successes with Herceptin and Imatinib have led to a widespread search for inhibitors of protein kinases and growth factor receptors as potential anticancer agents.

Additional layers of control impinge on the CDK/Cyclin complex. In order to be active, CDKs must be phosphorylated at a particular threonine residue. In CDK2, this activating phosphorylation occurs at T160, and in CDK1 at T161. These residues are phosphorylated by CDK-activating kinase (CAK), itself a complex of CDK7, Cyclin H, and the protein Mat1. Cyclin H is an example of a Cyclin that does not oscillate, and activates CDK7 throughout the cell cycle. CDKs are also inactivated by phosphorylation. These inhibitory phosphorylations provide an important mode of regulation when DNA is damaged. Since many chemotherapeutic agents induce DNA damage, inhibitory phosphorylation of CDKs is a common response to these drugs.

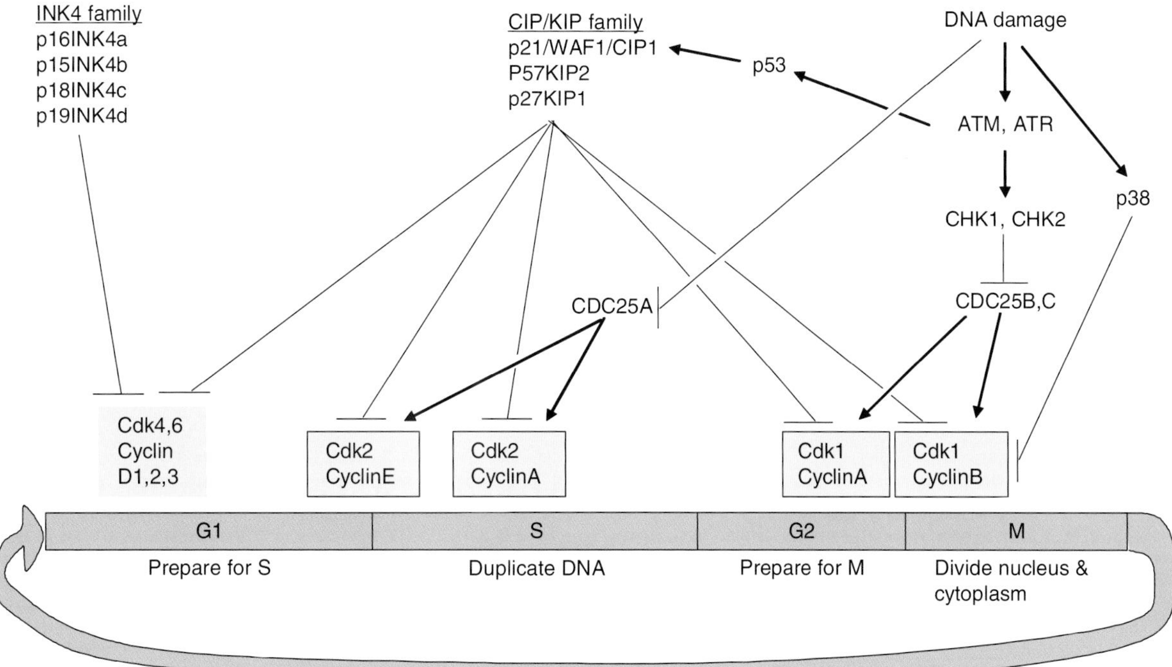

Figure 17.1 Control of cell cycle progression by CDKs, Cyclins, and CDKIs. Progression from G1 into S phase is controlled by CDK4/6 in combination with one of the D-cyclins and by CDK2 bound to Cyclin E and then Cyclin A. Progression from G2 into mitosis is controlled by CDK1 bound to Cyclin A and then Cyclin B. Proteins of the INK family inhibit CDK/6 bound to D-cyclins, whereas CIP/KIP proteins inhibit a wider range of CDKs. p53 links DNA damage to CDK inhibition through p21/WAF1/CIP1. DNA damage also inhibits CDKs by turning off its activators CDC25A, B, and C.

Inhibitory phosphorylation of CDK2 occurs primarily on Y15 and is catalyzed by the kinase Wee1. Dephosphorylation of this residue is catalyzed by the cell cycle regulated phosphatase CDC25A. Inhibitory phosphorylation of CDK1 is catalyzed by Wee1 and Myt1 kinases, which phosphorylate T14 and Y15. These phosphorylations ensure that CDK1 is turned off as Cyclin B accumulates during G2. Rapid dephosphorylation and activation of CDK1 is accomplished by the phosphatases CDC25B and CDC25C. The phosphorylation of inhibitory sites on CDK1 plays an important role in its regulation in response to genotoxic stress. When DNA is damaged, CDK1 cannot be dephosphorylated, resulting in cell cycle arrest.

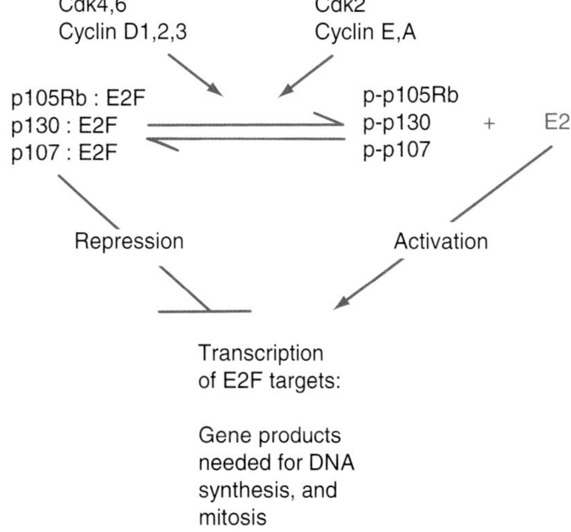

Figure 17.2 Control of transcription by Rb/E2F. CDKs phosphorylate Rb proteins releasing free E2F that binds to promoters of target genes and activates their transcription. E2F bound to Rb can still bind to promoters, however Rb causes the transcription of those same genes to be repressed.

17.2.2 RB/E2F

CDKs are needed for cell cycle progression. If CDK1 is inhibited, cells are blocked in G2; if CDK2 is inhibited, the block is in G1. One of the major substrates of the G1-S CDKs (CDK4/6, CDK2) is a family of proteins that regulate transcription. The three Rb family proteins, p107, p130, and p105Rb bind to promoters as a trimeric complex consisting of an Rb protein and a heterodimer of the proteins E2F and DP (Figure 17.2). E2F is a DNA binding protein that recognizes a specific sequence in the promoters of a number of genes. When it binds it activates the transcription of those targets. DP proteins are structurally related to E2F, and act as an obligate partner in DNA binding. E2F/DP heterodimers bind independently to E2F binding sites to activate transcription. When an Rb protein joins the complex, the heterotrimer still binds to DNA but no longer activates transcription; instead it actively silences the transcription of the target gene.

CDKs provide a major level of control over Rb/E2F complex formation by phosphorylating Rb and releasing it from the E2F/DP dimer. In general, when CDKs are active, E2F-mediated transcriptional activation predominates on target promoters. When CDKs are inactive, Rb-mediated transcriptional repression predominates. The types of genes that are under the transcriptional control of Rb/E2F are those that encode proteins that are needed for cell cycle progression. For example, the gene encoding dihydrofolate reductase, an essential enzyme involved in producing substrates required for DNA synthesis is transcriptionally upregulated by E2F. Also, the gene encoding Cdk1, required to drive cells into mitosis, is upregulated by E2F. The Rb/E2F system ensures that proteins needed for cell cycle events are present at the appropriate time and is a major mechanism by which CDKs drive cells through the cell cycle.

Many other CDK substrates must be phosphorylated to drive cells through the cell cycle. For example, CDK2 phosphorylates CDC6, protecting it from degradation. CDC6 is an essential component of the complex of proteins that associate with origins of replication and participate in the initiation of DNA replication during S phase. CDK1 phosphorylates a large number of substrates to bring about the many changes that occur in cells as they enter mitosis. For example the phosphorylation of nuclear lamins by CDK1 causes them to dissociate, which allows the nuclear membrane to disassemble during mitosis.

17.3 CELL CYCLE CHECKPOINTS

Cell cycle checkpoints originally were defined as pathways that ensure that cell cycle events occur only when previous cell cycle processes are completed successfully. Much of the groundwork for understanding cell cycle checkpoints was laid using genetically tractable systems including fission and budding yeast. The large oocytes of frogs and starfish also were exploited to make cycling extracts, which provided an innovative tool for unique biochemical experiments. These systems helped to illuminate the molecular basis of cell cycle transitions and the targets of cell cycle checkpoints.

17.3.1 G1-DNA Damage Checkpoint

There are a number of well-defined checkpoints that ultimately modulate CDK activity to ensure that cell cycle progression occurs only when previous events are completed. Some of these checkpoints are triggered by DNA damage, a by-product of many of the cancer treatments in use today. DNA damage leads to cell cycle arrest in cells from diverse organisms, and many of the proteins responsible are conserved. One of the early observations regarding the G1 checkpoint was that cells lacking the tumor suppressor protein p53 were unable to arrest in G1 when exposed to ionizing radiation. Instead, these cells were blocked in the G2 phase of the cell cycle. The p53 tumor suppressor had previously been implicated as a regulator of oncogenesis, first as an oncogene and later, in its actual role as an antioncogene (or tumor suppressor). In original experiments, mutants of p53 were unknowingly analyzed and when overexpressed they were effective dominant-negatives that eliminated wild-type p53 function.

It is now clear that p53 is a tumor suppressor of major importance. Mutational inactivation of p53 occurs in over half of all human cancers. Also, the cancer predisposition syndrome, originally described by Li and Fraumeni is due to heterozygous mutation of p53, with spontaneous loss of the other good allele occurring in cancers that arise at higher frequency and at an earlier age than the general population.

17.3.2 p21/WAF1/CIP1 and the CDKIs

The regulation of the G1/S transition by p53 involves an additional layer of CDK control, specifically involving one of the classes of CDK inhibitors (CDKIs). The CDKIs are a group of proteins that bind to the CDK/Cyclin heterodimer and inhibit the activity of the kinase. The two major families of CDKIs are the INK4 family and the CIP/KIP family (Figure 17.1). The specific targets and modes of action of these classes are distinct. The four INK4 proteins, p16INK4a, p15INK4b, p18INK4c, and p19INK4d inactivate the CDKs that drive early G1 events. These inhibitors bind to CDK4/CDK6 and block their ability to bind to D-type Cyclins. The CIP/KIP family includes p21/WAF1/CIP1, p27KIP1, and p57KIP2. These proteins bind to a wider range of CDKs, including the early G1 enzymes CDK4 and CDK6 as well as CDK2 and CDK1. CIP/KIP proteins do not disrupt Cyclin binding, but nonetheless inhibit CDK activity. An interesting variation on this theme is the fact that p21/WAF1/CIP1 can enhance assembly of CDK4/6-D-Cyclin complexes thereby functioning as an activator. Part of the inhibitory effect of the INK4 proteins is that by disrupting Cyclin binding to CDK4/6, these proteins can also displace CIP/KIP proteins already bound. These released inhibitors are then free to bind to CDK2/Cyclin complexes resulting in their inhibition as well. The fact that p16INK4a is a common target of inactivation in human cancer indicates that its role in inhibiting CDK activity is essential to prevent inappropriate progress of cells through the cell cycle.

p21/WAF1/CIP1 is a key factor in the p53-dependent cell cycle responses to stress because it is an essential downstream target of p53 activity (Figure 17.1). The function of p53 in cell cycle control and cancer progression is due to its ability to bind to DNA in a sequence-specific manner and activate transcription of genes with its target sequence in their promoters. p53 induces the transcription of many genes, several of which are essential for cell cycle control. p21/WAF1/CIP1 was one of the first two transcriptional targets of p53 identified, the other being hDM2 (described next). Without p21/WAF1/CIP1, cells have difficulty in responding properly to stimuli that induce p53, including DNA damage.

p53 activity increases in response to DNA damage and other stresses. This is due mainly to stabilization of the p53 protein as a result of inhibition of its ubiquitin-dependent degradation. In normal cells, p53 is ubiquitinated constantly and targeted for degradation by the proteasome. Adding ubiquitin to p53 is the job of hDM2, an E3 ubiquitin ligase. Not surprisingly, overexpression of hDM2 is observed in human cancer, particularly in sarcomas where high levels of the hDM2 protein keep p53 inactive and unable to respond to genotoxic insults.

A multitude of different stressors (arrest of DNA synthesis, blockade of transcription, hypoxia, DNA damage, nucleotide pool imbalance, oncogene activation) induce the activation of p53. When cells are stressed both p53 and hDM2 become phosphorylated, disrupting the interaction between the two and releasing p53 from constitutive proteasome degradation. p53 levels rise, leading to accumulation of its transcriptional targets including p21/WAF1/CIP1, which binds to and inhibits CDKs and blocks progression through the cell cycle. If the cell arrives in G1 with damaged DNA and high p21/WAF1/CIP1 it will not progress further and will be blocked in G1 until the DNA damage is repaired. If the damage can't be repaired, the G1 arrest is permanent, resembling the state of cells that exit the cell cycle due to replicative senescence.

When a cell does not have p53, which is the case for many tumor cells, the G1 arrest that normally is induced by DNA damage is severely reduced. However, there are at least two redundant pathways for G1 arrest that function in the absence of p53. One pathway leads to the rapid degradation of Cyclin D1, and the second pathway leads to rapid degradation of CDC25A. Stable G1 arrest requires p53 and without it, the next major DNA-damage-induced cell cycle block in G2 predominates.

17.3.3 S Phase Checkpoints

Another cell cycle phase under major checkpoint control is S phase. A cell in S phase can encounter various defects, including damaged DNA in the form of double strand breaks and stalled replication forks. S phase checkpoints cause a slowing of DNA replication as a result of the inhibition of the firing of late origins of replication in response to both double strand breaks and stalled replication forks. Also, checkpoints operating during S phase stabilize stalled replication forks, so that DNA synthesis can be restarted once the damage is repaired.

17.3.4 Antimetabolites and Damage During S Phase

Although many chemotherapeutic agents create strand breaks as a major form of damage, other classical drugs kill cells by inhibiting DNA synthesis. The antimetabolites hydroxyurea, methotrexate, and 5-fluorouracil target different points in nucleotide metabolism to starve cells of dNTPs required for DNA synthesis. Hydroxyurea depletes an essential iron atom from ribonucleotide reductase, the enzyme that reduces NDPs to dNDPs (which later are converted to their triphosphate forms). Methotrexate binds to and inhibits dihydrofolate reductase, an enzyme required for the synthesis of thymidine needed for DNA synthesis. 5-fluorouracil is metabolized to an inhibitor of thymidylate synthase also required for thymidine synthesis. Both methotrexate and 5-fluorouracil disrupt RNA synthesis through their effects on nucleotide metabolism. *N*-(phosphonacetyl)-L-aspartate (PALA) also disrupts pyrimidine biosynthesis, and although this drug currently is not used clinically the responses of cells to PALA *in vitro* have provided a wealth of information about the role of p53 in gene amplification and resistance to this class of drugs.

PALA effectively kills tumor cells, however resistant clones arise at a frequency of one in a thousand or less. However, PALA resistance has not been observed in normal human cells. An important determinant of whether cells can acquire resistance to PALA is the presence of p53. Inactivating p53 in normal human cells renders them permissive for PALA resistance. In many cases, cells that are resistant to killing by PALA have amplified the CAD gene, which encodes aspartate transcarbamoylase, the intracellular target of PALA. When resistant colonies are analyzed by fluorescence *in situ* hybridization, multiple large (tens of megabases) repeats of the chromosomal region containing CAD are observed. A likely scenario is that bridge-breakage-fusion cycles (BBF), initially described by Barbara McClintock, are responsible for these structures and the gene amplification. A BBF cycle can begin when telomeres of sister chromatids fuse (possibly as a result of telomere erosion). This fused chromosome can acquire bipolar attachment to the mitotic spindle and will likely break during telophase. If the break does not occur between the two homologous copies of the CAD gene, one daughter cell will inherit two CAD genes from a single chromosome. Repetition of this cycle can lead to amplification, creating hundreds of gene copies.

Important by-products of BBF cycles are double-strand DNA breaks. This DNA damage is detected early by pathways that induce p53, leading to cell cycle arrest. Cells lacking p53 will continue to replicate DNA and undergo repeated BBF cycles giving rise to amplified arrays. Investigation of PALA provides an example where gene amplification, allowed when the DNA damage response is disabled, can give rise to drug resistance. Resistance to hydroxyurea can also be overcome by amplification of its intracellular target, the R2 subunit of ribonucleotide reductase.

The short-term response of cells to antimetabolites is also controlled by p53. Cells lacking p53 die more rapidly than those with p53 function. Normal diploid fibroblasts with wild-type p53 arrest in G_0 for extended periods of time in the case of PALA. Removal of the drug allows reentry in the cell cycle. In this case, it is presumed that the imbalance of nucleotide pools is the trigger for p53 induction and cells do not necessarily enter S phase to initiate this response. In those cells that do enter S phase in the presence of PALA, p53 is still able to suppress killing by the drug, and there is evidence that this intra-S phase response is mediated by MIC1. MIC1 is a transcriptional target of p53 and a member of the TGFβ superfamily of cytokines. Adding MIC1 protein to p53-null cells is sufficient to suppress killing by PALA, indicating an important role for this protein. The effects of MIC1 on the response to other antimetabolites and its effect on drug resistance are not known and warrant further investigation.

Damage that occurs during S phase is recognized by a large group of proteins. These proteins are needed to coordinate repair, and initiate cell cycle checkpoint signals. Many of these proximal sensor/transducer proteins are also involved in responding to DNA damage at other times in the cell cycle. Before these proteins are discussed one additional major point of cell cycle arrest will be described.

17.3.5 DNA Damage G2 Checkpoint

Although DNA damage induces a slowing of DNA replication, under many conditions this response is transient and cells end up in G2 phase with damaged DNA. G2 is a major arrest point in response to damaged DNA. This response can be observed in many different types of organisms and utilizes highly conserved proteins, some of which are also utilized during the G1 and S phase response to damaged DNA.

Under normal conditions, cells arrive in G2 with abundant CDK1, but low levels of Cyclin B, which is degraded rapidly during G1 and S phases. For CDK1 to be active, it must be phosphorylated by CAK, a process that resides in the nucleus (Figure 17.3). The nuclear/cytoplasmic shuttling of the CDK/Cyclin B complex is an essential part of its regulation. Early in G2, CDK1/Cyclin B accumulates in the cytoplasm. The complex is imported into the nucleus, but is then rapidly exported. As mitosis ensues and cells enter prophase, nuclear export is turned off by phosphorylation of Cyclin B1, and the complex enters the nucleus to phosphorylate its substrates. CDK1/Cyclin B1 is also under the control of inhibitory phosphorylation. Myt1 and Wee1 phosphorylate T14 and Y15 of CDK1 to shut off the kinase (Myt1 works in the cytoplasm, Wee1 in the nucleus). Dephosphorylation is accomplished by CDC25C, which is activated abruptly at the G2/M transition. The rapid activation is aided by the phosphorylation of CDC25C by CDK1/Cyclin B, which forms a positive feedback loop. Aiding in the rapid activation of CDK1 is the protein TOME-1 (trigger of mitotic entry). TOME-1 becomes active as cells

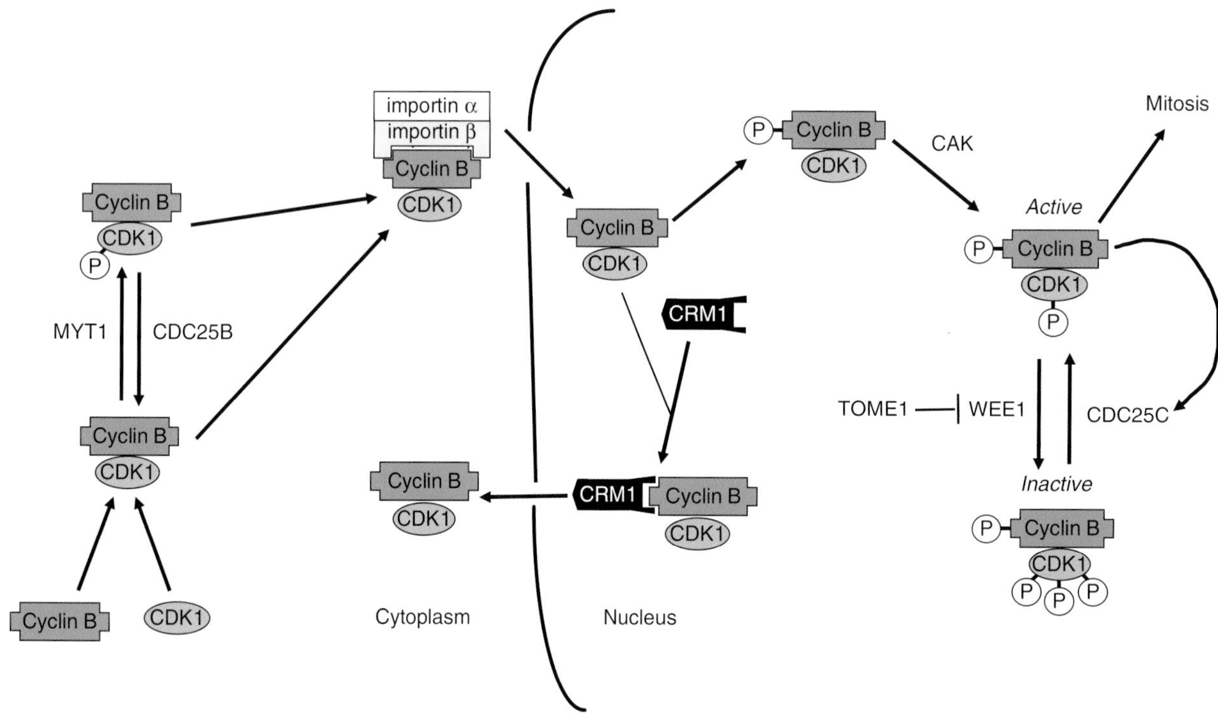

Figure 17.3 Multiple modes of regulation of CDK1/Cyclin B. Formation of the CDK1/Cyclin B complex occurs when Cyclin B levels accumulate during G2. This complex is phosphorylated at an inhibitory site by Myt1 in the cytoplasm and imported into nucleus via binding of Cyclin B to importin β. During G2, CDK1/Cyclin B is rapidly removed from the nucleus via CRM1-dependent export, however entry into the nucleus allows CAK to phosphorylate CDK1 at an activating site. At the G2/M transition, a pool of CDK1/Cyclin B is activated by CDC25B in the cytoplasm. Also, at the G2/M transition, Cyclin B becomes phosphorylated at a site that inhibits CRM1 binding, and nuclear export thereby concentrating the complex in the nucleus. CDK1/Cyclin B1 is also under the inhibitory control of Wee1 in the nucleus, which phosphorylates an inhibitory site of CDK1. Wee1 is targeted for degradation by Tome-1 when cells approach mitosis. At the right time, CDC25C becomes active, dephosphorylates nuclear CDK1 to activate it and drive cells into mitosis.

approach mitosis and functions by hastening the degradation of the CDK1 inhibitor Wee1. There is also an important role of CDC25B in the initial activation of a cytoplasmic pool of CDK1Cyclin B. This process occurs at the centrosome, presumably to kick-start the kinase.

Once the CDC25C/CDK1/Cyclin B feedback loop is initiated, the cell has no choice but to enter mitosis. If, however, the cell arrives in G2 with damaged DNA, activation of CDC25C will not occur. Under these conditions, CDC25C becomes phosphorylated and is bound to a 14-3-3 protein that will inhibit the phosphatase by stranding it in the cytoplasm. The activation of CDK1/Cyclin B1 requires active CDC25C in the nucleus, which is where CDK1 substrates reside. Binding of CDC25C to 14-3-3 depends on phosphorylation of CDC25C at serine 216, catalyzed by CHK1 and CHK2 kinases (Figure 17.1). This response keeps cells blocked in G2. However, G2 arrest is also enforced by activities under the control of p53. p53 is activated throughout the cell cycle and as described has a key role in G1 arrest. In cells arrested in G2, p53 still induces p21/WAF1/CIP1 resulting in CDK inhibition. As in G1, CDK inhibition leads to the assembly of Rb/E2F complexes that repress transcription of E2F targets. Key targets for G2 arrest are genes encoding proteins needed for cells to progress from G2 into mitosis. These included proteins needed to enter mitosis (CDK1, CYCLIN B1, CDC25C), formation of the mitotic spindle (Stathmin), attachment of chromosomes to the spindle (MCAK), and cytokinesis (ECT2, MKLP1) among others.

Therefore, the inactivation of CDC25C induces a rapid arrest in G2. However, cells arrested by this mechanism are prone to continue through the cell cycle. For example, when mouse fibroblasts lacking all three Rb family proteins are treated with doxorubicin to damage DNA they initially arrest in G2, presumably as a result of CDC25C inactivation. However, after several days cells are observed in all stages of the cell cycle and a large percentage of them die. Wild-type cells are blocked in G1 but mostly in G2. This arrest is stable and few cells die, at least during the first few days. Thus, loss of the Rb proteins reduces the strength of the cell cycle arrest and leads to cell death. Similar observations have been made in cells lacking either p53 or p21/WAF1/CIP1, suggesting that this pathway is essential to stabilize G2 arrest.

17.3.6 Proteins That Recognize and Respond to Altered DNA Structures

A large number of proteins recognize damaged DNA and transmit the signal to downstream effectors such as p53, which induces p21/WAF1/CIP1 for G1 arrest, and CHK1/CHK2, which phosphorylate CDC25C for G2 arrest. Many of the proximal damage response proteins are inactivated by mutation in cancer predisposition syndromes. One of the first of these response proteins to be described in human cells is Ataxia Telangiectasia Mutated (ATM). ATM belongs to the family of phosphatidylinositol 3-kinases (PI3K), and its closest relatives are Ataxia Telangiectasia and Rad3 Related (ATR) and DNA-PK, which also help cells respond to DNA damage. ATM and ATR directly phosphorylate p53 at residues in its N-terminus. Phosphorylation of these sites disrupts binding to hDM2, and is an important factor in the stabilization of p53 in response to DNA damage. DNA-PK associates with broken DNA by interacting with the KU antigens, which bind directly to broken DNA ends. This binding activates DNA-PK, which is essential for the process of DNA recombination in immune cells, a process that involves the controlled breakage of DNA and rejoining of ends. The mechanism by which ATM and ATR are recruited to sites of DNA damage is remarkably similar to the mode of DNA-PK recruitment (Figure 17.4).

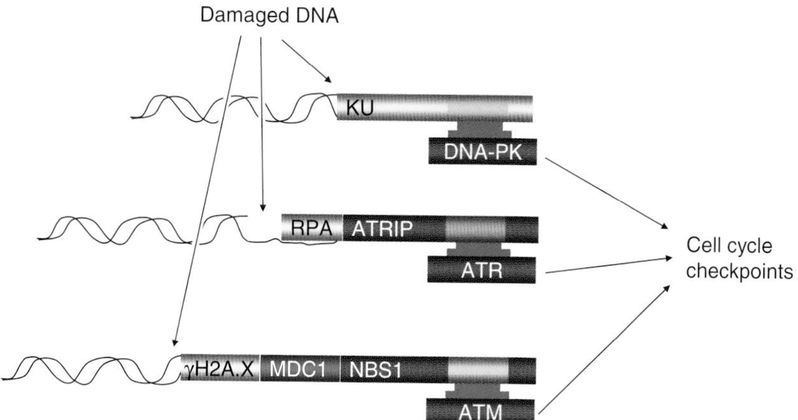

Figure 17.4 Common mode of recruitment of DNA damage response proteins to sites of damage. KU binds to broken DNA ends and recruits DNA-PK, which binds to a short stretch of amino acids in the KU protein. This stretch of amino acids has sequence similarity to a region of the ATRIP protein. This region in ATRIP binds to ATR, thus recruiting ATR to ATRIP found at sites of DNA damage. ATRIP does not bind directly to broken DNA ends but interacts with RPA associated with single-stranded DNA. The ATR-binding region of ATRIP has sequence similarity to a region of NBS1. This region in NBS1 allows it to bind to ATM, recruiting it to regions of DNA damage. NBS1 does not directly bind broken DNA but interacts with MDC1, which binds to γH2A.X, which is enriched at sites of DNA damage.

ATM is recruited to sites of DNA damage by binding to NBS1, a protein that forms a trimeric MRN complex with MRE11 and RAD50.

The MRN complex is essential for multiple responses to DNA damage. People with constitutive mutations in either NBS1 or MRE11 have been found, and they are predisposed to cancer, similar to people with ataxia telangiectasia. MRN is recruited to sites of DNA damage and the NBS1 component recruits the ATM protein. ATM binds to a short (~20 amino acid) region at the carboxyl-terminus of NBS1. This stretch of amino acids is similar to a region in the protein ATRIP, and this region in ATRIP binds to the kinase ATR. ATRIP binds to the protein RPA, which binds to single-stranded DNA created at sites of DNA damage. Furthermore, the ATR-binding region in ATRIP has amino acid similarity to a region in KU that binds to DNA-PK. Therefore, three DNA damage recognition proteins (NBS1, ATRIP, KU) share a region of similarity that allows them to bind to protein kinases (ATM, ATR, DNA-PK) that will transmit the signal to the rest of the cell. Although the regions are similar, they are different enough so that there is specificity in the interactions. For example, KU does not recruit ATM, and NBS1 does not recruit ATR.

An important and general finding is that cells lacking components of the DNA damage recognition and response process continue to progress through the cell cycle when DNA is damaged. The loss of normal checkpoint responses leads to a high degree of cellular sensitivity to DNA damage. Also, constitutive mutations that target these proteins in people confer hypersensitivity to conditions that cause DNA damage. For example, AT patients with homozygous inactivation of ATM are very sensitive to ionizing radiation. As described earlier, AT is also characterized by susceptibility to spontaneous tumors. AT heterozygotes are also radiosensitive, which presents a serious clinical challenge since these patients do not exhibit the characteristic symptoms of AT. AT heterozygotes that present with a tumor to be treated by radiation may succumb to radiation toxicity. This situation would be avoided by knowing either the genotype of the individual or the *in vitro* radiation sensitivity of cells from their tissues.

Numerous additional proteins are recruited to sites of DNA damage. One of the characteristics of chromatin in the vicinity of damaged DNA is the phosphorylation of the variant core histone H2A.X at serine 139 to create the γ-H2A.X isoform. Phosphorylation of H2A.X is catalyzed by ATM and ATR and forms a binding site for the protein MDC1. MDC1 acts as an adapter protein that recruits the MRN complex to sites of DNA damage. Other important adapter proteins include BRCA1 and p53BP1, both of which are required for optimal activation of ATM and ATR when DNA is damaged.

ATM plays a crucial role in the response to double-strand DNA breaks. However, ATR controls the cellular response to diverse forms of damage, including stalled replication forks and double-strand breaks. The order of events at these various DNA templates has not been determined; however, we now have a glimpse of some of the major components, as well as the complexity of converting a damaged DNA structure into a cellular response.

ATM activation has been linked to autophosphorylation at S1981, a reaction that disrupts inactive ATM dimers. This phosphorylation occurs when DNA is broken and even when chromatin architecture is disrupted. It has been suggested that the initial activation of ATM in response to broken DNA is due to the change in chromatin topology. There is evidence that further activation of ATM requires additional proteins that localize to specific sites of DNA damage (such as the MRN complex), indicating that the completion of the ATM activation process occurs at the site of DNA damage.

17.3.7 Claspin and RAD17 in ATR Signaling

Adapter proteins are key features of signaling in response to DNA damage and likely work by ensuring the proper localization of their binding partners, thereby allowing them to be efficiently phosphorylated by ATM and ATR, or other kinases. For example, the protein Claspin is essential for ATR to phosphorylate and activate its downstream target Chk1. Further, Claspin must be phosphorylated by ATR in order for it to help ATR phosphorylate CHK1. Claspin, phosphorylated by ATR, binds directly to CHK1, and this interaction is required for ATR to phosphorylate CHK1. Activation of CHK1 by ATR also requires the proteins RAD17, RAD1, HUS1, and RAD9. RAD1, HUS1, and RAD9 to form the trimeric "9-1-1" complex, a ring-shaped clamp that encompasses and slides along the DNA helix at sites of damage. This sliding clamp exhibits structural similarities to the PCNA sliding clamp that functions at replication forks. The 9-1-1 clamp appears to be loaded onto the DNA at sites of damage by RAD17 in association with RFC subunits. There is evidence that the requirement for RAD17 in activating CHK1 involves Claspin. RAD17 is phosphorylated by ATR, which allows RAD17 to bind to Claspin. When wild-type RAD17 in human cells is replaced by a mutant that cannot be phosphorylated, Claspin no longer binds, and there is a defect in the phosphorylation of CHK1. These cells are killed much more easily with hydroxyurea, likely due to a role for CHK1 function in stabilizing stalled replication forks. Interestingly, although RAD17-null cells are unable to arrest in G2 in response to DNA damage, the cells rescued with the nonphosphorylatable RAD17 are able to arrest.

RAD17 does not appear to be involved in ATM-dependent signaling. This suggests that depending on the specific downstream effectors (and depending on the checkpoint), RAD17 may coordinate ATR-dependent phosphorylation events via different modes. When the signal is stalled replication forks and the outcome is stable S phase arrest, phosphorylated RAD17 recruits Claspin to aid in downstream signal generation. When the outcome is G2 arrest in response to DNA damage, Claspin binding to RAD17 appears to be less important.

Experiments with Xenopus extracts have addressed the roles of the adapter protein BRCA1 and Claspin in the response to double-strand breaks. When Oocyte extracts are supplemented with sperm DNA, it is replicated. Stalling replication forks with the DNA polymerase inhibitor aphidicolin causes both Claspin and Chk1 to become phosphorylated. Immune depletion of Claspin or ATR abolishes CHK1 phosphorylation. Interestingly, cleaving the sperm DNA with the restriction enzyme EcoR1 before adding it to the extract also induces the phosphorylation of CHK1 and Claspin. Immune depletion indicated that CHK1 phosphorylation was catalyzed by ATR and not ATM. CHK1 phosphorylation is partially abrogated when Claspin is depleted, indicating a role for Claspin in the response to double-strand breaks. Also, depleting BRCA1 partially abrogates CHK1 phosphorylation in response to double-strand breaks and removing both Claspin and BRCA1 eliminates CHK1 phosphorylation. These experiments suggest that Claspin and BRCA1 work in parallel to allow ATR to phosphorylate CHK1 in response to double-strand breaks.

If wild-type Claspin is replaced with a mutant that cannot be phosphorylated at either T817 or S819, the phosphorylation of CHK1 in response to double-strand breaks induced by EcoR1 is inhibited. However, phosphorylation at these sites was not required for CHK1 to be phosphorylated in response to stalled replication forks (i.e., aphidicolin). Antibodies recognizing Claspin phosphorylated at S819 indicated that this site is phosphorylated in the extract in response to broken DNA (i.e., EcoR1) in an ATR-dependent manner. Therefore, similar to RAD17, the phosphorylation of Claspin appears to be required for it to send certain signals but not others. How these signals are differentiated are not known but may involve additional adapter proteins that allow CHK1 to be properly localized. ATR itself does not appear to show an increase in specific activity in response to the various stresses that it responds to. Therefore, specific localization to the vicinity of its substrates is likely to be the key to understanding how this protein signals.

ATR is needed for cell cycle arrest when DNA is damaged by various mechanisms, including ultraviolet radiation, ionizing radiation, alkylating agents, and nucleotide deprivation. These conditions create damaged DNA with very different chemical composition. One way that these different types of damage are converted into a coherent signal is through the stalling of replication forks. Exposure of cells to either ultraviolet radiation or the alkylating agent cisplatin blocked ongoing DNA synthesis. However, the stoppage of DNA synthesis by DNA polymerase was uncoupled from the unwinding of the DNA helix by MCM helicase proteins in front of the replication fork (a prerequisite for DNA synthesis). However, without the concomitant advance of DNA polymerase, long stretches of single-stranded DNA were formed, which became coated by the single-stranded binding protein RPA. Lowering the levels of RPA using siRNA inhibited ATR-dependent signaling, indicating that single-stranded DNA coated with RPA is an important trigger to activate ATR-dependent pathways. RPA is needed for RAD17 to load the 9-1-1 complex, providing a potential link between single-stranded DNA created at stalled replication forks and ATR signaling.

17.3.8 IRIF, Microfoci, and Flanking Chromatin

Various repair and response proteins concentrate at small subnuclear spots after DNA damage. These irradiation induced foci (IRIF) can be detected by immunofluorescence using antibodies to the specific repair/response protein, indicating that the binding of these proteins to sites of DNA damage is likely not stochiometric. Instead, many (likely thousands) of the individual protein molecules accumulate at these sites to facilitate signaling and repair. Careful examination of IRIF has suggested that the spatial organization of different repair and response proteins is diverse and complicated. By using laser microirradiation coupled with BrdU substituted DNA, single- and double-strand DNA breaks were created in small regions in a defined nuclear volume. This approach has facilitated a high degree of resolution of IRIF and microfoci within them. Within the microfoci were found single-stranded DNA, RPA (which binds ssDNA), proteins involved in homologous recombination repair (RAD51, RAD52, BRCA2, and FANCD2), and the signaling proteins ATRIP and ATR (Figure 17.5).

Spreading farther out from the microfoci was a region defined by the presence of γH2A.X, the so-called IRIF. In this region was found the signaling kinase ATM, the adapters MDC1, 53BP1, and BRCA1, as well as components of the MRN complex. MDC1 is known to bind directly to γH2A.X and NBS1, thereby acting as a bridge to bring the MRN complex to regions of chromatin containing γH2A.X. In turn, NBS1 binds directly to ATM, explaining the localization of ATM to regions of chromatin with γH2A.X. Suppressing H2A.X expression with siRNA resulted in the localization of both NBS1 and BRCA1 to the ssDNA containing microfoci. Other adapters (53BP1, MDC1) appeared to be restricted to the chromatin flanking the site of damage (i.e., the γH2A.X-stained regions). Also, microfoci were found predominantly in cells in either S or G2, and not during G1, consistent with recent work indicating that it is during these cell cycle phases that double-strand breaks are converted to large single-stranded regions, presumably as part of the repair process. Other key proteins required to send various checkpoint signals (for example, p53, Chk1, Chk2) do not concentrate in either microfoci or the chromatin flanking the damage. These proteins likely spend only enough time at these damaged regions to become phosphorylated and activated, and then diffuse to regions of the cell where they are needed to induce cell cycle arrest (Figure 17.5). DNA-PK was concentrated at irradiated sites in the nucleus but only after massive damage, which may reflect a more subtle mode of activation of this kinase that does not affect its local concentration in response to lower levels of damage.

17.3.9 Cell Cycle Responses to Cancer Therapies That Damage DNA

Any chemotherapeutic agent that damages DNA will invariably induce p53 activity leading to cell cycle arrest. Exactly where the cell arrests depends heavily

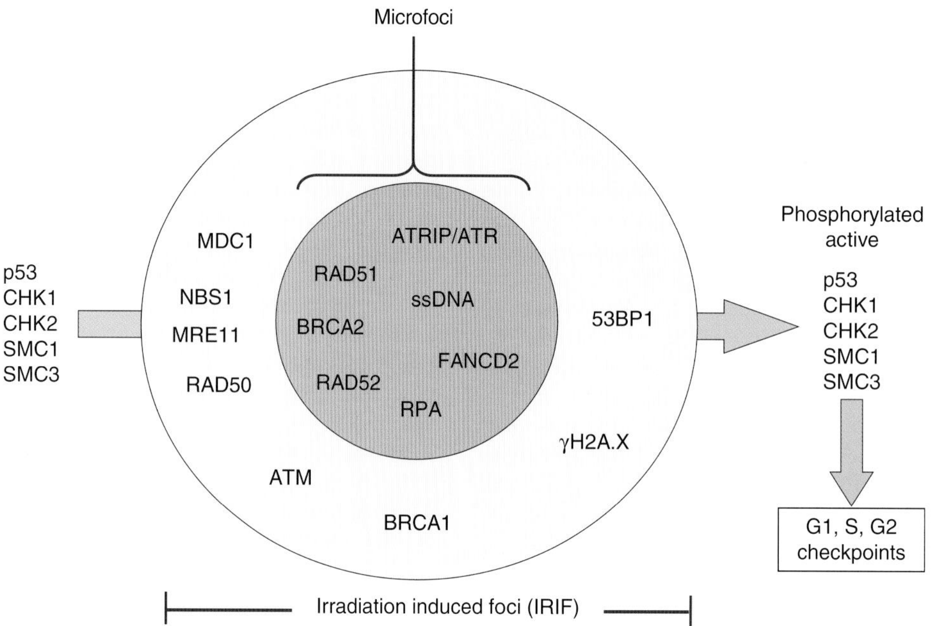

Figure 17.5 Recruitment of recognition/repair/response proteins to sites of DNA damage. Sites of DNA damage are characterized by microfoci, characterized by the presence of single-stranded DNA (ssDNA), ssDNA-binding protein RPA, and the ATRIP/ATR signaling kinase along with proteins involved in DNA repair such as RAD51. Spreading out from the microfoci is a larger region referred to as an irradiation induced foci (IRIF). IRIFs are characterized by the presence of H2A.X phosphorylated on serine 139 (the so-called γH2A.X isoform), the MRN complex, and the ATM kinase. Other damage response proteins (p53, CHK1, CHK2, SMC1, SMC3) travel to and from the sites of damage. While at the sites of damage, these proteins are phosphorylated and activated, after which they travel to other parts of the cell to activate the G1 (p53), S (SMC1, SMC3), and G2 (CHK1, CHK2) checkpoints. Overlap in the checkpoint pathways exist to allow p53 to stabilize S phase arrest under some conditions (pyrimidine depletion) and G2 arrest during prolonged damage.

on where the damage is incurred. For example, camptothecin creates DNA damage predominantly during S phase since it inhibits topoisomerase I, an enzyme needed to relax DNA as it is replicated. Camptothecin is an example of a topoisomerase poison that freezes the enzyme at a state in its catalytic cycle after it has created a single DNA nick (but before it is resealed). Camptothecin slows progression through S phase due to a checkpoint operating during S phase (see later). Cells that complete S phase and enter G2 with damaged DNA will arrest in G2 due to the DNA-damage G2 checkpoint. Ionizing radiation damages DNA independently of cell cycle position and since mammalian cells spend most of their time in G1, that is where most of them will encounter the damage. Therefore, in the presence of a normal p53 response, ionizing radiation imposes a strong G1 arrest in a population of mammalian cells. Bleomycin, commonly used in cancer therapy regimes, mimics the effects of ionizing radiation by creating double-strand DNA breaks.

One of the major targets of chemotherapy is topoisomerase II, an enzyme that like topoisomerase I, relaxes torsional strain in DNA. Topoisomerase II is a major component of the mitotic chromosome scaffold, and plays an important role in decatenating DNA during chromosome condensation at mitosis. Topoisomerase II is also active during S phase and is postulated to decatenate DNA behind the replication fork. As part of its mechanism of action, Topoisomerase II creates a double-strand DNA break, remaining covalently linked to both broken ends. Rotation of the two ends can relieve torsional strain in the DNA and allow decatenation. The end of the catalytic cycle involves sealing of the two broken ends by Topoisomerase II, an activity that has been exploited in recombinant DNA cloning reactions, replacing the need for DNA ligase. Most Topoisomerase II inhibitors in clinical use trap the enzyme at a stage in its catalytic cycle after the DNA breakage step, but before resealing. Etoposide and doxorubicin have this effect and lead to the creation of a large number of lesions in which broken DNA is covalently attached to topoisomerase II. These breaks can occur whenever Topoisomerase II is active. Cells that complete mitosis in the presence of these drugs arrive in G1 with broken DNA that can trigger a G1 arrest. However, many cells become arrested in G2 due to DNA breakage during S phase and G2.

Topoisomerase II poisons slow down progression through S phase via specific checkpoint responses. The complex of topoisomerase II linked to DNA in the presence of etoposide appears to induce unique signals different from a simple double-strand break. For example, etoposide disrupts the location of DNA ligase I and PCNA during S phase. During an unperturbed S phase, these two proteins localize to replication factories, specific regions of the nucleus that are visualized as subnuclear puncta. In response to etoposide, DNA ligase I and PCNA are localized heterogeneously in the nucleus. This disruption of replication factories requires ATR and NBS1. Furthermore, etoposide does not appear to immediately stop replication fork progression, however single-stranded DNA was observed at regions of the genome that were being duplicated at the time that etoposide was added. One possibility is that although DNA synthesis can continue immediately after adding etoposide, eventually replication forks slow down or stall. This would create a condition where uncoupling of helicases and DNA polymerase could generate the single-stranded DNA observed. Disruption of replication factories was not observed when DNA was damaged with bleomycin. Therefore, the topoisomerse-DNA covalent complex appears to disrupt DNA replication, leading to the creation of single-stranded DNA that is likely the signal to activate ATR and NBS1.

The DNA damage created by Topoisomerase II poisons invokes the highly conserved G2 checkpoint machinery (ATM/ATR-CHK1/2-CDC25C). However, a different class of Topoisomerase II inhibitors suggests that additional signals cooperate to cause cell cycle arrest. Catalytic inhibitors of Topoisomerase II (as opposed to poisons) inhibit the enzyme at a stage of its catalytic cycle where DNA is not broken. For example, some can inhibit binding of Topoisomerase II to DNA altogether, and others block the release of the enzyme from DNA after it has resealed the break. Exposure to these drugs induces a G2 arrest that has been attributed to a "decatenation checkpoint" that is proposed to sense when DNA has not been properly decatenated. This condition induces an arrest that can be overcome by exposure to inhibitors of ATM and ATR, indicating that there is overlap in the signaling pathways that are activated by DNA damage. Catalytic inhibitors of Topoisomerase II induce the phosphorylation of H2A.X similar to the effect of DNA damaging agents and consistent with their ability to activate ATR, an enzyme capable of phosphorylating this histone. In addition, catalytic inhibitors activate the p38 stress activated kinase, which contributes to G2 arrest. p38 is known to phosphorylate and inactivate the CDK1 activators CDC25B and CDC25C.

17.3.10 Spindle Checkpoint

If a cell enters mitosis without DNA damage another major checkpoint operates during M phase to ensure that chromosomes are properly segregated. This spindle assembly checkpoint (SAC) keeps cells in mitosis until all chromosomes have acquired a bipolar attachment to the spindle. The process of bipolar attachment starts in pro-metaphase, usually with the attachment of a single kinetochore on a sister chromatid to microtubules emanating from a single spindle pole. This monotelic attachment persists until the unattached kinetochore is captured by microtubules from the opposite spindle pole (amphitelic attachment). During this stage of mitosis, chromosomes are seen to oscillate to and from the spindle pole at which they are attached. Occasionally, both kinetochores will be captured by microtubules emanating from the same spindle pole to cause a syntelic attachment. Monotelic and syntelic attachments activate the SAC and delay exit from mitosis until these are resolved into amphitelic attachments (Figure 17.6).

There appears to be two main features at the kinetochore/spindle interface that can indicate a problem with proper chromosome attachment. First, kinetochores that are not occupied by microtubules can send a signal to activate the SAC and block further movement through mitosis. Second, chromosomes that are not under tension at the metaphase plate can signal to activate the SAC (Figure 17.6). The situation is complicated by the fact that tension appears to stabilize kinetochore/microtubule attachments. Some of the biochemical events that indicate the state of the kinetochore are being discovered. For example, 3F3/2 refers to an antibody that recognizes several proteins only when they are phosphorylated during mitosis. The 3F3/2 epitope can be generated by phosphorylation of specific proteins by the kinase PLK1, a protein that is active during mitosis and required for progression through this stage of the cell cycle. Immunofluorescence has indicated that the 3F3/2 epitope is sensitive to tension at the kinetochore. Exposing cells to taxol, a drug that stabilizes microtubules, allows kinetochores to attach to microtubules, but disrupts tension. Kinetochores in taxol-treated cells stain highly for the 3F3/2 epitope. Also, artificially applying tension to mono-attached kinetochores suppresses 3F3/2 staining.

Mad2 is one of the major targets of the events taking place at the kinetochore. Mad2 can be found at unattached kinetochores, and is able to diffuse away from the kinetochore presumably to carry the checkpoint signal to other places in the cell. If spindle pole separation is inhibited, cells enter mitosis with a mitotic spindle with one spindle pole. Syntelic attachments that occur under these conditions give rise to kinetochores with high levels of Mad2 staining. This suggests that tension may also trigger activation of Mad2 to engage the spindle checkpoint. An interesting variation occurs with merotelic attachments that occur early during mitosis. Merotelic attachments allow some tension to develop, as a single kinetochore is pulled simultaneously to both poles. Consistent with this is the absence of significant 3F3/2 staining on kinetochores participating in merotelic attachments. However, despite having mis-attached kinetochore, merotelic attachments do not appear to activate the spindle checkpoint (Figure 17.6). Unless these attachments are corrected, the sister chromatids of the improperly attached chromosome might not segregate from each other, leading to a loss or gain of a chromosome upon mitotic exit. An important surveillance system destabilizes these merotelic attachments and involves the recruitment of Aurora B kinase to kinetochores with this type of attachment. As described next,

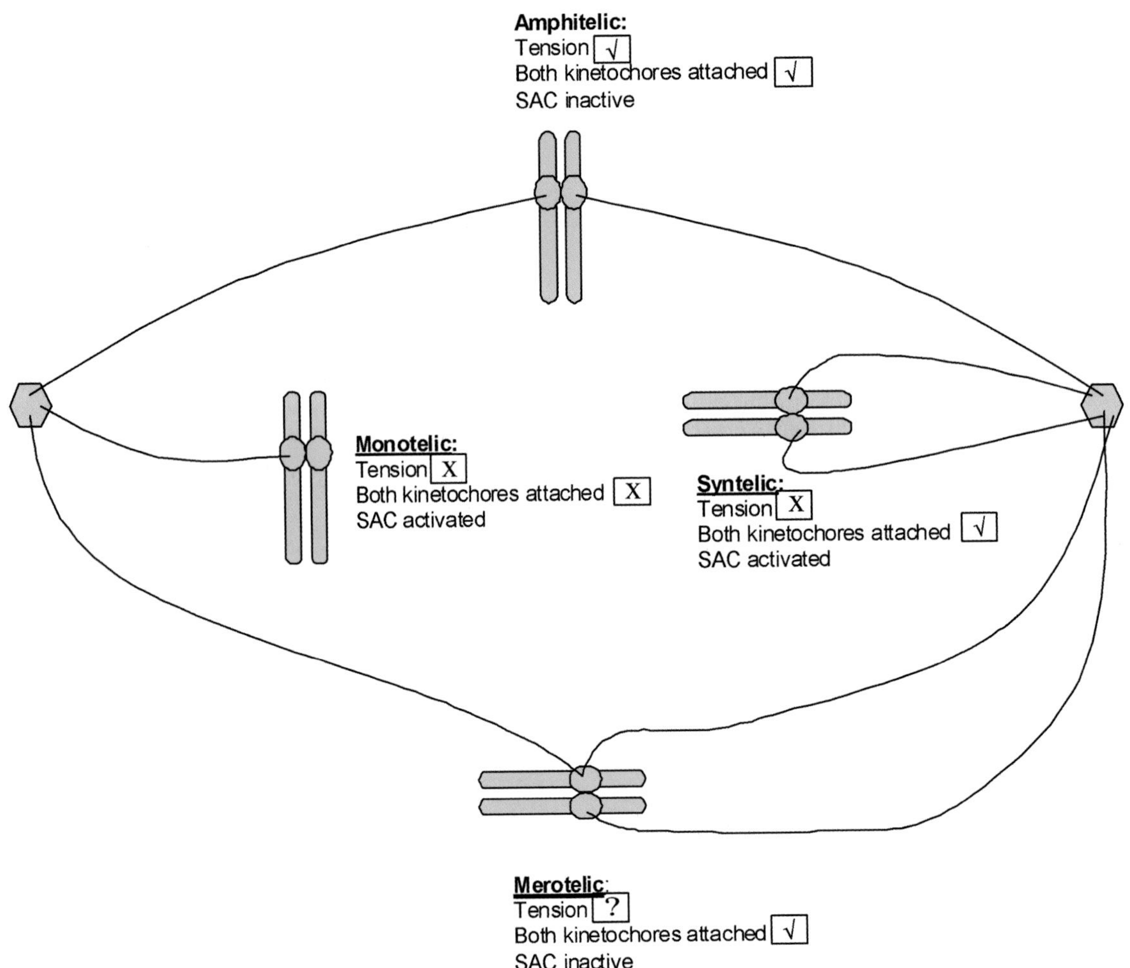

Figure 17.6 Attachment of kinetochores to the spindle. During prometaphase, kinetochores on chromosomes capture microtubules emanating from the spindle poles. Several types of attachments are possible, however only amphitelic (i.e., bipolar) attachment is compatible with segregation of chromosomes to opposite poles when anaphase begins. Monotelic and syntelic attachments trigger the spindle assembly checkpoint to give more time for them to be converted to amphitelic attachments. Merotelic attachments do not trigger the spindle assembly checkpoint but are corrected by a mechanism that requires Aurora B kinase.

Aurora B plays multiple roles in mitosis and is currently under investigation as a target for the development of novel anticancer drugs.

The ultimate job of the SAC is to ensure that cells enter anaphase only after all chromosomes have acquired a bipolar (i.e., amphitelic) attachment to the spindle. As described earlier, the checkpoint signal is initiated at kinetochores that either are not attached to the spindle or display a loss of tension. The kinetochore is composed of many specific proteins that play two crucial roles: (1) coordinate attachment to microtubules, and (2) send signals when attachments are incorrect. Kinetochores are assembled by a complicated process at the centromere, a specific region of the chromosome characterized by the presence of nucleotide repeats. Thus, it is the DNA sequence that ultimately determines where the kinetochore will assemble. Centromeric chromatin is also characterized by the presence of a variant histone, CENP-A, which takes the place of histone H3 in the nucleosome core. Kinetochores contain a number of microtubule-binding proteins, including those that regulate microtubule polymerization (for example, MCAK, CLASP1) and those that function as microtubule motors (for example, Kif4A). The oscillation of chromosomes during microtubule capture is dependent on the dynamic assembly and disassembly of the microtubule end to which the kinetochore is attached. There is evidence that stable attachments of kinetochores to microtubules do not occur via the end, but via the side of the microtubule. This implies that the connection must slide along the microtubule as it shrinks and grows. This sliding attachment appears to be mediated by microtubule motors that have the ability to bind to microtubules and at the same time translocate along the microtubule (Figure 17.7).

In addition to the constitutive components of the kinetochore are the proteins involved in signaling a troubled connection to the spindle. These include the protein Zwint1, which interacts with several of the

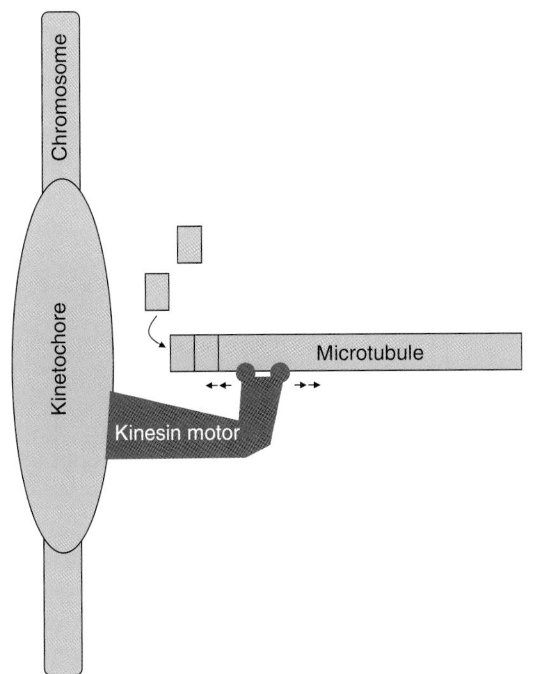

Figure 17.7 Kinesins at the kinetochore attach to the lateral surface of microtubules. Kinetochores attach to the plus ends of microtubules at which there is constant exchange for tubulin monomers. This exchange leads to growth and shrinkage. Attachment is maintained by kinesins that bind to the side of the microtubule, not the unstable end.

constitutive kinetochore proteins including NDC80, a protein that does not appear to interact with microtubules but is important in kinetochore structure. Zwint1 binds to a trimeric complex composed of the proteins ZW10, ROD1, and ZWILCH. This trimeric complex is required to communicate the presence of improper kinetochore attachment to MAD2 and MAD1. Thus, when the levels of ZW10 are suppressed using siRNA, there is a reduction in the association of MAD1 and MAD2 with kinetochores.

At unattached kinetochores, MAD1 and MAD2 engage in an intriguing reaction that ultimately activates MAD2 to carry the signal away from the kinetochore. MAD2 exists in two conformations, an open conformation (OMAD2) and a closed conformation (CMAD2). In the open conformation, a region of the MAD2 amino acid sequence is disordered, in the closed conformation this region encloses its binding partner to form a stable complex. Two important MAD2 binding partners are MAD1 and CDC20. Unattached kinetochores recruit MAD1 bound to CMAD2. This CMAD2 appears to convert cytosolic CMAD2 to OMAD2, a prerequisite for it to form a stable complex with CDC20. The CMAD2-CDC20 complex diffuses away from the unattached kinetochore to make sure the cell stays in mitosis until the kinetochore captures its microtubules and the chromosome is aligned at the metaphase plate.

Mad2/CDC20 keeps cells in mitosis by inactivating the anaphase promoting complex (APC). The APC is a ubiquitin ligase that initiates mitotic exit. It does so by degrading securin, an inhibitor of Separase, a proteolytic enzyme that degrades Cohesins, which are the proteins that hold sister chromatids together and oppose the force generated by the mitotic spindle at metaphase. This is why when cells enter anaphase, kinetochores are seen to move away from each other with their arms trailing behind. Additional proteins cooperate as part of the SAC machinery and include the kinases BUB1, BUBR1, and MPS1 as well as the BUB3 protein which forms a complex with BUBR1. Removal of any of these proteins results in cells that do not arrest in mitosis when kinetochore/spindle attachments are disrupted. BUBR1 and BUB3 have been found in a complex with MAD2/CDC20 that can inhibit the APC. The exact positions of MPS1 and BUB1 in the SAC pathway have not been determined, however, MPS1 itself is a target of the APC. This results in the inability of cells to turn the SAC back on once the APC is activated at metaphase, even if unattached kinetochores are present.

Degradation of cohesins in response to APC activation at anaphase allows the tension built up at the kinetochores to pull sister chromatids to the opposite pole of the cell. At the same time, the cell makes preparation to exit mitosis and enter a new G1. The process of mitotic exit is also initiated by the APC, which, in addition to being activated by CDC20 is activated by the protein CDH1. CDH1-APC, which forms at anaphase, ubiquitinates Cyclin B1 to extinguish CDK1 activity. The phosphatases CDC14A and B function during mitotic exit by dephosphorylating residues in proteins that were phosphorylated by CDK1 during mitotic entry. The CDC14 phosphatases are inactive during early mitosis but active during mitotic exit.

When all chromosomes achieve a bipolar attachment to the spindle, the APC is activated, sister chromatids separate, and the cell exits mitosis. The cell cycle is not over until cell division is completed to produce two daughter cells in G1. Recently, an additional checkpoint pathway has been discovered in budding yeast. This checkpoint, called the "nocut pathway," delays cytokinesis until all chromatin has cleared the cleavage plane. Mutants in Ipl1, an Aurora kinase inactivate this pathway resulting in cytokinesis before chromosome have cleared the cleavage plane. The lagging chromosomes become broken, illustrating the diversity of checkpoints that protect the integrity of the genome. Many of the proteins of the nocut pathway are present in mammalian cells, however it is not known whether the same pathway is functional.

17.3.10.1 Drugs That Target the Mitotic Spindle

The mitotic spindle has been a target of anticancer drugs for many years. The vinca alkaloids vincristine and vinblastine inhibit microtubule polymerization. These drugs trigger the spindle checkpoint, leading to a long-term arrest in mitosis. As long as the drug is present, the formation of the mitotic spindle will be blocked, and as long as the checkpoint is active, the cell will remain in mitosis. Some cells die when blocked for a long time in mitosis. Another phenomenon, termed checkpoint adaptation, may occur. This process inactivates the checkpoint arrest even though the damage persists. Adaptation of the spindle checkpoint results in cells exiting mitosis without forming a spindle or segregating their chromosomes. The cells arrive in G1 with twice the normal DNA content and twice the number of centrosomes. Centrosomes duplicated during S phase must be segregated by cytokinesis for daughter cells to maintain the normal number of 1 during G1, and 2 at mitosis. The cells that exit mitosis due to checkpoint adaptation may reenter S phase, a process called endoreduplication. If the drug is still present when the cell arrives at the next mitosis, spindle assembly will again be disrupted and the process of adaptation and endoreduplication may be repeated. Eventually these giant cells will die. Endoreduplication is suppressed by G1/S arrest if p53 and Rb pathways are intact.

As mentioned previously, many tumors have defects in these pathways, which is one way that tumor cells can be rendered susceptible to killing by agents that cause microtubule disassembly. Even in cells that do not endoreduplicate, it is difficult to recover from a single round of mitotic arrest and adaptation. For example, removal of the drug after a single round of adaptation may allow the cell to reenter the cell cycle; however, if the cell started out as diploid, it would have become tetraploid entering mitosis with four centrosomes that are able to direct the formation of spindles with three or four poles instead of two. These conditions can lead to loss of chromosomes and death. This recently was illustrated in experiments in which siRNA molecules that target either BUBR1 or MAD2 were used to inactivate the spindle checkpoint. Since the spindle checkpoint appears to operate even during unperturbed mitoses, loss of this checkpoint in normally growing cells leads to loss of chromosomes and eventual cell death. If cytokinesis is simultaneously blocked, the cells will survive longer as multinucleated giant cells. This rescue suggests that death upon inactivation of the spindle checkpoint is due to loss of chromosomes containing genes essential for survival. These chromosomes are lost when cells exit mitosis without properly segregating sister chromatids to the opposite poles of the cell.

17.3.10.2 Taxanes and the Spindle Checkpoint

The taxanes originally were extracted from the bark of the Pacific Yew tree and have found widespread use as anticancer agents. The structurally related taxanes, docetaxel and paclitaxel, bind to and stabilize polymerized microtubules. Cells that enter mitosis in the presence of paclitaxel attempt to assemble a spindle apparatus, however the inhibition of depolymerization renders this structure unable to properly position chromosomes at the metaphase plate. Therefore, although kinetochores bind to microtubules, there is insufficient tension to inactivate the SAC. Paclitaxel-treated cells become blocked in mitosis, and eventually die by the mechanisms just described. Currently, there is no consensus on whether cells with a weakened SAC are more or less susceptible to killing with drugs like paclitaxel. There is evidence that cells that exit from the mitotic arrest imposed by paclitaxel and enter G1 are destined to die by programmed cell death. Death in the postmitotic G1 was also observed when cells were treated with KSP1A, a small molecule inhibitor of KSP/EG5, a kinesin required for spindle pole separation. KSP1A causes cells to enter mitosis with monopolar spindles that trigger the SAC blocking the cell in mitosis. KSP1A represents a new class of drugs that can kill tumor cells by triggering the SAC. The potential benefit of this type of drug is that it will have its effects primarily in mitosis. In contrast, the vinca alkaloids and taxanes disrupt microtubule functions in mitosis but also in interphase. As such, these drugs can have side effects on treated patients such as damage to peripheral nerves, which results from disrupting interphase microtubule functions.

17.4 MITOTIC KINASES AS TARGETS OF NEW CHEMOTHERAPEUTICS

The orderly progression through mitosis relies on multiple cell cycle specific kinases, which are good targets for the development of small molecular inhibitors. Several of these kinases have received attention as potential targets of novel chemotherapeutics. Inhibitors of CDKs, such as flavopiridol, have been extensively investigated as anticancer agents. However, a number of clinical trials have indicated that flavopiridol may be of limited use in cancer treatment. For example, Phase II trials with patients diagnosed with mantle cell lymphoma, advanced colorectal cancer, or advanced gastric cancer showed only minimal responses. In general, the doses administered were based on data gathered from *in vitro* studies in which bovine serum was used for cell growth. It was later found that there is higher binding of flavopiridol to proteins in human serum compared to bovine serum. With this in mind, a Phase I trial was conducted with an altered dose schedule aimed at optimizing tumor cell exposure to the drug. In this trial, 43% of patients with chronic lymphocytic leukemia showed a partial response. Further research will help to determine the efficacy of flavopiridol and other CDK inhibitors as anticancer agents.

A new inhibitor of polo-like kinase 1(PLK1) named ON01910 has recently been discovered. PLK1 is one of four polo-like kinases (PLK1-4) that play multiple roles during mitosis. PLKs are essential for centrosome maturation, spindle pole separation, activation of CDC25 at the onset of mitosis, exit from mitosis, and cytokinesis. Furthermore, PLKs are commonly overexpressed in a number of different cancer tissues. Exposure of cells to ON01910 blocks progression through mitosis ultimately leading to programmed cell death. The combination of doxorubicin with ON01910 effectively blocked the ability of the human breast cancer cell line MCF7 to form tumors. The effects of this compound in humans are unknown.

The Aurora kinases are another group of enzymes that function during mitosis and have recently been investigated as cancer targets. The Aurora family consists of three proteins, Aurora A, B, and C. Aurora A appears to have a function independent of the B and C enzymes. Aurora A localizes on duplicated centrosomes from the end of S phase to the beginning of G1 and relocates to mitotic spindles during mitosis. When localized to the centrosome, Aurora A plays a role in CDK1 activation, as it phosphorylates and activates CDC25B. Aurora A has also been implicated in regulating p53 function. Aurora A phosphorylates p53 at ser-215, which inhibits p53 activity, and at 315, which enhances the ability of hDM2 to ubiquinate and inactivate the tumor suppressor protein. When Aurora A is suppressed with siRNA, p53 phosphorylation is inhibited and the levels of p53 rise, which causes G2 arrest. Both Aurora B and C function as components of the chromosomal passenger complex (CPC).

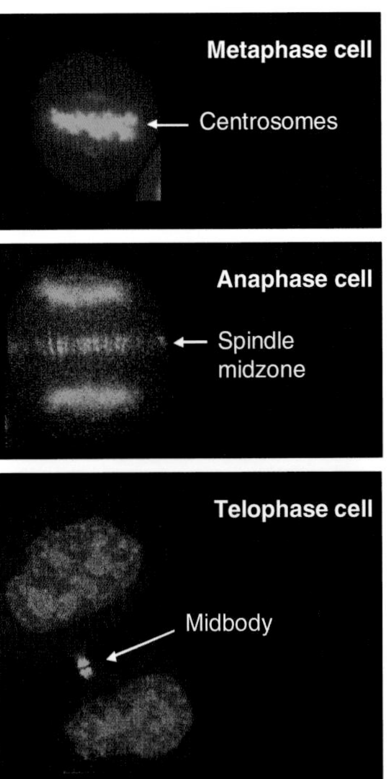

Figure 17.8 Localization of Borealin. A Hela cell clone stably transfected with a Borealin-GFP fusion was analyzed by confocal microscopy. Three cells in different stages of mitosis are shown with Borealin localized to centromeres, the spindle midzone, and the midbody.

17.4.1 The Chromosomal Passenger Complex

The chromosomal passenger complex (CPC) consists of at least four proteins, INCENP, Survivin, Borealin, and Aurora B. The best described function of this complex is to ensure that Aurora B kinase is properly localized and activated during mitosis. Activation of the Aurora B kinase occurs upon its interaction with the C-terminus of INCENP whereas the other passenger proteins ensure that Aurora B has access to its substrates at the right time. When CPC function is disrupted, mitosis cannot be properly completed and cells exhibit defects in chromosome segregation and cytokinesis.

17.4.2 CPC at the Inner Centromere

INCENP was the first component of the CPC to be identified, and an early study uncovered its dynamic subcellular localization pattern. Early in mitosis, INCENP is localized to chromosome arms after which it concentrates at the inner centromere, the central region between centromeres of the two sister chromatids. When cells entered anaphase and sister chromatids separated, INCENP was released from the inner centromere. It remained at the central plane of the cell where the metaphase chromosomes had earlier aligned even as sister chromatids retreated to their opposite poles of the cell. The positioning of INCENP at this central plane is mediated by its attachment to a structure called the spindle midzone, an overlapping group of microtubules that begin at the spindle poles, but do not attach to kinetochores. As the cleavage furrow constricts the cell membrane at the equator, it collects the midzone microtubules into a dense tubulin-rich structure called the midbody. The midbody persists until daughter cells are completely separated. INCENP is localized to the spindle midzone and the midbody.

All components of the CPC exhibit the pattern of localization observed for INCENP (Figure 17.8). The N-terminus of INCENP is important in centromere targeting but how it is achieved is not fully known. Interestingly, a small fragment of INCENP from amino acid 1 to 58, can bind to both Survivin and Borealin but not Aurora B, which instead binds to the C-terminus of INCENP. When the 1-58 fragment is expressed in cells in which endogenous INCENP is depleted by siRNA, the fragment, Borealin and Survivin all localize to the centromere. This suggests that Aurora B binding is not needed for the CPC to localize to the centromere.

Crystallographic studies have indicated that INCENP, Borealin and Survivin interact by forming a triple helical bundle (Figure 17.9). Consistent with this structure is the observation that the INCENP 1-58 fragment does not localize to the centromere when either Borealin or Survivin are targeted with siRNAs. Replacing the N-terminus of INCENP with Survivin creates a fusion protein that localizes to the centromere in the absence of Borealin. The components in the inner centromere to which Borealin and Survivin bind are not fully known, however Borealin can bind to DNA. Although this may stabilize binding of the CPC to the inner centromere, other targets must exist to specifically target the CPC to centromeric DNA.

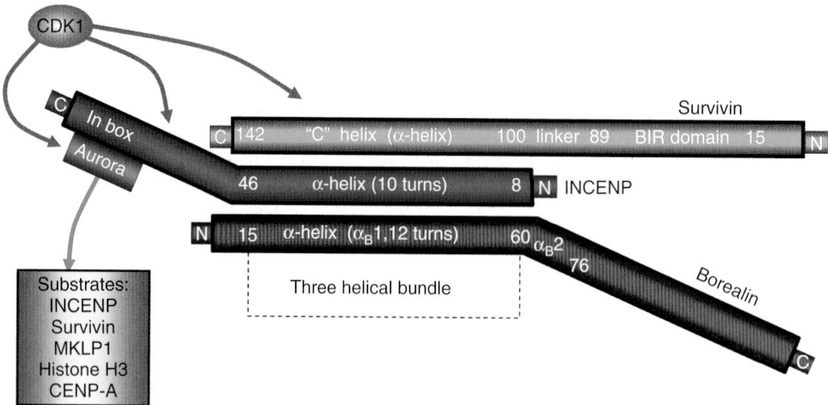

Figure 17.9 Model for the arrangement of the CPC proteins. Borealin, Survivin, and INCENP interact via a triple helical bundle. INCENP, interacting with both Borealin and Survivin recruits Aurora B, which phosphorylates Survivin, INCENP, CENP-A, Histone H3, and MKLP1. Aurora B, INCENP, and Survivin are also phosphorylated by CDK1.

17.4.3 Substrates of Aurora B at the Centromere

An important substrate of Aurora B is the histone H3. Serine 10 of histone H3 is phosphorylated in a localized manner during interphase specifically in regions of the genome encompassing actively transcribed genes. During mitosis, serine 10 of histone H3 becomes phosphorylated in a global manner: immunofluorescence with antibodies recognizing S10-phosphorylated H3 stain entire chromosomes. Aurora B appears to be the major mitotic S10 kinase. One function of the phosphorylation at S10 on H3 during mitosis is to disrupt binding of the heterochromatin protein family HP1. HP1 localizes to heterochromatin where it is involved in maintaining the transcriptionally inactive chromatin state. HP1 binds to histone H3 that is trimethylated, but not to H3 that is also phosphorylated at S10. Phosphorylation of H3 by Aurora B causes the removal of HP1 from chromatin during mitosis, which then rebinds after telophase when H3 is dephosphorylated. Inhibiting Aurora B kinase causes HP1 to persist on chromatin during mitosis, however the consequences of this are not known.

Additional substrates of Aurora B include CENP-A, a histone H3 variant found only in centromeric chromatin. This phosphorylation has been implicated in the translocation of the CPC to the spindle midzone. INCENP is also phosphorylated by Aurora B, which enhances the ability of INCENP to activate Aurora B. As described earlier, one of the important functions of Aurora B kinase is in the destabilization of inappropriate spindle-kinetochore attachments. Aurora B is also required for the SAC, however its targets in this checkpoint are not known.

17.4.4 CPC at the Spindle Midzone

When cells enter anaphase the CPC translocates from the inner centromere to the spindle midzone. The mitotic kinesin MKLP2 is required for the translocation of the CPC to the spindle midzone, possibly as a result of its binding to the phosphatase CDC14. In addition, CDK1 has been implicated in controlling the release of the CPC from the centromere. For example, persistent activation of CDK1 using a nondegradable Cyclin B1 inhibited the release of Aurora B from the centromere. Since CDC14 dephosphorylates many CDK1 targets, dephosphorylation of a component of the CPC or an associated protein may trigger the release of the CPC from the centromere.

When the CPC is released from the inner centromere, it is deposited on microtubules at the spindle midzone. Direct binding of INCENP to tubulin appears to mediate attachment of the CPC to this site. The CPC remains attached to the overlapping microtubules of the spindle midzone as the cleavage furrow progresses and the microtubules condense into the midbody. It is only when the two daughter cells separate from each other that both the midbody and the CPC are released from this location.

One important role of the CPC at the spindle midzone is to ensure that the cleavage furrow is properly positioned. Early experiments using a mechanical barrier in cultured cells indicated that the spindle midzone induces a signal that positions the cleavage furrow. Recent studies have implicated Aurora B in this positioning effect. Aurora B phosphorylates MKLP1, a kinesin that bundles microtubules to organize the spindle midzone. MKLP1 binds to the protein MgcRacGap, a GTPase activating protein, to form a binary complex called centralspindlin, which is essential for cytokinesis. Phosphorylation of MKLP1 by Aurora B kinase is required for centralspindlin to be localized to the spindle midzone. Centralspindlin recruits ECT2 to a region near the spindle midzone. ECT2 is a guanine nucleotide exchange factor (GEF) that activates the small GTPase Rho. Rho is found throughout the cell, but when it is activated by interaction with a GEF, it translocates to the membrane to activate its downstream effectors, one of which is Citron kinase. It is proposed that a high local concentration of ECT2 near the spindle midzone activates Rho, which travels to the nearest membrane surface, a ring that ultimately becomes the cleavage furrow. At the membrane, Rho activates Citron kinase, which activates myosin light chain kinase, which further activates the motor function of myosin II, leading to actin/myosin-mediated cleavage furrow formation (Figure 17.10).

17.4.5 Regulation of the CPC

Several components of the CPC are regulated by posttranslational modification (Figure 17.9). INCENP is phosphorylated not only by Aurora B but also by CDK1, which enhances its ability to activate Aurora B. Also, CDK1 phosphorylation of INCENP allows it to interact with PLK1 and recruit it to the centromere. There is also evidence that Survivin is regulated by phosphorylation. Aurora B is able to phosphorylate T117 of Survivin *in vitro*. Furthermore, the phosphomimic mutant of Survivin T117E did not properly localize during mitosis and was unable to efficiently interact with INCENP. Phosphorylation of Survivin by CDK1 has been implicated in regulating a second function of the protein in apoptosis. Based on domain structure, Survivin is predicted to be an IAP (inhibitors of apoptosis protein). Ectopic overexpression of Survivin inhibits apoptosis of some cell types, and many human cancers overexpress Survivin, which may suppress death of cancer cells. However, suppression of Survivin using siRNA did not induce apoptosis in normal human fibroblasts, but did induce defects in chromosome segregation. These results argue against a role for Survivin in counteracting a constitutive

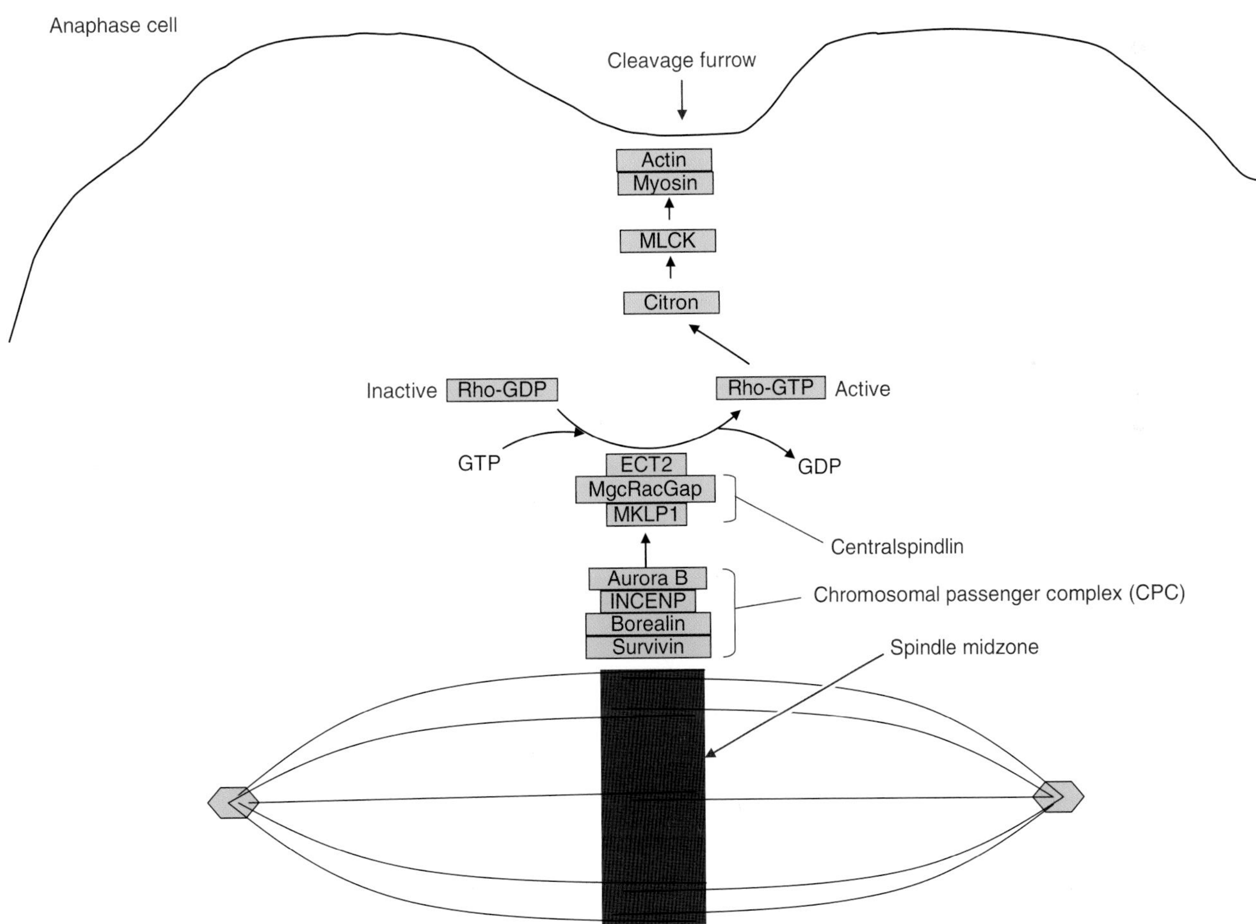

Figure 17.10 Model for the role of the chromosomal passenger complex in cleavage furrow specification. At anaphase, the chromosomal passenger complex localizes to the spindle midzone where Aurora B phosphorylates MKLP1. This event recruits the centralspindlin complex to the spindle midzone. Centralspindlin in turn recruits ECT2, a guanine nucleotide exchange factor for the small GTPase Rho. Rho activated in the vicinity of the spindle midzone diffuses to the nearest cell membrane where it activates Citron kinase. Citron kinase in turn phosphorylates and activates myosin light chain kinase (MLCK), which phosphorylates the myosin light chain leading to acto-myosin dependent furrowing of the membrane. This is one potential model for the role of the CPC in the regulating cleavage. This model is based primarily on siRNA and overexpression experiments in various model systems, and other regulators of cleavage furrow specification are likely at play.

pro-apoptotic signal in human cells. Additional modifications to CPC proteins have been implicated in their regulation. For example, Aurora B has been reported to be controlled by poly(ADP-ribosyl)ation in response to DNA damage.

17.4.6 Aurora Kinase Inhibitors as Anticancer Agents

The three Aurora kinases play multiple roles in cell cycle progression and cell proliferation and may be useful targets for cancer therapy. Also, Aurora kinases are often overexpressed in cancer. For example, Aurora A is overexpressed in breast cancer, and is found on chromosomal region (20q13.2), which is commonly amplified in tumors. Ectopic overexpression of Aurora A in Rat1 and NIH/3T3 cells gives rise to genetically unstable aneuploid cells with multiple centrosomes that are capable of forming tumors when injected into nude mice. Also, amplification and overexpression of Aurora A is associated with aneuploidy in human bladder cancer tissues.

The multiple roles of Aurora B and the CPC in chromosome segregation suggest an important role in maintaining ploidy. Aurora B is overexpressed in many cancers. For example, overexpressing Aurora B in hamster fibroblasts with defective p53 resulted in transformed cells that were able to form highly aggressive metastatic tumors when injected into mice. Also, Aurora B is overexpressed in human gastric cancer AGS cells. The suppression of Aurora B expression induced by RNAi or by an inhibitor of Aurora kinase activity significantly reduces the growth of thyroid anaplastic carcinoma cells. Additionally, microarray analysis of primary tumor samples showed that both Aurora A and B are overexpressed in parallel. For example, both Aurora A and B are overexpressed in breast, lung, colon, prostate, pancreas, liver, skin, stomach, rectum, esophagus, endometrium, cervix, bladder, ovary, and thyroid tumors. There is also evidence that Aurora C, which can substitute for Aurora B in the CPC, is overexpressed in human cancer tissues.

Currently, three Aurora kinase inhibitors, Hesperadin, ZM447439, and VX-680, have been most extensively characterized, however new compounds are still being developed. All three inhibitors specifically target the enzymatic activity of the Aurora kinases by occupying the catalytic ATP binding site. Additionally, all three inhibitors prevent phosphorylation of histone H3 and cell division. Hesperadin (a novel indolinone) primarily targets Aurora B, while ZM447439 (a quinazoline derivative) is a specific inhibitor of both Aurora A and B (IC_{50} value of 110 and 130 nM), and VX-680 (a 4,6 di-amino pyrimidine) inhibits Aurora A, B, and C (IC_{50} value of 0.6 nM, 18 nM, and 4.6 nM). The Aurora kinase inhibitors are not antimitotic agents; rather, following an aberrant mitosis, activation of the p53 post-mitotic checkpoint induces a "pseudo G1" cell-cycle arrest. Consistently, p53 is required to prevent endoreduplication in U20S cells following exposure to ZM447439. Cells exposed to Hesperadin or ZM447439 undergo anaphase and exit mitosis prematurely with altered chromosome morphology, indicating that the spindle checkpoint is compromised and proteins BUB1 and BUBR1 do not localize to kinetochores. It has been suggested that the SAC is composed of two arms, one dependent on BUB1, monitoring kinetochore-microtubule attachment, and the other on Aurora B, monitoring biorientation. When cells are exposed to Hesperadin, chromosomes are oriented syntelically, where both kinetochores are attached to the same pole. After Hesperadin treatment of MCF7 (breast cancer cells) and PC3 (prostate adenocarcinoma cells), cell proliferation is inhibited due to multiple mitotic defects caused by the reduction of Aurora B activity and elimination of checkpoint proteins (hBUBR1 and CENP-E) from kinetochores of mitotic chromosomes. VX-680 blocks cell-cycle progression and induces apoptosis in many human tumors. Nude mice harboring tumor xenografts derived from human colon tumor or leukemia cell lines undergo dose-dependent tumor growth inhibition and up to 98% regression when treated with VX-680. In addition, VX-680 exposure significantly reduces cell viability of C1A, PC3, LNCaP prostate cancer cells overexpressing Aurora kinases (C1A> PC3>LNCaP). When VX-680 was used in combination with doxorubicin, cell viability was reduced an additional two-fold, indicating that combination therapy might be possible. Further, VX-680 binds to the catalytic domain of BCR-ABL and inhibits its kinase activity, indicating that this drug may also be useful for treating patients with CML. The integrity of the p53-p21Cip1-dependent postmitotic checkpoint governs the response to Aurora kinase inhibition. Although cells with intact checkpoint function arrest with 4 N DNA content, those with compromised checkpoint function are more likely to undergo endoreduplication and apoptosis. Therefore, VX-680 exposure provides evidence that Aurora kinase inhibition will be selectively cytotoxic to malignant cells.

There are currently several clinical trials underway to test the effects of Aurora kinase inhibitors, and the results of most of these have not been published. Preliminary findings of Phase I trials with VX-680 and a new drug AZD1152 indicated that suppression of white blood cells in response to both drugs is a side-effect that will limit the dose of drug that can be used. Twenty-two patients with advanced tumors (colon, pancreas, lung, and other sites) were enrolled in the Phase I trial with VX-680, and two patients experienced disease stabilization. In the Phase I trial with AZD1152, 19 patients with colorectal, melanoma/schwannoma, prostate cancer, or cancers of other sites were treated and three patients had stable disease during the trial. Phase II trials for both drugs are currently underway.

17.4.7 Long-term Responses to Aurora Kinase Inhibitors *In Vitro*

The use of Aurora kinase inhibitors as anticancer drugs requires that they efficiently kill their target cells. Since they target mitotic processes, these drugs are predicted to be as specific as other drugs that rely on the uncontrolled cell cycle progression to kill cancer cells. As such, side effects due to depletion of rapidly growing host cells are expected to occur. Also, p53 appears to play a role in the initial response of cells to Aurora kinase inhibition. The effects of p53 are reminiscent of its influence on the cellular response to inhibitors of cytokinesis.

Initial studies used cytochalasin D to disrupt the actin cytoskeleton and probe the role of p53 in subsequent entry into the cell cycle. Cells treated with cytochalasin D enter and exit mitosis, segregate their chromosomes but are unable to divide. These cells eventually exit mitosis as a binucleated G1 cell. Initial studies indicated that this tetraploid state was sufficient to induce p53 and block entry into a new S phase. Cells lacking p53 did enter S phase, duplicated their genome, and became octoploid (i.e., via endoreduplication). More recent evidence suggests that the drug treatments themselves induce p53, and simply having a tetraploid DNA content is not sufficient for p53 induction.

As described earlier, similar results have been obtained with inhibitors of Aurora kinase. Inhibition of Aurora B blocks cell division but not progress into and out of mitosis. Therefore, when ZM447439 or VX-680-treated cells exit mitosis they enter a tetraploid G1. When p53-containing cells are exposed to ZM447439, they enter a tetraploid G1 state and have trouble in further duplicating their genome, likely as a result of induction of p53 and G1 arrest. In contrast, cells lacking p53 do reenter S phase, duplicate their DNA, enter mitosis, and if ZM447439 is still there, fail to divide and enter an octoploid G1. Analyzing cells after several days of treatment with VX-680 reveals the presence of cells with many times their normal complement of DNA.

Recent experiments indicated that tetraploid cells produced by treatment with the myosin inhibitor blebbistatin are highly susceptible to spontaneous apoptosis. However, in our time-lapse experiments using ZM447439, over the short term (3–4 days) very few cells die spontaneously. Nonetheless it seems reasonable that allowing cells to rereplicate their genome many times without dividing will be a lethal event and it is clear than many of the giant cells do die. In our experiments, with long-term observation, colonies of cells were seen to emerge after exposure to ZM447439. These colonies are heterogeneous in that some consist of mononucleated cells, whereas others contain cells with disorganized nuclear architecture. Whether these represent truly resistant clones is currently under investigation. The emergence of viable colonies after ZM447439 treatment occurs with a higher frequency in the absence of p53, possibly as a result of the cell cycle arrest. Currently, we do not know where the emergent colonies come from. Using time-lapse observation we have found that the multinucleated giant cells are able to enter mitosis, however many of them die in the process. In some rare cases, these mitotic events result in asymmetric division, and it is possible that this leads to the emergence of viable cells from a population of multinucleated giant cells. However, we currently have no direct evidence to support this idea. As with cytochalasin and blebbistatin, ZM447439 and VE induce p53. It is unlikely that the induction is due to the polyploid state per se, and whether DNA damage is responsible is currently under investigation.

17.5 CONCLUSIONS

The orderly progression through the cell cycle is controlled by CDK/Cyclin complexes that are under multiple levels of regulation. Subunit availability, subcellular localization, and inhibitory and activating phosphorylations are controlled dynamically to ensure that CDKs are active when needed. Cell cycle checkpoints feed into these various modes of regulation to ensure that cell cycle events occur only when all previous events have been properly completed. Many current treatments for cancer trigger cell cycle checkpoints and induce cell cycle arrest. Radiation therapy induces double-strand DNA breaks that are recognized by a series of recognition, response, and repair proteins that trigger the arrest. Cell cycle arrest can allow time for repair, or might be permanent, thereby eliminating the damaged cell. Bleomycin mimics the effects of ionizing radiation by inducing double-strand DNA breaks whereas doxorubicin and camptothecin damage DNA by inhibiting topoisomerases. Topoisomerase inhibition can induce stalling of replication forks, a condition that generates single-stranded DNA, a potent inducer of cell cycle checkpoint responses. In-depth analysis of the mechanics of mitotic progression has uncovered several protein kinases that are currently under investigation as novel drug targets in cancer. Drugs that inhibit PLK1, CDKs, and Aurora kinases are the subjects of a number of clinical studies and hold promise as new ways to treat cancer.

REVIEW QUESTIONS

1. What controls movement of cells from one phase of the cell cycle to another, and on what do they depend for activity?
2. Describe how phosphorylation affects the Rb/E2F system, and its ability to regulate transcription.
3. What are cell cycle checkpoints?
4. When DNA is damaged, CDK activities are inhibited much more efficiently if p53 is intact. Why?
5. Explain how the spindle assembly checkpoint ensures that chromosomes are equally segregated during mitosis.
6. Taxol stabilizes microtubules and disrupts the function of the mitotic spindle. Neurons are permanently blocked in G0. Therefore, taxol has no effect on neurons.
7. True or False? Explain your answer.
   The chromosomal passenger complex is found at the following locations (choose 3):
   A) mitochondria
   B) lamellopodia

   C) spindle midzone
   D) spindle pole
   E) midbody
   F) chloroplast
   G) inner centromere
8. Many different types of DNA damage can activate ATR. One way this is possible is that stalled replication forks lead to the production of what type of DNA? By what protein is it coated?
9. Inhibitors of Aurora kinases, PLK1 and CDK1, are good candidate anticancer drugs because these enzymes are active only during:
   A) apoptosis
   B) mitosis
   C) G0
   D) G1
   E) metastasis
10. Explain how the phosphorylation of the N-terminus of p53 by ATM or ATR leads to the accumulation of the p53 protein.

REFERENCES

Research Articles

Agarwal, M. K., Hastak, K., Jackson, M. W., Breit, S. N., Stark, G. R., & Agarwal, M. L. (2006). Macrophage inhibitory cytokine 1 mediates a p53-dependent protective arrest in S phase in response to starvation for DNA precursors. *Proceedings of the National Academy of Sciences of the United States of America, 103*, 16278–16283.

Agarwal, M. L., Agarwal, A., Taylor, W. R., Chernova, O., Sharma, Y., & Stark, G. R. (1998). A p53-dependent S-phase checkpoint helps to protect cells from DNA damage in response to starvation for pyrimidine nucleotides. *Proceedings of the National Academy of Sciences of the United States of America, 95*, 14775–14780.

Ainsztein, A. M., Kandels-Lewis, S. E., Mackay, A. M., & Earnshaw, W. C. (1998). INCENP centromere and spindle targeting: Identification of essential conserved motifs and involvement of heterochromatin protein HP1. *The Journal of Cell Biology, 143*, 1763–1774.

Aklilu, M., Kindler, H. L., Donehower, R. C., Mani, S., & Vokes, E. E. (2003). Phase II study of flavopiridol in patients with advanced colorectal cancer. *Annals of Oncology: Official Journal of the European Society for Medical Oncology / ESMO, 14*, 1270–1273.

Andreassen, P. R., Lohez, O. D., Lacroix, F. B., & Margolis, R. L. (2001). Tetraploid state induces p53-dependent arrest of nontransformed mammalian cells in G1. *Molecular Biology of the Cell, 12*, 1315–1328.

Bakkenist, C., & Kastan, M. (2003). DNA damage activates ATM through intermolecular autophosphorylation and dimer dissociation [In Process Citation]. *Nature, 421*, 499–506.

Banin, S., Moyal, L., Shieh, S., Taya, Y., Anderson, C. W., Chessa, L., et al. (1998). Enhanced phosphorylation of p53 by ATM in response to DNA damage. *Science, 281*, 1674–1677.

Bekker-Jensen, S., Lukas, C., Kitagawa, R., Melander, F., Kastan, M. B., Bartek, J., et al. (2006). Spatial organization of the mammalian genome surveillance machinery in response to DNA strand breaks. *The Journal of Cell Biology, 173*, 195–206.

Bischoff, J. R., Anderson, L., Zhu, Y., Mossie, K., Ng, L., Souza, B., et al. (1998). A homologue of Drosophila aurora kinase is oncogenic and amplified in human colorectal cancers. *The EMBO Journal, 17*, 3052–3065.

Booher, R. N., Holman, P. S., & Fattaey, A. (1997). Human Myt1 is a cell cycle-regulated kinase that inhibits CDC2 but not CDK2 activity. *The Journal of Biological Chemistry, 272*, 22300–22306.

Borel, F., Lohez, O. D., Lacroix, F. B., & Margolis, R. L. (2002). Multiple centrosomes arise from tetraploidy checkpoint failure and mitotic centrosome clusters in p53 and RB pocket protein-compromised cells. *Proceedings of the National Academy of Sciences of the United States of America, 99*, 9819–9824.

Borgne, A., Ostvold, A. C., Flament, S., & Meijer, L. (1999). Intra-M phase-promoting factor phosphorylation of cyclin B at the prophase/metaphase transition. *The Journal of Biological Chemistry, 274*, 11977–11986.

Bressan, D., Baxter, B., & Petrini, J. (1999). The Mre11-Rad50-Xrs2 protein complex facilitates homologous recombination-based double-strand break repair in Saccharomyces cerevisiae. *Molecular and Cellular Biology, 19*, 7681–7687.

Buffin, E., Lefebvre, C., Huang, J., Gagou, M. E., & Karess, R. E. (2005). Recruitment of Mad2 to the kinetochore requires the Rod/Zw10 complex. *Current Biology: CB, 15*, 856–861.

Bulavin, D. V., Higashimoto, Y., Popoff, I. J., Gaarde, W. A., Basrur, V., Potapova, O., et al. (2001). Initiation of a G2/M checkpoint after ultraviolet radiation requires p38 kinase. *Nature, 411*, 102–107.

Bunz, F., Dutriaux, A., Lengauer, C., Waldman, T., Zhou, S., Brown, J. P., et al. (1998). Requirement for p53 and p21 to sustain G2 arrest after DNA damage. *Science, 282*, 1497–1501.

Byun, T. S., Pacek, M., Yee, M. C., Walter, J. C., & Cimprich, K. A. (2005). Functional uncoupling of MCM helicase and DNA polymerase activities activates the ATR-dependent checkpoint. *Genes & Development, 19*, 1040–1052.

Canman, C. E., Lim, D. S., Cimprich, K. A., Taya, Y., Tamai, K., Sakaguchi, K., et al. (1998). Activation of the ATM kinase by ionizing radiation and phosphorylation of p53. *Science, 281*, 1677–1679.

Cao, L. G., & Wang, Y. L. (1996). Signals from the spindle midzone are required for the stimulation of cytokinesis in cultured epithelial cells. *Molecular Biology of the Cell, 7*, 225–232.

Carter, T. A., Wodicka, L. M., Shah, N. P., Velasco, A. M., Fabian, M. A., Treiber, D. K., et al. (2005). Inhibition of drug-resistant mutants of ABL, KIT, and EGF receptor kinases. *Proceedings of the National Academy of Sciences of the United States of America, 102*, 11011–11016.

Castedo, M., Coquelle, A., Vivet, S., Vitale, I., Kauffmann, A., Dessen, P., et al. (2006). Apoptosis regulation in tetraploid cancer cells. *The EMBO Journal, 25*, 2584–2595.

Cazales, M., Schmitt, E., Montembault, E., Dozier, C., Prigent, C., & Ducommun, B. (2005). CDC25B phosphorylation by Aurora-A occurs at the G2/M transition and is inhibited by DNA damage. *Cell Cycle (Georgetown, Tex.), 4*, 1233–1238.

Chang, B. D., Broude, E. V., Fang, J. V. K. T., Abdryashitov, R., Poole, J. C., & Roninson, I. B. (2000). p21Waf1/Cip1/Sdi1-induced growth arrest is associated with depletion of mitosis-control proteins and leads to abnormal mitosis and endoreduplication in recovering cells. *Oncogene, 19*, 2165–2170.

Chang, J. L., Chen, T. H., Wang, C. F., Chiang, Y. H., Huang, Y. L., Wong, F. H., et al. (2006). Borealin/Dasra B is a cell cycle-regulated chromosomal passenger protein and its nuclear accumulation is linked to poor prognosis for human gastric cancer. *Experimental Cell Research, 312*, 962–973.

Chaturvedi, P., Eng, W. K., Zhu, Y., Mattern, M. R., Mishra, R., Hurle, M. R., et al. (1999). Mammalian Chk2 is a downstream effector of the ATM-dependent DNA damage checkpoint pathway. *Oncogene, 18*, 4047–4054.

Chieffi, P., Cozzolino, L., Kisslinger, A., Libertini, S., Staibano, S., Mansueto, G., et al. (2006). Aurora B expression directly correlates with prostate cancer malignancy and influence prostate cell proliferation. *The Prostate, 66*, 326–333.

Cimini, D., Howell, B., Maddox, P., Khodjakov, A., Degrassi, F., & Salmon, E. D. (2001). Merotelic kinetochore orientation is a major mechanism of aneuploidy in mitotic mammalian tissue cells. *The Journal of Cell Biology, 153*, 517–527.

Cliby, W. A., Roberts, C. J., Cimprich, K. A., Stringer, C. M., Lamb, J. R., Schreiber, S. L., et al. (1998). Overexpression of a kinase-inactive ATR protein causes sensitivity to DNA-damaging agents and defects in cell cycle checkpoints. *The EMBO Journal, 17*, 159–169.

Clifford, B., Beljin, M., Stark, G. R., & Taylor, W. R. (2003). G2 arrest in response to topoisomerase II inhibitors: The role of p53. *Cancer Research, 63*, 4074–4081.

Coulonval, K., Bockstaele, L., Paternot, S., & Roger, P. P. (2003). Phosphorylations of cyclin-dependent kinase 2 revisited using two-dimensional gel electrophoresis. *The Journal of Biological Chemistry, 278*, 52052–52060.

De Souza, C. P., Ellem, K. A., & Gabrielli, B. G. (2000). Centrosomal and cytoplasmic Cdc2/cyclin B1 activation precedes nuclear mitotic events. *Experimental Cell Research, 257*, 11–21.

Deming, P. B., Cistulli, C. A., Zhao, H., Graves, P. R., Piwnica-Worms, H., Paules, R. S., et al. (2001). The human decatenation checkpoint. *Proceedings of the National Academy of Sciences of the United States of America, 98*, 12044–12049.

Deming, P. B., Flores, K. G., Downes, C. S., Paules, R. S., & Kaufmann, W. K. (2002). ATR enforces the topoisomerase II-dependent G2 checkpoint through inhibition of Plk1 kinase. *The Journal of Biological Chemistry, 277*, 36832–36838.

Ditchfield, C., Johnson, V. L., Tighe, A., Ellston, R., Haworth, C., Johnson, T., et al. (2003). Aurora B couples chromosome alignment with anaphase by targeting BubR1, Mad2, and Cenp-E to kinetochores. *The Journal of Cell Biology, 161*, 267–280.

Downes, C. S., Clarke, D. J., Mullinger, A. M., Gimenez-Abian, J. F., Creighton, A. M., & Johnson, R. T. (1994). A topoisomerase II-dependent G2 cycle checkpoint in mammalian cells. *Nature, 372*, 467–470.

el-Deiry, W. S., Tokino, T., Velculescu, V. E., Levy, D. B., Parsons, R., Trent, J. M., et al. (1993). WAF1, a potential mediator of p53 tumor suppression. *Cell, 75*, 817–825.

Eliyahu, D., Raz, A., Gruss, P., Givol, D., & Oren, M. (1984). Participation of p53 cellular tumour antigen in transformation of normal embryonic cells. *Nature, 312*, 646–649.

Falck, J., Coates, J., & Jackson, S. P. (2005). Conserved modes of recruitment of ATM, ATR and DNA-PKcs to sites of DNA damage. *Nature, 434*, 605–611.

Flatt, P. M., Tang, L. J., Scatena, C. D., Szak, S. T., & Pietenpol, J. A. (2000). p53 regulation of G(2) checkpoint is retinoblastoma protein dependent. *Molecular and Cellular Biology, 20*, 4210–4223.

Fontijn, R. D., Goud, B., Echard, A., Jollivet, F., van Marle, J., Pannekoek, H., et al. (2001). The human kinesin-like protein RB6K is under tight cell cycle control and is essential for cytokinesis. *Molecular and Cellular Biology, 21*, 2944–2955.

Fortune, J. M., & Osheroff, N. (1998). Merbarone inhibits the catalytic activity of human topoisomerase IIalpha by blocking DNA cleavage. *The Journal of Biological Chemistry, 273*, 17643–17650.

Furnari, B., Rhind, N., & Russell, P. (1997). CDC25 mitotic inducer targeted by CHK1 DNA damage checkpoint kinase. *Science, 277*, 1495–1497.

Gadea, B. B., & Ruderman, J. V. (2005). Aurora kinase inhibitor ZM447439 blocks chromosome-induced spindle assembly, the completion of chromosome condensation, and the establishment of the spindle integrity checkpoint in Xenopus egg extracts. *Molecular Biology of the Cell, 16*, 1305–1318.

Gassmann, R., Carvalho, A., Henzing, A. J., Ruchaud, S., Hudson, D. F., Honda, R., et al. (2004). Borealin: A novel chromosomal passenger required for stability of the bipolar mitotic spindle. *The Journal of Cell Biology, 166*, 179–191.

Girdler, F., Gascoigne, K. E., Eyers, P. A., Hartmuth, S., Crafter, C., Foote, K. M., et al. (2006). Validating Aurora B as an anti-cancer drug target. *Journal of Cell Science, 119*, 3664–3675.

Gizatullin, F., Yao, Y., Kung, V., Harding, M. W., Loda, M., & Shapiro, G. I. (2006). The Aurora kinase inhibitor VX-680 induces endoreduplication and apoptosis preferentially in cells with compromised p53-dependent postmitotic checkpoint function. *Cancer Research, 66*, 7668–7677.

Goto, H., Kiyono, T., Tomono, Y., Kawajiri, A., Urano, T., Furukawa, K., et al. (2006). Complex formation of Plk1 and INCENP required for metaphase-anaphase transition. *Nature Cell Biology, 8*, 180–187.

Graeber, T. G., Peterson, J. F., Tsai, M., Monica, K., Fornace, A. J., Jr., & Giaccia, A. J. (1994). Hypoxia induces accumulation of p53 protein, but activation of a G1-phase checkpoint by low-oxygen conditions is independent of p53 status. *Molecular and Cellular Biology, 14*, 6264–6277.

Green, C. M., Erdjument-Bromage, H., Tempst, P., & Lowndes, N. F. (2000). A novel Rad24 checkpoint protein complex closely related to replication factor C. [erratum appears in *Curr Biol* 2000 Feb 24;10(4):R171]. *Current Biology: CB, 10*, 39–42.

Griffiths, D. J., Barbet, N. C., McCready, S., Lehmann, A. R., & Carr, A. M. (1995). Fission yeast rad17: a homologue of budding yeast RAD24 that shares regions of sequence similarity with DNA polymerase accessory proteins. *The EMBO Journal, 14*, 5812–5823.

Gumireddy, K., Reddy, M. V., Cosenza, S. C., Boominathan, R., Baker, S. J., Papathi, N., et al. (2005). ON01910, a non-ATP-competitive small molecule inhibitor of Plk1, is a potent anticancer agent. *Cancer Cell, 7*, 275–286.

Guse, A., Mishima, M., & Glotzer, M. (2005). Phosphorylation of ZEN-4/MKLP1 by aurora B regulates completion of cytokinesis. *Current Biology: CB, 15*, 778–786.

Harper, J. W., Elledge, S. J., Keyomarsi, K., Dynlacht, B., Tsai, L. H., Zhang, P., et al. (1995). Inhibition of cyclin-dependent kinases by p21. *Molecular Biology of the Cell, 6*, 387–400.

Harrington, E. A., Bebbington, D., Moore, J., Rasmussen, R. K., Ajose-Adeogun, A. O., Nakayama, T., et al. (2004). VX-680, a potent and selective small-molecule inhibitor of the Aurora kinases, suppresses tumor growth in vivo. *Nature Medicine, 10*, 262–267.

Hauf, S., Cole, R. W., LaTerra, S., Zimmer, C., Schnapp, G., Walter, R., et al. (2003). The small molecule Hesperadin reveals a role for Aurora B in correcting kinetochore-microtubule attachment and in maintaining the spindle assembly checkpoint. *The Journal of Cell Biology, 161*, 281–294.

Hendzel, M. J., Wei, Y., Mancini, M. A., Van Hooser, A., Ranalli, T., Brinkley, B. R., et al. (1997). Mitosis-specific phosphorylation of histone H3 initiates primarily within pericentromeric heterochromatin during G2 and spreads in an ordered fashion coincident with mitotic chromosome condensation. *Chromosoma, 106*, 348–360.

Hirao, A., Kong, Y. Y., Matsuoka, S., Wakeham, A., Ruland, J., Yoshida, H., et al. (2000). DNA damage-induced activation of p53 by the checkpoint kinase CHK2. *Science, 287*, 1824–1827.

Hirota, T., Lipp, J. J., Toh, B. H., & Peters, J. M. (2005). Histone H3 serine 10 phosphorylation by Aurora B causes HP1 dissociation from heterochromatin. *Nature, 438*, 1176–1180.

Honda, R., Korner, R., & Nigg, E. A. (2003). Exploring the functional interactions between Aurora B, INCENP, and survivin in mitosis. *Molecular Biology of the Cell, 14*, 3325–3341.

Hsu, J. Y., Sun, Z. W., Li, X., Reuben, M., Tatchell, K., Bishop, D. K., et al. (2000). Mitotic phosphorylation of histone H3 is governed by IPl1/aurora kinase and GLC7/PP1 phosphatase in budding yeast and nematodes. *Cell, 102*, 279–291.

Ishida, S., Huang, E., Zuzan, H., Spang, R., Leone, G., West, M., et al. (2001). Role for E2F in control of both DNA replication and mitotic functions as revealed from DNA microarray analysis. *Molecular and Cellular Biology, 21*, 4684–4699.

Jackson, M. W., Agarwal, M. K., Yang, J., Bruss, P., Uchiumi, T., Agarwal, M. L., et al. (2005). p130/p107/p105Rb-dependent transcriptional repression during DNA-damage-induced cell-cycle exit at G2. *Journal of Cell Science, 118*, 1821–1832.

Jazayeri, A., Falck, J., Lukas, C., Bartek, J., Smith, G. C., Lukas, J., et al. (2006). ATM- and cell cycle-dependent regulation of ATR in response to DNA double-strand breaks. *Nature Cell Biology, 8*, 37–45.

Jeyaprakash, A. A., Klein, U. R., Lindner, D., Ebert, J., Nigg, E. A., Conti, E. (2007). Structure of a Survivin-Borealin-INCENP core complex reveals how chromosomal passengers travel together. *Cell, 131*, 271–285.

Jin, P., Hardy, S., & Morgan, D. O. (1998). Nuclear localization of cyclin B1 controls mitotic entry after DNA damage. *The Journal of Cell Biology, 141*, 875–885.

Kamijo, K., Ohara, N., Abe, M., Uchimura, T., Hosoya, H., Lee, J. S., et al. (2006). Dissecting the role of Rho-mediated signaling in contractile ring formation. *Molecular Biology of the Cell, 17*, 43–55.

Kastan, M. B., Onyekwere, O., Sidransky, D., Vogelstein, B., & Craig, R. W. (1991). Participation of p53 protein in the cellular response to DNA damage. *Cancer Research, 51*, 6304–6311.

Katayama, H., Sasai, K., Kawai, H., Yuan, Z. M., Bondaruk, J., Suzuki, F., et al. (2004). Phosphorylation by aurora kinase A induces Mdm2-mediated destabilization and inhibition of p53. *Nature Genetics, 36*, 55–62.

Khan, S. H., & Wahl, G. M. (1998). p53 and pRb prevent rereplication in response to microtubule inhibitors by mediating a reversible G1 arrest. *Cancer Research, 58*, 396–401.

Khanna, K. K., Keating, K. E., Kozlov, S., Scott, S., Gatei, M., Hobson, K., et al. (1998). ATM associates with and phosphorylates p53: Mapping the region of interaction. *Nature Genetics, 20*, 398–400.

Kharbanda, S., Saleem, A., Datta, R., Yuan, Z. M., Weichselbaum, R., & Kufe, D. (1994). Ionizing radiation induces rapid tyrosine phosphorylation of p34cdc2. *Cancer Research, 54,* 1412–1414.

Klein, U. R., Nigg, E. A., & Gruneberg, U. (2006). Centromere targeting of the chromosomal passenger complex requires a ternary subcomplex of Borealin, Survivin, and the N-terminal domain of INCENP. *Molecular Biology of the Cell, 17,* 2547–2558.

Knowlton, A. L., Lan, W., & Stukenberg, P. T. (2006). Aurora B is enriched at merotelic attachment sites, where it regulates MCAK. *Current Biology: CB, 16,* 1705–1710.

Kops, G. J., Foltz, D. R., & Cleveland, D. W. (2004). Lethality to human cancer cells through massive chromosome loss by inhibition of the mitotic checkpoint. *Proceedings of the National Academy of Sciences of the United States of America, 101,* 8699–8704.

Krystyniak, A., Garcia-Echeverria, C., Prigent, C., & Ferrari, S. (2006). Inhibition of Aurora A in response to DNA damage. *Oncogene, 25,* 338–348.

Lane, D. (1984). Cell immortalization and transformation by the p53 gene. *Nature, 312,* 596–597.

Lee, E. A., Keutmann, M. K., Dowling, M. L., Harris, E., Chan, G., & Kao, G. D. (2004). Inactivation of the mitotic checkpoint as a determinant of the efficacy of microtubule-targeted drugs in killing human cancer cells. *Molecular Cancer Therapeutics, 3,* 661–669.

Lee, E. C., Frolov, A., Li, R., Ayala, G., & Greenberg, N. M. (2006). Targeting Aurora kinases for the treatment of prostate cancer. *Cancer Research, 66,* 4996–5002.

Lindsey-Boltz, L. A., Bermudez, V. P., Hurwitz, J., & Sancar, A. (2001). Purification and characterization of human DNA damage checkpoint Rad complexes. *Proceedings of the National Academy of Sciences of the United States of America, 98,* 11236–11241.

Linke, S. P., Clarkin, K. C., Di Leonardo, A., Tsou, A., & Wahl, G. M. (1996). A reversible, p53-dependent G0/G1 cell cycle arrest induced by ribonucleotide depletion in the absence of detectable DNA damage. *Genes & Development, 10,* 934–947.

Liu, F., Stanton, J. J., Wu, Z., & Piwnica-Worms, H. (1997). The human Myt1 kinase preferentially phosphorylates Cdc2 on threonine 14 and localizes to the endoplasmic reticulum and Golgi complex. *Molecular and Cellular Biology, 17,* 571–583.

Liu, Q., Guntuku, S., Cui, X. S., Matsuoka, S., Cortez, D., Tamai, K., et al. (2000). Chk1 is an essential kinase that is regulated by Atr and required for the G(2)/M DNA damage checkpoint. *Genes & Development, 14,* 1448–1459.

Liu, Q., Kaneko, S., Yang, L., Feldman, R. I., Nicosia, S. V., Chen, J., et al. (2004). Aurora-A abrogation of p53 DNA binding and transactivation activity by phosphorylation of serine 215. *The Journal of Biological Chemistry, 279,* 52175–52182.

Livingstone, L. R., White, A., Sprouse, J., Livanos, E., Jacks, T., & Tlsty, T. D. (1992). Altered cell cycle arrest and gene amplification potential accompany loss of wild-type p53. *Cell, 70,* 923–935.

Lock, R. B., & Ross, W. E. (1990). Inhibition of p34cdc2 kinase activity by etoposide or irradiation as a mechanism of G2 arrest in Chinese hamster ovary cells. *Cancer Research, 50,* 3761–3766.

Lukas, C., Melander, F., Stucki, M., Falck, J., Bekker-Jensen, S., Goldberg, M., et al. (2004). MDC1 couples DNA double-strand break recognition by NBS1 with its H2AX-dependent chromatin retention. *The EMBO Journal, 23,* 2674–2683.

Mackay, A. M., Eckley, D. M., Chue, C., & Earnshaw, W. C. (1993). Molecular analysis of the INCENPs (inner centromere proteins): separate domains are required for association with microtubules during interphase and with the central spindle during anaphase. *The Journal of Cell Biology, 123,* 373–385.

Mailand, N., & Diffley, J. F. (2005). CDKs promote DNA replication origin licensing in human cells by protecting CDC6 from APC/C-dependent proteolysis. *Cell, 122,* 915–926.

Malkin, D., Li, F., Strong, L., Fraumeni, J., Nelson, C., Kim, D., et al. (1990). Germ line p53 mutations in a familial syndrome of breast cancer, sarcomas, and other neoplasms. *Science, 250,* 1233–1238.

Marumoto, T., Hirota, T., Morisaki, T., Kunitoku, N., Zhang, D., Ichikawa, Y., et al. (2002). Roles of aurora-A kinase in mitotic entry and G2 checkpoint in mammalian cells. *Genes to Cells: Devoted to Molecular & Cellular Mechanisms, 7,* 1173–1182.

Matsuoka, S., Rotman, G., Ogawa, A., Shiloh, Y., Tamai, K., & Elledge, S. J. (2000). Ataxia telangiectasia-mutated phosphorylates chk2 in vivo and in vitro [in process citation]. *Proceedings of the National Academy of Sciences of the United States of America, 97,* 10389–10394.

Mikhailov, A., Shinohara, M., & Rieder, C. L. (2004). Topoisomerase II and histone deacetylase inhibitors delay the G2/M transition by triggering the p38 MAPK checkpoint pathway. *The Journal of Cell Biology, 166,* 517–526.

Minoshima, Y., Kawashima, T., Hirose, K., Tonozuka, Y., Kawajiri, A., Bao, Y. C., et al. (2003). Phosphorylation by aurora B converts MgcRacGAP to a RhoGAP during cytokinesis. *Developmental Cell, 4,* 549–560.

Mishima, M., Kaitna, S., & Glotzer, M. (2002). Central spindle assembly and cytokinesis require a kinesin-like protein/RhoGAP complex with microtubule bundling activity. *Developmental Cell, 2,* 41–54.

Monaco, L., Kolthur-Seetharam, U., Loury, R., Murcia, J. M., de Murcia, G., & Sassone-Corsi, P. (2005). Inhibition of Aurora-B kinase activity by poly(ADP-ribosyl)ation in response to DNA damage. *Proceedings of the National Academy of Sciences of the United States of America, 102,* 14244–14248.

Moore, J. D., Yang, J., Truant, R., & Kornbluth, S. (1999). Nuclear import of CDK/cyclin complexes: identification of distinct mechanisms for import of CDK2/cyclin E and CDC2/cyclin B1. *The Journal of Cell Biology, 144,* 213–224.

Morrow, C. J., Tighe, A., Johnson, V. L., Scott, M. I., Ditchfield, C., & Taylor, S. S. (2005). Bub1 and aurora B cooperate to maintain BubR1-mediated inhibition of APC/Cdc20. *Journal of Cell Science, 118,* 3639–3652.

Murata-Hori, M., Tatsuka, M., & Wang, Y. L. (2002). Probing the dynamics and functions of aurora B kinase in living cells during mitosis and cytokinesis. *Molecular Biology of the Cell, 13,* 1099–1108.

Murata-Hori, M., & Wang, Y. L. (2002). The kinase activity of aurora B is required for kinetochore-microtubule interactions during mitosis. *Current Biology: CB, 12,* 894–899.

Palframan, W. J., Meehl, J. B., Jaspersen, S. L., Winey, M., & Murray, A. W. (2006). Anaphase inactivation of the spindle checkpoint. *Science, 313,* 680–684.

Parker, L. L., & Piwnica-Worms, H. (1992). Inactivation of the p34cdc2-cyclin B complex by the human WEE1 tyrosine kinase. *Science, 257,* 1955–1957.

Passalaris, T. M., Benanti, J. A., Gewin, L., Kiyono, T., & Galloway, D. A. (1999). The G(2) checkpoint is maintained by redundant pathways. *Molecular and Cellular Biology, 19,* 5872–5881.

Paull, T. T., Rogakou, E. P., Yamazaki, V., Kirchgessner, C. U., Gellert, M., & Bonner, W. M. (2000). A critical role for histone H2AX in recruitment of repair factors to nuclear foci after DNA damage. *Current Biology: CB, 10,* 886–895.

Peng, C. Y., Graves, P. R., Thoma, R. S., Wu, Z., Shaw, A. S., & Piwnica-Worms, H. (1997). Mitotic and G2 checkpoint control: regulation of 14-3-3 protein binding by phosphorylation of CDC25C on serine-216. *Science, 277,* 1501–1505.

Pines, J., & Hunter, T. (1991). Human cyclins A and B1 are differentially located in the cell and undergo cell cycle-dependent nuclear transport. *The Journal of Cell Biology, 115,* 1–17.

Polager, S., Kalma, Y., Berkovich, E., & Ginsberg, D. (2002). E2Fs upregulate expression of genes involved in DNA replication, DNA repair and mitosis. *Oncogene, 21,* 437–446.

Ren, B., Cam, H., Takahashi, Y., Volkert, T., Terragni, J., Young, R. A., et al. (2002). E2F integrates cell cycle progression with DNA repair, replication, and G(2)/M checkpoints. *Genes & Development, 16,* 245–256.

Rogakou, E. P., Pilch, D. R., Orr, A. H., Ivanova, V. S., & Bonner, W. M. (1998). DNA double-stranded breaks induce histone H2AX phosphorylation on serine 139. *The Journal of Biological Chemistry, 273,* 5858–5868.

Rossi, R., Lidonnici, M. R., Soza, S., Biamonti, G., & Montecucco, A. (2006). The dispersal of replication proteins after Etoposide treatment requires the cooperation of NBS1 with the ataxia telangiectasia Rad3-related/CHK1 pathway. *Cancer Research, 66,* 1675–1683.

Rudolph, N. S., & Latt, S. A. (1989). Flow cytometric analysis of X-ray sensitivity in ataxia telangiectasia. *Mutation Research, 211,* 31–41.

Sanchez, Y., Wong, C., Thoma, R. S., Richman, R., Wu, Z., Piwnica-Worms, H., et al. (1997). Conservation of the CHK1 checkpoint pathway in mammals: linkage of DNA damage to CDK regulation through CDC25. *Science, 277,* 1497–1501.

Sasai, K., Katayama, H., Stenoien, D. L., Fujii, S., Honda, R., Kimura, M., et al. (2004). Aurora-C kinase is a novel chromosomal passenger protein that can complement Aurora-B kinase function in mitotic cells. *Cell Motility and the Cytoskeleton, 59*, 249–263.

Savitsky, K., Bar-Shira, A., Gilad, S., Rotman, G., Ziv, Y., Vanagaite, L., et al. (1995). A single ataxia telangiectasia gene with a product similar to PI-3 kinase. *Science, 268*, 1749–1753.

Schwartz, G. K., Ilson, D., Saltz, L., O'Reilly, E., Tong, W., Maslak, P., et al. (2001). Phase II study of the cyclin-dependent kinase inhibitor flavopiridol administered to patients with advanced gastric carcinoma. *Journal of Clinical Oncology: Official Journal of the American Society of Clinical Oncology, 19*, 1985–1992.

Sen, S., Zhou, H., & White, R. A. (1997). A putative serine/threonine kinase encoding gene BTAK on chromosome 20q13 is amplified and overexpressed in human breast cancer cell lines. *Oncogene, 14*, 2195–2200.

Sen, S., Zhou, H., Zhang, R. D., Yoon, D. S., Vakar-Lopez, F., Ito, S., et al. (2002). Amplification/overexpression of a mitotic kinase gene in human bladder cancer. *Journal of the National Cancer Institute, 94*, 1320–1329.

Shieh, S. Y., Ikeda, M., Taya, Y., & Prives, C. (1997). DNA damage-induced phosphorylation of p53 alleviates inhibition by MDM2. *Cell, 91*, 325–334.

Siliciano, J. D., Canman, C. E., Taya, Y., Sakaguchi, K., Appella, E., & Kastan, M. B. (1997). DNA damage induces phosphorylation of the amino terminus of p53. *Genes & Development, 11*, 3471–3481.

Smith, K. A., Gorman, P. A., Stark, M. B., Groves, R. P., & Stark, G. R. (1990). Distinctive chromosomal structures are formed very early in the amplification of CAD genes in Syrian hamster cells. *Cell, 63*, 1219–1227.

Smith, K. A., Stark, M. B., Gorman, P. A., & Stark, G. R. (1992). Fusions near telomeres occur very early in the amplification of CAD genes in Syrian hamster cells. *Proceedings of the National Academy of Sciences of the United States of America, 89*, 5427–5431.

Sogo, J. M., Lopes, M., & Foiani, M. (2002). Fork reversal and ssDNA accumulation at stalled replication forks owing to checkpoint defects. *Science, 297*, 599–602.

Sorrentino, R., Libertini, S., Pallante, P. L., Troncone, G., Palombini, L., Bavetsias, V., et al. (2005). Aurora B overexpression associates with the thyroid carcinoma undifferentiated phenotype and is required for thyroid carcinoma cell proliferation. *The Journal of Clinical Endocrinology and Metabolism, 90*, 928–935.

Srivastava, S., Zou, Z., Pirollo, K., Blattner, W., & Chang, E. (1990). Germ-line transmission of a mutated p53 gene in a cancer-prone family with Li-Fraumeni syndrome. *Nature, 348*, 747–749.

Stewart, N., Hicks, G. G., Paraskevas, F., & Mowat, M. (1995). Evidence for a second cell cycle block at G2/M by p53. *Oncogene, 10*, 109–115.

Sudo, T., Nitta, M., Saya, H., & Ueno, N. T. (2004). Dependence of paclitaxel sensitivity on a functional spindle assembly checkpoint. *Cancer Research, 64*, 2502–2508.

Takizawa, C. G., Weis, K., & Morgan, D. O. (1999). Ran-independent nuclear import of cyclin B1-Cdc2 by importin beta. *Proceedings of the National Academy of Sciences of the United States of America, 96*, 7938–7943.

Tao, W., South, V. J., Zhang, Y., Davide, J. P., Farrell, L., Kohl, N. E., et al. (2005). Induction of apoptosis by an inhibitor of the mitotic kinesin KSP requires both activation of the spindle assembly checkpoint and mitotic slippage. *Cancer Cell, 8*, 49–59.

Tarnawski, A., Pai, R., Chiou, S. K., Chai, J., & Chu, E. C. (2005). Rebamipide inhibits gastric cancer growth by targeting survivin and Aurora-B. *Biochemical and Biophysical Research Communications, 334*, 207–212.

Taylor, W. R., DePrimo, S. E., Agarwal, A., Agarwal, M. L., Schonthal, A. H., Katula, K. S., et al. (1999). Mechanisms of G2 arrest in response to overexpression of p53. *Molecular Biology of the Cell, 10*, 3607–3622.

Taylor, W. R., Schonthal, A. H., Galante, J., & Stark, G. R. (2001). p130/E2F4 binds to and represses the CDC2 promoter in response to p53. *The Journal of Biological Chemistry, 276*, 1998–2006.

Thullberg, M., Bartkova, J., Khan, S., Hansen, K., Ronnstrand, L., Lukas, J., et al. (2000). Distinct versus redundant properties among members of the INK4 family of cyclin-dependent kinase inhibitors. *FEBS Letters, 470*, 161–166.

Tibbetts, R. S., Brumbaugh, K. M., Williams, J. M., Sarkaria, J. N., Cliby, W. A., Shieh, S. Y., et al. (1999). A role for ATR in the DNA damage-induced phosphorylation of p53. *Genes & Development, 13*, 152–157.

Tlsty, T. D. (1990). Normal diploid human and rodent cells lack a detectable frequency of gene amplification. *Proceedings of the National Academy of Sciences of the United States of America, 87*, 3132–3136.

Toczyski, D. P., Galgoczy, D. J., & Hartwell, L. H. (1997). CDC5 and CKII control adaptation to the yeast DNA damage checkpoint. *Cell, 90*, 1097–1106.

Toyoshima-Morimoto, F., Taniguchi, E., Shinya, N., Iwamatsu, A., & Nishida, E. (2001). Polo-like kinase 1 phosphorylates cyclin B1 and targets it to the nucleus during prophase. *Nature, 410*, 215–220.

Uetake, Y., & Sluder, G. (2004). Cell cycle progression after cleavage failure: mammalian somatic cells do not possess a "tetraploidy checkpoint". *The Journal of Cell Biology, 165*, 609–615.

Vader, G., Kauw, J. J., Medema, R. H., & Lens, S. M. (2006a). Survivin mediates targeting of the chromosomal passenger complex to the centromere and midbody. *EMBO Reports, 7*, 85–92.

Venclovas, C., & Thelen, M. P. (2000). Structure-based predictions of RAD1, RAD9, HUS1 and RAD17 participation in sliding clamp and clamp-loading complexes. *Nucleic Acids Research, 28*, 2481–2493.

Ward, I. M., & Chen, J. (2001). Histone H2AX is phosphorylated in an ATR-dependent manner in response to replicational stress. *The Journal of Biological Chemistry, 276*, 47759–47762.

Wheatley, S. P., Henzing, A. J., Dodson, H., Khaled, W., & Earnshaw, W. C. (2004). Aurora-B phosphorylation in vitro identifies a residue of survivin that is essential for its localization and binding to inner centromere protein (INCENP) in vivo. *The Journal of Biological Chemistry, 279*, 5655–5660.

Wheatley, S. P., Kandels-Lewis, S. E., Adams, R. R., Ainsztein, A. M., & Earnshaw, W. C. (2001). INCENP binds directly to tubulin and requires dynamic microtubules to target to the cleavage furrow. *Experimental Cell Research, 262*, 122–127.

Williams, B. C., Li, Z., Liu, S., Williams, E. V., Leung, G., Yen, T. J., et al. (2003). Zwilch, a new component of the ZW10/ROD complex required for kinetochore functions. *Molecular Biology of the Cell, 14*, 1379–1391.

Wolf, G., Hildenbrand, R., Schwar, C., Grobholz, R., Kaufmann, M., Stutte, H. J., et al. (2000). Polo-like kinase: a novel marker of proliferation: Correlation with estrogen-receptor expression in human breast cancer. *Pathology, Research and Practice, 196*, 753–759.

Wong, C., & Stearns, T. (2005). Mammalian cells lack checkpoints for tetraploidy, aberrant centrosome number, and cytokinesis failure. *BMC Cell Biology, 6*, 6.

Wright, J. A., Smith, H. S., Watt, F. M., Hancock, M. C., Hudson, D. L., & Stark, G. R. (1990). DNA amplification is rare in normal human cells. *Proceedings of the National Academy of Sciences of the United States of America, 87*, 1791–1795.

Xiong, Y., Hannon, G. J., Zhang, H., Casso, D., Kobayashi, R., & Beach, D. (1993). p21 is a universal inhibitor of cyclin kinases. *Nature, 366*, 701–704.

Yan, X., Cao, L., Li, Q., Wu, Y., Zhang, H., Saiyin, H., et al. (2005a). Aurora C is directly associated with survivin and required for cytokinesis. *Genes to Cells: Devoted to Molecular & Cellular Mechanisms, 10*, 617–626.

Yan, X., Wu, Y., Li, Q., Cao, L., Liu, X., Saiyin, H., & Yu, L. (2005b). Cloning and characterization of a novel human Aurora C splicing variant. *Biochemical and Biophysical Research Communications, 328*, 353–361.

Yang, D., Welm, A., & Bishop, J. M. (2004). Cell division and cell survival in the absence of survivin. *Proceedings of the National Academy of Sciences of the United States of America, 101*, 15100–15105.

Yang, J., Bardes, E. S., Moore, J. D., Brennan, J., Powers, M. A., & Kornbluth, S. (1998). Control of cyclin B1 localization through regulated binding of the nuclear export factor CRM1. *Genes & Development, 12*, 2131–2143.

Yin, Y., Tainsky, M. A., Bischoff, F. Z., Strong, L. C., & Wahl, G. M. (1992). Wild-type p53 restores cell cycle control and inhibits gene amplification in cells with mutant p53 alleles. *Cell, 70*, 937–948.

Young, M. A., Shah, N. P., Chao, L. H., Seeliger, M., Milanov, Z. V., Biggs, W. H., 3rd, et al. (2006). Structure of the kinase domain of an imatinib-resistant Abl mutant in complex with the Aurora kinase inhibitor VX-680. *Cancer Research, 66,* 1007–1014.

Yuce, O., Piekny, A., & Glotzer, M. (2005). An ECT2-centralspindlin complex regulates the localization and function of RhoA. *The Journal of Cell Biology, 170,* 571–582.

Zeitlin, S. G., Shelby, R. D., & Sullivan, K. F. (2001). CENP-A is phosphorylated by Aurora B kinase and plays an unexpected role in completion of cytokinesis. *The Journal of Cell Biology, 155,* 1147–1157.

Zhou, H., Kuang, J., Zhong, L., Kuo, W. L., Gray, J. W., Sahin, A., et al. (1998). Tumour amplified kinase STK15/BTAK induces centrosome amplification, aneuploidy and transformation. *Nature Genetics, 20,* 189–193.

Review Articles

Abraham, R. T. (2001). Cell cycle checkpoint signaling through the ATM and ATR kinases. *Genes & Development, 15,* 2177–2196.

Altieri, D. C. (2003). Validating survivin as a cancer therapeutic target. *Nature Reviews. Cancer, 3,* 46–54.

Appella, E., & Anderson, C. W. (2001). Post-translational modifications and activation of p53 by genotoxic stresses. *European Journal of Biochemistry / FEBS, 268,* 2764–2772.

Barbacid, M., Ortega, S., Sotillo, R., Odajima, J., Martin, A., Santamaria, D., et al. (2005). Cell cycle and cancer: genetic analysis of the role of cyclin-dependent kinases. *Cold Spring Harbor Symposia on Quantitative Biology, 70,* 233–240.

Bartek, J., Lukas, J., & Bartkova, J. (1999). Perspective: Defects in cell cycle control and cancer. *The Journal of Pathology, 187,* 95–99.

Bernhard, E. J., Maity, A., Muschel, R. J., & McKenna, W. G. (1995). Effects of ionizing radiation on cell cycle progression. A review. *Radiation & Environmental Biophysics, 34,* 79–83.

Bernhard, E. J., McKenna, W. G., & Muschel, R. J. (1999). Radiosensitivity and the cell cycle. *Cancer Journal from Scientific American, 5,* 194–204.

Bolanos-Garcia, V. M. (2005). Aurora kinases. *The International Journal of Biochemistry & Cell Biology, 37,* 1572–1577.

Boulaire, J., Fotedar, A., & Fotedar, R. (2000). The functions of the CDK-cyclin kinase inhibitor p21WAF1. *Pathologie-biologie, 48,* 190–202.

Brinkley, B. R., & Goepfert, T. M. (1998). Supernumerary centrosomes and cancer: Boveri's hypothesis resurrected. *Cell Motility and the Cytoskeleton, 41,* 281–288.

Brittle, A. L., & Ohkura, H. (2005). Centrosome maturation: Aurora lights the way to the poles. *Current Biology: CB, 15,* R880–R882.

Brown, J. R., Koretke, K. K., Birkeland, M. L., Sanseau, P., & Patrick, D. R. (2004). Evolutionary relationships of Aurora kinases: Implications for model organism studies and the development of anticancer drugs. *BMC Evolutionary Biology, 4,* 39.

Cam, H., & Dynlacht, B. D. (2003). Emerging roles for E2F: Beyond the G1/S transition and DNA replication. *Cancer Cell, 3,* 311–316.

Chan, G. K., Liu, S. T., & Yen, T. J. (2005). Kinetochore structure and function. *Trends in Cell Biology, 15,* 589–598.

Cortez, D. (2005). Unwind and slow down: Checkpoint activation by helicase and polymerase uncoupling. *Genes & Development, 19,* 1007–1012.

D'Amours, D., & Jackson, S. (2002). The MRE11 complex: at the crossroads of DNA repair and checkpoint signaling. *Nature Reviews. Molecular Cell Biology, 3,* 317–327.

Doggrell, S. A. (2004). Dawn of Aurora kinase inhibitors as anticancer drugs. *Expert Opinion on Investigational Drugs, 13,* 1199–1201.

Dong, Z., & Bode, A. M. (2006). The role of histone H3 phosphorylation (Ser10 and Ser28) in cell growth and cell transformation. *Molecular Carcinogenesis, 45,* 416–421.

Draetta, G., & Eckstein, J. (1997). CDC25 protein phosphatases in cell proliferation. *Biochimica et Biophysica Acta, 1332,* M53–63.

Ducat, D., & Zheng, Y. (2004). Aurora kinases in spindle assembly and chromosome segregation. *Experimental Cell Research, 301,* 60–67.

Elledge, S. J. (1996). Cell cycle checkpoints: Preventing an identity crisis. *Science, 274,* 1664–1672.

Froelich-Ammon, S. J., & Osheroff, N. (1995). Topoisomerase poisons: Harnessing the dark side of enzyme mechanism. *The Journal of Biological Chemistry, 270,* 21429–21432.

Gautschi, O., Mack, P. C., Davies, A. M., Lara, P. N., Jr., & Gandara, D. R. (2006). Aurora kinase inhibitors: A new class of targeted drugs in cancer. *Clinical Lung Cancer, 8,* 93–98.

Giet, R., Petretti, C., & Prigent, C. (2005). Aurora kinases, aneuploidy and cancer, a coincidence or a real link? *Trends in Cell Biology, 15,* 241–250.

Greenblatt, M. S., Bennett, W. P., Hollstein, M., & Harris, C. C. (1994). Mutations in the p53 tumor suppressor gene: Clues to cancer etiology and molecular pathogenesis. *Cancer Research, 54,* 4855–4878.

Hagan, R. S., & Sorger, P. K. (2005). Cell biology: The more MAD, the merrier. *Nature, 434,* 575–577.

Harbour, J. W., & Dean, D. C. (2000). Rb function in cell-cycle regulation and apoptosis. *Nature Cell Biology, 2,* E65–E67.

Hirano, T. (2000). Chromosome cohesion, condensation, and separation. *Annual Review of Biochemistry, 69,* 115–144.

Kadura, S., & Sazer, S. (2005). SAC-ing mitotic errors: How the spindle assembly checkpoint (SAC) plays defense against chromosome mis-segregation. *Cell Motility and the Cytoskeleton, 61,* 145–160.

Kastan, M. B., & Bartek, J. (2004). Cell-cycle checkpoints and cancer. *Nature, 432,* 316–323.

Katayama, H., Brinkley, W. R., & Sen, S. (2003). The Aurora kinases: Role in cell transformation and tumorigenesis. *Cancer Metastasis Reviews, 22,* 451–464.

Keen, N., & Taylor, S. (2004). Aurora-kinase inhibitors as anticancer agents. *Nature Reviews. Cancer, 4,* 927–936.

Lee, J. J., & Swain, S. M. (2006). Peripheral neuropathy induced by microtubule-stabilizing agents. *Journal of Clinical Oncology: Official Journal of the American Society of Clinical Oncology, 24,* 1633–1642.

Lowndes, N. F., & Murguia, J. R. (2000). Sensing and responding to DNA damage. *Current Opinion in Genetics & Development, 10,* 17–25.

Maity, A., McKenna, W. G., & Muschel, R. J. (1994). The molecular basis for cell cycle delays following ionizing radiation: A review. *Radiotherapy & Oncology, 31,* 1–13.

McGowan, C. H. (2002). Checking in on CDS1 (CHK2): A checkpoint kinase and tumor suppressor. *BioEssays: News and Reviews in Molecular, Cellular and Developmental Biology, 24,* 502–511.

Mistry, S. J., & Atweh, G. F. (2002). Role of stathmin in the regulation of the mitotic spindle: Potential applications in cancer therapy. *The Mount Sinai Journal of Medicine, New York, 69,* 299–304.

Molinari, M. (2000). Cell cycle checkpoints and their inactivation in human cancer. *Cell Proliferation, 33,* 261–274.

Momand, J., Wu, H. H., & Dasgupta, G. (2000). MDM2—Master regulator of the p53 tumor suppressor protein. *Gene, 242,* 15–29.

Nurse, P. (1990). Universal control mechanism regulating onset of M-phase. *Nature, 344,* 503–508.

O'Connell, M. J., Walworth, N. C., & Carr, A. M. (2000). The G2-phase DNA-damage checkpoint. *Trends in Cell Biology, 10,* 296–303.

Pines, J. (1995). Cyclins and cyclin-dependent kinases: a biochemical view. *The Biochemical Journal, 308,* 697–711.

Pinsky, B. A., & Biggins, S. (2005). The spindle checkpoint: Tension versus attachment. *Trends in Cell Biology, 15,* 486–493.

Prigent, C., & Dimitrov, S. (2003). Phosphorylation of serine 10 in histone H3, what for? *Journal of Cell Science, 116,* 3677–3685.

Reichard, P. (2002). Ribonucleotide reductases: The evolution of allosteric regulation. *Archives of Biochemistry and Biophysics, 397,* 149–155.

Smits, V. A., & Medema, R. H. (2001). Checking out the G(2)/M transition. *Biochimica et Biophysica Acta, 1519,* 1–12.

Stark, G. R., & Taylor, W. R. (2006). Control of the G2/M transition. *Molecular Biotechnology, 32,* 227–248.

Trimarchi, J. M., & Lees, J. A. (2002). Sibling rivalry in the E2F family. *Nature Reviews. Molecular Cell Biology, 3,* 11–20.

Vader, G., Medema, R. H., & Lens, S. M. (2006b). The chromosomal passenger complex: Guiding Aurora-B through mitosis. *The Journal of Cell Biology, 173,* 833–837.

Vagnarelli, P., & Earnshaw, W. C. (2004). Chromosomal passengers: The four-dimensional regulation of mitotic events. *Chromosoma, 113*, 211–222.

Vogelstein, B., Lane, D., & Levine, A. J. (2000). Surfing the p53 network. *Nature, 408*, 307–310.

Weaver, B. A., & Cleveland, D. W. (2005). Decoding the links between mitosis, cancer, and chemotherapy: The mitotic checkpoint, adaptation, and cell death. *Cancer Cell, 8*, 7–12.

Book Chapters

Dash, B. C., & El-Deiry, W. S. (2004). Cell cycle checkpoint control mechanisms that can be disrupted in cancer. *Methods in Molecular Biology (Clifton, N. J.), 280*, 99–161.

Nojima, H. (2004). G1 and S-phase checkpoints, chromosome instability, and cancer. *Methods in Molecular Biology (Clifton), 280*, 3–49.

Chapter

18

Programmed Cell Death

George S. Robertson . Eric C. LaCasse . Martin Holcik

OUTLINE

18.1 INTRODUCTION

18.1.1 Overview and History

It is now well established that programmed cell death (PCD, also referred to as cellular suicide, or apoptosis) is an essential part of the maintenance of cellular homeostasis and survival of multicellular organisms. Apoptosis is central to the smooth operation of a number of important cellular processes ranging from host defense against viral infections to the sculpting of organs and tissues during embryonic development. Given that apoptosis is a fundamental biological process essential for the systematic dismantling and elimination of unwanted cells it is not surprising that impaired apoptosis has been implicated in an increasing number of diseases. For example, excessive cell death resulting in the destruction of healthy cells is often associated with neurodegenerative disorders. Conversely, too little cell death is suspected to be partly responsible for the uncontrolled proliferation of cancer cells and the failure of auto-immune cells to be eliminated from the circulation contributing to diseases such as arthritis, multiple sclerosis, and lupus erythematosus. It therefore follows that tight control of the apoptotic machinery is absolutely critical for cellular survival. Realization in the mid-1980s that cells die by an active process that is genetically defined, changed not only our views on cell death and survival but led to a whole new discipline of biological study with significant implications for medicine. Indeed, several decades of research devoted to mechanisms of programmed cell death (PCD) have identified a large number of genes and pathways that control and influence, either positively or negatively, the progression of apoptosis from the initial death trigger to the final demise of a cell. Apoptosis research has advanced our understanding of a basic cellular biology, shed insight into many diseases, and is poised to affect the future practice of medicine by the introduction of rationally designed drugs targeting the apoptotic process.

The original anatomical characteristics of apoptosis were noted in the nineteenth century. However, it was not until publications in 1951 and in the 1960s, describing developmental cell death or shrinkage necrosis, in which the PCD concept was recognized, reintroduced, and formalized. The term apoptosis was coined in 1972, referring to this morphological form of cell death. The PCD concept did not, however, take hold until seminal studies performed by Horvitz and colleagues in the early 1980s demonstrated the molecular underpinnings of this process in the nematode, *C. elegans*. These discoveries recently were recognized with the awarding of the 2002 Nobel Prize in Physiology or Medicine to Sidney Brenner, John E. Sulston, and H. Robert Horvitz.

Apoptosis is characterized by the orderly dismantling of a cell without maintenance of plasma membrane integrity, displaying features listed in Table 18.1, and is distinct from an extreme type of cell death known as necrosis, that is characterized by disruption of the plasma cell membrane. In necrosis, loss of cellular plasma membrane

Table 18.1 Distinguishing Features of Apoptosis and Necrosis

	Apoptosis	Necrosis
Physiological/Pathological Features		
Cellular role	Normal	Abnormal, accidental
Process	Active, energy-dependent	Passive, results from lack of energy
Distribution	Dispersed, affection of individual cells	Contiguous, massive affection of tissue areas
Triggers	Various physiological and noxious stimuli, and during development	Severe stress, specific toxins, or ATP depletion
Induction	Slow (hours), stochastic	Rapid (seconds, minutes)
Tissue inflammation	Absent	Present
Cell removal	Rapid and discrete	Slow
Morphological features		
Cellular membranes	Preserved integrity, blebbing of intact plasma membrane	Loss of integrity, with extrusion of cell constituents
Cell volume	Decreased, as well as the formation of small, fragmented apoptotic bodies or inclusions	Increased
Organelles	Preserved	Swelling of nucleus and other organelles
Chromatin	Condensation (e.g., pyknotic nuclei)	
Biochemical and Molecular Features		
Mitochondrial permeability transition	Moderate	Severe
Mitochondrial membrane potential (delta psi-m)	Transient collapse	Permanent collapse
Requirement for ATP	Yes	No
Membrane phospholipid asymmetry	Exteriorization of phosphatidylserine from inner to outer leaflet of plasma membrane	
Cell pH	Acidification	
DNA cleavage	Initial specific large cleavage products of 50 kbp, then followed by internucleosomal cleavage leading to DNA ladder pattern of 180 bp unit repeats	Random DNA cleavage
Caspase dependence	Yes	No

integrity promotes an inflammatory response, whereas in apoptosis, preservation of plasma membrane integrity enables cells to be discretely phagocytosed without promoting an inflammatory response. Necrosis occurs in severe circumstances, such as stroke, blunt trauma, frost bite, or exposure to certain toxins, that rupture the plasma membrane or severely compromise the energy-producing respiratory process of a cell. The normal physiological route to cell death is, under most circumstances, apoptosis. Only under extreme conditions, when the cell is irreparably damaged and therefore cannot commit apoptosis, does the cell die by necrosis. Necrosis is a medically undesired form of cell death because the ensuing inflammatory response causes secondary cell death and tissue damage. For example, the acute use of high-dose steroid therapy to suppress inflammation in spinal cord injury has led to improvements in neurological outcomes by suppressing some of this secondary cell death. Arguments for a physiological and potentially beneficial role of necrosis have also been made.

18.2 MECHANISM AND REGULATION OF PCD

18.2.1 Pathways of PCD

There exist multiple cellular pathways triggering apoptosis, two of which, the extrinsic and intrinsic pathways, are the best studied (Figure 18.1). Both of these cell death pathways culminate in the activation of a proteolytic cascade involving a family of proteases, the caspases. The extrinsic pathway (e.g., receptor mediated) is initiated by an external stimulus (ligand) that acts on a membrane-bound receptor. An example of this pathway is activation of the Fas receptor by the Fas ligand, resulting in recruitment of the death-inducing signaling complex (DISC) on the cytoplasmic side of the Fas receptor. This leads to the recruitment and activation of caspase-8 and subsequent generation of active caspase-3, that ultimately results in cell death. In contrast, the intrinsic pathway(s) (e.g., mitochondria mediated) responds to various cellular stresses and some developmental apoptotic triggers that result in the release of cytochrome *c* from the mitochondria to the cytoplasm where it binds to a pro-apoptotic protein Apaf-1, resulting in the ATP-dependent oligomerization of Apaf-1 into a structure named the apoptosome. Apoptosomes further recruit and activate caspase-9 followed by activation of caspase-3.

In addition to cytochrome *c*, other factors such as apoptosis inducing factor (AIF), endonuclease G, and second mitochondria-derived activator of caspases (Smac/DIABLO) may also be released from the inter-mitochondrial membrane space to exert their pro-apoptotic effects (see later). Recently, the endoplasmic reticulum (ER) has been identified as another organelle that can initiate the intrinsic apoptotic cascade in response to cellular stress. The ER is essential for proper

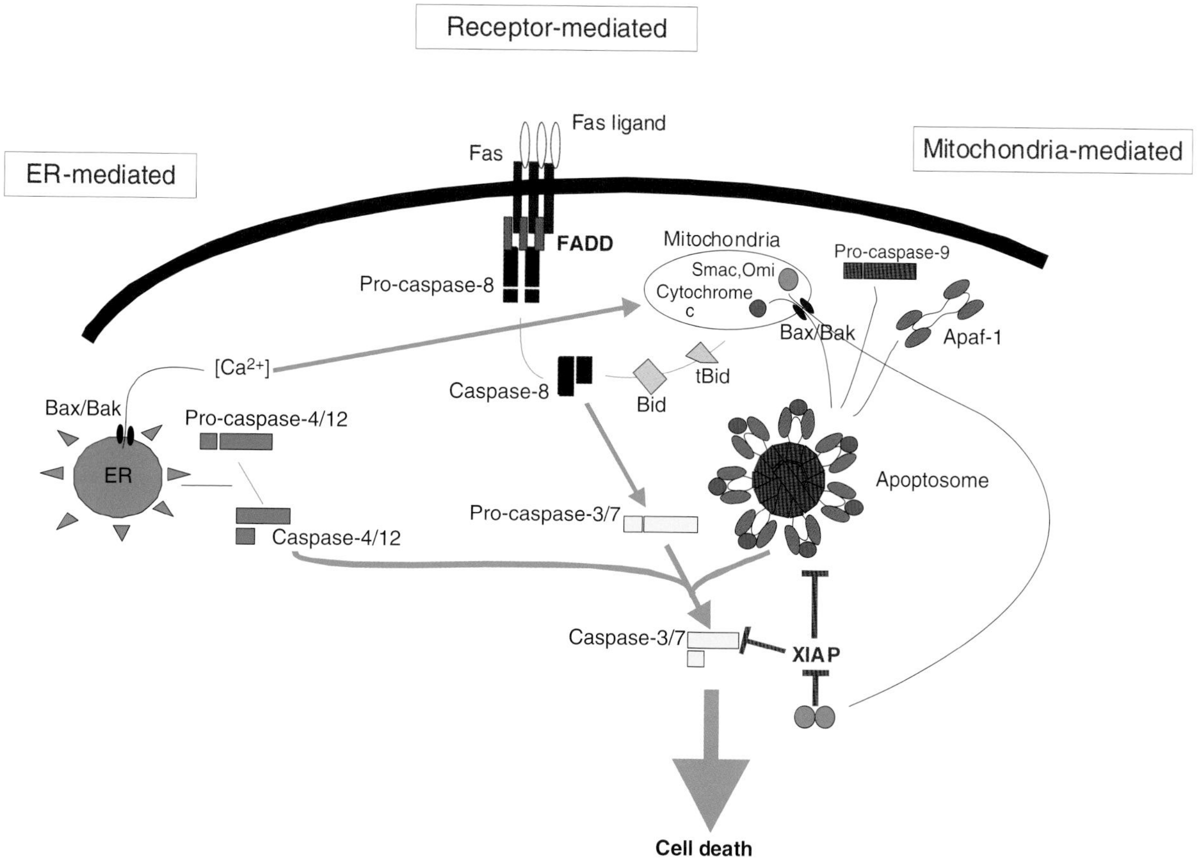

Figure 18.1 All known apoptotic signals converge on caspases that create a self-amplifying cascade. Apoptotic triggers can be either external or internal, and evoke distinct cellular responses. Intracellular stress (such as DNA damage) results in activation of the mitochondrial, or intrinsic, pathway. This pathway is characterized by cytochrome c release, formation of the apoptosome, and caspase-9 activation. Endoplasmic reticulum (ER) stress results in the activation of an ER-specific pathway as well as the mitochondria-dependent pathway. The ER-specific pathway activates caspase-12 (or a similar caspase in humans) and/or caspase-4 and, subsequently, caspase-3. Extracellular ligand binding to death receptors triggers the extrinsic pathways that can either directly result in activation of the caspases, or require further amplification through the mitochondrial pathway (dashed arrow), depending on the cell type. All apoptotic signaling pathways converge at the level of effector caspases, such as caspase-3 and -7. Multiple control points exist along these pathways, regulating either the release of cytochrome c and other apoptogenic factors from the mitochondria (by Bcl-2 family proteins such as Bax and Bak), or by regulating the levels or activity of caspase inhibitors, the inhibitors of apoptosis (IAPs, such as XIAP), through their antagonists (such as Smac/DIABLO or HtrA2/Omi) or through other regulatory mechanisms. Green lines represent positive, and red line the negative regulation. (Adapted from Holcik, M. (2004). Targeting endogenous inhibitors of apoptosis for treatment of cancer, stroke and multiple sclerosis. *Expert. Opin. Ther. Targets* **8**: 241–253.)

protein folding and the introduction of posttranslational modifications. As such, the ER is exquisitely sensitive to perturbations in cellular homeostasis triggered by different stimuli, that results in the induction of a stress response known as the unfolded protein response (UPR). The UPR is characterized by reduction of global protein synthesis and specific upregulation of stress-response genes such as ATF4 or BiP. The role of UPR is to protect cells from ER stress. Indeed, failure to alleviate this stress leads to the activation of apoptotic pathway(s) and cell death. Recent evidence suggests that there exists an ER-specific apoptotic pathway in which caspase-12 is activated in response to ER stress. Activation of caspase-12 leads to the activation of downstream caspase-9 and caspase-3, forming a caspase cascade analogous to the mitochondria-induced pathway. It is not clear, however, which caspase functions as an initiator caspase during the ER stress in human cells as caspase-12 is nonfunctional in most, but not all, humans.

18.2.2 Caspases

It is well understood that caspases are critical for the process of apoptosis. Caspases are cysteinyl-containing active center proteases with specificity for protein cleavage after aspartyl residues. Thus the term caspase is derived from *c*ysteinyl-containing *asp*artate-specific protein*ase*. The caspases are responsible for many of the hallmarks of apoptosis defined in Table 18.1, mediated through their cleavage of specific polypeptide substrates. The caspases (e.g., caspase-2, -3, -6, -7, -8, -9, -10, and -12 in the mouse) are not the only proteases involved in PCD, as calpains have also been shown to play a role, particularly in forms of death triggered by calcium overload within the cell. Caspases are, however, the prime effectors of apoptosis and promote apoptosis by cleaving a large number of cellular targets. Caspases are synthesized as inactive zymogens that are proteolyticaly processed to produce mature, active proteases. In addition, caspases are arranged into a cascade such that the upstream caspases (initiator caspases, such as caspase-9) activate downstream caspases (effector caspases, such as caspase-2, -3 and -7). Note that not all caspases are involved in apoptosis, and that certain caspases are involved in the processing of pro-inflammatory cytokines (e.g., caspase-1, -4, -5, -11) (Figure 18.2). In addition, certain caspases may play highly specific roles in normal cell differentiation and maturation, such as the enucleation of red blood cells, formation of lens cells of the eye, platelet formation from megakaryocytes, or in blast phase activation of lymphocytes, apparently without inducing apoptosis.

18.2.3 Activation of Caspases

Caspases exist within the cell as inactive zymogens, and their activation is controlled primarily by two distinct mechanisms involving protein–protein interactions within large complexes and proximity-induced processing of the caspases. One mechanism involves generation of the DISC, the death-inducing signaling complex, that is formed by the trimerization of plasma membrane death receptors upon binding of death ligands, such as TNFalpha or TRAIL, and the recruitment of adaptor molecules and caspases such as caspase-8 or -10 to the cytoplasmic portion of the death receptors. This induced proximity then allows for activation of the apical caspase, that can then in turn activate downstream effector caspases. The second mechanism involves the release of apoptogenic factors from the mitochondria, particularly cytochrome c, that results in the formation of the apoptosome, a large helical complex of apaf-1, cytochrome c, and caspase-9. This complex formation allows the proximity-induced activation of the apical caspase-9 that can then activate downstream effector caspases such as -3 and -7 by cleaving them. The intrinsic and extrinsic death pathways do not exist in isolation; there is crosstalk between them, and feed-forward circuits enabling exquisite regulation and rapid amplification of these two important pathways for cell death. In addition, other pathways and mechanisms for caspase activation have been described but are less well understood. A third characterized pathway of caspase activation is specific to cytotoxic T-cell mediated cell death. In this form of cell death, introduction of serine proteases, known as granzymes into the cytoplasm directly activates the caspase cascade by cleavage of the caspases at sites that activate them.

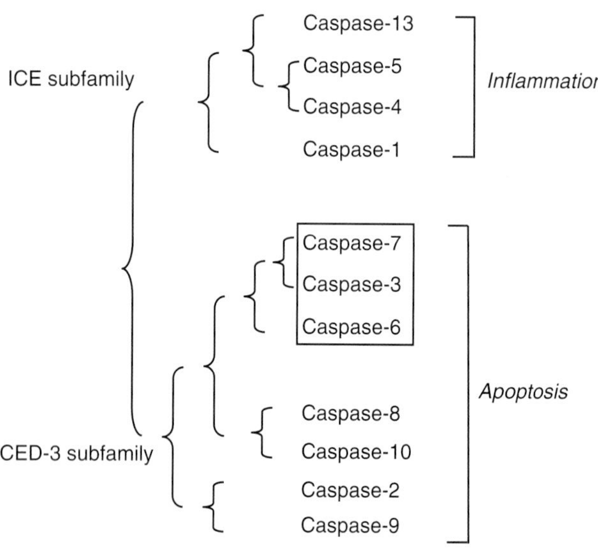

Figure 18.2 Phylogenetic analysis segregates the human caspases into two major subfamilies, one based on caspase-1 previously referred to as ICE, for interleukin-converting enzyme, and the other based on similarities to the *C. elegans* cell death gene, *ced-3*. Further classification of the caspases is possible: into those that mediate cytokine maturation that are involved in inflammation, those with a short prodomain involved in the effector phase of apoptosis (shown boxed), and those with a long prodomain that are involved in the initiator phase of apoptosis (not boxed). Note evolutionary distances are not accurately represented in this dendrogram. (Adapted from Nicholson, D.W. (1999). Caspase structure, proteolytic substrates, and function during apoptotic cell death. *Cell Death Differ* **6**: 1028–1042.)

18.2.4 Apoptosis Inhibitors

Since the cell is armed with elaborate mechanisms of self-destruction composed of inactive zymogens that can be rapidly activated by numerous stressors or triggers, these mechanisms must remain under tight control. Opposing the cellular destruction by caspases are two classes of cellular apoptotic inhibitors—members of the B-cell lymphoma 2 (Bcl-2) and inhibitor of apoptosis (IAP) gene families—that can completely block or at least significantly delay the execution of apoptosis. To maintain the life/death balance in the cell these anti-apoptotic factors are themselves controlled by several different mechanisms, including transcriptional and posttranscriptional regulation of gene expression, translational control of protein expression, as well as interactions with other proteins that control their activity by phosphorylation, proteolysis, and ubiquitin-mediated protein degradation. Thus within the cell there exist highly regulated and structured machinery to either induce or suppress cell death. The dynamics between these opposing forces that control the final life-or-death decision of a single cell is currently the focus of an enormous amount of basic and clinical research.

18.2.4.1 The Inhibitors of Apoptosis, IAPs

The Inhibitor of Apoptosis proteins are a family of intrinsic regulators of programmed cell death and are of particular interest since they are the most powerful inhibitors of cell death and could potentially be used for therapeutic intervention. IAPs were initially described in baculoviruses, where their role is to block the apoptotic response initiated as a defense mechanism in response to viral infection. The homologues of viral IAPs were soon discovered in metazoan species including *Caenorhabditis elegans*, yeast, *Drosophila*, and vertebrates. There are at present eight mammalian IAPs (Figure 18.3). IAPs are potent inhibitors of apoptosis induced by a variety of triggers both *in vitro* and *in vivo* by virtue of their ability to bind and inhibit distinct caspases. IAPs are the only endogenous inhibitors that block both initiator and effector caspases.

The IAP proteins are defined by a ~80 amino acid zinc finger motif called BIR (Baculovirus IAP Repeat). In fact, any protein that contained the BIR domain was considered to be an IAP. Reexamination of the BIR domains, however, identified differences in the BIR domains and, more importantly, in the function(s) of the IAP proteins carrying distinct BIR domain subtypes. Thus, a new subgroup of IAP proteins was identified as BIR domain containing proteins (BIRP) that include Bruce, survivin, as well as yeast and *C. elegans* BIR-containing proteins. Interestingly, these IAPs regulate mitotic spindle formation and cytokinesis.

The number of BIR domains in a given IAP is variable, ranging from one to three, but they are invariably present in the amino-terminus of the protein and mediate the interaction with caspases. Several, but not all, IAPs also contain a carboxyl-terminal RING (*r*eally *i*nteresting *n*ew *g*ene) zinc finger, that has E3 ubiquitin ligase activity. This modular structure of IAPs is reflected in their multifunctionality. In addition to regulating apoptosis, IAPs also play a role in other important cellular processes including receptor-mediated signaling, cell cycle, and ubiquitination.

The Mechanism of IAP Action The best characterized IAP is the X-chromosome linked IAP, XIAP, that is often used as a prototype for other IAPs in terms of mechanism of action. The initial genetic evidence implied that the BIR domains are essential for the caspase inhibitory function of XIAP since they directly bind to distinct caspases. XIAP inhibits both the initiator caspase-9 and the effector caspases-3 and -7. *In vitro* kinetic studies have shown that XIAP is the most potent caspase inhibitor in the IAP family, with K_i values of 0.2 to 0.8 nM as compared to the 1 to 20 nM range for other members of the IAP family. The caspases-3 and -7 inhibiting activity of XIAP is localized to the linker region that precedes BIR2 domain. It was shown that the isolated BIR3 domain is sufficient to potently inhibit caspase-9. Furthermore, although the three-dimensional structure of BIR2 and BIR3 of XIAP indicated that these two domains are quite similar, different sets of amino acid residues were found to be critical for the inhibition of distinct caspases. Structural data also support the concept that XIAP inhibits initiator and effector caspases by different means, and shed light on the mechanism of caspase binding and inhibition by discrete BIR domains of XIAP.

The crystal structure of caspase-7 in complex with the inhibitory fragment of XIAP (amino acid residues 124-240) shows the XIAP peptide binding to the catalytic groove of caspase-7, thus completely filling the active site and preventing the entry of other substrates. A similar structural arrangement was found between XIAP and caspase-3 (Figure 18.4). This observation is not surprising considering that caspase-3 and caspase-7 share 54% sequence identity and have nearly identical backbone structures. Despite the fact that XIAP does not share a sequence motif in common with natural caspase substrates, the physical interaction between caspases-3 and -7 and XIAP are similar to that

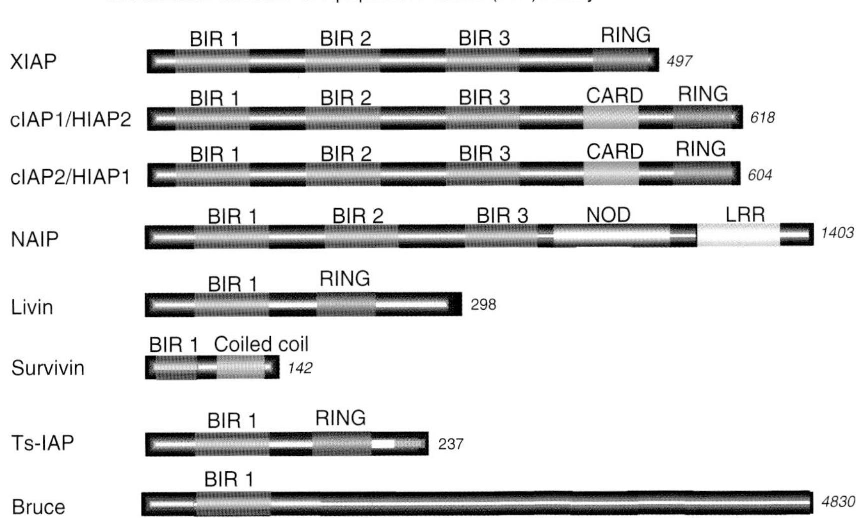

Figure 18.3 The mammalian IAP family. The distinct domains are shown for each IAP. (BIR—baculovirus IAP repeat; CARD—caspase activation recruitment domain; RING—really interesting new gene zinc finger; LRR—leucine rich repeat; NOD—nucleotide-binding oligomerization domain).

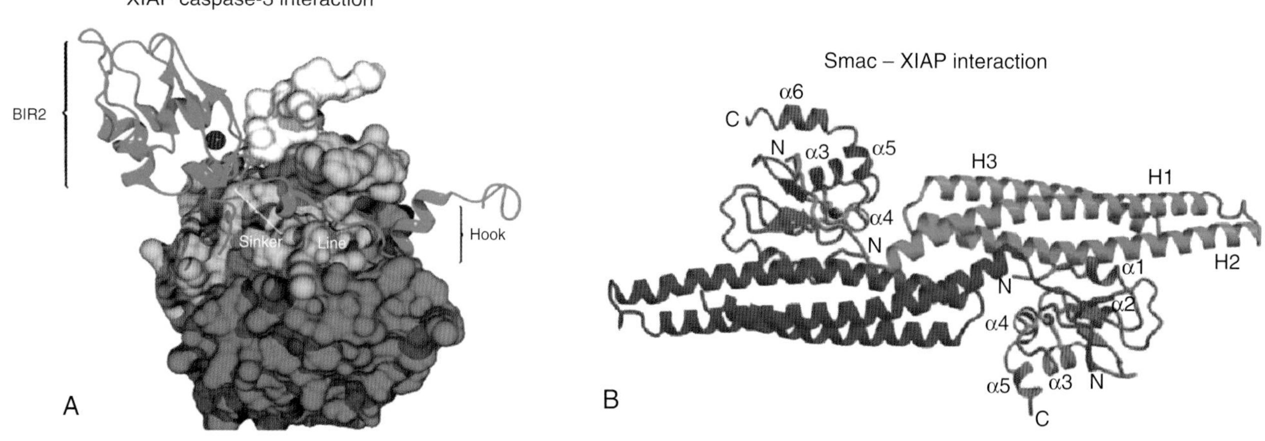

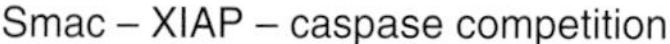

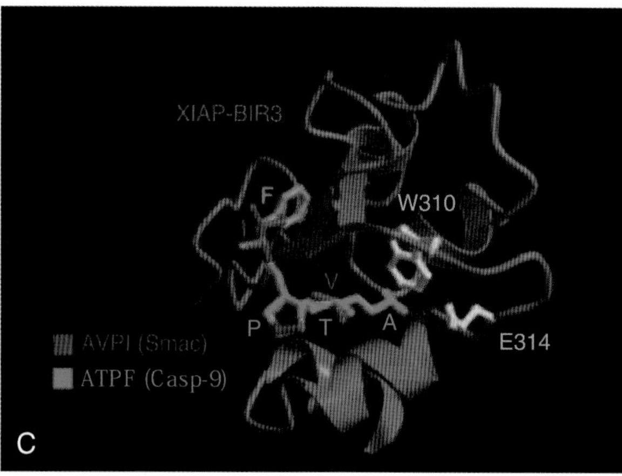

Figure 18.4 Key structural elements underlying the regulation of caspase activity by IAPs. A. Structural details of the contact between caspase 3 (dark and light blue) with XIAP BIR2 (green) in caspase-inhibited form. Distinct regions of the XIAP BIR2 linker region termed sinker, line, and hook are identified. (From Riedl et al. (2001). Structural basis for the inhibition of caspase-3 by XIAP. *Cell* **104**: 791–800; Figure 2A.) B. Interaction of Smac with XIAP BIR3. Ribbon representation of the complete structure of two Smac protomers (green and blue) with two BIR3 domains (pink and orange). Smac protomer utilizes the exposed N terminus to bind to BIR 3. (From Wu et al. (2000). Structural basis of IAP recognition by Smac/DIABLO. *Nature* **408**: 1008–1012, Figure 1B.) C. The XIAP inhibitory tetrapeptide motif (AVPI in Smac (red) or ATPF in caspase-9 (green)) binds to the same region of XIAP BIR3 (pink) in a competitive fashion. Thus, binding of Smac to XIAP BIR3 precludes binding and inhibition of caspases-9 by XIAP. (From Srinivasula, S. M. et al. (2001). A conserved XIAP-interaction motif in caspase-9 and Smac/DIABLO regulates caspase activity and apoptosis. *Nature* **410**: 112–116, Figure 5A.)

of other caspases and the synthetic tetrapeptide inhibitor DEVD-CHO. Interestingly, however, the binding of XIAP is antiparallel to the binding of most other caspase substrates. This allows the XIAP-caspase interaction to be reversible.

The caspase-interacting residues are conserved between XIAP and two other IAP proteins, human inhibitor of apoptosis-1 (cIAP1or HIAP2) and human inhibitor of apoptosis-2 (cIAP2 or HIAP1), that also inhibit the effector caspases-3 and -7. However, these critical residues are not found in the baculoviral inhibitor of apoptosis repeat-2 (BIR2) domain itself but in the short linker region that precedes BIR2. In fact, the BIR2 domain itself is dispensable and can be replaced with an unrelated protein such as GST (glutathione *S*-transferase). The BIR2 domain has been proposed to stabilize the interaction between XIAP and caspases inhibited by this protein and may mediate interactions with other IAP-binding proteins (see later).

A unique feature of the IAPs is that they inhibit both effector and initiator caspases. The mechanism, however, by which XIAP inhibits the initiator caspase-9 is fundamentally different from that used to inhibit the effector caspases-3 and -7. Genetic studies identified the BIR3 domain of XIAP as being solely responsible for the inhibition of caspase-9. Interestingly, XIAP binds only to processed caspase-9, not to the inactive procaspase-9. Autocatalytic processing of procaspase-9 at Asp315 (following recruitment of procaspase-9 to oligomerized Apaf-1 within the apoptosome) was found to liberate the p12 subunit of caspase-9 with a "new" free amino-terminus that directly interacts with the BIR3 domain of XIAP. Deletion or mutagenesis of the amino-terminal four residues of the p12 subunit

(Ala-Thr-Pro-Phe) of caspase-9 abolished binding to XIAP. Furthermore, when the amino terminal sequence of processed caspase-3 (which does not normally interact with XIAP BIR3) was changed to that of processed caspase-9, it then exhibited strong binding to XIAP BIR3, demonstrating that the tetrapeptide sequence of processed caspase-9 confers specificity for the BIR3 domain of XIAP.

Data from pull-down experiments suggests that XIAP associates with the apoptosome. In this complex, XIAP interacts with both caspase-9 and caspase-3 and it was proposed that the role of XIAP is not only to prevent activation of caspase-3 by caspase-9 but also to prevent caspase-3 release from the apoptosome. Since each caspase interacts with a different BIR domain of XIAP—specifically, caspase-3 and caspase-7 with BIR2 and caspase-9 with BIR3—the task of dual inhibition can be achieved more efficiently by one, rather than two proteins.

Although the BIR2 and BIR3 domains of IAPs bind to their respective caspases in a structurally different way, the interaction and subsequent caspase inhibition is, in both cases, reversible. This is in contrast to the broad-spectrum baculoviral caspase inhibitor protein p35, that does not discriminate among caspases and acts as a suicide inhibitor by forming a covalent thioester linkage with the target caspase. The structural difference between IAP- and p35-mediated caspase inhibition is probably explained by their different biological functions. p35 functions as an apoptotic OFF switch, blocking apoptosis that was triggered in response to viral infection (and is therefore designed to block virus multiplication). In contrast, IAPs are intrinsic caspase inhibitors that block initiation of the caspase cascade in response to divergent extra- and intracellular stimuli. By functioning more as a rheostat than an on/off switch to adjust the cellular apoptotic threshold, the reversibility of IAP-caspase interaction therefore allows fine-tuning of the cellular response to stimuli that may trigger apoptosis.

Regulation of IAPs Given the critical role IAPs play in the control of caspases it is not surprising that their expression and/or activity are controlled at multiple levels. So far, three distinct modes of IAP regulation—transcriptional/posttranscriptional, posttranslational, and regulatory proteins—have been described (Figure 18.5).

Transcriptional/Posttranscriptional Control Some IAPs proteins are subject to transcriptional control either during the cell cycle or by the stress-inducible transcriptional activator NF-κB.

In addition, some IAPs are translated by a cap-independent mechanism of translation. The majority of cellular mRNAs are translated by a so-called cap-dependent ribosome scanning mechanism. The m^7G-cap structure that is added in the nucleus onto the 5′ end of each newly synthesized mRNA is specifically recognized by a cap-binding protein, eukaryotic initiation factor eIF4E. The binding of eIF4E further facilitates binding of additional factors, ultimately forming an initiation complex and commencing translation of a given mRNA. In contrast, however, a relatively small number of cellular mRNAs are translated by a cap-independent mechanism of translation that is mediated by a specific RNA structure called IRES (Internal Ribosome Entry Site). Importantly, IRES-mediated translation escapes some of the control mechanisms that regulate cap-dependent translation. Therefore the translation of IRES-containing mRNAs can continue under conditions when cap-dependent translation is suppressed or attenuated. This is of particular importance during conditions of cellular stress, including apoptosis that frequently results in the inhibition of protein synthesis. Thus, the concept was proposed that selective regulation of IRES-mediated translation is critical to the regulation of cell death and survival.

Two IAPs, XIAP and cIAP1/HIAP2, contain IRES elements in their respective 5′ UTRs, and are translated by an IRES-mediated mechanism. Both XIAP and cIAP1/HIAP2 have been shown to be upregulated (as assessed by increasing the rate of translation of their mRNAs) in response to stress. However, the specific triggers that stimulate XIAP or cIAP1/HIAP2 IRES are distinct for each IAP. XIAP (and its IRES) is upregulated in response to serum starvation, low dose gamma irradiation, anoxia, and treatment of cells with FGF2 and IL-6. In contrast, activity of the cIAP1/HIAP2 IRES increases in response to ER stress, treatment with etoposide, and sodium arsenate. It has been proposed that the unique stress response of each IRES is mediated by specific RNA binding proteins, termed IRES trans-acting factors (ITAFs) that bind to XIAP and cIAP1/HIAP2 IRES elements. Indeed, the subsets of XIAP and cIAP1/HIAP2 ITAFs are distinct and include both hnRNPC1/C2 and the autoantigen La for XIAP and p97/DAP5 for cIAP1/HIAP2.

The regulation of XIAP and cIAP1/HIAP2 expression at the translational level is an important mechanism for rapid response to transient cellular stress. The fact that XIAP and cIAP1/HIAP2 translation is responsive to different stress signals also suggests that there are distinct pathways and/or proteins involved in the IRES-mediated translation of each of these proteins.

Posttranslational Control As mentioned previously, in addition to the obligatory BIR domain, several IAPs also contain a RING motif, typically at the C-terminus of the protein. This RING domain of XIAP, cIAP2/HIAP1, cIAP1/HIAP2, and Livin contain an E3 ubiquitin ligase (or a chimeric E2/E3 ligase in case of Bruce) activity that targets either themselves or other cellular proteins for ubiquitylation and subsequent proteosome-mediated degradation or altered cellular locations or functions. Ubiquitylation of proteins is now recognized as one of the main regulatory mechanisms that affects protein half-life in eukaryotic cells. The process of ubiquitylation utilizes concerted action of four enzymes known as E1, E2, E3, an E4 that conjugate the 76-amino-acid ubiquitin peptide to a protein substrate, thereby targeting it for proteosomal degradation and other cellular functions, such as signal transduction. The E3 ligases determine the target specificity of the ubiquitylation process.

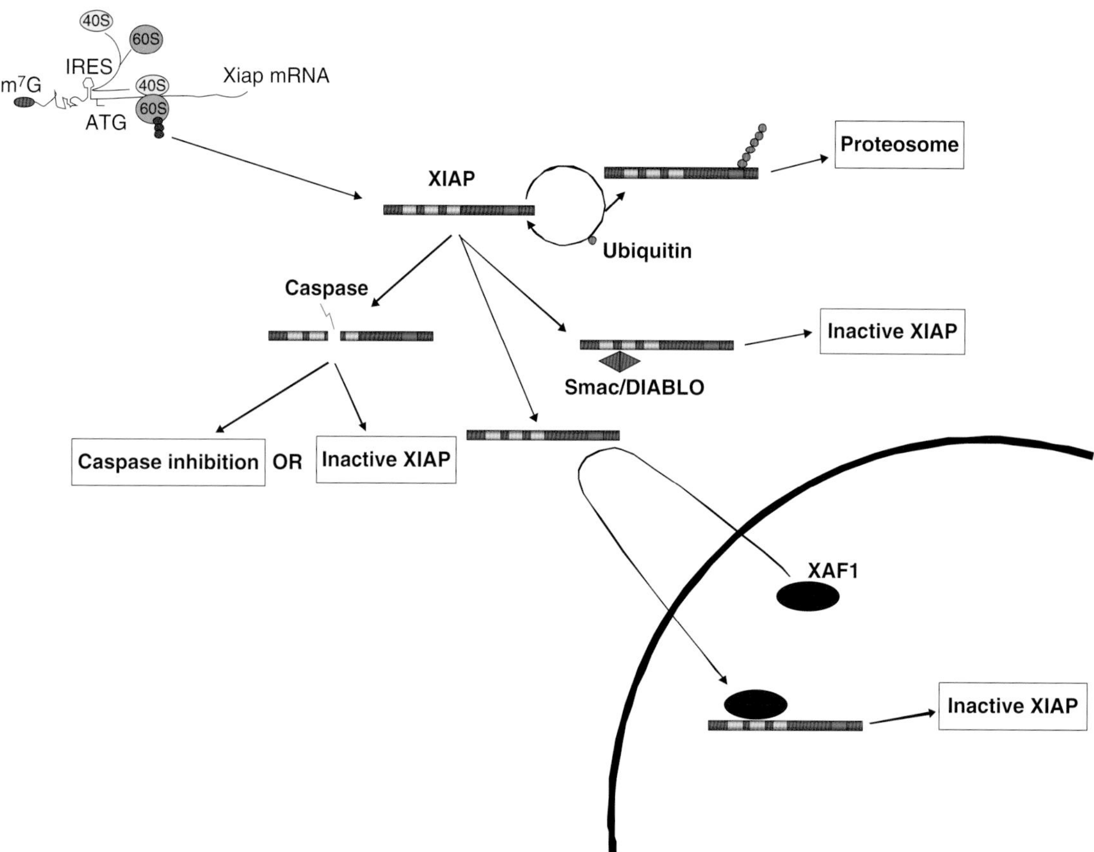

Figure 18.5 XIAP expression is regulated on different levels. The translation of XIAP mRNA is facilitated via an IRES element located in the 5′ UTR and is resistant to cellular stress. The levels of XIAP protein can be upregulated in response to low-dose γ irradiation or serum deprivation. The C-terminal RING zinc finger domain of XIAP possess E3 ubiquitin ligase activity that is involved in the auto-ubiquitination of XIAP and its targeting for removal in the proteosome. XIAP can also be specifically cleaved by caspases following apoptotic trigger in T lymphocytes, giving rise to two discreet fragments. The caspase-generated XIAP fragments retain their caspase-inhibiting activity, but they could also be targeted for proteolytic degradation. The activated Smac/DIABLO protein interacts with the BIR domains of XIAP and inactivates its caspase inhibiting activity. Another XIAP-binding protein, XAF1, facilitates translocation of cytoplasmic XIAP into the nucleus and neutralizes XIAP caspase-inhibiting activity. (Adapted from Holcik et al. XIAP: Apoptotic brake and promising therapeutic target. *Apoptosis* **6**: 253–261.)

Several targets of the IAP RING have been described. However, given the large number of E2s to which IAPs can recruit potential target proteins and given the diversity of ubiquitylation processes (mono-, multi-mono-, and poly-ubiquitylation) a comprehensive picture of the role of E3 ligase function of the IAPs still eludes us. Critically, however, pro-apoptotic proteins such as caspase-3, caspase-9, Reaper, and Smac are all targets of IAP-mediated degradation. Conversely, some of the IAP antagonists, such as Smac or GSPT1/eRF3, can promote autoubiquitylation and degradation of XIAP and cIAPs/HIAPs. In addition, it has emerged recently that IAPs can also regulate their abundance. For example, deletion of the cIAP1 gene resulted in marked elevation of cIAP2/HIAP1 protein levels without a concomitant increase in cIAP2/HIAP1 mRNA. Further investigation of this phenomenon revealed that cIAP2/HIAP1 is a direct target for cIAP1/HIAP2-mediated ubiquitylation and subsequent degradation. In addition, this process is enhanced by the adaptor function of the tumor necrosis factor receptor (TNFR) associated factor 2 (TRAF2). Thus, the cIAPs/HIAPs represent a pair of TNFR-associated ubiquitin protein ligases in which one regulates the expression of the other by a posttranscriptional and E3-dependent mechanism.

IAP Regulatory Proteins By far the most interesting and intricate regulation of IAP activity is by the IAP-binding proteins. The first such protein was discovered in mitochondria and termed Smac or DIABLO. Binding of Smac/DIABLO to IAPs disrupts the binding of IAPs to caspases and promotes apoptosis. Smac/DIABLO is synthesized as a precursor protein that is targeted into the mitochondria where its 55 amino acid NH_2-terminal targeting sequence is removed. The cleavage of the targeting sequence is essential for the pro-apoptotic role of Smac/DIABLO since it exposes a tetra-peptide sequence (Ala-Val-Pro-Ile) that is critical for Smac/DIABLO binding to IAPs. Mature Smac/DIABLO is released from mitochondria together with cytochrome *c* during mitochondria-induced apoptosis and has been shown *in vitro* to interact with several of the IAP proteins including XIAP, cIAP1/HIAP2, cIAP2/HIAP1, and survivin. The structural basis of the Smac/DIABLO interaction with XIAP has recently been elucidated and provides new insight into the regulation of the apoptotic process that is applicable to other IAPs as well. In addition, Smac/DIABLO connects, for the first time, IAPs with mitochondria controlled cell death.

Smac/DIABLO interacts with both the BIR2 and BIR3 domains of XIAP. The crystal structure of Smac/DIABLO revealed that it forms a homodimer via a large hydrophobic interface and that this homodimerization is essential for its binding to the BIR2, but not BIR3, domain of XIAP (Figure 18.4). The four amino-terminal residues of Smac/DIABLO (Ala-Val-Pro-Ile) make specific contact with a surface groove of the BIR2 and BIR3 domains, but not the BIR1 domain, of XIAP. Significantly, the conserved tetrapeptide motif has remarkable homology to the IAP-interacting motif found in the p12 amino-terminal sequence of caspase-9 (Ala-Thr-Pro-Phe) and the *Drosophila* proteins Hid (Ala-Val-Pro-Phe), Reaper (Ala-Val-Ala-Phe), and Grim (Ala-Ile-Ala-Tyr). Although Smac/DIABLO, by overall primary sequence structure is not a homologue of these *Drosophila* proteins, it clearly acts as their functional analogue. Indeed, an entire new class of proteins has now been described that harbors this IAP-binding motif (IBM) that regulates IAP functions. This family of proteins includes for example the mammalian proteins Smac/DIABLO, Omi/HtrA2, and *Drosophila* Hid, Reaper, Grim, Sickle, and Jafrac2. Remarkably, the fact that the processing of caspase-9 exposes the IAP-interacting motif suggests that this new class of proteins could be activated by caspases or other cellular proteases. If this is in fact the case, it would add a new dimension to the control and regulation of apoptosis.

The relieving of caspase-3/-7 inhibition by XIAP is mechanistically different and has been suggested to play a role in the sensitization of type II cells that are typically resistant to death receptor-induced apoptosis. Since XIAP binds caspase-3/-7 via its linker region, this binding does not involve the BIR2 domain, that is then free to bind Smac/DIABLO. The binding of Smac/DIABLO to XIAP is proposed to destabilize the XIAP/caspase interaction by steric hindrance that results in the disruption of the XIAP/caspase complex. In addition, the binding of Smac/DIABLO to the BIR2 domain of XIAP results in a conformational change in XIAP that leads to decreased affinity of XIAP for caspase-3/-7.

Interestingly, Smac/DIABLO can bind to only one BIR at a time and monomeric Smac/DIABLO does not interact with BIR2, only with BIR3. If these restrictions also exist *in vivo*, it would suggest additional mechanisms exist that regulate Smac/DIABLO-XIAP interactions. Furthermore, Smac/DIABLO displays a pro-apoptotic activity that is independent of its amino-terminal tetrapeptide sequence. The basis of this mechanism, that is likely independent of the binding to IAPs, remains unclear.

Two other proteins, XIAP associated factor 1 (XAF1) and neurotrophin receptor-interacting MAGE homolog (NRAGE) that modulate IAP activity but utilize different mechanism than Smac were also identified. XAF1 is a seven zinc-finger containing protein and was found to antagonize the ability of XIAP to suppress caspase activity and cell death *in vitro*. There are no structural data available on the mechanism of this inhibition and the interacting domains of XIAP and XAF1 have not yet been identified. In contrast to Smac/DIABLO, XAF1 does not need to be processed and appears to be constitutively able to interact with and inhibit XIAP. Significantly, XAF1 expression is low or missing in the majority of tumor cell lines, suggesting that XAF1 is a tumor suppressor. NRAGE was recently identified as an IAP-binding protein that requires the RING domain of IAP for this interaction. The mechanism of NRAGE inhibition of XIAP is not known. However, its binding to XIAP is inducible following growth-factor deprivation perhaps functioning through an inactivation/sequestration mechanism.

18.2.4.2 Bcl-2 Family

The members of the Bcl-2 family of pro- or anti-apoptotic proteins are critical regulators of cell death induced by distinct apoptotic triggers. Unlike the IAPs, Bcl-2 proteins are not direct caspase inhibitors but regulate pivotal steps leading to caspase activation (e.g., Bax, Bak, Bid) (Figure 18.1). Members of the Bcl-2 family are typified by the presence of a variable number of conserved domains termed Bcl-2 homology domains (BH domain; Figure 18.6). The role of these structural motifs is to support homodimeric and heterodimeric interactions between various members of this family, enabling the function of these proteins. Bcl-2 proteins can be divided into two distinct groups—the prosurvival and prodeath groups. The prosurvival members usually contain four BH domains (such as Bcl-2, Bcl-xL, Bcl-W) whereas the prodeath members contain either a variable number of BH domains (such as Bak, Bax, or Bok) or a single BH3 domain (such as Bad, Bid, Bim, Puma, or harakiri). The intricate interplay between various members of the Bcl-2 family members orchestrates a tight control over the intrinsic and, in some cases, extrinsic pathways of cell death.

Mechanisms of Action of Bcl-2 Protein The Bcl-2 proteins execute their effect at the level of mitochondria. Mitochondria are centrally involved in cell death pathways (in particular the intrinsic pathway; Figure 18.1) as they contain several pro-apoptotic factors that are released following recognition of a specific death stimulus by this organelle. Disruption of the outer mitochondrial membrane causes the release of cytochrome c that interacts with Apaf-1 to form caspase-9 activating multiprotein complex termed the apoptosome (see earlier). The release of cytochrome c is an early event during chemically induced apoptotic death that precedes the loss of plasma membrane integrity; it is rapid, complete, and kinetically invariant. Thus, it is generally accepted that the release of cytochrome c from mitochondria is the intracellular signal for apoptosome formation, caspase activation, and cell death.

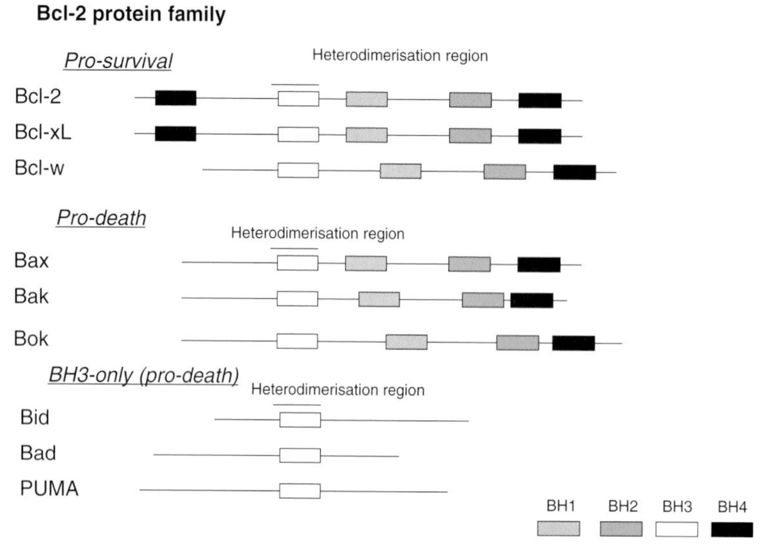

Bcl-2 protein family

Pro-survival — Heterodimerisation region

Bcl-2
Bcl-xL
Bcl-w

Pro-death — Heterodimerisation region

Bax
Bak
Bok

BH3-only (pro-death) — Heterodimerisation region

Bid
Bad
PUMA

BH1 BH2 BH3 BH4

Figure 18.6 The mammalian Bcl-2 protein family. The distinct BH domains are shown for each representative member of the family. In addition, heterodimerization regions are indicated.

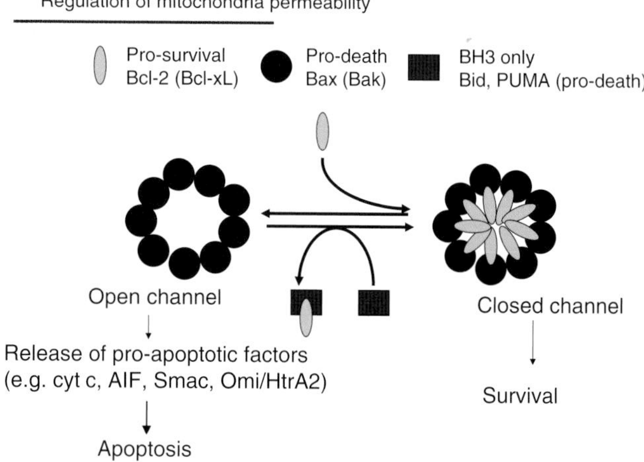

Figure 18.7 A model for regulation of mitochondrial permeability by proteins of the Bcl-2 family. The association of pro-survival and pro-death members will result in the formation of an opened or closed channel resulting in either sequestration or release of pro-apoptotic factors from mitochondria. The BH3-only proteins, such as Bid or PUMA, play a critical role in tipping the balance in favor of cell death.

Additional pro-apoptotic factors that are released from mitochondria are the Apoptosis Inducing Factor (AIF) and the inhibitors of IAPs-Smac/DIABLO and Omi/HtrA2 (see earlier).

The critical step in the initiation of intrinsic apoptosis pathways is the release of cytochrome c from mitochondria. There exist several models for the release of the pro-apoptotic mitochondrial proteins: (1) regulation of an existing pore (such as permeability transition pore, PTP) by Bcl-2 family members; (2) the formation of a channel by Bcl-2 proteins; or (3) oligomerization of apoptotic Bcl-2 family proteins to form a pore through which cytochrome c can be released.

Bcl-2 and Bcl-xL are proposed to modulate the PTP by maintaining it in a closed conformation whereas pro-apoptotic members such as Bax and Bak are thought to promote the opening of the PTP leading to mitochondrial membrane depolarization. In some cases, however, the release of cytochrome c precedes the membrane depolarization, suggesting the PTP is not always necessary for cytochrome c release.

Bcl-xL and Bax are structurally similar to the pore-forming diphtheria toxin and bacterial colicins. Moreover, Bcl-2, Bax, and Bcl-xL can form functional channels or pores in the outer mitochondrial membrane, lipid vesicles and planar lipid membranes supporting the notion that these pores may be utilized for the release of mitochondrial factors (Figure 18.7). Although Bax by itself may be too small to form a large enough pore to allow cytochrome c release, it does oligomerise with Bak to form a larger complex that may be sufficiently large for cytochrome c and other mitochondrial proteins to pass through. For this to occur, Bax must undergo a conformational change and translocation from cytoplasm to the outer mitochondrial membrane. The conformational change of Bax is facilitated by another BH3-only protein tBid. tBid is derived from full length Bid by caspase-3 or -8 cleavage. Once cleaved to tBid, it can interact with Bax resulting in oligomerization and integration into the outer mitochondrial membrane. This creates a pore large enough for cytochrome c to be released into the cytoplasm, promoting activation of the intrinsic cell death pathway. Since tBid is derived from truncation of Bid by caspase-8 (extrinsic pathway), tBid serves as an amplification loop connecting the extrinsic and intrinsic (mitochondrial) death pathways.

18.3 APOPTOSIS IN HEALTH AND DISEASE

18.3.1 Apoptosis in Health

Apoptosis is a normal physiological process that plays a critical role in day-to-day life by maintaining tissue homeostasis through the elimination of defective, infected, or auto-reactive cells. It is estimated that a trillion cells die every two weeks in the average adult human, thus allowing for the continued turnover of tissue, and removal of potentially harmful cells. Certain processes, such as B- and T-cell maturation or spermatogenesis, engender large waves of apoptosis during development to produce a small number of functional cells in the end. For the most part, apoptosis goes unnoticed because of its asynchronous nature (i.e., not all cells are committing suicide at the same time) and the fact that apoptotic cells or bodies are quickly engulfed and digested leaving little trace of these events. Another prime example of normal apoptosis is during morphogenesis, where apoptosis is responsible for the removal of superfluous cells during organ maturation such as the removal of cells that form the interdigital webbing in mammals. Apoptosis also plays remodeling roles in the adult, such as during follicular atresia of the postovulatory follicle, in mammary gland involution postweaning, during atrophy, and in other absorbtive processes. The orderly, noninflammatory removal of unwanted cells is necessary for life of the organism by allowing for tissue turnover and repair and in maintaining optimal cell population size. Depending on the brain region, as many as 50% of the neurons observed at birth fail to make functional connections during development, resulting in removal by apoptosis.

18.3.2 Apoptosis in Disease

The death of cells that causes, or results from, various disease states occurs, for the most part, by the normal route of apoptosis. This has been demonstrated by different means, and for a large number of distinct pathologies. In many diseases, necrosis also is often observed in tandem with apoptosis because the severity of the insult or pathology results in a loss of cellular integrity by shearing forces, or a massive compromise of energy production and osmotic balance that occurs so quickly apoptosis cannot be initiated. The release of cellular contents from necrotic cells leads to an inflammatory response at the site of injury that can cause secondary cell death by apoptosis in the surrounding tissue. Additional apoptotic death may occur in some injury states due to loss of trophic support or cell contact, such as seen in nerve transections. Therefore, the question arises whether cells that are destined to die by apoptosis in acute or chronic pathologies can be saved by inhibiting the apoptotic process. More importantly, if some or most of the cells can be saved by an appropriate intervention, then is the rescued cell completely functional, and not a simple living corpse? These questions are particularly germane to neurodegenerative disorders, such as in stroke and reperfusion injuries, spinal cord trauma, or chronic disorders like Parkinson's or ALS, because of the nondividing properties of a terminally differentiated neuron and the limited regenerative capabilities of the adult brain. The saved neuron would still have to function properly for any benefit to be seen. Indeed, this appears to be possible in proof of principle studies in animal models of neurodegenerative diseases and in cell culture experiments. The overexpression of caspase inhibitors by gene therapy or transgenic approaches, as well as the use of cell permeable small molecule caspase inhibitors, has clearly demonstrated that it is possible to save neurons and to derive functional benefits in some animal models of acute and chronic disorders. It should be noted, however, that it may not be possible to intervene with the execution of cell death if caspase-3 has been fully unleashed. Indeed in some cases, the interventions only delay cell death or show no such benefit at all. This is most likely because the severity of the insult and engagement of nonapoptotic cellular processes such as calpain activation may not be inhibited by an anti-apoptotic therapeutic approach. Nevertheless these highly promising animal studies suggest that it may be possible to limit cell death injury and disease to only those cells that are not too far gone, and if intervention is early enough then one may be able to save cells that will ultimately recover fully. The approach here is one of emergency medicine at a cellular level, that is to treat the life threatening sequelae (block caspases), stabilize the patient's vitals (the cell's mitochondrial respiration), and provide support (e.g., trophic factors) and time for recovery and return of normal biological parameters (e.g., reestablishment of synaptic connections in the case of neurons). Strategies attempting these anti-apoptotic approaches will be discussed in Section 18.4.

Although the inappropriate activation of apoptosis may contribute to neurodegenerative disorders, diabetes, myocardial infarctions, and many other diseases, it is the failure of apoptosis to occur that enables the massive expansion or survival of dangerous cells such as in cancer and auto-immune disorders, respectively. Resistance to apoptosis is considered a hallmark of cancer, and this property allows for many of the other malignant behaviors of a cancer cell to take place. One of the seminal discoveries of the late 1980s was that the Bcl-2 oncogene, originally identified as a prominent translocation in follicular lymphoma, was identified not as a growth stimulatory gene but as an apoptosis suppressing gene, thus defining the suppression of apoptosis for the first time as an oncogenic process.

Table 18.2 lists apoptosis genes directly involved in disease, and those that are merely implicated in disease. Genes directly involved in disease are identified through causative mutations, deletions, gene rearrangements (translocations), amplifications, or loss-of-heterozygosity (LOH). It should be noted that this direct evidence for apoptosis involvement in disease applies to only a small percentage of monogenic disorders, some with rare incidence or prevalence. However, these examples provide greater significance in terms of identifying apoptosis genes as causes of disease.

Also included in Table 18.2 are genes implicated in disease through associations, alterations in expression,

Table 18.2 Apoptosis Genes and Disease Associations[a]

Disease or Syndrome	Genes Directly Involved (through Mutations, Deletions, Translocations, LOH, or Amplifications)
ALPS (type 0 or Ia)	Fas/CD95/TNFRSF6
ALPS (type Ib)	Fas ligand
ALPS (type II)	Caspase-10
Blau syndrome	NOD-2/CARD15
BLS	CIITA
Crohn's disease	NOD-2/CARD15
CINCA/NOMID	NALP3/cryopyrin/PYPAF1/CIAS1
FCAS/FCU	NALP3/cryopyrin/PYPAF1/CIAS1
MWS	NALP3/cryopyrin/PYPAF1/CIAS1
FHL	Perforin
FMF	Pyrin/marenostrin
Familial cylindromatosis	CYLD
Follicular lymphoma	Bcl-2 (*T*)
HED/EDA	EDA1, EDAR, EDARADD
Incontinentia pigmenti	NEMO/IKKgamma
Li-Fraumeni syndrome	tp53
Cancer	tp53 (*LOH*)
MALT lymphoma	Bcl-10 (*T*)
MALT lymphoma	cIAP2 and MALT1/paracaspase (*T*)
MALT lymphoma	MALT1/paracaspase (*T*)
SMA (type 1)	NAIP (*D*)
TRAPS	TNFRSF1A/TNFR1
Cancer (esophageal, cervical, lung)	cIAP1 and/or cIAP2 (*A*)
NHL and CLL	Bcl-3
NHL	MALT1/paracaspase (*A*)
Primary macroglobulinemia	cIAP2 and MALT1 (*T*)
	Genes Implicated *(Through Altered Expression/Association)*
Cancer (many)	Survivin, XIAP, bcl-2, bcl-Xl, A1, cIAP2
Pancreatic cancer	Survivin (*A*)
Cancer (many)	XAF-1 (*LOH*)
Melanoma, renal cell carcinoma	Livin
Cancer (many or various specific forms)	Bax, apaf-1, caspase-8, CD95, DR4, DR5
Ovarian cancer	XIAP
Advanced cancer, multiple myeloma	Alterations in NFkB pathway/activity
Multiple sclerosis	XIAP, cIAP1, cIAP2, survivin, NAIP
Legionnaire's disease	NAIP5/bircle (in mice)
Colorectal cancer	cIAP2
Pancreatic cancer	cIAP2
Colon cancer	Bax
Rheumatoid arthritis	NFkB
Mycosis fungoides/CTCL	cIAP2
Diffuse large cell lymphoma (NHL), and Hodgkin's disease	cIAP2, A1, NFkB pathway

[a]**Legends and abbreviations:** ADULT, acro-dermato-ungual-lacrimal-tooth; AEC, ankyloblepharon, ectodermal dysplasia, clefting; ALPS, autoimmune lymphoproliferative syndrome (Canale-Smith syndrome); BLS, bare lymphocyte syndrome; CINCA, chronic infantile neurologic cutaneous articular syndrome; CLL, chronic lymphocytic leukemia; CTCL, cutaneous T-cell lymphoma; EDA, anhidrotic ectodermal dysplasia; EEC, ectrodactyly, ectodermal dysplasia, clefting; FCAS, familial cold autoinflammatory syndrome; FCU, familial cold urticaria; FHL, familial hemophagocytic lymphohistiocytosis; FMF, familial Mediterranean fever; HED, hypohidrotic ectodermal dysplasia; LMS, limb-mammary syndrome; MALT, mucosa-associated lymphoid tissue; MWS, Muckle-Wells syndrome; NHL, non-Hodgkin's lymphoma; NOMID, neonatal-onset multisystem inflammatory disease; SMA, spinal muscular atrophy; TRAPS, TNFRSF1A-associated periodic syndrome; *T* = translocation, *A* = amplification, *D* = deletion, LOH = loss-of-heterozygosity, * = strong or direct link, ** = causal relationship not conclusively proven.

and/or correlations that do not necessarily discriminate between cause and effect. These genes have been implicated in a large number of diseases, that are mostly polygenic or multifactorial in nature, and reflect the majority of diseases with significant morbidity and mortality. The burden of proof for direct gene involvement in these cases is more difficult to attain. For this reason, these genes are listed simply as implicated and not as causative, as this may require further validation to convincingly demonstrate a direct or causative role. For several of the genes listed in Table 18.2, there exists a corresponding model in the mouse, either through natural mutations (e.g., *gld* and *lpr* mice), or through gene knock-out or transgenic manipulations, all of which support a role for failed apoptosis in proliferative diseases.

The pivotal role apoptosis plays in a cell's demise, be it a primary cause or a secondary effect in a disease process, makes it an attractive approach for the development of novel therapeutics. Many different drug and gene therapy approaches targeting apoptosis are underway; success would validate specific proteins as drug targets. Therapeutic approaches attempted to date include traditional small molecules antisense oligonucleotides (ASOs), or monoclonal antibodies and recombinant proteins. More experimental approaches are underway using gene therapy or oncolytic viruses. Many of these compounds may never become drugs due to the many inherent problems in drug development (unexpected toxicities, poor pharmacokinetics, poor stability, poor oral bioavailability, etc.). However, they represent important first steps in demonstrating the validity of triggering apoptosis as a therapeutic approach for cancer or auto-immune disorders. These compounds may serve as gold standards in screening approaches, or as precursor molecules for more effective drugs, all aimed at developing clinically effective therapeutics targeting key apoptosis regulatory molecules that will impact on healthcare and society.

ASOs will most likely be the first 'apoptosis' drugs on the market. The bcl-2 antisense drug, GenasenseTM, developed by Genta is nearing completion of several pivotal phase III cancer trials. Caspase inhibitors hold promise for disorders such as sepsis, liver disease, acute neurological disorders, and myocardial infarctions, but have to overcome drug delivery (pharmacokinetic) problems. Biologics, such as monoclonal antibodies targeting TNFalpha and recombinant proteins such as interferon beta, are already on the market but are used mainly as immunomodulatory drugs, and are mentioned here for the sake of completeness. More direct applications targeting apoptosis, such as through the use of TRAIL as a cancer therapy, await further development and the clearing of toxicity and efficacy hurdles. Gene therapy and oncolytic viruses have to overcome even greater developmental hurdles, inherent to the manufacturing of live viruses for therapeutics, as well as overcoming some recent setbacks in gene therapy clinical trials, and other limitations. Oncolytic viruses are included as apoptosis modulatory drugs because they make use of apoptotic pathways and responses inherent to viral infection to kill cancer cells.

18.4 THERAPEUTIC STRATEGIES FOR TARGETING APOPTOSIS

18.4.1 Apoptosis Inhibition as Treatment Strategy for Neurodegenerative Disease

Apoptosis has been implicated in delayed neuronal death associated with many neurodegenerative disorders such as Parkinson's disease, stroke, Huntington's disease, traumatic head injury, Alzheimer's disease, motor neuron degeneration, spinal cord injury, and multiple sclerosis. Since an extensive description of the role of apoptosis in each of these disorders is beyond the scope of the present text, we shall focus on anti-apoptotic strategies for stroke, Parkinson's disease, and multiple sclerosis.

18.4.1.1 Caspase-3 Inhibitors for the Treatment of Stroke

In the case of stroke, a major source of blood supply to the brain is carried by the middle cerebral artery. Embolic strokes result when a blood clot or a piece of debris called plaque, which formed in another vessel in the body, breaks away and flows through the bloodstream blocking or occluding blood flow to the brain. Embolic strokes typically result from occlusion of the middle cerebral artery. Normal blood flow to the brain is about 50 ml/100g/min (Figure 18.8). As we age, blood flow gradually decreases over the years but there are no symptoms because of compensatory mechanisms such as increased efficiency in the extraction of oxygen and glucose from the blood. However, if the middle cerebral artery is partially blocked and blood flow becomes less than 20 ml/100g/min, signs of a transient ischemic attack occur such as difficulty speaking and understanding, headache, dizziness, inability to maintain balance or move a limb. If the restriction in blood flow does not decrease blood flow below 10 ml/100g/min, the affected brain region is know as a transition zone or penumbra in which neurons are electrically quiescent but still viable. In theory, this area may still be salvaged if blood flow is restored to near normal levels within a few hours. This is in contrast to brain areas where blood flow plummets below 10 ml/100g/min and neuronal cells become necrotic within minutes forming an infarct that cannot be rescued. The best available strategy for clinicians is to restore blood flow rapidly using drugs that dissolve the blot clot. Unfortunately, 15–20% of all strokes are hemorrhagic in nature (blood vessel tears) and the administration of clot busters to such patients would exacerbate bleeding resulting in further deterioration and perhaps death. As a result, attention has been focused on the development of drugs that will extend the survival time of neurons in the penumbral region until blood flow can be reinstated to near normal levels. One experimental strategy by which to achieve this goal is through the inhibition of apoptosis.

A large number of studies have shown that markers of apoptosis such as active caspase-3 and proteins that have been cleaved by this enzyme are displayed by neurons in the penumbra region. Detection of these markers in brain sections from animals subjected to an experimental stroke by a method known as immunohistochemistry suggests that a window of therapeutic opportunity extending to nearly 24 hours exits for the use of caspase-3 inhibitors. Unfortunately, such drugs are difficult to get into the brain and have a very short plasma half-life making them difficult to develop to the stage where they may be tested on people. All inhibitors include an aspartic acid-like moiety since caspase-3 has an absolute requirement for cutting proteins after this amino acid residue. The high abundance of acid transporters in the bile duct means that this chemical feature results in the rapid transport of such compounds from the circulation to the bile resulting in the short plasma half-life of caspase-3 inhibitors. A more serious shortcoming, at least for the

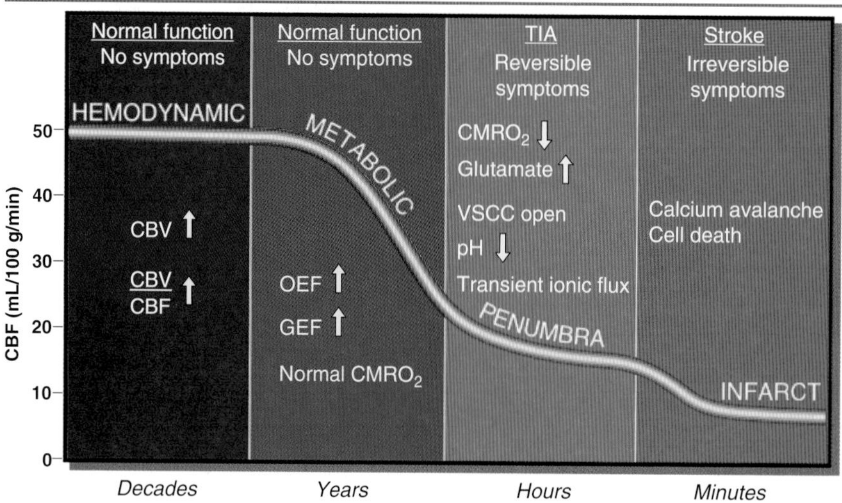

Figure 18.8 Progressive loss of neurological function associated with decreased cerebral blood flow (CBF) measured in millilitres (mL) per 100 grams (g) of brain tissue per minute (min). The brain normally receives about 50 (mL/100 g/min) and can tolerate a reduction in CBF to about 20 (mL/100 g/min) by increasing hemodynamic factors such as cerebral blood volume (CBV) or local cerebral blood flow (CBF). Beyond this point, transient ischemic attacks (TIA) occur, resulting in compensatory changes that maintain energy production in the brain. These consist of elevated oxygen extraction factor (OEF) and glucose extraction factor (GEF) that maintain a normal cerebral metabolic rate for oxygen (CMRO2). In brain regions where CBF drops below 20 ml/100 g/min, neurons are still viable but electrically quiescent. Due to the lack of energy in the absence of oxygen and glucose delivery, ionic pumps fail resulting in decreased pH, opening of voltage sensitive calcium channels (VSCC), and the release of excitatory amino acid transmitters (glutamate and aspartate) that over the space of hours can result in tissue injury if CMRO2 is depressed for hours. If blood flow falls further to 10 ml/100 g/min irreversible damage occurs within minutes due to the massive influx of calcium into neurons that results in protease activation and cell death.

treatment of adult stroke, is that there is a rapid reduction in the amount of caspase-3 detected in brain within three weeks after birth. Consequently, should caspase-3 inhibitors reach the point where they would be safe enough to be tested in humans it is more likely that such compounds would be used to treat fetal rather than adult stroke.

Despite the shortcomings of small molecule caspase-3 inhibitors for the treatment of adult stroke, treatments that increase levels of the caspase-3/-7 inhibitor XIAP have repeatedly been shown to improve both cellular and behavioural outcome in experimental models of stroke. In addition to being caspase inhibitors, at least two other activities of IAP proteins such as XIAP may account for the ability of these anti-apoptotic proteins to reduce stroke injury in experimental models. First, XIAP has been shown to possess E3 ligase activity enabling it to target a kinase known as TAK1 (mitogen-activated protein kinase 7) for degradation by ubiquitylating this enzyme. TAK1 inhibition blocks activation of the pro-apoptotic stress kinase JNK (c-Jun amino-terminal kinase) whereas small molecule inhibitors of JNK have been shown to be neuroprotective, suggesting that ubiquitination of TAK1 may account in part for the ability of XIAP to reduce neuronal loss in several neurodegenerative models. Another protective activity of IAPs such as NAIP is the ability to reduce neuronal injury associated with excessive increases in cytosolic calcium. Excitotoxicity resulting from the excessive activation of N-methyl-D-aspartate (NMDA) receptors is a common feature of many neurodegenerative disorders, particularly stroke. The excessive activation of NMDA receptors triggers a massive influx of calcium into the neuron that results in necrosis. Unfortunately, NMDA receptor antagonists have failed in clinical trials for stroke due at least in part to their psychotic side effects and short therapeutic time window. Functional studies using neuroblastoma and motor neuron cell lines have reported an interaction of NAIP with the calcium binding protein hippocalcin that renders cells more resistant to cell death induced by elevated $Ca2^{+}$ concentrations. Conversely mice that lack NAIP are most susceptible to the injurious effects of excitotoxins. Mutations in the NAIP gene are associated with a disease called spinal muscular atrophy (SMA) that is characterized by a loss of ventral motor neurons. NAIP is not the cause of SMA, that is caused by mutations in the survival motor neuron (SMN) protein on human chromosome 5 (adjacent to NAIP). Nevertheless, it is thought that the severity of the disease is correlated with mutations or lack of NAIP in these patients. The finding that NAIP can bind hippocalcin and protect against elevated $Ca2^{+}$ suggests that this interaction may be another mechanism by which IAPs such as NAIP are able to protect neurons.

18.4.1.2 Anti-Apoptotic Strategies for the Treatment of Parkinson's Disease

In the case of Parkinson's disease, there is a progressive loss of dopamine neurons that comprise the nigrostriatal pathway. If dopamine levels in the striatum are depleted by more than 80%, the cardinal features of Parkinson's disease become apparent: tremor of the hands, muscular rigidity, bradykinesia (slow movement), postural instability, or impaired balance and coordination. These symptoms increase in severity with the progressive loss of nigrostriatal dopamine neurons; however, since Parkinson's patients can survive for several decades after the initial diagnosis, there is a tremendous need and opportunity for therapeutic intervention.

Parkinson's disease can be modeled in rodents and primates by systemic administration of the selective dopaminergic neurotoxin MPTP (1-methyl-4-phenyl-1,2,3,6-tetrahydropyridine) or intracerebral administration of 6-OHDA (6-hydroxydopamine). In both young (7 days of age) and adult rats (over 70 days of age) intrastriatal injection of 6-OHDA results in the retrograde destruction of the nigrostriatal pathway; however, only in the former can active caspase-3 be detected in the degenerating cell bodies. Nevertheless, virally-mediated NAIP overexpression reduces the loss of nigrostriatal neurons in adult animals lesioned by intrastriatal administration of 6-OHDA. Hence, NAIP appears to have neuroprotective activities that extend beyond the inhibition of caspase-3. Given that NAIP may protect neurons by decreasing the impact of excessive calcium influx, we have determined whether calcium activated protease calpain plays a role in the loss of dopamine neurons produced by MPTP. Administration of MPTP at a dose of 25 mg/kg/day for five days (i.p.) resulted in the loss of nigrostriatal dopamine neurons that was accompanied by calpain activation. Intracerebral delivery of a calpain inhibitor (MDL-28170) or virally-mediated overexpression of the endogenous calpain inhibitor calpastatin significantly reduced the loss of dopamine neurons. Furthermore, immunohistochemical analysis of postmortem midbrain tissues from Parkinson's patients and age-matched controls also revealed evidence of calpain activation that was not present in the controls. These findings suggest that disturbed calcium homeostasis may be an important factor in idiopathic Parkinson's disease. Unfortunately, the clinical development of calpain inhibitors for the treatments of neurodegenerative disorders has been hampered by the fear of toxicities associated with the nonspecific inhibition of calpain activity such as deficiency in platelet aggregation, insulin secretion and muscular atrophy. Despite the broad utility of calpain inhibition in preventing neuronal death in a variety of neurodegenerative contexts, it is unlikely that such a strategy will have clinical utility.

JNK activation has also been implicated in dopamine neuron death in experimental models of Parkinson's disease. It is therefore not surprising that overexpression of XIAP is also neuroprotective in the MPTP model of Parkinson's disease whereas small molecule inhibitors of kinases that activate JNK have been shown to be effective in numerous models of Parkinson's disease and stroke. Despite these encouraging results, a compound capable of blocking JNK activity has not yet been advanced for phase III testing in humans.

18.4.2 Apoptosis Induction as a Novel Therapeutic Approach for Multiple Sclerosis

Multiple sclerosis (MS) is a progressive neurological disorder characterized by an autoimmune mediated attack against the myelin sheath surrounding axons in the central nervous system (CNS) resulting in inflammation, demyelination, gliosis, and ultimately axonal degeneration. Magnetic resonance imaging (MRI) with the contrast agent gadolinium often is employed during or following an initial attack, to identify lesions within the CNS and to confirm disease diagnosis. The initial symptoms of MS include difficulty in walking, unusual sensations including numbness or tingling in the upper and lower extremities, loss of balance, weakness, fatigue, pain, impaired vision, and bladder dysfunction, usually present as a direct result of active demyelination producing disrupted communication between neurons of the CNS and nerve impulses to the muscles and organs. With disease progression, MS patients may experience more severe symptoms including cognitive impairment, paralysis, and blindness corresponding to new demyelinated plaques in the brain and spinal cord.

The clinical course of MS has been divided into four major categories: relapsing-remitting (RRMS), secondary-progressive (SPMS), primary progressive (PPMS), and benign. Patients with RRMS have clinical relapses every few months or years, with intervening periods of clinically stability. RRMS is two to three times more common in females compared to males. In contrast to RRMS, patients with SPMS display progressive deterioration that may, or may not, be superimposed with clinical relapses. RRMS patients generally convert to SPMS over time, characterized by a gradual decline in neurological function. Approximately 15% of MS patients have PPMS characterized by late-onset and progressive deterioration of neurological function. There are currently no effective treatments for PPMS. In addition to RRMS, SPMS, and PPMS, there is a benign form of the disease that affects approximately 10 to 20% of RRMS patients. Benign MS is arbitrarily defined in RRMS patients who after more than 10 years following initial diagnosis, are still mobile and show only minor, if any, neurological deficits (Expanded Disability Status Scale [EDSS] 3–4). These patients generally show little or no progression after their initial attack. Moreover, patients with an EDSS score of ≤ 2 and disease duration of more than 10 years tend to maintain a low EDSS disability score for an additional 10 years. Benign MS requires no therapeutic intervention, and is generally not diagnosed until 10 to 15 years from disease onset.

18.4.2.1 Cellular Immunology of MS

Although the cause of MS is still unclear, this autoimmune disease is considered to be T cell-mediated and can be modeled in both rodents and nonhuman primates by experimental autoimmune encephalomyelitis (EAE). The clinical manifestations and neuropathology of EAE parallel many of the cardinal features of MS. Like MS, EAE is predominantly a Th1-cell mediated autoimmune disease. In the EAE model, animals are immunized with a specific myelin antigen adjuvant pertusis toxin that triggers an immune response against the recognized antigen. The first clinical signs of EAE generally become apparent 10–12 days post induction, beginning with loss of muscle tone in the tail followed by walking deficits and eventually progressing to ascending paralysis. Multiple myelin antigens, such as myelin oligodendrocyte glycoprotein (MOG), proteolipid protein (PLP), and myelin basic protein (MBP) all induce EAE. The combination of myelin antigen and animal species/strain often predicts the clinical course of EAE that can be either chronic, acute, or relapsing-remitting.

While $CD4^+$ T cells specific for myelin antigens are thought to initiate and exacerbate MS through the secretion of pro-inflammatory cytokines, activated macrophages also migrate into the CNS and release a variety of factors that directly cause nerve and tissue damage. Activated macrophages and microglia are consistently found in demyelinated plaques in MS patients, and probably serve as the major antigen-presenting cells (APCs) in the CNS. Moreover, the extent of axonal damage in demyelinated lesions of the CNS and the persistence of neurological deficits in MS are directly correlated with the number of activated macrophages/microglia and $CD8^+$ T cells within the margins of sclerotic plaques.

18.4.2.2 Failed Apoptosis as a Disease Mechanism in MS

Apoptosis is an important mechanism in immune system regulation, responsible for the elimination of auto-reactive T and B cells (lymphocytes) and macrophages from the circulation and preventing their entry into the CNS. It has been hypothesized that a failure of auto-reactive T and B lymphocytes, as well as activated macrophages, to undergo apoptosis contributes to the pathogenesis of MS. Consistent with this hypothesis, expression of members of the inhibitors of apoptosis (IAP) family of anti-apoptotic proteins such as XIAP, cIAP1/HIAP2, and cIAP2/HIAP1 are elevated in mitogen stimulated T cells from MS patients relative to neurologically healthy control subjects. It should be emphasized that while recent evidence from Sharief and colleagues suggests that the IAPs are involved in MS, these findings are based primarily on IAP expression in mitogen (PHA) stimulated T cells from RRMS patients. By comparison, we have recently expanded these findings to untreated PBMN (peripheral blood mononuclear cells) and T cells in other forms of MS. In more aggressive forms of MS, higher levels of XIAP expression were found in PBMN cells while both cIAP1/HIAP2 and cIAP2/HIAP1 were elevated in resting T cells relative to healthy controls.

In contrast to bcl-2, the IAPs directly block upstream triggers of apoptosis known as death receptors that initiate Fas mediated activation of caspase-8, the extrinsic cell death pathway. Like bcl-2, the IAPs also block the intrinsic cell death pathway, mediated by the release of pro-apoptotic factors from the mitochondria. Consequently, the anti-apoptotic activities of the IAPs can be distinguished from members of the bcl-2 family by their ability to block both of these cell death pathways. Elevated expression of XIAP, cIAP1/HIAP2, and cIAP2/HIAP1 in patients with active MS correlates with clinical features of disease activity, deficits in Fas mediated cell death, and T cell resistance to apoptosis. By contrast, protein expression of bcl-2 in activated T cells is similar in MS patients and normal controls. Basal levels of XIAP, cIAP1/HIAP2, and cIAP2/HIAP1 in B lymphocytes and macrophages obtained from MS patients are currently unknown; however, it has been reported that expression of bcl-2 proteins in B cells of RRMS patients, as well as patients with systemic inflammatory diseases, is elevated relative to normal control subjects. Transgenic mice that overexpress bcl-2 in T cells display a more severe form of EAE during the chronic phase, suggesting that increased survival of auto-reactive T cells enhances EAE pathogenesis supporting a role for elevated bcl-2 in MS. In macrophages, upregulation of XIAP also increases cell survival while XIAP knockdown, using antisense oligonucleotides, decreases cell viability and improves clinical outcome in models of MS. Taken together, these findings suggest that impaired apoptosis resulting from elevated IAP and/or bcl-2 family member expression contributes to MS.

18.4.2.3 IAP Downregulation as a Novel Treatment for MS

The goal of current MS therapies is to lengthen the time between relapses and thereby slow or perhaps even halt disease progression. Much of the work in the EAE model has led to the development of novel therapeutic strategies for treating MS. There are currently three categories of approved therapies for long-term treatment of RRMS, including three different preparations of interferon-beta (IFN-β; Avonex, Betaseron, and Rebif), glatiramer-acetate (Copaxone), and mitoxantrone (Novantrone). IFN-β has been shown to lengthen the time between relapses in individuals with MS. One mechanism underlying the propensity of IFN-β to lengthen the time between relapses in MS patients is its ability to promote the elimination of auto-reactive T and B cells through the reduction of anti-apoptotic proteins. IFN-β has been shown to reduce expression of the anti-apoptotic proteins XIAP, HIAP1/cIAP2, and HIAP2/cIAP1 in mitogen-stimulated T cells from MS patients, suggesting that IFN-β drugs may improve the symptoms of MS by promoting the elimination of auto-reactive T cells through IAP downregulation.

The anti-apoptotic activity of XIAP, cIAP1, and cIAP2 is opposed by a physical interaction with XIAP-associated factor-1 (XAF-1) (Figure 18.5). IFN-β has been shown to increase the expression of XAF-1 mRNA in a number of melanoma and myeloma cell lines, as well as dendritic and natural killer cells. A specific role for XAF-1 in programmed cell death was confirmed by showing that XAF-1 overexpression sensitized cells normally resistant to tumor necrosis factor-related apoptosis-inducing ligand (TRAIL)-induced apoptosis, whereas inhibition of XAF-1 expression prevented the sensitizing effects of IFN-β. Many cancer cell lines undergo apoptosis when exposed to TRAIL; however, several cancer cell lines that are resistant to TRAIL-induced apoptosis can be sensitized to this apoptotic trigger by exposure to IFN-β. In this case, there is a corresponding increase in levels of XAF-1 protein. The ability of IFN-β to sensitize auto-reactive T cells to TRAIL-induced apoptosis therefore appears to be mediated by the induction of XAF-1. In EAE, using TRAIL blockade, the disease is inhibited and activation of auto-reactive T cells is prevented. In addition, TRAIL has been correlated with IFN-β responsiveness and shown to influence disease severity in a murine model of EAE. If similar mechanisms are at play in MS, it is possible that induction of XAF-1 in auto-reactive T cells may be indicative of clinical responsiveness to IFN-β. In MS patients who do not respond to IFN-β, there may be a failure of IFN-β to induce XAF-1 in auto-reactive T cells.

18.4.2.4 IAP Associated Proteins as Diagnostic Markers in MS

IFN-β treatment has been associated with the development of neutralizing antibodies in MS patients 6 to 18 months following the initiation of treatment. The predictive value of such antibodies for IFN-β responsiveness remains controversial and there is an urgent need for more robust and reliable diagnostic markers. To this end, cDNA microarray studies have been performed to identify genes responsive to IFN-β in PBMN cells from MS patients. This work has lead to retrospective studies reporting a positive correlation between expression of TRAIL mRNA in PBMN cells or levels of this pro-apoptotic protein in the serum of MS patients responsive to IFN-β therapy. These findings encouraged us to explore the possibility that clinical disability, disease progression, and responsiveness to IFN-β may be predicted by the expression profile of apoptosis-related genes such as XIAP, HIAP-1, HIAP-2, and XAF-1 in immune cells from MS patients. Moreover, since XAF-1 has been implicated in the signaling mechanisms that mediate the apoptotic actions of IFN-β, we hypothesize that levels of XAF-1 in auto-reactive immune cells may represent a reliable biochemical index of IFN-β unresponsiveness. In comparison to T-cell apoptosis, little is known about the effects of IFN-β on XIAP, HIAP1/cIAP2, HIAP2/cIAP1, and XAF-1 levels in auto-reactive B cells or macrophages. By stark contrast, it has been reported that IFN-β treatment does not alter increased bcl-2 protein levels in auto-reactive B cells in patients with RRMS. Hence the IAPs may be more relevant to disease course than members of the bcl-2 family.

18.4.2.5 Therapeutic Prospects for IAP Downregulation in MS

In summary, we hypothesize that expression levels of the IAP family of anti-apoptotic genes may represent novel diagnostic markers predictive of disease severity, subtype, and IFN-β responsiveness in MS. In support of this hypothesis, knock-down of XIAP expression in PBMN cells by systemic administration of an antisense oligonucleotide, AEG35169, against XIAP recently has been reported to reduce the severity of EAE in a murine model. Furthermore, AEG35169 dramatically decreased the severity of EAE even when administration of this compound was delayed until the animals showed early signs of paralysis. It is now well established that knock-down of XIAP expression with AEG35169 also lowers the resistance of cancer cells to apoptotic triggers. A similar sequence, AEG35156 is currently in Phase I/II clinical trials in the United States and Canada for the treatment of leukemia. Success of this study would pave the way for clinical trials designed to assess the efficacy of XIAP knock-down in the treatment of MS.

18.4.3 Induction of Cell Death in Treatment of Cancer

Blocking cell death via the expression of apoptosis inhibitors has obvious selection benefits for the development of the transformed phenotype, as well as in the development of chemotherapy and radiation resistance. The prototype of this category of oncogene is Bcl-2, which can be translocated and transcriptionally activated in human follicular B cell lymphomas. Although Bcl-2 is not an inducer of cell proliferation, its suppression of normal cell death results in slow growing tumors. The development of more aggressive tumors occurs with the subsequent accumulation of additional genetic alterations. Although Bcl2 genetic rearrangement occurs in a very limited subset of cancers, Bcl-2 overexpression is a frequent occurrence, found in up to 50% of all human cancers, suggesting that upregulation of anti-apoptotic genes may be a common, if not a universal, factor in cancer development. Given the centrality of the IAPs in regulating cell death and the importance of suppressing apoptosis in the development of cancer, it long has been suspected that deregulated IAP expression will prove to be a common event in many cancer types. Indeed, there is now overwhelming evidence for the role of the IAP genes in cancer. For example, the analysis of XIAP (X-chromosome linked IAP) in 78 patients with acute myelogenous leukemia (AML) revealed a strong correlation between the XIAP levels and the patients' survival. Patients with lower levels of XIAP had significantly longer survival times than those with increased XIAP levels.

Similarly, Survivin levels were increased in 34 (out of 34) tumor samples (adenocarcinoma and squamous cell carcinoma) when compared with nontumor controls. Survivin expression is frequently observed in tumors from breast cancer patients. One study reported that 71% of breast carcinomas (stages I to IH) were positive for Survivin whereas no expression of Survivin was detected in adjacent normal tissues. In colorectal cancers the expression of Survivin is inversely correlated with the apoptotic index of transformed cells and is significantly related to an increased disease-free survival rate and to a reduced risk for distant metastases.

A direct role of XIAP in the resistance of cancer cells to radiation and chemotherapeutic intervention was demonstrated using a XIAP antisense approach. Low dose γ-irradiation was found to result in translational upregulation of XIAP in nonsmall cell lung carcinoma cells and that this upregulation correlated with enhanced resistance to radiation-induced apoptosis. Transduction of the nonsmall cell lung carcinoma line H661 with the adenoviral XIAP antisense vector resulted in decreased levels of XIAP protein, that was correlated with significant sensitization to low dose γ-irradiation. A similar approach was used to sensitize ovarian carcinoma cells to cisplatin-induced apoptosis. In addition to increasing the sensitivity of previously resistant cells to cisplatin, transduction with the XIAP antisense vector resulted in activation of caspase-3, caspase-mediated MDM2 processing, and accumulation of p53. Significantly, adenoviral XIAP antisense treatment resulted in the induction of apoptosis in ovarian cancer cells with wild-type p53, but not null or mutant p53. However, XIAP antisense oligonucleotides have induced apoptosis in various p53 backgrounds.

Additional direct genetic evidence is now emerging to support the contention that the IAPs function as oncogenes. The cIAP1/HIAP2 and cIAP2/HIAP1 locus on chromosome 11q22 is amplified in numerous cancers, including medulloblastomas, renal cell carcinomas, glioblastomas, and gastric carcinomas. Transcriptional analysis of esophageal squamous cell carcinomas and cervical carcinomas displaying the 11q22 amplification indicates that cIAP1 mRNA is the most frequently overexpressed gene within this region, suggesting that cIAP1 disregulation may be important in the development of certain cancer types. Genetic rearrangements within the cIAP1/cIAP2 locus also have been demonstrated in extranodal marginal zone mucosa-associated lymphoid tissue (MALT) B cell lymphomas. MALT B cells initially hyperproliferate in response to chronic inflammation, such as during persistent *Helicobacter pylori* infection or certain autoimmune diseases. These inflammatory responses lead to chronic NF-κB activation in B cells, resulting in the upregulation of the anti-apoptotic cIAP2/HIAP1 protein, and slow-growing tumors resulting from aberrant B cell survival. Antibiotic treatment of the underlying *H. pylori* infection leads to decreased inflammation, decline in NF-κB activation, downregulation of cIAP2/HIAP1, and tumor cell regression. Recently, direct evidence for an oncogenic role of cIAP1 has emerged demonstrating cooperativity between cIAP1 and YAP1 in cellular transformation resulting in hepatomas in mice. In addition, cooperativity has been demonstrated between cIAP1 and cMyc in cellular transformation, as cIAP1 acts as an E3 ligase for the Myc antagonist, Mad1.

Antibiotic therapy nonresponsive MALT lymphomas demonstrate two recurring translocation events involving genes in the TNF/MALT1 signaling pathway: Of the two common MALT B cell lymphoma translocations, the t(11;18)(q21;q21) translocation is the more frequent, occurring in greater than 50% of all extranodal MALT lymphomas. This translocation combines the *hiap1/cIAP2* and *mlt/malt1* genes and creates an in-frame fusion protein consisting of the cIAP2/HIAP1 BIR domains and the carboxyl terminus of the MLT/MALT1 protein. The cIAP2/MLT fusion protein activates the NF-κB pathway and upregulates its own transcription though the NF-κB responsive *cIAP2/HIAP1* promoter. This positive feedback loop continually stimulates NF-κB and may explain why the majority of antibiotic resistant gastric MALT lymphomas display the cIAP2/MLT translocation.

18.4.3.1 Targeting IAPs in Cancer—Proof of Principle Studies

Selective downregulation of IAPs using antisense targeting was successfully utilized in several models. Transduction of the nonsmall cell lung carcinoma line H661 with the adenoviral XIAP antisense vector resulted in decreased levels of XIAP protein that was correlated with significant sensitization to low dose γ-irradiation. Antisense XIAP cDNA also was used to sensitize ovarian carcinoma cells to cisplatin-induced apoptosis. Recently, combination of doxorubicin and antisense oligonucleotides targeted against XIAP were shown to significantly increase cytotoxicity of four bladder carcinoma cell lines by enhancing apoptosis. Similarly, antisense therapy to XIAP has proven effective in prostate cancer cells tumor xenografts either alone or in

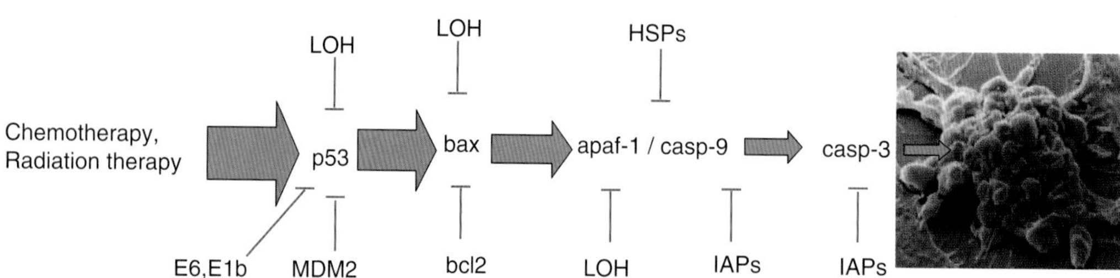

Figure 18.9 Apoptosis resistance is a hallmark of cancer. Multiple genetic lesions results in an increased apoptotic threshold that accompanies the cancerous phenotype. The relative resistance of cells to apoptosis is indicated by the thickness of the arrow and the key genes involved in setting the apoptotic threshold are shown. The function of these genes can be affected by either genetic mutations (such as loss of heterozygosity, LOH) or direct inhibition of their function by cellular inhibitors (such as Bcl-2, IAP, or heath shock (HSP) proteins). The ultimate outcome is the inability of cancer cells to undergo apoptosis despite exposure to potent cell death triggers (such as in case of therapeutic intervention with chemo- or radiation therapy).

combination with taxotere and is undergoing Phase I clinical trials. Antisense targeting of Survivin with antisense oligonucleotides or ribozymes led to the induction of apoptosis, reduced tumor growth in mouse models, and sensitized cancer cells to chemo- and radiation-therapies. Similarly, antisense targeting of cIAP2/HIAP1 in malignant pleural mesothelioma decreased basal cell viability and increase of cell sensitivity to cisplatin. Utilization of small molecules that mimic IAP binding partners (such as Smac) have been shown to promote the apoptotic sensitivity of the cancer cells in both *in vitro* and *in vivo* models. For example, a small molecule compound that inhibits XIAP activity was shown to induce apoptosis in tumor cell lines tested as well as to suppress growth of established tumors in xenograft models in mice, while displaying little toxicity to normal tissues. These compounds are also currently in phase I trials.

18.5 KEY POINTS AND CONCLUSIONS

Apoptosis is a fundamental process that is required for proper maintenance and survival of multicellular organisms. Thus, dysregulated apoptosis is associated with a number of human disorders and disease states ranging from autoimmune disorders to neurodegeneration to cancer. Understanding how apoptotic machinery works thus enables rational design for novel therapeutic approaches that will either activate apoptotic pathways (to eliminate cells, such as in cancer or autoimmune disorders) or to suppress excess apoptosis (to protect dying cells such as in neurodegeneration). We have focused here on several examples of targeting the key players of apoptotic pathways—caspases, IAPs, and Bcl-2—either by traditional pharmacological approaches (small molecules) or by novel biologics (antisense oligonucleotides). Several of these strategies are already in preclinical or clinical development phase and are showing therapeutic promise. However, many challenges remain that are associated with the concept of targeting cell death pathways to successfully modulate cellular survival.

REVIEW QUESTIONS

1. How does apoptosis differ from necrosis?
2. What three distinct pathways participate in the execution of apoptosis?
3. What are the executioners of apoptosis and how do they function?
4. Which two classes of proteins inhibit the progression of cell death?
5. How does the mechanism of action of IAPs differ from that of Bcl-2 proteins?
6. What are the morphological hallmarks of apoptosis?
7. Give examples of human disorders that are caused by dysregulated apoptosis.
8. Describe a therapeutic strategy that could be used to inhibit apoptosis, and explain why.
9. Give an example of a therapeutic strategy to promote apoptosis, and explain why.

ACKNOWLEDGEMENTS

We thank the members of our laboratories for fruitful and critical discussions. The work in author laboratories is supported by grants from Canadian Institutes of Health Research (MH, GSR), Genome Canada (GSR), MS Society of Canada (GSR), Nova Scotia Heart and Stroke Foundation (GSR), Canada Foundation for Innovation, Ontario Innovation Trust, and Ontario Research and Development Challenge Fund (MH).

KEY REFERENCES AND FURTHER READING

Aktas, O., Prozorovski,T., & Zipp, F. (2006). Death ligands and autoimmune demyelination. *Neuroscientist, 12*(4), 305–316.

Callus, B. A., & Vaux, D. L. (2006). Caspase inhibitors: Viral, cellular and chemical. *Cell Death and Differentiation*, Sept. 8, Epub ahead of print, doi: 10.1038.

Debatin, K. M., & Fulda, S. (Eds.). (2006). *Apoptosis and Cancer Therapy*. Wiley-VCH Verlag GmbH & Co. KGaA.

Igney, F. H., & Krammer, P. H. (2002). Death and anti-death: Tumour resistance to apoptosis. *Nature Reviews. Cancer, 2*, 277–288.

Inohara, N., & Nunez, G. (2003). NODs: Intracellular proteins involved in inflammation and apoptosis. *Nature Reviews. Immunology, 3*, 371–382.

Johnstone, R. W., Ruefli, A. A., & Lowe, S. W. (2002). Apoptosis: A link between cancer genetics and chemotherapy. *Cell, 108*, 153–164.

McDermott, M. F. (2002). Genetic clues to understanding periodic fevers, and possible therapies. *Trends in Molecular Medicine, 8*, 550–554.

Mullauer, L., Gruber, P., Sebinger, D., Buch, J., Wohlfart, S., & Chott, A. (2001). Mutations in apoptosis genes: A pathogenetic factor for human disease. *Mutation Research, 488*, 211–231.

Nathan, C. (2002). Points of control in inflammation. *Nature, 420*, 846–852.

Nicholson, D. W. (2000). From bench to clinic with apoptosis-based therapeutic agents. *Nature, 407*(6805), 810–816.

O'Brien, T., & Lee, D. (2004). Prospects for caspase inhibitors. *Mini Reviews in Medicinal Chemistry, 4*(2), 153–165.

Riedl, et al. (2001). Structural basis for the inhibition of caspase-3 by XIAP. *Cell, 104*, 791–800.

Robertson, G. S., Crocker, S. J., Nicholson, D. W., & Schulz, J. B. (2000). Neuroprotection by the inhibition of apoptosis. *Brain Pathology (Zurich, Switzerland), 10*(2), 283–292.

Robertson, J. D., Fadeel, B., Zhivotovsky, B., & Orrenius, S. (2002). 'Centennial' Nobel Conference on apoptosis and human disease. *Cell Death and Differentiation, 9*, 468–475.

Salvesen, G. S., & Duckett, C. S. (2002). IAP proteins: Blocking the road to death's door. *Nature Reviews. Molecular Cell Biology, 3*, 401–410.

Schulz, J. B. (2006). Anti-apoptotic gene therapy in Parkinson's disease. *Journal of Neural Transmission. Supplementum*, (70): 467–476.

Srinivasula, S. M., et al. (2001). A conserved XIAP-interaction motif in caspase-9 and Smac/DIABLO regulates caspase activity and apoptosis. *Nature, 410*, 112–116.

Tamm, I., Schriever, F., & Dorken, B. (2001). Apoptosis: Implications of basic research for clinical oncology. *The Lancet Oncology, 2*, 33–42.

Thompson, C. B. (1995). Apoptosis in the pathogenesis and treatment of disease. *Science, 267*, 1456–1462.

Tschopp, J., Martinon, F., & Burns, K. (2003). NALPs: A novel protein family involved in inflammation. *Nature Reveiws. Molecular Cell Biology, 4*, 95–104.

Wu, et al. (2000). Structural basis of IAP recognition by Smac/DIABLO. *Nature, 408*, 1008–1012.

Zhivotovsky, B., & Orrenius, S. (2003). Defects in the apoptotic machinery of cancer cells: Role in drug resistance. *Seminars in Cancer Biology, 13*, 125–134.

Zornig, M., Hueber, A., Baum, W., & Evan, G. (2001). Apoptosis regulators and their role in tumorigenesis. *Biochimica et Biophysica Acta, 1551*, F1–F37.

Chapter

19 Drug Discovery

Paul Erhardt

OUTLINE

19.1 INTRODUCTION

19.1.1 Overview

19.1.1.1 A Working Definition

Given the numerous disciplines involved in drug discovery and the wide range of perspectives that exist among its participants, it is important to begin by defining how we intend to consider the not-so-simple words in this chapter's title. Since confusion primarily arises around the word "drug," we will focus our attention on its meaning. The complexities associated with "discovery" should then fall properly into place as this chapter continues to unfold.

To this end, the dictionary indicates that the word "drug" is derived from the Old English *dryge*, which in turn, was reconstructed from the Primitive Germanic *dreug*. Because these older words meant "to dry," it has been suggested that the word "drug" originally was used to convey how herbs were commonly processed so as to produce "dried powders for administration as early medicinals." Even if historically correct, however, the field of medicine and the word "drug" have evolved well past this origin and a modern usage must be sought. In today's broadest sense, the term "drug" is often taken to include any nonfood substance that exhibits activity upon administration to any biological setting. The latter includes an *in vitro* test as well as an *in vivo* animal model or human subject. However, this definition also falls short of today's practice. It does not convey how the overall drug discovery process has so critically come to be a highly interdisciplinary effort all the way to its validated end-point within the clinic. Thus, the present chapter will specifically apply the term "drug" to include only single chemical substances that become marketed, albeit often then accompanied by added excipients, for use in human or veterinary medicine either by prescription (ethical pharmaceuticals) or as over-the-counter products (OTCs). Inherent to this modern definition while still connecting to the past is the continuum of interdisciplinary activities needed to actually produce marketed substances that eventually become "administered as [today's] medicinals."

It can be noted that this definition does not exclude recreational or abused substances. Because these chemicals involve nonconventional marketing strategies, to say the least, as well as nontherapeutic, if not harmful, applications, these "drug-shouldn't-be's" will not be considered further within this chapter. Alternatively, the definition does exclude both herbals and dietary supplements or nutraceuticals, even though some of these products may have a firmly established medicinal value. The latter are typically complex mixtures for which the complete range of components are not well understood and are not well controlled in their lot-to-lot content. Thus, although dietary supplements and herbals can serve as excellent sources for new drugs, they are not themselves drugs by today's standards. Though they may sometimes represent very popular consumer products, they too will not receive further attention. Finally, in line with the working definition and integral to fully appreciating how difficult it is to truly discover an actual drug substance, it will be important to keep in mind that all the compound libraries, hit, lead, preclinical, and clinical development compounds that you will soon be reading about should be regarded only as "drug-wannabes" since they all fall short of our strict definition.

A similar view should be extended to the participants who work in the field of drug discovery. Although investigators involved in studies at any given step in this process should be considered to be making very critical contributions, within the context of our definition the overall process of drug discovery entails numerous steps that need to be brought together as part of a much larger undertaking in order to eventually produce what we will be calling a true drug. The huge challenge associated with this undertaking is illustrated in the next section. Finally, in addition to the interdisciplinary emphasis afforded by this working definition, this chapter will focus primarily upon the process of drug discovery as it specifically pertains to the pursuit of small molecule agents. Although this will preclude in-depth consideration of biopolymers and vaccines, this division is commonly taken to separate these types of therapeutics from small molecule drugs. The development and production of biopolymers are achieved in a distinctly different manner that relies heavily upon biotechnology-driven methods. Summarizing, a drug is a single chemical substance marketed for use in human or veterinary medicine either by prescription or as an OTC.

19.1.1.2 A Glimpse of the Challenge

With the aforementioned definition in-hand, this chapter will proceed to convey how it becomes possible to convert a small molecule drug-related concept into a physical entity that is actually marketed for the medical benefit of human or veterinary populations. The most recent statistical trends associated with this process suggest that it is an enormously challenging and difficult undertaking. For example, Figures 19.1, 19.2, and 19.3, respectively, convey:

- That there is actually a downward trend in the number of new drugs entering the marketplace even though research and development (R&D) sophistication and expenditures have continued to climb
- That there is an extraordinarily high attrition rate for the specific molecules that are initially selected from the huge compound surveys that are conducted to ultimately launch just one new drug into the marketplace
- The reasons for such high attrition, which can in most cases be ascribed to specific shortcomings of the numerous drug "wannabes"

The numbers in Figure 19.1 refer to new molecular entities (NMEs). These figures represent a composite of both small molecule therapeutics, or NCEs (for new chemical entities), and large biopolymer products, or NBEs (for new biological entities) that entered the marketplace each year. Factors responsible for the trends shown in Figures 19.2 and 19.3 will be discussed in greater detail as this chapter proceeds.

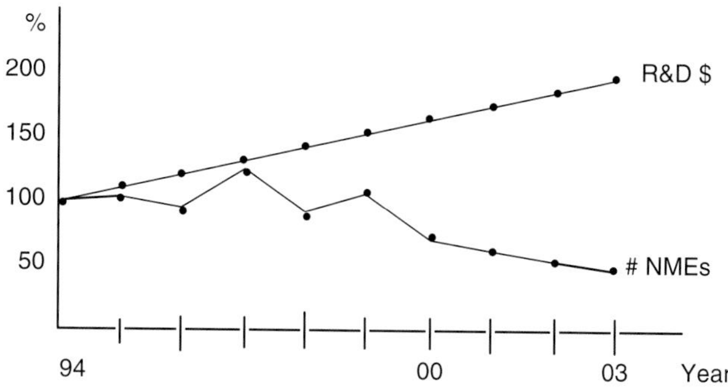

Figure 19.1 Diminishing returns (data reflects a collation from several surveys reported up to 2003). Note the downward trend in the number of new drugs entering the marketplace while drug research and development (R&D) expenditures continue to climb. NMEs are New Molecular Entities, which includes the sum of New Chemical Entities (NCEs) plus New Biological Entities (NBEs). More recent reports (2008) indicate that the decreasing trend in the number of NMEs may have begun to level off, whereas the rising costs of R&D have continued to accelerate, some suggesting that the latter has even become exponential.

19.1.1.3 Drug Discovery Starting Points

In general, the process of discovering new drugs can be thought of as beginning from either one of two distinct types of basic science starting points. The first starting point has a long-standing history associated

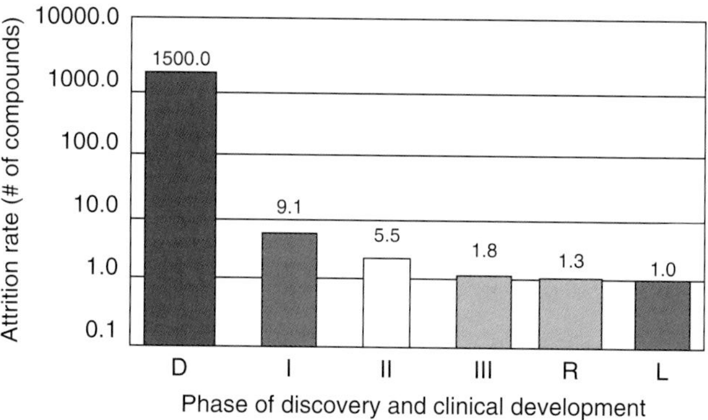

Figure 19.2 Drug candidate attrition numbers (data reflects a collation from several surveys reported prior to 2005). Bar graphs represent the numbers of compounds that typically are tested in order to advance to the next stage of the overall drug discovery process so as to ultimately achieve the successful market launch of one new product at the last step. Letters correspond to: D = Discovery and preclinical development stages; I, II, and III = Clinical development phases; R = Regulatory registration; and, L = Market launch. On average, only one marketed drug can be expected from nine drug-wannabes that enter clinical study at the Phase I stage. More recent reports (2008) suggest that this ratio may have widened even further, to about one out of 11 in general, although it should also be appreciated that the ratios from the more recent surveys are subject to considerable variance depending upon the different types of therapeutic classes from which they are derived.

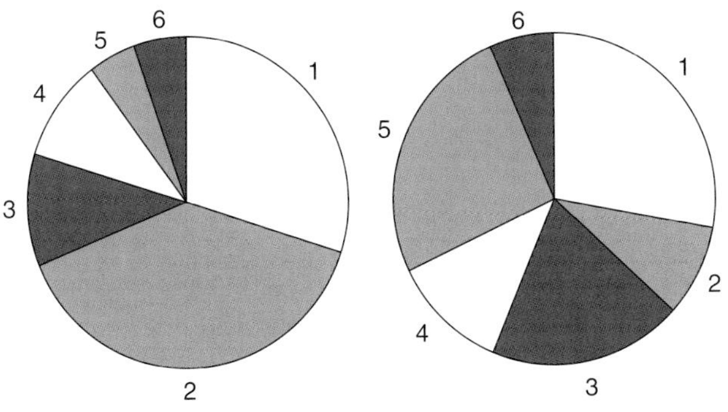

Figure 19.3 Drug candidate attrition reasons. The pie chart on the left depicts collated data from several surveys reported up to the year 2000. Several reasons for the high attrition rate are compared via their percentage of contribution. Numbers correspond to: (1) Lack of efficacy (30%); (2) Poor PK/ADME (39%); (3) Advanced animal toxicity observed in parallel to ongoing clinical studies (11%); (4) Adverse effects in humans (10%); (5) Commercial reasons (5%); and (6) Miscellaneous (5%). Note that although problems associated with the combined ADMET properties nearly doubled (60%) efficacy problems within surveys reported up to 2000, more recent reports (2008), as shown in the chart on the right, indicate that attrition percentages for PK/ADME appear to have been reduced to only about 9%, whereas animal toxicity and commercialization issues have both risen significantly to about 19% and 26%, respectively. Specific percentages for the same set of numbered factors within the pie chart on the right are: (1) 28%; (2) 9%; (3) 19%; (4) 12%; (5) 26%; and (6) 6%. ADMET = Drug Absorption, Distribution, Metabolism, Excretion and Toxicity. PK = Pharmacokinetic profile. See text for details.

with natural product chemistry. It begins with the chemical-related observation that a particular substance exhibits a biological activity that may be of potential therapeutic interest. This type of observation is typically pursued by trying to better understand the associated biology and by trying to further delineate the biology's chemical connection with the substance. Although the substances can be any chemical, their source has typically been small-molecule natural products (molecular weights of less than 1000 daltons) derived from plants, microbes, marine organisms, and even from animals. The identification of these substances typically has been prompted by either a general survey for active compounds or by an apparently successful traditional medicine or nutraceutical. The latter term comes full-circle to again link history with some of today's related jargon.

The second drug discovery starting point represents a somewhat more recent development. It begins with an interesting molecular biology or pharmacologic observation. In this case the observation, often involving very large biomolecules or entire physiological systems, serves to prompt the pursuit of a substance that can be used to modulate the biological activity in a potentially therapeutic manner. Today, these types of pursuits usually entail a survey of one or more compound libraries using high-throughput screening (HTS) methods to identify efficacious hit compounds and to generate initial structure-activity relationship (SAR) data. In line with today's terminology, it can be noted that when the biological-related observations originate within the clinic, the ensuing drug discovery process is often referred to as translational medicine. Alternatively, when these observations occur at the level of molecular biology or pharmacology, the ensuing drug discovery process is referred to as translational research. Accordingly, it may be useful to unify these two subclassifications of the biological drug discovery starting-point with that of the first fundamental division by thinking of the first as being that of translational chemistry, since it clearly distinguishes itself by originating from observations associated with a chemical substance. Figure 19.4 shows three drugs that can be considered to have been derived from each of these translational drug discovery paradigms. Also depicted is a fourth drug of considerable notoriety whose discovery is probably best thought of as drawing from a composite of all these starting points.

From Figure 19.4, d-tubocurarine (**1**) exemplifies a case where drug discovery began as translational chemistry. This drug's origin can be traced back to the initial observation that a natural product obtained from hot water extraction of a certain South American plant was used by natives during hunting to paralyze game after dipping their arrow heads into the extract. Indeed, the "tubo" portion of this drug's generic name is a constant reminder of this type of starting point in that it reflects the fact that the early supplies of (**1**) as a concentrated, white powder were obtained from South America in sealed tubes made from bamboo shoots. Given intravenously, (**1**) was later found to be a potent muscle relaxant that can be used to paralyze the diaphragm during open-chest surgery. Both its chemical structure as shown in Figure 19.4 and its pharmacological mechanism of action as a cholinergic neuromuscular junction blocking agent were eventually elucidated. Propranolol (**2**) exemplifies a case of translational research. Its origin can be traced to Black's early pharmacologic observation that activation of the beta-adrenergic system increases sympathetic drive and oxygen consumption within animal cardiac tissues. Black hypothesized that it might be possible to protect the ischemic (low oxygen) myocardium and alleviate angina pectoris in humans by administering a beta-adrenergic receptor blocking agent. Pursuit of compounds to modulate this pharmacologic pathway eventually led to (**2**), which has come to be regarded as the prototypical beta-blocker with a range of clinical indications that includes hypertension. For the latter, propranolol can be taken by the oral route (p.o.) and has a several-hour half-life in the body, which allows it to be used in a convenient manner with good compliance during chronic dosing. Esmolol (**3**) exemplifies a case of translational medicine that was inspired by the clinical observation that propranolol's long half-life was no longer a desirable feature when it was given by the intravenous route (IV) while attempting to modulate adrenergic tone during critical care situations. Pursuit of compounds that retained beta-adrenergic receptor blocking activity while

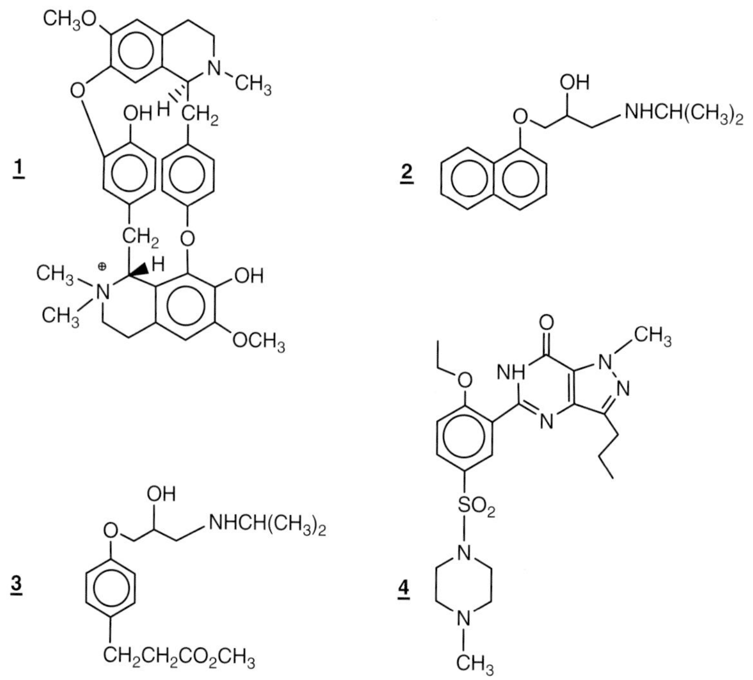

Figure 19.4 Examples of drugs that were derived from translational chemistry, translational research and translational medicine, respectively: (1) d-tubocurarine; (2) propranolol; and (3) esmolol. Also shown is sildenafil, (4), which is probably best considered to have been derived from a composite of all three of these drug discovery starting points. See text for details.

uniquely displaying an ultra-short duration of action for IV use in the emergency room eventually led to (3), which is now administered in critical care situations including use as an antiarrhythmic agent. Compound (4) combines all three translational drug discovery starting points. It will be discussed later in Section 19.1.1.6. Compounds (2) and (3) will also be discussed in greater detail within the Case Studies section as examples of how rational structural modifications can be done so as to modulate both the efficacious activity and the pharmacokinetic (PK; e.g., drug half-life in the body) properties of a drug-wannabe.

19.1.1.4 Credentializing Biological Targets and Lead Compounds

Regardless of starting point, all quickly converge onto a common pathway when drug discovery next deploys biological testing screens to assess a given compound's efficacy at the targeted biological surface. Today, screens that utilize HTS assay methods are established to be as close as possible to the biological mechanism that is thought to be responsible for the desired therapeutic effect. From this vantage point, the HTS methods can be utilized to clarify the underlying biology and its accompanying SAR for an interesting chemical observation, or to identify a new chemical substance that has acceptable efficacy within the context of an initial biological observation. For example, in the case where inhibition of a selected enzyme is thought to represent a mechanistic point of modulation that can lead to therapy, an inhibitor having activity at nanomolar concentration is generally sought in a biochemical assay of that particular enzyme's specific function. Substances and initial hit compounds are typically modified so as to achieve this level of potency as part of this early step in the overall process of drug discovery. Once a potent lead compound is in-hand, the next step generally involves its examination in one or more secondary pharmacology models that are thought to closely reflect the pathology that is to be rectified. A typical example of the latter for the case of a potential anticancer agent that works by inhibiting a specific enzyme would be to examine the lead compound's ability to inhibit the growth of a human cancer cell line in a cell culture assay and also when the cancer cells are implanted into a rodent animal model. When a direct correlation can be established between potency in the mechanism-based biochemical assay and efficacy in the pathology-based *in vitro* and *in vivo* models, the biological concept and the drug-wannabe can be thought of as a credentialized therapeutic target and a credentialized lead compound, respectively.

19.1.1.5 Optimizing Pharmacological Profile and Advancing a Preclinical Drug Development Candidate

Having reached the point of identifying one or more compounds that exhibit potent activity in a mechanistic assay that either correlates directly with the targeted human pathophysiology or has been indirectly credentialized as described earlier, it next becomes critical to fine-tune one of these compounds for its actual use as a potential drug in humans. The anticipated route of administration and dosage protocol as governed by PK profile must also receive attention at this point. The difficulty of this step has already been indicated in Figure 19.3, where it is clear that a significant attrition rate of potential new drugs when tested in humans can be accounted for by an inadequate pharmacologic profile associated with PK and toxicity related parameters, as well as with low potency and inadequate efficacy. Part of the reason for this attrition is that the studies needed to address these types of pharmacologic parameters can be extremely complex and often, in themselves, lack a solid credentialization relative to how the preclinical results actually correlate with their analogous endpoints in humans. As a result, addressing these types of parameters has long constituted a significant hurdle for progression of drug discovery into its final stages.

In addition to the noted shortcomings of some of the development-related assays and preclinical models, the chemical complexity rises suddenly at this point due to the need to simultaneously optimize all the secondary pharmacological-related parameters like drug absorption, distribution, metabolism, excretion, and toxicity (the so-called ADMET properties), while preserving the specific molecular features that enabled the initial substance to display its potentially therapeutic or efficacious attributes in the first place. The structural features needed for efficacy constitute what is called a pharmacophore. These key features need not necessarily reside in a contiguous arrangement within the overall molecule. Furthermore, given the flexibility of molecules to adopt different shapes in three-dimensional space, it becomes a significant challenge to define which features constitute the requisite pharmacophore versus those portions of the structure that can be modified to enhance the compound's overall ADMET profile. Because of this chemical complexity, a proactive approach is often adopted during the previous step where *in vitro* assessments of some of the ADMET factors are additionally undertaken as part of the prior, hit-to-lead survey. This is done in a complementary manner with the potency enhancement type of structural modifications being done on the initial hit compounds. In this way, a systematic and mutually knowledge-building SAR dataset can be assembled. This combination of data can then be used to more effectively contribute to the initial construction and selection of an improved lead compound, as well as during the next phase of serious drug design where continued attempts will be made to further optimize these types of complex ADMET-related parameters. Once a fully optimized lead is selected, the so-called preclinical development compound or preclinical drug candidate (PDC) needs to be scaled-up in quantity and thoroughly characterized analytically prior to undergoing an even more rigorous and final assessment of its efficacy and ADMET properties in advanced *in vivo* models.

Having crossed this hurdle, the penultimate stage of the overall drug discovery process entails addressing the specific regulatory mandates that seek to insure that a PDC can be examined safely during Phase I testing in humans. In order to conduct clinical testing within the United States, or to produce a material within the United States that will be tested in humans outside of the United States, an Investigational New Drug Application (IND) must first be approved by the U.S. Federal Drug Agency (FDA). Many of the studies to be done at this point will now be directed toward the MET portion of the ADMET profile with a major emphasis being placed on toxicity (T) in an attempt to predict and maximize human safety. The kilogram quantities of the PDC that are now needed for use in requisite multispecies toxicity studies intended to become part of the IND submission, along with the specific batch of raw drug that will be used in the actual human dosage formulations, all need to be produced according to FDA-mandated Good Manufacturing Processes (GMPs) accompanied by analytical quality control protocols conducted according to Good Laboratory Practices (GLPs).

The overall difficulty associated with reaching this point is reflected by Figure 19.2, where it was shown that approximately 166 compounds (1500 ÷ 9), on average, are studied in order to move one or more initial hit compounds forward so as to obtain just one PDC that is actually able to enter the first phase of clinical testing. However, since statistics then show that somewhere between one-in-nine to every one-in-11 of these clinical development compounds will actually make it to a market launch, most drug discovery efforts simultaneously seek to have at least one back-up PDC already in place at this step. Thus, not including the initial compound libraries that first might have been screened to produce one or more hits, nearly 332 analogs will likely have been surveyed at this point, or shortly thereafter, in order to provide one clinical candidate and a backup. Continuing to follow this statistically driven analysis, of five different drug discovery groups or companies who might have two compound chances in-hand for a given type of new therapy, today's average suggests that only one of these groups or companies is likely to actually achieve success. For the "losers" in this game, however, other options can sometimes present themselves at this point and these will also be elaborated later.

19.1.1.6 Validating Therapeutic Targets and the First Chance for a New Drug

Phase I testing is the first in a series of closely regulated clinical testing protocols that constitute the last sequence of steps in the overall process of drug discovery. Phase I generally involves a dose-ranging safety study in healthy human volunteers, however today it is quite common to also obtain a read-out of some biomarker that is indicative of the potential drug's desired efficacy. Further Phase II and III studies involve treatment of the indicated human pathophysiological conditions for which all the preceding efforts have been directed. Once potency and therapeutic effect have been discerned within the clinic, the initial biological mechanism that was previously credentialized can now be said to have truly become validated as a new therapeutic target. If all the clinical testing proves favorable and all the possible reasons for attrition shown in Figure 19.3 happen to be circumvented by either clever drug design, brute force numbers, or just plain luck, then the process of new drug discovery can now be said to be complete and a New Drug Application (NDA) can be submitted to the U.S. FDA. Once the latter becomes approved, an actual market launch can be effected.

If compound attrition occurs during clinical testing after validation of the therapeutic target, then according to our definition, the drug discovery process cannot be said to have been fully accomplished. However, at this point, reselection of a back-up PDC, or even a different hit or lead compound, can again be undertaken and similarly brought through the process with much greater ease and with a much higher degree of certainty about the efficacy-related biological variables than was present during the first attempt. Alternatively, if the biological mechanism is also not validated, then it becomes a much greater risk to reinvest the time and resources needed to make another pass through this process based upon the same starting-point strategy. Finally, having arrived in the clinic, it is also possible to fortuitously observe a different, potentially therapeutic application, which can then be considered as an alternative indication. Note that this new therapeutic indication will be able to be pursued with higher confidence and in an expedited version of the first pass through the overall drug discovery process, perhaps even by simply further deploying the compound in-hand toward the new clinical pathway and its associated protocols. Although this last possibility may seem somewhat remote, it does indeed occur and it is exactly what happened for the case of sildenafil, whose structure (**4**) was previously shown in Figure 19.4.

Sildenafil's discovery can be thought of as beginning with a combination of collaborative chemical and pharmacological findings (translational chemistry and translational research activities) that showed this particular structure to be an effective inhibitor of the enzyme Phosphodiesterase V (PDE V). The latter, in turn, was known to catabolize cyclic gaunosine monophosphate or cGMP, which is an intracellular second messenger associated with calcium homoeostasis and which can cause relaxation of certain vascular beds. Thus, inhibition of PDE V sustains higher levels of intracellular cGMP, which could be useful in the treatment of hypertension or angina pectoris. Indeed, (**4**) was taken into clinical testing twice—first to be examined as an antihypertensive and when that failed, second, to be examined as a therapy for angina pectoris, which also failed. Alternatively, another vascular bed was observed to be significantly dilated during these clinical studies (translational medicine) and hence sildenafil's eventual indication as a treatment for erectile dysfunction was identified and no less than a multibillion dollar market was born.

A schematic version for the overall process of drug discovery is provided in Figure 19.5. This figure emphasizes the three different types of translational drug discovery paradigms that are derived from either

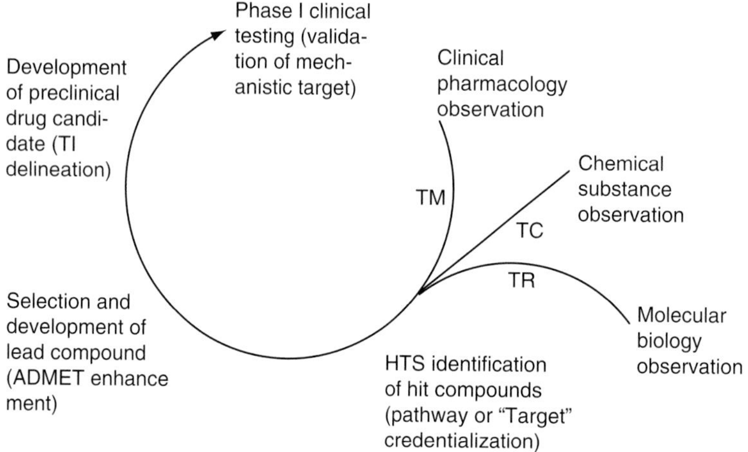

Figure 19.5 Schematic of the overall drug discovery process that emphasizes the types of starting points that can be pursued. When the starting point is a clinical pharmacology observation, the overall process is also referred to as translational medicine (TM). When the starting point is a nonclinical and nonchemical observation such as one associated with molecular biology or pharmacology, the overall process of drug discovery is also referred to as translational research (TR). By analogy to TM and TR, when the starting point is an observation associated with an interesting chemical substance, the overall process can be referred to as translational chemistry (TC). HTS refers to high-throughput screening, generally of compound libraries. ADMET refers to drug absorption, distribution, metabolism, excretion and toxicity. TI refers to the therapeutic index which is a ratio of toxicity over efficacy, generally expressed in units of dose required to cause noticeable toxicity compared to the dose required to evoke what is considered to be an efficaciously therapeutic effect, or in similar doses needed to cause 50% lethality of an animal model population compared to doses needed to evoke 50% of some desired effect in that same population (LD_{50}/ED_{50}). For both expressions of TI, a higher ratio is thus desirable.

a chemically-driven or a biologically-driven fundamental drug discovery starting point. Additional discussions for several of the steps in this overall process will convey a more chemically oriented perspective, which will then become the main technical thrust for the remainder of this chapter.

19.1.2 History

The highly collaborative nature of the drug discovery process from beginning to end should be apparent from the description provided in Section 19.1.1, and likewise upon consideration of Figure 19.5 in terms of the different onsets that are possible for the process followed by the same seamless progression across the various types of interdisciplinary activities that then ensue. From a historical perspective, however, it is the field of medicinal chemistry that stands out as being the most closely entwined with the overall conduct of drug discovery around this circle as well as across time. Thus, a brief account of this field's evolution will serve to provide a useful backdrop for further understanding and appreciating the overall process of interdisciplinary drug discovery as it has come to be practiced today. Toward that end, the following summary draws heavily from similar treatments of this topic within the recent edition of the series entitled "Comprehensive Medicinal Chemistry," and within a forerunner publication in *Pure and Applied Chemistry* that commemorated the arrival of the new millennium.

19.1.2.1 Medicinal Chemistry as an Academic Discipline and Its Adoption by the Industry

Medicinal chemistry's (MC's) roots can be found in the fertile mix of ancient folk *medicine* and early natural product *chemistry*, hence its name. That this field's solid foundation drawing from both applied and basic research has not only sustained itself, but continues to be enhanced in an interdisciplinary manner today, is captured nicely within Figure 19.6A. Figure 19.6 also conveys a similar relationship for the field of pharmacology (B), and finally, how both of these key disciplines unite in a complementary manner during the challenging ADMET optimization and development stages of drug discovery (C).

Responding to a growing appreciation for the links between chemical structure and observed biological activity, MC emerged from its fertile mix about 175 years ago as a distinct discipline intending to explore these relationships via chemical modification and structural mimicry of nature's materials, particularly with an eye toward enhancing the efficacy of substances thought to be of potential therapeutic value. In the United States, MC became formally recognized as a graduate level discipline nearly 100 years ago within the academic framework of pharmacy education. From

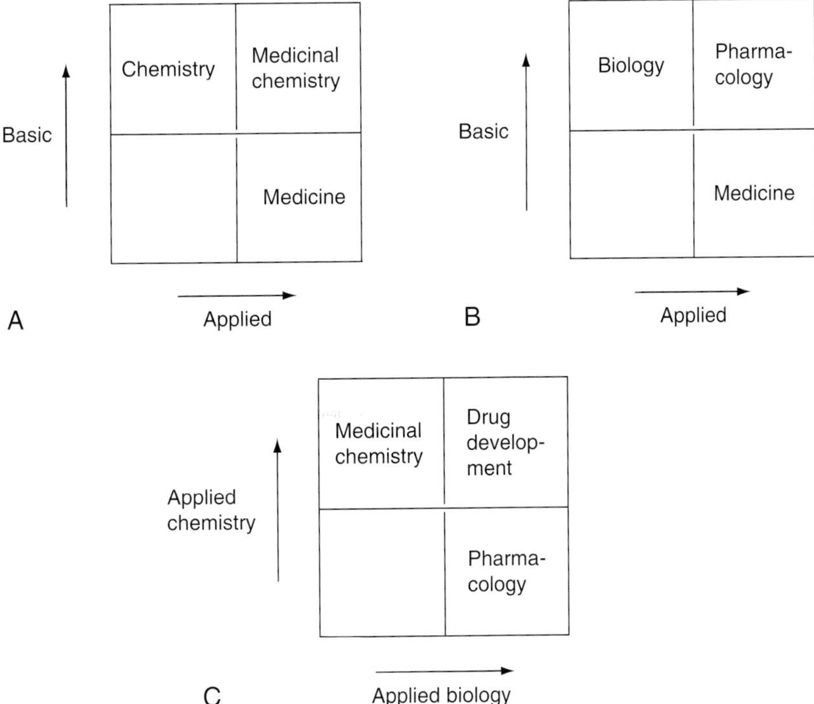

Figure 19.6 Relationships of medicinal chemistry (A) and pharmacology (B) to basic and applied research, as well as medicinal chemistry and pharmacology to the development stages of the overall process of drug discovery (C).

this setting, overviews of MC's subject matter have been offered to both undergraduate and graduate pharmacy students for many years.

Understanding the relationships between chemical structure and biological activity (SAR) at the level of inherent physical organic properties such as lipophilic, electronic, and steric parameters, coupled with consideration of molecular conformation, soon became the hallmark of MC research. This development further distinguished MC from its natural products predecessor, which instead, had begun to focus more upon understanding plant biochemistry (phytochemistry) as a source for new chemical structures in general. It follows that because fundamental SAR is useful during the design of new drugs, applications toward drug discovery became the principal domain for the still sprouting, basic science component of MC. Perhaps somewhat prematurely, MC's drug design role became especially important in the private sector where its practice quickly spread among the rich fields being staked out across the acres of intellectual property that were of particular interest to the pharmaceutical industry. This full-scale adoption into the industry provided a second home for the continued growth of MC, where critical influences important to the private sector would also serve to further shape its maturation.

19.1.2.2 An Adolescent Heyday of Rational Drug Design

As a comprehensive understanding about the links between observed activity and pharmacological mechanisms began to develop about 75 years ago, MC soon entered what can now be considered an adolescent phase. Confidently instilled with new knowledge about what was happening at the biomolecular level, MC wanted to respond more quickly to the pressing needs of its adopted home within the private sector. Rather than waiting for Mother Nature to reveal another natural product template, scientists began to envision being able to proactively design new drugs in a rational, *ab initio* manner. This adolescent "heyday of rational drug design" can be credited with having spurred significant advances in the methods that are used to consider molecular conformation. However, the rate of actually delivering useful therapeutic entities having novel chemical structures, referred to today as NCEs (Figure 19.1), was not significantly improved for most pharmacological targets. Some successes did occur but these were usually when the target's relevant biomolecules also lent themselves to rigorous structural analysis, such as obtainment of an X-ray diffraction picture of a crystallized enzyme's active site with or without a bound ligand.

One of the main reasons why rational drug design fell short of its promise was because without experimental data like an X-ray view of the drug's target site, MC's hypothetical SAR-derived models often reflected speculative notions that still required synthesis of a considerable number of molecular probes in order to assess a given model's associated hypotheses. Thus, with only a small number of clinical, true drug success stories, MC's "preconceived notions about what a new drug ought to look like" began to take on negative, rather than positive, connotations. This was particularly so when proposed within the results-oriented setting of a private sector drug discovery program. Importantly and key to this historical juncture, however, is the fact that even though the design of drugs in a rational manner had fallen short of the hyped expectation, MC continued to thrive quite well during this early period. Its maturation progressed as both a recognized academic discipline and as a central player for the drug discovery efforts taking place within the private sector.

19.1.2.3 High-Throughput Screening, Combinatorial Chemistry, and a Marriage Made on Earth, If Not in Heaven

Arriving at the next historical segment puts us at the time when the biotechnology rainfall began to hover over the field of drug discovery a little more than about 25 years ago. With this development, not only did the number of interesting biological targets begin to rise rapidly (translational research), but also the ability to assay targets in a high-throughput manner suddenly prompted the screening of huge numbers of compounds in very quick timeframes (HTS). Ultimately, the need to satisfy HTS's immense appetite for compounds was addressed not by any natural product, synthetic medicinal or organic chemistry, but instead by further developments within what had quickly become a flood-level, continuous downpour of biotechnology-related breakthroughs. Starting as gene-cassette-altered, biosynthetic peptide libraries and quickly moving into solid-phase, randomly generated peptide and nucleotide libraries, this novel technique soon spread across other disciplines to also spawn the new field of small molecule, combinatorial chemistry. Today, using equipment and platforms available from a variety of suppliers, huge libraries of small molecules can readily be produced in either a random fashion or in a directed manner based upon a structural template afforded by a suspected hit compound. Thus, the marriage of HTS with combinatorial chemistry soon would propagate a new approach toward implementing the discovery of drugs.

19.1.2.4 Birth of a New Drug Discovery Paradigm

When the marriage of compound library technologies to HTS became consummated, it quickly propagated a new paradigm for the discovery of NCEs across the entire big pharma segment of the pharmaceutical enterprise. Schemes 19.1 and 19.2 provide a side-by-side comparison of the old (classical) and new (today's) drug discovery paradigms, respectively.

Interestingly, the marriage of HTS with combinatorial chemistry and the latter's extended family of compound libraries has also led to a situation where identifying initial hit compounds is no longer considered to be a bottleneck for the overall process of drug discovery. Indeed, many of the programs within

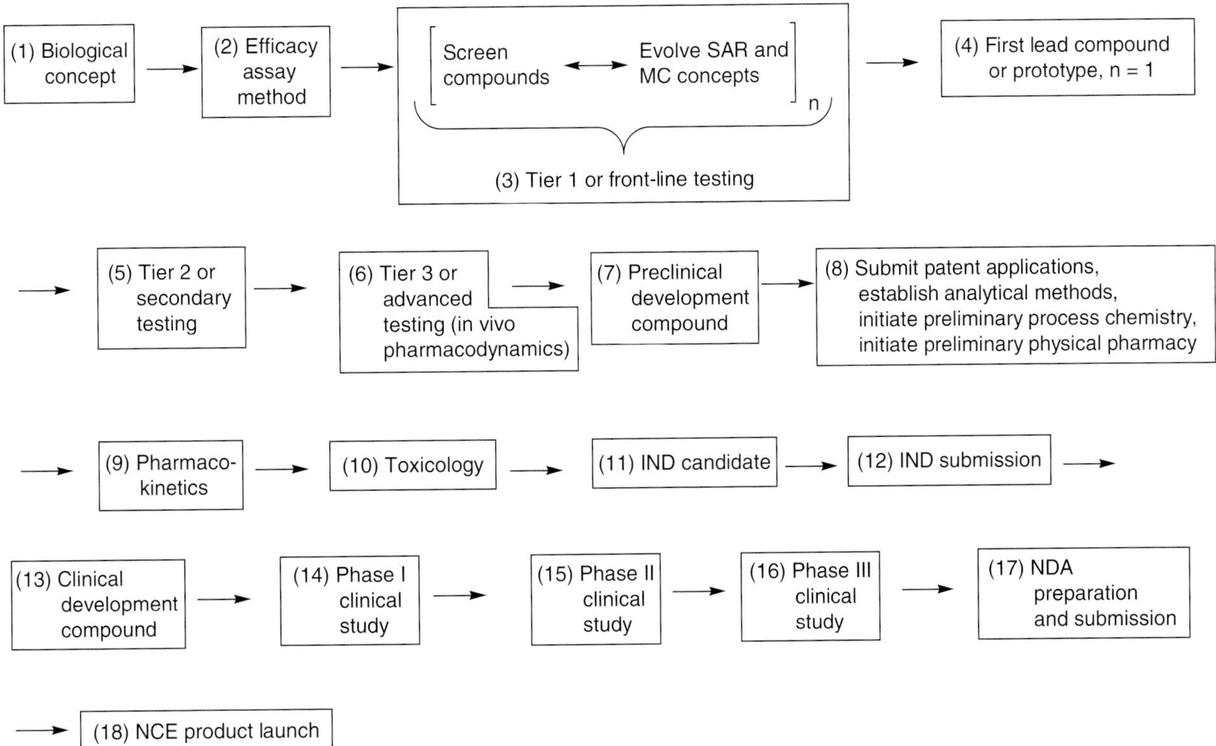

Scheme 19.1 Classical drug discovery and development paradigm. This model portrays interactions with U.S. regulatory agencies and uses terms related to those interactions for steps 11 to 17. All the other terms typify generic phrases that have been commonly adopted by the international pharmaceutical community. Although some of the noted activities can be conducted in parallel or in an overlapping manner, the step-wise, sequential nature of this paradigm's overall process is striking. Furthermore, whenever a progressing compound fails to meet criteria set at an advanced step, the process returns or draws again from step 3 for another reiteration. Numerous reiterations eventually identify a compound that is able to traverse the entire process. A successful passage through the entire process to produce just one product compound has been estimated to require about 15 years at a total cost of about $868 M (July, 2006). The largest share of these time and cost requirements occur during the later steps, although the identification of a promising preclinical development compound, step 7, can be estimated to take about 4 years from the time of initiating a therapeutic concept.
Step 1 is typically associated with some type of physiological or pharmacological notion that intends to amplify or attenuate a specific biological mechanism so as to return some pathophysiology to an overall state of homeostasis (see prior text for drug discovery starting points). Step 2 typically involves one or two biochemical level assay(s) for the interaction of compounds intending to amplify or attenuate the concept-related mechanism. Steps 3 and 4 historically have reflected key contributions from medicinal chemistry and typically use all sources of available information to provide for compound efficacy hits, e.g., everything from natural product surveys to rational approaches based upon X-ray diffractions of the biological target (also see Section 2.3.1). Step 5 generally involves larger *in vitro* models (e.g., tissue level rather than biochemical level) for efficacy and efficacy-related selectivity. Step 6 generally involves *in vivo* testing and utilizes a pharmacodynamic (observable pharmacologic effect) approach toward assessing compound availability and duration of action. Step 7 typically derives from a formal review conducted by an interdisciplinary team upon examination of a formalized compilation of all data obtained to that point. Step 8 specifies parallel activities that are typically initiated at this juncture by distinct disciplines within a given organization. Step 9 begins more refined pharmacokinetic evaluations (PK) by utilizing analytical methods for the drug itself to address *in vivo* availability and duration of action. Step 10 represents short-term (e.g., two-week) dose-ranging studies to initially identify toxic markers within one or more small animal populations. Expanded toxicology studies typically progress while overlapping with steps 11 through 14. Steps 11 to 13 represent formalized reviews undertaken by both the sponsoring organization and the U.S. Food and Drug Administration (FDA). Step 14 is typically a dose-ranging study conducted in healthy humans. Steps 15 and 16 reflect efficacy testing in sick patients, possible drug-interactions, etc. Step 17 again reflects formalized reviews undertaken by both the sponsoring organization and the FDA. The FDA's fast-track review of this information is now being said to have been reduced to an average of about 18 months. It is estimated that it costs a company about $200 K for each day that a compound spends in clinical development. Step 18 represents the delivery of a new chemical entity, NCE, to the marketplace wherein it can finally be stated that a new drug has been truly discovered.

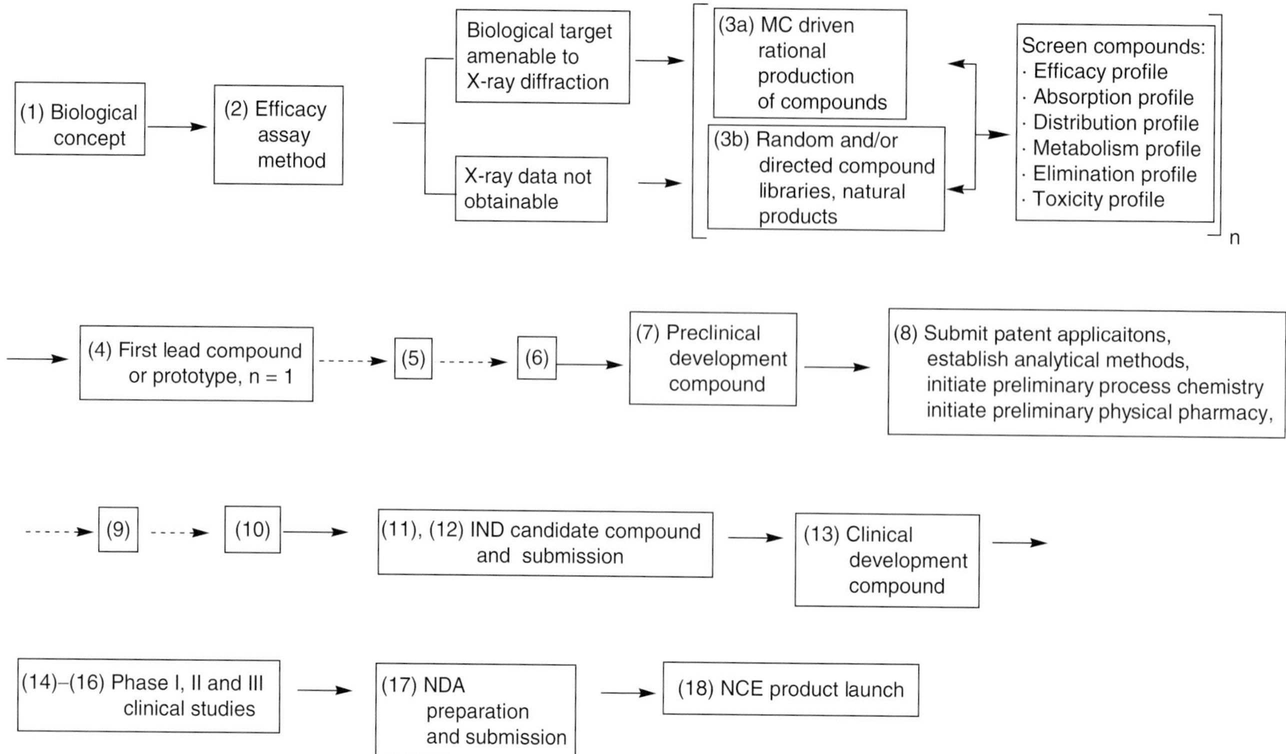

Scheme 19.2 Today's Drug Discovery and Development Paradigm. This model also portrays interactions with U.S. regulatory agencies and uses terms related to those interactions for steps 11 to 17. All the other terms typify generic phrases that are commonly used by the international pharmaceutical community. The battery of simultaneous profiling included in step 3 represents a striking contrast to the classical drug discovery paradigm (Scheme 19.1). Furthermore, all these screens are typically of a high-throughput nature such that huge numbers of compounds can be tested automatically in extremely short time periods. As the predictive value of the resulting profiles improve, selected compounds will have a higher and higher likelihood to successfully proceed through steps 5, 6, 9, and 10 (Scheme 19.1) to the point that these assays may become more of a confirmatory nature or may even be able to be completely omitted (hence their dotted lines in Scheme 19.2). The efficiency of successfully traversing the various clinical testing steps 14 to 16 will also be improved but their complete removal from the overall process is highly unlikely. After the initial investments to upgrade step 3 and enough time has passed to allow for the generation of knowledge from step 3's raw data results (see text for discussion), the overall timeframe and cost for a single NCE to traverse the new paradigm should be improved considerably from the estimates provided in Scheme 19.1. Step 1 is likely to be associated with some type of genomic and/or proteomic derived notion that intends to amplify or attenuate a specific biological mechanism so as to return some pathophysiology to an overall state of homeostasis. Step 2 is typically a high-throughput assay derived from using molecular biology and bioengineering techniques. Because step 3a exploits actual pictures of what type of structural arrangements are needed to interact with the biological targets, this approach toward identifying new compound hits will continue to operate with high efficiency. However, because of this same efficiency, the biological targets that lend themselves to such experimental depiction (by affording crystals suitable for X-ray diffraction) could become depleted much faster than the range of more difficult biological targets. Step 3b represents various combinatorial chemistry-derived libraries, natural product collections, and elicited natural product libraries (see text for discussion of this topic). Steps 4 to 18 are similar to the descriptions noted in Scheme 19.1.

pharmaceutical companies soon began to suffer from "compound overload" with far too many initial hits to effectively follow up. Shifting the rate-limiting step into development, a new situation was created where there was a need to move much more quickly toward characterizing a potential lead compound's pharmacokinetic (PK) and ADME profiles that would be anticipated upon administration to humans. When the latter are also combined with concerns about toxicity, the entire process of ADMET assessment became the new bottleneck for the overall process of drug discovery, along with the traditionally sluggish clinical and associated regulatory steps as shown near the end of Schemes 19.1 and 19.2. Responding to this pressure, an emphasis was also placed upon moving the challenging ADMET-related assessments into more of an HTS format that could be undertaken at earlier decision points associated with defining a lead compound. Thus, even though efficacy-related HTS and combinatorial chemistry reflect very significant incorporations of new methodologies, from a strategic point of view the most striking feature of today's drug discovery and development paradigm shown in Scheme 19.2 compared to the classical approach depicted in Scheme 19.1 actually becomes the movement of ADMET-related assays closer to the beginning of the overall process of drug discovery.

The plethora of biology-based therapeutic concepts can be expected to rise even further. Likewise, the identification of compounds capable of interacting with the biological surfaces associated with those concepts that become selected as therapeutic targets can also be expected to become quicker as the marriage of HTS to compound library and combinatorial chemistry technologies continues to enjoy each successive anniversary. In the end, a more efficient handling of ADMET-related concerns clearly represents one of the most significant challenges facing today's drug discovery enterprise, a situation that becomes exacerbated with each new day of HTS and the identification of a hit or lead compound that constitutes yet another drug-wannabe.

19.1.2.5 Solving an Identity Crises and Moving on to Play a Key Role as the Central Interpreter of Drug Discovery Information

The use of these new approaches toward identifying lead compounds and for studying SAR represent exciting developments that clearly had an invigorating effect upon the practice of MC in many areas. Alternatively, the SAR hallmark and drug design intellectual domains of MC, along with chemically servicing the experimental approaches toward identifying novel hit structures, had all been overrun by technologies derived from other disciplines. This, in turn, produced somewhat of an unnerving impact upon MC because it had previously been the nearly exclusive deliverance of these roles from a chemical orientation that had served to distinguish MC as a distinct discipline for so many years. Thus, as a field, MC moved from its disappointing adolescent heyday only to find itself in the middle of an identity crisis. Similarly, the new drug discovery paradigm supplanted MC's long-standing position where its practitioners have typically been regarded as the primary inventors of the composition of matter specifications associated with NCE patent applications. This situation further added to the critical need for MC to undergo a metamorphosis.

Fortunately for MC, as promising hits have continued to pile up from industry-based efforts and recent academic-based efforts promoted by the U.S. National Institutes of Health NIH Roadmap Initiative, it is now recognized that MC must even more heavily engage itself in the drug discovery process. Responding to this new challenge and picking up on today's themes of translational medicine and research as displayed in Figure 19.5, MC is beginning to fill the gap needed to move initial hits into legitimate leads and ultimately into high caliber preclinical development compounds (PDCs) that may have a lower attrition rate upon clinical testing. Furthermore, as MC continues to undergo this symbiotic metamorphosis with secondary pharmacology, where its distinctive pursuit of fundamental SAR principles are increasingly applied toward addressing ADMET issues (Figure 19.6, C), it is likely that a generally useful knowledge base will gradually accumulate in this area.

19.1.2.6 Medicinal Chemistry and the Process of Drug Discovery Today and into the Future

As the MC-derived SAR principles accumulate across the ADMET arena, we can expect this new bottleneck to become alleviated. Moving this theme into the future, it is hoped that these types of basic science activities (Figure 19.6, A) will eventually allow for a third version of the overall drug discovery process to be undertaken in much more of an *in silico* fashion where the latter can ultimately rest upon solid SAR principles established by the interdisciplinary experimental work of MC and pharmacology. This futuristic version of the overall process of drug discovery is depicted in Scheme 19.3, which has been laid out in close juxtaposition to the classical and present-day processes of drug discovery so that it can be readily contrasted to both of these versions as its immediate predecessors (Schemes 19.1 and 19.2).

19.2 UNDERLYING PRINCIPLES

19.2.1 Pharmacological Media and Biological Surfaces

As discussed earlier, a chemical substance on the way to becoming a drug often starts by demonstrating a favorable interaction with a biological surface associated with therapeutic efficacy, such as inhibition of a particular enzyme required for growth of a cancer cell. However, this is only the first aspect of the overall profile that a drug must display if it is ultimately to become successful. The remaining aspects involve interactions with a diverse array of other pharmacological media and biological surfaces that, when taken together, result in the drug's ADMET profile. The high attrition rate during drug discovery was discussed in Section 19.1, where it was emphasized that numerous drug-wannabe compounds fail in the clinic because they display an inadequate ADMET profile (Figure 19.3). Likewise, the complexities of trying to better address these issues prior to clinical testing have also been alluded to. Taking as an example an orally administered central nervous system (CNS) drug that has a targeted site of efficacious action within the brain, Scheme 19.4 depicts the various pharmacological media and biological surfaces that this drug will have to favorably traverse if it ultimately is to display its desired effect.

Although we shall come to see that these additional factors are governed by both the overall physicochemical properties and the specific chemical structural detail of the drug, the process of traversing the body to arrive at a targeted site of action was initially described by Hansch as a "random walk." From our prior discussion we have come to appreciate that this

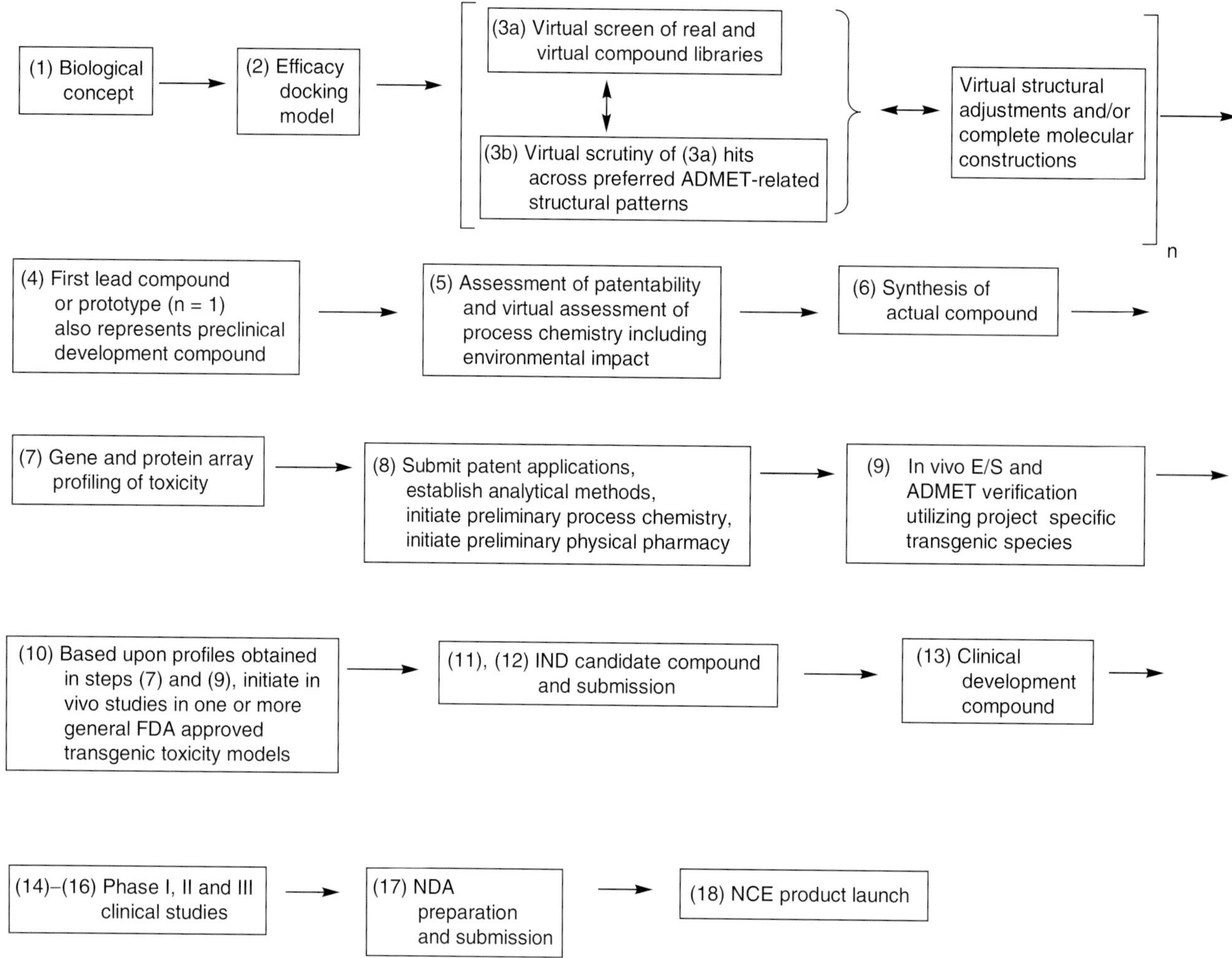

Scheme 19.3 Future Drug Discovery and Development Paradigm. This model also portrays interactions with U.S. regulatory agencies and uses terms related to those interactions for steps 11 to 17. *Future* implies about another 75 to 100 years. The most striking feature of this paradigm compared to Schemes 19.1 and 19.2 is the considerable number of decisions that will be made from virtual constructs rather than from experimental results. Confidence in the virtual decisions will be directly proportional to the level of knowledge that is learned from the huge amounts of drug screening data being amassed during the next 50 years, coupled with the overall ability to predict clinical outcomes. Step 1 is likely to be associated with some type of genomic and/or proteomic derived notion that intends to amplify or attenuate one or more specific biological mechanisms so as to either return some pathophysiology to an overall state of homeostasis, or to modify some system in a manner that prevents or provides prophylaxis toward an otherwise anticipated pathophysiological development. Note that a growing emphasis of drug usage will be directed toward prevention rather than toward treatment. Step 2 may be based upon an actual X-ray diffraction version of the biological target or upon a computationally constructed version derived from similar known systems that have been catalogued for such extrapolations. In either case, ligand-receptor docking studies will be conducted in a virtual mode. Steps 3, 4, and 5 will also be conducted in a virtual mode, and steps 6 and 7 represent the first lab-based activities. After submission of patents, it is proposed that *in vivo* testing involving steps 9 and 10 will be able to take advantage of project specific and FDA approved generic toxicity model transgenic species. Steps 11 to 18 are similar to those in Schemes 19.1 and 19.2 except that the likelihood for a compound to fall short of the desired criteria will be significantly reduced. Due to advances in analytical methodology, the first exposure of the potential drug to humans is likely to involve micro-dosing so as to ascertain preliminary human PK data. Larger dose studies will be able to take advantage of subject inclusion/exclusion criteria that will be much more refined and based upon advances in the field of pharmacogenetics.

walk can also be likened to an exceedingly difficult race involving an array of ADMET hurdles that can quickly eliminate a new drug-wannabe before it even becomes a competitive contender. Furthermore, because of the likelihood that other research groups may be circling the same technology track, the resulting competition to be the first to succeed can often turn into an outright sprint down the final lap of the race to the market with the potential new drug in the hands of the clinical "anchormen" like the baton of an interdisciplinary relay. Thus, in addition to the difficulties associated with the ADMET hurdles

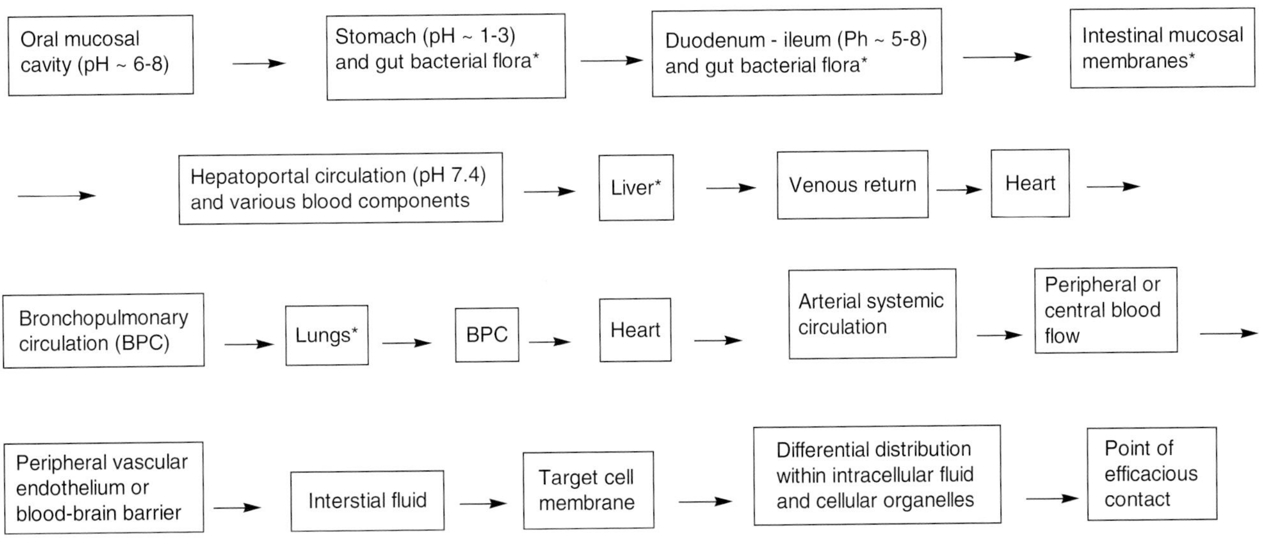

Scheme 19.4 Random walk taken by an oral drug en route to its point of efficacious interaction within a human target cell, such as within the brain for a CNS drug. This continuum of interactions between a drug and various biological surfaces within the human biological realm is typically divided into categories associated with ADMET and efficacy. Biological milieu marked with an asterisk (*) represent compartments having particularly high drug metabolizing capabilities in general. Blood is notably high in only esterase capability. More and more, drug discovery teams are utilizing knowledge about ADMET-related SARs to more effectively identify the best drug leads and to further enhance the therapeutic profiles of selected compounds.

of drug discovery, the highly competitive nature of the overall business at this particular juncture should likewise be fully appreciated. That five to 25% of the attrition during clinical testing is thought to be associated with business rather than technical concerns (Figure 19.3) likely also reflects this highly competitive aspect of the overall process of drug discovery.

19.2.1.1 The Oral Cavity and Gastro-Intestinal (GI) Tract

Turning to Scheme 19.4 and beginning immediately after administration by the oral route, we find that our exemplary CNS drug is immediately exposed to a dynamic pharmacologic media that spans a range of strongly acidic pH within the stomach to somewhat basic pH as it continues to proceed down the intestinal tract. In addition, the GI-tract is rich with two main groups of metabolizing enzymes. The first group is excreted by the body primarily to hydrolyze chemical bonds present in the foods of our normal diets in order to expedite the absorption of key nutritional components. However, in this case the ready hydrolysis of exogenous peptides and proteins by these enzymes often renders the latter types of biotechnology-derived substances and drug candidates very difficult to be successfully administered by the oral route. The second group of metabolizing enzymes is contributed by the microorganisms living within the GI tract. This population is capable of causing various biotransformations on small molecule drug substances, particularly the rather unique reactions related to metabolic reduction. Interestingly, this unique type of microorganism-derived metabolism can play a role during the discovery of new drugs as well as during their development, an example being the sulfonamide antibiotics.

The prototypical sulfonamide antibiotic, sulfanilamide, is shown in Scheme 19.5 as structure **6**. Its activity was discovered in the mid-1930s by Domagk, a German physician who was studying a series of bright-red, azo-linked dyes and their effects upon streptococcal infections. Domagk noted that one of these dyes, prontosil (shown as structure **5** in Scheme 19.5), was very active when administered orally to streptococcal-infected mice. However, he was not able to confirm this activity in an *in vitro* experiment when the streptococcal bacteria were systematically studied within the well-controlled environment of a culture dish. Unable to impress pharmaceutical companies, such as Bayer, into further exploring these ambiguous findings, Domagk took a huge leap across all of today's drug development paradigm steps and, as a last resort for his own daughter who was succumbing to an incurable streptococcal infection, administered prontosil to her on his own. She, in turn, is said to have undergone a "miraculous recovery" from which further research then showed that this chemical substance has valuable efficacious properties.

As shown in Scheme 19.5, however, prontosil is itself an inactive prodrug that, upon oral administration, requires metabolic reduction by the gut microflora to become sulfanilamide, **6**. The latter is an active antimicrobial that is very effective against streptococcal infections upon its absorption into the body. Once this was understood, the birth of the sulfonamide antibiotics can be said to have occurred and both Domagk and his daughter lived "happily-ever-after." It was later shown that the structure of **6** resembles that of para-aminobenzoic acid (PABA) because

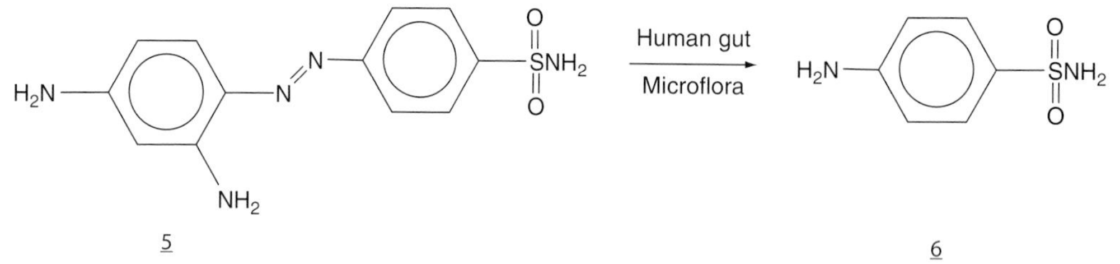

Scheme 19.5 Landmark experiment leading to the birth of the sulfonamide antibiotics. Prontosil, **5**, is itself inactive but upon oral administration **5** is metabolized by gut microflora to **6**, sulfanilamide, which exhibits excellent activity against streptococcal infections. **6** has gone on to become the prototypical sulfonamide antibiotic from which numerous other successful antibiotic drugs have been designed.

its sulfonamide group has a weakly acidic proton that mimics PABA's carboxylic acid. PABA is a requisite biochemical building block for folic acid (FA), which microorganisms are forced to biosynthesize. Unlike humans, microorganisms are not able to absorb this key vitamin intact. Thus, when **6** blocks the synthesis of FA, its toxicity is directed exquisitely toward the infecting microorganisms rather than their human host (thanks, Domagk, for taking this chance, although we, as well as the FDA, would certainly never want you to try to do so today).

19.2.1.2 Absorption and the First-Pass Effect

Drug absorption can occur anywhere along the GI tract. For example, ethanol's absorption begins immediately within the mouth. In general, however, drug absorption is usually greatest across either the stomach or the small intestine, for which a chemistry-derived differential will be described later. Interestingly, the GI-tract epithelial lining is also a rich source of localized metabolizing capability and active transport systems that work to pump materials back into the GI tract. Likely evolving in response to the human consumption of foods that contain a wide variety of potentially toxic natural product xenobiotics, these enzymes are particularly well situated to metabolize small molecule substances via hydrolytic, oxidative, and conjugation reactions that can alter a parent molecule so as to render it inactive upon absorption. Thus, these enzymes and the accompanying transporter systems serve as a front-line defensive barrier or "home security force" toward allowing xenobiotic substances to enter the body when they are present as part of the diet. Unfortunately, our small molecule CNS agent example, like all drugs taken by the oral route (p.o.), is also subject to possible metabolism by these enzymes and transport back to the GI tract. To make matters worse, upon passage through this epithelial barrier, the drug then enters the hepatoportal circulation rather than the general circulation.

Although this vascular bed has evolved to provide a massive net over the GI-tract so that it effectively captures nutrients as they are degraded and thereby made available for absorption into the body, it also delivers its entire blood supply with its pick-up of exogenous materials exclusively to the liver. The liver is the body's clearing house for unwanted substances that might have gained access to the blood as part of the food-capturing process, and in turn, for our model CNS drug when administered p.o. Of all tissues in the body, the liver is the richest in its overall composite of drug metabolizing enzymes, particularly those associated with the cytochrome P450 family, which performs oxidative biotransformations, and those associated with formation of glucuronide conjugation. The specific details for these types of metabolism are described in another chapter.

When the metabolism capabilities of the GI tract, particularly those of the gut wall, are coupled with those of the liver and blood, which itself has a very significant esterase compliment, this entire composite of metabolism capability is referred to as the first-pass effect. All drug molecules taken p.o. will first have to traverse this inherent hurdle in order to gain access to the general circulation. Drug design directed toward circumventing too rapid metabolic degradation upon absorption is a common activity that is frequently prompted by this hurdle. Alternatively, it is probably fortunate that most natural product xenobiotics do not present themselves in high concentrations when accompanying the normal diet. As a result, the body's first line of defense has evolved to handle their presence in comparatively low concentrations. Thus, when more concentrated formulations of a drug are administered, the drug's levels can exceed the liver's extraction capability during the first pass so that in most cases a significant portion of the drug proceeds to reach the general circulation. This fortuitous situation is depicted in Figure 19.7 (A versus B).

19.2.1.3 The Bronchopulmonary Circulation and the Second-Pass Effect

Having survived the liver, our model CNS drug will now make a short run through the venous return to the heart where it will next be pumped through the bronchopulmonary circulation to the lungs. Though primarily intended to exchange oxygen for carbon dioxide in the blood, the huge biological surface displayed by the lungs is also rich in drug metabolizing enzymes, vying with the gut wall for second place in this regard relative to the liver, which stands alone in a distant first place for overall drug metabolizing capability. Given this high propensity for continued metabolism, the lungs are generally considered to be part of the first-pass

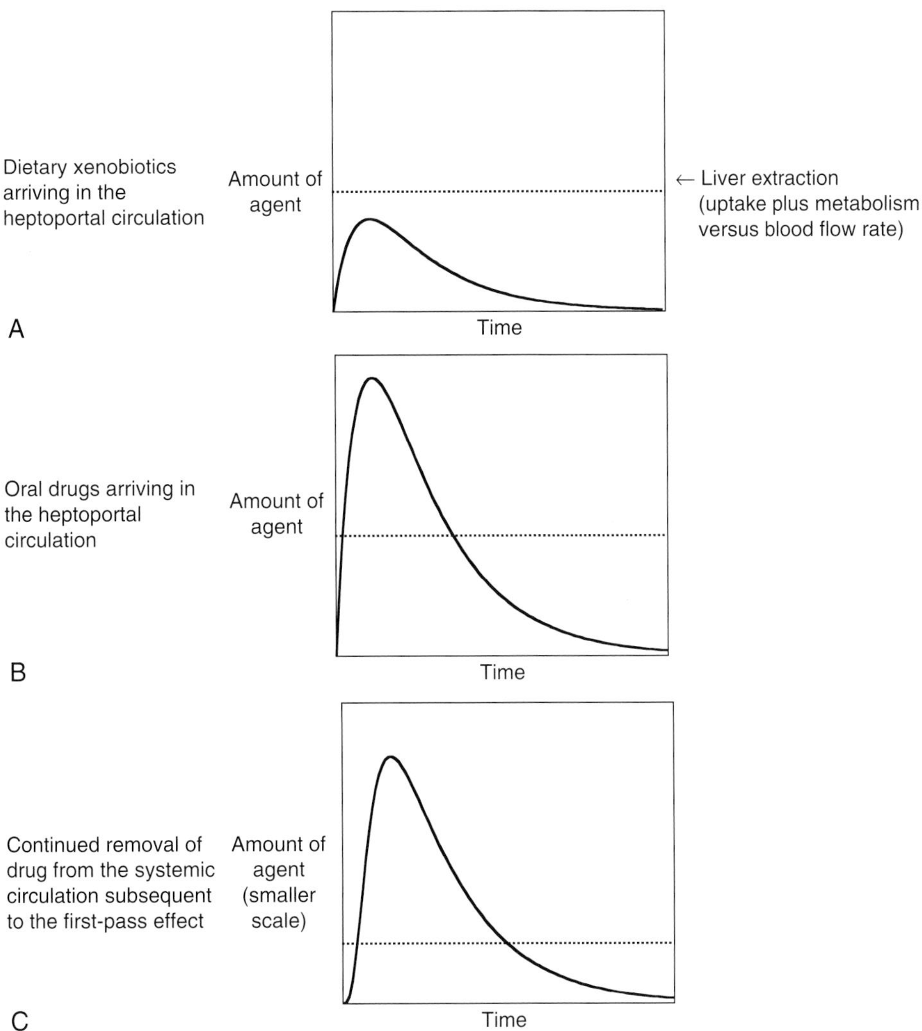

Figure 19.7 Liver extraction of dietary xenobiotics and drugs from the hepatoportal circulation after their absorption from the GI-tract (A and B, respectively) and liver's subsequent drug extraction from the systemic circulation (C). Note that because drugs are often administered in much higher concentration than what is present for natural products normally found in the diet, they can surpass the liver's initial extraction capability and first-pass effect so as to eventually deliver at least some portion of the dose to the general systemic circulation. For C note: (1) Smaller scale for y-axis because concentration in the general circulation will be less than initially present in the hepatoportal circulation during drug absorption; (2) Slight lag in drug appearance and peak concentration times compared to the hepatoportal circulation; and (3) Decreased liver extraction capability (lower dotted line) because a much smaller percentage of the overall arterial blood flow traverses the liver.

effect since at this point, the p.o. administered drug still has not made it to the general, systemic circulation.

Alternatively, emphasizing the distinct anatomical difference, I prefer that the lungs be considered to provide for a second-pass effect, which still precedes a drug's entry into the general systemic circulation after oral absorption. Following this type of compartmental distinction, the lungs thus would provide for a pseudo-first-pass effect after administration of a drug by any route other than p.o. and intra-arterial, because all of these other routes will place the drug directly into the venous return to the heart while bypassing the GI tract and liver hepatoportal circulation completely. Intraperitoneal administration (i.p.), often used in dosing animals, bypasses the GI tract and gut wall but not the liver, so it can still be thought of as being subject to a portion of the first-pass effect and then a full second-pass effect.

19.2.1.4 The Systemic Circulation and Blood–Brain Barrier

Assuming that our model CNS drug has survived and exited the lungs, it will next proceed back to the heart where it will finally be pumped to the general systemic circulation so that it can be distributed throughout the body and thereby to its desired sites of action. However, even though this is generally true for most of the body's tissues, it is not such a simple case for the brain, which has an additional barrier. Consisting of tightly packed, specialized endothelial cells that protect the brain from certain components of the vascular contents, this specialized arrangement is referred to as the blood–brain barrier (BBB). The BBB was discussed in Chapter 7. Although not highly active in terms of metabolizing enzymes, like the gut wall the BBB is very rich in active transporters that pump drugs out of the edothelial cells and back into the cerebral vasculature.

19.2.1.5 Efficacy Surfaces: Receptors, Active Sites, and Cell Signaling Clusters

Having managed to traverse the BBB and to avoid the outward transporters, our model CNS drug will have finally reached the desired compartment, where its efficacious receptors or active sites reside. Passage across the interstial fluid and brain cell membranes followed by equilibration within the target cells will occur as the drug finally approaches its distinct, efficacious biological surface. Note that a distinction is typically drawn between enzyme active sites and all other types of ligand-biological surface interactions, which, in turn, are then referred to as receptor interactions. One notable exception is that of the various transporter systems. Their cargo ligands are usually regarded as substrates, even though no structural changes on the cargoes actually ensue. For example, the neurotransmitter norephinephrine (NE; **14** in Scheme 19.7) should be thought of as binding like an agonist onto its postsynaptic receptor, whereby it activates the receptor prior to binding as a substrate within the active sites of either MAO enzyme (Scheme 19.7) or its reuptake transporter located in the sympathetic nerve ending. NE either undergoes a biodegradative metabolic reaction prompted by MAO, or transports into the nerve terminus without undergoing any change. Likewise, a distinction in the terminology for drugs that block one or the other of these types of biological surfaces is also generally utilized, namely that of receptor antagonists versus active site inhibitors. A brief consideration of different types of efficacious targets is provided next, particularly with regard to future possibilities based upon the present emphasis within molecular pharmacology and protein chemistry to interrogate cell signaling pathways.

In terms of drug targets within the body, the major neurochemical pathways like the parasympathetic and sympathetic nervous systems have probably received the most attention to date, particularly with regard to their cell surface receptors. These areas are probably closely followed by the major hormone pathways. In terms of targets distinct from the body, the ever-continuing war against infectious microorganisms and viruses likewise has been raging for a long time. No matter what the pharmacologic or therapeutic area, however, numerous new targets continue to present themselves as our detailed knowledge about their related biological systems continues to grow. Figure 19.8 attempts to convey just some of the types of targets that can be readily pursued today. The intracellular nature of most of these targets is noteworthy, although novel systems exposed on the outer surfaces of cells also continue to be uncovered as well.

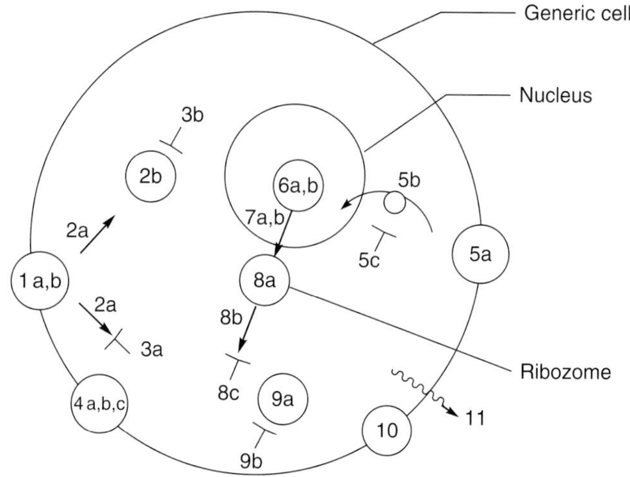

Figure 19.8 Generalized version of the numerous target surfaces that are presenting themselves today. This schematic diagram attempts to convey just some of the types of biological surfaces that can be pursued as potential therapeutic targets by trying to modulate their functions in either a positive or a negative manner. To date, only type 1a might be thought of as being reasonably well worked-over in terms of drug discovery. Designations for the benefit of this figure are: 1(a) Permanent cell-surface receptors, (b) Signal amplification; 2(a) Second messenger system, (b) Subsequent intracellular processes; 3(a) Messenger control systems, (b) Subsequent processes control systems; 4(a) Gated channels, (b) Transporters, (c) Control systems; 5(a) Internalizing receptors, (b) Signal transduction, (c) Control systems; 6(a) Nuclear receptors, (b) Gene regulation; 7(a) Signal translation, (b) Control systems; 8(a) Signal transcription, (b) Signal transduction, (c) Control systems; 9(a) Other intracellular receptors, (b) Control systems; 10 Cell-surface receptors whose messages largely involve externally-directed communications; and, 11 Released materials whose messages largely involve externally directed communications.

Completion of the human genome project has ushered in the new field of proteomics, which now seeks to define which of all the potentially codable proteins are actually expressed in a relevant manner pertaining to either homeostasis or a given pathology. When these factors are considered further at different time-points during each of our lives, proteomic studies merge with the field of pharmacogenetics. The functional proteomics task dwarfs that of defining the genome. In this regard, the current emphasis on cell signaling pathways suggests that this type of biological target class will greatly expand in the near future. Unlike the case for a simple neurotransmitter like NE, however, the cell signaling types of pathways generally involve one or more large biopolymeric molecules interacting with one or more additional large biopolymeric molecules as a key part of their dialogue. This type of interaction makes the derivation of SAR applicable to small molecule-related therapeutic interventions difficult to achieve and perhaps not even possible in some cases. Nevertheless, cell signaling clusters can still be thought of as having receptors or active sites for their specific contact points, and this at least offers the tantalizing opportunity for drug intervention. Thus, as the sophistication and complexity of future targets continues to rise and no matter what the biological surfaces are, efforts to establish useful SAR for the subsequent pursuit of potential drugs are likely to occur in parallel every time any type of target becomes credentialized, let alone validated within the clinic. In addition, credentializing these complex pathways will be able to exploit new technologies such as a genetic knockout or an inhibited RNA (RNAi for RNA interference) study in a model species. The latter models can implicate a given pathway to be associated with an undesirable deviation from homeostasis. As soon as an assay for some critical step within the implicated pathway becomes available, the pursuit of new substances to modulate that step will undoubtedly begin.

19.2.1.6 Drug Metabolism and Excretion versus Side-Effect Toxicity

Since lipophilic xenobiotics generally tend to more readily traverse membranes and reside in the body for longer durations than do more polar xenobiotics, they also have a greater propensity to result in toxicity. This is particularly so for toxicity that results from an accumulation of the xenobiotic upon repeated exposure or dosing. Thus, it is not surprising that the first and foremost theme of human drug metabolism can be thought of as increasing the polarity and water solubility of lipophilic xenobiotics so that they might be excreted more quickly from the body into the urine or bile. As mentioned earlier, a separate chapter will discuss drug metabolism in detail, including the various nuances that can lead to numerous exceptions to the aforementioned generalization. Thus, only a very brief discourse about drug metabolism will be offered at this point so that its intimate relationship with the overall drug discovery process can be demonstrated within the context of the chemical structures that are being advanced toward an NCE.

Drug metabolism often utilizes a two-step process to increase a drug's polarity. The first step generally involves a phase 1 metabolic reaction that typically utilizes one of several cytochrome P450 metabolizing enzymes to perform an oxidation reaction on the parent drug substance so as to either add or expose a functional group. The latter is then used as a further metabolic handle for a phase 2 metabolic reaction. By definition, the phase 2 process involves a drug conjugation reaction by coupling the phase 1 metabolite to an extremely polar biomolecule such as a glucuronic acid moiety. This fundamental, two-step or tandem drug biotransformation pathway is illustrated in Scheme 19.6.

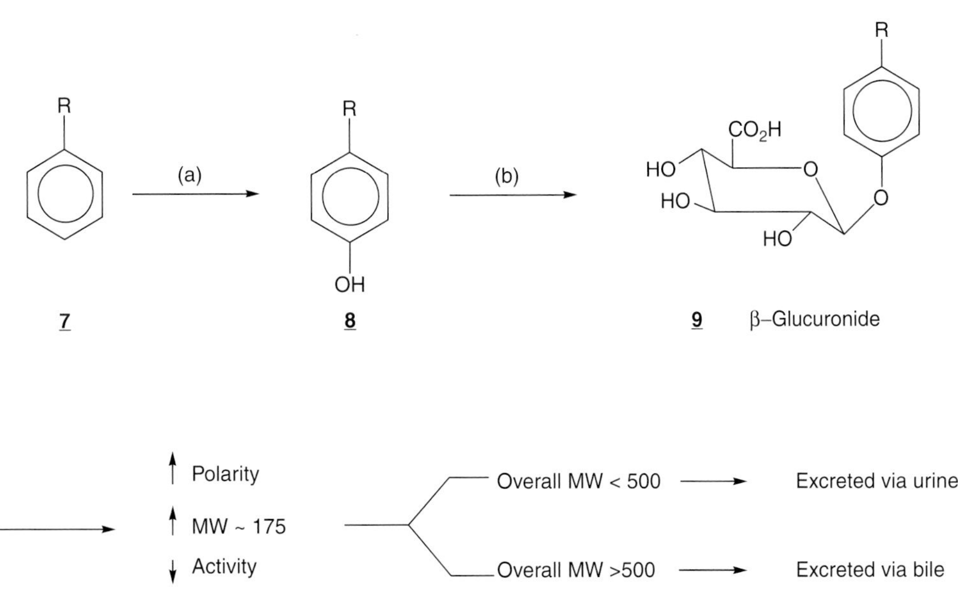

Scheme 19.6 Example of classical phase 1, 2 drug metabolism conducted in a tandem manner. In this case **7** is the parent drug that is relatively lipophillic and **8** is the metabolite from a common, aromatic hydroxylation phase 1 oxidation reaction mediated by a CYP450 enzyme (a). Compound **9**, in turn, is a β-glucuronide metabolite resulting from a common phase 2 conjugation reaction mediated by Uridinediphosphoglucuronic Acid Glycosyltransferase (UGT) (b). Also indicated is the change in polarity, molecular weight (MW) and the typical consequence that the parent drug's activity and any side-effect toxicity are generally reduced after glucuronidation. The final set of parallel arrows indicate the two common excretion pathways available to exogenous materials and their metabolites wherein one will generally have preference over the other depending upon the molecular weight of the xenobiotic.

It should be noted that a phase 2 conjugation reaction does not always follow a phase 1 oxidation reaction, and that even after a phase 2 conjugation has occurred, it is still possible sometimes to observe a phase 1 reaction at another locale on the molecule. Likewise, if an appropriate functional group is already present on the parent drug, then a phase 2 biotransformation presents itself as an immediate metabolic possibility without the need for a phase 1 reaction. Finally, it should be noted that the most prevalent type of phase 1 metabolizing enzymes are actually the Esterases. When a nonsterically hindered ester is present in a parent molecule, the Esterases will typically degrade them in a very aggressive manner. Figure 19.9 provides a structure-oriented summary for six of the most common drug biotransformation pathways. It is meant to serve only as an introduction to this topic so that drug metabolism can be considered again later as part of the overall drug discovery process when its discussion turns toward addressing this particular ADMET hurdle.

If not apparent from Scheme 19.4, upon reaching the general systemic circulation the exemplary CNS drug will now be delivered throughout the body. This includes the arterial blood supply leading to the liver so that the aforementioned biotransformations can still be effected even if the drug managed to survive the first-pass and second-pass events described earlier. In this regard, however, it can be noted (Figure 19.7, C) that there is no longer a 100% dedicated blood-flow to the liver. Thus, while the liver's subsequent attempts to extract drugs from the systemic circulation are more efficient (lower drug concentration), they are significantly less predominant overall compared to drug removal from the original hepatoportal circulation. Likewise, the CNS drug will now make a pass through the kidneys where the chance for renal excretion will present itself either on the parent molecule or on a more polar metabolite for which an enhanced water solubility can serve to effectively decrease the possibility for metabolite reabsorption through the renal tubular membranes. The two major pathways for drug excretion, namely the liver and the kidney, are also shown in Scheme 19.6, where it can be seen that, in addition to lipophilicity, the molecular weight of the xenobiotic plays a role in determining which pathway will be followed. Smaller compounds and volatiles may also be excreted through the skin and via the lungs, respectively. Ethanol serves as an example for elimination by the lungs where it can be readily measured by a breathalyzer.

The last factor, but certainly not the least of concerns, within the random walk theme is that of toxicity (the "T" among the ADMET hurdles). Toxicity can sometimes be a reflection of too much of an efficacious action, an example being too great or too prolonged inhibition of the target enzyme, which was supposed to be only partially or moderately attenuated in order to produce an optimal therapeutic effect. This type of toxicity can be very difficult to address since its removal can also reduce the desired effect. A well-known example is the class of coumarin anticoagulants. Warfarin (Structure **10** in Figure 19.10) requires careful titration into patients initially and then periodic monitoring of the patients' coagulation levels throughout the course of drug use so as to avoid a potentially serious overdose toxicity associated with excessive bleeding or hemorrhage.

A second and even more common type of toxicity reflects that of unwanted side-effects where the loci for the observed toxicity is at some other biological surface than that of the targeted therapeutic site. An example of this type of toxicity can be found in aspirin (structure **11** in Figure 19.10), which long has been used to treat headache, fever, and several other short-term maladies without significant incidence of side

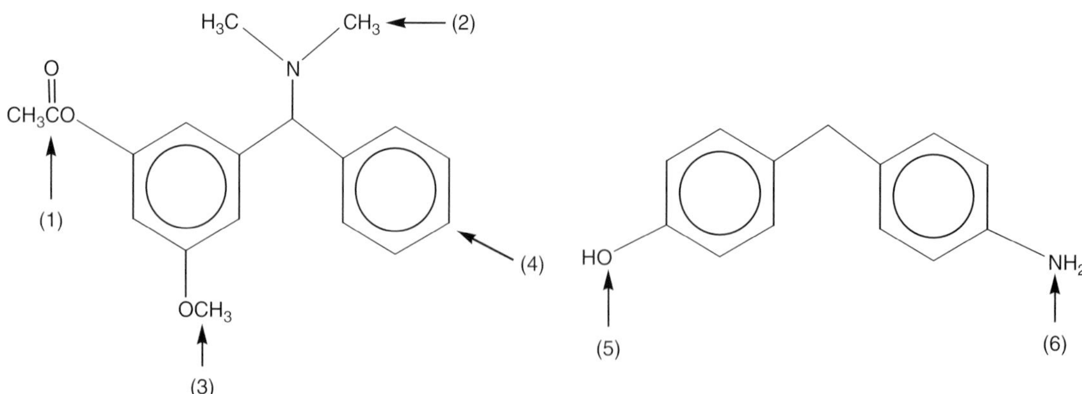

Figure 19.9 Metabolic possibilities for model compounds having representative functionality. Selected phase 1 reactions: (1) Hydrolysis of various types of esters, in this case mediated by a carboxylesterase; (2) N-dealkylation mediated by certain of the Cytochrome P-450 (CYP) enzymes; (3) O-dealkylation mediated by certain of the CYPs; and (4) Aromatic hydroxylation also mediated by certain of the CYPs. Depending upon the subtleties of their electronic and steric environments, the relative competitive biotransformation rates for these processes will generally be (1) $>>$ (2) $>$ (3) $\sim$ (4). Selected phase 2 reactions: (5) Formation of a glucuronic acid conjugate (or in some cases a sulfate conjugate); and (6) N-acetylation. In terms of relative biotransformation rates in general: (5) $>>$ (6).

effects. However, longer-term use of aspirin for arthritis and most recently for use in a prophylactic manner to avoid heart attack and stroke, now has demonstrated a reasonably prevalent toxicity. Arising separate from any of its efficacious sites, is the potential upon chronic administration of aspirin to elicit toxicity associated with irritation of the GI tract lining. Fortunately, the prophylactic indications require a much lower dose and hence the proliferation of numerous low-dose products for this particular use. These products do indeed have a lower incidence of GI-tract-related side-effects. They serve to illustrate a key pharmacologic/toxicologic point, namely that both efficacy and toxicity are a matter of dose or, even better, of concentration achieved at each of their given loci. Even water is toxic when too much is present within the alveolar sacs of our lungs where it can take only a few milliliters to drown.

An example of toxicity that can be thought of as representing a mix of these first two categories is displayed by many of the cancer chemotherapeutic agents such as paclitaxel (**12** in Figure 19.10), which essentially rely on the rate of cellular division to exert some degree of selectivity to kill rapidly dividing cancer cells compared to slower growing normal cells. In this case, toxicity resulting from the same mechanism that is desired in cancer cells is now readily observed at other healthy cells that also happen to be undergoing rapid cell division, like hair follicles, various epithelial linings, and the blood cell forming system. A final type of potential toxicity can occur at the level of a drug–drug or drug–xenobiotic interaction. A classic example for this last type of toxicity involves the monoamine oxidase (MAO) inhibitors, which have been used as antidepressant drugs. Because of their blockade of certain biodegradative enzymes, however,

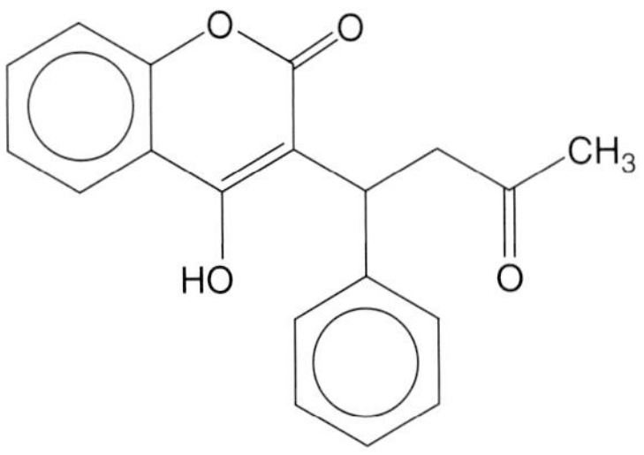

10

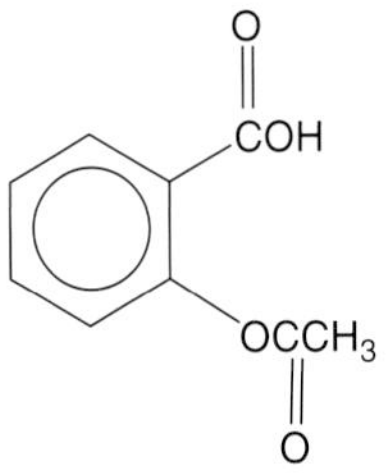

11

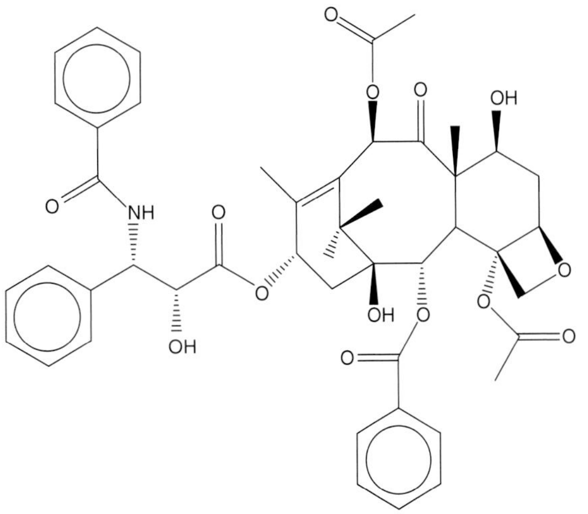

12

Figure 19.10 Selected drugs to exemplify different types of toxicities. **10** is warfarin, an anticoagulant that is marketed as the sodium salt of the vinylogous carboxylic acid (present as an –OH attached to a carbonyl group via a double-bond) so as to enhance its aqueous solubility. **11** is acetylsalicylic acid or aspirin which, in addition to its many long-standing indications, is now being used prophylatically as an OTC to deter cardiovascular disease. **12** is paclitaxel, an anticancer chemotherapeutic agent whose selective toxicity relies upon the rapid rate of cancer cell replication. Note that the selection of these particular drugs should not be taken to mean that they have toxicity issues that are greater than that for other drugs in their respective therapeutic classes. Nearly all drugs will display toxicity of some type at some point as their doses are increased. See text for discussion of the therapeutic index (TI).

the MAO inhibitors can also attenuate the body's clearance of tyramine, which, in turn, can become toxic at high levels. The latter is typically not a problem unless the person also happens to indulge heavily in a diet that is rich in tyramine. Thus, the patient walking away with a prescription for a MAO inhibitor in one hand and a grocery bag with cheese and a bottle of wine in the other, could be heading for a problem since such dietary items are rich sources of tyramine. The pathway for this last example of toxicity is shown in Scheme 19.7.

Because they can lower drug concentration, metabolism and excretion become closely entwined with how much toxicity may be observed. Although it is apparent that drug excretion will serve to decrease the potential for toxicity, this benefit must be balanced during drug design and discovery with the desire to retain the intact drug in the body so that it can display its efficacy for whatever period may be desired. For an oral drug to be taken for several days or more, the latter duration is generally for as long a period as possible. Alternatively, drug metabolism can sometimes lead to active compounds that either retain or display new toxicity. In this regard, phase 1 reactions typically decrease activity (metabolic detoxification), but they can also cause metabolism-related bioactivation, the latter being a particularly predominant pathway for many carcinogens. Alternatively, phase 2 reactions typically lead to inactivation even for those cases where a less polar, acetylation reaction has taken place (entry 6 in Figure 19.9), let alone for those cases where an extremely polar glucuronide has been formed. However, again there are selected exceptions that can be cited for phase 2 reactions, the active morphine glucuronide adducts being one of particular note.

Given the complexity of the possibilities for toxicity, this final ADMET parameter is truly a daunting hurdle for those involved in drug discovery. It is also a challenge for investigators within the federal agencies trying to regulate the final stages of the overall process so as to insure the public's safety while striving for the most rapid approval possible for new agents that are likely to alleviate significant health maladies. As mentioned earlier, for these last stages of the drug discovery process, acute and repetitive-dosing toxicity studies are typically conducted in several animal species as a mandate prior to examining a potential new drug in humans. Whenever possible, specific species are selected for these studies based upon their perceived sensitivity to an anticipated or suspected type of toxicity that the candidate drug may exhibit in humans. Dosing is intentionally scaled-up past what is considered to be an efficacious level until overt signs of toxicity are observed or until an extremely high margin of safety can be predicted with high certainty. Calculations for toxicity compared to efficacy, the so-called therapeutic index (TI) generally take the form already conveyed in the caption to Figure 19.5. Since the dose required for toxicity is always expressed as the numerator and that for efficacy as the denominator, the higher the TI the better, no matter what the end-points of the toxicity study may have been.

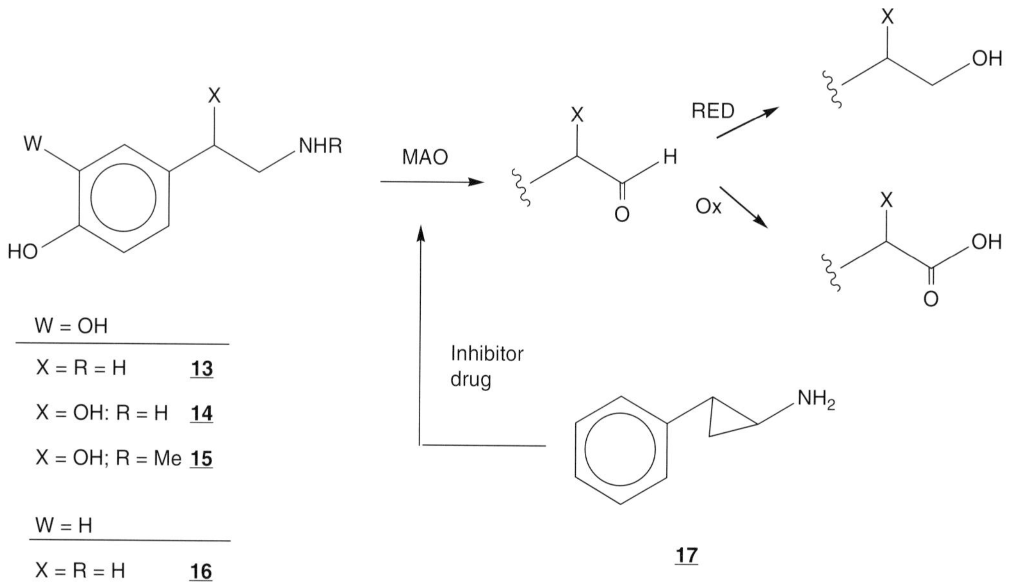

W
HO
X
NHR
MAO
X
H
O
RED
Ox
X
OH
X
OH
O

W = OH

X = R = H 13

X = OH: R = H 14

X = OH; R = Me 15

W = H

X = R = H 16

Inhibitor drug

NH_2

17

Scheme 19.7 Role of Monoamine Oxidase (MAO) in the biodegradation of the body's common adrenergic substances (first reaction only). The resulting aldehyde is quickly further metabolized by either a Reductase (RED) or by an Oxidase (Ox). The 'squiggle-line' indicates that the structural portion to its left remains the same as that in the original. Although not depicted here, Catechol O-Methyl Transferase (COMT) is another major biodegradative pathway for all of these substances except **16**. Also shown is one of the older inhibitors of MAO, namely tranylcypromine **17**. **13** is dopamine, **14** is norepinephrine, **15** is epinephrine and **16** is tyramine. Since **16** is a potent vasoconstrictor that largely relies upon this pathway for its biodegradation, inhibition of MAO can become problematic and lead to hypertensive crisis if large amounts of **16** happen to be simultaneously consumed via the diet.

Finally, despite all the aforementioned concerns and related efforts, it must be appreciated that there is always a chance for a low-level of toxicity that can gradually accumulate upon continued usage, perhaps even within just a specific genetic segment (pharmacogenetic) of the population in a manner or association that could not be predicted beforehand. Thus, the ultimate clinical test for any new drug finally occurs when it is first market-launched for the broadest possible, FDA-approved use within the specified population (both of the latter constituting the approved indication). Recognizing this, formal mechanisms are also in place for the continued surveillance of the new drug and for the mandated reporting of any adverse reactions to the FDA. Given the long-term nature for this type of insidious toxicity to become manifest, it can be noted that even our strict working definition for what we are considering to be a true drug within this chapter, has stopped short of expecting the drug to also have to prove its sustainability within the clinic, perhaps well past its initial market launch and into some arbitrary point of the future. Thus, in our definition, the chemical substance becomes a drug upon market launch even if at some point thereafter it must be withdrawn for any reason whatsoever, such as a low-level but underlying insidious toxicity.

19.2.2 Consideration of the Ten Most Prescribed Drugs

Before turning to a discussion about key chemical parameters, Table 19.1 provides a summary for Sections 19.1 and 19.2 by listing the 10 most commonly prescribed drugs in the United States during 2005, and itemizing the drug discovery starting points and biology-related factors for each entry. Chemical structures for these drugs are shown in the accompanying Figure 19.11. From Table 19.1, it is interesting to note that seven of these compounds are analogs of a previously known substance, if not the exact structure reproduced as a single stereoismer (enantiomer of the original racemic form) or as a single component from an endogenous hormone mixture. Furthermore, the remaining three compounds, although seemingly more distinct chemically, still represent structural alternatives to a prior drug that already exists in their pharmacological class.

Although this might lead us to suspect that the starting point for drug discovery is usually translational chemistry, this would be an erroneous conclusion for at least two reasons. First, essentially all these big-sellers happen to be second- or third-generation agents. The incremental improvements in therapy achieved by these compounds as true new drugs (according to our definition) are extremely important. For example, most of these second-generation compounds have led to a significant improvement compared to the original or pioneer drug's overall ADME or PK profile, if not also to an entirely new indication. These types of improvements generally reflect clinical observations stemming from initial deployment of the pioneer drug. Thus, the second reason for not concluding that translational chemistry is the most common starting point for drug discovery is because the further evolution of such second- and third-generation compounds generally reflects translational medicine just as much as it reflects the fact that there is an efficacious substance already in hand for further modification. Supported by a validated therapeutic target these types of improved drug discoveries reflect new clinical observations coupled to a validated drug and, as you will see in a later section, this common situation can be classified as a special case of ligand-based drug design that typically yields second- and third-generation agents having significantly enhanced therapeutic profiles for one or more specific indications.

Pushing further into the history of the previous drugs that have led to those listed in Table 19.1 via the footnotes, it is additionally interesting to note that six of the initial pioneer compounds appear to have been delivered by Mother Nature as either microbial/fungal natural products or as endogenous ligands. The remaining four sources reflect more of a chemical synthesis or compound library source. All three translational drug discovery starting points become well represented upon considering the earlier entries for the tabulated drugs. Exemplifying translational chemistry, products deriving from the Hantzch reaction were observed to have interesting biological activity. Upon further pursuit, this eventually led to nifedipine and the entire calcium-channel blocker class of drugs where amlodipine (**20**), with its number three ranking, is one of today's prescription favorites in Table 19.1. Alternatively, with a specific HTS assay in-hand for measuring the ability to inhibit Hydroxymethylglutaryl-Coenzyme A Reductase (HMG-CoA Reductase), a translational research campaign prompted the survey of approximately 8000 microbial broths that eventually uncovered mevastatin, the HMG-CoA Reductase inhibitor class of drugs, and ultimately both atorvastatin (**18**) and simvastatin (**27**) with their number one and 10 rankings within Table 19.1, respectively. Finally, the synthesis of the specific thyroid hormone levothyroxine (**21**), with a number four ranking, was clearly prompted by translational medicine when attempts to administer the body's natural hormone mixture could not be accomplished with an adequate degree of quality control.

Another important observation deriving from Table 19.1 that has general applicability is that 80% of these compounds are inhibitors or antagonists at some biological surface. Indeed, of the two remaining drugs, one is a hormone replacement agent (**21**) and the other (**24**) is a modulator of an inhibitory pathway. That most drugs are receptor antagonists or enzyme inhibitors certainly holds true well beyond the arena of chemotherapeutics, which tend to all be inhibitors except for the immune enhancers. Aside from the more frequent demands for inhibitors dictated by the specific biological targets, in general it is also a much easier undertaking to produce antagonists than agonists at any given biological receptor surface. The structural requirements for agonist binding are typically much

Table 19.1 Ten Most Commonly Prescribed Drugs within the United States during 2005[a] (Chemical Structures are Shown in Figure 19.11)

Drug	Efficacy Biological Surface (Mechanism)	Discovery Starting Point	Source of Initial Compound	Most Significant ADMET Hurdle	Principal Clinical Indication	Toxicity Biological Surface
Atorvastatin **18**	HMG-CoA Reductase[b] (inhibitor)	Analog of mevastatin	Microbial metabolite (mevastatin)	First pass (issues still linger)	Lower cholesterol and triglycerides	Muscle myosin
Metoprolol **19**	Beta-l-Adrenergic receptor (blocker)	Analog of practolol	Endogenous ligand (Epinephrine) →→→→ practolol[c]	First pass (issues still linger)	Angina and hypertension	Cardiac[d] beta-1
Amlodipine **20**	Calcium-channel (blocker)	Analog of nifedipine	Synthetic compound libraries derived from the Hantzch reaction[e]	Overcame short duration[f]	Angina and hypertension	Peripheral vasculature
Levothyroxine **21**	Thyroid hormone receptor (agonist)	Specific form of thyroid hormones, namely T_4, which has 4 iodines	Endogenous hormone family (thyroid hormones T_4, T_3, where T_3 has 3 iodines)[g]	–[h]	Hypothyroidism	Overextensison of thyroid hormone activity
Sertraline **22**	Serotonin transporter protein or SERT (inhibitor)	Alternative to fluoxetine[i]	Targeted compound library[j]	Overcame drug–drug interactions	Antidepressant	GI tract
Escitalopram **23**	SERT (inhibitor)	Alternative to fluoxetine[i]	(S)-Enantiomer of citalopram, which is racemic and, in turn, was derived like **22**[j]	Overcame drug–drug interactions	Antidepressant	GI tract
Zolpidem **24**	GABA Receptor[k] (modulator)	Alternative to benzodiazepines[l]	Ring-opened analog of the general benzo-diazepine compound class	Optimized onset and half-life	Insomnia	CNS-related
Azithromycin **25**	50S subunit of bacterial ribosomes (inhibits protein synthesis)	Semi-synthetic analog of erythromycin	Microbial metabolite (erythromycin)	Optimized for once/day dosing	Antibiotic	GI tract
Esomeprazole **26**	Gastric proton pump[m] (inhibitor)	Analog of omeprazole	(S)-Enantiomer of omeprazole, which is racemic[n]	Enhanced oral bioavailability	Esophagitis	GI tract
Simvastatin **27**	HMG-CoA Reductase[b] (inhibitor)	Methylated analog of lovastatin	Fungal metabolite (lovastatin)[o]	First pass (issues still linger)	Lower cholesterol and triglycerides	GI-tract

[a]Ranked according to their total number of prescriptions with **18** having the highest ca. 63 million (M) for Lipitor® and **27** having the lowest at ca. 22 M for Zocor®, both of which happen to be HMG-CoA Reductase inhibitor or statin drugs.b **19** was tallied from Toprol XL®, **20** from Norvasc®, **21** from Synthroid®, **22** from Zoloft®, **23** from Lexapro®, **24** from Ambien®, **25** from Zithromax-Z-Pak®, and **26** from Nexium®.

[b]HMG-CoA is hydroxymethylglutaryl – Coenzyme A that is converted by the Reductase to mevalonate, which, in turn, is a biochemical precursor for the sterols including cholesterol.

[c]Practolol can be thought of as deriving from propranolol, which, in turn, was sequentially derived from pronethalol and dichloroisoproterenol, respectively. Dichloroisoproterenol is an analog of epinephrine.

[d]Overextension of therapeutic effect resulting in bradycardia (too much slowing of heart rate).

[e]This reaction produces symmetrical dihydropyridines whose chemistry can be traced back to the late 1800s, biochemistry shortly thereafter, and pharmacology relevant to the present indication to the early 1970s.

[f]Although its precursor nifedipine suffered from too short a half-life, if anything, **20** may now have too long a half-life.

[g]T_4 and T_3 ratios can vary in the natural hormone.

[h]The main challenge was chemical quality control of the natural hormone so a synthetic T_4-only product was developed. Also note that T_4 is metabolized by removal of one iodine to T_3 in the periphery and that T_3 is the principal hormone responsible for activity.

[i]Fluoxetine is a potent inhibitor of CYP2D6 and CYP 3A4 and is subject to considerable drug–drug interactions.

[j]Screening compounds having SERT pharmacophore (i.e., 3D beta-arylamino-like group plus an "extra" aryl).

[k]Gama-aminobutyric acid (GABA) alpha-subunit or omega- or benzodiazepine-receptor. Modulation is toward enhanced function of this inhibitory CNS pathway.

[l]Subject to muscle relaxation and used for other CNS indications.

[m]$(H,^{+} K^{+})$-ATPase enzyme pump that acidifies the stomach.

[n]Omeprazole, in turn, was derived from the family of substituted benzimidazole synthetic compounds that had been found to display activity.

[o]Isolation of mevastatin preceded that of lovastatin, so the former can be thought of as the first agent to establish this general class of compounds (also then called the pioneer drug).

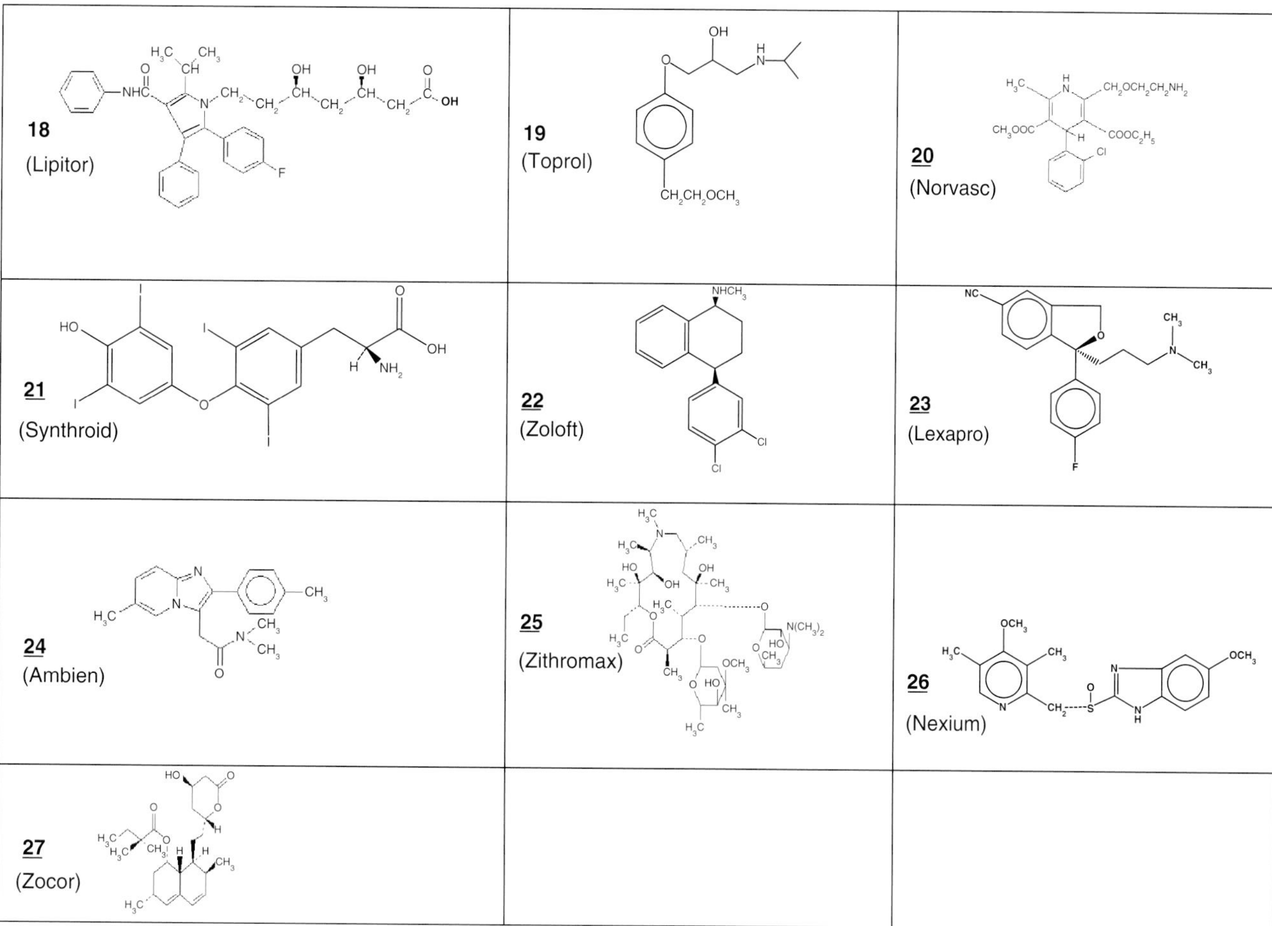

Figure 19.11 Chemical structures for drugs listed in Table 19.1 (various proprietary names are given in parentheses). The specific marketed products listed in Table 19.1's footnote (a) actually utilize the following salt forms: **18** Compound dimer with one Ca^{++}; **19** Compound dimer with one succinic acid; **20** Benzenesulfonate salt; **21** Sodium salt; **22** Hydrochloride salt; **23** 1:1 Oxalate salt; **24** 1:1 Tartrate salt; 25 Free base (as shown); 26 Compound dimer with one Mg^{++} and three water molecules (• 3 H_2O); and, **27** No salts (as shown). Note that although several of these compounds also have active metabolites, **27** is an example of a true prodrug (inactive until its lactone ring is opened) while **21** can be considered to also be a prodrug in that its deiodinated T_3 form is thought to be the active species at the thyroid hormone receptor.

more stringent than for receptor antagonists and, in addition, the agonist must accomplish two events during its visit, namely to trigger the receptor as well as to initially associate or bind with it. Alternatively, the situation is often not nearly as stringent for designing substrates versus inhibitors at various enzyme active sites. For example, the cytochrome P450 drug metabolizing enzymes and the numerous transporter systems generally tend to be quite promiscuous about which molecules they will bind. They usually demonstrate little regard for any strict structural arrangements.

19.2.3 Chemical Parameters

This section will consider some of the drug-associated chemical parameters that are related to the various pharmacological media and biological surfaces discussed earlier. Manipulation of these parameters becomes the basis for optimizing a potential drug's ADME profile while simultaneously reducing its toxicity (T) and, of course, enhancing its potency at efficacious receptors. Because the latter typically marks the onset for new drug discovery, it will be discussed first. Bear in mind, however, that it is the composite of eventually addressing all the ADMET parameters that constitutes the field of drug design today.

19.2.3.1 Identifying Hits and Producing Lead Compounds

Experimental Strategies Assuming that an HTS type of assay for a selected biological target is in hand, today's scientist embarking on a drug design expedition can choose from the list of strategies conveyed in Table 19.2. These strategies are ranked in an inverse manner to how much information is already available about the target surface. Since we are generally on firmer ground when there is more known about any given scientific endeavor, it becomes less risky to operate within the context of Table 19.2's entry III.D.

Table 19.2 Chemically Oriented Experimental Strategies That Can Be Pursued during Drug Design[a]

I. Library-based Drug Design	II. Ligand-based Drug Design	III. Structure-based Drug Design
A. Random library	A. Endogenous-based drug design	A. Receptor or active site hypothetical picture
B. Directed library	B. Prototype-based drug design	B. Receptor or active site prototype picture
C. Fragment library	C. Analog-based drug design	C. Receptor or active site actual picture
		D. Receptor or active site actual picture with and without ligands present

[a]Site-directed mutagenesis is an additional experimental strategy that can be undertaken during drug design. It has more of a biological orientation and is discussed separately, later.

Conversely, although we have the lowest percentage for producing active compounds when operating within the context of I.A, there is a higher chance of identifying a completely novel structural hit relative to all the other methods since there is no structural bias present at this level other than that bestowed by the compound library itself.

In addition to these experimentally driven approaches, computational and *in silico* screening can also be pursued. For the latter, virtual compounds can be docked into models or pictures of the target surface to determine how well they might fit or bind in advance of synthesizing them for an experimental assessment. Several docking programs are available to survey an unending number of virtual compounds at quick throughput rates. It will be shown later that the binding interaction energies can be tallied across a molecule in a simple algebraic manner. Alternatively, it becomes a more difficult situation to derive just how the two partners may be lined up in 3D space. Thus, like all computational approaches, *in silico* binding or docking studies are subject to the nature of the mathematical approximations that necessarily will have been made in a given software program. In this regard it is typically difficult to discern how a particular mathematical shortcut may translate from one set of potential ligand structures to that of another set. Therefore, it still becomes necessary to validate a given *in silico* approach by actually testing at least a few members of a selected series thought to be of interest so as to insure that the computational predictions match experimentally derived results. Finally, the various experimental strategies listed in Table 19.2 and the computational and *in silico* approaches are not mutually exclusive. All these strategies can be mixed in any manner that seems appropriate during the pursuit of a given target molecule. Indeed, an overall strategy that simultaneously combines several of these approaches can provide the best chance for an eventual success. For the purpose of clarity, however, each approach is discussed separately, next.

Library-based Drug Design In order to be successful when undertaking a random library approach (I.A in Table 19.2), the compound library itself must reflect a high degree of structural diversity and be large enough in its compound membership to allow for the survey of a wide range of structural space. As suggested in the Introduction, Mother Nature's natural products represent a continuing source of molecular diversity. However, these materials must be harvested from their natural habitats and fractionated, if not individually isolated, prior to testing. Harvesting and purification steps can be very time-consuming and costly. Thus, compound libraries that already have been preassembled are typically sought for HTS campaigns. The typical library for this purpose requires several thousands of diverse compounds, if not several hundred thousands of compounds. Commercially available compound libraries can be obtained from private vendors. A limited number of libraries, such as those from the NIH Roadmap Initiative, are also available from the public sector by request. To date, few suppliers of preassembled libraries, however, are able to provide follow-up supplies for any compound member deemed to be of interest as a hit. Most of the larger pharmaceutical companies, therefore, have assembled their own libraries, which then contain a mix of natural products, commercial source members, and a large segment of their own proprietary compounds.

Assuming its biological relevancy has been credentialized already, the faster the bioassay component of this approach, the better, reflecting that this strategy is a low-percentage, high-test-numbers proposition for success in the first place. Toward that end, HTS methods have now gone to ultra-HTS methods within the industry, where several tens-of-thousands of compounds can be assayed each day in a robotic manner from beginning to end of an entire survey of massive compound libraries that are kept on stock. Interestingly, once churning away, this type of discovery step requires little human intervention of any sort. However, when one or more hits are obtained, this process must immediately move into more of a compound design mode that is driven by human-implemented rationale.

Directed libraries (I.B in Table 19.2) represent one of the immediate follow-up approaches when a hit has been obtained. Representing an extension of the former approach, a small family of compounds is assembled around the basic structural template afforded by the initial hit compound. Although the nature of these members is often dictated by what types of chemistry are allowed to be performed on the hit compound's template, ideally a systematic attempt is made to map out the structural space in all directions from the hit template. Unlike a random compound library, a directed library can often be very effective with less than 100 compound members in that it is now intentionally biased along the structural theme of the hit compound. It seeks to rationally derive discrete SAR details rather than continuing to strive for a high degree of diversity in a random manner. As shown in Figure 19.2, although a given hit may be able to be hybridized all the way to a clinical development compound via an examination of only another approximately 150 compounds, the attrition rate thereafter prompts the need, on average, to bring nearly 10 hybridized compounds into Phase I clinical testing. Further discussions in this chapter will focus upon how to advance just a single hit or lead, but the reality of these statistics generally demands that several hits will likely have to be taken forward in order to achieve success in the overall game.

Fragment libraries (I.C in Table 19.2) represent a relatively new strategy that attempts to identify more than one HTS hit from a library of smaller and more discrete functional group arrangements that can be pieced together to construct larger, drug-like molecules that possess multiple binding regions. Since the combinations can potentially lead to enhanced binding, the criteria for the initial round of hits can be softened. Less potent species can be acceptable for moving forward in this manner. Although this approach has yet to prove itself by producing an actual new drug, several examples of drug candidates do appear to have been derived from this strategy. In addition, this stepwise strategy may provide a reasonable path for probing the previously mentioned biological targets involving protein–protein interactions for which small molecule SAR can be particularly difficult to discern when attempted in an all-or-none fashion with rigorous potency criteria.

Ligand-based Drug Design This approach takes advantage of an initial hit compound or of some other compound that is already known to interact favorably, if not ideally, with the biological surface of interest. In this sense, the directed library strategy mentioned earlier is a form of this approach although it also represents a continuum of the compound library-HTS theme. If the ligand to be used is an endogenous material known to interact with the targeted biological surface in a manner that does not actually bestow the desired efficacy, then at least the initial drug design process can be considered to be proceeding by endogenous-based drug design. An example of the latter would be the case where it is desirable to inhibit a particular enzyme, but the only known ligands are the enzyme's specific endogenous substrates and perhaps a closely-related structural family of substrate analog compounds. Given today's huge influx of genetic, proteomic, and biological-related data in general, this situation (II.A in Table 19.2) is probably already the most common scenario from which to enter drug design. This situation can also be expected to proceed even more dominantly into the future. Also note that this common level of knowledge about the target opens up the possibility of taking at least three strategic experimental approaches, namely:

- Random library in search of an efficacious hit by an HTS survey of a huge compound library
- Directed library by screening a limited compound series selected from a larger collection to resemble the endogenous ligand, perhaps with the additional aid of a computational structure-matching or structure-similarity program, or by simple visual inspection
- Endogenous-based by design and procurement from commercial sources or from chemical synthesis, of a systematic SAR probe series using the endogenous ligand as a lead template

Alternatively, if the ligand is a hit from prior screening accomplished either internally or gleaned from the published literature, and its activity reflects at least some modest level of what is desired, then the subsequent process can be further classified as prototype-based drug design (II.B in Table 19.2). An example of this strategy would be the case where it is again desirable to inhibit a particular enzyme and a known, weak inhibitor exists that can serve as the starting-point ligand for further design. The latter could be either an exogenous or an endogenous material, although the former is by far the more common case. Finally, if the ligand that is known to interact with the efficacy surface happens to be a clinically used drug, then the proceeding effort can be classified as analog-based drug design (II.C in Table 19.2). Taking propranolol (**2** in Figure 19.4), which represents the pioneer drug for the general class of beta-adrenergic receptor blocking agents, as the clinical agent, the elaboration of esmolol, **3**, can be considered to have been initiated according to an analog-based drug design strategy. It should be noted that the systematic structural investigation and modification of a clinically used agent for a new pharmacological indication also constitutes a situation of analog-based drug design. Thus, this last category, just like all the preceding chemically-oriented categories, is defined by the chemical structure and not by the biological activity.

Structure-based Drug Design This approach requires a high level of knowledge about the biological surface that the drug is supposed to interact with. The word "structure" refers to the structure of the biological surface's receptor or active site rather than to the structure of the ligand, although at the highest level for this approach a considerable knowledge about both receptor and ligand may exist. In the receptor or active site hypothetical picture or model approach (III.A in Table 19.2), an accumulated body of SAR will have evolved to the point where a hypothetical construct for at least some of the types of amino acids or types of binding regions that may be present on this surface can be placed in a three-dimensional, spatial model. This can be done even if the connections between these various regions cannot yet be accounted for in a contiguous manner. In the receptor or active site prototype picture approach (III.B in Table 19.2), a similar biological surface from another species or human tissue has been fully characterized by an x-ray diffraction so that it can be used as a prototype for analogous consideration of how ligands might be interacting with the targeted biological surface. For entry III.C in Table 19.2, an X-ray of the actual efficacious site has become available and in entry III.D the pictures also include one or more snap shots showing the specific relationship with a given ligand while it is binding to the site. At this highest level of knowledge about the system, hybridization of an early-ligand-lead to an actual clinical candidate compound can be accomplished upon examination of a number of related compounds that is far less than 100, assuming that no extraordinary ADMET hurdles are present. Several examples with accompanying figures for this strategy are shown in the third case study near the end of this chapter.

Site-directed Mutagenesis One final technique, most closely related to the structure-based drug design strategy, that can contribute knowledge to all these approaches is that of site-directed mutagenesis, or SDM. SDM begins from more of a biological orientation although its ultimate goals become the same. To undertake these types of studies, all that is needed is the amino acid sequence of the target protein, although a knowledge of the protein's actual receptor pocket or active site is additionally useful, as would be any higher level of structure-based drug design information. Within the context of drug design, SDM involves making systematic point mutations directed toward selected sites on genes that translate to specific amino acid residues within the proteins associated with enzyme active sites or ligand receptor pockets so that the specified changes can be used to study SAR details while holding one or more active site/receptor ligands constant during the assessment. This approach is depicted in Scheme 19.8.

Numerous investigators are now utilizing this reverse SAR technique to explore both enzyme- and receptor-ligand interactions. It is called a reverse SAR technique because the variables become each of the modified biological surfaces, but the small molecule ligands

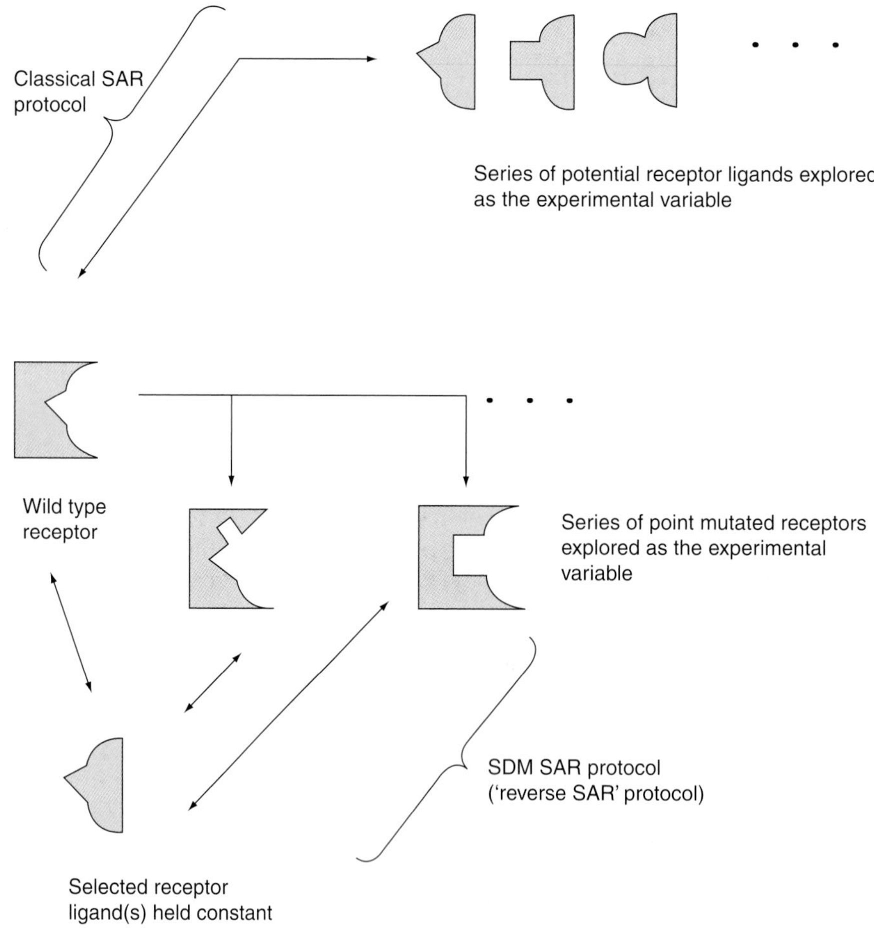

Scheme 19.8 Classical ligand exploration versus site-directed mutagenesis (SDM) exploration of structure-activity relationships (SAR). In the classical approach, various ligands are presented to the same receptor or active site of interest. In SDM, one or more ligands of merit are held constant and used as standards whereas various mutated forms of the receptor or active site are presented for interaction. Both approaches can produce useful SAR data and when used simultaneously, they can be highly complimentary.

remain the same during the analysis. Eventually the data obtained in this manner can help to identify the key binding features within an enzyme active site or receptor. The latter, in turn, can be used to guide further structural modifications on various hit and lead compounds. Examples and figures for SDM are also shown in the third case study near the end of this chapter.

Once an enzyme's peptide sequence is in hand, it is not uncommon that transformation of a bacterial host with an appropriate gene copy plasmid can allow at least one point-mutated and overexpressed protein to be examined per month in an associated functional biochemical assay. Although still very much slower than HTS, this clearly demonstrates that SDM need not be considered to be lengthy and tedious compared to classical SAR studies undertaken by rational synthetic modifications of an enzyme's substrates or inhibitors. Random mutations can sometimes also be accomplished in an even faster mode of operation, and when these are combined with SDM, production of a receptor/active site library can be undertaken in a very practical manner to also assist further drug design. The analogous use of today's phraseology for the receptor libraries should be noted as should the accompanying desire to also bring the SDM approach into an HTS mode.

Considering Chemical Space No matter what the therapeutic target, moving from an initial hit to an actual lead compound typically requires improving potency to the nanomolar (nM) level within the efficacy screen. In addition, looking forward to the ADMET hurdles that loom just ahead, this becomes a critical time to establish discrete SAR data directed toward ascertaining what changes can and cannot be made on the hit template while retaining the desired activity. Likewise, no matter what strategy or combination of strategies are adopted to couple the continuing compound survey to an efficacy-related HTS, the aforementioned goals remain the same. For example, data obtained from a directed library-based drug design effort can be sorted with these goals in mind, or the goals can themselves be used in a proactive manner to optimally design ligand-based analogues that will probe structural space in the most efficient manner possible.

Using Functional Group Interactions to Track Ligand Binding The SAR data typically obtained from HTS at this point is generally related to how well the compounds interact or bind with the biological surface associated with efficacy. Binding strength, in turn, can be related to the strength of the interactions between functional groups on the compound and functional groups displayed by the amino acids present within the biological surface's receptor pocket or enzymatic active site. Thus, continuing structural exploration typically involves attempts to define not only what sections of the initial hit compound's overall framework may be important for activity, but also what are the specific SAR details associated with the hit's display of distinct chemical functional groups. For example, taking again the structure of the natural

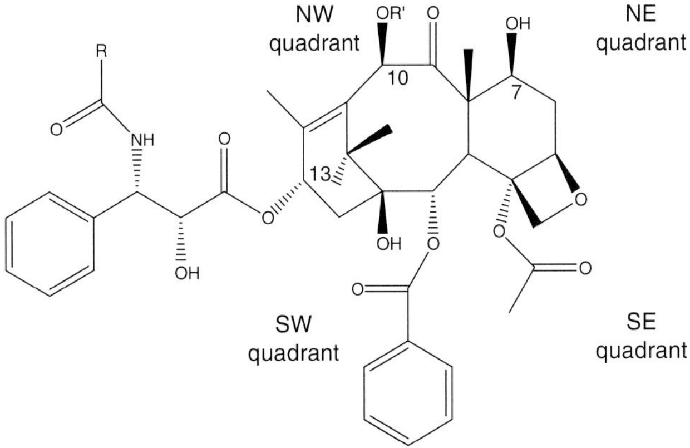

Figure 19.12 Example of how an initial hit's structural space can be explored (see text for corresponding discussion). Actual structures are: Paclitaxel, **12**, where R = phenyl and R' = acetyl (also see Figure 19.10); and docetaxel, **28**, where R = t-butoxy and R' = hydrogen.

product compound paclitaxel (PAC; **12** in Figure 19.10 and as redrawn in Figure 19.12), it was determined that the side-chain at position **13** on the main PAC template is requisite for activity. The same was found for the carbon skeleton defining PAC's main template since all efforts to selectively fragment this portion also led to complete loss of potency.

Assigning the structural space around PAC's main template into four quadrants and taking advantage of PAC's hydroxyl groups and esters to readily explore chemical modifications, next it was determined that any alteration of the original types of functionalities displayed along the southern edge of PAC also leads to significant losses in potency. Finally it was found that the functional groups residing along the northern edge are quite tolerant toward change. It should be noted that PAC was rather unique as a hit because it already possessed low nM potency. Alternatively, PAC's distinct action to overstabilize microtubules was not initially appreciated, which caused a gap to occur in the normal discovery process. Once its novel mechanism was elucidated, PAC's development was suddenly catapulted all the way into the clinic to validate this therapeutic approach with little additional structural modification efforts being undertaken.

Alternatively, a second-generation compound has taken advantage of the structural tolerance afforded by the northern edge so as to replace PAC's 10-position acetoxy-group with a hydroxyl-group. This simple structural manipulation improves PAC's extremely low aqueous solubility and avoids the necessity of using a Tween-solubilizer. The latter is significant because PAC's intravenous solution formulation otherwise requires that this excipient's level be so high that it, in itself, can lead to potential side-effect toxicity. The second generation compound also replaced one of the aromatic groups present in PAC's 13-position side chain with a tertiary-butoxy-group, but this may reflect more of an artifact created during chemical synthetic manipulations than the actual pursuit of an SAR goal to improve aqueous solubility. This second generation compound, namely docetaxel (**28**), is also shown in Figure 19.12.

A listing of some of the common functional groups that can be substituted or attached onto the various quadrants during these types of SAR assessments is provided in Table 19.3, which also details some of their relative physicochemical properties. Replacement of a group that is initially present on the hit compound with a group that has very similar physicochemical properties is obviously less likely to result in a change in activity than when a substitution is done with a group having significantly different physicochemical properties. In addition, the listed properties can be used to probe the nature of the interaction between the hit compound and the biological surface. That knowledge, in turn, allows for a more rationally devised change to be made next. For example, if an aliphatic hydroxyl-group is present in one of the quadrants of the hit compound and its complete removal (replacement by a hydrogen) leads to a dramatic reduction in potency, then the hydroxyl must be regarded as doing something favorable during the interaction. But what is the nature of that favorable interaction, and can it be further manipulated to enhance potency? Perhaps the hydroxyl-group forms a hydrogen-bond with the receptor, a likely event for this type of a group. But is this done as a donor (with the hydroxyl group supplying the hydrogen to its partner) or as an acceptor (with the biological surface supplying an appropriate hydrogen to one of the hydroxyl-groups oxygen atom's lone-electron pairs)?

Substitution of a methoxy-group for the hydroxyl on the hit compound can begin to shed light on these possibilities. If the methoxy version is still highly active, then the original hydroxyl is likely to have been behaving as a hydrogen-bond acceptor since that's all the methoxy-group can do (as indicated in Table 19.3 by having only an "A"). Alternatively, if the methoxy-analog leads to significantly less activity, then it may be that the original hydroxy-group was serving as a hydrogen-bond donor, although this negative result could also mean that there is simply not enough room (steric hindrance) allowed for the methoxy-group compared to the hydroxyl-group since the methoxy's larger size ("8" compared to "3" with all steric values being relative to a hydrogen set at "1") also demands more room for a potential fit. Returning to the first and positive consequence, if hydrogen-bonding as an acceptor seems likely, then perhaps this interaction might be enhanced

Table 19.3 Common Functional Groups and a Simplified Version of Their Approximated Physicochemical Properties (adapted from Hansch and Leo)

Functional Group	Relative Size (Steric Effect)[a]	Relative Lipophilicity[b]	Hydrogen Bonding[c]	Relative Electron Donation[a,d]
H	1	0.0	0	0
CH_3	5	0.6	0	0.1
CH_2CH_3	10	1.0	0	0.1
$CH_2CH_2CH_3$	15	1.6	0	0.1
$CH(CH_3)_2$	15	1.5	0	0.1
C_6H_5	25	2.0	0	−0.1
OH	3	−0.7	A,D	−0.1
OCH_3	8	0.0	A	−0.1
NH_2	5	−1.2	A,D	0.1
$NHCH_3$	10	−0.5	A,D	0.3
$N(CH_3)_2$	16	0.2	A	0.2
$N(CH_3)_3^{\oplus}$	21	−6.0	0	−0.9
CO_2H	7	−0.3	A,D	−0.4
$CO_2^{\ominus}$	6	−4.4	A	0.1
CO_2CH_3	13	0.0	A	−0.4
$CONH_2$	10	−1.5	A,D	−0.3
$CONHCH_3$	15	−1.3	A,D	−0.4
Br	9	0.9	0	−0.4
Cl	6	0.7	0	−0.4
F	1	0.1	0	−0.3
I	14	1.1	0	−0.4
CF_3	5	0.9	0	−0.4

[a]These values have their origins in studies related to their effects when present on standard aromatic systems. Thus, their simple algebraic relationships (see text for examples) are most accurate when used as aromatic substituent modifications. Nevertheless, they can likewise be used in a general manner across various other molecular contexts to provide at least crude approximations for the relative changes that ensue upon similar modifications.

[b]These values can be used directly with Log P (partition coefficient) data and just like for properties (a), their simple algebraic relationships are most useful in a relative sense when considering different substituent possibilities on the same template.

[c]0 indicates no hydrogen-bonding, A indicates hydrogen-bond accepting capability, and D indicates hydrogen-bond donating capability.

[d]The indicated electronic effects pertain only to induction; i.e., electronic resonance effects are not shown here. A positive value indicates electron donation and a negative value indicates electron withdrawal; i.e., the electron withdrawing nature of a quaternary ammonium ion is quite distinctive with a value of −0.9.

by replacement with an amino-group since the nitrogen's lone-electron pair would be even more favorably inclined to enter a hydrogen-bond relationship. In this case, however, care must also be exercised not to provide too aggressive of a hydrogen-bond acceptor like a highly basic amine. The latter could simply remain protonated at physiological pH only to have its lone-electron pair so heavily tied up with a water molecule that it can no longer become accessible to the biological surface's hydrogen-donating partner, thus behaving like a quaternary ammonium species (Table 19.3).

If, in turn, an attenuation of the amine's basicity is needed, then this might be further attempted by substitution with a trifluoromethylamino-group, although this will also decrease the amine's ability to accept a hydrogen-bond from the biological surface's partner and, likewise, it would add more steric bulk to the new substituent. Thus, from this short discourse pertaining to the exploration of just a single functional group, it should be apparent that several different types of substitutions are typically required at any given point on a hit compound in order to effectively probe the SAR for that spot, and to ultimately optimize what might be able to be placed at just that one location. Furthermore, even a single, small functional group change can cause several different types of physicochemical-related properties to change in that location and sometimes across the overall structure as well. Because of the latter, the results from one spot must be rechecked whenever another location has likewise been changed.

Nevertheless, with enough iterations of this process, an entire compound having numerous functional groups can eventually become completely optimized. Table 19.4 lists the general types of functional group interactions that can occur. It also indicates the energies that are associated with each type of interaction. The accompanying Figure 19.13 displays these same types of functional group interactions by using the terminal amino-group of a lysine residue's side-chain to exemplify just one type of amino acid partner that may be present within the biological surface's receptor pocket or enzymatic active site. Negative energy values indicate that a favorable interaction has occurred (the less energy in the system then the more stable). In the end, it will be the lowest summation of all of the energies associated with all of the functional group interactions that can take place, that will ultimately provide for the most strongly bound ligand-biological surface interaction.

The simple algebraic summation of binding interaction energies across an entire compound also forms the basis for more sophisticated computational paradigms where ligands can be docked into binding pockets as a way to screen potential compounds in a virtual mode. This is because higher binding usually provides for higher potency, at least when simple inhibitors of the biological surface's function are being sought. Agonists must bind and then also rely on another set of SAR properties to additionally activate a receptor, so their potency need not necessarily correspond directly with just the binding energy portion of their interaction.

Table 19.4 Types of Functional Group Interactions and Their Related Energies

Molecular Interaction	ca. Δ Energy (–Kcal/lmole)
1. Covalent bond	70–80
2. Ionic or electrostatic	7–9
3. Ion-dipole	4–6
4. Dipole-dipole	3–5
5. Hydrogen bond	3–5
6. Charge-transfer	3–5
7. Hydrophobic	
One small group (Methyl)	2
Two or more small groups; one or more large groups (Phenyl)	4
8. van der Waals (per each pair of atoms)	0.5

Note that energy values are in negative Kcal/mole. Also see Figure 19.13 and the text for related details.

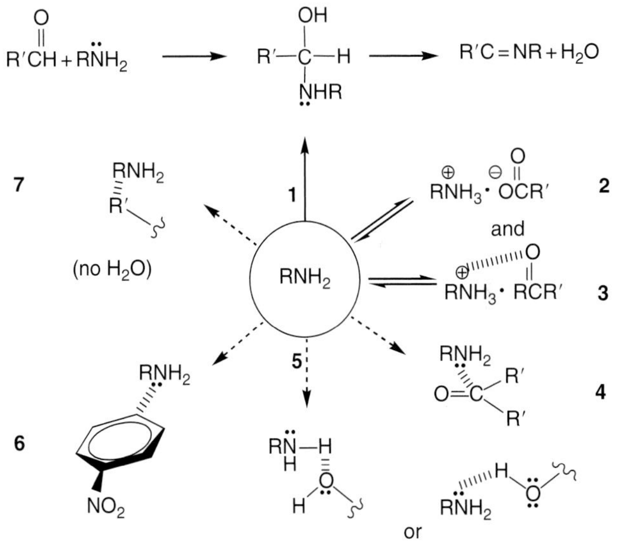

Figure 19.13 Examples of the types of functional group interactions listed within accompanying Table 19.4. A single terminal amino-group of a lysine residue's side-chain has been used to exemplify these interactions. In actuality, numerous possibilities present themselves for each of the amino acid residues that are present within a receptor pocket or enzyme active site. Examples include: 1 covalent bonding shown here by formation of a Schiff base; 2 Ionic or electrostatic; 3 Ion-dipole; 4 Dipole-dipole; 5 Hydrogen bonding where the amine serves as a donor or as an acceptor; 6 Charge transfer; and 7 Hydrophobic bonding. Not depicted are van der Waals interactions (one atom's electrons being attracted to another nonbonded atom's protons). Even though the latter provide only very small attractions energetically, their summation across the entire surface of a given chemical structure can become very significant.

From a basic science point of view, these types of medicinal chemistry efforts can also be considered to be comparable to that of an explorer who, for the first time, is mapping out the rivers and mountains within a virgin region of the wilderness. Thus, they are sometimes referred to as receptor or active site topographical mapping studies that are performed at the molecular level rather than at the continental level. Finally, although a functional group categorization for these types of interactions is a useful conceptual tool to manipulate SAR and track topographical mapping studies, both the biological surface and the compound surface actually relate to each other as overall electrostatic surface potential maps; that is, neither surface has any idea of what a functional group is, and instead reacts only to a continuum of varying electronic density and its distribution in space. An appreciation of this broader reality of a functional group will become even more important for the later section of this chapter pertaining to toxicity and the deployment of biososteric functionalities.

The Importance of Ligand Alignment No matter how energetically favorable a given pairing of a ligand's functional group may be with a receptor/active site's reciprocal functional group, unless these two functionalities are able to find each other, this interaction will not occur. Thus, the spatial orientation adopted by a ligand becomes critical as it begins to enter and associate with the binding pocket so that it can arrange as many of these introductions as possible. In the end, preference will be given to those relationships that can ultimately deliver the greatest energy stabilization. That this is an energy-driven (net lowering) process that occurs in a continuum of accommodating steps and adjustments by both parties via a process that has been called mutual molding, is probably an accurate way to imagine this event. It is a more dynamic process than Ehrlich's original declaration of haptophores capable of fixation (binding) to receptors in a lock-and-key arrangement, which connotes a more rigid behavior by both parties. In accord with the intended specificity implied by the latter phrase, however, is the fact that the range for mutual molding will still have constraints that become precisely dictated by each system in a distinct manner. And therein lies the possibility also to use conformational considerations to advantage when further optimizing hit compounds. Thus, in addition to delineating the SAR associated with the various functional groups present on a hit compound, an exploration of the hit compound's display of its groups in three-dimensional space is also undertaken. This generally is done with an eye toward subsequently freezing that display in an arrangement that is so highly preferred by the biological surface of interest that it becomes possible to achieve selectivity for just that desired surface (like a perfect-fit key for the desired lock that then does not work well for any of the locks associated with the numerous other biological surfaces present in the body). Conformational explorations can be attempted by pursuing drug design and synthesis strategies that produce compounds referred to as semi-rigid analogs. This strategy is exemplified within Figure 19.14 and Scheme 19.9, along with their accompanying text. It is also appropriate to again note Ehrlich's very early and imaginative phraseology where chemotherapeutic "arrows" might be aimed toward microorganism "bull's-eyes" just like magic bullets that can selectively wipe out only the enemy.

Within Figure 19.14, the far-left column depicts two possible conformations of dopamine **13**, namely an extended or "E" conformation in Panel A and a folded or "F" conformation in Panel B. Prior analog work, conducted along the strategies described earlier, has shown that the two hydroxyl- and amino-functional groups present in **13** are all requisite for activity. Two diagrams showing how the biological surface's three reciprocal partners would have to be arranged in either case so as to optimally interact with **13**'s three groups also are provided in the far-right column of Panels A and B. Inspection of these conformations when displayed in their Newman Projection formulas (middle column) suggests that "E" should be more stable (of lower energy) than the crowded (eclipsed) atom arrangement that occurs in "F." Assuming that the energy difference between these two possibilities is about 5 Kcal, most of the population of molecules for **13** will be residing in the "E" conformation.

Now turning to the energetics that are likely to result during **13**'s interaction with its biological surface, namely a dopamine receptor pocket (DARP), we can reasonably assume that each of the requisite hydroxyl groups, (a) and (b) in Figure 19.14, is involved in a hydrogen-bond relationship with an appropriate partner at the DARP. Likewise, a common interaction for the requisite amine (c) would be as an ionic bond since (c) is very likely to be protonated under these conditions; that is, exist as $-NH_3^+$ even if not depicted in this manner within the figure. Assuming that these three interactions can be optimally positioned so that the higher-end ranges listed within Table 19.4 should be used, the favorable energy reduction from binding becomes –5 Kcal + (–5 Kcal) + (–9 Kcal) for a total of –19 Kcal. However, before using this sum directly, it must be additionally noted that in the general systemic circulation, **13** will already be associating with a pharmacological media where at physiological pH 7.4 the amine will be largely protonated and all three functional groups will likely be involved with mobile hydrogen bonds supplied by various solvating water molecules. Since these types of random or weak hydrogen bonds within the quickly moving circulatory system will not be as ideally partnered as a series of receptor-related events, all three of these hydrogen-bonding interactions can be given values from the lower-end range specified within Table 19.4. The total for **13**'s favorable solvated energy reduction when likewise compared to our bare structure **13** as depicted in Figure 19.14 thus becomes $3 \times (-3\ \text{Kcal}) = -9$ Kcal. Before **13** can enter into any of its desired relationships with the DARP, it must first shed these three water molecules. This temporarily causes an energy gain in the system of + 9 Kcal that

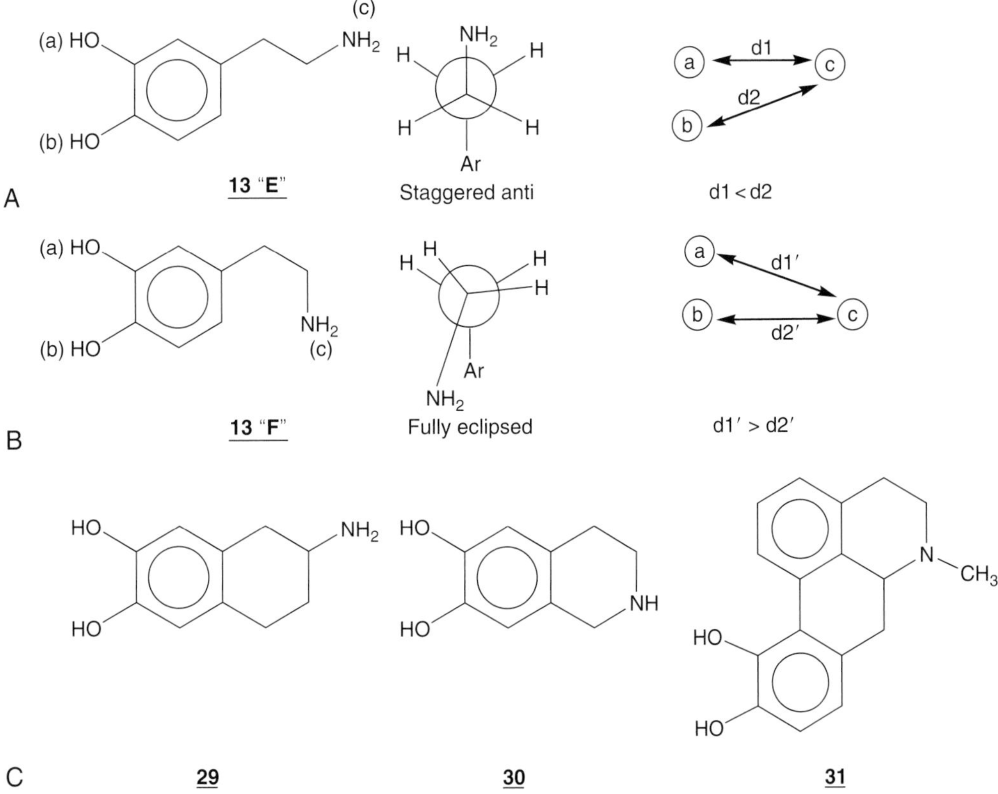

Figure 19.14 Panel **A** shows dopamine, **13** from prior Scheme 19.7, in its 'extended' or (E) conformation, which allows for a staggered anti-Newman Projection formula (Ar = 3,4-dihydroxyphenyl). Panel **B** shows **13** in its folded or (F) conformation, which leads to a fully eclipsed Newman Projection formula of higher energy. Panel **C** shows ADTN **29**, THIQ **30** and apomorphine **31**. d1, d2, d1' and d2' (in the far-right column) refer to distances between the partners for groups (a), (b), and (c) that would exist on the dopamine receptor in order to accommodate dopamine's E or F conformation, respectively. The different spatial arrangements for these two sets of partnering groups are apparent.

must be subtracted from the favorable energy reductions calculated earlier. Ignoring 3D shape for the moment, the net energy reduction for **13** to leave its aqueous milieu, enter into the DARP, and associate with its receptor-related partners becomes –19 Kcal – (–9 Kcal) = –10 Kcal.

Turning next to the conformation of **13**, if the DARP binding scheme requires the more favorable "E" 3D shape as depicted in the far-right column of Panel A, the value of –10 Kcal remains the same because it is essentially the most heavily populated shape of **13** and little more needs to be adjusted for the DARP receptor pockets to greet the vast majority of their guests. Alternatively, if the DARP binding scheme requires the less favorable "F" 3D shape as depicted in the far-right column of Panel B, then not very many suitable guests will even be showing up, unless they first undergo a conformational rotation from "E" to "F." As stated at the beginning of this example, this rotation can be assumed to require about + 5 Kcal and the net energy for binding in this second 3D case will become only –10 Kcal + (+5 Kcal) = –5 Kcal. Since the latter is still a significantly favorable net reduction in energy, either binding scenario could be operative as a successful, energy-driven biological process. Although the scheme requiring the "E" conformation clearly would lead to the larger net reduction in energy and thus seemingly reflect a better one for the body to have evolved, this need not be the case and, as mentioned earlier, distinct 3D constraints will be dictated by each system in a unique manner.

To continue with the example, at this point during drug discovery a synthetic medicinal chemist might make semi-rigid analogs of the "E" and "F" conformations and have each of them tested for their binding with the desired biological surface, namely the DARP. If the DARP required the "E" conformation, then only a modest gain in binding would be expected for its semi-rigid analog since **13** largely presents itself to the receptor in this conformation naturally. At the same time, if other non-DARP-related receptors preferred the "F" conformation, perhaps some leading to an unwanted toxicity when bound by a suitable ligand, then the semi-rigid "E" analog would not be able to interact with these other receptors and their associated toxicity could be avoided. Alternatively, if the DARP required the "F" conformation, a significant gain in binding energy (i.e., ca. –5 Kcal) accompanied by a gain in potency could be expected for a rigid form of folded **13** because all the guests would be arriving already locked into the requisite 3D conformation with no need to expend any energy. Note that if the same

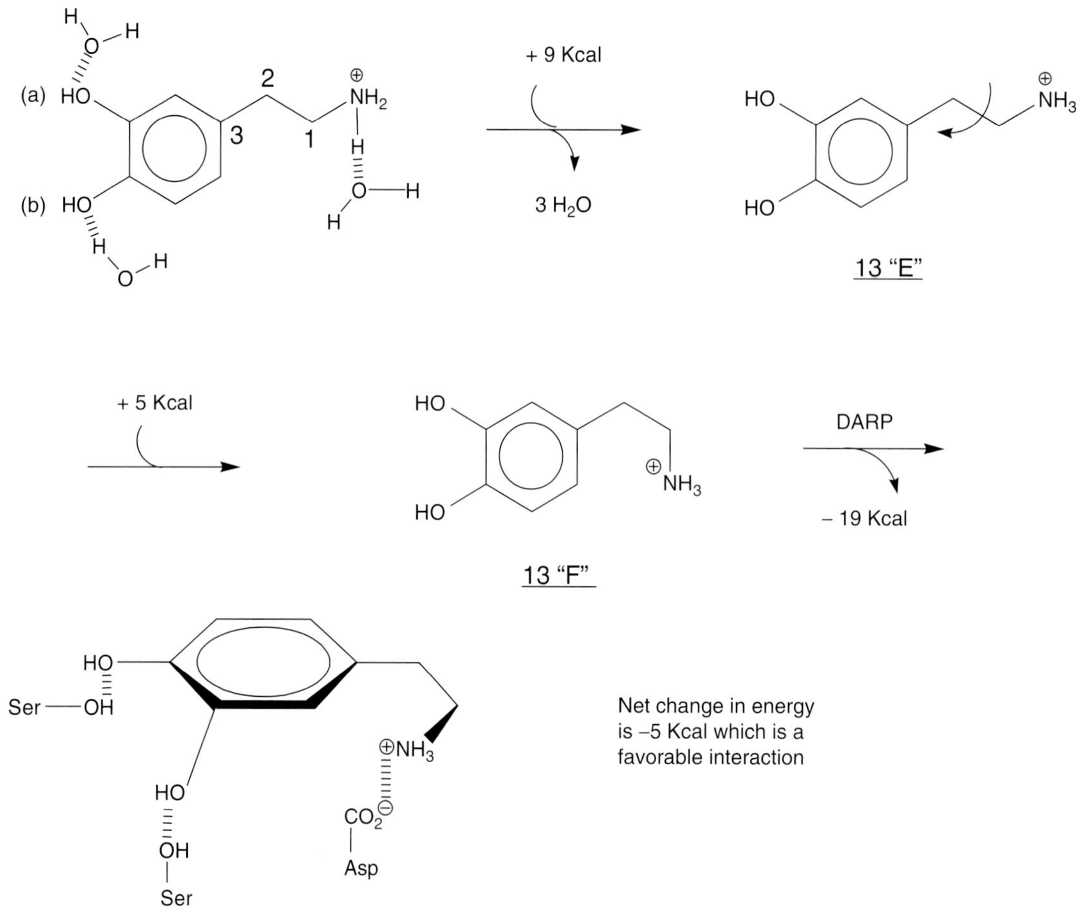

Scheme 19.9 Summary of exemplary case where **13** ultimately binds to the dopamine receptor pocket (DARP) in a folded conformation (**13 F**) (see text for details). Note that in reality, the extended conformation (**13 E**) is actually preferred. Also note that (a) attempts to exemplify the situation where **13**'s hydroxyl-group is serving as a hydrogen-bond donor to water while (b) attempts to exemplify **13**'s other hydroxyl-group serving as a hydrogen-bond acceptor from water. A protonated ammonium system can only serve as a donor during hydrogen bonding. In the final arrangement the roles for **13**'s hydroxyl-groups are similar when interacting with the DARP, which is shown to be utilizing two serine amino acid residues for its partners. Finally, a depronated aspartic acid present within the DARP is depicted to be interacting with the protonated ammonium group within **13** so as to form a very favorable (−9 Kcal) ionic bond relationship. Since no X-ray pictures for any of these interactions are yet available, they are meant to be used only in an exemplary manner. Also note that although bond rotation between carbons 1 and 2 has been considered within this example, for simplicity the additional bond rotation between carbons 2 and 3 has been ignored. A similar analysis would need to be conducted to ascertain the conformational possibilities resulting from rotation between carbons 2 and 3.

non-DARP-related and toxicity-associated receptors were again present, this analog could also be expected to exacerbate side-effect toxicity. If the potency for our example was so important to achieve that the "F" analog became selected for further development, then other means would have to be explored to avoid the toxicity possibility. Additional measures to avoid toxicity will be described in a subsequent section. Scheme 19.9 summarizes this binding scenario and all its related energy calculations, assuming that the final association with the DARP prefers the "F" conformation.

In reality, however, when the extended analog known as ADTN and the folded analog abbreviated herein as THIQ (structures **29** and **30**, respectively, in Figure 19.14) were prepared and tested for activity at the DARP, only **29** showed activity. Although this suggests that it is the "E" conformation that is probably preferred by the DARP, as we have seen from the preceding discussion about functional groups, even one small change in a hit molecule generally leads to several types of physicochemical changes locally, and sometimes also has a significant tumbling effect that is felt across the entire molecule. In the case of **30**, the seemingly simple methylene unit (i.e., only one additional -CH_2-) that was used to tether the side-chain back toward the ring, also causes the amino functionality in **13** to be changed from a primary amine to a secondary amine. Because of the latter, there is the possibility that it is this type of change that is the reason for the dramatic loss of potency rather than anything to do with the change in its 3D shape. However, noting that the tertiary-amine compound **31**, which is a natural product known as apomorphine, also exhibits potent activity at the DARP, clearly indicates that the change in **30**'s level of amine substitution is not the reason for the fall in activity. Finally, although **31**'s nonsubstituted aromatic ring is in an "F" relationship to the amine, its key (requisite) catechol ring is held in a reasonably rigid "E" relationship with the amine.

It should be noted that the complexity of these types of considerations does not necessarily go up as a hit compound's size and molecular weight increase. Indeed, the difficulty is often less for larger molecules because they tend to form intramolecular interactions that can stabilize certain conformations. In addition, they often have ring-forming bond relationships that inherently rigidify certain conformations. The case of large protein systems serves to exemplify both relationships, where specific runs of amino acid sequences tend to repeatedly adopt distinct structural motifs like alpha-helices or beta-sheets, and intramolecular disulfide bonds tend to draw strands together into reasonably stable, ring-like conformations. Thus, the tougher challenges associated with assessing the importance of molecular conformation upon biological activity often reside with smaller molecular systems that have a high degree of energetically allowed flexibility (rotatable single bonds) and that do not contain contiguous aromatic ring systems, the latter falling to the much simpler case of a largely planar arrangement. In terms of studying conformation with analytical approaches, it should be apparent that structure-based drug design strategies at their higher levels of knowledge about the system (i.e., X-ray diagrams with and without bound ligands) represent the ideal case. However, even then it becomes dangerous to speculate what the 3D conformation of a ligand might look like in a solution compared to the environment within the active site as captured by the X-ray that was likely obtained in the crystalline, solid-state phase.

Nuclear magnetic resonance spectroscopy (NMR) can be used to deduce the conformations of molecules while in solvents. This technique primarily focuses upon just the locations and interactions of hydrogens within a given molecule and so it is not nearly as rich in information as an X-ray. Similarly, computational paradigms can be used to calculate the energies of small molecule systems, and these can be done with specified numbers of accompanying solvation molecules.

Conformational explorations during structure-based drug design are on the most solid ground when all three of these techniques can be used to address 3D spatial arrangements within a series of hit compounds. Figure 19.15 is meant to depict how these tools can be used simultaneously while also listing some of the strengths and weaknesses for each method.

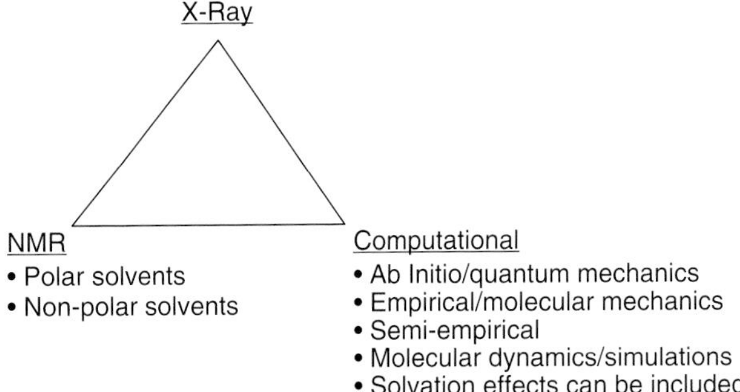

Figure 19.15 Complementary techniques that can be employed individually or simultaneously to assess conformational detail. X-ray diffraction requires a suitable crystal and its results are subject to solid-state interactions. Computational paradigms are most accurate when done at the highest levels of calculation but these types of calculations become prohibitively computer-time intensive. NMR requires that the molecule be soluble in the chosen solvent and that adequate compound supplies be available. Mass spectrometry is also becoming an important tool for larger molecules although it provides smaller amounts of descriptive conformational data. A composite of all approaches provides for the best possible assessment of molecular conformation.

Design of Irreversible Inhibitors This specific strategy merits a brief consideration because it can lead to extremely potent molecules when inhibition of a given biological process is desired. It is a very aggressive approach toward inhibition in that rather than establishing functional groups to form the favorable but reversible interactions discussed earlier, a chemically reactive functional group is added to the hit compound so that it will form a covalent bond with the desired biological surface. Indeed, referring again to Table 19.4, it can be noted that this type of energy change can be favorable by as much as –80 Kcal. Its downside, however, is that unless the chemical reaction that produces the irreversible interaction is specific for the desired biological surface, a high degree of toxicity may ensue. This approach became practical for therapeutic agents when Baker proposed the concept of active site-directed alkylating agents. A good way to illustrate the type of chemical principles that are utilized during this strategy is to convey the early history around the so-called nitrogen mustard family of compounds.

These types of compounds initially were designed as chemical warfare agents about the time of World War I. Shown as **32** in Scheme 19.10, they possess simple alkyl R groups that do not attenuate either the formation or reactivity of the aziridinium functional group, **33**, that is spontaneously formed *in vivo* and is central to their reactivity. When these simple compounds are taken up by humans, they quickly form the aziridinium species and react with the first suitable partner they came across, namely the biological surfaces of the ubiquitous Acetylcholine Esterases. These enzymes contain a binding pocket that has evolved to accommodate the quaternary ammonium functionality present in acetylcholine, **34**, which is their normal biological substrate.

An example of this approach applied to drug discovery is provided by the alpha-adrenergic antagonist drug, phenoxybenzamine, shown as **35** in Scheme 19.11. The construction of **35** actually borrowed from the nitrogen mustards. However, **35** was designed

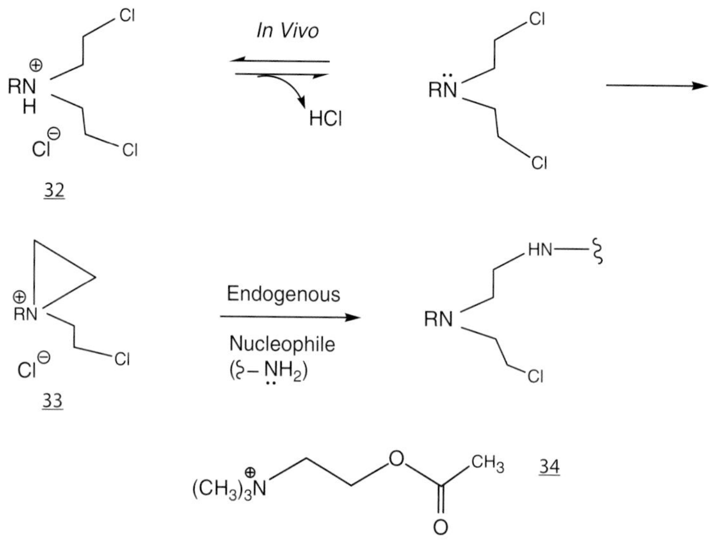

In Vivo

HCl

32

Endogenous

Nucleophile

33

34

Scheme 19.10 Reaction of a nitrogen mustard (**32**) with an endogenous nucleophile to form a covalent, irreversible bond. When the hydrochloride salt is buffered by the physiologic media of the body, a small equilibrium fraction will become deprotonated. In this state, spontaneous cyclization to the aziridium species **33** can occur. Because **33** is a highly-strained, three-membered ring and a high energy ammonium ion system, it is extremely reactive toward nucleophiles which can open it up and also lead to a neutral species. The body's numerous free-amine nucleophiles are glad to oblige the ring-opening reaction but, in the process, they become alkylated in an irreversible manner. When this happens, it becomes difficult for the endogenous material to continue to perform its normal functions and in the case of an enzyme's active site, the latter will be completely shut down (irreversibly inhibited). Ultimately, catabolic turnover and biochemical resynthesis of the enzyme is required to restore functional activity to this system. Acetylcholine, **34** (shown separately), is also a quaternary ammonium ion, but it is not reactive because it lacks the strained three-membered-ring. Since **34** resembles the nitrogen mustards, Acetylcholine Esterase which normally recognizes **34** as its substrate, becomes fooled and is the principle toxic site for the nitrogen mustards.

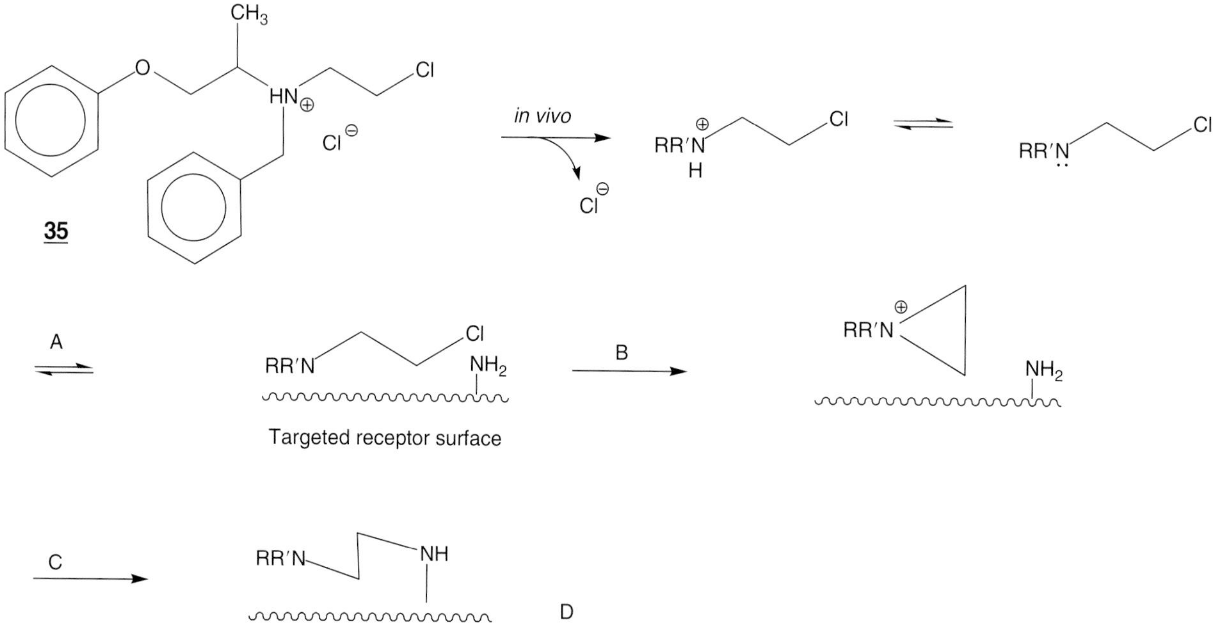

35

in vivo

Targeted receptor surface

Scheme 19.11 Phenoxybenzamine's (**35**) irreversible interaction with its targeted biological surface, namely that for treating pheochromacytoma. Note that while this is analogous to the mechanism of the nitrogen mustards displayed in Scheme 19.10, in this case the rate of formation of the aziridinium species has been attenuated by the steric features of the N-benzyl group. This feature, in turn, allows **35** to first associate with its target biological surface (A). Once bound at this intended destination, formation of an aziridinium does occur (B) and this is rapidly followed by a reaction with an endogenous nucleophile located within this immediate locale (C). Ultimately, this biological surface is selectively shut down (D).

further to have R and R groups that endow selectivity for the alpha-adrenergic receptor while also sterically attenuating the rate of formation of the aziridinium functional group. In this way, **35** is encouraged to first find its desired biological surface before forming an aziridinium intermediate. Once bound with the alpha-adrenergic receptor, the aziridinium is formed, and this is immediately followed by irreversible reaction with an endogenous nucleophile located in this vicinity. Note that complete selectivity for the alpha-adrenergic receptor is not achieved. Because of side-effect toxicity, this type of drug design strategy is often confined to the pursuit of anticancer agents.

In an attempt to further enhance the selectivity for this type of approach, subsequent strategies have been devised where the reactive functional group requires a metabolic bioactivation either for its generation or for its adequate exposure in an *in vivo* setting. When this bioactivation is selectively accomplished by an enzyme that is also the efficacy-related biological surface target, and the latter immediately succumbs to the irreversible chemical reaction, this type of drug-wannabe is called a suicide enzyme inhibitor since the enzyme is conducting a bioactivation process that then serves to kill itself. An example of a successful suicide inhibitor drug can be found in the prototype MAO-B inhibitor deprenyl. This drug is shown as **36** (also see prior discussion about MAO inhibitors in Section 19.2.1.6). After recognizing **36** as a potential substrate, MAO-B begins to metabolize it by oxidative degradation. However, the chemically reactive intermediate that is formed during this conversion immediately reacts with MAO-B in a covalent manner so as to irreversibly inhibit the enzyme. In this particular case, it is the N-propargyl that endows the chemical reactivity, itself being inert until the metabolic activation occurs. In general, suicide inhibitors are also referred to as enzyme activated, mechanism-based, or Kcat inhibitors, the latter deriving from their effect upon enzyme kinetic parameters.

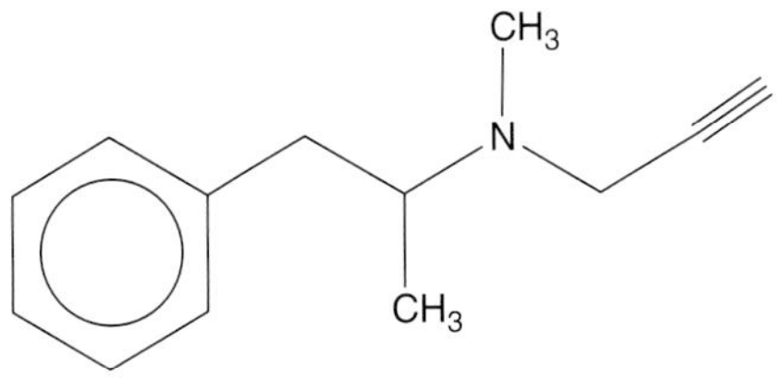

CH_3
N
CH_3

36

Inhibiting Proteases It was mentioned in the Introduction that today's emphasis upon proteomics coupled with the present interrogation of cell signaling processes will likely feed heavily into tomorrow's categories of new drug targets. It was also noted that the SAR associated with the protein–protein interaction aspects of cell signaling is likely to be difficult to ascertain relative to small molecule drug approaches. Alternatively, the control mechanisms for production and maintenance of these cell signaling components represent viable small molecule approaches, namely their anabolic biosyntheses and their catabolic turnover. Thus, a brief section covering at least the primary aspects associated with the specific design of drugs intended to modulate proteinases is appropriate at this juncture.

Active-site directed irreversible inhibitors and mechanism-based inhibitors or suicide inhibitors have already been adequately exemplified in the preceding section relative to biological surfaces in general and also with respect to a couple of specific examples. Another approach, namely that of substrate analog inhibitors, has also been described within the prior discussion pertaining to analog-based drug design (see earlier). Thus, only one other major strategy for inhibiting enzymes remains. It involves what are called transition-state analogs or inhibitors. Focusing upon the various proteinases, it becomes important to understand that there are four types of proteinase mechanisms as defined by the chemical components participating in what is considered to be the transition state during hydrolysis of a protein's amide linkage. Table 19.5 lists the divisions of proteinases according to the now well-accepted transition-state or mechanistic criteria referred to earlier. Table 19.5 also conveys a specific endogenous substrate for each classification and a common chemical substance that can selectively inhibit each type of proteinase.

Figure 19.16 depicts the chemical details of these mechanistic classifications and highlights the transition state ($\neq$) for each.

With this level of knowledge in hand it becomes common practice to modify initial hit compounds that are targeted for a specific type of protease along the lines of their corresponding transition states ($\neq$). Thus, tetrahedral carbons are typically used to replace the carbonyl group in compounds seeking to inhibit serine, cysteine and aspartic proteases by using neutral systems like a simple methylene for either of the first

Table 19.5 Classification of the Common Proteases[a]

Protease	Active Site Machinery	Exemplary Member	Exemplary Endogenous Substrate	Common Inhibitor
Serine	Ser hydroxy	Plasmin	Fibrin	Diisopropyl-fluorophosphate
Cysteine	Cys sulfhydro	Cathepsin B	Insulin	Iodoacetate
Aspartic	Asp carboxylate	Renin	Angiotensinogen	Pepstatin
Metallo	Zn or Cu, etc.	Angiotensin converting Enzyme (ACE)	Angiotensin I	Enalaprilat

[a]This classification is based upon catalylic mechanisms originally proposed by Hartly and further modified by Barrett.

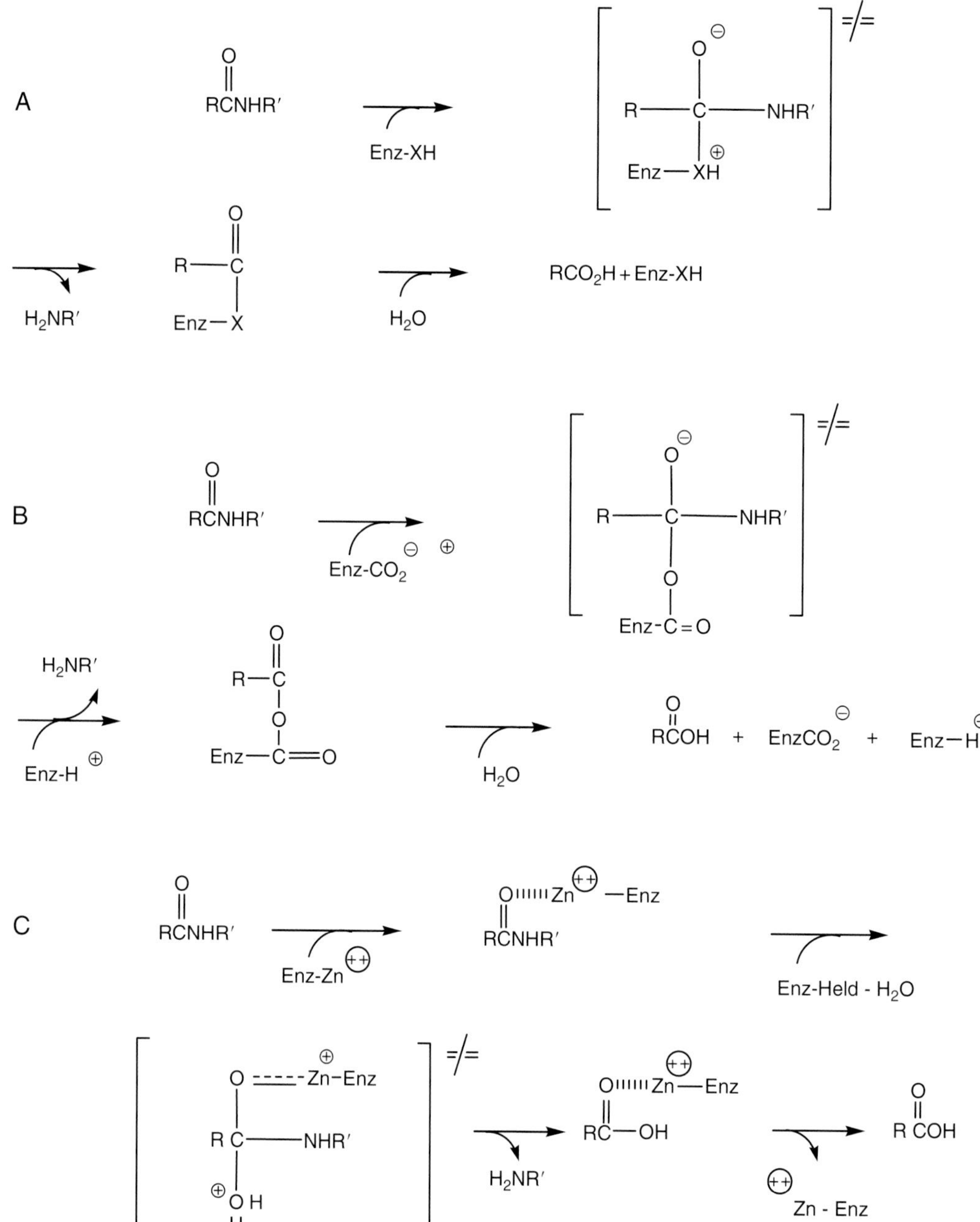

Figure 19.16 Chemical depiction of the protease classification system showing both the metabolic machinery and the transition state that is thought to be operative for each case. (A) represents both serine (X=O) and cysteine (X=S) proteases with each of these specific amino acids being implicated, respectively. (B) exemplifies an aspartic protease with the latter playing a key catalytic function within the active site. (C) depicts the metallo proteases with Zn^{++} representing one of the most common. Suspected transition states ≠ for each protease reaction are shown within brackets.

two, and perhaps a methylene-hydroxy for a more polarized version of the aspartic case. Alternatively, metal chelator functional groups are typically added to hit compounds that are intended to target metallo proteases. One classic example for this type of strategy is afforded by the Angiotensin Converting Enzyme (ACE) inhibitor enalaprilat. Figure 19.17 depicts the binding interactions thought to occur during the inhibition of ACE by enalaprilat, **37**. Without going into any of the details for how **37** was designed historically, suffice it to say that a combination of ligand-based drug design and structure-based drug design was used accompanied by knowledge about Zn^{++} proteases. With regard to the latter and pertinent to the present discussion, a free carboxyl group was ultimately selected to chelate with Zn^{++} as a characteristic type of active site interaction. This became the most important component eventually contributing to a highly potent inhibitor of ACE. Also note that the free carboxyl group was positioned on a tetrahedral carbon

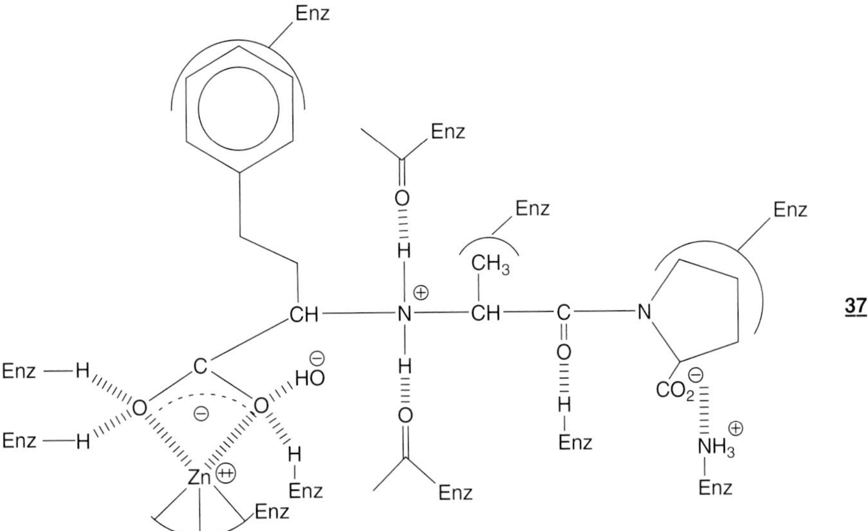

Figure 19.17 Hypothetical interaction of enalaprilat (**37**) with the Angiotensin Converting Enzyme (ACE) active site (Enz). Note that a free carboxylate functional group was added so as to chelate with the Zn^{++} known to be present in this particular protease. A prodrug ester of this drug is also marketed since it has improved bioavailability after oral administration.

atom (also bearing the phenethyl-group in Figure 19.17) so as to additionally mimic the transition state for when this position normally would be the carbonyl of a typical amide bond.

19.2.3.2 Traversing ADMET Hurdles and Producing Preclinical Development Compounds

Assuming that from some combination of the drug design strategies and chemical alterations discussed earlier, a high potency (low nanomolar), lead compound becomes identified that, if needed, also seems suitable for further structural modification, then this compound becomes a good candidate for entrance into more advanced, in-depth study. As discussed in the Sections 19.1 and 19.2.1, the next studies will typically entail secondary biological models for efficacy and, importantly, preliminary models of anticipated human ADMET properties. Chemical principles and potential structural adjustments that pertain to each of the ADMET areas are discussed separately, later. The same composite of drug design strategies and chemical manipulations already described will continue to be employed while also encompassing each of these additional principles as may be applicable to solving a given compound's unique set of ADMET-related shortcomings. Since this phase of structural modification is so heavily directed toward enhancing the ADMET properties and overall profile of a given lead compound, it has also been referred to as property-based drug design.

Assuring Absorption This section will focus upon oral dosing since that is by far the most frequently sought administration protocol for new drugs in general. In this regard, aside from drug metabolism issues and the previously discussed first-pass effect, three primary features of a dosage form can be thought of as dictating its ability to be absorbed from the GI tract after oral administration. The first is its dissolution rate because it will be the finely dispersed, if not completely solubilized, form of any molecule that will be required for reasonable absorption to occur. If necessary, formulation excipients can be added to the drug-wannabe even at this early point of investigation so as to promote dispersion or, ideally, a rapid dissolution. Likewise, an enteric coated formulation that is resistant to breakdown under acidic conditions while still being susceptible to breakdown under more neutral and basic conditions can be readily devised as a means to protect a lead compound that is inherently unstable under the acidic conditions that will be encountered in the stomach (Scheme 19.4). At first glance, this initial aspect of addressing a lead compound's absorption can seemingly be handled by pharmaceutical manipulation of the dosage form. However, pharmaceutical properties are not typically elaborated during early drug development and a poorly absorbed lead compound can sometimes be cast aside even though its fix may have been reasonably straightforward.

Typically, formulation properties and preliminary dosage forms are not considered seriously until the next stage for the overall process of drug discovery, namely that of preclinical compound development (Section 19.2.3.3). In addition, to avoid solubility issues altogether, initial administration to rodents during secondary efficacy testing and *in vivo* ADMET assessments often takes advantage of presolubilized dosage forms. In this regard, the use of dimethylsulfoxide (DMSO) as a universal solvent has become popular. However, the question still remains as to how solubilized the compound is once the DMSO solutions begin to mix with a given biological media. Indeed, this is a fundamental question that particularly applies to the initial, front-line screening process when HTS surveys of huge compound libraries are still attempting to identify initial hit compounds.

The second principle chemical feature associated with a substance relative to its absorption is the overall hydrophilic-to-lipophilic balance. This property can be divided into two major categories, the first being the overall charge situation for compounds capable of being ionized, and the second being a composite of lipophilicity-related parameters applicable to neutral molecules and to the ionizable molecules when in their noncharged state. Scheme 19.12 depicts the importance of the first category of behavior by demonstrating this situation for lead compounds that contain either an acid or a basic functional group, which is likely to be highly ionized under various biological environments.

As shown in Scheme 19.12, only the unionized equilibrium species is able to be absorbed through the gut wall by passive diffusion. As a general rule, acidic drugs tend to be better absorbed from the stomach whereas both acidic and basic drugs tend to be similarly absorbed from the intestine where the local pH at the surface of the gut wall is about 5 and is thus midway between that of the stomach and the intestinal lumen (pH ca 8). However, since equilibration between the ionized and unionized species is very fast compared to the rate of movement through the GI tract's huge surface area, the preferred locations for absorption of different types of ionizable substances are not absolute. Nevertheless, these are processes that sometimes can be enhanced by using simple chemical principles to adjust the acidity or basicity of an ionizable functional group, namely its pKa. This was also mentioned previously when examining the role of a suspected hydrogen-bond formation between a ligand and a biological surface of interest. Recall that if an amino-group is utilized to explore this relationship, care must be taken to insure that it does not simply result in a protonated ammonium group presenting itself to the biological surface, because the latter may actually be looking to partner with a hydrogen-bond accepting moiety.

Table 19.6 provides a very abbreviated listing of a few common types of carboxylic acid and amino group arrangements that may be present in a drug-wannabe molecule. If needed, their degree of ionization can be readily attenuated by taking advantage of the electronic effects conveyed in Table 19.3. For example, if a methlyamino-containing compound is found to be poorly absorbed due to the fact that it is too ionized while traversing the GI-tract, then its basicity (and thereby its protonation and ionization) could be dramatically reduced by substituting its methyl-group with a strongly electron withdrawing trifluoromethyl-group. As a useful rule-of-thumb for appreciating just how ionized a given functional group might be at a pH that is of biological interest, first remember that the pKa value also represents that pH where the two equilibrium species will be equally represented (i.e., at their 50/50 point). Then, depending upon whether the group is an acid or a base, if the actual pH environment is lowered (becomes more acidic), the group will ionize less or more, respectively, and vice versa for the acids and bases if the pH is raised. The greater this change in pH (from that represented by the pKa) to reach an actual biologically relevant value, the greater the aforementioned directional shift in their equilibria. Finally, since the pH scale is logarithmic (numbers reflect

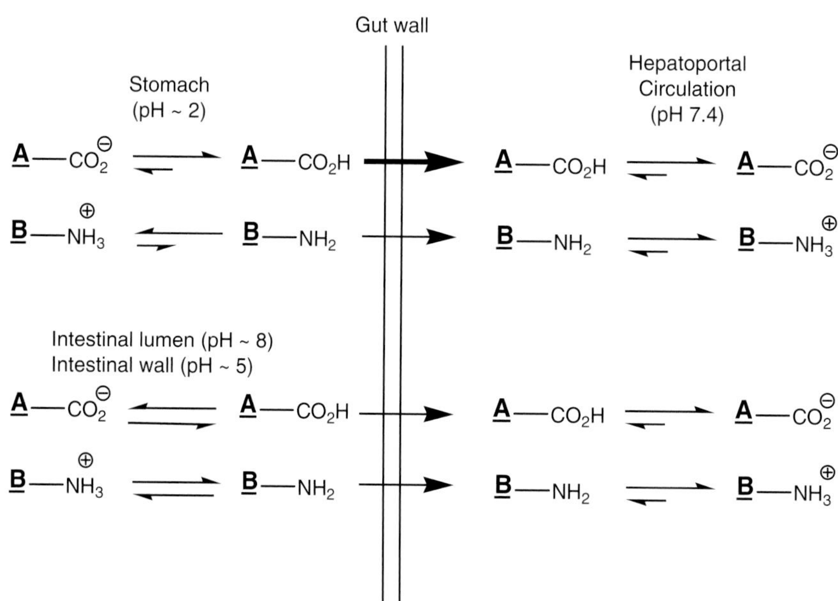

Scheme 19.12 Impact of ionization upon drug absorption. Only the unionized species are absorbed by passive diffusion through the gut wall. **A** represents an acidic drug and **B** represents a basic drug. Note the difference in their equilibrium ratios (half-arrows) and in their degree of absorption (heavy arrow versus lighter arrow) when in the stomach and when in the intestine. The local pH (~5) dictates behavior in the intestine during absorption.

Table 19.6 pKa Values for Selected Functional Groups and Impact upon Their Equilibrium Ratios at the Principal Site for Their Absorption after Oral Administration and within the Blood

Functional Group	Exemplary Compound	pKa[a]	Principal Site for Absorption[b]	Blood[c]
Conjugated acid	$-CO_2H$	4.2	(S) U $\rightleftharpoons$ I	U $\rightleftharpoons$ I
Nonconjugated acid	CH_3CO_2H	4.8	(S) U $\rightleftharpoons$ I	U $\rightleftharpoons$ I
Conjugated amine	$-NH_3^{\oplus}$	4.6	(IN) I $\rightleftharpoons$ U	I $\rightleftharpoons$ U
Nonconjugated amine	$CH_3CH_2NH_3^{\oplus}$	10.7	(IN) I $\rightleftharpoons$ U	I $\rightleftharpoons$ U

[a]This value represents the dissociation equilibrium constant (release of a proton) for the species shown in the Exemplary Column. Thus, acids become ionized when they dissociate and bases (as conjugate acids) become neutral when they dissociate.
[b](S) indicates stomach (pH ~ 1 or 2) and (IN) indicates intestine (local wall pH~5) as the principal site for absorption. U indicates unionized species and I indicates ionized species.
[c]Blood pH of 7.4 typically is cited to be the physiological pH, although this can vary slightly for discrete locations and very dramatically within the binding pocket of a receptor or enzymatic active site where bulk solution properties like pH may no longer be applicable.

powers of 10), even fractional pH changes can have a significant impact upon the equilibrium ratio of the ionized to unionized species.

The other major category associated with this second chemical principle for drug absorption is that of the overall physicochemical properties of the substance when it is in a neutral state or in the form that can pass through the gut-wall membrane via passive diffusion. In this regard, Lipinski has reviewed a huge sampling of marketed drugs and devised a set of chemical property rules that suggest that as these rules' limits are broken by a given substance, that substance's chances for having acceptable oral bioavailability go down. Since the values associated with each of Lipinski's four rules are simple multiples of the number 5, they have come to be called the Rule-of-5. These rules are listed as follows, and it is important to appreciate that they should be applied only to passive diffusion process and not to active transport.

The Rule-of-5 stipulates that a drug's ability to permeate membranes by passive processes will be reduced when:

- Molecular weight is greater than 500.
- There are more than five hydrogen-bond donors.
- There are more than 10 hydrogen-bond acceptors.
- The drug's calculated octanol-water partition coefficient log value (cLog P) is greater than 5.

At this point in the chapter, you should be familiar with all these chemical properties except for the partition coefficient. Experimentally, partition coefficient values (P) are determined by measuring the amount of a given substance in each layer of a partition media between water and n-octanol, the latter "oil" being chosen historically to resemble how a substance might partition between the lipophilic nature of a lipid bilayer or biological membrane versus that of the highly polar, aqueous phase. The log of this concentration ratio is the Log P value. Since the lighter "oil" value is placed on the top-side of this math expression, the greater the number, the more lipophilic the compound and the more of it that will reside in the "oil" or membrane-mimic phase compared to the aqueous phase. Computational schemes also have been devised to calculate (c) partition coefficients, and although they can be subject to various types of critique, the most common of these computational methods is used in the Rule-of-5 so that an experimental value doesn't have to be determined for each compound in question.

Not just randomly walking through these rules, it should be clear that too much molecular weight (or overall size) will deter compounds from sneaking between the junctions of gut-wall membrane cells and also from muscling through pores that may be able to be stretched (recall the concept of mutual molding) to allow for their passage. Likewise, too much hydrogen bonding with the aqueous phase, particularly as a donor species, is going to cost high energy to break these up since the lipid layer will not allow the substance to cross while carrying a baggage of highly polar water molecules still attached (recall our earlier example of a substance's need to likewise shed solvent molecules when entering a receptor pocket or enzymatic active site). Finally, what about the Log P preference: why should too high a value (i.e., too high lipophilicity) deter movement of a substance out of the polar, aqueous phase and into the nonpolar, lipophilic membrane-like phase? This may seem opposite to what we might predict based upon the logic of like-dissolving-like. In fact, increased Log P values don't act as a deterrent for entry into the lipid membrane. Instead, a Log P that is too high begins to encourage too much penetration, to the point that the substance does not

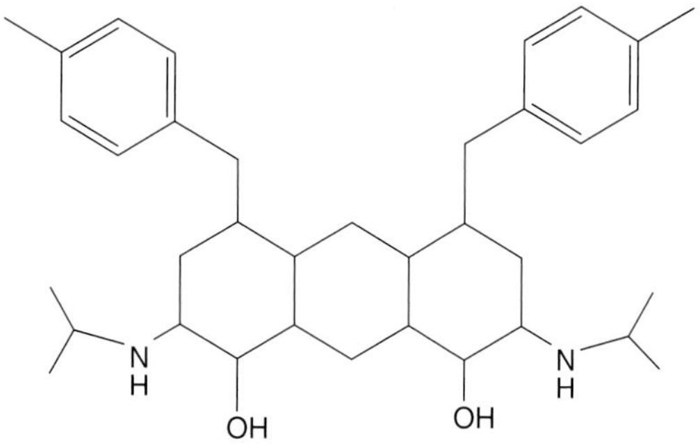

38

mw 547
cLog P 7

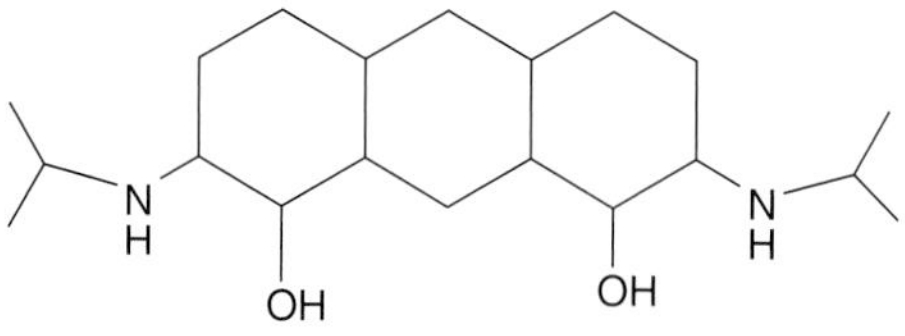

39

mw 338
cLog P 2

Figure 19.18 Example compound **38** having low oral bioavailability in a rodent model due to poor passage across the gut-wall, i.e. essentially all of a presolubilized dose was recovered unchanged in the feces. Previous SAR studies suggest that the northern edge is not a critical face of the molecule for binding to the efficacy-related receptor pocket because structural changes in this region had little impact upon the desired activity. A proposed analog, **39**, that may address the bioavailability issue is shown to the right.

want to leave the membrane on the other side. Thus, substances with high Log P values tend to dissolve and stay within the membranes and are not readily released in an equilibrium manner to the other side so that they can enter the largely aqueous hepatoportal circulation.

In addition to solvation energies per se, what type of functional group binding energies might be thought of as contributing to a highly lipophilic substance's tendency to stay embedded within a biological membrane? This answer lies within Table 19.4, where hydrophobic binding becomes a dominating factor when numerous alkyl and/or aryl groups present in a molecule serve to multiply binding energy values as part of the overall structure's interactive process.

Figure 19.18 conveys a model compound that is meant to exemplify some of these physicochemical properties in action. It also serves as a demonstration of how drug design might proceed at this juncture. Assume that oral bioavailability has been determined to be problematic for compound **38** because of poor passage across the gut-wall membrane. Also assume that it has been determined previously that considerable structural modification can be done to the northern edge of this molecule without diminishing its desired activity. How might you proceed toward potentially remedying its low bioavailability issue?

A quick inspection of structure **38** and its related data indicates that its molecular weight (MW) is greater than 500 and that its cLog P value is greater than 5. Taken together within the context of the Rule-of-5, this suggests that these factors probably contribute significantly to the lack of oral bioavailability if not being the sole reason for the problem. Alternatively, the number of hydrogen-bond donors is 4 and the number of hydrogen-bond acceptors is also 4, so the solvation energetics for these types of parameters are probably okay. Two choices present themselves to lower the lipophilicity of **38**: add polar functional groups along the northern edge, or remove some of the highly non-polar groups presently located on the northern edge. Given the prior SAR data, either approach should be tolerable from an efficacy point of view. and if hydrogen-bond accepting, rather than donating groups, are utilized as polar adducts, then this approach would not run the risk of adding too many hydrogen-bond donating groups. However, since the MW is already fairly high, it makes more sense to remove some of the lipophilic groups and at the same time reduce molecular weight. A reasonable, appropriately stripped-down target molecule thus becomes compound **39**, which is also shown in Figure 19.18. Removal of the two methyltoluyl-groups (each being C_8H_9 and having an MW of 105) will reduce MW by 208 ($2 \times [-105 + 1$ for their replacement with a hydrogen]), and should reduce the cLog P by about 4 to 6 units ($2 \times$[ca. 2 units for the phenyl ring plus ca. 1 unit for the methylene and methyl combined contribution as estimated from Table 19.3]). The result is shown under compound **39** in Figure 19.18. Synthesis of this compound followed by actual biological testing then would be undertaken to verify if the approach was leading in the right direction and should be pursued further.

The third and final feature to be considered for any substance relative to its oral absorption is that of active transport. In this case specific structural details, just like for interacting and binding with any other biological surface in a specific manner, become very important. Toward this possibility, SAR for transport phenomena need to be ascertained to see if the lead structure is subject to these types of processes and if so, to determine if alterations in structure might be able to use the transporters to better advantage. Also appreciate, however, that at least one major transporter in the GI-tract, namely a P-glycoprotein or Pgp transporter, works in the wrong direction because it serves to pump drugs entering the gut-wall epithelial cells back into the stomach and intestine rather than into the hepatoportal circulation. Alternatively, numerous other transporters, like those for the amino acid nutrients, may be able to be exploited to potentially improve the oral bioavailability of a lead compound. *In vitro* test systems, such as a human epithelial cancer cell line called Caco-2 that expresses high levels of Pgp, can be used to assess analogs that are being designed and synthesized in an attempt to explore possible improvements of oral bioavailability. Certain of these cell membrane transporters will be discussed further in the next session relative to directing distribution since they will again be prominent players in that regard. Likewise, aggressive drug metabolism that can occur within the gut-wall will be addressed within the subsequent section as part of the strategies that are described to avoid too fast of a metabolism.

A different strategy that also needs to be mentioned within this section, is that of taking a prodrug approach toward improving oral bioavailability. Scheme 19.13 contrasts the prodrug design motif to that of a regular drug's behavior, as well as to a soft drug design strategy (the latter will be discussed in a subsequent section). As mentioned in the Introduction during the discussion about prontosil and the discovery of the sulfonamide antibiotics, prodrugs are inactive substances until they undergo conversion in the body to their active forms. Although the prontosil case was accidental, this can also be intentionally arranged as a specific design strategy to enhance the features of the parent substance so as to improve its absorption. Note that the prodrug strategy can be used to either increase or decrease the lipophilicity of a substance depending upon what degree of polarity the component to be attached is endowed with. A classic example of increasing lipophilicity is the successful masking of the acidic moiety present in the ACE inhibitor enalaprilat shown previously as **37** in Figure 19.17. By making the simple, lipophilic ethyl ester enalapril or **40** as shown, compound **37**, which is otherwise not orally bioavailable, then could be administered effectively by the p.o. (oral) route as its ester. From

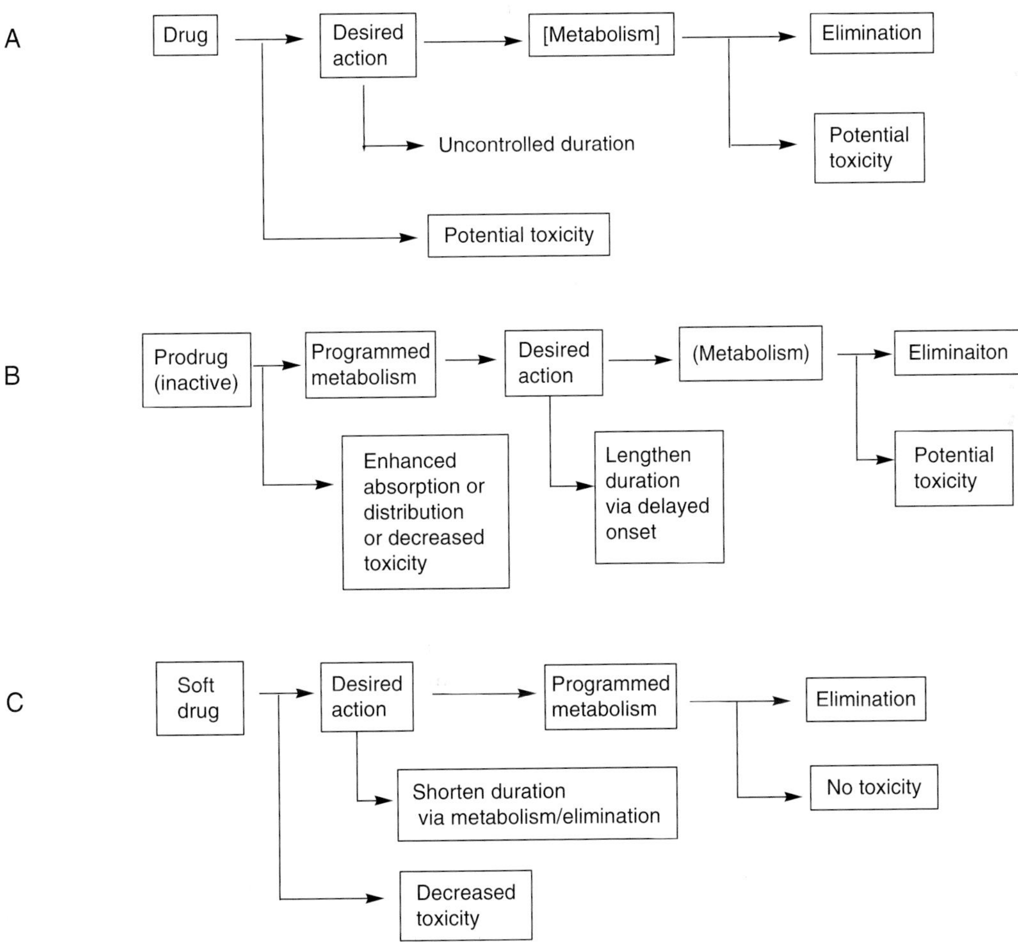

Scheme 19.13 Contrasting dispositions of a drug, prodrug, and soft drug. (A) depicts a generalized version of a standard drug's pattern of observed activities. (B) depicts how a prodrug approach can be used to modify the entry-side portion of a given drug's overall profile of actions. (C) depicts how a soft drug approach can be used to modify the elimination-side portion of a given drug's overall profile of action. Both prodrugs and soft drugs can be used to decrease toxicity.

Table 19.3 we can estimate the increase in lipophilicity for **40** to be rather dramatic, namely about + 5 units (CO_2^- when ionized in the gut to instead be CO_2CH_3 is worth + 4.4 units since we're removing a – 4.4, and then the additional methylene of an ethyl versus a methyl [$CH_3 \rightarrow CH_2CH_3$] being worth another ca. + 0.6). Once the more lipophilic prodrug is absorbed into the gut wall, it is quickly metabolized by esterase enzymes present in that location and during the subsequent attacks by the first- and second-pass-effect from the numerous esterases present in the blood, liver, and lungs. These attacks quickly release and deliver the parent drug **37** into the systemic circulation.

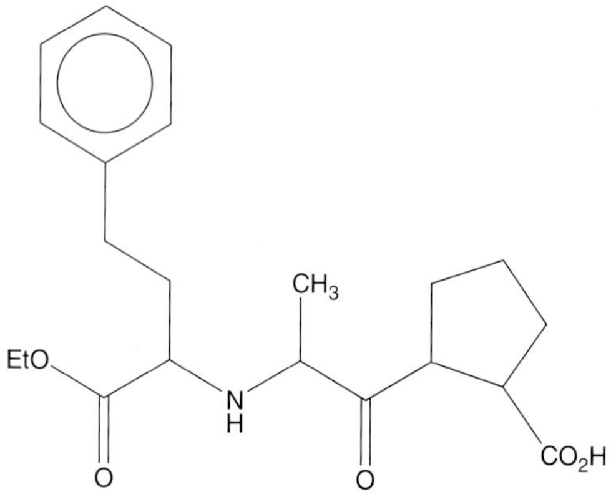

As a summary to this section, drug design to improve oral bioavailability will often need to simultaneously account for adequate dissolution; minimal ionization; balanced hydrophilic-to-lipophilic ratio; low solvation energetics; desirable interaction or lack of interaction with influx and efflux transporters, respectively; and, the possibility that a prodrug approach may become a ready fix toward accomplishing the desired goal and thus not to be taken as only a backup or last resort strategy to situations where structural modifications haven't been able to do the job. All these parameters, of course, need to be optimized without losing the potent and selective efficacious activity that is requisite for the final product.

Directing Distribution Assuming that we have traversed the oral bioavailability hurdle and that we have managed to retain high potency in our *in vitro* models for the desired efficacy-related biological surface, our next challenge will be to insure that our drug-wannabe is delivered to the appropriate tissues where it is supposed to be efficacious *in vivo*. If an intended drug never arrives at the requisite locale in adequate concentration, there can be no therapy. When the lead compound has distribution issues that relate to the same types of physicochemical property considerations described earlier, then similar types of modifications must be reexamined within the context of this next step.

One of the first set of surfaces that the substance will encounter immediately after absorption will be those present within the blood, namely the latter's cell constituents and plasma proteins (PP). Blood cells will have membrane penetration barriers akin to those described for the gut-wall epithelium. Given an appropriate blend of physicochemical properties, penetration of blood-borne substances into these cells can occur. Likewise, significant association with these cells' surfaces along with the blood's PP components can occur. Indeed, it is this type of early, chemical sentinel system that forms the basis of the body's immune-response system. The latter has been posted to guard against foreign protein and peptide invaders that have managed to penetrate the first line of defense set up by the gut wall and liver. Although this is generally not a problematic situation for a small molecule drug-wannabe, it can be devastating to peptidic and biopolymer NBE-wannabes (recall Figure 19.1). As a result, the latter may be very effective during initial treatment but then become much less effective, or perhaps even toxic, upon subsequent treatments.

Alternatively, PP represent a huge compartment within the flowing blood where the drug-wannabe will have free access and binding (PPB) that can sometimes be useful to avoid the first- and second-pass effect. In order to hide out in this or any other type of drug depot, however, binding has to be extremely high. This is because the equilibration rates for PPB and localization versus residence in the blood's aqueous milieu are typically very rapid. Thus, PPB usually is not considered to be a major influence upon a substance's distribution unless it occurs at the level of 90% or more (see Chapter 12 for a more detailed discussion of this topic).

As a xenobiotic substance proceeds along its random walk (Scheme 19.4), literally all the body's inner surfaces eventually become accessed and unless a drug-wannabe has an inherent selectivity for just the desired biological surface that is the target for its therapeutic mechanism, Erhlich's so-called magic bullet for a therapeutic effect is likely to be sprayed more like a shot gun in a random manner throughout the body that can potentially create more toxicity than actual therapy. This is the reason that both selectivity and high potency for the mechanistic target utilized in the front-line HTS process is so very important to achieve at the onset of drug discovery. Both factors can now serve to limit the desired effect to the proper tissue, the first by the drug-wannabe's inherent selectivity for binding with just that biological surface in a unique manner, and the second by allowing the overall concentrations of the drug-wannabe in the body to be kept to a minimum.

Here also lies another drug design strategy that can be undertaken, which is essentially to preclude or limit the drug-wannabe from being allowed to wander around the body during the entire course of therapy. This can be done in a proactive manner by orchestrating two approaches. The first is to build recognition for selected tissue-related components or transporters directly onto the parent substance's structure in a manner that remains compatible with retaining the molecule's desired efficacy. When this cannot be accomplished, a second approach is to build this same type of recognition into an appendage that is part of a prodrug system (Scheme 19.13) that then becomes cleaved before the drug-wannabe's targeted interaction with the desired efficacy-related biological surface. This release is sometimes accomplished locally in an additionally selective manner. This strategy to bias the random walk and to enhance the delivery of a drug-wannabe to the desired target tissue has been referred to by Portoghese as deploying an address (molecular delivery) component attached to the (molecular therapeutic) message component. This approach has a long-standing history in both small molecule and bioconjugate techniques, the latter typically representing a prodrug strategy where a biopolymer that displays a very selective address recognition for a certain tissue or cell type is coupled with a small molecule message compound that, once released from the conjugate within that specific locale, can freely interact with the efficacious mechanism's receptor or enzyme active site. A few examples are provided next to further display how drug distribution can be biased in a proactive manner by undertaking various molecular design strategies.

Scheme 19.14 conveys a case where an all-or-nothing shortcoming in the distribution of a drug-wannabe absolutely had to be addressed. Enhancing the concentration of dopamine (DA), **13** (Scheme 19.7), in certain brain pathways can alleviate the debilitating effects of Parkinson's disease and thus provide for at least palliative therapy. However, when dopamine is introduced into the systemic circulation, it will not cross the blood–brain barrier (BBB). Alternatively, as shown within Scheme 19.14, when levodopa, **40**, is administered, it can take advantage of the specific amino acid influx-transporter to cross the BBB. It is then converted in the brain to DA by DOPA Decarboxylase. Thus, a prodrug strategy was used to successfully deliver DA to the brain, although even with this strategy rather large doses of **40** (i.e., ca. 5 grams per day) still have to be administered. In another situation involving the BBB, an opposite goal was desired, namely to keep antihistamines out of the brain so that their inherent sedating properties would not be so prominent. In this case several analog-based drug design programs (Table 19.2) were able to be undertaken and, even though at the time that these studies were conducted they did not know exactly what the phenomena responsible for their successful brain exclusion was, several nonsedating antihistamines were able to reach the status of true drugs, (i.e., were able to reach the marketplace). Figure 19.19 depicts just a few of the compounds related to this area. It is now known

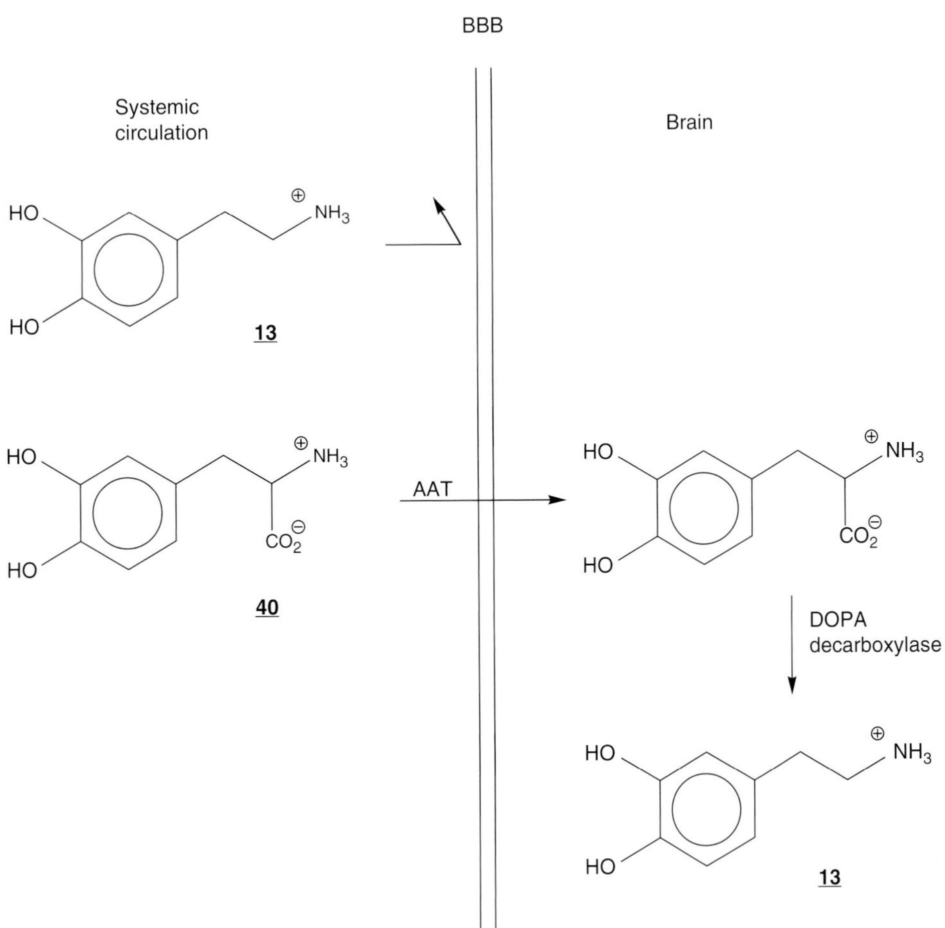

Scheme 19.14 Prodrug approach toward delivering dopamine, **13**, into the brain. Although **13** cannot itself cross the blood–brain barrier (BBB), levodopa, **40**, is able to take advantage of a specific amino acid transporter (AAT). Once inside the CNS, **40** undergoes biochemical conversion to **13** via DOPA Decarboxylase.

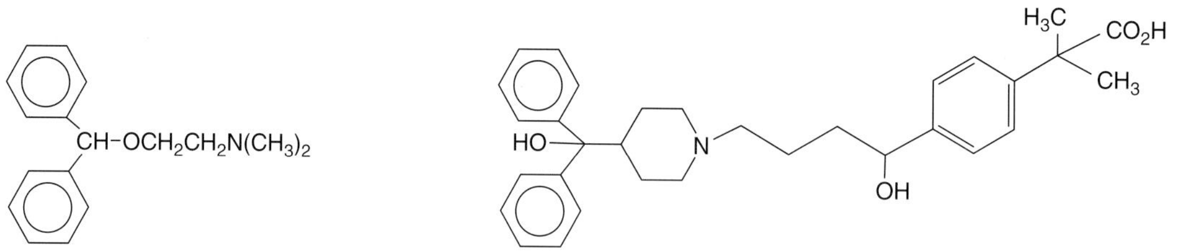

Figure 19.19 Compounds related to the antihistamine arena. Compound **41**, diphenhydramine (Benadryl®) is an older antihistamine that exhibits considerable sedating side-effects. Analogs **42** to **44** (fexofenadine (Allegra®), loratadine (Claritin®), cetirizine (Zyrtec®), respectively) are newer, nonsedating antihistamines. Many of the newer agents are now thought to be good substrates for P-glycoprotein (Pgp), which is situated within the BBB and serves to pump drugs out of the CNS and into the cerebral circulation (brain capillaries).

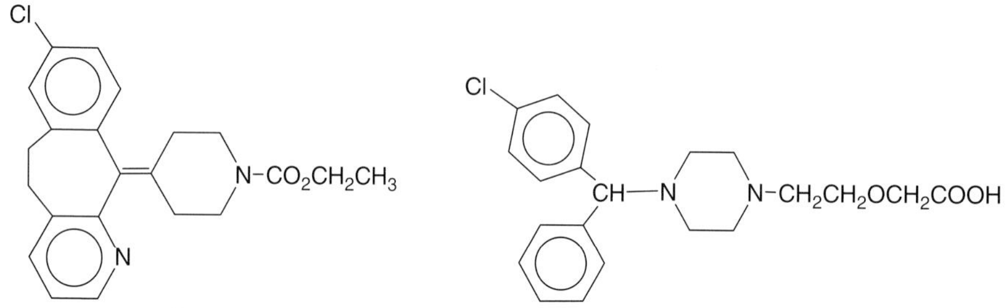

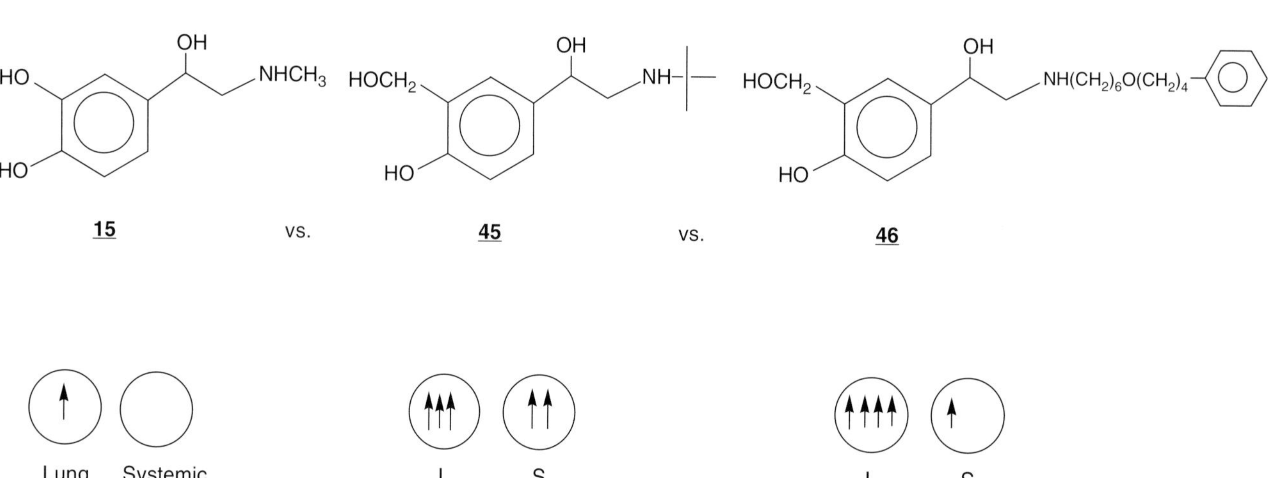

Figure 19.20 Localizing activity to the lung. When epinephrine, **15**, is delivered to the lungs via an inhaler device, its rapid metabolism limits its effectiveness as a bronchodilator (note only a single arrow in the lung compartment). Albuteral, **45**, has been modified to prevent metabolic breakdown (see text for details) but it then also shows considerable systemic side-effects (shown as two arrows in the circle representing the systemic circulation). Finally, salmeterol, **46**, has been modified to sustain its presence within the lung and to further enhance its activity in that compartment compared to the systemic circulation (note several arrows within the circle representing the lung compartment compared to the single arrow in the systemic circulation compartment).

that many of these newer structures are good substrates for Pgp, which serves as an efflux-transporter component of the BBB (see Chapter 7 for a more detailed discussion of this topic).

Figure 19.20 conveys an example where it was desirable to localize the vasodilation properties of epinephrine, **15** (Scheme 19.7), to be confined to the bronchial tissue after self-administration with an inhaler during the treatment of asthmatic episodes. Although the quick metabolism of epinephrine can be relied upon to essentially prevent any significant systemic side-effects, in this case the pseudo-first-pass effect by the lungs also decreases the activity precisely within the locale where it is wanted. In order to slow down **15**'s metabolism, analog-based drug design first produced albuterol, **45** (Figure 19.20), which has a sterically-demanding tertiary-butyl group in place of the N-methyl-functional group so it slows down all N-dealkylation metabolism (metabolic reaction number 2 in Figure 19.9), and a methylene-hydroxy functional group in place of **15**'s meta-hydroxy-group, which is otherwise subject to a rapid methylation reaction by Catechol-O-methyl-transferase (COMT) to form an OCH_3 group (not shown in Figure 19.9, but covered in the chapter that is dedicated to the topic of drug metabolism).

Although this improves upon the bronchodilating activity, **45** now also begins to exhibit systemic side-effects, particularly on cardiac tissue. This problem was addressed by limiting the distribution of an analog of **45** by further building upon the N-alkyl functionality in such a manner that salmeterol, **46** in Figure 19.20, essentially remains deposited in lung tissue (drug depot as well as the destination for its efficacy). From there, it is only slowly released into the systemic circulation where its metabolism can keep pace and, in this manner, the slow-release is relied upon to minimize systemic side-effects. At this point you should be able to appreciate some of the structural subtleties that went into the design of **46**. For example, how lipophilic do you think **46** is compared to **15**, and do you think that this may be the basis for its tendency to stay within the lung tissue as opposed to quickly equilibrating into the aqueous media of the broncho-pulmonary circulation (Scheme 19.4)? From Table 19.3 this difference is about 6.8 Log P units. Nearly a 10^7-fold difference, this is indeed a large enough change to significantly drive the compound into the lipid (membrane-like) phase rather than the aqueous phase. For this calculation, removal of **15**'s N-methyl group and addition of a methylene group between the phenyl-ring and the hydroxyl-oxygen atom strike a near balance so that we need only to add-up the Log P contribution from the elongated aralkyl-group that is added to **15's** nitrogen: -$(CH_2)_6$- approximated by two sets of 3 C methylene chains for a value of approximately 3.2; an -OCH_2- approximated by Table 19.3's OCH_3, which then contributes nothing in this regard; -$(CH_2)_3$- approximated by one set of a 3 C methylene chain for an approximate value of 1.6; and finally, the phenyl ring for which an exact value in the table is 2.0. Thus, the total change becomes $3.2 + 0.0 + 1.6 + 2.0 = 6.8$.

Figure 19.21 conveys a final example of a specific address and message system where the address portion of the conjugate molecule, **47**, hones to the reduced folate transporter system that becomes overexpressed in certain types of cancer, likely occurring in response to the cancer's rapid growth placing a higher demand upon the cancer cells' needs for the required folic acid vitamin. After preferentially entering cancer cells over-expressing folate transporters, this conjugate is cleaved to release the cargo drug, doxorubicin (**48**), which is an effective anticancer agent that has thus been designed to be more selectively delivered to cancer cells compared to normal cells in the body. Although **48** is indeed a marketed drug, the conjugate prodrug is still under experimental study and so, in this particular case, it does not yet constitute a real drug example.

Modulating Metabolism As can be seen from the preceding sections, drug metabolism (DM) can play a significant role within all the other ADMET parameters as well as being something to be concerned about in itself during drug design. By far the most common hurdle is when metabolism occurs too quickly. Just like

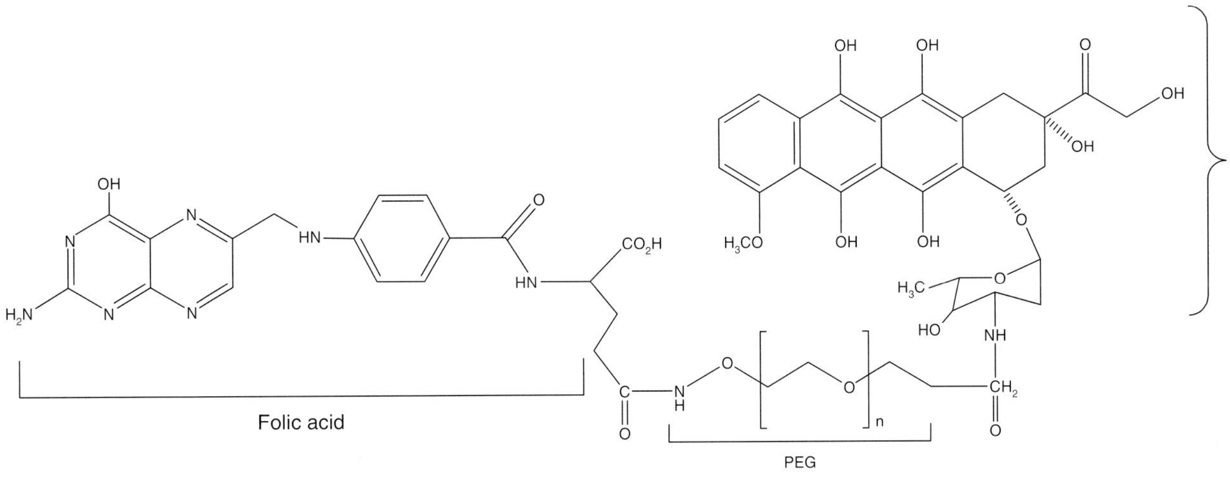

Figure 19.21 Folate address system attached to an anticancer agent cargo. The folic acid (FA) component is indicated in the western edge of this overall conjugate prodrug **47**. A polyethylene glycol or (PEG) connecting chain was then used to connect the FA address to the anticancer drug doxorubicin (message) shown in the eastern sector as **48**. After taking advantage of the FA transporter to selectively hone to cancer cells that overexpress this particular transporter, the doxorubicin is metabolically cleaved to liberate the active anticancer agent.

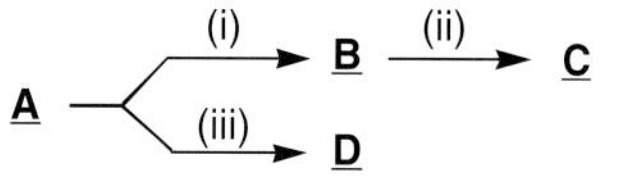

Scheme 19.15 Key relationships between metabolism and prodrugs. Prodrug **A** and metabolites **C** and **D** represent molecules that are not active at the desired site. **B** represents an active drug. Conversion (i) represents a metabolic pathway that accomplishes the desired bioactivation and (ii) and (iii) represent other metabolic conversions and/or elimination pathways. The goal in any prodrug design strategy is to have the rate of (i) > (ii) + (iii).

the drug-wannabe that never arrives at its biological target because it isn't absorbed in the first place or because it randomly distributes in a noneffective manner, too rapid DM can altogether eliminate the chance for activity. For example, unless simple carboxylic ester groups are sterically hindered, they are usually so metabolically labile that they cannot be deployed effectively as a useful functional group while investigating SAR for a drug-wannabe. Instead, as we have already seen, simple esters do find utility in the area of prodrugs, where it becomes desirable to have a rapid metabolic conversion occur so as to produce the active compound in preference to any other type of metabolic activity that might detract from the bioactivation process (Scheme 19.15). Several examples of prodrugs have been cited previously within this chapter.

A very common situation pertaining to DM is when an efficacious response is initially obtained after administration but can't be sustained for an adequate duration needed for therapy because the drug-wannabe's half-life is too short due to rapid metabolic degradation. Furthermore, for oral administration, a convenient once-a-day dosing regimen is often desirable from a patient compliance point of view, and this usually requires an even longer metabolic stability and delayed excretion of the exogenous material. Typically, a four- to six-hour half-life or longer is required for a once-a-day drug target. There are four drug design strategies that can be pursued to slow down the metabolism of a drug-wannabe. Because this is a very common problem during drug discovery, each of these strategies is discussed briefly and exemplified in the following.

The first and by far the most reliable structure metabolism relationship (SMR) that can be pursued to slow down DM utilizes steric effects to advantage. Simply put, two bodies cannot occupy the same space at the same time. Thus, blocking the site that is metabolized in a lead compound with a steric impediment placed at that site or very closely nearby, is almost guaranteed to deter the enzyme from being able to arrange its particular chemical machinery around that site. As a result, the initial type of metabolism becomes blocked. Since it is not uncommon for DM to occur at multiple sites on a given xenobiotic (Figure 19.9 and Scheme 19.16), this type of structural manipulation needs to be done at every site where metabolism occurs rapidly. It is also important to emphasize that only the initial type of metabolism will be blocked, and what can sometimes happen next is for the body to move its metabolism to yet another site on the molecule, perhaps even onto the group that was utilized as a steric impediment. This behavior can be referred to as DM switching by analogy to the older use of this phrase in the context of nutrition. Despite these types of continuing complexities that DM can often display, the steric impediment approach is still the most reliable SMR to exploit. Examples of successfully deploying this approach during drug design include the steric impediment toward what would otherwise be rapid N-dealkylation, by substituting the simple N-methyl-group on epinephrine, **15**, with the bulkier N-isopropyl- or N-tertiary-butyl-groups as present in propranolol, **2**, and in albuterol, **45**, respectively. An even more dramatic example is afforded by the natural product paclitaxel, **12**. In this case even the normally labile carboxylic esters present in **12** become quite stable when juxtaposed by nature unto the sheer bulk provided by paclitaxel's huge, central scaffold system.

The second most reliable SMR that can be utilized to slow down DM during drug design relates to electronic effects. This can be approached from two aspects, where both pertain to modifying a site that is too rapidly attacked by a cytochrome P450 (CYP450)

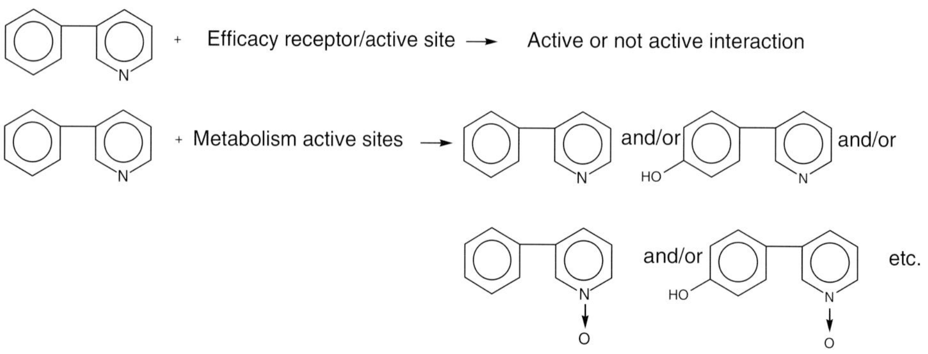

Scheme 19.16 The promiscuous nature of drug metabolism results compared to those obtained for interaction at a typical efficacy-related biological surface. In both cases a graded response is also possible for each outcome (also see Figure 19.9 and text for details).

enzyme. The first involves making a molecular substitution on the lead compound that causes electron withdrawal from the metabolic reaction site, a strategy that is most applicable to metabolic aromatic hydroxylation (event 4 in Figure 19.9) but is of less value for O- and N-dealkylation biotransformations (events 2 and 3) and is generally fruitless for trying to manipulate ester hydrolysis (largely a non-CYP-mediated process shown as event 1 in Figure 19.9). The second electronic manipulation involves removing the hydrogen atom that is necessary in the alpha-position to either a N or an O during N- and O-delakylations because it is the abstraction of such a hydrogen by CYP that is the first step toward the eventual cleavage reaction. In this case, substitution of hydrogens with fluorine atoms can be quite effective because the hydrogen is normally abstracted in a radical form that most closely resembles the electronic state of a proton, and a fluorine atom cannot adopt such a quasi-positive species. Note that all the hydrogens must be removed, however, or the CYP will simply grab one of the remaining hydrogens while ignoring the fluorine atoms that may have been placed there; that is, a N-CH_2F and a N-CHF_2 can still be N-dealkylated but a N-CF_3 cannot. An example of advantageously changing the electronic state of the biotransformation site relative to a non-CYP-mediated pathway, namely that of slowing down rapid attack by COMT, is again provided by albuterol, **45**. In this case the placement of a methylene between the phenyl-ring and the hydroxyl-group insulates the latter from the electronics of the phenyl-ring so that it is no longer recognized as a suitable substrate for O-methylation.

The third SMR that can be manipulated is much less predictable. It involves changing the overall physicochemical properties and plotting each variable against the observed biotransformation rates to discern if a favorable direction can be obtained that can then be further exploited. In general, moving toward more polarity will decrease metabolism and vice versa.

The final approach toward deterring metabolism involves use of a separate inhibitor compound. This should be regarded as a last resort in terms of a lead compound where all attempts toward self-adjustment of the lead will have already been attempted. Nevertheless, it can sometimes "save the day" to produce a successful clinical outcome. For example, recalling that the delivery of dopamine to the brain by administering the prodrug levodopa, **40**, still requires doses of several grams, investigation of this problem within the clinic (translational medicine) revealed that it results from peripheral DOPA Decarboxylase also attacking levodopa to produce dopamine in the systemic circulation before the levodopa has had a chance to cross the BBB. Coadministration of a peripheral DOPA Decarbxylase inhibitor, namely carbidopa, allows the levodopa dose to be reduced by nearly one-half and much less side-effects are observed. Eventually, a marketed product containing a fixed ratio of 1 part carbidopa to 10 parts levodopa was developed.

As a continuation of this same theme, it also was found that a centrally acting MAO inhibitor (Scheme 19.7) can further improve the effectiveness of levodopa by prolonging the activity of the centrally produced dopamine. The MAO inhibitor used in this case is selegiline. The structures for carbidopa and selegiline are shown here as **49** and **50**, respectively. Note the interesting interplay of the intentionally directed distribution away from the brain for **49** and into the brain for **50**, as well as noting the double success of these last resorts toward attenuating unwanted metabolism. However, this example relies upon very selective metabolic biotransformations for a rather specific biochemical pathway. As a more general approach involving promiscuous enzymes like the CYP450s, extreme care would have to be exercised so as to insure that one was not opening the door to a multitude of drug–drug interactions upon inhibition of a given CYP, hence the relegation to a last resort nature for this approach.

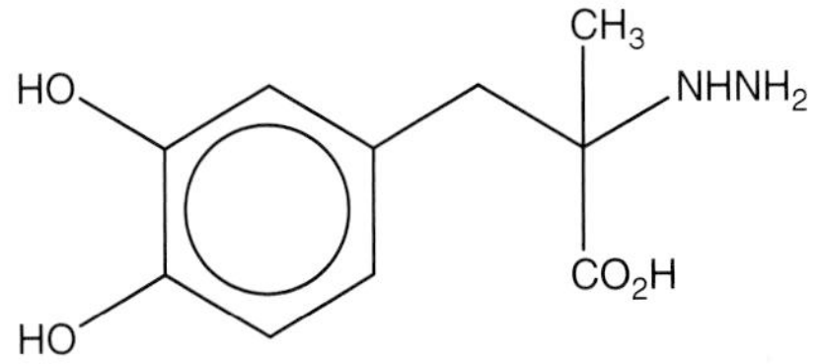

HO, HO, CH_3, $NHNH_2$, CO_2H

49

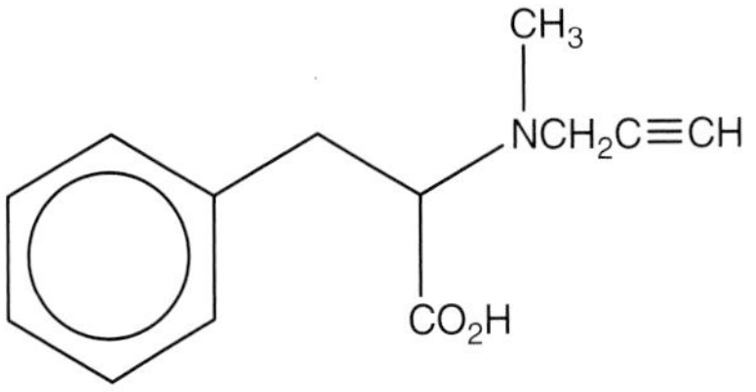

CH_3, $NCH_2C{\equiv}CH$, CO_2H

50

Modulation of DM can also be undertaken to encourage the elimination of a substance's activity and to avoid toxicity. These approaches generally fall within a strategy called soft drug design and they will be further discussed within the next section. As a summary for this section, it may be useful to frame some of these DM design principles into a simple set of rules that can be contemplated as a guide that is analogous to the previous Rule-of-5 for drug absorption behavior. These rules, as we understand them today, are listed as follows. Given that the manipulation of steric effects stands alone in its near guarantee for being able to successfully modulate essentially every metabolic event possible, this set of rules should be called metabolism's Rule-of-1, to emphasize that steric effects will always represent the most consistent and predominant factor among any array of additional parameters that we may be able to compile today or further devise in the future.

Metabolism's Rule-of-1 indicates that:

- If there is a simple ester present in the molecule, it will typically get hydrolyzed as the predominant metabolic pathway unless it is sterically hindered.

- All metabolic processes are exquisitely sensitive to steric features, where the rate for any given event is inversely proportional to the immediate steric environment at its biotransformation site.
- Decreasing the electron density at the site of a CYP450-mediated biotransformation will generally attenuate aromatic hydroxylation but have little impact upon N- and O-dealkylation processes.
- Replacing all the hydrogens alpha to a heteroatom by fluorine atoms can block CYP450-mediated N- or O-dealkylation processes completely but the similar replacement of hydrogen by fluorine atoms on an aryl-system will have little impact upon aromatic hydroxylation beyond that of electron withdrawal.
- As a very general and often excepted parameter, increasing a substrate's overall polarity will tend to decrease its metabolism and vice versa.

Engaging Excretion and Tending to Toxicity With absorption and distribution bringing a lead compound into the whole biological system, metabolism and excretion can generally be thought of as eliminating the compound from the system and thereby ending its actions including any toxicity, exceptions being the case of prodrugs and of inadvertent metabolic activation. The goal is to strike a balance between the desired efficacious action, a therapeutic and user-friendly (compliant) duration of action, and the eventual elimination (metabolism and excretion) while minimizing any toxicity inherent to the intact parent compound and to any of its metabolites that, without elimination, will otherwise build up in concentration upon continued use of the compound.

As we have seen previously, drug-related excretion generally utilizes either the renal or biliary pathway (Scheme 19.6) although other routes such as exhalation and the skin are also possible. The renal system tends to clear smaller compounds whose molecular weights are not much higher than 500 daltons and are reasonably polar and water soluble in the acidic urine so that they are not readily reabsorbed. Knowing this, do you think that amine-containing or carboxylic acid-containing compounds would be subject to higher clearance by the kidneys? Referring to Scheme 19.12, you should conclude that compounds having an amino-group, such as present in the common molecular motif of numerous drug substances, would make better candidates for renal clearance based just upon pH considerations. Alternatively, biliary excretion tends to excrete larger compounds whose weights can go well past 500 daltons and are much less polar in general. Interestingly, to handle carboxylic acids, which would tend to ionize to their respective anions at physiological pH and thus likely become too polar for the liver to want to deal with, the liver is also rich in Organic Anion Transporters (OATs) whose mission is to excrete just such compounds. Perhaps it is no coincidence, then, that one of the human body's main metabolic-conjugates, namely the formation of a glucuronide metabolite as shown in Scheme 19.6, happens to add not only a polar sugar molecule but also a carboxylic acid functional group to the xenobiotic that it is trying to eliminate from the system. When this fact is coupled with the glucuronide's hefty addition of about 175 daltons of molecular weight, we can understand how this particular metabolic pathway and this particular aspect of biliary excretion likely coevolved to work in tandem to rid the system of nonamine-containing xenobiotics. Knowing this level of detail about these processes allows for drug design to either play toward more or less excretion through the same types of functional group manipulations that have been delineated to this point.

The purposeful inhibition of metabolic-related elimination or clearance has already been discussed. By applying these same principles in reverse it becomes possible to accelerate drug metabolism and clearance. For example, in the prior situation conveyed in Figure 19.20 and its accompanying text, why do you suppose that salmeterol, **46**, was constructed so as to not contain the gem-dimethyl arrangement depicted as follows, that had worked so well to avoid CYP450-mediated N-dealkylation when placed in albuterol, **45**, in the form of a tertiary-butyl group?

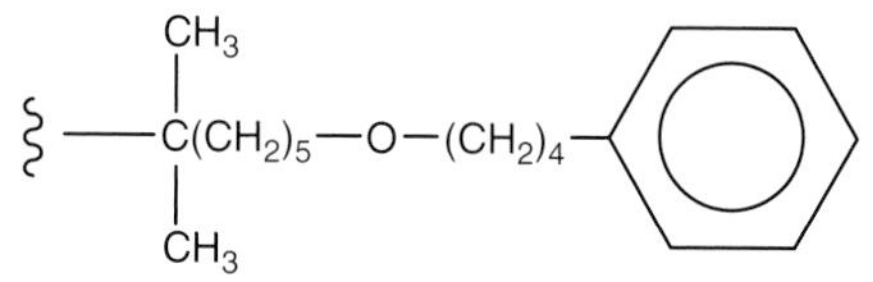

CH_3
$-C(CH_2)_5-O-(CH_2)_4-C_6H_5$
CH_3

"gem-dimethyl" version of salmeterol's N-substituent

Because of a highly lipophilic depot effect, salmeterol is retained in the lungs where its actions are desired. After it has finally been released into the systemic circulation, it then becomes very desirable to have CYP450 aggressively attack the molecule by N-dealkylation so as to eliminate it and avoid potential toxicity. Thus, use of a gem-dimethyl arrangement, as depicted earlier, would attenuate the desired N-dealkylation reaction and the desired clearance from the systemic circulation (i.e., thin rather than bulky works best to accelerate a desired metabolism-driven clearance).

An even more proactive approach toward controlling excretion and reducing toxicity is to undertake a soft drug design strategy (Scheme 19.13). In this case a specific, metabolically susceptible, if not highly labile functional group, is added to the parent compound and then its immediate steric environment is finely adjusted so as to program both a preselected metabolic pathway and specified degradation rate for the resulting compound where ideally, the programmed metabolic event also leads to an inactive and innocuous (totally nontoxic) metabolite. Unlike a prodrug, however, this strategy requires that the soft drug's additional functional group does not alter the desired efficacy of the parent compound, a situation that is often not easy to achieve during drug design. Just like for prodrugs, the soft drug strategy generally employs esters as the metabolically susceptible linkage. There are numerous indications where deployment of a soft drug strategy would be appropriate, just a couple being to limit the duration of action of a drug and to localize a given drug's action to a given physiological compartment whenever it can be administered either selectively or in a depot manner. An example of this approach will be given in the Case Studies section, where the discovery of esmolol, the prototypical example of a soft drug, will be outlined in detail.

One final drug design tool that can be mentioned at this point is that of using bioisostere functional group replacements to avoid toxicity while retaining the desired efficacious activity. Although this strategy can be deployed across any of the ADMET parameters analogous to any other type of functional group modification, it is a particularly useful exercise to undertake when trying to avoid toxicity. Therefore, its description has been reserved until this section. As implied by the term, this strategy uses functional groups that are expected to have similar (isostere) biological (bio) behaviors. Recall that the structural demands placed upon a given ligand by the efficacy-related receptor or enzyme active site are regarded as being uniquely specific to that system (see earlier discussions about mutual molding phenomena). Likewise, the structural aspects of the same ligand when it interacts with another biological surface to display some type of unrelated toxicity will likely have a different set of unique requirements. Thus, the goal of this strategy is to replace any structural feature, including even a key pharmacophore element, with one or more bioisosteres that will still allow the new analogue to work at the efficacious site but will, hopefully, no longer allow it to work at the surface responsible for the toxicity.

Table 19.7 lists just a few bioisosteric groups and the type of property that they are thought to be mimicking. As mentioned, the use of these groups is just like functional group replacements in general. Both can be undertaken to address toxicity per se or to explore and probe SAR at any given type of biological surface including all the other surfaces associated with the various ADME parameters as well as the original efficacy surface. A few points of interest can be mentioned about Table 19.7 to further illustrate the bioisosteric strategy. First, rows can be used in either direction and in some cases, like that for amides and esters, column entries may also be interchangeable. An example of the latter would be bioisosteric replacement of the ester moiety present in the short-acting local anesthetic drug procaine, **51**, with an amide to provide the long-acting compound procainamide, **52**, which finds use as an antiarrhythmic agent. Another interesting example is afforded by sulfanilamide, **6**, which was described previously. The sulfonamide's acidic proton (pK ~ 10 when R = H) is close enough in acidity to mimic the carboxylic acid group present in the endogenous para-amino-benzoic acid (PABA) building block (**53** pKa ~ 5) of folic acid. As a result, **6** inhibits utilization of **53** during a bacterium's attempted biochemical construction of this key biochemical. Both of these examples also demonstrate the use of bioisosteric replacements within the context of efficacy-related manipulations, again emphasizing the general utility of this strategy beyond that of avoiding toxicity.

Table 19.7 Bioisosteres[a]

Functional Group		Bioisosteres	
Carbonyl	—C(=O)—	—S(=O)—	—CH(CN)—
Carboxylic acid	—C(=O)OH	—S(=O)(=O)NHR	3,5-difluoro-4-hydroxyphenyl (F, OH, F)
Amide	—C(=O)NHR	—NH—C(=O)R[b]	—C(=O)OR
Ester	—C(=O)OR	4-OR-1,2,5-oxadiazol-3-yl (N—O—N ring, OR)	
Ether	—O—R	—CH_2—R	
Hydroxyl	—OH	—NHC(=O)NH_2	—CH_2OH
Halogen	—X[c]	—CF_3	
Hydrogen	—H	—F	

[a]This list is meant only to be exemplary; more exhaustive tables can be found elsewhere.
[b]Reverse amide (also applicable to esters).
[c]X = halogen such as Cl, Br, and I.

p-H_2N—C_6H_4—C(=O)R

51 R = $O(CH_2)_2NH(CH_2CH_3)_2$

52 R = $NH(CH_2)_2NH(CH_2CH_3)_2$

53 R = OH

54 p-H_2N—C_6H_4—R

55 R-substituted imidazole (N, NH)

In both cases R not being a carbonyl system like the compounds above

On the other side of these desirable replacements lie toxicophore arrangements or functional groups that should be avoided in order to circumvent toxicity. Highly reactive chemical species like an acid chloride (RCOCl) are obvious drug no-no's. Compounds containing these types of groups are removed (filtered) altogether from compound libraries prior to HTS. Functional groups that can demonstrate toxicity of a less dramatic nature, if not also removed entirely, are likewise flagged within compound libraries destined to join a HTS campaign. Examples of the latter include the anilines **54** and the imidazoles **55**, the first sometimes undergoing a metabolic bioactivation process that leads to highly reactive and toxic species, and the second sometimes causing severe inhibition of certain of the CYP450 metabolizing enzymes such that there is a high potential for drug–drug related interactions and an indirect toxicity.

In the end, the balance of desired activity versus potential toxicity where each can be subject to its own distinct process for elimination comes down to the experimental assessment of risk as defined by the therapeutic index (TI). This term has been defined previously in terms of both overt toxicity (e.g., LD_{50} data) and more subtle forms of toxicity. Again, since the toxic dose is always expressed as the numerator and the efficacious dose as the denominator, in all cases the larger the TI the better.

19.2.3.3 Summary For Predevelopment-Related Activities

Before moving into the advanced stages of the drug discovery process, a brief summary point is in order. Although the various drug design and lead optimization activities described to this stage have each been delineated in a step-wise manner for the sake of clarity, it is important to appreciate that their considerations are actually undertaken in a simultaneous manner. Thus, the impact upon efficacy and all the ADMET parameters are simultaneously considered with each structural change, and the challenge becomes to move across all these hurdles as quickly and efficiently as possible. For the medicinal chemist, this means trying to simultaneously bridge properly derived structural assessments associated with various functional group changes, to all the results obtained from various biological tests associated with efficacy and ADMET. Given that the same functional group can behave differently in different biological settings and then again change its behavior in all regards when another alteration is made on the parent compound at even a remote location, the task of bridging chemical structure to biological activity becomes a challenging one that is exacerbated by the need to derive these relationships quickly within a competitive environment. Figure 19.22 attempts to capture the thought processes and activities needed to be undertaken in a simultaneous manner by an investigator involved in a typical lead optimization program.

19.2.3.4 Drug Development-Related Multitasking

The seamless nature of today's drug discovery paradigm is a natural consequence of moving what used to be later ADMET considerations into earlier time-points of the overall process. Likewise, the distinct types of chemical-related activities that need to be addressed when a lead compound progresses to advanced stages of development are also being contemplated at earlier time-points. Several of these activities are worth mentioning within their own category. Like the close interplay of medicinal chemistry and the new era of efficacy and ADMET biological assessments discussed to this point, most of the chemical-related activities conveyed by Figure 19.23 are also best undertaken in a simultaneous and close interdisciplinary manner. These activities are briefly discussed within the context of the most recent trends applicable to each case.

Analytical Chemistry Briefly, of foremost importance is the preparation and complete characterization of an analytical standard for each preclinical development compound. All process chemistry-related activities and advanced biological testing activities, particularly those associated with toxicological assessments, will rely on the analytical standard for verification of substance and solution integrity. As part of the characterization of the high purity standard, chemical precursors along with deliberately synthesized reaction side-products and potential chemical breakdown products, are typically utilized to establish that they can be unambiguously distinguished, for example by HPLC, from the desired material. Since this same type of characterization is typically mandated by government regulatory bodies to validate an analytical assay for a new drug substance, the complimentary relationship between synthetic medicinal chemistry and analytical chemistry becomes quite clear at this particular juncture of the overall drug discovery paradigm. Validations of analytical methods to be used for raw drug substance, various formulations and for support of biological studies represent a rigorous undertaking in themselves. Accuracy, precision and ruggedness, as well as several other criteria must be established by repetitive runs using the refined assay method. Each parameter is required to lie within regulated specifications in order for the method to be regarded as acceptable. For example, the documented report for a single GLP-validated analytical method can easily reach 100 pages, thus becoming a small technical thesis in itself.

Interplay of Synthetic Chemistry and Advanced Pharmacology Similar to the demands prompted by rigorous analytical chemistry, the need for syntheses of both anticipated metabolites and experimentally derived metabolite possibilities serves to maintain the complimentary relationship between medicinal chemistry and the biologically oriented disciplines working in the field of drug metabolism and toxicology. This is a valuable relationship where the medicinal chemist

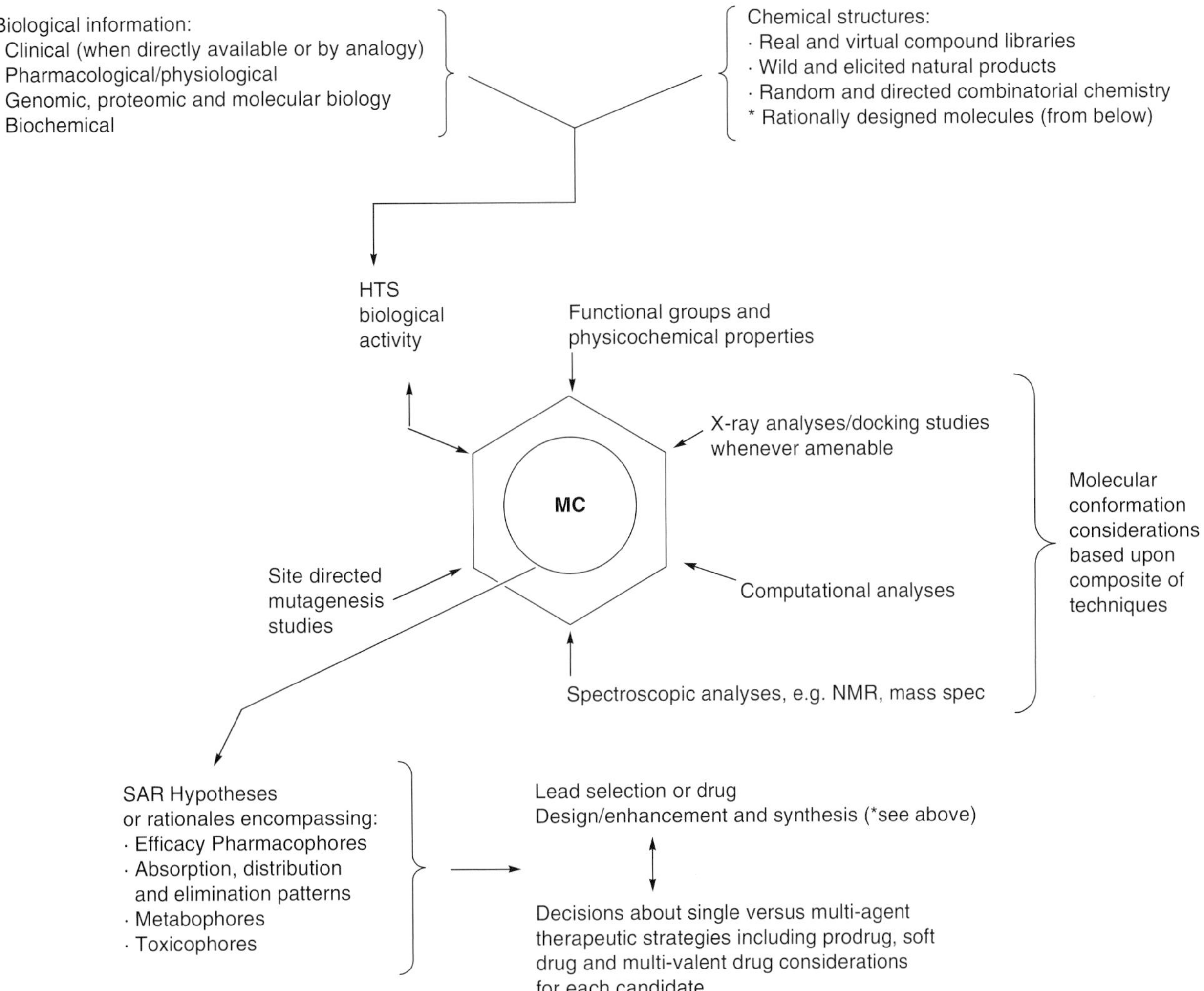

Figure 19.22 Today's practice of medicinal chemistry: Drug design-related multitasking during lead optimization. The most striking differences from the long-standing practice of medicinal chemistry (MC) are: (1) data reduction of huge amounts of rapidly derived HTS biological results; (2) greater emphasis upon multitechnique chemical structure considerations; and most importantly, (3) the simultaneous attention given to all of the ADMET-related parameters along with efficacy and efficacy-related selectivity during lead compound selection and further design or enhancement coupled with an expanding knowledge base. The latter also offers the possibility for achieving synergistic benefits by taking advantage of various combinations of multiagent, prodrug, soft drug and/or multivalent drug strategies.

can continue to contribute knowledge about the nuances of chemical structure relative to metabolism and/or toxicity. It becomes imperative when the preclinical development compound itself prompts an even further prolongation of a very tightly focused, additional analog program specifically directed toward the final refinement of drug metabolism-related PK properties or the remediation of a distinct toxicity concern.

Process Chemistry Process chemistry also becomes important at this point, not just for longer-range thinking in terms of an eventual product cost, but because several hundred grams will be needed immediately for preliminary formulation and toxicology studies. The need for multikilograms will soon follow if the compound does indeed undergo Phase I clinical testing, the latter usually also accompanied by extended toxicity testing. Four key issues pertaining to the interplay of medicinal chemistry with process chemistry relative to current developments are mentioned next. Like the trend for the ADMET-related assessments, all these issues are moving toward earlier consideration points within the overall process of drug discovery.

First, issues pertaining to intellectual property (IP) involve both the structural novelty of biologically interesting compositions of matter and the latter's synthetic accessibility via practical process chemistry routes that do not infringe patent-protected technologies. Furthermore, both the compound itself and the methods that will be used to synthesize it can be more strongly protected when they are both distinctly novel over the prior art. With regard to patentability, it should be noted that today's fixation upon emphasizing compound library members that have drug-like properties

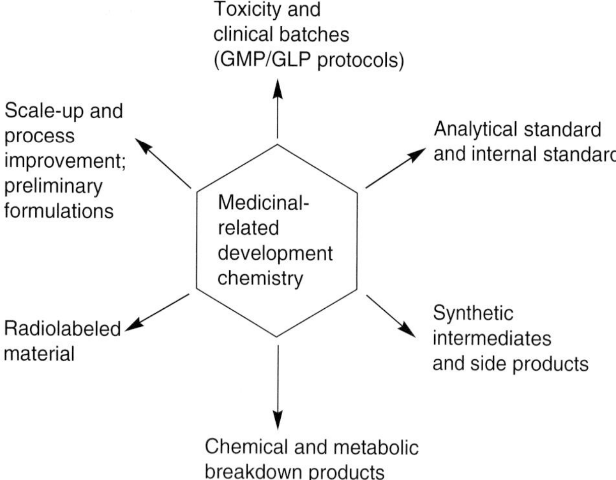

Figure 19.23 Drug development-related multitasking. Although big pharma typically has specialized teams of pharmaceutical chemists dedicated to various of these activities, it is not uncommon in small pharma for drug discovery medicinal chemists to become actively involved with several (or all) of these tasks relative to each final lead compound that may progress into development. Note that the final toxicity and clinical batches must be prepared and formulated according to Good Manufacturing Practices (GMP) accompanied by Good Laboratory Practices (GLP) analytical support.

and the future possibility for further instillation of additionally preselected molecular arrangements that can endow preferred metabolic profiles, in some ways become contradictory to enhancing the future molecular diversity, and thereby patentability, of the overall drug discovery structure landscape. A further discussion of IP and the pharmaceutical patenting process is offered in a later section.

A second point for process chemistry is that of the eventual production cost for a new therapeutic agent, an issue that has become much more important today than it has been in the past. The sentiment of today's consumers demands that pharmaceutical companies must now garner their profits from a marketplace that, right or wrong, has become sensitized about the cost of ethical pharmaceutical agents. The days of simply raising the price of pharmaceutical products in parallel with the increasing costs associated with discovering and developing new drugs have been over for quite some time. In this regard, the cost-effectiveness of small molecule drugs will probably maintain an edge over biotechnology-derived therapeutic agents for at least the near term.

A third point to be mentioned pertains to the impact of the "green chemistry" movement. This movement has prompted pharmaceutical companies to insure that their productions of drugs are friendly toward the environment in terms of all materials and methods that may be used during the process. Although unquestionably a good thing, the downside is that these efforts further add to the overall cost of discovering a new drug, sometimes in a very significant manner.

Finally, the U.S. FDA's initiative to have all stereoisomers present within a drug defined both chemically and biologically has prompted industry's pursuit of drugs that either do not contain asymmetric centers or are enantiomerically pure. This, in turn, has prompted the need for better stereocontrolled synthetic processes during chemical production. Stereocontrol has always represented an extremely interesting area for synthetic chemistry exploration and now for biotechnology-derived chemistry and reagent research as well (e.g., exploitation of enzymes at the chemical manufacturing scale). Considerable progress is being made toward developing asymmetric methods on many fronts including enzymatic and microarray technologies. Oftentimes, however, the new laboratory techniques do not readily lend themselves toward inexpensive, scale-up/manufacturing types of green chemistry. Thus, of the various challenges facing medicinal chemists also involved in drug development, devising practical routes to single stereoisomer compounds that are both cost effective and conducive toward green chemistry probably represents one of the more significant.

Formulation Chemistry As analytical methods and scaled-up quantities of raw drug-wannabes become available, serious formulation studies can begin. At this stage of the discovery process the formulations are called preliminary dosage forms, with development of the final forms being reserved until the results from initial clinical testing are in hand. The nature of the raw drug-wannabe material and its reproducibility need to be characterized in terms of solid state physical properties and inherent stability; crystal polymorphism; dissolution, solubility profiles, and solution stabilities; characteristics important for manufacturing steps; and compatibility with potential formulation excipients. A variety of salt forms may need to be explored at this point to further optimize one or more of these properties. In addition to the formulations anticipated to be required for the Phase I studies, the types of materials used in the prolonged toxicity studies and in any other key *in vivo* experiments to be done during these late stages of discovery also need to receive the same level of scrutiny in terms of GMP production supported by validated GLP analytical quality control and stability assessments. The reason that this level of rigor is required is because the concern is now focused as much upon potential toxicity as it is upon achieving efficacy. Failure to observe efficacy due to any of these factors in all the previous work would have led to a false-negative that would have caused the drug-wannabe developers to stop the progression of their lead. Alternatively, failure to observe toxicity due to any of these factors will lead to a dangerous false-negative that will encourage the drug-wannabe developers (and the FDA as a regulatory body) to continue developing the compound for human testing under the erroneous assumption that it is safe. Thus, to prove that a drug-wannabe is not toxic at a given dose in a given model, the compound integrity of that dose/formulation all the way into the model must be verified via validated GLP assays. In summary, formulation studies become requisite at this point to cap the overall drug discovery process in terms of toxicity and clinical testing, while also beginning to lay plans for what physical form a marketed product might be able to ultimately assume.

Protecting the Corporate Checkbook No matter how clever and industrious a team may have been in order to arrive at this point in the overall process of drug discovery, and no matter how promising the potential technology is for alleviating even some major human malady, it will never reach the consumer unless there is a financial backer willing to market it and to undertake the costs associated with mass producing and distributing it. Whether in academia, a nonprofit research institute, research foundation or a government laboratory, just like working within a private sector biotech or full-fledged pharmaceutical company, it becomes critical to secure a patent position on the new technology and ideally, the broadest field possible for its closely-related intellectual property (IP). Gaining a patent position assures a company or potential backer that they can attempt to recoup their expenses while not having to immediately engage in a price war with generic competitors who will not have borne any of the discovery costs associated with all the various activities that have been discussed to this point. In this same regard, also realize that unlike a generic, where patent protection for the given therapeutic agent has typically already run its course, there is still no clinical or market performance record for how well the still evolving technology is actually going to fare as either a problem-free therapy or as a well-accepted agent by the consumers. In the end, it is the latter who will ultimately have to bear the cost for all the activities and failed drug-wannabes that eventually lead to any technology's end-stage product. Thus, picking up the technology at this point is still a gamble for someone.

Accepting that procuring patent protection is yet another very important facet of the overall process of drug discovery, it is being mentioned at this point in the chapter not because it is necessarily a chemical-related activity, but because it is usually at the point of having a preclinical drug candidate in hand, if not somewhat sooner, that it becomes imperative for patent protection to be sought. Since issued patent life spans are now 20 years from the date of a submitted patent application and because there are still several years to go (perhaps as many as 10) before a marketed product will actually be in hand, filing patent applications prior to this stage further cuts down on the duration of remaining protection that a backer will have once the technology does become marketed. Also recalling our earlier discussion about the oftentimes highly competitive nature of drug discovery, however, a balance must be sought between not really wanting to patent prior to this point in discovery but perhaps having to do so due to the threat that there may be one or more competitors also on the same technology race track and that as a result, all of your team's efforts to this time-point could be lost with just one more quick lap of passed time (i.e., should someone else then be able to file and eventually gain protection for the same technology in advance of your team's effort to do so).

You should already appreciate that the patenting process and designation of inventorship for drug-related technologies have also become very interdisciplinary. For example, in order to obtain a patent for any technology, the technology must be new, novel (nonobvious over the close art) and reduced to practice within the context of a given utility that is actually useful in some real sense. Indeed, after submission of a patent application there is typically a one- to two-year period (and hopefully not longer although this can certainly happen as well) called the prosecution phase. During prosecution there is a burden of proof placed on the submitters to definitively establish that the written commentary within their application (patent specification) and the related claims for the specific technology's protection, not only meet these criteria but are not too broad in scope. Claims drafted beyond what the submitters have actually found and clearly demonstrated according to these same criteria will not be allowed. Thus, in the eyes of a government Patent Examiner (e.g., working within the U.S. Patent and Trademark Office, or US PTO), the key chemical, molecular biology, or clinical observation that can serve as a starting-point for drug discovery remains only an idea for a potential drug until, much like our own definition, it truly has been reduced to practice in the form of a real physical entity (drug substance) that actually has demonstrated itself to be useful for the intended indication. In our case the indication would be a human or veterinary, ethical or OTC pharmaceutical agent. Patent applications can be written to protect both "compositions of [chemical] matter "(i.e., the drug substance) and the "use [of such]" (i.e., the intended clinical or marketplace indications). It is also possible to obtain a new use patent on an existing pharmaceutical agent whose composition of matter protection may already reside with some other company. In this case, both parties would have to come to an agreement as to how to proceed with the new indication since the first party's patent would bar the use of that composition for any indication that they did not grant, and the second party's patent would bar the deployment of the compound in the new use that only they can grant.

At this point you should have a serious question about how this requisite business consideration of the overall drug discovery scenario appears to be contradictory to the still-evolving technology: namely, if a reduction to practice is absolutely required for a patent and, as has been indicated continuously from the onset of this chapter, it truly does not occur for a drug technology until it becomes successfully approved for marketing, then how can any team or company involved in drug discovery expect to be granted a patent allowance before it has even entered its technology into clinical testing, particularly with the failure rate that must still be overcome? This seeming contradiction is actually a major ideological concession. It is a concession made long ago by patent-granting, governmental agencies across the world who quickly came to realize that because the development costs for pharmaceuticals is so enormously high, no business entity would even embark on this exercise unless they felt reasonably certain that they could recoup their investment on the backside by also having an allowed patent in-hand with its guarantee for their exclusivity of the market. This is not a minor point in that there is no other technological field that has been afforded such a patenting concession. Thus, for a pharmaceutical-wannabe, it is necessary to have only one example of an actual physical compound that displays desirable activity in a biochemical or in an *in vitro* model perceived (and not necessarily credentialized or validated as we have previously discussed) to be predictive of benefit in humans or animals depending upon the intended indication.

Actually, most pharmaceutical patents begin with their broadest use claim being directed toward mammals in general. This strategy can indeed provide adequate protection for the intended use, but given the vagaries of the discovery process yet ahead, it would certainly be foolish to patent just one compound at such an early point of exploring the technology. Instead, a family of potential compounds (compositions of matter) is usually sought. This, in turn, requires that a representative sampling of the variously possible family members actually be prepared and tested in the relied-upon biological model. The longer the lack of a threat from competition, the further the technological exploration can occur and the more matured the technology can become, so that an optimal patent can then be devised to better protect the corporate checkbook around any new technology moving through the overall process of drug discovery.

A quick word about the assignment of inventorship is also in order as this section is brought to a close. Certainly the person(s) responsible for the initial observation and idea (concept) about a new drug should be regarded as part of the inventors' pool. Then comes the long stream of individuals associated with reducing the idea to practice. In this case, however, if only routine or standard approaches and methods are utilized, none of these individuals is likely to be regarded as an additional inventor. Alternatively, if nonroutine or nonstandard methods become necessary to move the technology forward, then the individuals associated with these steps are typically added to the inventor's pool. This also occurs if new ideas or concepts are required along the way. The design of new chemical constructs (new compositions of matter) to ultimately accomplish the job, precisely along the lines that have been described in the preceding chemical principles sections, typically constitute an inventive process. Thus, for determining inventorship beyond the individual(s) that conceived of the novel idea in the first place, it is not the amount of work that a given person may have contributed, but rather the level of creative thought and novel problem-solving that any person may have had to devise in order to accomplish one or more of the requisite steps on the path of reducing the idea to practice.

19.2.3.5 Clinical Testing

The importance of delivering the GMP-produced raw drug for clinical study within an appropriate, GMP-produced preliminary dosage form devised during the preclinical development stage has already been mentioned. The rigorous GLP analytical chemistry requirements for these production activities were emphasized as well. During clinical study, the drug-wannabe samples that are administered and the biological samples that are withdrawn for analysis will continue to use the GLP analytical chemistry methods. Another important aspect pertaining to chemical principles at this point entails the same thought processes that have been described across all the earlier sections for efficacy and ADMET considerations except that they are now directly relevant to the human case. For example, the question can be asked if there is a medicinal chemical basis for a difference being observed in the human half-life of the drug-wannabe versus that which was previously observed in one or more animal models. If so, can this be best dealt with by further molecular adjustments, formulation adjustments, or administration protocols?

The initial Phase I study will primarily involve establishing human safety via the enrollment of healthy volunteers, however more advanced studies will need to optimize the dosage protocols for delivering therapy to sick individuals. All the aforementioned questions are important to consider during optimization, as well as the pharmacogenetics of each individual enrolled in a given study. Among several other goals the field of pharmacogenetics seeks to optimize each patient to a given therapy based upon the patient's genetic predispositions. This can pertain to having distinct ADMET-related behaviors as well as to inherent efficacy-related-response differences. Hopefully, the drug-wannabe works well in a large enough segment of a particular pharmacogenetically characterized population so that it can then be expected to be marketed to a large enough audience to recoup all its discovery costs. A drug that works even very well in only a small segment of the population will likely have difficulty finding a backer to bring it to the marketplace. These types of markets are in need of so-called orphan drugs, and special governmental programs are in place to at least partially assist in fulfilling this need.

Driven by the flood of genome-derived knowledge, the phrase individualized therapy may be appealing to both the patient and health-care provider but, strictly speaking and for the same reasons mentioned earlier, this will not likely be pursued per se by the drug discovery process in a proactive manner. Instead, pharmacogenetics will more likely be used within the context of patient selection and enrollment criteria to screen out individuals who are not likely to respond to the drug-wannabe during its clinical trials. Alternatively and on a more positive note, adopting the best drug from an armamentarium of available agents and then individualizing its dosage regimen for each patient based upon his or her pharmacogenetic profile is a very realistic goal. But again note that this would then occur after clinical testing when the drug-wannabe has finally made it to becoming a true drug.

19.2.4 Reconsideration of the Ten Most Prescribed Drugs

Returning to this topic for the purpose of summarizing some of the chemical principles that have been delineated earlier, let us together examine the first structure in Figure 19.11 and see what we might be able to say about the various functional groups that are present in **18**. The most striking feature that literally jumps out from this HMG-CoA Reductase inhibitor is the terminal carboxylic acid group. We know that this group distinguishes itself by being highly ionized at physiological pH, and that it will likely form a large cluster with water molecules as it embarks on its random walk throughout the body. Although it will be much less ionized under the acidic conditions of the stomach and thus be more compatible with membrane passage and oral absorption within that particular locale, a carboxylic acid's overall behavior at physiologic pH is simply not all that user-friendly from a broader ADME perspective, particularly with regard to a drug's further distribution and the need to avoid Organic Anion Transporters that will notice the carboxylate anion and try to dump it into the bile for quick excretion. So what is it doing on **18**—why wasn't it excised during lead compound optimization? Even without knowing for sure, it's a reasonably safe bet to say that this particular functional group is likely present because it is a key component of the efficacy-related pharmacophore where its ability to associate with the desired biological surface is not only a requisite feature for such recognition, but where it can then also endow a rather unique advantage in its highly favorable reduction in energy during ionic binding.

Although not as dramatic, the same scenario can be said for the rather unique sequential arrangement of two hydroxyl-groups that appear along the aliphatic carbon chain leading to the carboxylic acid; their interesting display is likely an additional requirement for efficacy. Alternatively, since the remainder of the molecule (i.e., the western hemisphere) tends to be lipophilic, perhaps these hydroxyl-groups simply have been placed on the molecule in an innocuous (nonefficacy-related) location so as to better balance the overall Log P value and to enhance water solubility. In this regard, a quick calculation of three phenyl-rings plus one heterocyclic ring plus nine methylene groups versus a carboxylate anion plus an amide (that you should spot in the northwest corner of the molecule) can provide a crude assessment of where the overall lipophilicity would reside for this system without the two hydroxyls. That comparison becomes [3 × 2 units] + [1 × ca. 2 units (using a phenyl-ring as the closest comparable entry)] + [3 × ca. 1.5 units (using the isopropyl value as an average)] = 12.5 units of lipophilicity versus [ca. – 4.4] + [ca. – 1.3] = –5.7 units of hydrophilicity (note negative values). This then turns out to be a net value that is near 6.8. Thus, there would be a considerably higher distribution of our model des-hydroxyl-compound in a layer of n-octanol (Log P media for a water-membrane interface) versus that within the aqueous media (at pH 7.4). Since this value is considerably more to the lipophilic-side than an average drug molecule (and notably above the Rule-of-5 limit, i.e., cLog P = 5), we probably would want to add more polarity; the two hydroxyl-groups present in the actual structure **18** may be there simply as a result of trying to enhance water solubility and improve upon the overall ADME profile of some precursor or lead compound that initially lacked these groups. Adding in the contribution from the two hydroxyl-groups reduces our estimated cLog P value to a more reasonable number near 5. Therefore, we should be open to this possibility, as well as to the possibility that these two hydroxyl groups are present because they are part of the requisite, efficacy-related pharmacophore.

One proviso to this assessment, however, is to additionally appreciate that other factors do come into play once the model compound enters a membrane where the immediate environment need not follow bulk-solution pH properties. Within a given local environment, it may also be appropriate to consider the unionized form of the carboxylic acid to be a predominant chemical species. When this is done, this group's contribution is about –0.3 and the overall lipophilicity for our model compound (again lacking the two hydroxyl-groups) jumps to a very high value that approaches 10.9 units. Perhaps without these hydroxyl groups, the compound would gradually accumulate within membranes or, in particular, some unwanted lipophilic depot such as adipose tissue.

This is meant to be an exercise and we shall check to see how these drugs actually perform later. For now, let us complete our analysis of **18** by recognizing that the isopropyl is also a rather interesting group, as is the presence of a fluorine atom. The former is a common building block in biochemistry as well as an element of peptide-related function (i.e., valine and leucine), but when present in small molecule drugs it is nearly always there to do something specific or else it will represent only a potential metabolic weak-link for a CYP450-mediated oxidative degradation process. Thus, we can assume that the isopropyl is either providing a steric shield for an even quicker metabolism that might otherwise occur, or that it is establishing a hydrophobic core for binding in an appropriate hydrophobic locale within the efficacy-related biological surface. However, knowing that amides are reasonably stable and that no other metabolic weak link appears to be present in this immediate locale, we might think that the isopropyl's presence is more for efficacy than for anything else. Either way, its presence should not be regarded as just circumstantial. Finally, a fluorine atom is not a typical element to find in the general realm of biochemical reactions and its presence is also not likely to be just circumstantial. Recalling that aromatic hydroxylation is a major route for drug metabolism, and that it can be impeded by withdrawing electrons from the subject aryl-system, we might knowledgably speculate that the fluorine is playing this protective role within **18**.

The same analysis of functional groups and chemical principles can be applied to the rest of the drugs in Figure 19.11. Leaving the detailed examinations up to you, I will highlight just some of the key features that you should immediately spot while you then, hopefully, have some fun by continuing to ponder each structure on your own. Beta-adrenergic receptor blocking agent structures like that present in **19** will receive attention in a subsequent case study so that you can readily check whatever you might come up with at that time, particularly with what you might determine to be the requisite pharmacophore. For now, you should immediately appreciate that the isopropyl-group, as just discussed, is indeed there to do something, in this case to prevent the rapid N-deakylation reactions that otherwise take place on the less strerically-hindered endogenous primary and N-methyl-secondary amines (recall **14** and **15** in Scheme 19.7). Alternatively, you should likewise recognize that the terminal methoxy-group probably still represents a metabolic weak link (which indeed it does in practice). In **20** you might spot the esters and think that they represent prodrug moieties because they are likely to be rapidly hydrolyzed after absorption to one or even to two carboxylic acid groups that may then constitute the actual portions of the requisite pharmacophore. However, looking more closely at **20** and recalling the metabolism Rule-of-1 you should further note that these esters are very sterically crowded and so they may actually be stable. In practice, they do indeed turn out to be quite stable and are themselves an inherent part of the calcium-channel blocker pharmacophore. The primary amine side-chain in **20** stands out as a metabolic weak link, although in practice oxidation of the unique dihydropyridine system (obviously also a key part of the pharmacophore) is a major route of degradative metabolism for this class of compounds in general. Finally, just in case you're looking at it suspiciously, in this case the electron-withdrawing halide relates to a pharmacophore requirement rather than to any need for a reduction in aromatic hydroxylation.

In **21** we are dealing with replacement therapy for the endogenous thyroid hormone, particularly its T_4 or tetra-iodo component, so drug design was not really a factor in this particular drug discovery situation. However, it is certainly interesting to note that in a highly uncommon fashion for biochemistry, the body has chosen to use several iodine atoms as key substituents in what might otherwise resemble a more mundane elaboration of a typical amino acid building block. Although one of these iodine atoms is eventually removed by metabolism in the periphery to produce the most active T_3 form of the hormone, the sheer bulk of the remaining three iodines still dictates a 3D conformation of the bi-aryl system that causes the planes of the two aromatic rings to reside in a skewed relationship that is, in turn, requisite for proper 3D alignment and binding with the thyroid hormone receptor.

Turning to **22**, you should recognize that it has several adrenergic features. Whatever you may decide represents the key pharmacophoric elements that make it a selective serotonin re-uptake inhibitor or SSRI drug, you should be able to check out your predictions by again relying upon the same beta-adrenergic receptor blocking agent case study that follows this section. For example, be alert for the interesting dichloro-aryl moiety in that section and be prepared to reconsider **22**, where at least one of the chlorines might be trying to model something in serotonin (shown as **56**). Likewise, look at the semi-rigid ring that extends the amine from one of the aryl rings and recall what was discussed previously about the importance of extended versus folded conformational aspects. Finally, the extra-ring may also be of interest compared to the endogenous material, and indeed it is in practice since it serves to establish selectivity.

Compound **23** is another SSRI drug and so it can be considered in the same manner. As a hint for this case, however, recall that once the tertiary amine is protonated at physiological pH, the resulting ammonium system now has a hydrogen that can form a hydrogen-bond donating-relationship with the neighboring ether oxygen. The latter, in turn, establishes a new conformation for the molecule that is thought to place its nitrogen atom in a 3D space arrangement relative to the aryl moiety that becomes very similar to that for other agents in this class, like **22**, and that is thought to be significant for interaction with the biological transporter surface. Again, there is an extra aromatic ring and the presence of electron withdrawing groups on the aryl rings. By comparison to serotonin itself, **56**, can you determine which ring in **23** is the extra one needed for selectivity? Having done that, what do you think the role of the fluorine atom might be in this overall molecule? If it's not mimicking serotonin's hydroxyl, like the cyano-group is likely to be doing (to answer the first question), then perhaps it's serving as an electron withdrawing substituent to deter aromatic hydroxylation on the extra ring so as to slow down the first of a two-step metabolic process that might otherwise lead to quick excretion of the drug as a glucuronide conjugate.

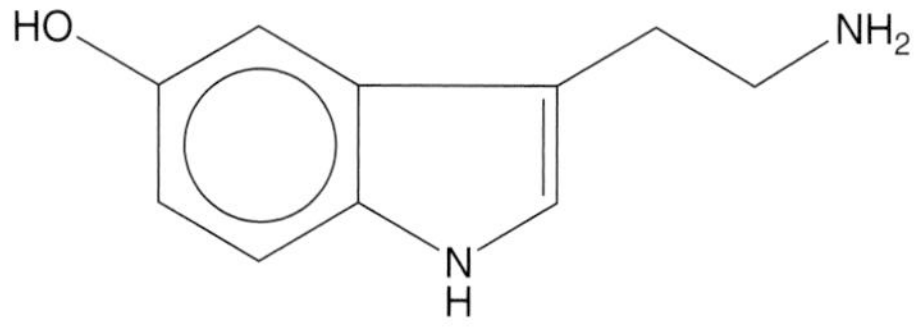

HO NH2 N H

56

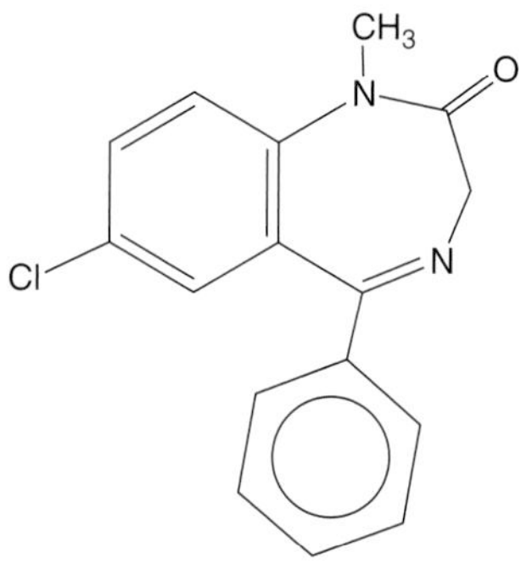

CH3 N O Cl N

57

Compound **24** is a gamma-aminobutyric acid (GABA) receptor modulator that interacts with the GABA-A subtype which is, in turn, the same locale where the classical benzodiazepine anxiolytics are also thought to interact (diazepam or Valium® being a common benzodiazepine structure shown above as **57**). Although **24** is classed as a nonbenzodiazepine sedative-hypnotic because it has a different structure, you should be able to discern some similar chemical features even though the scaffolds are indeed quite different between **24** and **57**. In terms of ADMET parameters, oxidation of the aryl-methyl groups appears to be the only major metabolic pathway available for clearing **24** from the body.

Compound **25** is a semisynthetic antibiotic that belongs to the general class of macrolide (large ring-containing) antibiotics. Other than spotting its 15-membered ring that so clearly establishes its categorization, there may not be much you can do with this structure in terms of defining the pharmacophore that is requisite for its efficacy toward inhibiting the 50S subunit on the ribosomes of bacteria. Alternatively, given its size (MW ca. 750) and its vast array of hydrogen-bonding functionality, this molecule represents a good exercise for applying the Rule-of-5 to see if anything might be suggested about its absorption after oral administration. Toward this end, you should discern that there are five hydrogen-bond donor atoms, 14 hydrogen-bond acceptor atoms, and an estimated cLog P value of about 2.5 resulting from −6 [two 3° amines that are ca. 50% protonated for an averaged value of ca. −3 for each and which will account for 2 nitrogens and 6 carbons] + −3.5 [five hydroxyl-groups] + 0 [accounts for one ester totaling 2 carbons and five ethers with 1 carbon each] + 12 [using 8 isopropyl values as an average way to account for the remaining 24 various carbon atom types]. Thus while the estimated cLog P value and number of hydrogen-bond donating atoms are okay, the other two Rule-of-5 parameters have been surpassed and your educated guess should be that this molecule should not exhibit good absorption after oral administration.

Importantly, however, Lipinski was quick to point out when first formulating his general set of rules that they often are not applicable to the antibiotic, antifungal, vitamin, and cardiac glycoside natural product types of compounds. Azithromycin is an antibiotic compound. Its oral bioavailability has actually been determined to be about 45% from a capsule formulation that is now no longer commercially available. You should also be able to discern numerous sites for metabolic degradation. Interestingly, the sugar moiety attachments are reasonably stable as is the lactone (cyclic ester), which you should spot as part of the large ring system. Also note again the steric crowding that is likely responsible for this esters high degree of metabolic stability (both an ethyl- and a methyl-group pointing down from the ring in this immediate vicinity to protect the lactone from a bottom-side attack while another nearby methyl-group points up to shield the lactone from a top-side assault).

Without reviewing the specific efficacy-related SAR, just like for **25**, it becomes difficult to discern the pharmacophoric components in compound **26**, which is a proton pump inhibitor (PIP) used to decrease gastric acid secretion. However, in this case the weak metabolic links are likely to be involved in efficacy, or they likely would have been excised during the lead optimization of this nonnatural product. Thus, the pyridine's para-methoxy group is likely to be requisite for activity, particularly since it appears that two methyl groups have been placed immediately on each side of it so as to conceivably provide a steric shield and thus serve as an impediment to rapid metabolism. The other methoxy-group, however, looks wide open for an O-demethylation reaction. It may be just fortuitous that this is apparently not too much of a metabolic weak point. This brings us to the last compound, **27**, which, in terms of its mechanism of efficacious action, is another HMG-CoA Reductase inhibitor exactly like **18**, which we have already covered in detail and only need to check our predictions. But recall that in **18** we ultimately implicated both the carboxylic acid moiety and the two sequential hydroxyl groups as being likely functional-group features of the pharmacophore requisite for efficacious activity. If that's so, then where are these requisite groups in **27** since it is supposed to be interacting at the exact same biolocial surface in exactly the same manner? Looking at this lactone you should note that unlike **25**, its ester is sterically hindered to an attack from only the bottom-side of its ring. Upon its metabolism from the top-side (or perhaps even spontaneous chemical hydrolysis at physiologic pH) and concomitant ring opening, both a carboxylic acid moiety and a second hydroxyl group are revealed. Furthermore, the sequence of these three functionalities becomes exactly analogous to the series present in **18**. This is such a remarkable coincidence that our confidence in the initial set of predictions about the pharmacophore-related importance of these three groups might be strengthened even further. Similarly, the presence of an isopropyl-group near an amide-link in **18** that we also deduced to likely be an additional part of the efficacy pharmacophore is at least mimicked to a certain extent by the presence of a sec-pentyl-group near an ester-link within **27**. This aliphatic ester is now rather sterically hindered in that its alcohol component is part of a bicyclic-ring system and its acid component has the aforementioned sec-pentyl group attached so as to have a gem-dimethyl group present in the most immediate, alpha-position to the esters's carbonyl.

Let's check our predictions for **18** and **27** to see if these molecules are really behaving according to what we have speculated from just an assessment of functional groups and application of drug discovery-related chemical principles. First, **27** is indeed a prodrug with little or no activity of its own until its six-membered lactone is hydrolyzed *in vivo* to generate what can be considered to be a mevalonic acid-like component that is thus present in the metabolite, and in **18** as an inherent component from the start. This component, in turn, resembles both the metabolic product mevalonic acid (**58**) endogenous hydoxymethylglutaryl CoA or HMG-CoA substrate for the enzyme (shown as **59**) HMG-CoA Reductase. Interference with the activity of this enzyme by either **18** or **27** reduces the quantity of mevalonic acid, which is the enzyme's normal metabolic product. Mevalonic acid, in turn, is required as a precursor or building block for cholesterol and its formation is the rate-limiting step in cholesterol synthesis. Thus, we appear to have nailed the key, efficacy-related pharmacophoric elements rather well.

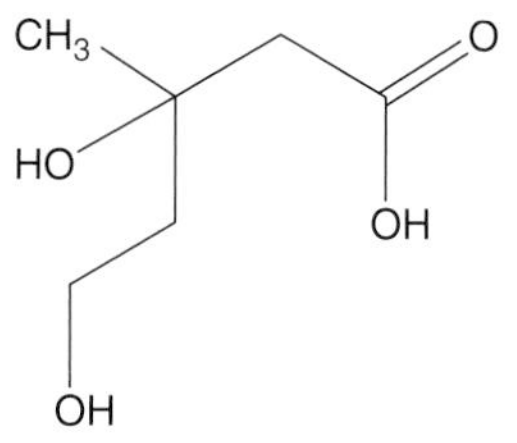

CH3 HO OH OH O

CH3 HO O OH S-CoA O

58

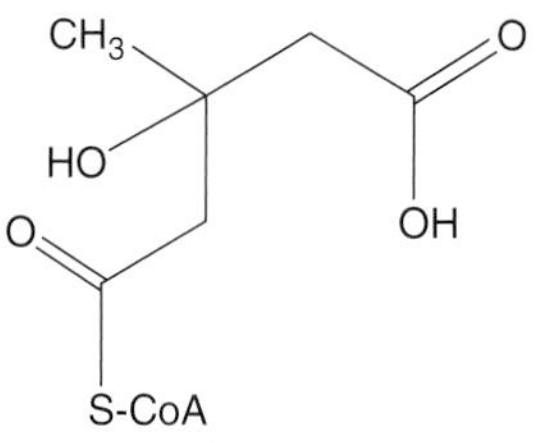

59 (Co-A = Coenzyme A)

What about these compounds' *in vivo* disposition, particularly that of **18**? In the different *in vivo* compartments we might imagine that various equilibrium ratios between the open and closed lactone may occur and this too appears to have some literature precedent. HMG-CoA Reductase is a hepatic microsomal enzyme, so distribution to the liver is imperative for action. We know that this is typically not a problem for any drug, but where else might **18** tend to distribute and what is its half-life? The half-life for **18** turns out to be a remarkable 14 to 19 hours, much longer than any of the other HMG-CoA Reductase inhibitor drugs and even for most drugs in general. When this is coupled to the fact that its systemic bioavailability is only about 30% due largely to an aggressive first-pass metabolism, it implies that subsequent distribution into peripheral depots may be taking place. By residing in depots, the drug may be able to linger for a longer period than what might normally be expected for typical compartment equilibrations, just like we suspected that **18** might be able to do based upon a change in its equilibrium species at a different pH within lipophilic tissues. A reported Log P value of approximately 4 is close to our rough estimate of 5. Finally, that this drug undergoes extensive CYP450-mediated aromatic hydroxylation as the main biotransformation pathway en route to its excretion is also in line with our prior speculation.

Hopefully, you will fare equally well upon checking the answers to your own predictions for the remainder of these drugs' actual behaviors within the clinic. However, each functional group can display a variety of size, lipophilic/hydrophilic and electronic properties for which any one or all may or may not be operative in a relevant manner within a given drug structure. Likewise, each drug can distinctly interact with its particular set of relevant efficacy and ADMET-related biological surfaces. Thus, do not feel disappointed if your predictions are often incorrect. This section is meant to be only an exercise about how we can think about drug structures in a chemically knowledgeable fashion. When further structural modifications are then coupled with actual experimental assessments, a progression of optimized properties and desirable pharmacologic behavior can ultimately be achieved in an expeditious manner and, hopefully, the high attrition rate for drug-wannabes during early clinical testing can ultimately be reduced. Furthermore, by analogy to the harsh reality of the latter, you should be able to take considerable comfort in knowing that your predictions did not cost about $868 M after contemplating them over the course of 15 years only to find out that you were right for just one out of the approximately nine compounds that you have just worked on from Figure 19.11. Working together, we did reasonably well on one compound. Thus, if you can add just one more successful prediction of overall clinical efficacy and PK-related behavior, in a certain sense you will have already beat the odds of today's prevailing average for the industry.

19.3 DRUG DISCOVERY CASE STUDIES

19.3.1 From the Early Days of Working with Mother Nature (Penicillins)

This first case study will review some of the interesting aspects about the early discovery and continued evolution of the overall class of penicillin drugs as we know them today. Attention is directed to various steps and principles that we discussed in the preceding sections with a special emphasis placed upon some of the chemical phenomena. Presently used terms and strategies have been inserted into what is otherwise a retrospective analysis of what these scientists were able to accomplish in a very remarkable fashion before the categorizations and accompanying tools that we have today were even in place.

19.3.1.1 Background

The story of the penicillins begins from a translational chemistry starting point with an observation that was made by a microbiologist named Fleming in 1929. Working in a damp, London laboratory, Fleming noticed that an inadvertent mold (Penicillium notatum, or PN) that managed to land in his staphylococci cell cultures was able to lyse and kill them. In a very elegant manner using simple filter materials of various pore sizes, he later deduced that a low molecular weight chemical substance was being released by these PN invaders. Almost 10 years later Florey and Chain isolated, purified, and identified this substance as penicillin G (PENG) for which they, along with Fleming, received the 1945 Nobel Prize in Medicine. The term antibiotics was coined shortly thereafter by Brotzu. Initially thought to be produced by microorganisms to fend off their competitors for local nutrient supplies, this term is now regarded as a misnomer since these substances actually appear to play a crucial role in normal cellular metabolism, namely as controlling signals to attenuate a microorganism's fast growth phase. Thus, the concentrations and excretion of antibiotics typically occur at their highest levels during the stasis period that follows the fast, logarithmic growth phase of a given microorganism. This early finding has become important during commercial manufacturing of the penicillins (PENs) where the microorganism manufacturers are manipulated to reach stasis rapidly and then held there for as long as possible to achieve maximum production levels.

A chemical diagram that encompasses many of the PENs is shown as **60**. Several analogs are recorded in the accompanying Table 19.8. Four areas within this general structure are of practical interest. First, the

Table 19.8 Selected Penicillin Analogs (R-groups refer to structure **60** as shown within the text)

#	R	Name	Comment
61	C_6H_5–CH_2–	Penicillin G	Natural product
62	C_6H_5–CH(NH_2)–	Ampicillin	Acid stable
63	HO–C_6H_4–CH(NH_2)–	Amoxicillin	Acid stable
64	2,6-(OCH_3)$_2$$C_6H_3$–	Methicillin	Resists penicillinases
65	C_6H_5–CH(CO_2H)–	Carbenicillin	Broad or extended spectrum

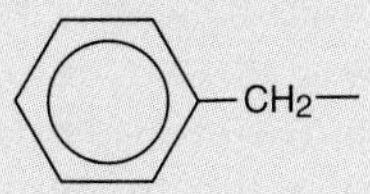

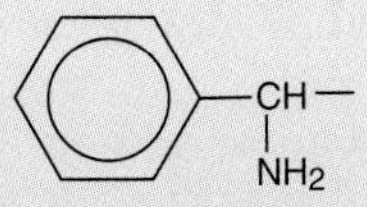

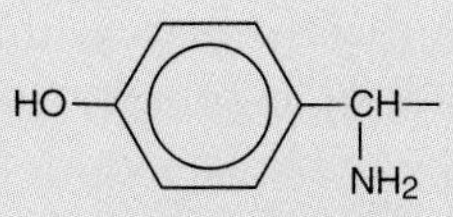

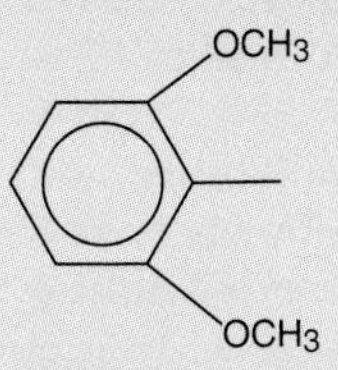

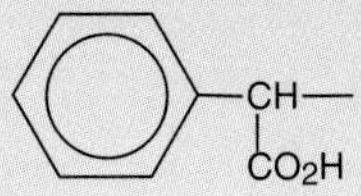

central scaffold that is comprised of a bicyclic (two fused rings) system having a thiazolidine ring (*thia* for sulfur, *azo* for nitrogen, and *olidine* for a five-membered saturated or nonaromatic system) fused to a beta-lactam ring (four-membered cyclic amide system). Other than catabolism by peptidases, amides are normally unreactive under physiological conditions. However, recall that a four-membered ring causes a strained-bond relationship to exist among its members that would rather be associated with a larger group of atoms in five- or six-membered rings, or to not even be cyclized at all under such tight circumstances. Thus, this particular amide arrangement is sitting in the PEN's structure like a loaded spring ready to undergo reaction with any nucleophile that is willing to attack the carbonyl and uncoil or pop open the strained beta-lactam ring. This is shown in Scheme 19.17 for an endogenous nucleophile that may be

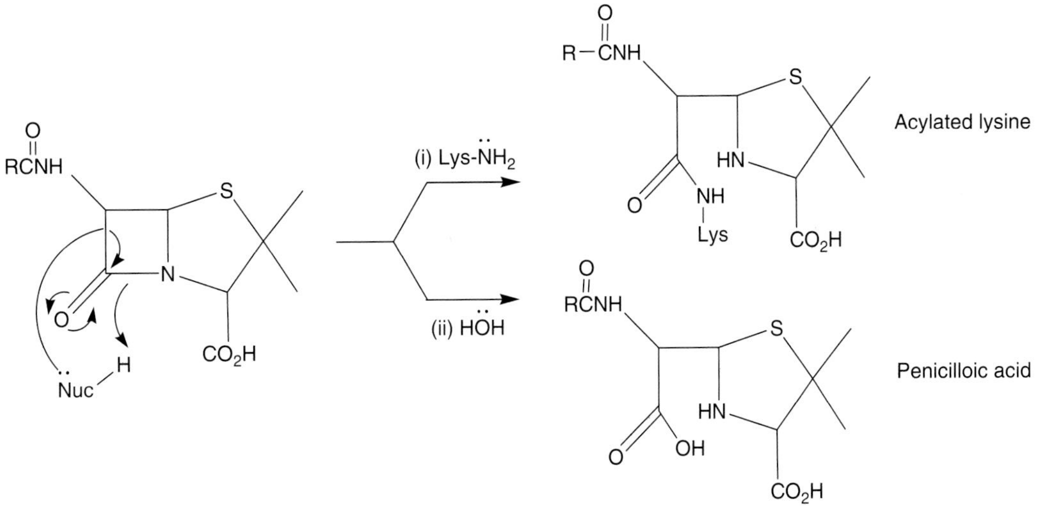

Scheme 19.17 Nucleophilic opening of penicillin's beta-lactam. This process occurs under basic conditions and is driven by the energetics associated with relieving the considerable bond-angle strain present in the 4-membered-ring. Two pathways are shown: (i) The top results in acylation of a biological surface that has a good nucleophile such as the terminal amino-group on a lysine amino acid residue; and, (ii) The lower represents a ready hydrolytic ring-opening by a water molecule to produce an inactive degradation product called penicilloic acid.

present on a biological surface such as the terminal amino group of a lysine residue.

If you are beginning to think about the possibility for an acylation reaction that we know to be so highly stable energetically (Table 19.4) that it can lead to irreversible inhibition of a biological surface, then you are indeed correct and you should hold onto this thought until just a bit later. For the moment, there is something else that this reactivity causes and it needs to be addressed first. Another nucleophile, even though less reactive than lysine's amine, is so prevalent in the body or in just moist air, that it takes precedent in opening the ring, namely a water molecule, which also is shown in Scheme 19.17 as a simple base-catalyzed hydrolysis reaction. Thus, the first formulations of the PENs required them to be produced as solids, which had to be kept very dry until just prior to use, whereupon they could be dissolved in aqueous media buffered between six and eight where, even when kept in the refrigerator, a physician could expect to have only a few days worth of product stability. In these early days, the formulations were generally freshly prepared and then had to be administered by injection within a doctor's office. And why not make the solutions even more acidic ($pH < 6$) so as to further improve stability? Because there is another pathway that causes significant decomposition to occur under acidic conditions, particularly when the pH is less than 5. This decomposition pathway will be discussed further as the PEN's history later unfolds into having orally bioavailable medications.

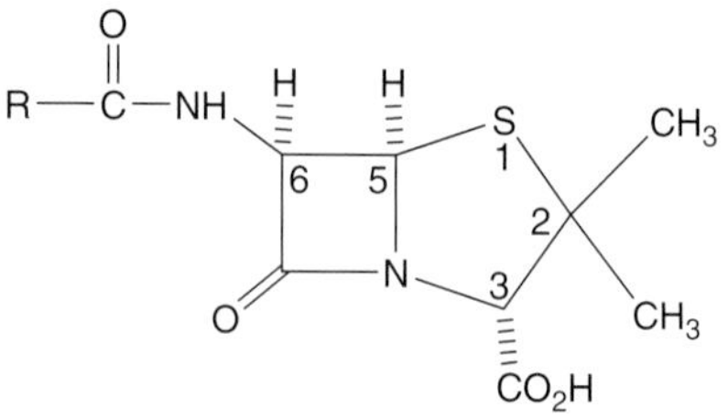

R—C(=O)—NH ... CO_2H ... CH_3 ... CH_3 **60**

Returning to the interesting chemical features inherently present in **60**, the next functional group that catches our eye is the carboxylic acid moiety at position 3. As discussed earlier, this type of group will tend to be largely deprotonated and thus highly ionized at physiological pH. In this regard it was quickly found that the Na^+ and K^+ salts with this carboxylate anion could be exploited to form crystalline solids, which are much easier to purify and formulate than when attempted from the natural form. It is these types of salts that are stable as solids for months when kept dry. Next comes the northwest-quadrant amide (at position 6 in **60**) where, among the various PEN products, its R-group has been varied across a wide range of substituents (see Table 19.8 for just a few selected examples). Among these products, the specific nature of the R-group can affect a given agent's:

- Spectrum of activity (i.e., broad or narrow spectrum antibiotic)
- Aqueous solubility
- Stability
- Oral bioavailability
- Resistance by bacteria
- Plasma protein binding

The last aspect of interest on this natural product's structure involves its distinct stereochemistry as indicated across the three asymmetric centers at positions 3, 5, and 6 in **60**. It was soon found that this exact stereochemistry is required in order for the PENs to properly display their functional groups in 3D space and thereby interact with their biological target in an optimal manner. Unfortunately, this specific 3D pharmacophore requirement makes the compound very difficult to synthesize in the large-scale required for drug manufacturing processes. Instead, PEN G (**61** in Table 19.8) is isolated from PN in industrial quantities by employing manufacturing-sized fermentation equipment. For the various analogs with different R groups, or the so-called semisynthetic penicillins, PEN G is first converted to 6-aminopenicillanic acid (6-APA) by enzymatic cleavage using an isolated Amidase enzyme called Penicillin Acylase. This process is depicted in Scheme 19.18. 6-APA, in turn, can be readily reacted with different acid chloride functional groups so as to produce the various R-substituted PENs that we have today.

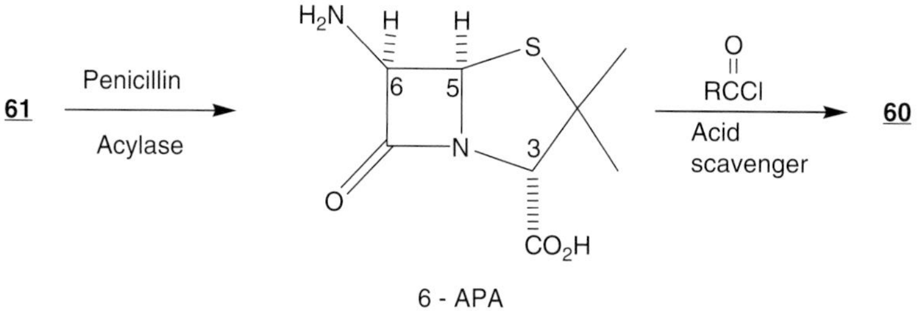

61 —Penicillin Acylase→ 6 - APA —RCCl(=O), Acid scavenger→ **60**

Scheme 19.18 Production of the semisynthetic penicillins. This process takes advantage of large-scale fermentation to obtain penicillin G (**61**) from microbes in order to establish the requisite stereochemistry at positions 3, 5, and 6 as indicated on 6-APA. An isolated enzyme (Penicillin Acylase) is then used to cleave the phenylacetic acid group off of the 6-position amide in **61**. The resulting 6-amino-penicillanic acid (6-APA) can then be readily acylated with any acid chloride under buffered conditions so as to prevent a build-up in acidity during the reaction. Table 19.8 lists some representative semi-synthetic penicillins.

19.3.1.2 Mechanism of Action

Turning next to the simultaneously evolving knowledge about the PEN's biological mechanism of action, it was known that bacteria have high internal osmotic pressure and rely on their cell walls to keep them from swelling and rupturing. Human cells do not have a high intracellular pressure and can rely upon their cell membranes to establish a demarcation from their extracellular (interstitial fluid) environments (i.e., human cells do not have cell walls). Since the PENs lyse (rupture) bacteria but not human cells, the locale or biological surface that immediately became implicated for their site of action was that of the bacterial cell wall. With time it became clear that the PENs precise 3D display of its two amide groups and various other appendages mimics the shape of one of the key building block polysaccharides within a bacterium's cell wall, namely the (D)-alanine-(D)-alanine tail of a peptidoglycan that is unique to bacteria. Bacteria synthesize this unusual pair of (D)-stereochemistry amino acids onto these terminal chains so as to make them more resistant to attack by Lysozymes, which is one of the human's enzymatic defense systems in tears and nasal fluid that works against bacterial insults by aggressively hydrolyzing the bacterium's natural peptides when they do have the normal (L)-amino acid members. These peptidoglycans dangling from the initial structure of a bacterium's cell wall undergo further cross-linking to form a more rigid framework. This occurs in a two-step process where the third amino acid from the peptidoglycan terminus, namely a lysine, is first coupled with a five-glycine sequence so that this extended appendage's amine can reach over to attack the second-position (D)-alanine in an enzyme catalyzed transamidation reaction that kicks-out the terminal (D)-alanine. This two-step, cross-linking process is shown in Scheme 19.19.

The key enzyme responsible for the second step is called (D)-Alanyltranspeptidase. The PENs 3D display is able to so closely mimic the peptidoglycan sidechain's terminal pair of (D)-alanines [(D)-Ala^1-(D)-Ala^2 in Scheme 19.19] that (D)-Alanyltranspeptidase is fooled into binding with PEN as a prelude to what it thinks is going to be just another uneventful cross-linking reaction. However, once inside the enzyme's pocket, PEN's beta-lactam beckons for a reaction with any nucleophile located on the enzyme's surface that can allow its strained ring to spring open. Thus, after allowing this Trojan Horse to enter its gates, the (D)-Alanyltranspeptidase falls victim to an acylation reaction that is of such a highly stable, covalent nature that it cannot rid itself of this enemy and its own enzymatic function succumbs to an irreversible inhibition. Since humans do not conduct this biochemical process in their cell membrane barriers, the penicillins might be thought of as having an exquisite selectivity toward bacteria that is based solely upon their pharmacodynamic

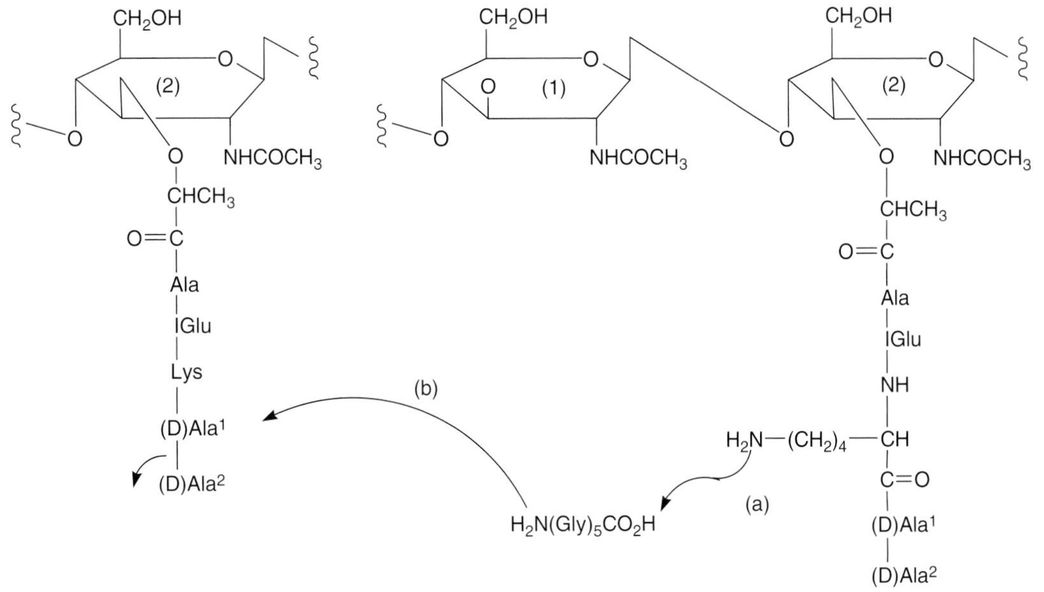

CH$_2$OH O (2) O O NHCOCH$_3$ CHCH$_3$ O=C Ala IGlu Lys (D)Ala^1 (D)Ala^2
CH$_2$OH O O (1) O NHCOCH$_3$
CH$_2$OH O (2) O O NHCOCH$_3$ CHCH$_3$ O=C Ala IGlu NH H$_2$N—(CH$_2$)$_4$—CH C=O (D)Ala^1 (D)Ala^2
(b) (a) H$_2$N(Gly)$_5$CO$_2$H

Scheme 19.19 Bacterial cell wall peptidoglycan cross-linking reaction. N-Acetylglucosamine (1) and N-acetylmuramic acid (2) with its specified side-chain that terminates in a pair of (D)-alanine amino acids (Ala^1 and Ala^2), together constitute a monomeric, peptidoglycan building block of a bacterium's polymeric cell wall. The side-chains undergo periodic cross-linking in order to strengthen the overall cell wall architecture. Cross-linking begins according to reaction arrow (a) by attaching a pentapeptide of five glycines (H$_2$N(Gly)$_5$CO$_2$H) onto the side-chain amino group of the lysine residue (Lys shown in-full in far-right structure) located three amino acids away from the peptidoglycine's side-chain terminus. The extended free amine from the terminal (Gly)$_5$ addition then attacks via reaction arrow (b) a neighboring peptidoglycan side-chain at its (D)-alanine located in the second position from this side-chain terminus [(D)-Ala^1]. The terminal (D)-alanine residue serves as a leaving group [(D)-Ala^2] during the transamidation reaction (b). The key enzyme required for this second transamidation step is called (D)-Alanyltranspeptidase. IGlu is an isoglutamic acid residue located in the fourth position from the side-chain terminus.

mode of action rather than upon any bias in their pharmacokinetic-related distribution, and so on. However, the penicillins also react with several other bacterial biological surfaces and furthermore, as we shall see in a few moments, they are not without similar types of mechanism-based side-effect problems when used within humans. Additional target surfaces for the penicillins include certain binding proteins that have come to be called penicillin binding proteins; various other transpeptidases involved in cell elongation, maintaining rod-shape, and formation of septums during cell replication; (D)-Alanine-(D)-alanylcarboxypeptidases, which are responsible for trimming the terminal peptide bonds of cross-linked peptidoglycans (i.e., removing left-over (D)-Ala^2 units); and likely several other targets as well. Fortuitously, these multiple sites of action make it more difficult for bacteria to become resistant to the penicillins by simply modifying their (D)-Alanyltranspeptidase to be a bit more fussy about its recognition of the peptidoglycan's terminus.

19.3.1.3 The Need for Better Analogs

Despite this impressive start, there were also problems with the penicillins that merited further drug design efforts. These additional drug design efforts have significantly changed the second- and third-generation agents that have subsequently entered the marketplace. In this regard, three problems can be mentioned, the first being stability, which has already been discussed relative to the basic side and has been alluded to relative to the acid side. The instability in acid was particularly problematic because this precluded administration by the oral route; that is, the early PENs readily decomposed when confronted with the acidity of the human stomach. Although Mother Nature had cleverly devised these compounds for use by bacteria, she clearly had not intended for them to be utilized by humans. Eventually, the mechanism for the collapse of the PENs under acidic conditions was also deduced. It is depicted in Scheme 19.20.

Once this knowledge was in hand, it was noted that the decomposition process begins with a nucleophilic attack (sound familiar?) by the 6-position amide's oxygen atom onto the carbonyl-carbon of the beta-lactam system so as to relieve the latter's ring strain (sure does, even though it is now an intramolecular process utilizing a poor nucleophile compared to those able to be enlisted from the environment in an intermolecular manner during decomposition under basic conditions). Thus, an answer became apparent, namely to substitute PEN G's simple benzyl-group by a functional group, which could deter this first step. Two choices are possible, one of which should be readily apparent. The more obvious is to deploy a bulky group that makes this a reaction too jammed-up to accomplish (i.e., a simple steric effect). The second, more subtle but still very effective, is to undertake an electronic approach where an electron withdrawing group would be expected to likewise impede this reaction. Note the direction of the electron flow for the first step in Scheme 19.20 and decide which way you would want to cause an electron withdrawal effect to take place: hopefully you'll agree

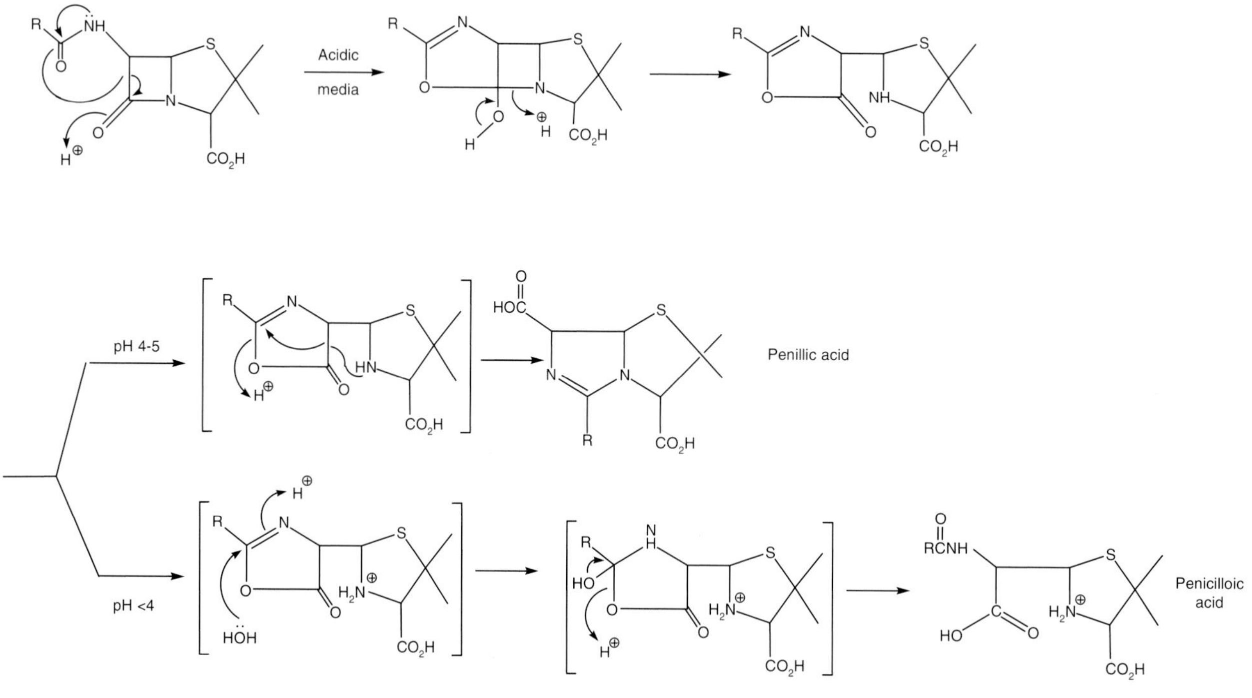

Scheme 19.20 Intramolecular opening of penicillin's beta-lactam. This process occurs under acidic conditions and is driven by the energetics associated with relieving the considerable bond-angle strain present in the 4-membered beta-lactam ring.

that this should be done so as to take electron density away from the nitrogen and its lone pair so as to make it less aggressive.

An example of an analog that reflects the first approach is methicillin (**64** in Table 19.8) although it actually came later. Examples of the second approach are ampicillin and amoxicillin, **62** and **63**, respectively. Looking at these structures and viewing the entries for amines on Table 19.3, you might wonder how placing an additional nitrogen-containing-group in this location can cause electron withdrawal. However, also realizing that these free amines will be highly protonated in the stomach (Scheme 19.12), the more appropriate functional group to refer to in Table 19.3 is the quaternary ammonium entry that models a protonated amine electronically and whose value is –0.9 (highly electron withdrawing). Indeed, these types of drug design enhancements in the PEN's overall technology work very well. For example:

- The first PENs had to be solubilized and administered within a doctor's office or hospital by intramuscular injection, typically into the buttock where their Na^+ and K^+ salt forms provided the prerequisite aqueous solubility but also caused pain on injection.
- Within 10 years, the next generation of orally available agents could be taken home from a pharmacy as thick, flavored suspensions that could be kept in the refrigerator for several days between reasonably well-tolerated oral dosing to children home from school with bacterial upper respiratory-tract infections.
- Within another 10 years, today's versions of tablets became available, which can be taken to school or to work for self-administration.

The last option has such a prolonged shelf half-life that patients sometimes stop taking their medicine as soon as they feel better so that they can save the rest for some future cold. This situation serves to demonstrate that advancing technology does not always equate to better drug usage since prematurely stopping a PEN dosing regimen can promote the development of resistant bacteria and because the next, self-diagnosed bout with a cold may be completely viral in nature for which the PENs would have no effect.

The next major problem of the PENs that has received considerable drug design attention is that of bacterial resistance. In this case, resistance by bacteria has been shown to occur by at least four different mechanisms:

- Bacterial production of Penicillinases or beta-lactamases, which attack the beta-lactam ring to form penicilloic acid
- Decreased permeability to the PENs at their immediate locale for activity
- Altered affinity for the PENs by the various Transpeptidases and PEN-binding proteins associated with their multiple mechanisms of action
- Increased bacterial production of Amidases capable of hydrolyzing the 6-position amide to form 6-APA.

Of these mechanisms, the first is the most significant and it has received the most attention. As a class, the Penicillinases are Serine Proteases (Table 19.5), which, by definition, utilize a serine residues side-chain hydroxyl-group to attack the beta-lactam to first form an acylated enzyme intermediate that results in an ester. Unlike an amide that results from the unwitting (and suicidal as described earlier) nucleophilic attack of the beta-lactam by (D)-Alanyl Transpeptidase, the ester that results from attack by a Penicillinase can be readily hydrolyzed by a water molecule. The Penicillinases intentionally hold a water molecule within their active sites to specifically accomplish this task. The water molecule spits out an inactivated penicilloic acid molecule analogous to a simple hydrolysis reaction (Scheme 19.17) while also serving to rejuvenate the active (nonacylated) form of the Penicillinase so that it can attack and inactivate another penicillin molecule. This knowledge has been used in drug design by making R-group analogs that contain large and hydrophobic substituents so as to decrease their access to the Penicillinases active site, which tends to be rather narrow and somewhat polar in nature with both a serine hydroxyl and a water molecule being present. Methicillin, **64**, again represents just such an analog that has much less of a problem with bacterial resistance.

Pursuit of this type of physicochemical profile, however, soon revealed a SAR paradox where although the larger, nonpolar types of R-groups could be relied upon to decrease Penicillinase-derived resistance problems, they also led to a narrower range of efficacy against bacterial invaders. This is because gram-negative bacteria have a membrane layer laced with pores that allow only the smaller, more polar R group PENs to enter. Thus, it became difficult to achieve both a broad or extended PEN in terms of efficacy (e.g., as with **65** in Table 19.8) that is simultaneously less subject to resistance by Penicillinases.

Another approach to avoiding such metabolic degradation while retaining a smaller and more polar type of R group utilizes an auxiliary compound to separately inhibit the Penicillinase, much as we saw for the case of the earlier levodopa example. For the PENs, the auxiliary compound is clavulanic acid, shown as **66**. When the beta-lactam moiety in **66** is being attacked by the Penicillinases, its unique hydroxymethylene-alkenyl system serves to further alkylate this enzyme in an irreversible manner at some other nucleophile. Hence, the enzyme cannot regenerate itself for a new attack of a beta-lactam system of any type. Thus, coadministration of **66** with a broad- or extended-spectrum PEN derivative is ultimately able to overcome the SAR paradox that is otherwise difficult to achieve within just a single molecule.

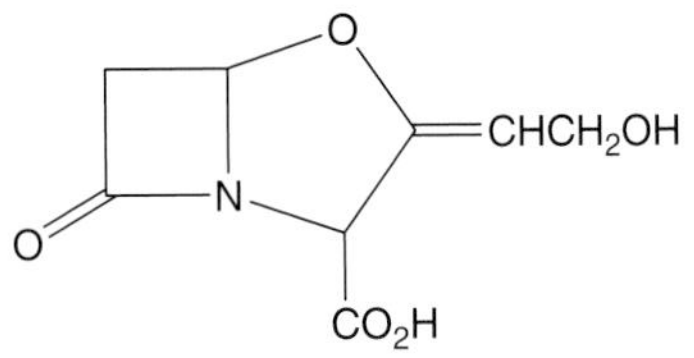

66

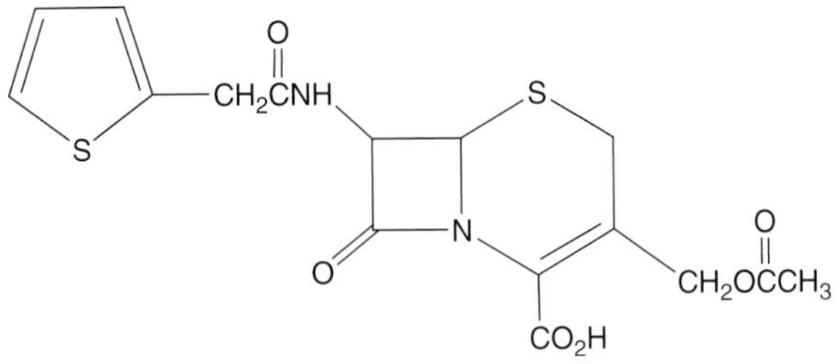

67

A third problem that can be observed with use of the PENs is that of penicillin allergy. This pharmacogenetic syndrome effects about 6 to 8% of the U.S. population. These individuals have an endogenous protein that aggressively interacts with the penicillins via a similar nucleophilic attack of the beta-lactam, likely via a lysine residue's terminal amino-group. Irreversibly acylated, these proteins now look like a foreign, invading protein and they proceed to trip the body's natural immune response mechanisms; that is, the acylated protein serves as an antigen to evoke the production of antibodies. This, as well as the always evolving bacterial resistance problem, has prompted the exploration of other penicillin-like analogs and natural products that have a different central core ring-system so that they must be recognized in a somewhat different manner at all biological surfaces. Of the natural products, the closely related cephalosporins should be mentioned as this case study is drawn to a close. An example of an early cephalosporin, namely cephalothin or **67**, with its six-, rather than five-membered ring, can be seen to stand out as being different from the PENs' central core. The cephalosporins are different from the PENs and only 8 to 10% of the population allergic to the PENs will also happen to be cross-allergic to the cephalosporins.

19.3.1.4 Summary

From a natural product starting point, this example conveys the important contributions that can result when biology and pharmacology are coupled in a synergistic manner with chemistry during further drug design (Section 19.1.2.1). Drug design was applied toward improving the overall properties and routes of administration for the initial compound and toward discovering an entire armamentarium of mechanistically related new drugs. The latter provided several different profiles for use in different clinical settings—various types of infection and degrees of bacterial resistance—as well as for specific pharmacogenomic aspects like individual variation toward therapy or the potential to develop an allergy response.

19.3.2 Across the Heydays of Rational Drug Design (Esmolol)

This case study will convey how esmolol, **3**, was discovered by a rational strategy characteristic of medicinal chemistry's heyday era. In addition, esmolol incorporated significant considerations of ADMET parameters into the design of its initial target structures and in that sense, its discovery process was ahead of its time. For this same reason, the case study serves as a rather unique example for much of today's efforts directed toward addressing PK problems in drug-wannabe's. To establish the backdrop for the discovery of esmolol, the earlier developments that lead up to beta-1-selective beta-adrenergic receptor-blocking agents will be conveyed first. Considerable portions of this case study have been borrowed from the author's treatment of this same topic in the text entitled *Analog-based Drug Discovery* and in a preceding series entitled *Chronicles of Drug Discovery*.

19.3.2.1 Background

Norepinephrine and epinephrine, **14** and **15**, are the endogenous receptor ligands that respectively serve as the neurotransmitter- and endocrine-derived agonists for both alpha- and beta-adrenergic receptors associated with the mammalian sympathetic nervous system. Isoproterenol is a long-standing, racemic derivative of these endogenous ligands whose (R)-enantiomer, **68** (shown below with **14** and **15**), demonstrates potent agonist properties at beta-receptors while exhibiting only minimal activity at alpha-receptors, the latter owing to the α-receptor's intolerance of steric bulk near the vicinity of the requisite amino-group. Still used as a bronchodilator, isoproterenol was the first synthetic catecholamine derivative to achieve clinical prominence. It should be noted that while the distinct enantiomeric spatial orientation depicted in these sympathomimetic amine agonists is required for the hydroxy-group to bind with beta-receptors, the vast majority of ligands that have been studied within this field, especially the numerous beta-blocker antagonists, have been prepared as their racemates. Thus, for convenience, the remaining compounds to be discussed within this section should be considered to be racemic unless stipulated to be otherwise.

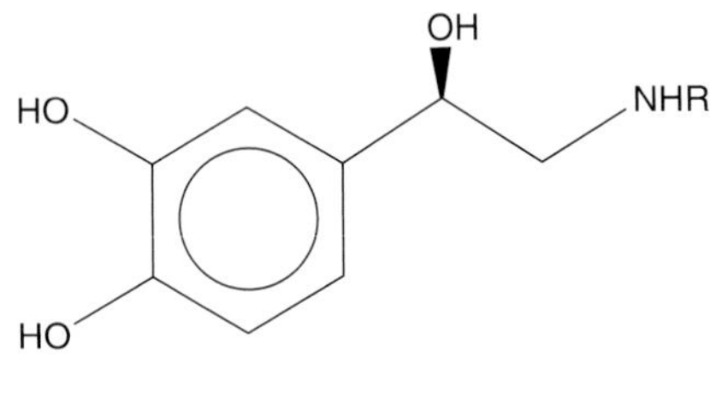

14 R = H

15 R = CH_3

68 R = $CH(CH_3)_2$

As part of initial efforts to define SAR for these types of compounds and to identify more chemically stable replacements for the air-sensitive catechol moiety, the dichloro-containing derivative shown as **69** was prepared. Although this modification did not prove to be a useful bioisosteric substitution in that agonist activity was largely lost, **69** was instead found to be a weak partial agonist that could be used to block the effects of the sympathomimetic amines on bronchodilation, uterine relaxation, and cardiac stimulation. This key, medicinal chemistry observation, coupled with Black's earlier pharmacological suggestion that beta-adrenergic receptor antagonists might protect the ischemic myocardium from sympathetic drive during angina pectoris, served to usher in the era of beta-blocker research. Subsequent replacement of the dichloro-substituents with an unsaturated carbon bridge afforded a naphthyl moiety that, in terms of seeking beta-blockade, did prove to be an effective bioisosteric replacement. The resulting beta-blocker pronethalol, **70**, was taken into the clinic where it was indeed shown to be effective in the treatment of angina pectoris. However, after having clearly validated beta-blockade as a useful therapeutic target by establishing clinical proof of principle in line with today's phraseology, within a year pronethalol had to be withdrawn due to inherent carcinogenicity (a case of insidious toxicity observed subsequent to marketing).

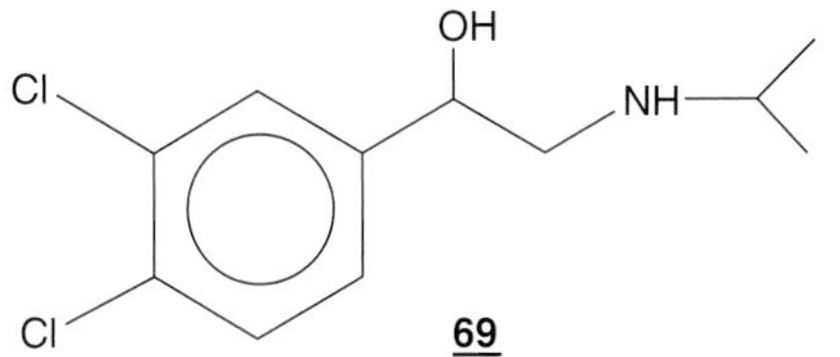

OH

Cl

NH

Cl

69

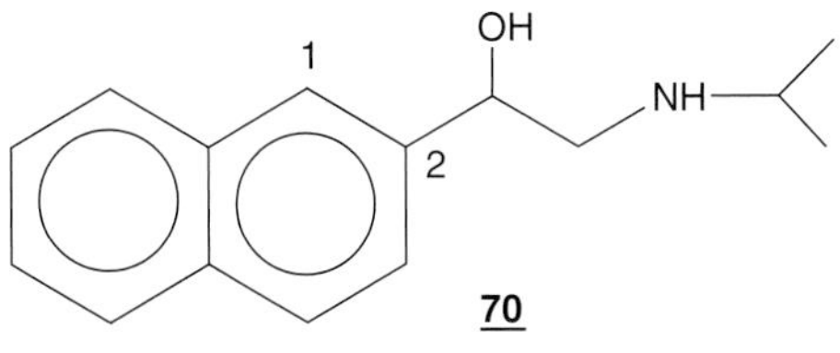

OH

1

NH

2

70

The insertion of an oxymethylene bridge, $-OCH_2-$, into the ethanolamine C2-substituent of pronethalol so as to form an oxypropanolamine, was found to retain beta-blocking activity, particularly when the entire oxypropanolamine appendage was also moved to the C1-position of the naphthyl ring. The resulting compound, propranolol (**2**), does not exhibit carcinogenicity and it soon became the first clinically sustained, successful beta blocker. Thus, subsequent to its own history of ligand-based drug design, propranolol should be considered to be the pioneer drug that, as we shall see, has gone on to inspire numerous other scenarios of analog-based drug-discovery including that of esmolol. For example, during its initial evaluation as a treatment for angina pectoris, propranolol was also found to have useful antiarrhythmic and antihypertensive properties, both of which represented new indications that needed significantly different pharmacologic profiles and, thereby, represented ideal pharmacological targets for further drug design and tailoring.

The next major development during the evolution of this field involved Lands' classification of beta-receptors into two distinct subclasses, namely beta-1 and beta-2 receptors. This key pharmacological finding prompted medicinal chemistry's drug design activities to turn toward the pursuit of compounds having beta-1 selectivity for the various cardiac-related indications. Selectivity was regarded as being particularly important for an antianginal drug to be used by patients prone to bronchospasm because of the preponderance of beta-2 receptors in bronchial tissue. In addition, ADMET-related properties to be generally enhanced included lowering lipophilicity as it specifically pertained to removing side-effect membrane stabilizing activity (MSA), and prolonging *in vivo* half-life as it specifically pertained to achieving convenient once-a-day dosing. Residual partial agonist properties called intrinsic sympathomimetic activity (ISA) and mixed patterns of selectivity between alpha- and beta-receptors, as well as among the two known beta-receptor subtypes, represented indication-dependent features that could also be further manipulated. Thus, as the era of beta-blocker research unfolded, numerous compounds became available that afforded a wide range of pharmacodynamic profiles. That nearly all these structures are aryloxypropanolamines that can be traced back to the pioneer drug, **2**, clearly underscores the important role that analog-based drug design can play during the overall course of drug discovery for a given pharmacological class, or in clarifying a distinct biochemical mechanism.

Although selective for beta- over alpha-receptors, propranolol is classified as a nonselective beta blocker in that it has nearly equipotent actions at both beta-1 and beta-2 receptors. In addition, **2** can cause cardiac depression by MSA-related mechanisms that are independent from its actions at beta-receptors. Thus, despite the significant pioneering role that **2** has played in the overall field of beta blockers, in terms of treating angina there remained an immediate need for more selective beta-1 blockers that could be used in patients with obstructive airway diseases so as to avoid blockade of bronchial beta-2 receptors and concomitant bronchoconstriction. It was at this stage of the beta-blocker field's overall development that a second, important medicinal chemistry observation relating to a key SAR would occur, namely that the para-substituted phenyl derivative, practolol (shown as **71**), was found to block cardiac beta-1 receptors at lower doses than those at which it blocked beta-2 receptors located within the bronchi and vascular beds. Thus, **71** became the first selective beta-1 adrenergic receptor blocking agent.

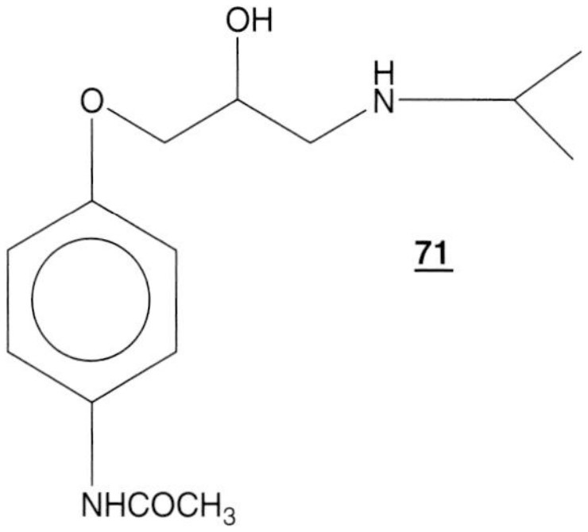

OH
H N
O
71
$NHCOCH_3$

Clinically, **71** initially proved to be a valuable antianginal agent that was much better tolerated by patients also suffering from obstructive airway disease. Unfortunately, just like the earlier experience with pronethalol, **70**, practolol also had to be quickly withdrawn from the clinic due to side-effects that this time were related to an occulomucotaneous syndrome. In concluding this Introduction, it should be appreciated that beyond the beta-1 selective compounds that are primarily directed toward cardiac-related indications like angina and myocardial infarction as well as hypertension, the overall family of beta-blockers has found a much wider range of therapeutic applications using nonselective beta blockers including hypertension, arrhythmias, glaucoma, migraine, anxiety, tremor, drug dependence, thyrotoxicosis, schizophrenia, and mania.

As mentioned, it was recognized that it would be beneficial to further tailor the overall profile of propranolol, **2**, for use as an antianginal agent within the setting of obstructive airway disease. Toward this end, Imperial Chemistry Industries, Inc. (ICI) immediately embarked on a program that sought to identify a compound with the following profile:

- Possess a potency equivalent to **2** at cardiac, beta-1 adrenoceptor sites
- Possess a greater affinity for cardiac beta-1 adrenoceptors than for beta-2 adrenoceptors in the bronchial tree, peripheral vasculature and coronary circulation, or for those involved in sugar metabolism where an additional receptor subclass at the time had not yet been identified
- Be devoid of partial agonist activity (ISA)
- Be free of membrane-depressant or -stabilizing activity (MSA)

Taking advantage of the beta-1-selectivity afforded by practolol, **71**, two structural features of **71**'s acetylamino functionality were considered for further exploration on propranolol's aryloxypropanolamine template:

- That the electron withdrawing effect of the carbonyl on imparting acidity to the proton of the –NH-CO-group might be mimicked by a $-CH_2-$CO- group
- That the hydrogen bonding capability might be retained by incorporating it into the preceding, even if in an extended manner, involving a $-CH_2CONHR$ arrangement

Approximately 5000 compounds were prepared and tested within the screening tree depicted in Scheme 19.21. Note, however, that this directed library chemistry campaign was not accompanied by today's benefit of also having combinatorial chemistry and HTS technologies available. Indeed, the front-line screen actually employed an *in vivo* model. From this brute force effort, atenolol, **72**, ultimately was identified as the compound that came closest to the desired pharmacological profile.

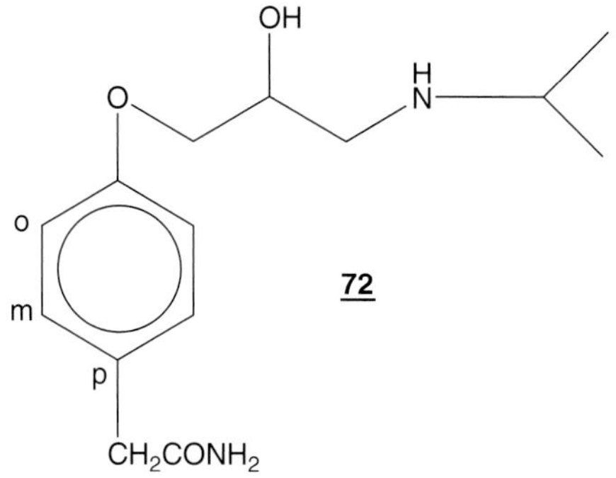

OH
H N
O
o
m
p
72
CH_2CONH_2

The production of a rich and useful SAR dataset also accompanied the selection of **72**. For example, the para-acetamido moiety gives rise to beta-1 selectivity with the amide –NH– group apparently playing an important role in this activity since the tertiary amide versions were found to be much less active. Likewise, though the methylene group does not appear to play a major role in activity or selectivity, it does have an important impact upon ISA, namely to reduce ISA to negligible levels. Thus, while para-amides with either the nitrogen or carbonyl group attached to the aromatic nucleus have varying levels of ISA, insertion of a methylene group between the phenyl-ring and the amide substituent significantly reduces this property. Interestingly, extension of a spacer beyond one methylene group

Anesthetized rats (beta-blocking activity) ⟶ Anesthetized cats (beta-blocking selectivity: cardiac versus vascular) ⟶ Guinea pigs (beta-blocking selectivity: cardiac versus bronchial)

⟶ Anesthetized rats (ISA) ⟶ Frog sciatic nerve (MSA)

Scheme 19.21 Biological screening sequence utilized by ICI during the discovery of atenolol **72**. ISA = Intrinsic (beta-agonist) activity. MSA = Membrane stabilizing (local anesthetic) activity. Note the use of an *in vivo* model for the front-line screen, as well as thereafter.

leads to a fall-off in inherent activity. Finally, although additional substituents can be present on the phenyl-ring, these are best tolerated when placed in an ortho-relationship to the ether rather than when in a meta-relationship, the latter perhaps reflecting steric interference with the hydrogen-bonding role that the amide wants to play.

19.3.2.2 Accumulated Structure-Activity Relationships

Although X-ray diffraction and/or detailed NMR studies are still not yet available to allow for explicit structure-based drug design or for precise topographical maps from which to orient SAR data, conceptual models based upon the known amino acid sequences for these well-established G-protein-coupled receptors are available. In this regard, the beta-2 receptor has received the most attention and its models can be used to assist in categorizing SAR that pertains to beta-receptors in general. Taking this approach, three principal binding domains need to be considered, namely an aromatic region, a specific interaction with the alkyl-hydroxy group, and a likely ionic bond area since the amino group is thought to be protonated during receptor interaction. These three pharmacophoric elements are shown within the generalized beta-blocker structure **73** in Figure 19.24 as bolded atoms in the ring, and as enlarged and bolded atoms on the oxypropanol side-chain.

The key atoms in **73** should be considered to be discretely displayed in 3D space via the oxypropyl-connecting chain, so as to be able to dynamically occupy a specified residence within the beta-receptor pocket after mutual molding, rather than to be merely residing in a static manner on the rigid plane that becomes defined by three points. For example, in the prior background section a surprising enhancement in beta-blocking potency occurred when an oxymethylene unit was inserted into the ethyl connecting chain that characterizes the endogenous agonists. From this, two salient SAR features should be emphasized. This can be done by also referring to two model structures, namely **74** and **75**, shown side-by-side.

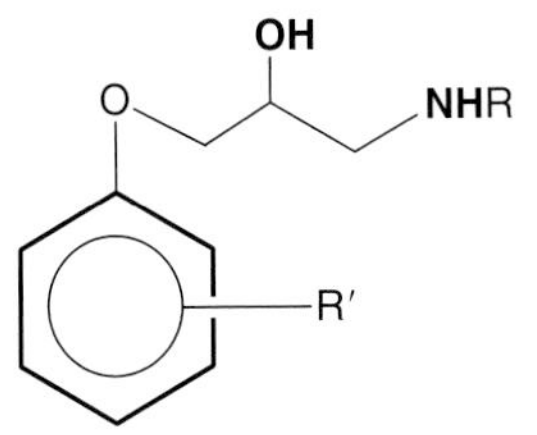

OH NHR O R′ 73

Figure 19.24 Generalized beta-blocker structure. The three key pharmacopheric components are shown as bolded and enlarged atoms, namely the phenyl-ring, the beta-hydroxy-group, and the amino-group. The amino-group is thought to be protonated during receptor interaction.

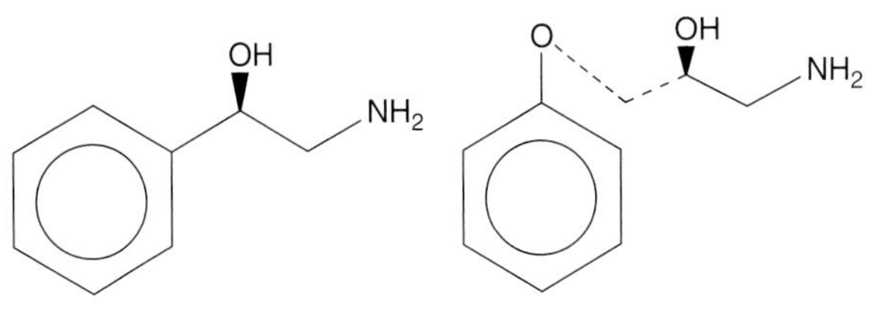

OH NH_2 74   O OH NH_2 75

First, as suggested by computational studies, the oxypropanolamine system present in **75** can adopt a conformation that places its hydroxy and amino groups into nearly the same 3D space relative to the aryl moiety, as that occupied by the ethanolamine system's analogous groups relative to **74**'s aryl moiety. Second, it is clear that in both cases, the hydroxyl-group resides in the same spatial orientation relative to the asymmetric carbon present in each system, namely (R)-**74** and (S)-**75**, where the designated switch from (R) to (S) reflects only a switch in the nomenclature-associated group priorities made during their assignments; that is, the C-O ether group present in **75** gains nomenclature priority over the C-N amino group that is present in both structures even though all these groups are still displayed in identical 3D space. Coupled with these chemical findings is the biological observation that while the (R)-arylethanolamine and (S)-aryloxypropanolamine systems produce active beta-receptor ligands, their enantiomeric counterparts are essentially inactive, being comparable to when no hydroxyl-group is present. Likewise, attempts to substitute the secondary hydroxyl group with other functionality that can form hydrogen bonds either as a donor, acceptor, or both have proven to be highly detrimental for activity.

Referring again to **73**, it is interesting to note that although these secondary amines show good activity as beta-blockers, neither primary or tertiary amines exhibit much activity, the primary amines likely being subject to rapid metabolism and the tertiary amines being outright unacceptable to the receptor. In terms of selectivity, although the oxypropanolamine system itself serves to reduce binding with alpha-receptors, it can be noted further that in general, as the steric bulk of R is increased, interaction with alpha-receptors is decreased while interaction with beta-receptors is increased. The latter is presumably due to association with an auxiliary lipophilic binding pocket lying adjacent to an ionized Asp (e.g., Asp 113 in the beta-2 receptor) residue that is thought to form an ionic bond with the protonated amine. Steric bulk near the amine also avoids the rapid metabolic degradation alluded to earlier, namely by Monoamine Oxidase (MAO). Likewise, steric bulk in this area helps to retard CYP450-mediated oxidative dealkylations. The N-dealkylation metabolic pathways commonly encountered by aryloxpropanolamines are the same as those for the arylethanolamine systems as shown in the prior Scheme 19.7. The importance of having a bulky R group to minimize these pathways is apparent.

For the last pharmacophoric element, a simple phenyl ring is all that's needed to serve as the aromatic system. However, when a phenyl ring is not further substituted (e.g., R′ = H in **73**), the compounds also demonstrate significant partial agonist effects or ISA. The latter is probably due to uptake into the presynaptic neuron followed by release of norepinephine, an indirect rather than a direct receptor-related mechanism, although this has yet to be established in a definitive manner. Interestingly, substitution with just about anything in any location on the ring appears to eliminate ISA, with the exceptions, of course, being the placement of an alcohol in the 3′ or 4′ position or of bioisosteric functionality that mimics one or the other of the endogenous sympathomimetic amines' two phenolic hydroxyl groups that constitute the catechol moiety. Once R′ groups are placed on the phenyl-ring, the following distinct trend is observed repeatedly as we move from the ortho- to meta- to the para-positions: decreased potency overall but significantly more so on beta-2 receptors. Thus, para-substituted systems generally yield weaker but more beta-1 selective beta-blockers. Multiple substitution on the ring can lead to variable effects and in some cases has proven to be quite useful.

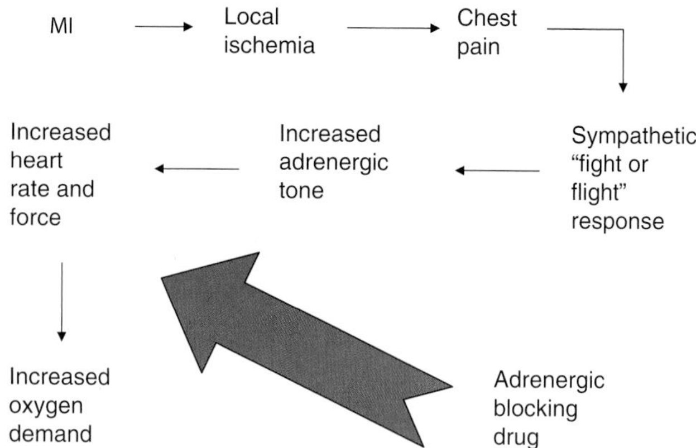

Figure 19.25 Pathophysiology of acute myocardial infarction (MI) and its potential treatment with a beta-adrenergic receptor blocking agent. Note that the body's natural fight-or-flight response can exacerbate the ischemic (low oxygen) damage during an MI because it increases the cardiac muscles' demand for oxygen. Alternatively, by attenuating heart rate and force, a beta-blocker drug may be able to preserve cardiac tissue because oxygen demand will also be reduced.

19.3.2.3 Esmolol Stat

As conveyed earlier, the clinical success of propranolol, **2**, served to establish it as the pioneer drug from which numerous companies undertook analog-based drug discovery to pursue additional compounds having enhanced pharmacological profiles. For most cardiac indications, the preferred profile typically sought was:

- Selectivity for beta-1 receptors over alpha- and beta-2 receptors
- Low partial agonist or intrinsic sympathomimetic activity (ISA)
- Low membrane depressant or stabilizing activity (MSA)
- A long duration of action conducive to once-a-day dosing

One cardiac indication that was particularly appealing involved the potential emergency treatment of heart attacks or acute myocardial infarctions (MIs). This seemingly ideal situation for using beta-blockers is depicted in Figure 19.25. Within the setting of MI, however, the full-scale adoption of beta blockers to preserve ischemic cardiac tissue by lowering the heart's energy and oxygen requirements was accompanied by considerable reservation. This is because a sickened cardiac muscle oftentimes has to rely upon beta-1 adrenergic drive to sustain its otherwise inherent contractility. Indeed, the early use of beta-1 blockers had occasionally resulted in heart-block and even death. Thus, in this case the clinical challenge became the need for an effective level of drug-induced beta-receptor antagonism to be finely balanced against the need to have a critical level of inherent, endogenous-driven beta-agonism, with the combination in a dynamic state of flux associated with an emergency situation where the precise level of adrenergic tone across the heart is very difficult to ascertain.

From this backdrop, in the late 1970s Arnar-Stone Laboratories, whose niche, strategic focus was directed toward emergency medications, set out to discover a beta-blocker compound that could be used safely in the critical setting of MI. It was clear that the desired balance between inherent adrenergic tone and its antagonism could be best achieved and continually adjusted by titrating the beta blocker's effects against some readily measurable parameter of cardiac function like heart rate. Thus, an ultra-short acting compound (e.g., with half-life of about 10 minutes) that could be administered by the intravenous (IV) route was called for. Not only could the level of blockade be adjusted for the compound, if it was given in too large an amount for a given patient, its ultra-short duration would allow for the antagonistic effects to be quickly removed by simply stopping the IV infusion. Interestingly, another pioneer drug served as an additional starting point to pursue an ultra-short acting compound. As shown in Scheme 19.22, procaine, **51**, is an ultra-short acting anesthetic agent that is rapidly deactivated by esterase-mediated hydrolysis because its aryl (**51a**) and amino (**51b**) pharmacophoric elements become severed from their requisite contiguous arrangement.

Combining these two pioneer drugs, namely **2** for its efficacy and **51** for its ultra-short duration, resulted in the target compound **76**. By analogy to procaine, it was anticipated that metabolic hydrolysis of the ester within **76** would fragment the requisite beta blocker pharmacophore and rapidly deactivate these types of compounds. This unique situation is depicted in Scheme 19.23.

Because an ester linkage had been incorporated within the oxypropanol connecting chain, these types of target molecules were called internal esters. SAR from the literature suggested that an increase in the oxypropyl chain's length by one carbon did not dramatically alter the interaction with beta receptors. Unfortunately, however, these types of structures proved difficult to synthesize, owing in part to their

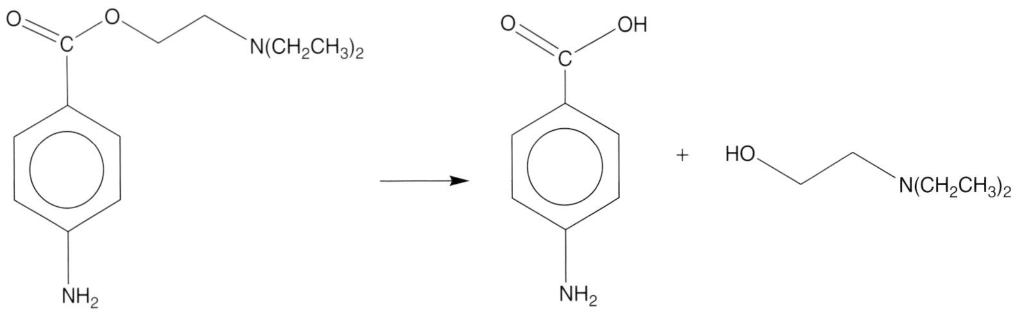

$N(CH_2CH_3)_2$ OH HO $N(CH_2CH_3)_2$

NH_2 NH_2

51 51a 51b

Scheme 19.22 Metabolic hydrolysis of procaine, **51**. Esterases convert **51** into two inactive fragments **51a** and **51b**. Since this process is accomplished very rapidly in the body by these ubiquitous enzymes, procaine exhibits an ultra-short duration of action (USA) after intravenous administration.

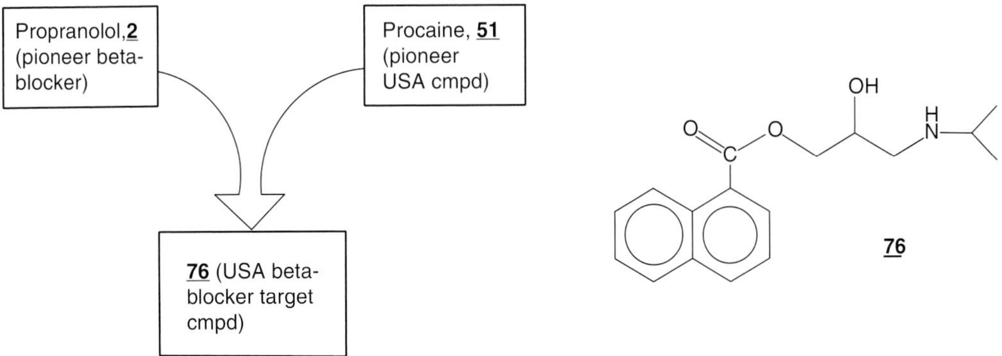

Scheme 19.23 Unique starting point for the rational design of beta blockers containing an internal ester moiety as shown in **76**. USA: ultra-short-acting; cmpd: compound.

propensity to undergo rapid side-product reactions that become problematic whenever the amine is not protonated.

Although these side-product problems eventually would be solved, at this early point in esmolol's history an alternate chemical strategy was proposed. By virtue of their lipophilic nature, it was assumed that the aryl and typical N-aliphatic substituent groups interacted with the beta-receptor in a hydrophobic manner, or within a pocket that at least preferred lipophilic groups. Thus, while the presence of an ester placed in either of these areas of the parent drug molecule might still be tolerated, the acid resulting from hydrolysis, upon further ionization at physiological pH accompanied by solvation with water molecules, should not be well tolerated. The new target molecules are shown as **77** and **78**. Since their ester moieties had now been placed outside of the requisite beta-blocking pharmacore, these compounds were called aryl-external esters and N-external esters, respectively. It is important to emphasize that this critical aspect of the overall strategy pertaining to the discovery of esmolol was based exactly upon the stated lipophilic versus hydrophilic hypothesis, and that it had nothing to do with the metabolism observed by others for various beta-blockers or with any resemblance to external amide appendages as present in practolol.

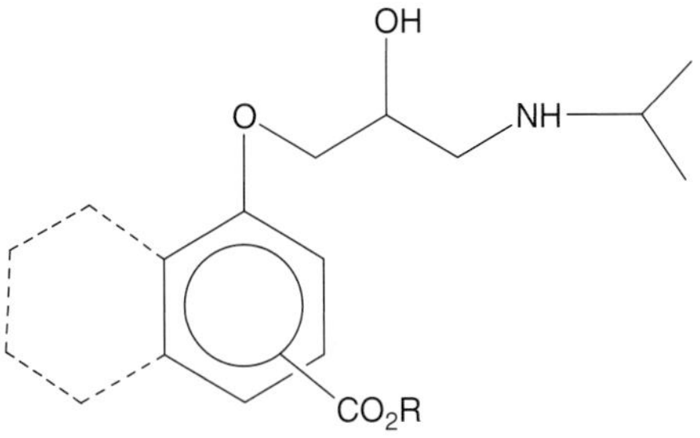

OH O NH CO_2R

77

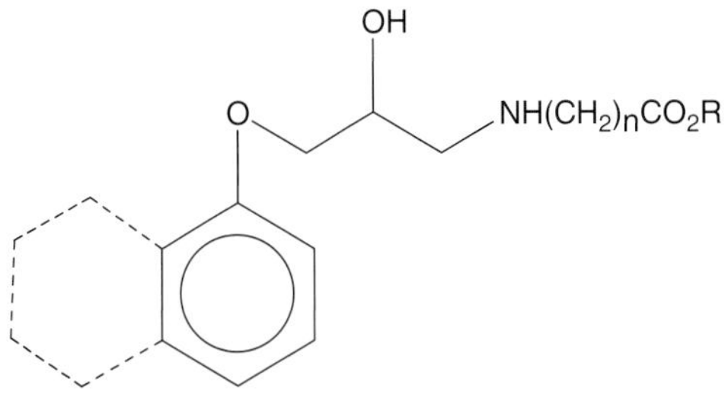

OH O $NH(CH_2)_nCO_2R$

78

Although **78** provided certain synthetic challenges in terms of controlling the degree of N-alkylation, several representatives for both series were prepared reasonably quickly. Interestingly, the resulting increase in the overall lipophilicity for these types of esters when first placed on a naphthyl system analogous to **2** (shown as dotted-line aryl systems), proved to lower aqueous solubility to the point that biological assessment became problematic. Thus, the single, phenyl-ring system was immediately explored as an alternative that provided an aryl pharmacophoric element with much less of an effect toward lowering overall aqueous solubility. However, when a single-ring system was unsubstituted, significant ISA became problematic. Given the earlier synthetic difficulties encountered with the internal esters ("strike one"), at this point the poor behavior toward testing encountered with the first, low-aqueous-solubility series immediately followed by the second, ISA-problem series of external esters ("strikes two and three") almost caused the entire ultra-short acting beta-blocker program to be dropped.

Finally, after quickly exploring a series of substituted phenyl rings to identify a suitable scaffold for use with the N-external ester targets, an ortho-methyl-phenyl ring was utilized for series **78** (**77**'s ring being inherently substituted via the ester placement was not showing problems with ISA). Importantly, in both **77** and **78**, these types of esters were found to retain their potency as beta blockers. Even more important for the hypothesis and novel design strategy, however, the carboxylic acid versions were found to be essentially inactive, just what was needed. As mentioned for **78**, a substituted phenyl-ring was required to eliminate ISA for the N-external esters, and in both **77** and **78** the effects of aromatic substitution followed the pattern where ortho-substituents enhanced potency greater than meta-substituents, which, in turn, were more active than those placed in a para-position. Furthermore, the fall-off in potency was much greater at beta-2 receptors than at beta-1 receptors. Thus, although the para-substituted series had lower potency overall, it was also much more beta-1 selective in its actions. This was analogous to the summary SAR recited earlier for non-USA beta blockers. Another important medicinal chemistry derived hypothesis stemming from these early observations was associated with a comparison of some of the initial aryl external ester compounds, namely **79** and **80**, as shown.

OH
O
NH
CO_2R

79 R = CH_3

80 R = CH_2CH_3

For **79** and **80**, the half-lives for beta-blocking activity in an *in vivo* dog model were found to be 30 minutes and 60 minutes, respectively. Assuming that this difference reflected simple steric effects, it was speculated that hydrolysis might be even quicker for esters placed further from the bulky phenyl ring. To address this hypothesis, compound series **81** was prepared. These compounds and their corresponding half-life data are shown in Figure 19.26. The "Goldilocks" nature of **81**, where the just-right half-life of 10 minutes is found only when n = 2, likely reflects the removal of the steric impediment caused by the aryl-ring. This further supports the hypothesis behind the design of this series. Likewise, the seeming paradox observed for **81** when n = 3 probably reflects conformational folding of the para-substituent so that its ester group tends to again reside closer to the overall bulk displayed by the entire aryloxypropanolamine system. Ultimately, the desired 10-minute half-life was reproduced in humans, and **81** where n = 2 became esmolol (also shown previously as **3**). Further illustrating the importance of the exquisite inverse relationship that was uncovered between enzymatic hydrolysis

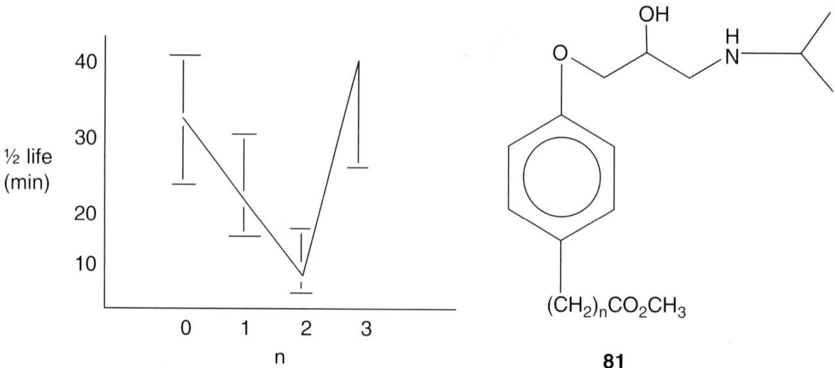

Figure 19.26 Correlation between biological half-life and added methylene units assessed by measuring 80% recovery from 50% beta-blockade of isoproternol-induced tachycardia after IV administration to anesthetized dogs (n = 5). Error bars indicate 1 SD from the mean. Note that when n = 0, then **81** = **79** and when n = 2, then **81** = **3** (esmolol).

rates and steric bulk, is the fact that all attempts to increase metabolic hydrolysis by the construction of good leaving group esters had only a negligible influence upon this process. Presumably, once Mother Nature is freed from steric constraints and gains access to a given site, she needs no further assistance toward lowering the transition state energy for effecting an enzymatic conversion.

19.3.2.4 Pharmacology and Clinical Profile of Esmolol

The required pharmacological profile as ultimately obtained by esmolol, **81** (n = 2), is depicted in Figure 19.27, which also clearly shows its superiority over propranolol, **2**, as an ultra-short acting agent. Upon IV infusion, esmolol quickly produces a pseudo-steady state of beta-blockade and when the infusion is stopped, the effects of esmolol rapidly disappear with a half-life of about 10 minutes. Alternatively, propranolol requires nearly two hours just to reach a pseudo-steady state of beta-blockade. It then dissipates only very slowly with a half-life of nearly four hours.

In the clinic, esmolol's distribution half-life is two minutes and its elimination half-life is nine minutes. According to its package insert, "esmolol hydrochloride is rapidly metabolized by hydrolysis of the ester linkage, chiefly by esterases in the cytosol of red blood cells and not by plasma cholinesterases or red cell membrane acetylcholinesterase." Its volume of distribution is 3.4 L/Kg and its total clearance is 285 mL/Kg/min "which is greater than cardiac output; thus the metabolism of esmolol is not limited by the rate of blood flow to metabolizing tissues such as the liver or affected by hepatic or renal blood flow." As expected from such a "high rate of blood-based metabolism, less than 2% of the drug is excreted unchanged in the urine." Within 24 hours after infusion, approximately 73 to 88% of the total dose can be accounted for in the urine as the acid metabolite. Esmolol is about 55% bound to plasma proteins, whereas the acid metabolite is only 10% bound. "The acid metabolite has been shown in animals to have about 1/1500 the activity of esmolol and in normal volunteers its blood levels do not correspond to [any significant] level of beta blockade. The acid metabolite has an elimination half-life of about 3.7 hours and is excreted in the urine with a clearance approximately equivalent to the glomerular filtration rate." The other metabolic by-product is methanol. Monitoring the latter in subjects receiving esmolol for up to six hours at 300 mcg/kg/min and 24 hours at 150 mcg/kg/min, approximated endogenous levels and were still less than 2% of those usually associated with methanol toxicity.

Esmolol is used to control adrenergic tone across the heart in emergency situations during critical care medicine of very young, as well as adult and elderly patients. It also finds use for alleviating the adrenergic-burst-prompted trauma that can be experienced during intubation prior to surgery. During the later stages of esmolol's clinical development, this type of drug (i.e., drugs having a deliberately appended functional group that is constructed to program a specified metabolic deactivation pathway and rate) came to be known as soft drugs, a phrase coined by Bodor who was working on similar technologies within an academic environment. Thus, in the end, esmolol itself has become the pioneer soft drug for which the template portrayed in bold-faced atoms can now serve as an effective starting point for soft analog-based drug discovery.

OH
O
NH
$CH_2CH_2CO_2CH_3$

Esmolol (**3**)

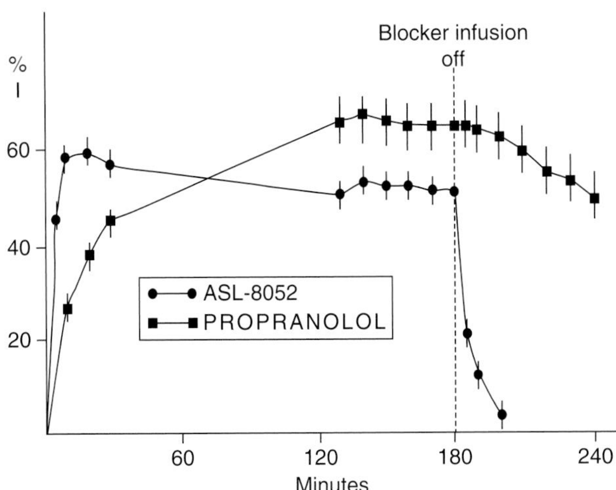

Figure 19.27 Three-hour intravenous infusion of esmolol versus propranolol in dogs (n = 5), where percentage inhibition (% I) of isoproterenol-induced tachycardia was measured against time (min). Error bars indicate 1 SD from the mean.

19.3.2.5 Summary

The discovery of esmolol took advantage of a combination of analog-based drug design from two different types of pioneer drugs, namely propranolol for efficacy and procaine for an ultra-short duration of action. However, a novel medicinal chemistry hypothesis led to a significant departure from procaine's internal ester structure and instead prompted the external ester arrangement. The latter, rational drug design approach eventually led to esmolol upon subsequent exploration of the relationship between enzymatic ester hydrolysis rates and steric factors. It can be noted that the rational design of esmolol simultaneously drew upon several of medicinal chemistry's basic science principles:

- Negative SAR, where it was envisioned that only lipophilic or, at most, moderately polar groups could be tolerated in the aryl-portion of the aryloxypropanolamine pharmacophore if activity was to be retained
- Electronic physicochemical properties operative within a biological matrix, where it was imagined that although an ester would be permissible in the aryl-portion (neutral SAR), a carboxylic acid moiety placed within the same aryl-portion would become too foreign to be recognized by β-adrenergic receptors upon ionization of the carboxylic acid at physiological pH
- General structure-metabolism relationships (SMR), where it was appreciated that an ester linkage might be relied upon to program a quick metabolism
- Steric physicochemical properties, where it was imagined that the metabolic hydrolysis rate could be quickened by extending the initial ester linkages away from the bulky aryl-group such that the sterically unhindered methyl 3-arylpropionate metabophore was finally identified
- Appreciation for the physiologic, drug excretion structural relationship (SER), where there is a general propensity to excrete low-molecular-weight acids, probably via the Organic Anionic Transporters (thus itself a useful transportophore relationship for excretion)

These are all fundamental physical organic principles applied in a straightforward manner within very specific contexts of the biological realm. Indeed, many of the hurdles traversed during the discovery of esmolol provide useful lessons for today's medicinal chemists who often become immersed in problems associated with a lead compound's overall pharmacokinetic profile. Taken together, the various aspects of this case study convey the important roles that analog-based drug design and rational-based drug design can play toward contributing to fundamental (basic science) medicinal chemistry principles, as well as toward the practical improvement or specified tailoring (applied science) of selected therapeutic entities (Figure 19.6).

19.3.3 Into Today and the Future for HTS of Compound Libraries (Anti-AIDS Drugs)

This case study has been adapted from its original version, written by Proudfoot, which previously appeared within the recent edition of the series entitled *Comprehensive Medicinal Chemistry* (Erhardt and Proudfoot 2006). Despite the noted decrease in recent NCEs (Figure 19.1), one area where implementation of modern technology has been enormously successful has been in the discovery of drugs to treat acquired immune deficiency syndrome (AIDS). Many of the new drugs in this area have come from the application of HTS and structure-based drug design approaches, with advances in molecular biology providing the molecular assays used to drive many of the medicinal chemistry efforts. Interestingly, since drugs for the treatment of AIDS typically have been approved more rapidly than is usual, it is possible that the success in this particular area serves to presage what we can also expect to see in the coming years as these newer technologies are further applied to the discovery process across various other therapeutic classes.

Although the earliest cases of AIDS occurred in the 1950s, the first documented cases came to the attention of the U.S. Centers for Disease Control (CDC) in 1981. Within just a few years it was discovered that AIDS is caused by a retrovirus, subsequently named human immunodeficiency virus type 1 (HIV-1). By 1985 there were 12,000 new cases and 7000 deaths from AIDS in the United States. In 2004, the World Health Organization (WHO) estimated that over 30 million people were infected with the AIDS virus worldwide and that 20 million people had died from AIDS since the start of the epidemic. Major drug discovery efforts were soon launched to identify antiviral agents to combat the disease. Arising mostly within big pharma, this drug discovery effort coincided with dramatic changes in the technologies and science available for medicinal chemistry. Thus, an overview of this area becomes particularly instructive with regard to the impact of these new technologies on modern drug discovery.

19.3.3.1 Background

HIV-1 invades and destroys the CD4 positive cells of the immune system. Like other retroviruses, the life cycle requires incorporation of viral genetic material into the host genome. Subsequent transcription and translation events generate virus progeny. Release of the new virus particles is fatal to the host CD4 positive cell. A gradual depletion of immune cells occurs over a period of years and compromises the immune response to the extent that infections that normally would be relatively benign can become life threatening and deadly.

Drug discovery efforts have focused on interfering with the various processes in the virus life cycle. As a retrovirus, the genetic material of HIV-1 is RNA. Two enzymes not found in human cells, Reverse Transcriptase (RT) and Integrase, are essential for incorporating the information from this genetic material into the host genome. RT has multiple catalytic activities, namely an RNA Dependent DNA Polymerase, a DNA Dependent DNA Polymerase, and an RNA Hydrolase. It transforms the virus RNA into double-stranded DNA. Subsequently, this viral DNA is incorporated into the host genome by the Integrase enzyme. After transcription provides new viral RNA and the template for the synthesis of new virus proteins, the activity of one additional virus enzyme, HIV Protease, is essential for the production of new, infectious viral progeny. To date, the Reverse Transcriptase enzyme (RT) and the protease enzyme have proven to be the most druggable targets in the virus life cycle and have yielded most of the drugs currently used to combat the virus and treat AIDS. More recently, effective inhibitors of the Integrase enzyme have been discovered and some have proceeded to clinical evaluation. There has also been success in targeting the processes required for the virus to recognize and enter host cells with one FDA-approved polypeptide drug acting by this mechanism and several small molecule clinical candidates under evaluation.

Some of the first efforts to identify anti-HIV agents involved assaying molecules for the prevention of virus replication in cell culture. Zidovudine (AZT) (**82** in Figure 19.28) is the first antiviral drug approved for the treatment of AIDS and it was discovered by this approach. The discovery process represents an example of knowledge and experience-based drug discovery similar to the esmolol case study previously provided. Analogs of the natural nucleosides have been used successfully for many years in the clinic as antiviral agents (e.g., acyclovir or **83** in Figure 19.28). AZT, first synthesized in the mid-1960s, was known to possess anticancer and antiviral properties, and in 1985 was demonstrated to have activity against HIV-1 replication in cell culture. AZT is an analog of the endogenous nucleoside deoxythymidine (**84** in Figure 19.28) and so it is converted by endogenous kinases into the active triphosphate derivative, which is recognized by RT and incorporated into the growing strand of viral DNA. However, because AZT lacks the 3′-OH group necessary for the attachment of additional nucleotides, further elongation of the DNA is impossible and the viral replication cycle is disrupted. AZT, **82**, proved effective in the clinic in suppressing the virus and prolonging the life of AIDS patients and was approved in 1987.

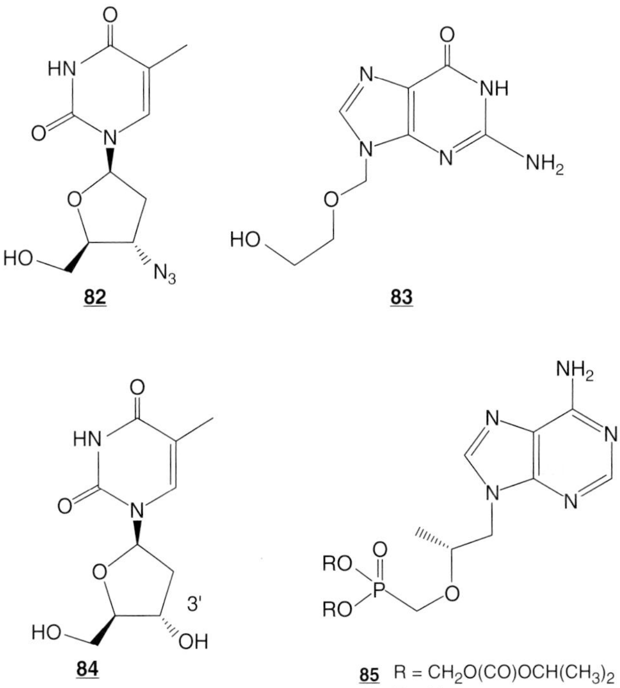

HN O O N O HO N3 82

N NH N N NH2 O HO 83

HN O O N O 3' HO OH 84

NH2 N N N N RO O P RO O

85 R = $CH_2O(CO)OCH(CH_3)_2$
86 R = H

Figure 19.28 Zidovudine or AZT (**82**) and related nucleoside analogs. An early nucleoside analog antiviral drug, acyclovir **83**, and the endogenous nucleoside deoxythymidine **84**, from which **82** was designed are also shown. Tenofovir disoproxil, **85**, is an orally bioavailable prodrug of tenofovir, **86**, which was also designed from **83**. (With permission from Proudfoot.)

The discovery of AZT as an effective therapeutic agent validated RT as a target in the virus life cycle and several additional nucleoside analogs that act in a similar manner have since been approved. They are analogs of the endogenous nucleosides with deoxythymidine and deoxycytosine representing the pyrimidines, and deoxyadenosine and deoxyguanosine representing the purines. In addition to lacking the 2′-OH group making them by definition deoxy nucleosides, all lack the 3′-OH group of the natural nucleosides that is necessary for DNA strand elongation. All resemble the endogenous nucleosides, and this structural similarity to the natural substrates is required since they must be recognized not only by RT but also by the kinases that first transform them into the active triphosphates.

Since the first phosphorylation step that produces the nucleoside monophosphates is the slow step in the activation of nucleoside analogs, it was also suspected that the monophosphate derivatives might be more effective therapeutic agents. However, phosphates as drug substances have two major liabilities: metabolic instability due to the action of phosphatase enzymes and poor cell permeability due to the two negative charges which then result at physiological pH. The design of tenofovir disoproxil, **85** in Figure 19.28, provided a creative solution to both of these issues. Susceptibility to phosphatase activity was solved by incorporation of a noncleavable phosphonate moiety (note the phosphorous-carbon bond rather than a phosphorous oxygen bond) appended to a modified sugar ring system also precedented by acyclovir, to give tenofovir, **86**. Although this provided proof of concept in the clinic (mechanistic validation) it was not orally bioavailable and could be delivered only by the IV route. To achieve oral bioavailability and cellular penetration, the phosphonate group was modified to **85**, which is a double ester prodrug (Scheme 19.13) that is rapidly cleaved by intracellular esterases to give **86**.

After its approval in 1987, it became apparent that prolonged use of AZT (and indeed any other anti-AIDS drug) as a monotherapeutic agent results in a resistant virus. RT lacks the transcriptional fidelity of mammalian DNA polymerases and no correction/editing features are involved in virus replication. Transcriptional errors occur at a rate as high as 1 per 2000 bases transcribed. Thus, several mutations may be introduced during each replication cycle and the virus can be described as a quasispecies with many variants present at any time. Given the facility with which mutations may be generated, it was clear that agents from a single therapeutic class would probably not be sufficient to suppress the virus indefinitely and prevent disease progression. Additionally, since nucleoside inhibitors are analogs of natural cellular components, they have the potential to interact with endogenous DNA polymerase enzymes. Some of the toxicities seen with AZT and other nucleoside analogs are thought to arise from their lack of selectivity. Therefore, many efforts were subsequently directed toward identifying structurally and mechanistically novel RT inhibitors. Whereas the discovery efforts in the area of nucleoside inhibitors can be characterized as a rational-based analog approach to drug design, the identification of nonnucleoside reverse transcriptase inhibitors (NNRTIs) hinged on the success of HTS to generate novel lead structures.

19.3.3.2 Today's Approaches

As mentioned in the previous sections of this chapter, over the past decade HTS technology has advanced to the extent that hundreds of thousand of compounds can be screened in a short period of time. The drugs shown in Scheme 19.24 came from earlier screening campaigns involving the evaluation of hundreds or perhaps thousands of compounds per month. They constitute early examples of the impact of HTS on the drug discovery process. Three successfully launched NNRTI drugs, nevirapine, delavirdine, and efavirenz, shown respectively as **87**, **88** and **89** in Scheme 19.24, as well as numerous additional clinical candidates, arose from these compound library-based screening campaigns.

The three efforts that resulted in drugs all dealt with similar issues during compound optimization. As is expected for hit optimization beginning from HTS-derived structures, improvement in potency was a common first goal. In contrast to the nucleoside inhibitors described earlier, the nonnucleoside inhibitors were generally first optimized for inhibition of RT in a molecular assay and then tested for antiviral activity in cell culture assays. In addition to improving potency and in line with the earlier discussions within this chapter that relate to the challenges of addressing inadequate PK and ADMET-related properties, attaining metabolic stability (and also chemical stability in the case of the efavirenz lead structure) proved to be critical. Optimization of the efavirenz lead structure also required replacement of a metabolically labile thiourea motif. The first NNRTI inhibitor class described in the literature, namely tivirapine (structure not shown), contained a similar thiourea motif, and although these molecules proceeded into clinical study, they failed to progress beyond Phase I.

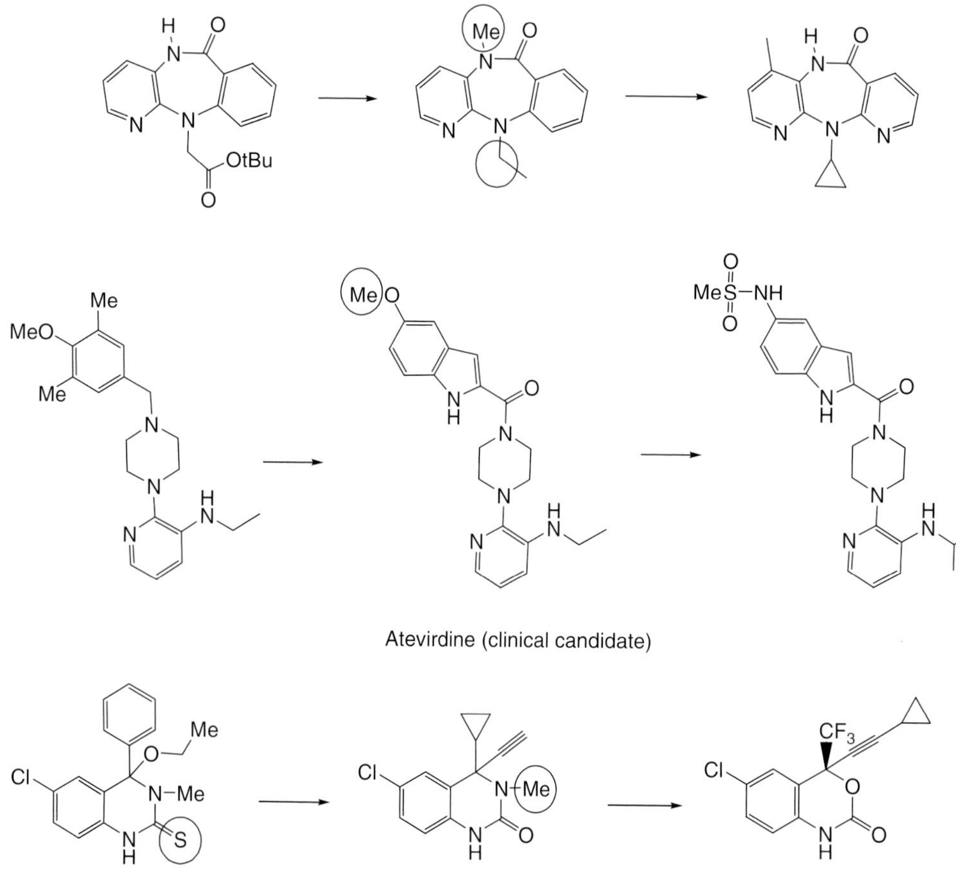

87

88

Atevirdine (clinical candidate)

89

Scheme 19.24 Non-nucleoside reverse transcriptase inhibitors (NNRTIs): Nevirapine **87**; Delavirdine **88**; and Efavirenz **89**. Circled portions of lead structures represent areas having problematic metabolism that were addressed during continued optimization to achieve the final drug compounds. (With permission from Proudfoot.)

One remarkable feature of the nonnucleoside RT inhibitors when compared to their nucleoside counterparts is the selectivity they exhibit for HIV-1 RT compared to HIV-2 RT. They are typically inactive against HIV-2 RT whereas nucleoside inhibitors (as their triphosphates) are usually equally effective against both enzymes. Efforts to understand this phenomenon involved biophysical and structural studies to identify the binding site occupied by NNRTIs. Biochemical studies showed that the NNRTIs are noncompetitive inhibitors of RT, thus indicating that they do not compete with substrates at the enzyme active site. Photoaffinity labeling experiments identified two tyrosine residues, namely tyrosines 181 and 188 as components of the NNRTI binding site. In sequence, these tyrosine residues are close to aspartic acid residues 185 and 186, which constitute part of the enzyme active site. Subsequently, cocrystal X-ray pictures of RT with nevirapine (Figure 19.29) and with other inhibitors provided a more detailed structural perspective on the interactions of the NNRTIs and RT.

The NNRTIs all bind to the same hydrophobic pocket on the enzyme and moderate the activity of RT through inhibition of a neighboring (allosteric) site that serves as a metabolic controlling unit to switch on the enzyme's activity. A comparison of the HIV-1 and HIV-2 protein sequences in the region of the binding pocket helped to rationalize the different efficacy of NNRTIs against HIV-1 and HIV-2. Sequence information showed positions 181 and 188, which contain tyrosine residues in HIV-1 RT are occupied by isoleucine and leucine residues in HIV-2 RT. Site-directed mutagenesis (SDM) studies confirmed that mutation of even the single amino acid tyrosine 188 in HIV-1 RT to leucine 188 abolished the effects of the drug nevirapine. These mutagenesis studies were the precursor to cell passaging studies of the wild-type virus in the presence of nevirapine that generated resistant virus carrying the mutation Y181C (tyrosine to cysteine at amino acid residue position 181) in HIV-1 RT. This ready generation of resistant virus was confirmed for nevirapine in the clinic. Unfortunately, this meant that the drug likely could not be used as a monotherapeutic agent. However, subsequent clinical studies showed that nevirapine and other NNRTIs are effective antiviral agents when used in combination with nucleoside or protease inhibitors. Although structural information on RT was available at an early stage, it was not a driving force in the design of the first generation NNRTI compounds. It did, however, allow for a better understanding of resistance at the molecular level. Even though mutations conferring resistance may be far apart in the primary sequence of the protein sequence, when the mutations are mapped on to the 3D X-ray structure of the enzyme, they all cluster around either the NNRTI binding pocket or regions important for substrate binding.

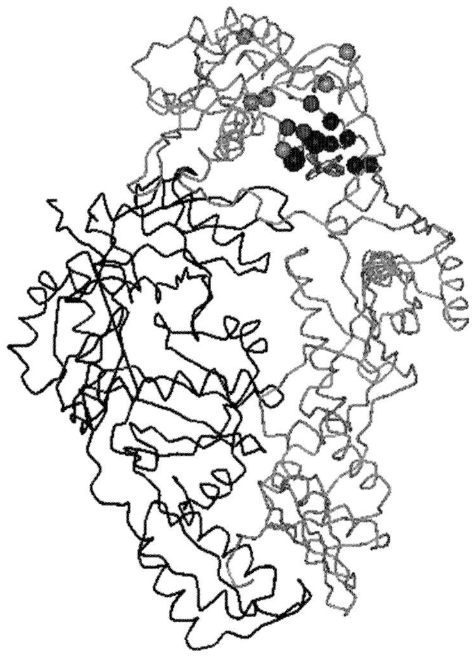

Figure 19.29 X-ray diffraction picture of nevirapine (**87**) bound to HIV-1 reverse transcriptase (RT). The alpha-carbons of the key aspartic acid residues of the active site are represented by red spheres. The blue spheres represent sites of mutation that confer resistance to nevirapine and other NNRTI drugs (the larger blue spheres represent the positions of tyrosines 181 and 188). The orange spheres represent sites that confer resistance to nucleoside inhibitors. See text for additional discussion. (With permission from Proudfoot.)

The ready emergence of resistance to NNRTIs is a consequence of the relative inefficiency of RT mentioned earlier and the fact that the NNRTI binding pocket can accommodate many different amino acid side-chain changes and still yield a functional enzyme. Efforts to design second-generation, more effective NNRTIs have focused on attaining efficacy against many of the resistant mutant RT enzymes along with the wild-type enzyme. The ability to generate and provide mutant enzymes for molecular assays and for structural studies has been an enabling force for compound optimization and would not have been possible without the techniques of modern molecular biology. Requirements for second-generation PK properties conducive to once-a-day dosing and compatibility of compounds with multidrug regimens soon became important issues as well. Indeed these two features have become a critical part of all current AIDS drug discovery efforts. Since patients often take many drugs as part of a therapeutic regimen, any drug features that accommodate patient compliance lessen the likelihood for emergence of resistant virus. There are several new drugs currently under evaluation as second-generation NNRTIs. Of interest here because it returns to the early roots of medicinal chemistry (Section 19.1.2.1) is calanolide A, which was discovered through bioassay directed fractionation of a tropical rainforest tree organic extract.

Shown as **90**, it is the only unmodified natural product currently progressing in the clinic as a treatment of AIDS.

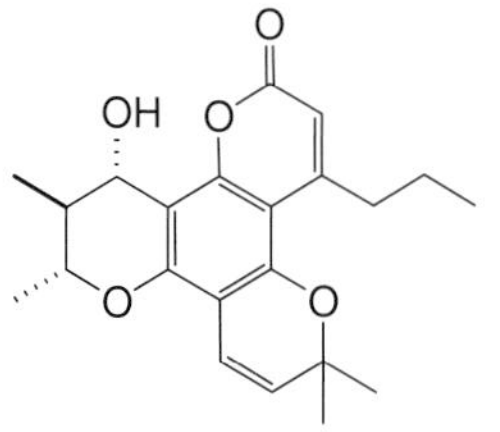

In contrast to these successes in the RT inhibitor area that were enabled through analog-based discovery approaches and HTS, success in the area of HIV-1 Protease inhibitors has been achieved mostly through rational, structure-based drug design (Table 19.2). Early confusion about the mechanism of action of HIV-1 Protease was clarified when it was recognized that the enzyme is an Aspartic Protease (Table 19.5) and functions as a dimer. The first X-ray crystal structures were published in 1987. This information, in combination with an experience base in the drug discovery community targeting other proteases (particularly the Aspartic Protease, Renin), laid the foundation for success in the area of HIV-1 Protease inhibitor design. Alternatively, enzyme structural information was not a factor in the design of the first protease inhibitor to reach the market, namely saquinavir shown as **91** in Scheme 19.25. This drug was derived from a ligand-based drug design strategy (Table 19.2) where peptidic substrates were modified to incorporate noncleavable peptide bond bioisosteres in order to attain potent enzyme inhibition. As shown in Scheme 19.25, incorporation of a hydroxyethylene peptide bond surrogate (bioisostere) into the substrate analog gave the lead structure with moderate potency against the protease (IC_{50} of 140 nM). Stepwise modification of the western and eastern sides of the lead structure led to significant improvements in potency and ultimately, combination of the preferred modifications gave saquinavir. Several additional marketed protease inhibitors, like nelfinavir, amprenavir, and atazanavir (structures not shown), also incorporate the hydroxyethylene bioisostere. One of these, amprenavir, has additionally been developed as a phosphate prodrug that has improved solubility. The phosphate group is readily cleaved in the gut to release amprenavir for absorption.

In an alternative approach to lead generation, researchers at Abbott hypothesized that since the protease enzyme functions as a dimer possessing C2 symmetry, inhibitors could also be designed based partially on symmetry considerations. Modification of the symmetrical lead compound (Scheme 19.26) ultimately led, after two clinical candidate casualties, to ritonavir, **92**, which finally became an approved drug in 1996. Efforts to generate a second generation inhibitor based on ritonavir focused on addressing two issues: (1) achieving potency against resistant proteases where Val 82 in the active site is mutated and (2) attenuating the significant CYP450 inhibition seen with ritonavir (unwanted drug–drug interaction issues as discussed in this topic's previous chapter). Analysis of structure-based drug design information (e.g., Figure 19.30) indicated that the resistance of the mutant enzymes was due to interactions with the isopropyl group on the thiazole ring. Subsequent modification of the eastern region of ritonavir to incorporate a smaller heterocyclic system gave activity against the mutant enzymes. The CYP450 issue was localized to the western-side thiazole ring. Modification of this ring system to the dimethylphenylether gave lopinavir, **93,** as shown in Scheme 19.26. Interestingly, the CYP450 inhibition properties of ritonavir appear to make it a useful partner in various cocktail regimens of AIDS drugs. For drugs that are metabolized by CYP450, coadministration with ritonavir can provide a significant boosting of plasma levels and efficacy (intentional drug–drug interaction strategy). Lopinavir, for example, has been approved in a fixed-dose formulation with ritonavir (Kaletra).

Two HTS-based approaches also have been successful in generating effective protease inhibitors. Screening of a collection of Renin inhibitors at Merck provided a peptidic lead structure (Scheme 19.27), which was modified to produce indinavir, **94**, in a process that also involved the use of X-ray derived crystal structure information and competitor structural information as part of the optimization process. In comparison, screening at Upjohn provided warfarin as a low molecular weight hit compound. Evolution of this structure proceeded across two clinical candidates with increasing molecular complexity to finally yield tipranavir, **95**. This design effort was also guided significantly by the availability of X-ray-derived structural information.

19.3.3.3 Future Approaches

In addition to the marketed inhibitors of RT and HIV protease, researchers have recently been successful in generating inhibitors of the Integrase enzyme. This enzyme is responsible for incorporating the double-stranded DNA virus genetic material into the host genome and has always been a promising target for AIDS drug discovery. Since combined inhibition of RT and HIV Protease is the mainstay of current therapies, and drug combinations are superior to the actions of individual drugs alone, an effective inhibitor of other key targets in the life cycle could provide substantial therapeutic benefit. Like the RT enzyme, Integrase has no host counterpart and offers the potential for a selective and safe therapeutic mechanism. After many years of effort and the report of several unattractive structures as inhibitors, a series of ketoacid derivatives discovered through HTS was recently disclosed to effectively inhibit the enzyme (Scheme 19.28). Optimization of this lead structure, particularly with regard to the metabolically unstable ketoacid moiety, has yielded very effective *in vitro* inhibitors of the enzyme. A molecule with similar structural features, namely S-1360 or **96** in Scheme 19.28, has progressed to clinical trials. An X-ray diffraction picture of an analog of S-1360 bound to Integrase is provided in Figure 19.31. As with the other classes of AIDS therapeutics,

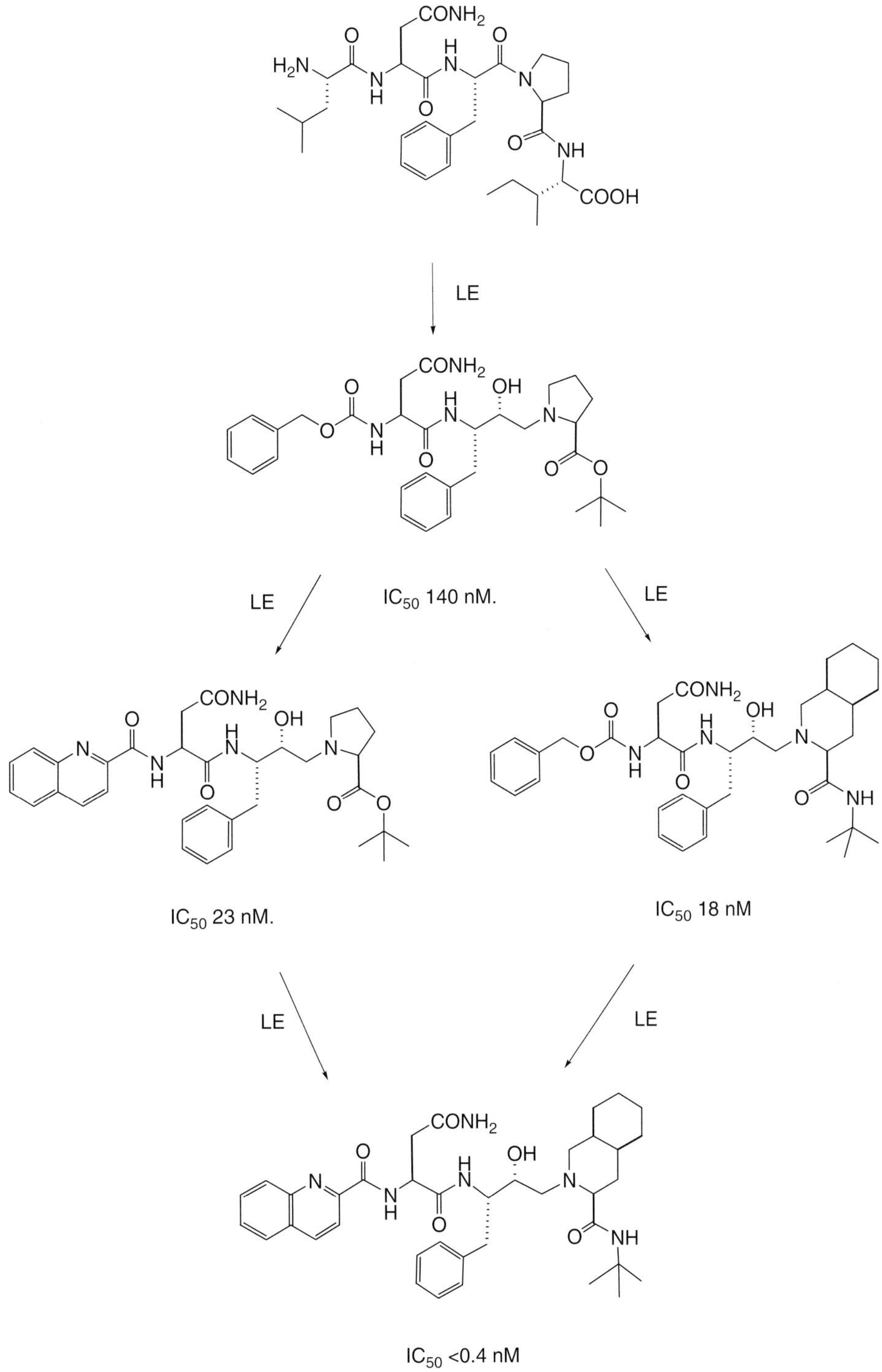

LE

IC_{50} 140 nM.

LE

LE

IC_{50} 23 nM.

IC_{50} 18 nM

LE

LE

IC_{50} <0.4 nM

91

Scheme 19.25 Molecular design strategies leading to a representative HIV-1 Protease inhibitor drug, namely saquinavir **91**. LE = Lead enhancement where synthesis of numerous analogs eventually led to the next depicted molecule. Note replacement of an initial peptidic linkage with a hydroxyl-ethylene bioisoster. The latter has also become a key functional group in many of the other newer HIV-1 Protease inhibitors. (With permission from Proudfoot.)

however, there is already evidence that therapeutic agents individually targeting Integrase will also be subject to resistance.

One additional area of AIDS drug discovery that has shown progress recently has been the field of viral entry inhibitors. The prototype proof of concept molecule for this class, enfuvirtide, has been approved for marketing. Enfuvirtide is a polypeptide derived from the C-terminal domain of the HIV-1 fusion protein, and prevents fusion of the virus with the cell and

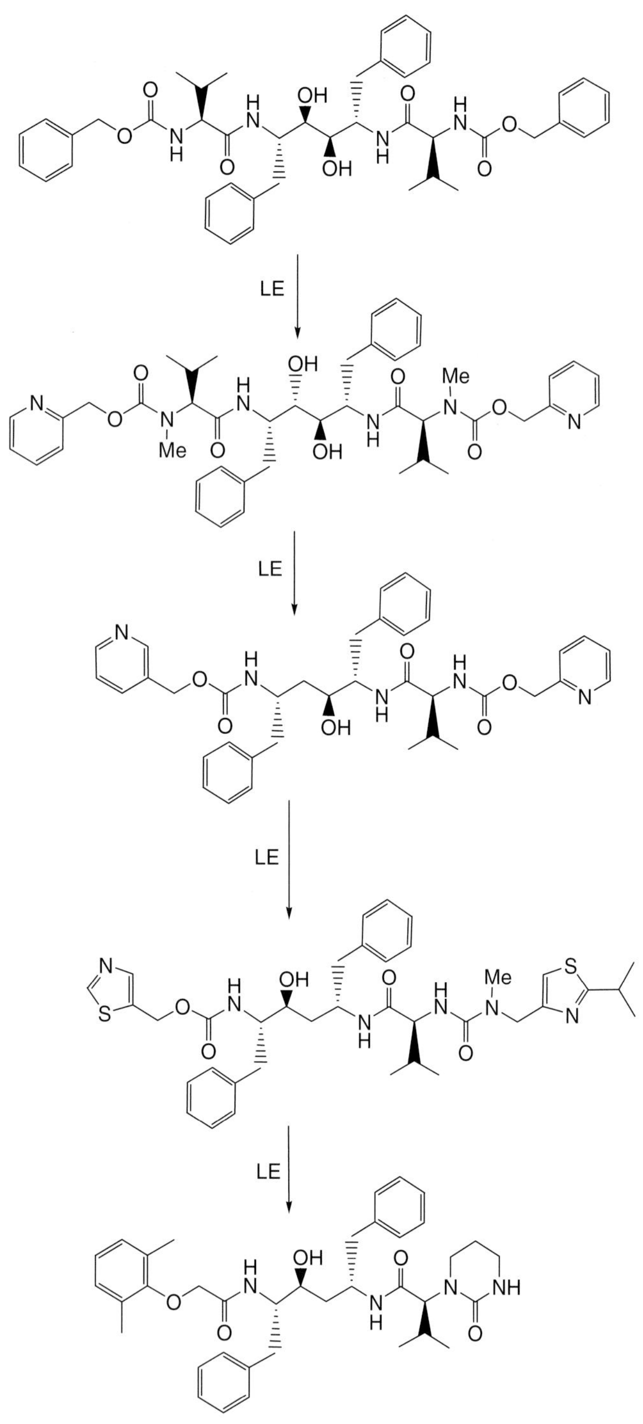

Lead structure

LE

Clinical candidate

LE

Clinical candidate
Better physical properties
Good oral bioavailability, low $t_{1/2}$ due to metabolism

LE

92

LE

93

Scheme 19.26 Dimeric molecular design strategy leading to two HIV-1 Protease inhibitor drugs, namely ritonavir, **92**, and lopinavir, **93**. LE = Lead enhancement wherein synthesis of numerous analogs eventually led to the next depicted molecule. Note that in this case two clinical candidate casualties were traversed in order to eventually obtain these successful drugs. (With permission from Proudfoot.)

subsequent entry. The drug is somewhat remarkable due to the fact that its synthesis requires 106 steps (99 on solid phase peptide support matrix). Although enfuvirtide did not come from a classical medicinal chemistry design effort, it provided evidence that prevention of virus entry constituted a validated therapeutic approach to combating HIV infection. More recently, additional opportunities for preventing virus entry were identified with the recognition that HIV-1 makes use of the chemokine coreceptors to enter cells. It is remarkable that in the relatively short period from this disclosure, chemokine receptor antagonists have already progressed from screening to clinical evaluation.

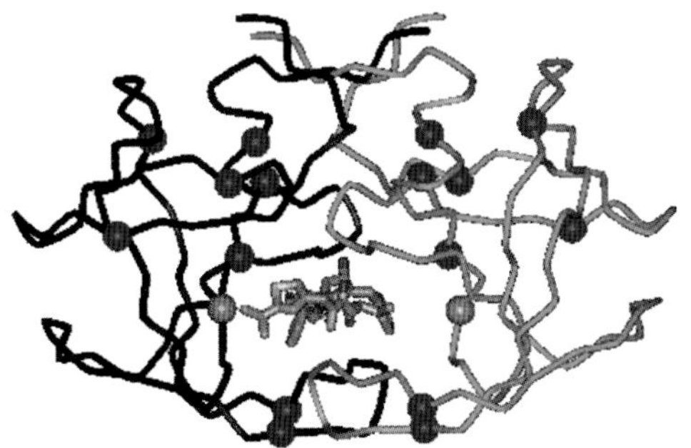

Figure 19.30 Ritonavir **92** bound to HIV Protease with resistance mutation sites also noted. The orange spheres represent the alpha-carbons of Val 82 and the blue spheres represent additional mutations in the protease enzyme that confer resistance to other protease inhibitors. The CYP450 issue was localized to the left-hand side thiazole ring. Modification of this ring system to the dimethylphenyl ether gave lopinavir. (With permission from Proudfoot.)

19.3.3.4 Summary

In the 20 years after recognizing that AIDS is caused by human immune deficiency virus, the drug discovery community has provided some 20 antiviral agents targeting various components of the virus life cycle. These drug discovery efforts have made use of historical knowledge, HTS of compound libraries, and structure-based drug design. All these strategies have been facilitated by advances in molecular biology. Significant ADMET hurdles have been addressed repeatedly by knowledge-driven SAR molecular modification. Finally, despite all the advanced technologies being implemented into today's drug discovery process, it is interesting to close this last case study by acknowledging that we can still become indebted to Mother Nature for supplying us with the just-right natural product that not only serves as an optimal lead compound, but may sometimes move all the way into the marketplace without additional modification (e.g., compound **90**).

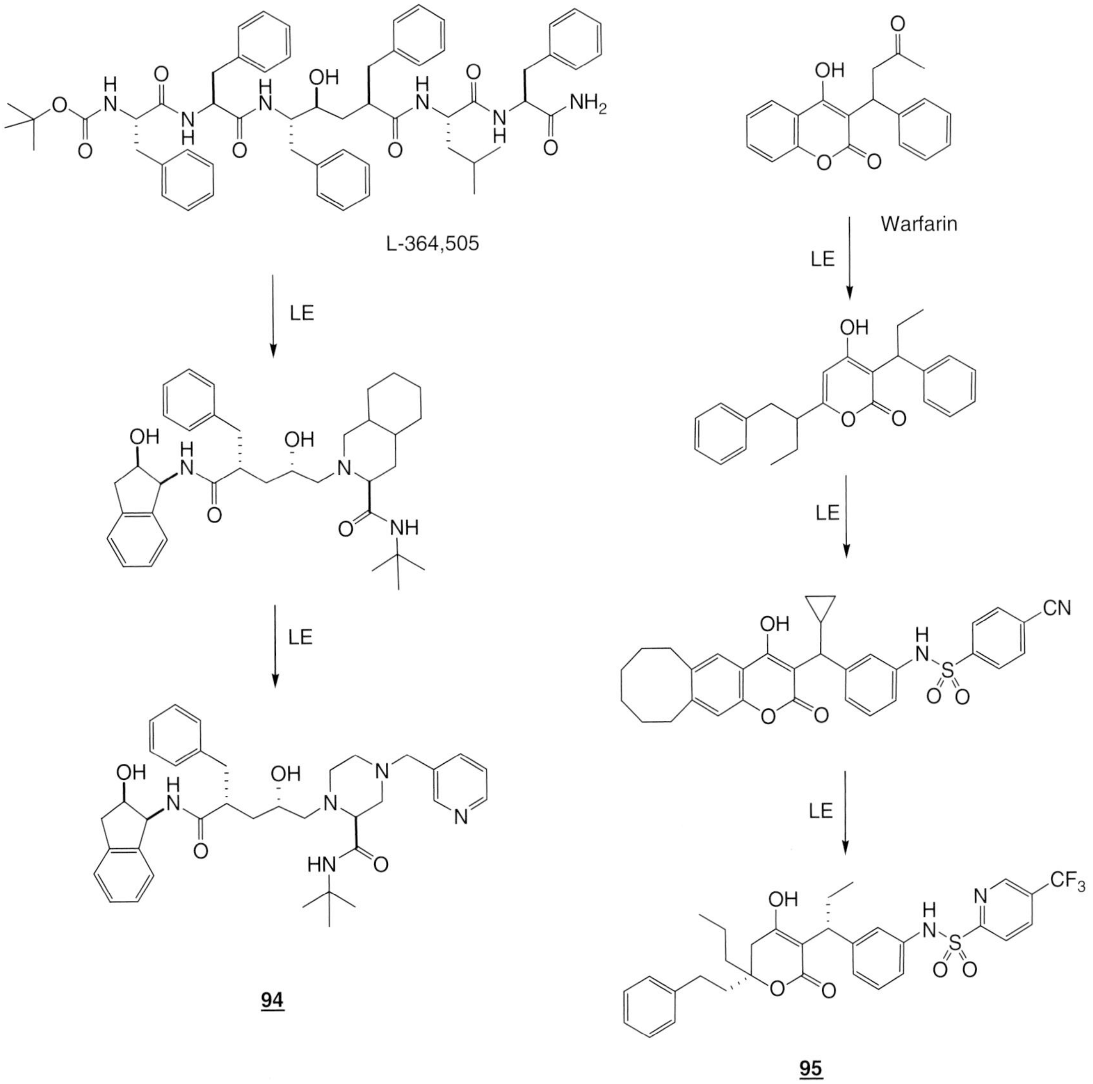

Scheme 19.27 Additional HTS-derived HIV-1 Protease inhibitors and their initial hit compounds. **94** is indinavir and **95** is tipranavir. LE = Lead enhancement wherein synthesis of numerous analogs eventually led to the next depicted molecule. (With permission from Proudfoot.)

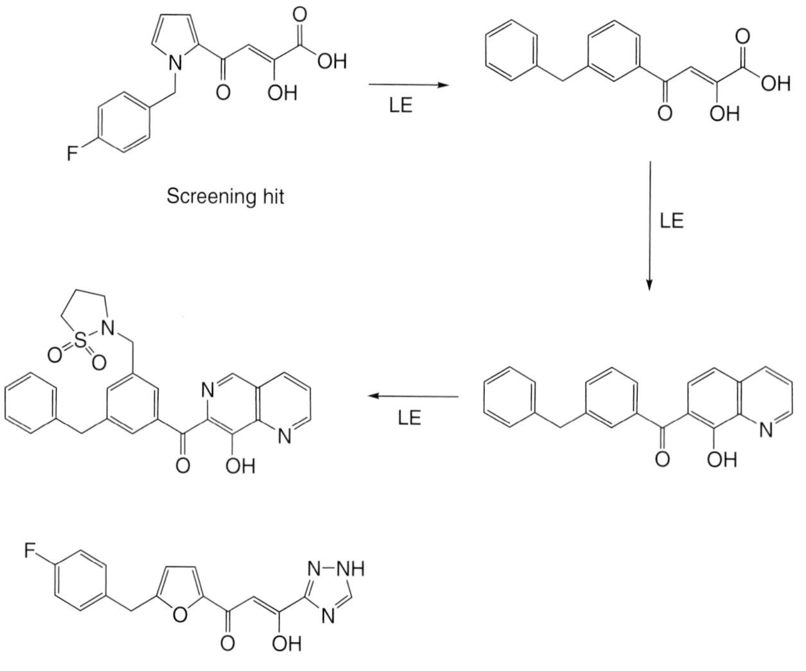

Screening hit

LE

LE

LE

96

Scheme 19.28 Potential, new HIV drugs that inhibit Integrase enzyme. Exemplified here is S-1360 **96**, which is undergoing clinical testing. LE = Lead enhancement where synthesis of numerous analogs eventually led to the next depicted molecule. Note that the keto-acid arrangement in the initial hit proved to be a metabolic liability and needed to be replaced. The three-nitrogen heterocycle has one residual proton that is very acidic, i.e., like a carboxylic acid. It thus serves as a useful bioisostere within this particular molecular context. (With permission from Proudfoot.)

19.4 SUMMARY

Within the context of this chapter's focus upon small molecule drug discovery, a working definition for the term "drug" was devised that stipulates that the drug has actually made it to the marketplace for a given set of indications. We have seen that it is not an easy matter for any molecule to achieve this status and that the overall process is not only lengthy and costly, but is accompanied by an extremely high compound attrition rate. Although the drug discovery process can be thought of as originating from a chemical, biological, or clinical observation starting point, it quickly becomes a highly interdisciplinary undertaking where both efficacy-related mechanistic concepts and drug-wannabes need to become credentialized during preclinical development and validated during initial clinical testing while en route to the marketplace. Historically, it has been the discipline of medicinal chemistry that has been most closely entwined with this challenging field of human endeavor, an association that we have seen at times to have led to rather stressful situations for this field. As part of the evolution of the drug discovery process, we have witnessed a marriage of HTS to combinatorial chemistry that provided new tools for finding efficacious molecules more quickly, and that subsequently gave birth to a new drug discovery paradigm. However, we have also learned that despite the adoption of these new technologies, it is really the consideration of ADMET properties at an earlier time-point of the overall process that more distinctly defines what we can call today's new strategy for drug discovery.

In terms of the biological and chemical principles that become important for drug discovery, we have seen that the efficacious interaction of a molecule with a biological surface is but only the beginning of several other factors that will need to be addressed if the molecule or one of its structural analogs is ultimately to become a drug. Usually presenting themselves as hurdles to be overcome during the advancing stages of drug discovery, these other factors pertain to the ADMET parameters that are encountered as any given compound embarks on what has been called a random walk throughout the body while in search of its efficacious site. Each ADMET parameter will have its own SAR, and a given compound must therefore be prepared to compromise its overall display of chemical functional groups so as to best accommodate or avoid these various parameters while maintaining enough of its own structural integrity to still be able to act appropriately upon finally reaching the desired address for its efficacious message. We have also noted, in turn, that the various chemical functional groups, while working together from a central molecular scaffold to constitute a given chemical structure, likewise display their own distinct blend of physicochemical properties, namely steric, lipophilic, and electronic. Through

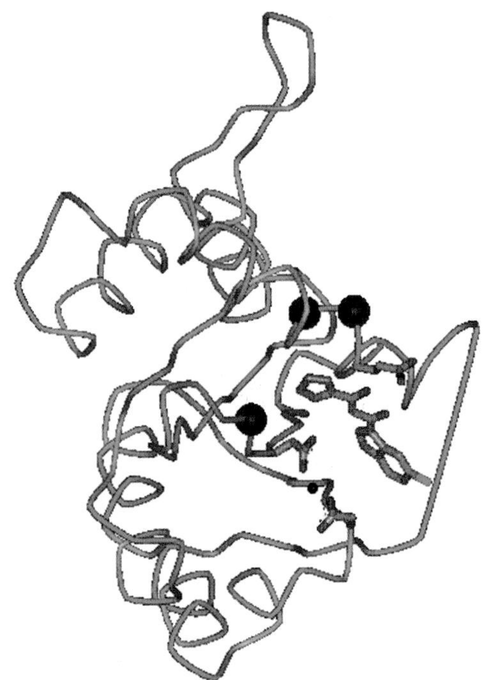

Figure 19.31 X-ray crystal structure of an analog of S-1360 bound to Integrase with resistance mutation sites also noted. Only that portion of the protein is shown so as to depict how the inhibitors bind close to three carboxylates of the active site. In addition, the sites of resistant mutations that have arisen *in vitro* are illustrated by the blue spheres. This structural information should provide additional guidance in the optimization of additional Integrase inhibitors. (With permission from Proudfoot.)

any combination of several drug design experimental strategies, the individual functional group properties and their displays in 3D space can be advantageously constructed so as to optimize a compound's overall interaction with a given biological surface and, when taken as an even broader composite across an entire chemical structure, to optimize the overall behavior of a compound in terms of its entire efficacy and ADMET profile.

We have listed the relative values for various properties for selected functional groups, and you have seen that their composite on any given compound can be tracked and roughly quantified by following simple algebraic relationships while paying attention to both pH and nonbulk solution considerations. The same was shown for the binding energies associated with the possible interactions between a compound and a biological surface. In addition, certain general rules, such as the absorption's Rule-of-5 and the metabolism's Rule-of-1, may often be applicable and these can be of assistance during compound hit or lead selection and structural optimization. However, all these approaches and general rules are only a guideline, and from our own exercise of predicting the clinical behaviors from the corresponding chemical structures for the 10 most prescribed drugs, we see that the prediction aspect of the overall drug discovery process is not at all an easy matter, a fact that is reinforced by the high attrition rate for drug-wannabes during clinical testing. Thus, even the best designed approaches toward structural optimization must also be closely coupled to biological experiments during the fine-tuning and tailoring of a compound's final blend of overall properties. In regard to biological testing we have seen that although efficacy models are often predicative of clinical behavior and therefore generally relied upon to procure patent protection, the entire array of ADMET-related preclinical models are still in their early stages of evolving into a clinically validated state of high predictability.

Despite the challenges, shortcomings and the sheer complexity of trying to simultaneously optimize the coupling of various chemical properties to all the efficacy and ADMET related biological surfaces, we have still seen that very clever efforts in essentially all regards have been achieved so as to have periodically produced numerous success stories across the entire history of drug discovery. Within just this chapter, examples included one from the very early days of drug discovery that pertained to the penicillins; one that happened to run across a historical period that otherwise had been rather traumatic for medicinal chemistry, namely the case study pertaining to the beta-adrenergic receptor blockers and the rational design of esmolol; and finally, one that was accomplished and is still ongoing via today's newest drug discovery paradigm, namely the case study pertaining to the anti-AIDS drugs.

REVIEW

Terms

You should be fully conversant with all the terms, phrases, and acronyms conveyed within this chapter. As an exercise, distinguish and compare the selected items gathered as a string behind each of the numerical entries listed. Include specific examples lifted from the chapter whenever possible. Note that this practice list is not meant to be inclusive of all the chapter's terms.

1. Hit, lead, preclinical development (PDC), and clinical development compounds; drug-wannabe, drug no-no, true drug, herbal remedy, dietary supplement (or nutraceutical) and drug shouldn't be; ethical pharmaceutical and OTC.
2. Drug-wannabe attrition numbers and reasons; NCE, NBE, and NME.
3. Drug discovery starting points (two- and three-type classifications); translational chemistry (TC), research (TR), and medicine (TM).
4. Combinatorial chemistry, compound libraries (three types), HTS, enhancing efficacy, and optimizing ADMET parameters; SAR and pharmacophores; credentializing and validating biological targets and drug candidate compounds.
5. U.S. FDA, GLP, GMP, IND; Phase I, II, and III; NDA and product launch.

6. Medicinal chemistry's roots, heyday, identity crisis, and key role in today's drug discovery process; basic versus applied research and the importance of interdisciplinary efforts.
7. Old, new, and future drug discovery paradigms (strategic orientations, specific steps, limiting factors, durations, and costs); U.S. NIH Road Map Initiative; treatment and preventative use of drugs.
8. Random walk, relay/hurdle race; pH variation across stomach, intestine, systemic circulation (physiologic), intramembrane, and receptor or active sites; first-pass, second-pass, and pseudo-first-pass effect; metabolizing enzymes' distributions.
9. Receptors, agonists, and antagonists; enzyme active sites, substrates, and inhibitors; proteomics, cell signaling pathways (signal transduction) and protein clusters; pharmacogenetics; micro-dosing.
10. The importance of the following molecular weights within the context of drug elimination (phase 1 and 2 metabolism plus excretion): plus ca. 175, < ca. 500 and > ca. 500.
11. Six common metabolic reactions (enzyme, type of structural change, and relative rates).
12. General types of toxicity (three); metabolic detoxification and activation.
13. The importance of second-, third-, and extended-generations of a parent (or pioneer) drug.
14. Experimental strategies that can be used during drug design (3) plus their subcategories (10); SDM and reverse SAR; in silico docking, screening, and filtering; *in vitro* and *in vivo* testing.
15. Deployment of functional groups to assess and optimize: steric, lipophilic, and electronic features; hydrogen-bond acceptor versus donor; electron withdrawal versus enrichment (impact upon acidity and basicity of neighboring groups).
16. Types of intermolecular interactions (8) and a general appreciation for their relative energies; the need for desolvation.
17. Importance of 3D conformation, lock-and-key versus mutual molding, semi-rigid analogs.
18. Irreversible antagonists or inhibitors; active site-directed alkylating agents, suicide enzyme inhibitors; Types of proteases (4); transition state (or mechanism-based) inhibitors.
19. Primary chemical features of a drug and its dosage form that can dictate oral bioavailability (3); DMSO; relationship between pH, ionizable groups and membrane permeation; absorption Rule-of-5, active transport (in and out), Pgp, OAT; prodrugs and soft drugs.
20. PPB, BBB; address and message strategy; drug depot; metabolism Rule-of-1 and its accompanying guidelines.
21. Bioisosteres, metabophores, toxicophores.
22. Validated GLP analytical method, green process chemistry, single stereoisomer compounds; preliminary dosage forms.
23. IP: inventors pool, types of patents and their requirements, seeming contradiction with drug discovery, patent application process, U.S. PTO, relationship to business concerns.
24. Enrollment of healthy volunteers; pharmacogenomics (again), micro-dosing; orphan drugs.
25. Resistance (within the contexts of the penicillins and the anti-AIDS drugs), ISA and MSA (within the context of the beta-blocker drugs); MI (as in myocardial infarct) and USA (as in ultra-short acting) agents; CDC, WHO, HIV-1, CD4, retrovirus and Y181C.

Chemical Structures

Rather than memorizing the details for a given drug's structure in an abstract and static manner, you should be considering these molecules as a dynamic composite of their functional groups and the potential structure-activity relationships (SAR) that can ensue within various biological media and across all biological surfaces including those associated with the ADMET parameters as well as with efficacious activity. Thus, upon looking at any new, small molecule drug-like structure even for the first time, you should be able to knowledgably engage in the following thought processes. As an exercise in this regard, there are about 100 chemical structures for true drugs conveyed in this chapter that you can ponder, and if definitive answers to your propositions for each compound are not also contained here or within any of the other chapters of this text, then they can readily be obtained from the existing literature.

1. Identify what appears to be the compound's central molecular scaffold and estimate how flexible or inflexible that system may be in terms of adopting different shapes or movements in 3D space; locate any asymmetric centers and if stereochemical information is displayed in the structure then discern the R or S absolute configuration nomenclature for each of these sites.
2. Identify all functional groups present in the structure including those that are embedded within your notion of what constitutes the molecule's central scaffold, as well as those that are appended or dangling off so as to assume more peripheral 3D arrangements; discern how flexible all the latter groups may be able to be displayed in 3D space; that is, is it possible to imagine some quadrant of allowable space that they might prefer to reside in or perhaps a trajectory of space that they might be able to move through without distorting appropriate bond angles or causing steric-related collisions with other chemical groups?
3. Assess each functional group's physicochemical attributes, namely:
   (a) Ability to ionize across a range of relevant pH conditions
   (b) General steric demands
   (c) Ability to engage aggressively or passively in hydrogen-bonding as either a donor or an acceptor
   (d) Contribution toward the hydrophobicity of their immediate molecular environment and toward the overall lipophilicity of the entire structure
   (e) Influence on the electron density of the immediate and any conjugated (through double bonds) molecular regions

4. Apply notions derived from 1 to 3 toward formulating SAR possibilities applicable to a potential activity-related pharmacophore and toward each of the ADMET-related parameters as appropriate.
5. Deduce and rank (by favorable energy) potential binding-type interactions for each of the functional groups when the molecule is in an aqueous phase and when it may be associating with a complete set of appropriate partners present within a receptor pocket or enzyme active site; determine how energetically favorable this process might be overall.
6. Apply the Rule-of-1 and the Rule-of-5 and pass judgment on the molecule's metabolic liabilities (earmarking at least a couple of reasonable sites for metabolism) and upon its potential for oral bioavailability (assuming for the moment that active transporters are not significant in either regard). Determine if steric shielding is inherently present across selected areas of the molecule or if that might be a useful addition to think about (see next) relative to potential drug metabolism issues.
7. Suggest further structural modifications to address any molecular regions that you deem to be potentially problematic for a completely optimized profile (assuming for the moment that a once-a-day orally bioavailable product is a crucial part of the desired indication).
8. Suggest appropriate prodrug and soft drug strategies that might be taken to optimize the molecule for various types of indications; if appropriate and as a last resort, consider concomitant administration of another agent for which the combination might be able to address a noted shortcoming in overall profile.
9. Be careful not to take any of your assessments, speculated SAR proposals, or suggestions too seriously until you have actually checked the existing literature for that exact structure whenever available or for the closest structural analog when not available.
10. Also take care not to enjoy this type of overall paper exercise too much. You may run the risk of pursuing a career in medicinal chemistry, for which each structure will also need to be additionally scrutinized with thoughts about how it might actually be synthesized in the most efficient and cost-effective manner possible. This is coupled with the frustration that when actually embarking upon SAR studies as part of any lead compound optimization campaign, each single change in a molecule generally leads to multiple changes in physicochemical parameters that can be displayed differently within different biological environments so that the experimental testing results are often confounded and it becomes a rather complicated matter to draw firm conclusions even from real data.

Specific Problems

1. Explain with words and an accompanying diagram why d-tubocurarine does not cause muscle paralysis in humans upon eating the meat from hunted game that was taken by use of this drug as a poison.
2. Provide a diagrammatic scheme detailing the steps undertaken during today's drug discovery paradigm and briefly contrast with words how the various activities have changed from the past and are expected to evolve into the future. What have been and are anticipated to be the consequences of these changes and evolution in terms of the duration, cost, and attrition rate for the overall process of drug discovery?
3. Assume that the mock natural product shown in the following diagram as **A** is efficaciously active and that in an attempt to define the minimally required pharmacophore, the two analogs **B** and **C** were synthesized and tested for activity. If only **B** was found to be active, what would you deduce to be the active pharmacophore present in **A** (key functional groups and their 3D spacing without necessarily including any scaffold-related atoms that are otherwise noncontributory)? Which, if any, of the additional analogs shown as **D** through **I** would you then predict also to be active? Alternatively, if only **C** were found to be active, what would you deduce to be the active pharmacophore present in **A** and which, if any, of the additional analogs shown as **D** through **I** would you then predict to be active?
4. Returning to Figure 19.17 from this chapter:
   (a) Identify the types of functional groups being used by enalaprilat to bind with ACE.
   (b) Define each type of binding interaction in both a chemical sense and lowering of energy.
   (c) Redraw enalaprilat as it might exist in the aqueous phase and define any hydrogen-bonds that you think might predominate within that milieu in both a chemical sense and lowering of energy.
   (d) Determine what the net energetics are for when enalaprilat leaves an aqueous environment to bind with the ACE active site. For simplicity, use the face of ACE as shown in this diagram also to be the same when no ligand is present even though we know that this may not be the case. Thus, there will also be one HO^- present before enalaprilat arrives and it will be associated with one of the two possible cationic species, namely the Zn ++ as an inherent component of this enzyme's active site and the indicated nitrogen, which is already protonated.
5. Review all the biochemistry associated with a bacterium's synthesis of a cell wall lattice and determine which alanine (Ala) in Scheme 19.19 will be cleaved by a (D)Alanine-(D)-alanylcarboxypeptidase and at what point during cell wall construction.

Structures for Problem 3

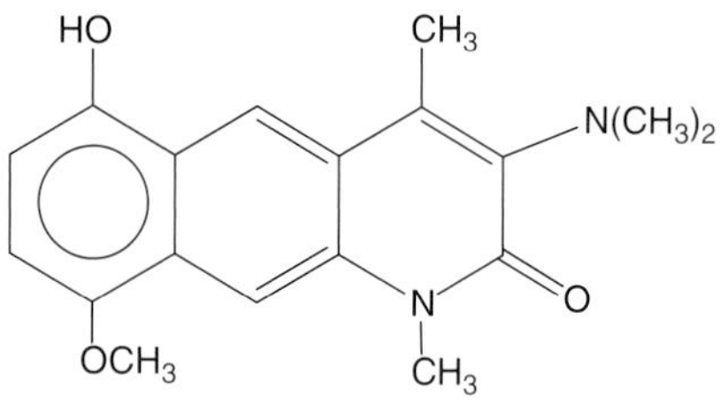

A 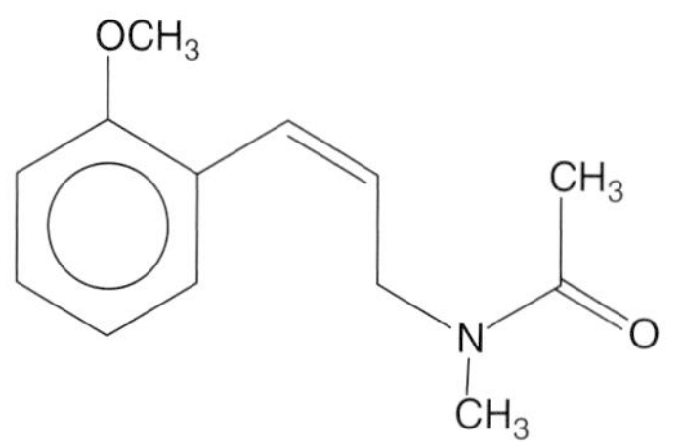 B 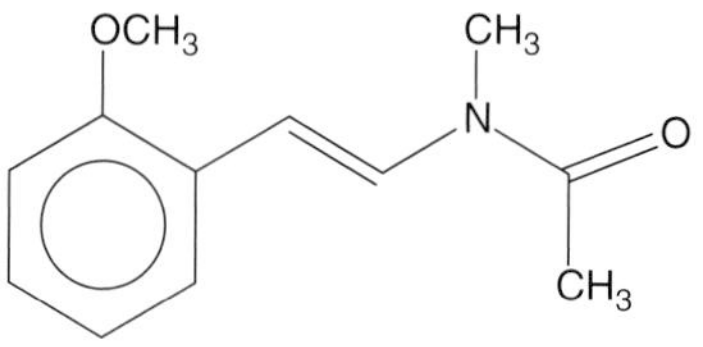 C 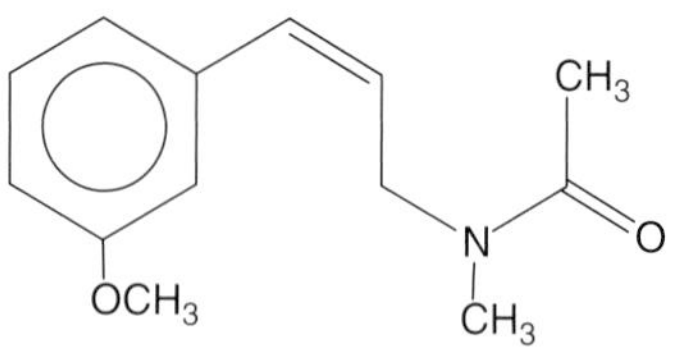 D 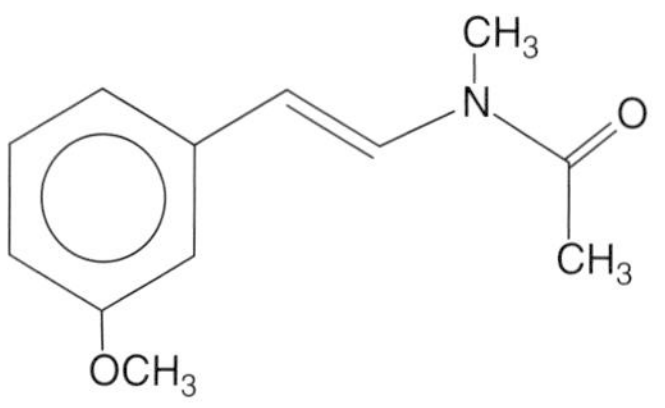 E 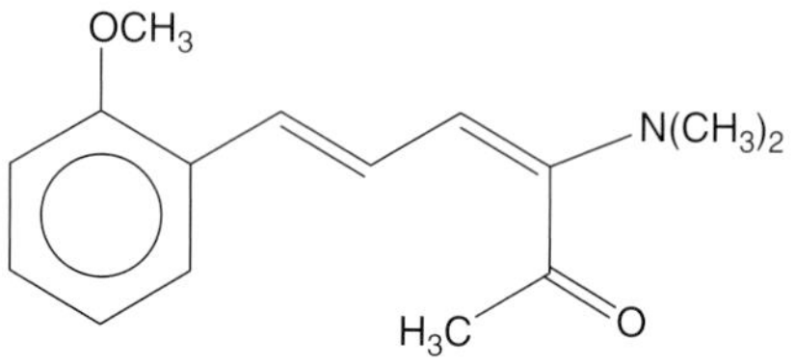 F 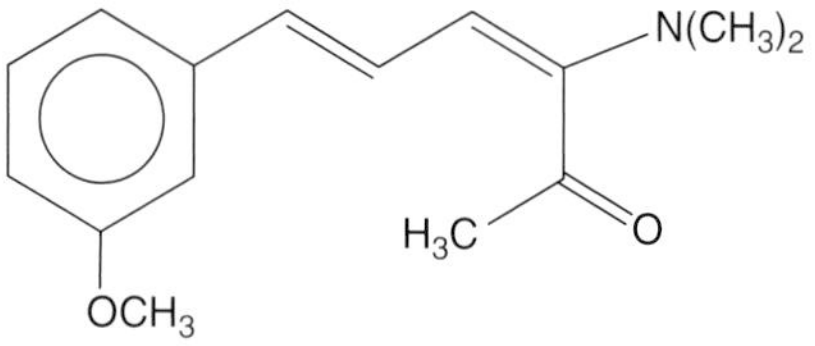 G 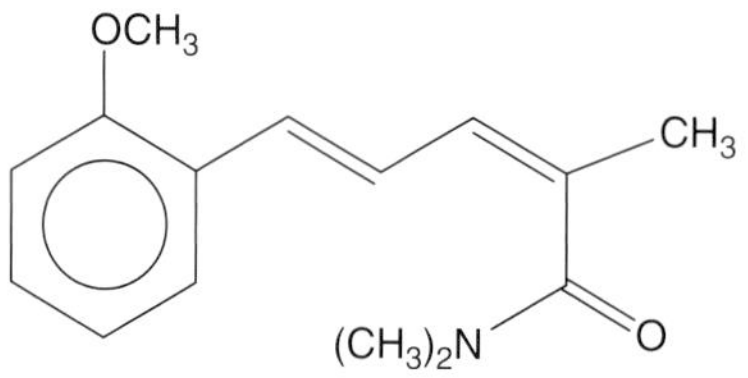 H 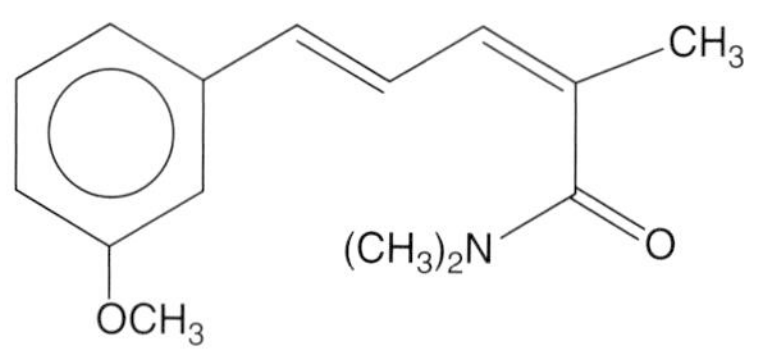 I

REFERENCES

Books

Anastas, P. T., Heine, L. G., & Williamson, T. C. (Eds.). (2000). *Green Chemistry Syntheses and Process (Part 1); Green Engineering (Part 2).* Cary, NC: Oxford Univ Press.

Block, J. H., & Beale, J. M. (Eds.). (2004). *Wilson and Gisvold's Textbook of Organic Medicinal and Pharmaceutical Chemistry* (11th ed.). Baltimore, MD: Lippincott Williams & Wilkins.

Bundgaard, H. (Ed.). (1985). *Design of Prodrugs.* Amsterdam, The Netherlands: Elsevier.

Chorghade, M. S. (Ed.). (2006). *Drug Discovery and Development, Volume 1 Drug Discovery.* Hoboken, NJ: John Wiley & Sons.

Duffus, J. H., & Worth, H. G. (Eds.). (2006). *Fundamental Toxicology.* Cambridge, United Kingdom: RSC Pub.

Ekins, S. (Ed.). (2006). *Computer Applications in Pharmaceutical Research and Development.* Hoboken, NJ: John Wiley & Sons.

Erhardt, P. W. (Ed.). (1999). *Drug Metabolism – Databases and High-Throughput Testing During Drug Design and Development.* Geneva, Switzerland: IUPAC/Blackwell.

Fischer, J., & Ganellin, C. R. (Eds.). (2006). *Analog-based Drug Discovery.* Wenheim, Germany: IUPAC/Wiley-VCH Verlag GmbH.

Hansch, C., & Leo, A. (1979). *Substituent Constants for Correlation Analysis in Chemistry and Biology.* New York, NY: John Wiley & Sons.

LaDu, B. N., Mandel, H. G., & Way, E. L. (Eds.). (1971). *Fundamentals of Drug Metabolism and Drug Disposition.* Baltimore, MD: Williams & Wilkins.

Lednicer, D. (Ed.). (1993). *Chronicles of Drug Discovery* (Vol. 3). Washington, DC: ACS.

Silverman, R. B. (Ed.). (2004). *The Organic Chemistry of Drug Design and Drug Action,* (2nd ed.). Oxford, United Kingdom: Elsevier.

Taylor, J., & Triggle, D. (Eds.). (2006). *Comprehensive Medicinal Chemistry* (Vol. 1). Oxford, United Kingdom: Elsevier.

Williams, D. A., & Lemke, T. L. (Eds.). (2002). *Foye's Principles of Medicinal Chemistry* (5th ed.). Baltimore, MD: Lippincott Williams & Wilkins.

WolffM. E. (Ed.). (1997). *Burger's Medicinal Chemistry and Drug Discovery, Volume 4 Therapeutic Agents* (5th ed.). New York, NY: John Wiley & Sons.

Monographs, Review Articles, and Original Papers

Archer, R. (1999). The drug discovery factory—An inevitable evolutionary consequence of high-throughput parallel processing. *Nature Biotechnology, 17,* 834.

Bachmann, K. A., Ring, B. J., & Wrighton, S. A. (2003). Drug-drug interactions and the cytochromes P450. In J. S. Lee, R. S. Obach, & M. B. Fisher (Eds.), *Drug Metabolizing Enzymes—Cytochrome P450 and Other Enzymes in Drug Discovery and Development* (pp. 311–336). Lausanne, Switzerland: Fontis Media.

Bemis, G. W., & Murcko, M. A. (1996). The properties of known drugs 1 molecular frameworks. *Journal of Medicinal Chemistry, 39,* 2887–2893.

Bemis, G. W., & Murcko, M. A. (1999). Properties of known drugs 2 side chains. *Journal of Medicinal Chemistry, 42,* 5095–5099.

Bodor, N., & Buchwald, P. (2000). Soft drug design—General principles and recent applications. *Medicinal Research Reviews, 20,* 58–101.

Bohm, H-J., & Stahl, M. (2000). Structure-based library design—Molecular modeling merges with combinatorial chemistry. *Current Opinion in Chemical Biology, 4,* 283–286.

Bondy, S. S. (1998). The role of automation in drug discovery. *Current Opinion in Drug Discovery & Development, 1,* 116–119.

Borman, S. (2000). Combinatorial chemistry—Redefining the scientific method. *Chem Eng News, 78,* 53–65.

Brennan, M. B. (2000). Drug discovery—Filtering out failures early in the game. *Chem Eng News, 78,* 63–73.

Bristol, D. W., Wachsman, J. T., & Greenwell, A. (1996). The NIEHS Predictive-Toxicology Evaluation Project. *Environmental Health Perspectives, 104,* 1001–1010.

Chen, X., & Wang, W. (2003). The use of bioisosteric groups in lead optimization. *Ann Rep Med Chem, 38,* 333–346.

Cheng, S., Comer, D. D., Williams, J. P., Myers, P. L., & Boger, D. L. (1996). Novel solution phase strategy for the synthesis of chemical libraries containing small organic molecules. *Journal of the American Chemical Society, 118,* 2567–2573.

Dantzig, A. H., Hillgren, K. M., & Alwis, D. P. Drug transporters and their role in tissue distribution. *Ann Rep Med Chem, 39,* 279–291.

Davies, K., & White, C. (1999). Managing combinatorial chemistry information. In P. M. Dean & A. L. Lewis (Eds.), *Molecular Diversity in Drug Design* (pp. 175–196). Dordrecht, The Netherlands: Kluwer Academic Pub.

DesJarlais, R. L., Sheriden, R. P., Seibel, G. L., Dixon, J. S., & Kuntz, I. D. (1988). Using shape complementarity as an initial screen in designing ligands for a receptor binding site of known three-dimensional structure. *Journal of Medicinal Chemistry, 31,* 722–729.

Drews, J. (2000). Drug discovery—A historical perspective. *Science, 287,* 1960–1969.

Eddershaw, P. J., Beresford, A. P., & Bayliss, M. K. (2000). ADME/PK as part of a rational approach to drug discovery. *Drug Discovery Today, 5,* 409–414.

Ehrlich, P. (1913). Chemotherapeutics—Scientific principles, methods and results. *The Lancet,16,* 445–451.

Erhardt, P. W., Gorczynski, R. J., & Anderson, W.G. (1979). Conformational analogus of dopamine—Synthesis and pharmacological activity of (E)- and (Z)-2-(3,4-dihydroxyphenyl)-cyclopropylamine hydrochlorides. *Journal of Medicinal Chemistry, 22,* 907–911.

Erhardt, P. W. (1983). Renal vascular dopamine receptor topography—Structure-activity relationships that suggest the presence of a ceiling. In C. Kaiser, & J. W. Kebabian (Eds.), *ACS Symposium Series, 224, Dopamine Receptors* (pp. 275–280). Washington, DC: ACS.

Erhardt, P. W. (1987). In search of the digitalis replacement. *Journal of Medicinal Chemistry, 30,* 231–237.

Erhardt, P. W., Hagedorn, A. A., & Sabio, M. (1988). Cardiotonic agents 3—A topographical model of the cardiac c-AMP phosphodiesterase receptor. *Molecular Pharmacology, 33,* 1–13.

Erhardt, P. W., & Chou, Y-L. (1991). A topographical model for the cAMP phosphodiesterase III active site. *Life Sciences, 49,* 553–568.

Erhardt, P. W. (1993). Esmolol. In D. Lednicer (Ed.), *Chronicles of Drug Discovery* (pp. 191–206). Washington, DC: ACS.

Erhardt, P. W. (1997). Chemotherapeutic agents—Lecture 1. *American Journal of Pharmaceutical Education 61,* 192–196.

Erhardt, P. W. (1999). Case studies—A prodrug and a soft drug. In P.W. Erhardt (Ed.), *Drug Metabolism—Databases and High Throughput Testing During Drug Design and Development,* (pp. 62–69). Geneva, Switzerland: IUPAC/Blackwell.

Erhardt, P. W. (2002). Medicinal chemistry in the new millennium—A glance into the future. *Pure and Applied Chemistry, 74,* 703–785.

Erhardt, P. W., & Matos, L. (2006). Selective beta-adrenergic receptor blocking agents. In J. Fischer & C. R. Ganellin (Eds.), *Analog-based Drug Discovery* (pp. 193–232). Weinheim, Germany: IUPAC/ Wiley-VCH Verlag GmbH.

Erhardt, P. W. (2006). Case study 'Esmolol Stat'. In J. Fischer & C. R. Ganellin (Eds.), *Analog-based Drug Discovery* (pp. 233–246). Weinheim, Germany: IUPAC/Wiley-VCH Verlag GmbH.

Erhardt, P. W. (2006). Medicinal chemistry in the new millennium—A glance into the future. In M. S. Chorghade (Ed.), *Drug Discovery and Development Volume 1 Drug Discovery* (pp. 17–102). Hoboken, NJ: John Wiley & Sons.

Erhardt, P. W., & Proudfoot, J. R. (2006). Drug discovery—Historical perspective, current status and outlook. In J. Taylor & D. Triggle (Eds.), *Comprehensive Medicinal Chemistry* (Vol. 1). Oxford, United Kingdom.

Floyd, C. D., Leblanc, C., & Whittaker, M. (1999). Combinatorial chemistry as a tool for drug discovery. *Progress in Medicinal Chemistry, 36,* 91–168.

Gillespie, P., & Goodnow, R. A., Jr. (2004). The hit-to-lead process in drug discovery. *Ann Rep Med Chem, 39,* 293–304.

Goodford, P. J. (1985). A computational procedure for determining energetically favorable binding sites on biologically important macromolecules. *Journal of Medicinal Chemistry, 28,* 849–857.

Grimley, J. (2006). Pharma challenged—Market shifts and generic competition create dynamic environment for drug developers. *Chem Eng News, 4,* 17–28.

Hansch, C., & Fujita, T. (1964). ρ-σ-π Analysis—A method for the correlation of biological activity and chemical structure. *Journal of the American Chemical Society, 86,* 1616–1625.

Herzberg, R. P., & Pope, A. J. (2000). High-throughput screening—New technology for the 21st century. *Current Opinion in Chemical Biology, 4,* 445–451.

Hopkins, A. L., & Polinsky, A. (2006). Knowledge and intelligence in drug design. *Ann Rep Med Chem, 41,* 425–437.

Houghten, R. A., Pinilla, C., Blondelle, S. E., Appel, J. R., Dooley, C. T., & Cuervo, J. H. (1991). Generation and use of synthetic peptide combinatorial libraries for basic research and drug discovery. *Nature, 354,* 84–86.

Horl, W. H., George, P. M., Carrell, R. W., Powers, J. C., Zimmerman, M., Markwardt, F., et al. (1989). Inhibition of proteinases. In M. Sandler & H. J. Smith (Eds.), *Design of Enzyme Inhibitors as Drugs* (pp. 573–649). Oxford, United Kingdom: Oxford Univ Press.

Jacobs, M. (Ed.). (2000). Challenging times for patent office. *Chem Eng News, 10,* 39–44.

Kuntz, I. D. (1992). Structure-based strategies for drug-design and discovery. *Science, 257,* 1078–1082.

Lau, K. F., & Sakul, H. (2000). Pharmacogenetics. *Ann Rep Med Chem, 35,* 261–269.

Lipinski, C. A., Lombardo, F., Dominy, B. W., & Feeney, P. J. (1997). Experimental and computational approaches to estimate solubility and permeability in drug discovery and development settings. *Advanced Drug Delivery Reviews, 23,* 3–25.

Lumley, C. (1990). Clinical toxicity—Could it have been predicted? Premarketing experience. In C. E. Lumley & S. R. Walker (Eds.), *Animal Toxicity Studies. Their Relevance for Man* (pp. 49–57). Lancaster, PA: Quay Pub.

Martin, Y. C. (1997). Challenges and prospects for computational aids to molecular diversity. *Perspect Drug Discov Res, 7/8,* 159–172.

Merritt, A. T. (1998). Uptake of new technology in lead optimization for drug discovery. *Drug Discovery Today, 3,* 505–510.

Metzger, T. G., Paterlini, M. G., Portoghese, P. S., & Ferguson, D. M. (1996). Application of the message-address concept to the docking of naltrexone and selective naltrexone-derived opioid antagonists into opioid receptor models. *Neurochemical Research, 21,* 1287–1294.

Milne, G. M., Jr. (2003). Pharmaceutical productivity—The imperative for new paradigms. *Ann Rep Med Chem, 38,* 383–396.

Mitscher, L. A., & Dutta, A. (2006). Contemporary drug discovery. In M. S. Chorghade (Ed.), *Drug Discovery and Development Volume 1 Drug Discovery* (pp. 103–128). Hoboken, NJ: John Wiley & Sons.

Nirmala, N. R. (2006). Genomic data mining and its impact on drug discovery. *Ann Rep Med Chem, 41,* 319–330.

Ohlstein, E. H., Ruffolo, R. R., & Elliott, J. D. (2000). Drug discovery in the next millennium. *Annual Reviews of Pharmacology and Toxicology, 40,* 177–191.

Patchett, A. A., & Nargund, R. P. (2000). Privileged structures—An update. *Ann Rep Med Chem,35,* 289–298.

Pickering, L. (2001). ADME/tox models can speed up development. *Drug Discovery & Development, 1,* 34–38.

Rodrigues, A. D. (1998). Rational high-throughput screening in preclinical drug metabolism. *Med Chem Res, 8*, 422–433.
Sadowski, J., & Kubinyi, H. (1998). A scoring scheme for discriminating between drugs and nondrugs. *Journal of Medicinal Chemistry, 41*, 3325–3329.
Sarshar, S., Zhang, C., Moran, E. J., Krane, S., Rodarte, J. C., Benbatoul, K. D., et al. (2000). 2,4,5-trisubstituted imidazoles—Novel nontoxic modulators of P-glycoprotein mediated multidrug resistance—Part 1. *Bioorganic & Medicinal Chemistry Letters, 10*, 2599–2601.
Schmid, E. F., & Smith, D. A. (2005). Trends in pharmaceutical innovation. *Ann Rep Med Chem, 40*, 431–441.
Seelig, A., & Landwojtowicz, E. (2000). Structure-activity relationship of P-glycoprotein substrates and modifiers. *European Journal of Pharmaceutical Sciences, 12*, 31–40.
Smith, P. W., Lai, J. Y. Q., Whittington, A. R., Cox, B., Houston, J. G., Stylli, C. H., et al. (1994). Synthesis and biological evaluation of a library containing potentially 1600 amides/esters—A strategy for rapid compound generation and screening. *Bioorganic & Medicinal Chemistry Letters, 4*, 2821–2824.
Tomizawa, K., Sugano, K., Yamada, H., & Hori, I. (2006). Physicochemical and cell-based approach for early screening of phospholipidosis-inducing potential. *The Journal of Toxicological Sciences, 31*, 315–324.
Veber, D. F., Johnson, S. R., Cheng, H.-Y., Smith, B. R., Ward, K. W., & Kopple, K. D. (2002). Molecular properties that influence the oral bioavailability of drug candidates. *Journal of Medicinal Chemistry, 45*, 2615–2623.
Walters, W. P., Stahl, M. T., & Murcko, M. A. (1998). Virtual screening—An overview. *Drug Discovery Today, 3*, 160–178.
Waring, J. E., & Ulrich, R. G. (2000). The impact of genomics-based technologies on drug safety evaluation. *Annual Review of Pharmacologys, 40*, 335–352.
Waterbeemd, H., van de, Smith, D. A., Beaumont, K., & Walker, D. K. (2001). Property-based design—Optimization of drug absorption and pharmacokinetics. *Journal of Medicinal Chemistry, 44*, 1313–1333.
Weir, M. P., Overington, J. P., & Schwarz, M. (2002). Expanding and exploring cellular pathways for novel drug targets. *Ann Rep Med Chem, 37*, 187–196.
Wermuth, C. G., Ganellin, C. R., Lindberg, P., & Mitscher, L. A. (1998). A glossary of terms used in medicinal chemistry. *Pure and Applied Chemistry, 70*, 1129–1143.
Yoo, H. S., & Park, T. G. (2004). Folate-receptor-targeted delivery of doxorubicin nano-aggregates stabilized by doxorubicin-PEG-folate conjugate. *Journal of Controlled Release, 100*, 247–256.
Zhang, C., Sarshar, S., Moran, E. J., Krane, S., Rodarte, J. C., Benbatoul, K. D., et al. (2000). 2,4,5-trisubstituted inmidazoles—Novel nontoxic modulators of P-glycoprotein mediated multidrug resistance—Part 2. *Bioorganic & Medicinal Chemistry Letters, 10*, 2603–2605.

WEB DATABASES OR GENERAL INFORMATION STARTING-POINTS

Bioinformatics: www.ncbi.nlm.nih.gov
Chemoinformatics: www.chemfinder.com
Clinical Pharmacology (Drugs): www.cpip.gsm.com
Clinical Trial Information (Drugs): www.centerwatch.com
Dietary Supplements (Herbals et al.): www.dietary-supplements.info.nih.gov
Drug–drug Interactions: www.fda.gov/cder/advisory
Drug Topics (Prescription patterns etc.): www.drugtopics.com
Toxicology: www.ciit.org

Chapter

20

Genomics and Proteomics in Drug Design and Discovery

Ying Wang ▪ Jen-Fu Chiu ▪ Qing-Yu He

OUTLINE

20.1 INTRODUCTION

The recently developed genomic and proteomic technologies feature high-throughput parallel analysis of all genes and proteins in a given genome and proteome, and thus opens up the possibility of providing details on the molecular mechanisms on a global level. Genomic and proteomic approaches combined with other biochemical methods can reconstruct regulatory networks, signaling cascades and metabolic pathways upon drug treatment. In this chapter, an overview will be given on recent progresses in genomic and proteomic research strategies that have an impact on drug discovery and their applications in identification and validation of drug targets, illustrating drug action mechanisms, prediction of drug resistance, and biomarkers discovery for determining clinical effects. This chapter concludes by exemplifying concrete data-driven studies in pharmaceutical research, which demonstrate the value of integrated genomic and proteomic platforms for drug target identification and validation, screening assay development, as well as the evaluations of drug candidate efficacy and toxicity.

20.2 GENOMICS AND PROTEOMICS

When we define success in science, we would always like to coin new words ended with the related suffix *-some* or *-ome*, meaning "body," which has been used to name various intracellular particles. "Chromosome" dates back more than 100 years, "ribosome" and "lysosome" are nearly half a century old, and "nucleosome" and "replisome" originated more than a quarter century ago. Even "splicesome" and "proteasome" are approaching two decades of service. Although "genome" was coined by German scientists (*genom*) in 1920 and first used in English in 1930, none of the other *-omes* can lay claim to more than a few years of history. However, it was only a quarter of a century after *Nature* published the structure of the DNA helix in 1953, that the advent of new methods to analyze genomes directly changed the field of genetics. When the genome of bacteriophage lambda was first sequenced, it allowed the enumeration of all the open reading frames (DNA sequences that potentially can be translated into protein). Over the past few years, more than 30 organisms have had their genomes completely sequenced, with another 100 or so in progress (see genomes@ncbi.nlm.nih.gov for a list).

Unfortunately, the billions of bases of DNA sequence do not tell us what all the genes do, how cells work, how cells form organisms, what goes wrong in disease, how we age, or how to develop a drug. The purpose of genomics is to understand biology, not simply to identify the component parts, and the experimental and computational methods take advantage of as much sequence information as possible. In this sense, the goal of genomics is not simply to provide a catalogue of all the genes and information about their functions, but to understand how the components work together to comprise functioning cells and organisms. Proteins are the workhorses encoded by the genome, thus like its precursor genomics, proteomics represents the emergence of a new way of doing research that is not dependent on the testing of specific models of cellular behavior. This style of science obviously does not replace, but rather will increasingly operate in tandem with, traditional biological research methods.

At present, biology is in the midst of an intellectual and experimental sea change; the data are coming from the fortuitous confluence of technological advances in DNA and protein analysis as well as imaging advances in cell biology. Using genomic and proteomic methods, we are starting to improve substantially our knowledge in drug design and development on a global scale, which is totally different from other well-developed molecular biological and biochemical methods that can only study potential key targets one by one.

20.2.1 Definition of Genomics and Proteomics

The genome refers to all the genes, including chromosome DNA, all forms of RNA, and transcriptional variants in a certain biological unit. The gene expression profiles generated from DNA microarrays of over 225,000 transcripts as a whole are commonly utilized in classification and predictive models. The genomic codes are translated to protein languages after transcription (Figure 20.1). Now as the complete human genome and many other genomes have been deciphered, we have to face the fact that the genomic sequence and protein function cannot be directly correlated. Proteins are the key components of the cellular machinery responsible for processing changes that are ordered by genomic information. Proteins can be modified at posttranscriptional level, and many different protein isoforms can be generated from even a single gene (Figure 20.1). In addition, proteins can also be regulated by proteolysis and compartmentalization. Since the statement of "one gene, one protein" is an oversimplification, the average number of protein isoforms per gene was predicted as one or two in bacteria, three in yeast, and three or more in humans. The proteome, therefore, is defined as all expressed protein complement of a cell, organ, or organism, and it includes all isoforms and posttranslational variants.

Proteomic technology, first coined in 1995, attempts to separate, identify, and characterize a global set of proteins in an effort to provide information about protein abundance, location, modification, and protein–protein interaction in a proteome of a given biological system. This postgenomic technology provides a direct measurement of the presence and relative abundance of proteins, and reveals the consequence of protein functioning in establishing the biological phenotype of organisms in healthy and disease states. By studying interrelationships of protein expressions and modifications in health and disease or drug treatment, proteomics contributes important insights into determining the pathophysiological basis of disease, validating drug targets, and illustrating drug action, toxicity, and side effects. Milestones in genomics and proteomics are listed in Table 20.1.

20.2.2 Subdisciplines of Genomics and Proteomics

20.2.2.1 Computational Proteomics

Computational proteomics refers to the large-scale generation and analysis of 3D protein structural information. Accurate prediction of protein contact maps is the beginning and essential step for computational proteomics. The major resource for computational proteomics is the currently available information on protein and nucleic acid structures. The 3D-GENOMICS (www.sbg.bio.ic.au.uk/3dgenomics/) and PDB (http://www.rcsb.org/pdb/), and other databases provide a broad range of structural and functional annotations for proteins from sequenced genomes and protein 3D structures, which make a solid foundation for computational proteomics.

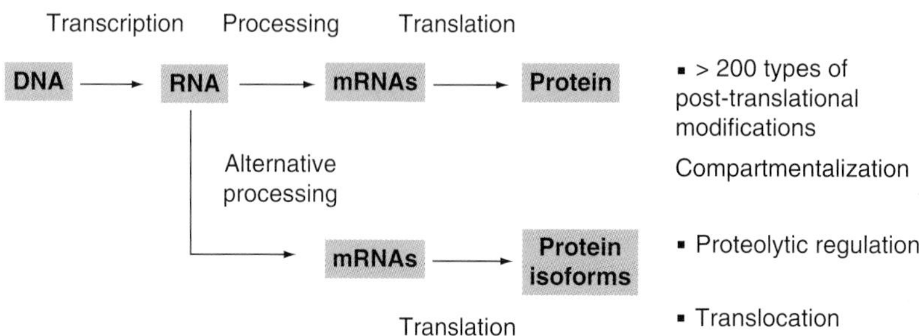

Figure 20.1 The flow of genomic information to protein products.

Table 20.1 Milestones in Genomics and Proteomics

	Year	Achievements	References
Genomics	1983	Invention of the PCR technology	(Mullis et al., 1986)
	1990	Beginning of the human genome project	(Watson, 1990)
	1995	Introduction of the high-throughput cDNA microarray technology	(Schena et al., 1995)
	1996	The genome of the yeast saccharomyces cerevisiae has been completely sequenced	(Goffeau et al., 1996)
	1998	Complete analysis of the caenorhabditis elegans genome	(Kamath et al., 2003)
	2001	Established the sequence of the human genome	(Venter et al., 2001)
Proteomics	1975	Introduction of 2DE technology	(O'Farrell, 1975)
	1981	Construction of the 2DE gel image analysis packages	(Anderson et al., 1981)
	1985	Utilization of electrospray ionization (ESI) for mass spectrometry (MS) of large biomolecules	(Fenn et al., 1989; Whitehouse et al., 1985)
	1987	Introduction of ionization of protein molecules by soft laser desorption, which is basic theory for MALDI-TOF MS and SELDI-TOF MS	(Karas and Hillenkamp, 1988)
	1995	Definition of proteomics was first coined	(Wasinger et al., 1995)

20.2.2.2 Chemical Proteomics

Chemical proteomics makes use of synthetic organic chemistry, cell biology, biochemistry, and mass spectrometry (MS) to design specific protein-modifying reagents that can be used for functional studies of distinct proteins within a certain proteome. The most important tools of this field are the carefully designed chemical probes that can specifically target diverse sets of enzyme families. A chemical probe contains three parts: a reactive ligand that can covalently bind to the target protein/enzyme, a linker region modulating the reactivity and specificity of the reactive ligand, and a tag for identification and purification of the target protein/enzyme. Several kinds of chemical probes have been used in proteomic study, for example, serine hydrolase probes, S-transferase probes, and phenyl sulfonate probes.

20.2.2.3 Structural Genomics and Proteomics

Structural genomics determines the structure of almost all the proteins in a cell or organism. Three-dimensional structures are important for the functional analysis of proteins in a cell and for rational drug design. Theoretically, genomic sequence databases allow cloning, expression, and purification of all encoded proteins in a certain genome. At present, it is difficult to determine the structures of all the proteins in a cell or organism in order to understand protein function and protein–protein interactions at molecular level, whereas structural genomics can overcome such difficulties of different protein variants due to alternative splicing or posttranslational modifications.

Structural proteomics is the determination of the relationship of all the proteins or protein complexes in a specific cellular organelle and the establishment of the relationship of these proteins in a proteome-wide scale. Combining structural biology with computational and medicinal chemistry, structural proteomics can help design drugs effectively. The important goal of structural proteomics is to determine the 3D structures of as many proteins as possible, so that other proteins in an organelle can be computationally modeled on the basis of similarity of their amino acid sequences.

20.2.2.4 Topological Proteomics

Topological proteomics aims at localizing and characterizing entire protein networks within a single cell, providing quantitative insights into their basic organization, which provides valuable information in identifying new drug targets and selecting potential lead compounds. The proprietary technology Multi-Epitope-Ligan Kartographie (MELK) is an ultra-sensitive topological proteomics technology for analyzing proteins on a single cell level. MELK can trace out large scale subcellular protein patterns simultaneously within a cell, and hence unravels hierarchies of proteins related to particular cell functions or dysfunctions. Another topological proteomic program, TopNet, is an automated web tool designed to facilitate the analysis of interaction networks, which is available from http://networks.gersteinlab.org/.

20.3 MAJOR TECHNOLOGICAL PLATFORMS OF GENOMICS AND PROTEOMICS

20.3.1 Microarrays

Microarrays, also referred as DNA chips, are powerful and versatile tools for genome analysis, and exploit the specific binding of complementary single-stranded nucleic acid sequences. A schematic plot of a cDNA microarray is shown in Figure 20.2. Use of gene chip microarrays provides a global profiling of RNA expression. There are two array-based technologies, cDNA and oligonucleotide arrays, to analyze patterns of gene expression. cDNA microarrays usually contain double-stranded cDNA sequences of interest that have been synthesized by PCR, which are capable of profiling gene expression patterns of tens of thousands of genes in a single experiment. Oligonucleotide microarrays

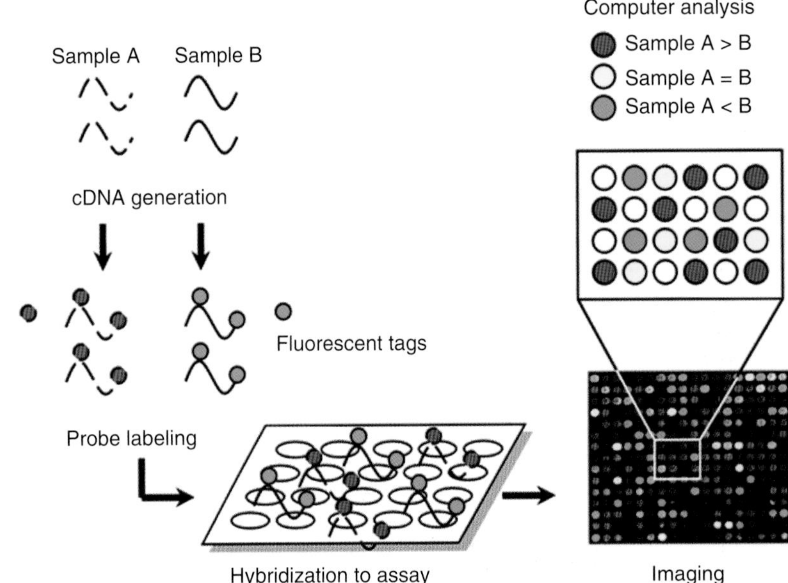

Figure 20.2 cDNA microarray schema.

are prepared using specific oligonucleotides synthesized directly onto a quartz or silicon wafer using combinatorial chemistry and photolithography.

RNA isolated from cells or tissue of interest and control samples are labeled with a fluorescent dye and allowed to bind in a quantitative manner to complementary sequences on the microarray. Relative expression fold of difference of the sequences in the test samples can be estimated by comparing the fluorescence intensities, measured by laser scanner, with those of the control samples. Data management and mining methods applied to microarray data analysis essentially have been correlation-based approaches that apply methods developed for the analysis of data that are more highly constrained than at the transcriptional level.

20.3.2 Quantitative Real-time PCR (RT-PCR)

Differentially expressed genes in treated groups compared with control groups can be analyzed further in more detail and in larger number of samples using RT-PCR. RT-PCR can analyze hundreds of genes in a more quantitative fashion than microarrays. Results from RT-PCR can provide information on the time course of the changes in expression of the target genes during treatment, compared to untreated control samples.

20.3.3 Separation Methods in Proteomics

Several technological platforms have been developed utilizing the separation efficiency of two-dimensional electrophoresis (2DE) and high performance chromatography (HPLC) in offline or online combinations with MS in proteomics.

2DE has been the main method available to routinely separate thousands of proteins, and thus is the dominant technique in the field of proteomics. The first 2DE apparatus was established by Patrick H. O'Farrell through combining the two most powerful electrophoresis methods available. 2DE separates protein complexes according to their isoelectric points and molecular weights (Figure 20.3). This technique is suitable for analyzing proteomes of cell, tissue, and serum, and can detect proteins with posttranslational modification, including phosphorylation, glycosylation, and such. However, low abundance proteins are always beyond the separation limit of 2DE. Numerous prefractionation methods can be applied prior to 2DE analysis; for example, sample prefractionation via multicompartment electrolyzers with isoelectric membranes, use of immobilized metal affinity chromatrography (IMAC) to enrich metal-associated proteins and peptides, subcellular fractionation, and affinity purification.

Complex protein mixture can also be separated by HPLC. Recent publications reported the successful utilization of one- or two-dimensional chromatographic approaches for proteomics such as cation exchange followed by online HPLC-MS to identify proteins in complex mixtures after tryptic digestion. Generally, larger polypeptides can frequently not be separated by HPLC; however, some low-abundant serum proteins in the nanogram per milliliter-range were found in HPLC-MS analysis, including human growth hormone and interleukins. Combined ion exchange and reverse phase chromatography, termed 2D-HPLC, can successfully separate complex peptide mixtures rather than protein mixtures. In the first dimension, peptides are separated by ion exchange chromatography. Each fraction obtained is then separated in the second HPLC-dimension. The collected fractions are identified by MS to constitute a complete peptide map.

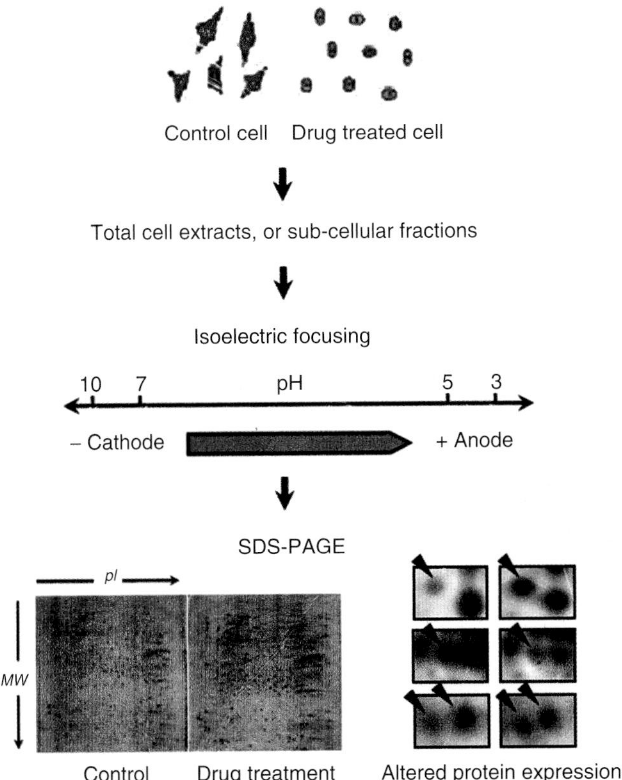

Figure 20.3 A general scheme for 2DE.

20.3.4 Protein Identification by Mass Spectrometry (MS)

The techniques of matrix-assisted laser desorption/ionization-time of flight (MALDI-TOF) and electrospray/ionization (ESI) have revolutionized biological MS since 1989. All state-of-the-art biochemistry and biology laboratories possess at least one of these ionization techniques and, in general, have access to both of them. Both ionization techniques are applicable to peptides and proteins, DNA and RNA, glycoconjugates, and synthetic polymers.

Differently expressed protein samples are subjected to digestion with a protease that yields peptides prior to MALDI-TOF MS. MALDI-TOF MS enables peptides to be ionized at high sensitivity without excessive fragmentation. Two steps in MALDI-TOF MS are peptides ionization by a laser coupled with time of flight and detection as ion mass to charge (m/z) ratio with a mass analyzer. The ionized and separated peptides can be further characterized by tandem mass spectrometry (MS/MS) through a second MS analyzer to generate an MS/MS spectrum representing a series of ion fragments of the specific peptide, which can construct a partial amino acid sequence according to the MS/MS spectrum. MS/MS based protein identification is often more accurate with higher outputs, since it provides information not only about peptide masses but also peptide sequences.

In ESI MS, the analyzed sample molecules are dissolved in water/methanol or water/acetonitrile mixture, and continuously injected into an electric field via a metal capillary with flow rates of 1 to 5 μl per minute or via a metal-coated glass capillary (nanoelectrospray source) with flow rates in the low nanoliters per minute range. The electric field generates a mist of charged droplets containing analyte molecules. The droplets move down a potential gradient and a pressure gradient, which both finally liberate analyte molecules from solvent molecules toward the mass analyzer. Quadrupole mass filters coupled to ESI sources, therefore, were the workhorses for ESI approaches. Triple quadrupole instruments offer the opportunity to obtain tandem MS (MS/MS).

Besides these two kinds of ionization techniques, surface-enhance laser desorption/ionization-time of flight (SELDI-TOF) is an approach that tries to overcome the requirement for purification and separation of proteins prior to mass spectrometry analysis. SELDI-TOF MS employs a variety of selective chips that can identify altered proteins by surface affinity and molecular weight, namely protein chip array (Figure 20.4). This is a very useful technique since the experimental conditions can be well controlled. For example, different cofactors or inhibitors such as hydrophobic, anionic exchanger, cationic exchanger, or metal chelate surface can be introduced in the binding assays to adjust the stringency of the binding activities. Another advantage of this technique is that these highly parallel assays are suitable for analysis of low abundant proteins. In addition, with proper detection methods, protein chip arrays can be used to identify the downstream targets of various enzymes such as kinases, phosphatases, methyl transferases, and proteases. SELDI-TOF MS is highly sensitive to analyze small amounts of raw protein samples, and can detect proteins with molecular weights lower than 6 kDa (the lowest detection range of 2DE). However, it is not a quantitative approach and protein identification cannot be directly determined through this method.

In addition, protein chip arrays can be multifaceted by changing the capture ligand on the protein chip surface. For example, small molecule array is used to investigate small-molecule-protein interaction, AB array uses specific antibody as the capture ligand to study cell-signaling, and peptide array uses peptides as capture ligands to study protein–protein interaction.

20.4 CURRENT ACHIEVEMENTS AND POTENTIAL APPLICATION OF GENOMICS AND PROTEOMICS IN DRUG DESIGN AND DISCOVERY

20.4.1 Identification and Validation of Drug Targets

Drug target discovery, which involves the identification and early validation of disease-associated targets, is the first step in the drug discovery pipeline. Disease involves alterations in gene and/or protein expression and

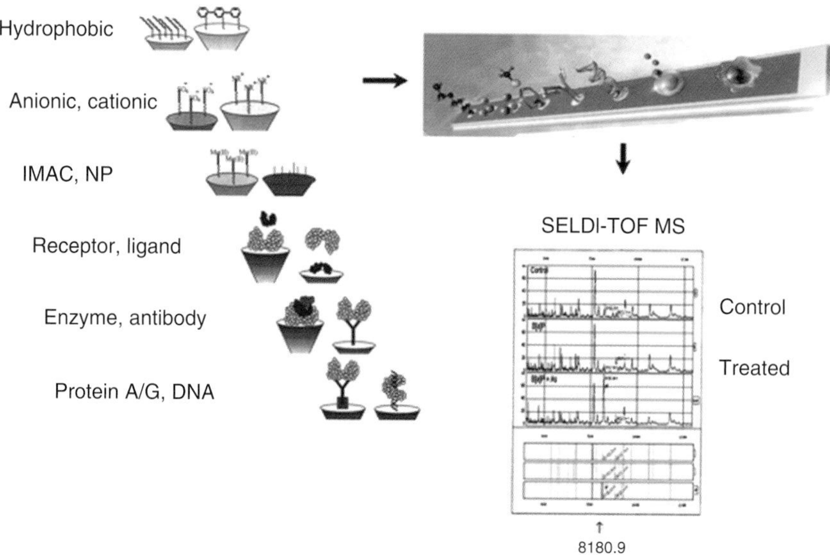

Figure 20.4 Schematic representation of protein chip array with examples of chemical functions responsible for protein category capture.

modification and thus offers a basis for detection of drug targets through examining the gene or protein expression profiles. Altered proteins in disease are candidates of drug targets that can be validated by modulating the proteins' activities in a model system to determine the outcome on disease phenotype (target validation). Genomics and proteomics are effective means to globally view and detect protein expression alterations in disease and drug treatment and thus serve in both processes of target identification and validation.

Examples using genomic and proteomic approaches for target protein discovery include the investigation of bengamides as a new class of methionine aminopeptidase inhibitors, the identification of transforming growth factor-β in lung epithelial cells and pancreatic carcinoma cells, plasma membrane proteins in breast cancer, BCNP1 and MIG2B in chronic lymphocytic leukemia, and heat shock protein 90 alpha (HSP 90) for tumor cell invasiveness. Others have applied preprecipitation prior to proteomic approach to identify targets in signaling pathways or certain cellular reactions. By using tandem affinity purification and nanospray microcapillary tandem mass spectrometry together with 2DE, Kumar et al. reported their comprehensive analysis of thioredoxin-targeted proteins in *Escherichia coli.* They found a number of proteins associated with thioredoxin that either participate directly (SodA, HPI, and AhpC) or have key regulatory functions (Fur and AcnB) in the detoxification of the cell. The thioredoxin targets in the unicellular photosynthetic eukaryote chlamydomonas reinhardtii also have been identified by proteomic approaches. With an efficient proteomic method, Godl et al., identified the cellular targets of protein kinase inhibitors, and this target may have significant implications on the development of p38 MAPK inhibitors as inflammatory drugs.

Genomics and proteomics can also be used to validate potential protein targets for those highly effective, widely used, or newly available drugs with unknown action mechanisms. For instance, HSP 70 has been reported as a target of farnesyl transferase inhibitor in ovarian cancer 2774 cell line and HSP 90 as a direct target of the anti-allergic drugs disodium cromoglycate and amlexanox. Cellular response of yeast cells to lithium and the enzyme active sites through labeling enzyme targets by sulfonate ester probes also have been investigated by proteomic approaches.

Functional proteomics is particularly useful for mapping protein–protein interaction in identifying potential targets. Protein–protein interaction, or receptor-ligand interaction, plays a critical role in cellular processes such as signal transduction, and thus is essential for the understanding of basic biological processes. In this regard, proteomics is often combined with other methods to study protein–protein interaction in developing suitable drug targets. Serebriiskii et al. used an enhanced Dual Bait two-hybrid system together with proteomic approaches to detect peptides, proteins, and drugs that selectively interact with protein targets. Other researchers applied luciferase complementation imaging together with proteomics to study kinetic regulation of protein-protein interactions. Rodriguez and his colleagues reported an oriented peptide array library approach to facilitate high throughput proteomic analysis of protein–protein interactions. The interaction of the SCF-like ubiquitin ligase was demonstrated as a potential target of drugs to control differentiation.

20.4.2 Actions of Anticancer Drugs

The growing knowledge about the close connection between apoptosis and cancer has led to an explosion of research revolving around apoptotic induction with chemotherapeutic agents and small molecule inhibitors.

Identification of cellular proteins that mediate apoptosis is a critical step toward the development of drug targets and new drug candidate screening. Genomics and proteomics present an overview of gene and protein alterations in both whole cell and subcellular fraction levels. Increasing efforts have been made to illustrate drug action mechanisms by genomics and proteomics.

Recently we have applied 2DE and MALDI-TOF MS based proteomic approach to identify cellular response and cytoplasmic protein alterations on cancer cells upon treatment of gold(III) porphyrin 1a, a potential anticancer drug lead. Anticancer drugs usually exhibit functions by initiation of apoptosis. Apoptosis, or programmed cell death, is a tightly controlled multistep cell death involving characteristic morphological and biochemical changes. This process is achieved via the aggregation and multimerization of the upstream molecules of the death effectors that activate sequential pathways. Major pathways involved in apoptosis include mitochondrial and/or cell membrane receptors activated caspase cascades, active oxygen species triggered cellular damages, cytoplasmic protein alteration, endoplasmic reticulum stress, and others.

In our studies, we have identified the upregulation of voltage-dependent anion channel 1 and the underexpression of mitochondrial single-stranded DNA binding protein as markers of mitochondria-mediated apoptosis pathways. A number of downregulated cytoplasmic proteins involved in cellular energy production were also found under gold(III) porphyrin 1a-induced apoptosis, including 3-phosphoglycerate dehydrogenase, glutamate dehydrogenase 1, actin-related protein 1 homologue A, sorbitol dehydrogenase, and glucose-6-phosphate dehydrogenase, further suggesting that mitochondrial damage is involved in gold(III) porphyrin 1a-induced cell death. Additionally, differentially expressed proteins including thioredoxin peroxidase, peroxiredoxin 1, peroxiredoxin 3, and peroxiredoxin 6, were potential markers for induction of reactive oxygen species.

Based on the results obtained in this study and biochemical characterization, we constructed a mode of action as shown in Figure 20.5. Gold(III) porphyrin 1a caused depletion of mitochondrial transmembrane potential ($\Delta\Psi_m$) soon after cellular uptake (within 3 h) with suppression of Bcl-2. $\Delta\Psi_m$ depletion facilitated the release of apoptosis-inducing factor (AIF) and cytochrome *c* from mitochondria. Subsequently, AIF activated the process of nuclear condensation, and cytochrome *c* activated the following caspases and caused oligonucleosomal DNA fragmentation and PARP-1 cleavage. Oxidative stress was likely to affect the cytotoxicity of gold(III) porphyrin 1a by regulating $\Delta\Psi_m$. Mitochondria are the major cellular target of gold(III) porphyrin 1a. However, the detailed mechanisms by which gold(III) porphyrin 1a targets mitochondria remain to be determined.

Increasing efforts have been made in exploring anticancer drug action mechanism by proteomic approaches. Proteomic profiling of drug-induced apoptosis in nonsmall lung carcinoma revealed that RS/DJ-1 (RNA-binding regulatory subunit/DJ-1 PARK7) and RhoGDI alpha (Rho GDP-dissociation inhibitor alpha) were uniquely altered in paclitaxel and MAPK inhibitor treatment. Proteomic analysis of protein kinase Raf-1 signaling complexes showed that Raf-1 counteracted apoptosis by suppressing the activation of mammalian sterile 20-like kinase (MST2), and that

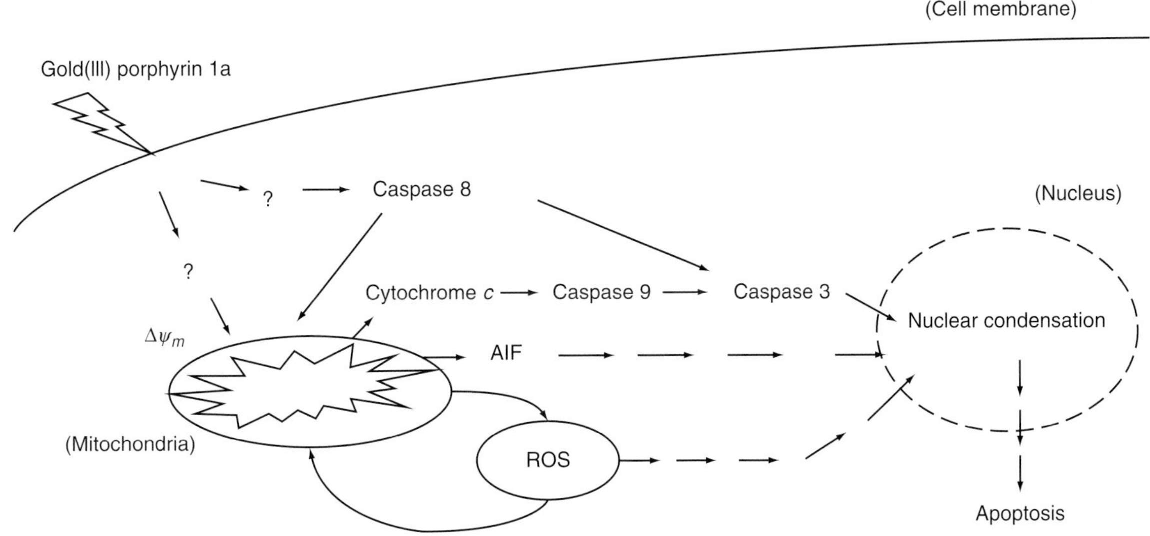

Figure 20.5 Proposed model for the cellular mechanisms of gold(III) porphyrin 1a induced apoptosis in HONE1 cells. Gold (III) porphyrin 1a directly caused depletion of $\Delta\Psi_m$, leading to the alteration of Bcl-2 family proteins, AIF nucleus translocation, and cytochrome c release, which further activated caspase-9 and caspase-3, and subsequently caused PARP-1 cleavage. ROS were also generated. The altered cellular oxidative state affected cytotoxicity of gold(III) porphyrin 1a by regulating mitochondrial permeabilization.

the concomitant depletion of both Raf-1 and MST2 prevented apoptosis. Another study used a proteomic method to profile the cellular targets of the clinical epidermal growth factor receptor kinase inhibitor gefitinib and determined alternative cellular modes of action for gefitinib, providing rationales for the development of related protein kinases targeted inhibitors.

Comparative proteomic studies have been used to identify the dynamic proteome changes upon ligand activation of Trk-receptors, direct induction of the mitochondrial chloride ion channel by Myc-induced apoptosis, and early changes in protein expression induced by erbB receptor inhibitors Tarceva (OSI-774) and herceptin. Global effects of diallyl trisulfide induced apoptosis in human gastric cancer cells, and 5-fluorouracil initiated cell death in cervical cancer cells were also analyzed with efficient proteomic method. Taken together, these studies revealed that interesting proteins identified by proteomics in the intracellular pathways targeted by anticancer drugs can be classified into several categories, including proteins related to mitochondrial function, endoplasmic reticulum (ER) stress proteins, oxidative stress and heat shock proteins, and nuclear proteins involved in signaling transduction. Further investigations can be carried out with prefractionated or purified proteins, or subcellular fractions, in order to reveal detailed protein alterations for the study of drug mechanism.

In addition to the sole use of proteomic methods, some studies have also applied combinational techniques to their investigation. By coupling 2D HPLCMS/MS with amino acid-coded mass tagging (AACT), Gu recently increased the analytical throughput and sequence coverage of MS-based methods for proteome-wide quantitation. Other investigators have employed the method to examine the anticancer effects of cyclin-dependent kinase inhibition. These researchers investigated the early stage of apoptosis by inducing the p53 upregulated modulator of apoptosis (PUMA) through the analyses of the relative ratios of the pairwise isotope signals that were originated from the control and labeled PUMA-induced cells. Integrated with transcriptomics, proteomics with simulation strategy have been used to profile the induction of apoptosis in mouse liver by microcystin-LR model.

Yan and his colleagues used a stable isotope labeled proteome internal standard to analyse protein expression alterations during oxidative stress in breast epithelial cells. Affinity chromatography was combined with MS/MS in the proteomic analysis of human O6-methylguanine-DNA methyltransferase. These studies demonstrated that proteomics can elucidate protein expre-ssions associated with the pharmacological and toxic effects of an anticancer drug when integrated with other biochemical methods.

20.4.3 Prediction of Drug Resistance

Drug resistance is a major problem that limits the effectiveness of chemotherapies used to treat cancer. Acquired drug resistance refers to the problem that tumors not only become resistant to the drugs originally used to treat them, but can also become cross-resistant to other drugs with different mechanisms of action. Cancer cell resistance to chemotherapy can occur at many levels, including increased drug efflux and decreased drug influx, drug inactivation, alterations in drug target, processing of drug-induced damage, and evasion of apoptosis. With the rapid accumulation of genomic and proteomic databases for complex biological systems, together with advances in technology platforms, functional proteomics offers more predictive "fingerprints" that can provide information about the responses upon therapeutic agents treatment. However, comparative transcriptional profiling alone is unlikely to predict drug sensitivity and/or resistance, a dynamic process where protein phosphorylation, protein trafficking, and protein–protein interactions with secondary effectors play key roles in the fate of cancer cells following therapeutic stress.

Genomic and proteomic approaches have been used to identify the underlying mechanisms for chemotherapeutic agents-induced resistance, including cisplatin, deoxycholate, incristine and vinblastine. Vincristine and vinblastine, two *vinca* alkaloids, are natural product drugs used extensively in the treatment of acute lymphoblastic leukemia. Previous studies have identified that these agents targeted beta-tubulin subunit alpha/beta-tubulin heterodimers, inhibiting the addition of heterodimers onto growing microbutules and hence, resulting in depolymerization of microtubules. However, this may not be the only reason leading to resistance of these agents. Alterations in tubulins, and/or tubulin-like proteins and tubulin-associated proteins may also be associated with *vinca* alkaloid resistance. Verrills examined the alterations of cellular protein expression in the drug-sensitive and drug-resistant cell lines using a differential proteomic approach to identify protein changes associated with *vinca* alkaloid resistance. A number of cytoskeleton proteins and their related proteins were expressed differentially in response to vincristine and vinblastine in *vinca* alkaloid-resistance cells, including downregulated cytoskeletal proteins class I beta-tubulin, alpha-tubulin, and actin, suppressed molecular chaperone HSP90, which serves as a tubulin-binding protein, decreased cell signaling regulators 14-3-3 epsilon and 14-3-3 tau associated with actin cytoskeleton, and some other proteins related to apoptosis process. In addition, to improve their understanding of the action mechanisms and cellular response to these agents, they also analyzed protein expression alterations in leukemia cells treated with vincristine.

Other studies suggested that alterations on actin cytoskeleton was an early event in apoptosis, with cytoskeletal disruption promoting damage of the mitochondrial membrane resulting in mitochondria-initiated apoptosis. Furthermore, disruption of the actin cytoskeleton can induce apoptosis with actin depolymerization triggered clustering and activation of Fas ligand. Together with results obtained from the study in *vinca* alkaloid resistance, it was most likely to predict that the changes in tubulin-binding proteins were responsible for drug resistance. Based on these results, prefractionation of cellular skeleton proteins or tubulin-binding proteins can be applied to further proteomics study on drug resistance.

20.4.4 Biomarkers for Determining Clinical Effects

Biomarkers are usually genes and proteins with their expressions altered in response to a disease condition. Biomarkers can be used as signatures to determine drug efficacy and clinical effects. Biomarkers can also be drug targets and serve as optimized selection of molecules that interact with these targets for further development. In genomics and proteomics, the challenge is to identify unique molecular signatures in complex biological mixtures that can be unambiguously correlated to biological events in order to validate novel drug targets and predict drug response.

Genomics and proteomics have emerged to be powerful approaches for directly identifying highly predictive pharmacogenomic markers in blood or tissues. Previously, we have reported the proteomic analysis of oral tongue carcinoma to globally search for tumor-related proteins. A number of tumor-associated proteins were consistently found to be significantly altered in their expression levels in tongue carcinoma tissues, compared with their paired normal mucosae. These proteins are potential biomarkers for tongue carcinoma diagnosis and therapeutic monitoring. A similar analysis for buccal squamous cell carcinoma also produced biomarker candidates that can be the proteomic signature for diagnostic and treatment. Hepatocarcinoma is another cancer that has received much attention recently. Several biomarkers have been identified by proteomic approaches, such as aldose reductase-like protein, cytokeratin 19, ferritin light chain, vitronectin, and serum associated fucosylated glycoproteins. Proteomic approaches have also been applied to biomarker or antigen identification for other cancers, including prostate cancer, bladder cancer, and ovarian cancer.

Advances of genomic and proteomic technologies also hold great promise for improvements in the understanding, diagnosis, and therapy of central nervous system disorders. Jin revealed a role of stathmin in adult neurogenesis by proteomic and immunochemical characterization. Others have reported that collapsin response mediator protein was a marker of changes developed in rat hippocampus. Great efforts have been made in searching for new and accurate biomarkers for cardiovascular system disease, HBV, and HCV infections.

Biomarker discovery could make great contributions to the characterization of the pharmacology of drug candidates and to the understanding of disease subtypes to which a therapeutic intervention applies. Proteomic approaches have been proved to be promising techniques in the process of biomarker discovery.

20.5 CONCLUSION AND FUTURE PROSPECTS

The potential value of genomics and proteomics in drug development, especially in mapping drug action mechanisms, has been demonstrated in many successful examples. Genomics and proteomic approaches have been recognized as promising techniques facilitating the systematic characterization of a drug targets' physiology, thereby helping to reduce the typically high attrition rates in discovery projects, and improving the overall efficiency of pharmaceutical research processes. A general strategy of genomics and proteomics in drug discovery and development is shown in Figure 20.6. However, at the present stage, the bottleneck for taking full advantage of these new experimental technologies are the rapidly growing volumes of automatically produced biological data, and technical challenges with regards to sampling, tumor heterogeneity, and lack of standardized methodologies. In addition, to complement the limitation of current genomic and proteomic technologies, other technological advances should be integrated with genomics and proteomics to better serve the purpose of illustrating the action mechanism of drugs and thus contribute to the success in drug development.

REVIEW QUESTIONS

1. What is genomics? List the milestones in the development of genomics.
2. What is proteomics? List the milestones in the development of proteomics.
3. How can microarrays be used to identify differentially regulated genes?
4. What is the principle of 2DE to separate protein mixtures?
5. In which aspects can genomic and proteomic approaches be integrated into drug discovery and development?
6. Describe the general strategy in illustration of drug actions by genomic and proteomic methods.
7. List a number of potential drug targets identified by genomic and proteomic approaches.
8. How can biomarker identification contribute to drug discovery and development?
9. What are limitations of genomics and proteomics at the present stage?
10. How can you confirm the vast number of data from genomic and proteomic studies?

ACKNOWLEDGEMENTS

This work was partially supported by Hong Kong Research Grants Council Grants HKU 7227/02M and HKU 7512/05M (to Q.Y.H.), HKU 7218/02M and HKU 7395/03M (to J.F.C.).

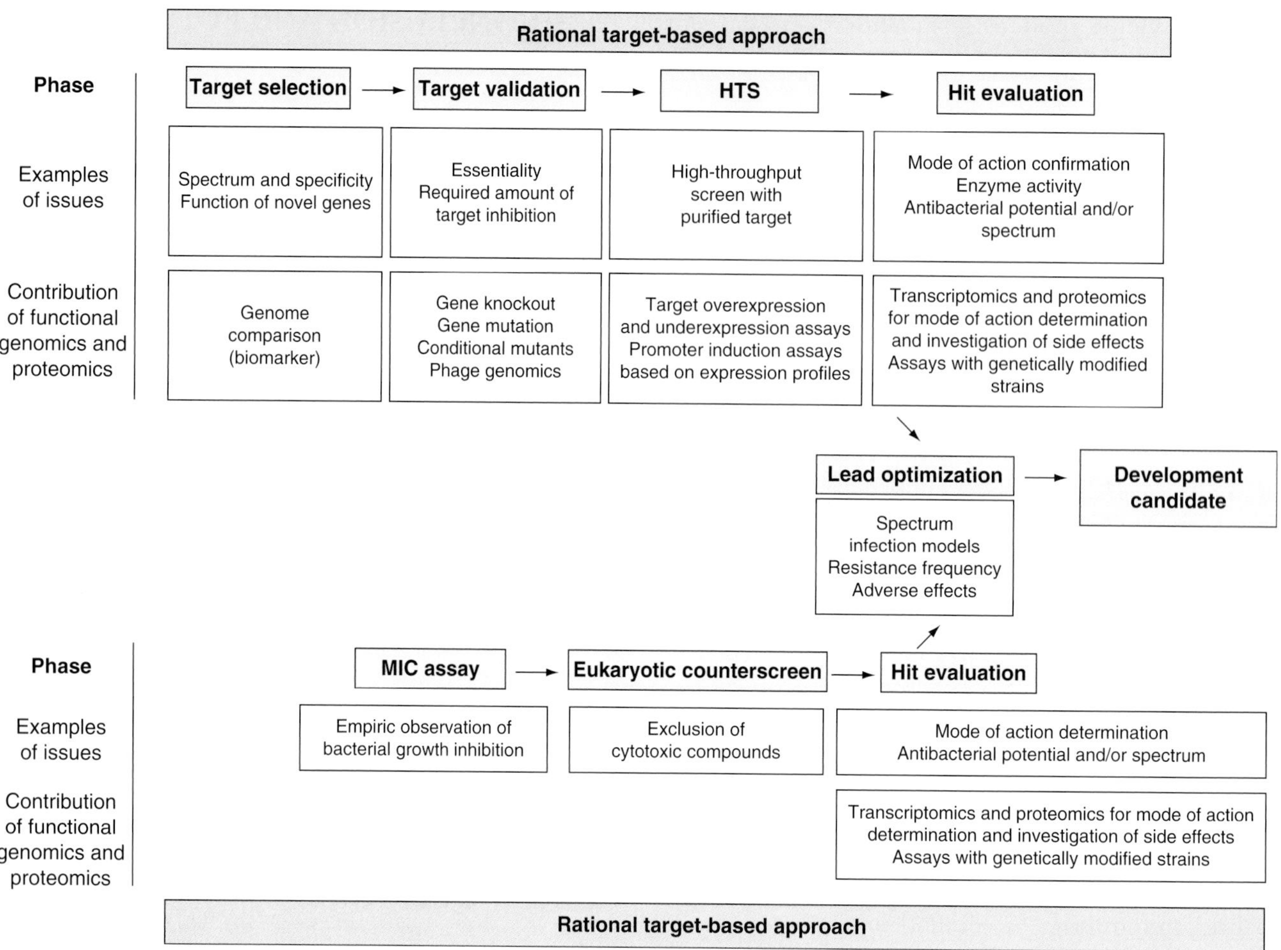

Figure 20.6 The overall contribution of genomics and proteomics to the drug discovery process. Abbreviation: MIC, minimal inhibitory concentration as a measure for drug activity.

REFERENCES

Adam, B. L., Vlahou, A., Semmes, O. J., & Wright, G. L., Jr. (2001a). Proteomic approaches to biomarker discovery in prostate and bladder cancers. *Proteomics, 1,* 1264–1270.

Adam, G. C., Burbaum, J., Kozarich, J. W., Patricelli, M. P., & Cravatt, B. F. (2004). Mapping enzyme active sites in complex proteomes. *Journal of the American Chemical Society, 126,* 1363–1368.

Adam, G. C., Cravatt, B. F., & Sorensen, E. J. (2001b). Profiling the specific reactivity of the proteome with non-directed activity-based probes. *Chemistry & Biology, 8,* 81–95.

Adam, G. C., Sorensen, E. J., & Cravatt, B. F. (2002a). Proteomic profiling of mechanistically distinct enzyme classes using a common chemotype. *Nature Biotechnology, 20,* 805–809.

Adam, G. C., Sorensen, E. J., & Cravatt, B. F. (2002b). Trifunctional chemical probes for the consolidated detection and identification of enzyme activities from complex proteomes. *Molecular & Cellular Proteomics: MCP, 1,* 828–835.

Adam, P. J., Boyd, R., Tyson, K. L., Fletcher, G. C., Stamps, A., Hudson, L., et al. (2003). Comprehensive proteomic analysis of breast cancer cell membranes reveals unique proteins with potential roles in clinical cancer. *The Journal of Biological Chemistry, 278,* 6482–6489.

Adkins, J. N., Varnum, S. M., Auberry, K. J., Moore, R. J., Angell, N. H., Smith, R. D., et al. (2002). Toward a human blood serum proteome: analysis by multidimensional separation coupled with mass spectrometry. *Molecular & Cellular Proteomics: MCP, 1,* 947–955.

Alonso, J. M., & Ecker, J. R. (2006). Moving forward in reverse: Genetic technologies to enable genome-wide phenomic screens in Arabidopsis. *Nature Reviews. Genetics, 7,* 524–536.

Amaral, L. A., Scala, A., Barthelemy, M., & Stanley, H. E. (2000). Classes of small-world networks. *Proceedings of the National Academy of Sciences of the United States of America, 97,* 11149–11152.

An, H. J., Kim, D. S., Park, Y. K., Kim, S. K., Choi, Y. P., Kang, S., et al. (2006). Comparative proteomics of ovarian epithelial tumors. *Journal of Proteome Research, 5,* 1082–1090.

Anderson, N. L., Taylor, J., Scandora, A. E., Coulter, B. P., & Anderson, N. G. (1981). The TYCHO system for computer analysis of two-dimensional gel electrophoresis patterns. *Clinical Chemistry, 27,* 1807–1820.

Archakov, A. I., Govorun, V. M., Dubanov, A. V., Ivanov, Y. D., Veselovsky, A. V., Lewi, P., & Janssen, P. (2003). Protein-protein interactions as a target for drugs in proteomics. *Proteomics, 3,* 380–391.

Arthur, J. M. (2003). Proteomics. *Current Opinion in Nephrology and Hypertension, 12,* 423–430.

Bernstein, H., Payne, C. M., Kunke, K., Crowley-Weber, C. L., Waltmire, C. N., Dvorakova, K., et al. (2004). A proteomic study of resistance to deoxycholate-induced apoptosis. *Carcinogenesis, 25,* 681–692.

Boyd, R. S., Adam, P. J., Patel, S., Loader, J. A., Berry, J., Redpath, N. T., et al. (2003). Proteomic analysis of the cell-surface membrane in chronic lymphocytic leukemia: Identification of two novel proteins, BCNP1 and MIG2B. *Leukemia: Official Journal of the Leukemia Society of America, Leukemia Research Fund, U. K, 17*, 1605–1612.

Braddock, M., & Quinn, A. (2004). Targeting IL-1 in inflammatory disease: New opportunities for therapeutic intervention. *Nature Reviews. Drug Discovery, 3*, 330–339.

Brehmer, D., Greff, Z., Godl, K., Blencke, S., Kurtenbach, A., Weber, M., et al., (2005). Cellular targets of gefitinib. *Cancer Research, 65*, 379–382.

Castagna, A., Antonioli, P., Astner, H., Hamdan, M., Righetti, S. C., Perego, P., et al. (2004). A proteomic approach to cisplatin resistance in the cervix squamous cell carcinoma cell line A431. *Proteomics, 4*, 3246–3267.

Celis, J. E., Wolf, H., & Ostergaard, M. (2000). Bladder squamous cell carcinoma biomarkers derived from proteomics. *Electrophoresis, 21*, 2115–2121.

Chen, J., He, Q. Y., Yuen, A. P., & Chiu, J. F. (2004). Proteomics of buccal squamous cell carcinoma: The involvement of multiple pathways in tumorigenesis. *Proteomics, 4*, 2465–2475.

Chen, T., Wang, Q., Cui, J., Yang, W., Shi, Q., Hua, Z., et al. (2005). Induction of apoptosis in mouse liver by microcystin-LR: A combined transcriptomic, proteomic, and simulation strategy. *Molecular & Cellular Proteomics: MCP, 4*, 958–974.

Cho, A., & Normile, D. (2002). Nobel Prize in Chemistry. Mastering macromolecules. *Science, 298*, 527–528.

Collins, M. O., Yu, L., Coba, M. P., Husi, H., Campuzano, I., Blackstock, W. P., et al. (2005). Proteomic analysis of in vivo phosphorylated synaptic proteins. *The Journal of Biological Chemistry, 280*, 5972–5982.

Comunale, M. A., Lowman, M., Long, R. E., Krakover, J., Philip, R., Seeholzer, S., et al. (2006). Proteomic analysis of serum associated fucosylated glycoproteins in the development of primary hepatocellular carcinoma. *Journal of Proteome Research, 5*, 308–315.

Ding, S. J., Li, Y., Tan, Y. X., Jiang, M. R., Tian, B., Liu, Y. K., et al. (2004). From proteomic analysis to clinical significance: Overexpression of cytokeratin 19 correlates with hepatocellular carcinoma metastasis. *Molecular & Cellular Proteomics: MCP, 3*, 73–81.

Duggan, D. J., Bittner, M., Chen, Y., Meltzer, P., & Trent, J. M. (1999). Expression profiling using cDNA microarrays. *Nature Genetics, 21*, 10–14.

Dyment, D. A., & Ebers, G. C. (2002). An array of sunshine in multiple sclerosis. *The New England Journal of Medicine, 347*, 1445–1447.

Eustace, B. K., Sakurai, T., Stewart, J. K., Yimlamai, D., Unger, C., Zehetmeier, C., et al. (2004). Functional proteomic screens reveal an essential extracellular role for hsp90 alpha in cancer cell invasiveness. *Nature Cell Biology, 6*, 507–514.

Fenn, J. B., Mann, M., Meng, C. K., Wong, S. F., & Whitehouse, C. M. (1989). Electrospray ionization for mass spectrometry of large biomolecules. *Science, 246*, 64–71.

Fleming, K., Muller, A., MacCallum, R. M., & Sternberg, M. J. (2004). 3D-GENOMICS: A database to compare structural and functional annotations of proteins between sequenced genomes. *Nucleic Acids Research, 32*, D245–D250.

Girvan, M., & Newman, M. E. (2002). Community structure in social and biological networks. *Proceedings of the National Academy of Sciences of the United States of America, 99*, 7821–7826.

Godl, K., Wissing, J., Kurtenbach, A., Habenberger, P., Blencke, S., Gutbrod, H., et al. (2003). An efficient proteomics method to identify the cellular targets of protein kinase inhibitors. *Proceedings of the National Academy of Sciences of the United States of America, 100*, 15434–15439.

Goffeau, A., Barrell, B. G., Bussey, H., Davis, R. W., Dujon, B., Feldmann, H., et al. (1996). Life with 6000 genes. *Science, 274*, 546, 563–566, 567.

Graves, P. R., Kwiek, J. J., Fadden, P., Ray, R., Hardeman, K., Coley, A. M., et al. (2002). Discovery of novel targets of quinoline drugs in the human purine binding proteome. *Molecular Pharmacology, 62*, 1364–1372.

Grossman, H. B., Soloway, M., Messing, E., Katz, G., Stein, B., Kassabian, V., et al. (2006). Surveillance for recurrent bladder cancer using a point-of-care proteomic assay. *JAMA: The Journal of the American Medical Association, 295*, 299–305.

Gu, S., Du, Y., Chen, J., Liu, Z., Bradbury, E. M., Hu, C. A., & Chen, X. (2004). Large-scale quantitative proteomic study of PUMA-induced apoptosis using two-dimensional liquid chromatography-mass spectrometry coupled with amino acid-coded mass tagging. *Journal of Proteome Research, 3*, 1191–1200.

Hanash, S. (2003). Disease proteomics. *Nature, 422*, 226–232.

He, Q. Y., Chen, J., Kung, H. F., Yuen, A. P., & Chiu, J. F. (2004). Identification of tumor-associated proteins in oral tongue squamous cell carcinoma by proteomics. *Proteomics, 4*, 271–278.

He, Q. Y., & Chiu, J. F. (2003). Proteomics in biomarker discovery and drug development. *Journal of Cellular Biochemistry, 89*, 868–886.

He, Q. Y., Lau, G. K., Zhou, Y., Yuen, S. T., Lin, M. C., Kung, H. F., et al. (2003). Serum biomarkers of hepatitis B virus infected liver inflammation: A proteomic study. *Proteomics, 3*, 666–674.

Heine, G., Raida, M., & Forssmann, W. G. (1997). Mapping of peptides and protein fragments in human urine using liquid chromatography-mass spectrometry. *Journal of Chromatography. A, 776*, 117–124.

Hock, D., Magerlein, M., Heine, G., Ochlich, P. P., & Forssmann, W. G. (1997). Isolation and characterization of the bioactive circulating human parathyroid hormone, hPTH-1-37. *FEBS Letters, 400*, 221–225.

Hu, W., Wu, W., Verschraegen, C. F., Chen, L., Mao, L., Yeung, S. C., et al. (2003). Proteomic identification of heat shock protein 70 as a candidate target for enhancing apoptosis induced by farnesyl transferase inhibitor. *Proteomics, 3*, 1904–1911.

Hughes, D. (2003). Exploiting genomics, genetics and chemistry to combat antibiotic resistance. *Nature Reviews. Genetics, 4*, 432–441.

Humphery-Smith, I., Cordwell, S. J., & Blackstock W. P. (1997). Proteome research: Complementarity and limitations with respect to the RNA and DNA worlds. *Electrophoresis, 18*, 1217–1242.

Imamura, T., Kanai, F., Kawakami, T., Amarsanaa, J., Ijichi, H., Hoshida, Y., et al. (2004). Proteomic analysis of the TGF-beta signaling pathway in pancreatic carcinoma cells using stable RNA interference to silence Smad4 expression. *Biochemical and Biophysical Research Communications, 318*, 289–296.

Jacobs, I. J., & Menon, U. (2004). Progress and challenges in screening for early detection of ovarian cancer. *Molecular & Cellular Proteomics: MCP, 3*, 355–366.

Jeffery, D. A., & Bogyo, M. (2003). Chemical proteomics and its application to drug discovery. *Current Opinion in Biotechnology, 14*, 87–95.

Jensen, O. N. (2006). Interpreting the protein language using proteomics. *Nature Reviews. Molecular Cell Biology, 7*, 391–403.

Jin, K., Mao, X. O., Cottrell, B., Schilling, B., Xie, L., Row, R. H., et al. (2004). Proteomic and immunochemical characterization of a role for stathmin in adult neurogenesis. *The FASEB Journal: Official Publication of the Federation of American Societies for Experimental Biology, 18*, 287–299.

Jordan, M. A., & Wilson, L. (1998). Microtubules and actin filaments: Dynamic targets for cancer chemotherapy. *Current Opinion in Cell Biology, 10*, 123–130.

Jung, J. W., Jung, S. H., Kim, H. S., Yuk, J. S., Park, J. B., Kim, Y. M., et al. (2006). High-throughput analysis of GST-fusion protein expression and activity-dependent protein interactions on GST-fusion protein arrays with a spectral surface plasmon resonance biosensor. *Proteomics, 6*, 1110–1120.

Kageyama, S., Isono, T., Iwaki, H., Wakabayashi, Y., Okada, Y., Kontani, K., et al. (2004). Identification by proteomic analysis of calreticulin as a marker for bladder cancer and evaluation of the diagnostic accuracy of its detection in urine. *Clinical Chemistry, 50*, 857–866.

Kamath, R. S., Fraser, A. G., Dong, Y., Poulin, G., Durbin, R., Gotta, M., et al. (2003). Systematic functional analysis of the Caenorhabditis elegans genome using RNAi. *Nature, 421*, 231–237.

Karas, M., & Hillenkamp, F. (1988). Laser desorption ionization of proteins with molecular masses exceeding 10,000 daltons. *Analytical Chemistry, 60*, 2299–2301.

Kebarle, P. (2000). A brief overview of the present status of the mechanisms involved in electrospray mass spectrometry. *Journal of Mass Spectrometry: JMS, 35*, 804–817.

Khawaja, X., Xu, J., Liang, J. J., & Barrett, J. E. (2004). Proteomic analysis of protein changes developing in rat hippocampus after chronic antidepressant treatment: Implications for depressive disorders and future therapies. *Journal of Neuroscience Research, 75*, 451–460.

Kopec, K. K., Bozyczko-Coyne, D., & Williams, M. (2005). Target identification and validation in drug discovery: The role of proteomics. *Biochemical Pharmacology, 69*, 1133–1139.

Kopf, E., Shnitzer, D., & Zharhary, D. (2005). Panorama Ab Microarray Cell Signaling kit: a unique tool for protein expression analysis. *Proteomics, 5*, 2412–2416.

Kramer, R., & Cohen, D. (2004). Functional genomics to new drug targets. *Nature Reviews. Drug Discovery, 3*, 965–972.

Kumar, J. K., Tabor, S., Richardson, C. C. (2004). Proteomic analysis of thioredoxin-targeted proteins in Escherichia coli. *Proc Natl Acad Sci USA, 101*, 3759–3764.

Kulms, D., Dussmann, H., Poppelmann, B., Stander, S., Schwarz, A., & Schwarz, T. (2002). Apoptosis induced by disruption of the actin cytoskeleton is mediated via activation of CD95 (Fas/APO-1). *Cell Death and Differentiation, 9*, 598–608.

Labugger, R., McDonough, J. L., Neverova, I., & Van Eyk, J. E. (2002). Solubilization, two-dimensional separation and detection of the cardiac myofilament protein troponin T. *Proteomics, 2*, 673–678.

Lau, A. T., He, Q. Y., & Chiu, J. F. (2004). A proteome analysis of the arsenite response in cultured lung cells: Evidence for in vitro oxidative stress-induced apoptosis. *The Biochemical Journal, 382*, 641–650.

Li, N., Guo, R., Li, W., Shao, J., Li, S., Zhao, K., et al. (2005). A proteomic investigation into a human gastric cancer cell line BGC823 treated with diallyl trisulfide. *Carcinogenesis.*

Liao, E. H., Hung, W., Abrams, B., & Zhen, M. (2004). An SCF-like ubiquitin ligase complex that controls presynaptic differentiation. *Nature, 430*, 345–350.

Linding, R., Jensen, L. J., Diella, F., Bork, P., Gibson, T. J., & Russell, R. B. (2003). Protein disorder prediction: implications for structural proteomics. *Structure (Camb.), 11*, 1453–1459.

Liu, Y., Patricelli, M. P., & Cravatt, B. F. (1999). Activity-based protein profiling: The serine hydrolases. *Proceedings of the National Academy of Sciences of the United States of America, 96*, 14694–14699.

Lockhart, D. J., Dong, H., Byrne, M. C., Follettie, M. T., Gallo, M. V., Chee, M. S., et al. (1996). Expression monitoring by hybridization to high-density oligonucleotide arrays. *Nature Biotechnology, 14*, 1675–1680.

Longley, D. B., & Johnston, P. G. (2005). Molecular mechanisms of drug resistance. *The Journal of Pathology, 205*, 275–292.

Luker, K. E., Smith, M. C., Luker, G. D., Gammon, S. T., Piwnica-Worms, H., & Piwnica-Worms, D. (2004). Kinetics of regulated protein-protein interactions revealed with firefly luciferase complementation imaging in cells and living animals. *Proceedings of the National Academy of Sciences of the United States of America, 101*, 12288–12293.

MacKeigan, J. P., Clements, C. M., Lich, J. D., Pope, R. M., Hod, Y., & Ting, J. P. (2003). Proteomic profiling drug-induced apoptosis in non-small cell lung carcinoma: Identification of RS/DJ-1 and RhoGDIalpha. *Cancer Research, 63*, 6928–6934.

Maggio, E. T., & Ramnarayan, K. (2001). Recent developments in computational proteomics. *Drug Discovery Today, 6*, 996–1004.

Mayr, M., Zhang, J., Greene, A. S., Gutterman, D. D., Perloff, J. K., & Ping, P. (2006). Proteomic based development of biomarkers in cardiovascular disease: Mechanistic, clinical, and therapeutic insights. *Molecular & Cellular Proteomics: MCP.*

Montaudo, M. S. (2002). Mass spectra of copolymers. *Mass Spectrometry Reviews, 21*, 108–144.

Mullis, K., Faloona, F., Scharf, S., Saiki, R., Horn, G., & Erlich, H. (1986). Specific enzymatic amplification of DNA in vitro: The polymerase chain reaction. *Cold Spring Harbor Symposia on Quantitative Biology, 51*(Pt 1), 263–273.

Nawrocki, S. T., Carew, J. S., Pino, M. S., Highshaw, R. A., Dunner, K., Jr., Huang, P., et al. (2005). Bortezomib sensitizes pancreatic cancer cells to endoplasmic reticulum stress-mediated apoptosis. *Cancer Research, 65*, 11658–11666.

Nielsen, U. B., Cardone, M. H., Sinskey, A. J., MacBeath, G., & Sorger, P. K. (2003). Profiling receptor tyrosine kinase activation by using Ab microarrays. *Proceedings of the National Academy of Sciences of the United States of America, 100*, 9330–9335.

Niture, S. K., Doneanu, C. E., Velu, C. S., Bailey, N. I., & Srivenugopal, K. S. (2005). Proteomic analysis of human O6-methylguanine-DNA methyltransferase by affinity chromatography and tandem mass spectrometry. *Biochemical and Biophysical Research Communications, 337*, 1176–1184.

Norell, H., Carlsten, M., Ohlum, T., Malmberg, K. J., Masucci, G., Schedvins, K., et al. (2006). Frequent loss of HLA-A2 expression in metastasizing ovarian carcinomas associated with genomic haplotype loss and HLA-A2-restricted HER-2/neu-specific immunity. *Cancer Research, 66*, 6387–6394.

O'Farrell, P. H. (1975). High resolution two-dimensional electrophoresis of proteins. *The Journal of Biological Chemistry, 250*, 4007–4021.

O'Neill, E., Rushworth, L., Baccarini, M., & Kolch, W. (2004). Role of the kinase MST2 in suppression of apoptosis by the proto-oncogene product Raf-1. *Science, 306*, 2267–2270.

Okada, M., Itoh, H., Hatakeyama, T., Tokumitsu, H., & Kobayashi, R. (2003). Hsp90 is a direct target of the anti-allergic drugs disodium cromoglycate and amlexanox. *The Biochemical Journal, 374*, 433–441.

Paradis, V., Degos, F., Dargere, D., Pham, N., Belghiti, J., Degott, C., et al. (2005). Identification of a new marker of hepatocellular carcinoma by serum protein profiling of patients with chronic liver diseases. *Hepatology (Baltimore, Md.), 41*, 40–47.

Park, K. S., Kim, H., Kim, N. G., Cho, S. Y., Choi, K. H., Seong, J. K., et al. (2002). Proteomic analysis and molecular characterization of tissue ferritin light chain in hepatocellular carcinoma. *Hepatology (Baltimore, Md.), 35*, 1459–1466.

Petricoin, E. F., Ardekani, A. M., Hitt, B. A., Levine, P. J., Fusaro, V. A., Steinberg, S. M., et al. (2002). Use of proteomic patterns in serum to identify ovarian cancer. *Lancet, 359*, 572–577.

Petricoin, E. F., Ornstein, D. K., & Liotta, L. A. (2004). Clinical proteomics: Applications for prostate cancer biomarker discovery and detection. *Urologic Oncology, 22*, 322–328.

Pinet, F., Poirier, F., Fuchs, S., Tharaux, P. L., Caron, M., Corvol, P., et al. (2004). Troponin T as a marker of differentiation revealed by proteomic analysis in renal arterioles. *The FASEB Journal: Official Publication of the Federation of American Societies for Experimental Biology, 18*, 585–586.

Qiao, J., Kang, J., Cree, J., Evers, B. M., & Chung, D. H. (2005). Gastrin-releasing peptide-induced down-regulation of tumor suppressor protein PTEN (phosphatase and tensin homolog deleted on chromosome ten) in neuroblastomas. *Annals of Surgery, 241*, 684–691.

Rai, A. J., & Chan, D. W. (2004). Cancer proteomics: Serum diagnostics for tumor marker discovery. *Annals of the New York Academy of Sciences, 1022*, 286–294.

Renfrey, S., & Featherstone, J. (2002). Structural proteomics. *Nature Reviews. Drug Discovery, 1*, 175–176.

Reyzer, M. L., Caldwell, R. L., Dugger, T. C., Forbes, J. T., Ritter, C. A., Guix, M., et al. (2004). Early changes in protein expression detected by mass spectrometry predict tumor response to molecular therapeutics. *Cancer Research, 64*, 9093–9100.

Righetti, P. G., Castagna, A., Antonioli, P., & Boschetti, E. (2005). Prefractionation techniques in proteome analysis: The mining tools of the third millennium. *Electrophoresis, 26*, 297–319.

Rodriguez, M., Li, S. S., Harper, J. W., & Songyang, Z. (2004). An oriented peptide array library (OPAL) strategy to study protein-protein interactions. *The Journal of Biological Chemistry, 279*, 8802–8807.

Rosamond, J., & Allsop, A. (2000). Harnessing the power of the genome in the search for new antibiotics. *Science, 287*, 1973–1976.

Sali, A., Glaeser, R., Earnest, T., & Baumeister, W. (2003). From words to literature in structural proteomics. *Nature, 422*, 216–225.

Sanishvili, R., Yakunin, A. F., Laskowski, R. A., Skarina, T., Evdokimova, E., Doherty-Kirby, A., et al. (2003). Integrating structure, bioinformatics, and enzymology to discover function: BioH, a new carboxylesterase from Escherichia coli. *The Journal of Biological Chemistry, 278*, 26039–26045.

Sauer, S., Lange, B. M., Gobom, J., Nyarsik, L., Seitz, H., & Lehrach, H. (2005). Miniaturization in functional genomics and proteomics. *Nature Reviews. Genetics, 6*, 465–476.

Schena, M., Shalon, D., Davis, R. W., & Brown, P. O. (1995). Quantitative monitoring of gene expression patterns with a complementary DNA microarray. *Science, 270*, 467–470.

Schubert, W. (2003). Topological proteomics, toponomics, MELK-technology. *Advances in Biochemical Engineering/Biotechnology, 83*, 189–209.

Serebriiskii, I. G., Mitina, O., Pugacheva, E. N., Benevolenskaya, E., Kotova, E., Toby, G. G., et al. (2002). Detection of peptides, proteins, and drugs that selectively interact with protein targets. *Genome Research, 12*, 1785–1791.

Shiio, Y., Suh, K. S., Lee, H., Yuspa, S. H., Eisenman, R. N., & Aebersold, R. (2006). Quantitative proteomic analysis of myc-induced apoptosis: a direct role for Myc induction of the mitochondrial chloride ion channel, mtCLIC/CLIC4. *The Journal of Biological Chemistry, 281,* 2750–2756.

Sielaff, I., Arnold, A., Godin, G., Tugulu, S., Klok, H. A., & Johnsson, K. (2006). Protein function microarrays based on self-immobilizing and self-labeling fusion proteins. *Chembiochem: A European Journal of Chemical Biology, 7,* 194–202.

Sitek, B., Apostolov, O., Stuhler, K., Pfeiffer, K., Meyer, H. E., Eggert, A., et al. (2005). Identification of dynamic proteome changes upon ligand activation of Trk-receptors using two-dimensional fluorescence difference gel electrophoresis and mass spectrometry. *Molecular & Cellular Proteomics: MCP, 4,* 291–299.

Skalnikova, H., Halada, P., Dzubak, P., Hajduch, M., & Kovarova, H. (2005). Protein fingerprints of anti-cancer effects of cyclin-dependent kinase inhibition: Identification of candidate biomarkers using 2-D liquid phase separation coupled to mass spectrometry. *Technology in Cancer Research & Treatment, 4,* 447–454.

Song, K. H., An, H. M., Kim, H. J., Ahn, S. H., Chung, S. J., & Shim, C. K. (2002). Simple liquid chromatography-electrospray ionization mass spectrometry method for the routine determination of salmon calcitonin in serum. *Journal of Chromatography. B, Analytical Technologies in the Biomedical and Life Sciences, 775,* 247–255.

Stasyk, T., & Huber, L. A. (2004). Zooming in: Fractionation strategies in proteomics. *Proteomics, 4,* 3704–3716.

Stoughton, R. B., & Friend, S. H. (2005). How molecular profiling could revolutionize drug discovery. *Nature Reviews. Drug Discovery, 4,* 345–350.

Sun, X., Chiu, J. F., & He, Q. Y. (2005). Application of immobilized metal affinity chromatography in proteomics. *Expert Reviews of Proteomics, 2,* 649–657.

Takashima, M., Kuramitsu, Y., Yokoyama, Y., Iizuka, N., Fujimoto, M., Nishisaka, T., et al. (2005). Overexpression of alpha enolase in hepatitis C virus-related hepatocellular carcinoma: Association with tumor progression as determined by proteomic analysis. *Proteomics, 5,* 1686–1692.

Takashima, M., Kuramitsu, Y., Yokoyama, Y., Iizuka, N., Toda, T., Sakaida, I., et al. (2003). Proteomic profiling of heat shock protein 70 family members as biomarkers for hepatitis C virus-related hepatocellular carcinoma. *Proteomics, 3,* 2487–2493.

Towbin, H., Bair, K. W., DeCaprio, J. A., Eck, M. J., Kim, S., Kinder, F. R., et al. (2003). Proteomics-based target identification: Bengamides as a new class of methionine aminopeptidase inhibitors. *The Journal of Biological Chemistry, 278,* 52964–52971.

Valianpour, F., Wanders, R. J., Barth, P. G., Overmars, H., & van Gennip, A. H. (2002). Quantitative and compositional study of cardiolipin in platelets by electrospray ionization mass spectrometry: Application for the identification of Barth syndrome patients. *Clinical Chemistry, 48,* 1390–1397.

Vaux, D. L., & Korsmeyer, S. J. (1999). Cell death in development. *Cell, 96,* 245–254.

Venkatraman, A., Landar, A., Davis, A. J., Chamlee, L., Sanderson, T., Kim, H., et al. (2004). Modification of the mitochondrial proteome in response to the stress of ethanol-dependent hepatotoxicity. *The Journal of Biological Chemistry, 279,* 22092–22101.

Venter, J. C., Adams, M. D., Myers, E. W., Li, P. W., Mural, R. J., Sutton, G. G., et al. (2001). The sequence of the human genome. *Science, 291,* 1304–1351.

Verrills, N. M., Walsh, B. J., Cobon, G. S., Hains, P. G., & Kavallaris, M. (2003). Proteome analysis of vinca alkaloid response and resistance in acute lymphoblastic leukemia reveals novel cytoskeletal alterations. *The Journal of Biological Chemistry, 278,* 45082–45093.

Vivanco, F., Martin-Ventura, J. L., Duran, M. C., Barderas, M. G., Blanco-Colio, L., Darde, V. M., et al. (2005). Quest for novel cardiovascular biomarkers by proteomic analysis. *Journal of Proteome Research, 4,* 1181–1191.

Wang, Y., He, Q. Y., Sun, R. W., Che, C. M., Chiu, J. F. (2005). Gold(III) Porphyrin 1a induced apoptosis by mitochondrial death pathways related to reactive oxygen species. *Cancer Research, 65,* 11553–11564.

Wang, Y., Cheung, Y. H., Yang, Z., Chiu, J. F., Che, C. M., & He, Q. Y. (2006a). Proteomic approach to study the cytotoxicity of dioscin (saponin). *Proteomics, 6,* 2422–2432.

Wang, Y., Hanley, R., & Klemke, R. L. (2006b). Computational methods for comparison of large genomic and proteomic datasets reveal protein markers of metastatic cancer. *Journal of Proteome Research, 5,* 907–915.

Wang, Y., He, Q. Y., Che, C. M., & Chiu, J. F. (2006c). Proteomic characterization of the cytotoxic mechanism of gold (III) porphyrin 1a, a potential anticancer drug. *Proteomics, 6,* 131–142.

Wasinger, V. C., Cordwell, S. J., Cerpa-Poljak, A., Yan, J. X., Gooley, A. A., Wilkins, M. R., et al. (1995). Progress with gene-product mapping of the Mollicutes: Mycoplasma genitalium. *Electrophoresis, 16,* 1090–1094.

Watson, J. D. (1990). The human genome project: Past, present, and future. *Science, 248,* 44–49.

Whitehouse, C. M., Dreyer, R. N., Yamashita, M., & Fenn, J. B. (1985). Electrospray interface for liquid chromatographs and mass spectrometers. *Analytical Chemistry, 57,* 675–679.

Yamazaki, Y., Tsuruga, M., Zhou, D., Fujita, Y., Shang, X., Dang, Y., et al. (2000). Cytoskeletal disruption accelerates caspase-3 activation and alters the intracellular membrane reorganization in DNA damage-induced apoptosis. *Experimental Cell Research, 259,* 64–78.

Yan, Y., Weaver, V. M., & Blair, I. A. (2005). Analysis of protein expression during oxidative stress in breast epithelial cells using a stable isotope labeled proteome internal standard. *Journal of Proteome Research, 4,* 2007–2014.

Yates, J. R., III. (1998). Mass spectrometry and the age of the proteome. *Journal of Mass Spectrometry: JMS, 33,* 1–19.

Yim, E. K., Lee, K. H., Bae, J. S., Namkoong, S. E., Um, S. J., & Park, J. S. (2004). Proteomic analysis of antiproliferative effects by treatment of 5-fluorouracil in cervical cancer cells. *DNA and Cell Biology, 23,* 769–776.

Yu, H., Zhu, X., Greenbaum, D., Karro, J., & Gerstein, M. (2004). TopNet: A tool for comparing biological sub-networks, correlating protein properties with topological statistics. *Nucleic Acids Research, 32,* 328–337.

Zeindl-Eberhart, E., Haraida, S., Liebmann, S., Jungblut, P. R., Lamer, S., Mayer, D., et al. (2004). Detection and identification of tumor-associated protein variants in human hepatocellular carcinomas. *Hepatology (Baltimore, Md.), 39,* 540–549.

Zhu, W., Wang, X., Ma, Y., Rao, M., Glimm, J., & Kovach, J. S. (2003). Detection of cancer-specific markers amid massive mass spectral data. *Proceedings of the National Academy of Sciences of the United States of America, 100,* 14666–14671.

Chapter

21

The Future of Pharmacology

John S. Lazo

OUTLINE

21.1 INTRODUCTION

It is interesting to speculate as to whether or not this is the most interesting period that has ever existed for Pharmacology. The Human Genome Project was completed with great fanfare, and now the genomes of thousands of species are being assembled, offering a profound view of who we are and how we evolved. We are at the confluence of enormous advancements in our understanding of Human Biology and Pathogenesis, in the application of novel methods in Synthetic Bioorganic and Medicinal Chemistry, and in the introduction of innovative approaches in Computational Chemistry. These powerful products of the last half-century of public investment in biomedical research offer wonderful opportunities for future therapies and will have a profound impact on how we find and use the drugs of the past and future. This chapter seeks to outline just a few of these issues and opportunities that might reasonably be predicted to occur in the next decade. Of course, as with any prediction, there is always the possibility that unpredicted observations will completely reorient our pharmacological thoughts or new tools will permit unimagined treatments. Let us hope so.

21.2 THE PROBLEM

If we objectively examine the process by which contemporary therapies are discovered and developed, it is obvious there is no one linear pathway. Indeed there are many roads to a successful new human therapy. Perhaps this is obvious when we think of all the peoples in the world and the history of drug discovery and development. In the ancient times, human remedies were derived largely from extracts of local plants, animals, or minerals. Prior to 1800, herbal listings or pharmacopeia could be found in China (*Materia Medica*), India (*Ayuryedic system*), or Greece (*De Materia Medica*). Even today in some cultures, such as the Chinese or American Indians, traditional medicines remain a central component of the healthcare system. Paracelsus urged alchemists to extract the pharmacological essence of mixtures, but it was the chemists of the eighteenth and nineteenth centuries that provided the first defined small molecules demonstrating drug-like activity.

Perhaps the most profound modifier of therapeutics in the Western world was the invention of aspirin, which remains today the most widely used drug in the world. The discovery of aspirin was serendipitous like almost all of its predecessors (Figure 21.1). Nonetheless, the popular adoption of this analgesic encouraged others to discover and develop the wonder drugs of the early twentieth century, including the sulfa drugs. The substantial developments in new synthetic and analytical chemical methodologies were particularly influential (Drews 2000) but the contributions of physiology, biochemistry, and molecular biology cannot be overstated. The increased complexity of new agents has led to problems that were never anticipated in the early years of drug discovery and development including the high cost of new pharmacological agents.

Pharmaceutical innovation has almost always been associated with higher costs for several reasons. First, there are many diseases for which we continue to require new treatments. For example, Alzheimer's disease and most adult cancers are not adequately treated by contemporary medicines. Second, resistance to antibiotic, antimalarial, and anticancer drugs renders previously active agents inactive. In the case of antibacterial drugs, the emergence of resistance can be traced to overusage and the rapid reproductive capacity of bacteria. This reduces the life cycle of effective drugs

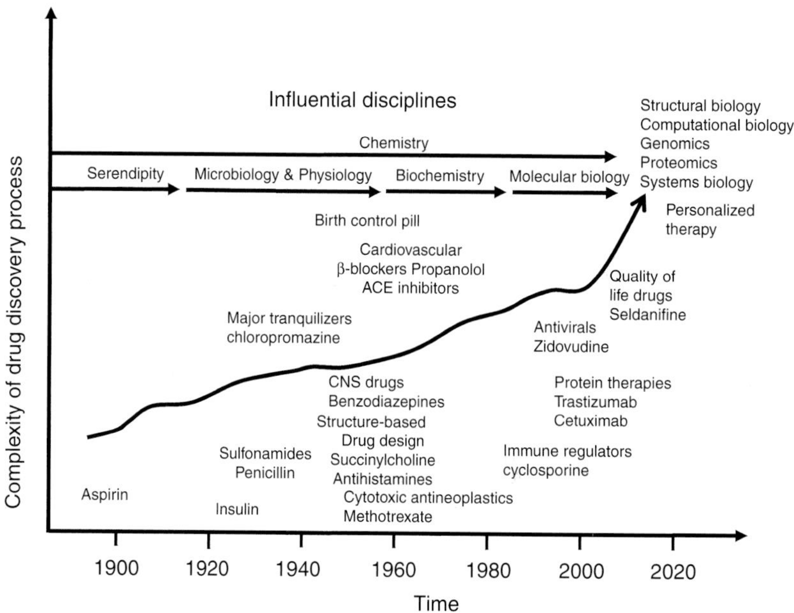

Figure 21.1 Timeline of new drugs. Some of the major classes of drugs discovered and developed in different periods are noted. The dominant influential disciples affecting the drug discovery and development process are listed above the timeline.

and encourages restricted use of newer drugs, all of which decreases the potential profits for commercial providers. A third cause for increased costs is the increased complexity of new agents. In some cases peptides and proteins including antibodies are emerging as potent drugs. These are generally expensive to produce and are not orally active. The development of innovative drugs is generally a high-risk venture that requires the combined efforts of chemists, biologists, pharmacologists, and clinicians. Historically, the success rate from first-in-human to registration has been approximately 10 percent with some areas such as oncology being as low as five percent (Kamb et al. 2007). The inefficiencies of the drug discovery and development process contribute to the cost of new drugs.

21.3 STRATEGIES FOR SEARCHING FOR FUTURE DRUGS

The search for new pharmacological agents historically has followed two general pathways: forward pharmacology and reverse pharmacology (Figure 21.2). As illustrated in Figure 21.1, the early days of discovery and development of new pharmaceutical agents was dominated almost completely by the use of empirical approaches that capitalized on enlightened serendipity. Potential drugs were identified using physiological methods with animals, isolated organs, or tissue preparations, and little or no understanding of the mechanism of action of the compound. This forward pharmacology approach had the advantage of knowing that the compound acted *in vivo* or *in situ*, enhancing the likelihood that the compound would produce the desired physiological effect in humans. If an animal model was being used, there was the added benefit that the investigator might be able to deduce some information about the duration of action, safety, and possibly metabolism of the drug. The approach was unbiased in that the investigator had no preconceived molecular target. The approach achieved success, however, generally only when good animal models or tissue preparations were available that replicated the human disease. Regrettably, for many diseases these do not exist, making forward pharmacology challenging.

An alternative approach, which has become increasingly popular with the advent and growth of molecular biology, is reverse pharmacology. This reductionist approach relies on the isolation of an identified molecular target, often an enzyme, and seeking a small molecule that affects the target's known or predicted function. Inhibitors are generally more attractive than enzyme activators because of the belief that gain-of-function is a much more challenging task for a small molecule than loss-of-function. Highly simplified test systems are designed to allow a deep understanding about the nature of the inhibition, including kinetics and site of inhibition. Armed with structural information about the target, sometimes at the atomic level, scientists can design even more potent and selective inhibitors. Although compelling at an intellectual level, reverse and computational pharmacology approaches can fail because the compounds are unable to reach the target, are rapidly metabolized, or are highly toxic. Moreover, the target may not be rate-limiting for the disease or the disease may be multifactorial. Some targets may not be readily obtained or functional in a highly simplified *in vitro* system. Demonstration of

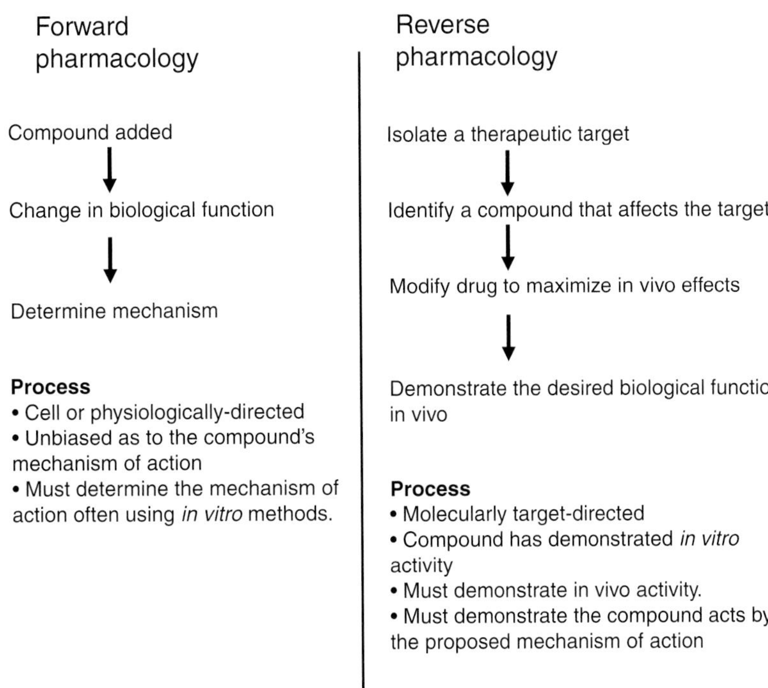

Forward
pharmacology
Compound added
Change in biological function
Determine mechanism
Process
• Cell or physiologically-directed
• Unbiased as to the compound's mechanism of action
• Must determine the mechanism of action often using in vitro methods.
Reverse
pharmacology
Isolate a therapeutic target
Identify a compound that affects the target
Modify drug to maximize in vivo effects
Demonstrate the desired biological function in vivo
Process
• Molecularly target-directed
• Compound has demonstrated in vitro activity
• Must demonstrate in vivo activity.
• Must demonstrate the compound acts by the proposed mechanism of action

Figure 21.2 The two fundamental approaches to drug discovery.

in vivo activity becomes an essential component of this approach.

Knowledge of the molecular targets enables one to practice computational pharmacology, in which we first seek desired pharmacological agents *in silico* with subsequent confirmation with *in vitro* assays. Although there are no obvious examples of clinically used compounds that have been discovered entirely by this approach, a number of newer agents have been assisted by computational methodologies. The increasing availability of high-resolution crystal and NMR structures for potential drug targets makes it likely that this innovative method will become an important platform for future drugs. Obviously, compounds first identified by *in silico* methods will require *in vitro* and *in vivo* validation, but programs that predict "drug-like" properties and toxicological propensity are increasingly being applied to reduce the likelihood of failure in preclinical and clinical trials.

A critical and perplexing question that frequently occurs in the search for new agents is the locus in a signaling pathway that we should target (Figure 21.3). For example, for a typical ligand-mediated signal transduction pathway, should we target the ligand-receptor interaction (Figure 21.3, pathway A), which will affect the entire distal process or further down the pathway, such as pathways B through D, to influence only a portion of the process? In many situations, the detailed kinetics of the pathway and the collateral signaling effectors are unknown, making a decision problematic. In some cases, it may be desirable to disrupt the pathway at several levels to ensure effective disruption and to reduce the likelihood of pathway disruption compensation or drug resistance.

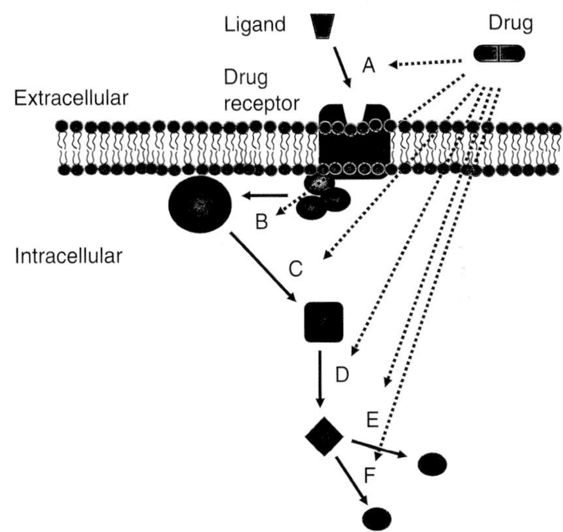

Figure 21.3 Potential targeting of receptors and signaling pathways. This schematic illustrates potential sites of intervention of drug in a cell. In pathway A, the drug blocks the ligand interaction with the receptor. In pathways B–D, different sites in the bifurcating signal transduction pathway are inhibited.

21.4 TOOLS FOR SEARCHING FOR FUTURE DRUGS

It is obvious that computational pharmacology will require more powerful computers, programs, and functional databases with new targets. Public and private efforts to produce new predictive software and to determine the structures of all the major disease-associated proteins seem likely to provide the tools required to undertake innovative searches. Moreover, these computational improvements may allow individuals conducting high throughput screening to narrow the number of compounds initially evaluated, thus permitting more productive screening. For reverse pharmacology, major tools have been the availability of automated protein production facilities, liquid handling systems, and detectors. These have enabled high throughput screening of molecular targets sometimes with millions of compounds in a single day. Assay miniaturization can often permit higher throughput, smaller compound consumption, and reagent usage.

A growing appreciation of the complexity of disease processes has stimulated an increased interest in the use of systems biology for forward pharmacology. Improvements in microscopic platforms, biosensors, and fluorescent probes now permit multiparametric analyses in cells and some lower organisms. The application of high content screening allows us to begin to examine several events simultaneously in cells such as signaling pathways, cell cycle movement, or death processes. These tools can be applied as a primary method to identify new agents or as secondary assays to confirm the desired biological activity. Equally important is the growing number of animal models designed to recapitulate human diseases. The availability of genetic methods to delete, mutate, or express genes that are thought to be associated with human diseases provide powerful tools for experimentalists. Cells can be isolated, that can be combined with the aforementioned high content methods for drug screens. Genetically altered bacteria, yeast, mice, or rats can also be employed for evaluation of compounds.

The number and types of compounds that can be investigating continues to expand because of efforts to increase the types of molecules that can be generated by combinatorial and diversity-oriented synthesis. There are now millions of compounds that are commercially available for interrogation. Natural products, which typically have benefited from evolutionary influences, provide bioactive, albeit often complex, chemical skeletons that can be probed for new uses. It is almost axiomatic that medicinal chemists increase rather than decrease the mass of analogs in their search for more potent and selective agents. Thus, fragment-based chemical libraries are emerging, which allow us to identify a weak perturbing agent, which can be further refined. New chemical approaches such as dynamic chemical libraries may provide even greater access to chemical space.

21.5 THE DRUGS OF THE FUTURE

So what will the drugs of the future look like? Of course, it is always dangerous to speculate about future therapies because of the complexities of the process. Nonetheless, the success of small molecules in the last century suggests they will be the dominant form of therapeutic intervention for the foreseeable future. A high premium will be placed on drugs that are orally active due to ease of administration and convenience. Compounds that are difficult to formulate may benefit from materials emerging from such fields as Material Sciences and Nanotechnology. The design of delivery systems that improve absorption and optimize release also seem likely. The development of closed loop or smart delivery systems that detect when a drug is needed for diseases such as diabetes and release drugs accordingly might emerge as transformational approaches. There is no doubt that large molecular entities will continue to be developed and used. Protein therapies in the form of humanized antibodies or naked proteins can provide highly selective approaches to treating human diseases. Although these are often expensive to produce, have limited body distribution, and are not orally active, they provide access to gain-of-function processes and molecular targets that can be difficult for small molecules. Nucleic acid-or protein-nucleic acid-based therapies may increase as newer chemical methods to improve delivery and stability are identified.

There continues to be considerable interest in using liposomes as a method to target specific tissues or tumors. Modification of the surface of the liposomes may enable investigators to improve delivery and efficacy. These same strategies are also being applied to genes in an effort to replace missing or altered endogenous genes. The challenges for gene therapy continue to be effective and complete delivery with durable expression and minimal toxicity so it is difficult to predict if these will become viable clinically used therapeutics. Vaccines represent attractive treatment approaches for a limited number of diseases, but there have been aggressive efforts to expand their use, especially for cervical cancer and malaria.

During the past decade progress in genome sequencing has exposed some of the genetic bases for human disease and for interpatient differences in drug metabolism. For example, we know there are many polymorphisms in the more than 220 drug metabolizing enzymes and drug transporters. This knowledge provides the foundation for the growing interest in applying genomic tools for highly individualized medicine. This could be in the form of using the presence of a specific mutated gene or elements of an individual's genome as diagnostic for determining the drug to be prescribed for that person. We know, for example, the CYP2D6 allelic composition can markedly influence the metabolic activity in individuals (Cai, Zhang 2007). Alternatively, we might use genetic information to design preventative therapeutic measures. There are already examples of gene-based individualized therapies. For example, irinotecan is a widely used anticancer drug for the treatment of advanced colorectal cancer and its toxicity is profoundly influenced by genetic variants in the promoter of UDP glucuronosyltransferase isoforms. Genetic tests have been developed that reveal the presence of dinucleotide insertions in the TATA-box that alter expression and thus, drug toxicity.

Nonetheless, there are considerable challenges for the more widespread use of diagnostics with drugs to permit truly individualized medicine. First, the true cause of a disease may not be reflected directly in an individual's genome, making it impossible to detect the relevant marker for drug treatment. DNA must be transcripted into RNA, which can be subjected to splicing leading to different transcripts, which are transcripts into proteins with distinct functions. Furthermore, the proteins themselves are subject to multiple posttranslational processes, which are not encoded in the DNA. Finally, proteins can be sequestered into specific regions of a cell and this spatial localization, which is not necessarily encoded in the genome, determines functionality. Thus, detecting the appropriate biomarker for proper therapy may require a proteomic approach. For some diseases the important determinant may not even be associated with a protein but a lipid, metabolite, or carbohydrate. Therefore, there remains considerable controversy about the detection systems that will provide the optimal information needed for true personalized medicine. Some investigators believe noninvasive molecular imaging in the form of computed tomography (CT), positive emission tomography (PET), or magnetic resonance imaging (MRI) have the greatest potential for allowing personalized therapy. Regardless, it seems likely that the drugs of the future will benefit from the use of new methodologies that will help guide a more effective patient selection and drug administration.

REFERENCES

Cai, W. M., Chen, B., & Zhang, W. X. (2007). Frequency of CYP2D6*10 and *14 alleles and their influence on the metabolic activity of CYP2D6 in a healthy Chinese population. *Clinical Pharmacology and Therapeutics, 81*, 95–98.

Drews, J. (2000). Drug discovery: A historical perspective. *Science, 287*, 1960–1964.

Kamb, A., Wee, S., & Lengauer, C. (2007). Why is cancer drug discovery so difficult? *Nature Reviews Drug Discovery, 6*, 115–120.

Note: Page numbers followed by *f* indicates figure and *t* indicates table.

A

B

C

D

E

F

G

H

I

J

K

L

M

N

O

P

Q

R

S

W

X

Z